Management of the HIV-infected patient

Management of the HIV-infected patient

Second edition

Edited by

Suzanne Crowe
Macfarlane Burnet Centre for Medical Research
Melbourne, Victoria, Australia

Jennifer Hoy
Alfred Hospital
Melbourne, Victoria, Australia

John Mills
Macfarlane Burnet Centre for Medical Research
Melbourne, Victoria, Australia

MARTIN DUNITZ

© 2002 Martin Dunitz Ltd, a member of the Taylor & Francis group

First published in the UK in 1996
Second edition published 2002 by Martin Dunitz Ltd,
The Livery House, 7–9 Pratt Street, London NW1 0AE

Tel.:	+44 (0) 20 74822202
Fax:	+44 (0) 20 72670159
E-mail:	info.dunitz@tandf.co.uk
Website:	http://www.dunitz.co.uk

Although every effort has been made to ensure that all owners of copyright material have been acknowledged in this publication, we would be glad to acknowledge in subsequent reprints or editions any omissions brought to our attention.

The Author has asserted his right under the Copyright, Designs and Patents Act 1988 to be identified as the Author of this Work.

Although every effort has been made to ensure that drug doses and other information are presented accurately in this publication, the ultimate responsibility rests with the prescribing physician. Neither the publishers nor the authors can be held responsible for errors or for any consequences arising from the use of information contained herein. For detailed prescribing information or instructions on the use of any product or procedure discussed herein, please consult the prescribing information or instructional material issued by the manufacturer.

A CIP record for this book is available from the British Library.

ISBN 1 901865 28 2

Distributed in the USA by
Fulfilment Center
Taylor & Francis
7625 Empire Drive
Florence, KY 41042, USA
Toll Free Tel.: +1 800 634 7064
E-mail: cserve@routledge_ny.com

Distributed in Canada by
Taylor & Francis
74 Rolark Drive
Scarborough, Ontario M1R 4G2, Canada
Toll Free Tel.: +1 877 226 2237
E-mail: tal_fran@istar.ca

Distributed in the rest of the world by
ITPS Limited
Cheriton House
North Way
Andover, Hampshire SP10 5BE, UK
Tel.: +44 (0) 1264 332424
E-mail: reception@itps.co.uk

Produced and typeset by Gray Publishing, Tunbridge Wells, Kent
Printed and bound in Spain

Dedication

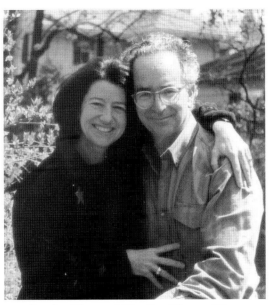

Jonathan Mann and Mary Lou Clements-Mann

The second edition of *Management of the HIV-infected patient* is dedicated to Jonathan Mann and Mary Lou Clements-Mann – two outstanding leaders of the global fight against HIV infection – whose lives were tragically ended by the crash of SwissAir Flight 111 on 2 September 1998. Jonathan and Mary Lou were flying together to Geneva, where she was to lecture on AIDS vaccines at a meeting of the World Health Organization, and Jonathan was to renew his long-dormant association with WHO and the United Nations Combined AIDS Programme.

This dedication is also particularly fitting, as Professor Mann, a valued friend and colleague, wrote the preface to the first edition of this text.

Following graduation from the Washington University School of Medicine and Harvard University School of Public Health, and employment with the US Centers for Disease Control and as State Epidemiologist in New Mexico, Jonathan Mann began his involvement with the HIV epidemic by starting Project SIDA – one of the first compre-

hensive HIV/AIDS research and prevention programmes in a developing country – in Zaire in 1984.

Two years later, in 1986, Mann was appointed as the first Director of the newly formed Global Programme on AIDS (GPA) of the WHO. Under Mann's extraordinary leadership the GPA grew from a staff of two to 280 over 4 years, and it led the first truly worldwide response to the HIV epidemic. At GPA, Mann challenged the world's nations to mobilize for control of the AIDS epidemic and to fulfil their commitment to world health.

As the result of a bitter philosophical dispute with the then Director-General of WHO, Hiroshi Nakajima, Mann left GPA in 1990 to assume a faculty position at the Harvard School of Public Health. There, Mann developed a theme he had begun while at GPA: that of the importance of respect for human rights in the battle against AIDS. This commitment culminated in his founding of the François-Xavier Bagnoud Center for Health and Human Rights at Harvard in 1993, a centre that was to be a world leader in the campaigns for equal rights for people with HIV infection, and for the empowerment of women as a means of controlling the spread of HIV. While at the centre, Mann also founded the influential journal, *Health and Human Rights*, born of his conviction that health and human rights were indivisible. In 1997, he resigned from his endowed professorship at Harvard to become the inaugural Dean of the newly formed Allegheny University School of Public Health, the position he held at the time of his death.

For those who have not met Jonathan Mann, it is diffi-cult to describe the force of his personality and the breadth of his vision. In addition to being a wonderful and caring person, he was an inspiring and gifted leader who catalysed both deep thought and concerted action in all who had contact with him. His concern for the disadvantaged was personal and deeply felt, and fully reflected in his words and deeds.

Jonathan was a crafter of visions, which he was able to shape to ensure their relevance, clarity and intellectual beauty. Then, in his uniquely eloquent way, he would present them to the world. In his many addresses to large international audiences, he would speak of AIDS and discrimination, of dignity and tolerance, of the mediocrity of traditional public health thinking, of the criminal indifference of governments and of the fragmentation of their response to this relentless global epidemic, of the grow-ing gap between the northern and southern hemispheres, and of the world's evolution towards a better future. His lis-teners would be filled with the courage and inspiration they needed to carry on with their work and their life.

Jonathan Mann married Mary Lou Clements on Boxing Day, 1996, public recognition of a powerful relationship that had begun several years previously. For all who knew them, theirs was an incredible love story, making their simultane-ous deaths all the more tragic. There is no doubt that they were holding hands in their final moments together.

After receiving her medical degree from the University of Texas Southwestern, Mary Lou Clements-Mann went on to further study at the London School of Tropical Medicine and Hygiene and the Johns Hopkins University School of Hygiene and Public Health. She had a lifelong interest in vaccines to prevent viral infections, beginning with her work with D.A. Henderson in India on the smallpox erad-ication campaign, and continuing as Professor of Interna-tional Health at Johns Hopkins University, where, after founding the Centre for Immunization Research, she worked on vaccines for influenza, respiratory syncytial, parainfluenza and rotaviruses. Professor Clements-Mann conducted over 100 vaccine research studies, involving thousands of volunteers. Her special genius was in the design and conduct of studies of experimental vaccines in healthy volunteers, in such a way that safety was always paramount but that scientific yield was maximized. She pos-sessed an unparalleled understanding of how vaccines react in normal people, and was in demand as a consultant by the pharmaceutical industry, regulatory agencies, and scientific institutions.

However, it was in the field of AIDS vaccines that Mary Lou emerged as a global figure. As a Principal Investigator for the National Institutes of Health AIDS Vaccine Evaluation Group (AVEG), she was instrumental in the selection of promising candidate vaccines and trials of those vaccines in healthy volunteers. Students came from around the globe to study the design and conduct AIDS vaccine trials with her, and then returned to Thailand, Uganda and a dozen other countries to set up their own national vaccine trial units. As a Scientific Advisor for the International AIDS Vaccine Initiative (IAVI), Mary Lou was a zealous advocate of the controversial idea that every promising new AIDS vaccine should be immediately and thoroughly evaluated in human studies. She and her husband fomented a healthy debate by publicly criticizing the slow pace of the US government AIDS vaccine research and development efforts.

There are only two means of controlling the HIV epidemic: social change, and development and distribution of an HIV vaccine. In the death of this wonderful couple, we have lost global leaders. Jonathan Mann was the foremost proponent of social change, and especially the importance of human rights, as the basis for interrupting transmission of HIV, and Mary Lou Clements-Mann was a leader of the HIV vaccine development effort. We must ensure that their philosophy and work is continued.

JOHN MILLS
MacFarlane Burnet Centre for Medical Research

DANIEL TARANTOLA and SOFIA GRUSKIN
Harvard School of Public Health

DONALD S. BURKE
Johns Hopkins University School of Hygiene and
Public Health

JOHN BARTLETT
Infectious Diseases Society of America

Contents

Contributors

Anuradha Aggarwal
Alfred Hospital, Prahran, Victoria, Australia

Francesca Aweeka
Associate Clinical Professor, San Francisco, California, USA

Roberto Badaró
Chief of Infectious Diseases Unit, Federal University of Bohia, Bohia, Brazil

S. Eralp Bellibas
Associate Clinical Director, Hoffmann-La Roche Inc., Department of Clinical Pharmacology, 340 Kingland Street, Nutley, New Jersey, USA

Constance Benson
University of Colorado Health Sciences Center, Denver, Colorado, USA

Chris Birch
Victorian Infectious Diseases, Reference Laboratory, Melbourne, Victoria, Australia

Bruce James Brew
Associate Professor of Medicine, University of New South Wales, National Centre in HIV Epidemiology and Clinical Research, Sydney, Australia

Pedro Cahn
Director, Fundación Huesped, Buenos Aires, Argentina

Christopher Carpenter
Senior Fellow, Division of Infectious Diseases, Johns Hopkins University, Baltimore, Maryland, USA

Richard Chaisson
Professor of Medicine, Epidemiology and, International Health, Johns Hopkins University, Baltimore, Maryland, USA

Kate Clezy
Staff Specialist, Department of Infectious Diseases, Prince of Wales Hospital, Randwick, New South Wales, Australia Head, Hospital Network, National Centre in HIV Epidemiology and Clinical Research, Darlinghurst, New South Wales, Australia

Nathan Clumeck
Professor of Medicine and Infectious Diseases, Division of Infectious Diseases, CHU Saint-Pierre, Brussels, Belgium

David Cooper
Professor of Medicine and Director, National Centre in HIV Epidemiology and, Clinical Research, University of New South Wales, Sydney, Australia

Suzanne Crowe
Head, AIDS Pathogenesis Research Unit, Macfarlane Burnet Centre for Medical Research, Melbourne, Victoria, Australia; Professor of Medicine Monash University, Melbourne, Victoria, Australia

Stéphane de Wit
Assistant Professor, Division of Infectious Diseases, CHU Saint-Pierre, Brussels, Belgium

Dominic E. Dwyer
ICPMR, Westmead Hospital, Westmead, New South Wales, Australia

Claudia Estcourt
Consultant Physician/Head of Department, Bart's Sexual Health Centre, St Bartholomew's Hospital, London, UK

Peter Frame
Director, Infectious Diseases Center, Holmes Hospital, Cincinnati, Ohio, USA

Hector Freilij
Chief of Parasitology and Chagas Disease Laboratory, Paediatrics Hospital Ricardo Gutierrez, Buenos Aires, Argentina

Martin French

Head, Communicable Diseases Service, Royal Perth Hospital, Perth, Australia

Julie Louise Gerberding

Head, Hospital Infections Program, National Center for Infectious Diseases, National Centers for Disease Control and Prevention, Atlanta, Georgia, USA

Mitchell Goldman

Associate Professor of Medicine, Division of Infectious Diseases, Indiana University School of Medicine, Wishard Hospital, Indianapolis, USA

Deborah Greenspan

Professor of Clinical Oral Medicine, Department of Stomatology, School of Dentistry, University of California, San Francisco, USA

John Greenspan

Professor of Clinical Oral Medicine, Department of Stomatology, School of Dentistry, University of California, San Francisco, USA

Marc Hellerstein

Associate Professor, Department of Nutritional Sciences, University of California, Berkeley, California, USA

David Ho

Professor, The Rockefeller University and Director, Aaron Diamond AIDS Research Centre, New York, USA

Masato Homma

Drug Research Unit, San Francisco General Hospital, San Francisco, California, USA

Jennifer Hoy

Head, Clinical Research Unit, Alfred Hospital, Melbourne, Victoria, Australia

Laurence Huang

AIDS Program, San Francisco General Hospital, San Francisco, California, USA

Fiona Judd

Professor of Rural Mental Health, Monash University, Professional Fellow, University of Melbourne, Department of Psychiatry, Centre for Rural Mental Health, Bendigo, Victoria, Australia

Christine Katlama

Professor, Assistance Hôpitaux, Publique de Paris, Paris, France

Gilbert Kaufmann

National Centre in HIV Epidemiology and Clinical Research, University of New South Wales, Sydney, Australia

Brian Kaye

Associate Clinical Professor of Medicine/University of California, San Francisco, Clinical Assistant Professor of Medicine, Stanford University, The Arthritis Center, Berkeley, California, USA

Alison Kesson

Head, Departments of Virology and Microbiology, The Children's Hospital, Westmead, New South Wales, Australia

N. Kumarasamy

YRG Centre of AIDS Research and Education, T. Nagar, Madras, India

Sharon Lewin

Ian Potter Research Fellow in Infectious Diseases and Infectious Diseases Physician, Victorian Infectious Diseases Service, The Royal Melbourne Hospital, Melbourne, Victoria, Australia

Brian McDonald

Director of Palliative Care, Peninsula Health, Frankston, Victoria, Australia

Ross McKinney Jr

Associate Professor, Pediatrics, Assistant Professor, Microbiology, Division Chief, Pediatric Infectious Diseases, Duke University School of Medicine, Duke South Hospital, Durham, North Carolina, USA

Anne Mijch

Alfred Hospital, Prahran, Victoria, Australia

Sam Milliken

St Vincent's Hospital, Darlinghurst, New South Wales, Australia

John Mills

Director, MacFarlane Burnet Centre of Medical Research; Director, (Australian) National Centre for HIV Virology Research; Consultant Physician in Infectious Diseases, Alfred Hospital, Melbourne, Victoria, Australia

Adrian Mindel

Head, Academic Unit of Sexual Health Medicine, University of New South Wales, Sydney Hospital, Sydney, Australia

Ronald Mitsuyasu
Director, UCLA Center, CARE, University of California, Los Angeles, California, USA

Alison Morris
AIDS Program, San Francisco General Hospital, San Francisco, California, USA

Robert Murphy
Associate Professor of Medicine, Northwestern University, Infectious Diseases Division, Evanston, Illinois, USA

Mark Newell
HIV-NAT Program II on AIDS, Thai Red Cross Society, Thailand

Daniel O'Brien
Infectious Diseases Physician, The Geelong Hospital, Geelong, Victoria, Australia

Carolyn Petersen
Associate Professor, Agouron Pharmaceuticals, Inc., La Jolla, California, USA

Alice Reier
UCLA Center, CARE, University of California, Los Angeles, California, USA

Tilman Ruff
Director, Clinical Medical Affairs for Australia/New Zealand/Oceania, Glaxo SmithKline Biologicals, Melbourne, Victoria, Australia

Kiat Ruxrungtham
Faculty of Medicine, Chulalongkorn Hospital, Bangkok, Thailand

William Sievert
Gastroenterologist, Monash Medical Centre, Melbourne, Victoria, Australia

Suniti Solomon
Director, YRG Centre for AIDS Research and Education, T. Nagar, Madras, India

Alan Street
Deputy Director, Victorian Infectious Diseases Service, The Royal Melbourne Hospital, Melbourne, Victoria, Australia

Alison Street
Clinical Associate Professor and Head, Haematology Unit, Alfred Pathology Service, Melbourne, Victoria, Australia

Russell van Dyke
Tulane University Medical Center, New Orleans, Louisiana, USA

Charles van der Horst
Professor of Medicine, Director, UNC AIDS Clinical Trials Unit, University of North Carolina at Chapel Hill, North Carolina, USA

Joe Wheat
Professor of Medicine and Pathology, Division of Infectious Diseases, Indiana University School of Medicine, Wishard Memorial Hospital, Indianapolis, Indiana, USA

Margot Whitfeld
Visiting Dermatologist, St Vincent's Hospital Skin and Cancer Foundation, Sydney, Australia

Aimee Wilkin
Fellow in Infectious Diseases, Holmes Division/Infectious Diseases Center, University of Cincinatti, Ohio, USA

Alex Wodak
Alcohol and Drug Service, St Vincent's Hospital, Sydney, Australia

David Wohl
Associate Professor, Department of Infectious Diseases, University of North Carolina ACTU, North Carolina, USA

Foreword

Sir William Osler once said that the physician who knew syphilis – in all its manifestations – knew medicine. Today, AIDS clearly occupies this same, unique position. (It is curious that two sexually transmitted diseases have acquired this particular stature in medical history.)

Yet what a challenge it is to 'know AIDS'. For as this excellent book demonstrates, the clinician caring for people with HIV infection and AIDS must be aware of at least three elements: the realities of disease, the diagnostic and therapeutic capacity of modern scientific medicine, and the psychologic and social dimensions that AIDS manifests and reflects.

Crowe, Hoy, and Mills have assembled a world-class group of authors – specialists in their domains. These authors describe the realities of the disease through a focus on systems; the diagnostic and therapeutic challenges are presented both broadly and within each constituent system-related chapter. Then, while maintaining a resolutely clinical and pragmatic focus, the psychologic and social dimensions of HIV/AIDS in the modern world and explored.

What emerges? From our medical education, we are familiar with the necessary process of disaggregation and reaggregation: we divide learning into many component pieces, which we later reassemble into a coherent whole. There is no substitute for this active process through which information becomes knowledge.

Therefore, this book is more than a useful reference and a practical guide for clinicians. This book provides the critical ingredients and the intellectual foundation for the physician who seeks, or has already engaged in the complex, envolving, and creative process of 'knowing AIDS' – which is to 'know medicine' in the modern world.

JONATHAN MANN

(Professor Mann wrote the foreword to the first edition of this book in 1996. He died in September 1998 in an aeroplane crash.)

Preface to the second edition

It is fitting that this guide to managing patients with HIV infection should be produced in the year marking the twentieth anniversary of the discovery of AIDS.

In 1981 the June 5 edition of the US Communicable Disease Center's epidemiology newsletter, Morbidity Mortality Weekly Report (MMWR), featured a front-page article describing a mysterious series of homosexual men from Los Angeles and New York with acquired immunodeficiency, *Pneumocystis carinii* pneumonia and Kaposi's sarcoma. In the space of only a further decade the HIV/AIDS epidemic would become a global pandemic despite the discovery of the etiologic agent, the development of an extraordinarily sensitive and specific diagnostic test, the formulation of strategies to treat and prevent the opportunistic infections associated with HIV disease, and the discovery of drugs to treat HIV infection itself.

In the second decade of the HIV epidemic we have seen continued spread of the virus, especially in economically and socially disadvantaged populations, despite efforts to control the spread by education, behavior modification, testing the blood supply and chemoprophylaxis to prevent mother-to-child transmission. In rich countries, patients with HIV infection have benefited from close monitoring of CD4 lymphocyte numbers and HIV plasma RNA concentrations ('viral load') and initiation of combination anti-retroviral therapy and comprehensive prophylaxis for opportunistic infections at appropriate points in the course of disease. Despite many efforts, a vaccine to prevent HIV infection still eludes us.

This text, the Second Edition of this successful book, aims to provide a clear overview of all the major issues surrounding the care of patients with HIV infection for clinicians in the third decade of the HIV epidemic. It has been comprehensively re-written and re-edited, and many new chapters have been added.

The authors and editors provide sound, practical information about the management of HIV-infected patients, with sufficient pathophysiology and basic science to for the health care provider to understand the rationale of the management strategies. The authors are all internationally-known experts in their respective areas, and the text has been rigorously edited for consistency of style, format and content.

We would like to acknowledge Kathy Tolli for assistance with manuscript preparation, Lesley Gray of Gray Publishing for expert help in editing and preparing the text, and all the authors for providing outstanding material for the book.

Suzanne Crowe, Jennifer Hoy and John Mills
Melbourne, Australia, 2001

Primary HIV-1 infection

1

DAVID COOPER AND GILBERT KAUFMANN

The first encounter of HIV-1 with the human immune system provides valuable information regarding the immunopathogenesis of HIV-1 infection and the host response to HIV-1. The increasing recognition of this early stage of infection has allowed the definition and investigation of its characteristic clinical, serological and immunological features. The identification of subjects at this stage of infection affords the opportunity to institute early counselling and to commence an early therapeutic intervention, thus avoiding further dissemination of HIV-1 infection within the community.

Epidemiology

Symptomatic primary HIV-1 infection has been reported in persons from each of the major groups affected, including homosexual men and women, heterosexual men and women, injecting drug users, persons with haemophilia, recipients of contaminated blood, blood components or organs and health-care workers associated with significant occupational injuries.

An acute clinical illness associated with HIV-1 seroconversion has been reported with a variable frequency ranging between 53 and 92% (Fox *et al.*, 1987; Tindall *et al.*, 1988; Keet *et al.*, 1993). In a prospectively studied group of homosexual men, primary HIV-1 infection was in frequency to influenza as the second cause of an acute febrile illness lasting more than 3 days (de Wolf *et al.*, 1988). However, a much lower frequency of symptoms of 4–10% has been reported for injecting drug users (Sinicco *et al.*, 1993b; Dorrucci *et al.*, 1995). The true proportion of asymptomatic primary HIV-1 infection may be difficult to estimate, since symptomatic individuals are more likely to come to the attention of clinicians (Fox *et al.*, 1987; Tindall *et al.*, 1988).

It is not yet clear which factors influence the occurrence or lack of symptoms during primary infection. Possible viral factors include inoculum size, cell tropism and virulence of the HIV-1 strain. The quantitative and qualitative response of the immune system may also contribute to the severity of symptoms.

A high index of clinical suspicion is needed to recognize primary HIV-1 infection. In one prospective study, primary HIV-1 infection was correctly diagnosed only in 25% of patients during the first encounter (Schacker *et al.*, 1996). Indeed, many patients are now more aware of the symptoms associated with primary HIV infection and present during the course of an illness suggesting HIV infection.

HIV-2 infection is prevalent mainly in West Africa. However, only two cases of symptomatic primary HIV-2 infection have been reported in the rest of the world (Besnier *et al.*, 1990; Ritter *et al.*, 1990). It is not possible from these to determine whether the clinical manifestations of primary HIV-2 infection are similar to those of primary HIV-1 infection.

Clinical presentation

The time from exposure to HIV-1 until the onset of the acute clinical illness is typically between 2 and 4 weeks, although incubation periods as short as 6 days and as long as 6 weeks have been reported (Tindall and Cooper, 1991). The clinical illness is acute in onset, lasts for a median of 2–3 weeks and is generally self-limited. In a multicentre investigation including 218 subjects, a median duration of 20 days with a range of 3–184 days has been noted (Vanhems *et al.*, 1997). However, 75% of subjects had a symptomatic period of 30 days or less and 26% had a duration of 10 days or less. Symptoms may be associated with an appreciable morbidity, requiring hospitalization. In one study, 42% of patients were hospitalized for an average duration of 10 days (Kinloch-de Loes *et al.*, 1993).

The main clinical features of primary HIV-1 infection reflect the broad cell and tissue tropism of this virus. The most frequently reported physical signs and symptoms include fever, fatigue, lymphadenopathy, pharyngitis, rash, myalgia or arthralgia, diarrhoea, headache, weight loss and mucocutaneous ulceration (Table 1.1).

Fever may be accompanied by night sweats and has been found in 53–94% of patients (Gaines et al., 1988b; Tindall et al., 1988; Kinloch-de Loes et al., 1993; Schacker et al., 1996; Vanhems et al., 1997). Fatigue, lethargy and malaise are common and are observed in 60–90% of individuals. Those symptoms are often severe and may persist for several months following resolution of other clinical manifestations of primary HIV-1 infection.

Enlarged lymph nodes have been reported in 39–55% of patients. They are detected generally in the second to the third week of the illness, usually concomitant with the development of peripheral blood lymphocytosis. Axillary, occipital, and cervical nodes are most commonly affected, but lymphadenopathy may also be generalized. Enlarged lymph nodes remain soft and are non-tender. Although the size tends to decrease with time, lymphadenopathy usually persists following the acute illness. In a small percentage of patients splenomegaly may accompany lymphadenopathy.

An erythematous macular or maculopapular rash has been observed in 23–68% of patients with primary HIV-1 infection and is the most frequently reported dermatological feature (Figure 1.1, in the colour plate section). It develops within 1–5 days during the acute illness and fades spontaneously after 5–8 days. Usually, upper trunk, neck and face are affected with a symmetrical distribution (Lapins et al., 1996). Less commonly, extremities, including the palms and soles, are involved. The rash is generally non-pruritic, but mildly pruritic lesions have also been reported. The single lesion is a macule or maculo-papule, round or oval, non-confluent and well demarcated. The colour is dull-red to deeply red and the diameter can range from a few mm to 1 cm. Similar lesions are observed in other viral

Table 1.1 Clinical manifestations of primary HIV-1 infection in 218 patients with primary HIV-1 infection

Clinical manifestation	Frequency (%)	Median duration – days (range)
Fever > 38°C	77	14 (3–184)
Fatigue	66	18 (1–184)
Exanthem	56	11 (1–73)
Myalgia	55	11 (2–184)
Headache	51	13 (2–⇒)
Pharyngitis	44	8 (1–51)
Cervical lymphadenopathy	39	12 (3–32)
Arthralgia	31	15 (3–184)
Oral ulcers	29	8 (1–85)
Odynophagia	28	14 (2–48)
Axillar lymphadenopathy	24	14 (1–⇒)
Weight loss	24	19 (3–⇒)
Nausea	24	14 (2–109)
Diarrhoea	23	8 (1–39)
Night sweats	22	10 (3–57)
Cough	22	13 (2–184)
Anorexia	21	10 (2–68)
Inguinal lymphadenopathy	20	9 (7–10)
Abdominal pain	19	12 (1–73)
Oral candidiasis	17	8 (1–34)
Vomiting	12	10 (1–31)
Photophobia	12	10 (2–39)
Sore eyes	12	12 (3–36)
Genital ulceration	7	12 (3–35)
Tonsillitis	7	10 (1–41)
Depression	6	7 (3–76)
Dizziness	6	10 (2–26)

⇒ The symptom never disappeared during the study period (adapted from Vanhems et al., 1997).

diseases or drug eruptions. The histopathology is identical with morphological skin alterations in morbilliform drug eruptions and other viral exanthemas (Balslev *et al.*, 1990). A sparse perivascular infiltrate is found, consisting of histiocytes, CD8 and CD4 T lymphocytes. The epidermis is minimally affected or not at all and can show a slight spongiosis, parakeratosis and vacuolar alteration of the basal layer.

Other skin lesions noted during primary HIV-1 infection include a roseola-like rash, diffuse urticaria (Ho *et al.*, 1985), a vesicular and pustular exanthem, desquamation of the palms and soles and alopecia (Kieff *et al.*, 1989). The desquamation and alopecia typically occur after resolution of other symptoms in the second month following the onset of primary HIV-1 infection. Erythema multiforme has also been reported in primary HIV-1 infection (Lewis and Brook, 1992).

Mucocutaneous manifestations include an asymmetrically distributed spotty enanthem of the hard and soft palate. Mucocutaneous ulcers are a distinctive feature of primary HIV-1 infection, occurring in 30–40% of patients. The round or oval ulcers are shallow and 5–10 mm in diameter with a surrounding thin red mucosal zone. Ulcers are localized on the buccal mucosa, gingiva, palate or tonsils. Other sites affected by ulcers include the oesophagus, anus, and penis (Gaines *et al.*, 1988b; McMillan *et al.*, 1989; Bartelsman *et al.*, 1990; Rabeneck *et al.*, 1990). The pathogenesis of ulcers is unknown. In one series, 50% of subjects who presented with odynophagia during primary HIV-1 infection had virus particles that morphologically resembled human retroviruses in specimens of oesophageal ulcer tissue as examined by electron microscopy (Rabeneck *et al.*, 1990). Bacteriological, mycological and other virological cultures of ulcer tissue are usually negative, suggesting a direct cytopathic effect of HIV-1. Pharyngitis occurs in 36–70% of patients and may be accompanied by an exudate, pharyngeal oedema and tonsillitis (Valle, 1987). Between 20 and 60% of patients suffer from arthralgia and myalgia. Myalgia may be associated with muscle weakness and serum creatinine kinase elevations.

The recovery of HIV-1 from cerebrospinal fluid (CSF) during primary HIV-1 infection indicates that the infection of the central nervous system occurs soon after exposure (Hardy *et al.*, 1991). In one series, HIV-1 could be cultured from CSF in 12 of 24 patients (Schacker *et al.*, 1996). In the CSF analysis, a pleocytosis with elevated protein levels as

well as elevated neopterin and beta2-microglobulin levels can be found in subjects with and without clinical meningitis (Sonnerborg *et al.*, 1989).

Neurological symptoms have been reported in 17–56% (see Chapter 10). The most common symptoms include headache, retro-orbital pain (generally exacerbated by eye movement) and photophobia, which may reflect an underlying aseptic meningitis (Carne *et al.*, 1985; Ho *et al.*, 1985; Hardy *et al.*, 1991). Cognitive or affective impairment expressed by mood changes, depression and irritability is frequently observed during primary HIV-1 infection and may indicate an early CNS involvement (Carne *et al.*, 1985; Tindall *et al.*, 1988). These changes may last from weeks to months following the resolution of other symptoms (Biggs and Newton-John, 1986). Acute encephalitis is a rare consequence of primary HIV-1 infection. After a non-specific prodrome lasting up to 2 weeks, mood changes, confusion and seizures may herald the onset of overt encephalitis (Carne *et al.*, 1985). Other more unusual neurological conditions that have been associated with primary HIV-1 infection include myelopathy, peripheral neuropathy, meningoradiculitis, brachial neuritis, facial palsy, cauda equina syndrome and Guillain-Barré syndrome. Although a persistent neurological deficit has been reported in some individuals, neurological manifestations generally last for 1–4 weeks. It is unknown which factors determine whether neurological involvement will occur during primary HIV-1 infection. It is conceivable that some strains of HIV-1 may be more neurotropic than others (Strizki *et al.*, 1996).

Gastrointestinal symptoms include anorexia, nausea, vomiting and diarrhoea. Significant weight loss was noted in 13–70% of patients with a median decline of 5 kg (range 1.4–10 kg) of weight in one series (Schacker *et al.*, 1996).

Respiratory manifestations are uncommon among homosexual men with primary HIV infection, although some subjects may have acute pneumonia or a dry cough (Ong and Mandal, 1991). A higher prevalence of respiratory symptoms has been reported among injecting drug users with primary HIV-1 infection. In one series, 28% of those patients suffered from bacterial pneumonia (Mientjes *et al.*, 1993). *Pneumocystis carinii* pneumonia (PCP) has also been observed in association with primary HIV-1 infection (Vento *et al.*, 1993). Each subject had severe CD4 lymphopenia (range of nadir 62–91 cells/μl). Also, the occurrence of oral and oesophageal candidiasis reflects the sometimes severe immunodeficiency associated with primary infection (Pena et al., 1991; Tindall et al., 1989).

Rare manifestations of primary HIV-1 infection include cardiomyopathy, renal failure, vasculitis, rhabdomyolysis, haemophagocytic syndrome, aplastic anaemia and epiglottitis (Bernard et al., 1990; Samuel et al., 1988; Del Rio et al., 1990; Pedersen et al., 1990; Pedersen and Pedersen, 1994; Martinez-Escribano et al., 1996).

Laboratory findings

Primary HIV-1 infection causes rapid changes in several laboratory parameters. Following an early transient lymphopenia, lymphocytosis develops generally in the second to third week of infection. Atypical lymphocytes are found in less than 50% of subjects concomitant with the lymphocytosis (Gaines et al., 1988b). During the first week of illness the white blood lymphocyte count may be low and the proportion of banded neutrophils increased. Mild thrombocytopenia is common in the first 2 weeks of illness, but has no clinical significance (Gaines et al., 1988b). The detection of antiplatelet antibodies that indicates that auto-immune mechanisms may be involved in the pathogenesis of thrombocytopenia. However, the infection of mega-karyocytes by HIV-1 also suggests a virus-mediated mechanism. No characteristic alterations in haemoglobin levels have been reported. Elevated serum levels of hepatic transaminases (e.g. aspartate aminotransferase (AST) as high as 865 IU/l) have been noted in association with tender hepatomegaly (Boag et al., 1992). These generally return to a normal range within 3 months of presentation. Clinically evident hepatitis is rare. The erythrocyte sedimentation rate (ESR) and C-reactive protein are raised in about 50% of subjects (Gaines et al., 1988b).

Symptomatic primary HIV-1 infection and disease progression

Several reports suggest that clinical symptoms at the time of primary HIV-1 infection may be useful to predict the subsequent course of disease. Pedersen et al. (1989a) found that the 3-year progression rate to symptomatic HIV-1 disease was eight times higher among subjects with a primary illness that lasted longer than 14 days. CD4 T lymphocytes declined more rapidly to levels below 500 cells/µl and the recurrence of HIV-1 antigenaemia was also more frequent in those subjects who had a longer-lasting primary HIV-1 infection. Similarly, reports of Sinicco et al. (1993b) and Lindback et al. (1994) indicate that symptomatic HIV-1 infection is associated with a more rapid progression towards AIDS. Boufassa et al. (1995) showed that neurological manifestations during primary HIV-1 infection are similarly associated with an accelerated disease progression. In a large series of 259 subjects with primary HIV infection, the association between individual symptoms and disease progression was evaluated (Vanhems et al., 1998). Oral candidiasis was most strongly associated with a more rapid disease progression, followed by skin rash, lethargy, odynophagia, abdominal pain and fever. The total number of symptoms and signs (excluding pharyngitis) was also associated with disease progression. These findings suggest that primary illness may reflect the early interaction between the virus and the host's immune response, which determines the course of the disease.

Pathogenesis

Immunological changes

Primary HIV-1 infection is characterized by rapid changes in peripheral T-cell subsets (Cooper et al., 1988; Gaines et al., 1990; Pedersen et al., 1990). During the first 1–2 weeks following the onset of symptoms lymphopenia is observed affecting CD4 and CD8 T lymphocytes (Figure 1.2). This may be profound, with levels of CD4 lymphocytes occasionally falling as low as those in advanced HIV-1 disease. The nadir of total lymphocytes occurs a median of 9 days following onset of illness (Cooper et al., 1988). This transient lymphopenia is followed by a peripheral lymphocytosis 2–3 weeks after the onset of illness. While mainly CD8 lymphocytes contribute to this lymphocytosis, CD4 lymphocyte numbers may also increase slightly, but they usually do not return to their initial values. CD8 lymphocyte numbers peak at a median of 33 days following onset of illness (Cooper et al., 1988). The changes of CD4 and CD8 lymphocytes result in an inversion of the CD4:CD8 ratio, which is maintained during the illness. The analysis of subsets of CD4 lymphocytes shows a reduction of both naive and memory cells, as defined by antigens CD45RA+ and CD45RO+, respectively (Zaunders et al., 1995). In CD8 lymphocytes, the CD45RO+ subset may be more increased than the CD45RA+ subset, especially among subjects with severe symptomatic primary HIV-1 infection (Brunngaard et al., 1995). An extensive activation of CD8 lymphocytes, as defined by the expression of cell surface antigens CD38 and HLA-DR, has been reported (Roos et al., 1992; Cossarizza et al., 1995; Zaunders

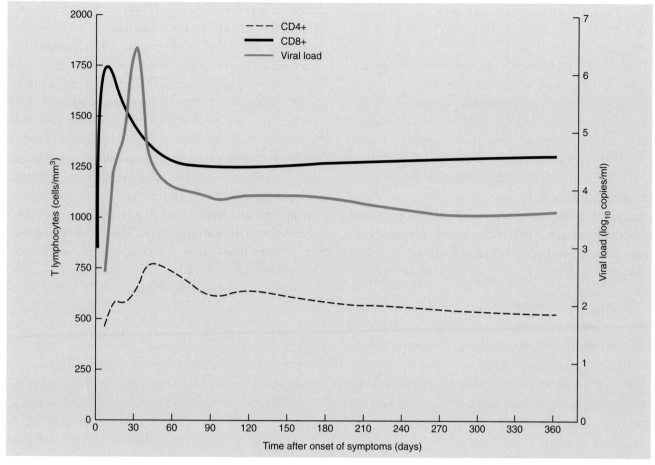

Figure 1.2 *Typical course of plasma HIV-1 RNA, CD4 and CD8 T lymphocytes in 41 patients with primary HIV-1 infection.*

et al., 1995). Subjects with a persistent elevation of the HLA-DR+CD38 negative CD8 lymphocyte subset during the first year after seroconversion appear to have more stable levels of CD4 lymphocytes (Giorgi *et al.*, 1994).

Cell-mediated immune responses

A CD8 T lymphocyte-mediated non-cytotoxic virus suppressor activity has been documented before HIV-1 seroconversion, associated with a decline in plasma viraemia (Mackewicz *et al.*, 1994). Moreover, virus-specific cytotoxic T lymphocytes (CTL) appear early during primary HIV-1 infection, coinciding with the decline of HIV-1 plasma viraemia (Borrow *et al.*, 1994; Koup *et al.*, 1994). In one series, the predominant CTL response was directed against HIV Env proteins (Musey *et al.*, 1997). CTLs directed against Gag and Pol proteins were found less frequently. A higher frequency of Env-and Gag-specific memory CTLs was associated with a lower HIV-1 plasma viraemia. The pressure exerted by CTLs may select for subpopulations of HIV-1 strains with altered epitopes, which escape from

the recognition of CTLs. This mechanism of immune escape has been demonstrated as early as in primary HIV-1 infection, as well as later in the course of the disease (Borrow *et al.*, 1997; Price *et al.*, 1997). Moreover, initially expanded HIV-1-specific CD8 T lymphocyte clones may disappear rapidly, possibly due to clonal exhaustion during primary infection, and further facilitate the immune escape of HIV-1 (Pantaleo *et al.*, 1997b). Recently, it has been shown that a polyclonal expansion of CD8 lymphocytes is associated with a more favourable clinical course and a slower decline of CD4 lymphocytes than a mono- or oligoclonal CD8 lymphocyte expansion (Pantaleo *et al.*, 1997a).

Cytokine responses

Concentrations of several cytokines are increased during primary HIV-1 infection including interferon (IFN)-α, IFN-λ, tumor necrosis factor (TNF)-α, TNF receptors, interleukin (IL)-1 and soluble CD30 (von Sydow *et al.*, 1991; Sinicco *et al.*, 1993a; Cossarizza *et al.*, 1995; Rizzardi *et al.*, 1996). The expression of mRNA for a cytokine panel

infection (Cooper et al., 1988; Pedersen et al., 1990). In a series of seven patients, Pedersen et al. (1990) found that pokeweed mitogen (PWM) responses were depressed in each patient at some time during the acute illness, and in most patients reached the lowest level 6–8 weeks after onset of illness. Responses subsequently improved but did not return to normal levels at 1-year follow-up. The reactivity to phytohaemagglutinin (PHA) was similarly reduced, but the response was less affected than the response to PWM. A rapid and persistent impairment of immunoglobulin synthesis and a decreased proliferation response of B lymphocytes has also been reported following primary HIV-1 infection (Terpstra et al., 1989; Gaines et al., 1990).

Virological changes

Primary HIV-1 infection is characterized by high levels of infectious virus in plasma and peripheral blood mononuclear cells (PBMCs) during the first weeks following infection (Clark et al., 1991; Daar et al., 1991; Piatak et al., 1993). Plasma viraemia reaches peak levels of 10^5–10^7 HIV-1 RNA copies/ml (Figure 1.2). Approximately 2 weeks after onset of symptoms, the viral burden decreases spontaneously by 10^1–10^3 HIV-1 RNA copies/ml (Schacker et al., 1998). After 3–6 months, the viral load approaches stable values between 10^4 and 10^5 HIV-1 RNA copies/ml, although this varies widely from patient to patient, and a number of individuals have viral load levels below the limits of detection. The magnitude of plasma viraemia 6 months after seroconversion has been shown to have prognostic significance for subsequent disease progression (Mellors et al., 1995). Earlier levels of viraemia (before 6 months) demonstrate a high variability and appear not to be predictive of the further course of the disease (Schacker et al., 1998). The rapid decay of viral load after an initial peak is probably the result of the immune response (Borrow et al., 1994; Koup et al., 1994). However, a lack of target cells susceptible to HIV-1 infection during the initial time of low circulating CD4 lymphocytes has been proposed as one factor leading to the rapid decline of plasma HIV-1 RNA (Phillips, 1996).

In several studies, the predominant virus phenotype in primary HIV-1 infection was a non-syncytium-inducing (NSI), macrophage (M-) tropic strain, now known to use the chemokine receptor CCR5, which suggests a possible role of mucosal macrophages or dendritic cells during the transmission (Roos et al., 1992; Nielsen et al., 1992; Zhu et al., 1993). However, the isolation of syncytium-inducing (SI), T-cell line tropic strains, which use the chemokine

including IL-2, IL-4, IL-6, IL-10, TNF-α and IFN-γ has been determined longitudinally using peripheral mononuclear cell samples obtained at different time points during primary HIV-1 infection (Graziosi et al., 1996). A significant number of patients had an early peak of IFN-γ mRNA expression, which coincided with the expansion of CD8 lymphocytes. IL-2 and IL-4 mRNA expression were barely detectable and IL-6 mRNA was demonstrated in PBMC from a minority of patients. However, substantial levels of IL-2 expression were found in mononuclear cells isolated from lymph nodes. IL-10 and TNF-α mRNA were detected in all patients, showing either a stable expression or an increase during the transition from acute to the chronic stage. It is conceivable that high levels of circulating cytokines may cause some of the clinical symptoms such as fever, chills, myalgia, headache, fatigue and weight loss.

Recently, chemokine receptors have been identified as HIV co-receptors. Chemokines such as RANTES, MIP1-α and MIP1-β can block HIV-1 co-receptors and may play a role in primary HIV infection (Alkhatib et al., 1996; Cocchi et al., 1996; Deng et al., 1996; Dragic et al., 1996). However, the significance of chemokines in primary HIV-1 infection needs further investigation.

Humoral immune responses

Although antibodies against several HIV-1 proteins appear early in primary infection, their role in controlling initial viraemia is uncertain (Moore et al., 1994). Neutralizing antibodies that may be protective against HIV-1 appear usually several weeks or months after seroconversion (Connick et al., 1996; Pellegrin et al., 1996; Moog et al., 1997; Pilgrim et al., 1997). In contrast, antibody-dependent cellular cytotoxicity (ADCC) against virally infected target cells has been demonstrated early in primary infection and may play a role in reducing initial viraemia (Connick et al., 1996). Early antibodies may also form immune complexes with HIV antigens, which are trapped in the follicular dendritic cell network or in the reticulo-endothelial system. Such immune complexes have been observed in blood during the period of declining concentrations of p24 antigen and increasing concentrations of IgM and IgG antibodies (von Sydow et al., 1988).

Lymphoproliferative responses to mitogens and antigens

A severe reduction of lymphocyte responsiveness to both mitogens and antigens occurs during primary HIV-1

receptor CXCR-4, has been reported in 33% of individuals in another study (Fiore *et al.*, 1994). Moreover, the analysis of 10 virus isolates with known index cases showed that the phenotype was usually retained during transmission. However, a switch from T-cell tropic to M-tropic strains was observed in one patient. The demonstration of CXCR-4-using variants during primary infection is associated with a more rapid decline of CD4 lymphocytes (Roos *et al.*, 1992; Nielsen *et al.*, 1993).

There is limited evidence that individuals who acquire HIV-1 infection from an index case with late stage HIV-1 disease may have a higher incidence of symptomatic primary HIV-1 infection and subsequent accelerated development of severe disease than those who acquire infection from an index case who is at an earlier stage of disease (Ward *et al.*, 1989; van Griensven *et al.*, 1990; Keet *et al.*, 1993). Patients in advanced stages of the disease may have a greater diversity of viral quasispecies and more frequently virulent strains such as CXCR-4-using virus (Ho *et al.*, 1989). Moreover, the transmitted inoculum size may be larger.

Several studies have reported the isolation of zidovudine-resistant virus during primary HIV-1 infection (Erice *et al.*, 1993; Fitzgibbon *et al.*, 1993; Imrie *et al.*, 1996; Briones *et al.*, 2001). In one series, zidovudine-resistant virus was found in 5 of 61 isolates (Imrie *et al.*, 1996). After 1 year, 2 of 5 zidovudine-resistant strains reverted to wild type. No association between zidovudine resistance and CD4 lymphocyte decline was found. However, the transmission of zidovudine-resistant strains may reduce the efficacy of subsequent therapy. In a more recent study in the UK, up to 27% of people infected in 2000 harboured resistant HIV (UK Collaborative Group, 2001). Also, the transmission of strains resistant to the non-nucleoside reverse transcriptase inhibitor (NNRTI) nevirapine and to protease inhibitors (PIs) has been reported (Imrie *et al.*, 1997; Hecht *et al.*, 1998a).

Lymph nodes are the primary sites of viral replication (Pantaleo, 1993). HIV-1 can be detected in lymph nodes early before seroconversion (Ferbas *et al.*, 1996). Within the first 3 months of HIV infection virus is mainly present in individual, virus-expressing cells. The entrapment of virions in the follicular dendritic network is minimal (Pantaleo *et al.*, 1998). After 3 months virus entrapment increases, coinciding with the rapid decline of plasma HIV-1 RNA. The structure of the germinal centres is relatively preserved during primary HIV-1 infection and contrasts with the follicular hyperplasia associated with established HIV-1 infection.

Diagnosis

Primary HIV-1 infection is confirmed serologically by the appearance of serum antibodies that are directed against HIV-specific proteins. Antibodies are generally detected by enzyme-linked immunosorbent assay (ELISA) and immunoblotting (Western blot) (Table 1.2) (see Chapter 4).

Table 1.2 Diagnostic tests for HIV-1 infection

Test	Detection	Sensitivity	Application	Comment
ELISA	HIV-1/2 antibodies	99%	HIV-1 screening	Negative in early primary HIV-1 infection
Immunoblot (Western blot)	HIV-1 antibodies	99%	Confirmation of ELISA result	Negative or indeterminate in early primary HIV infection Detects HIV-2 inconsistently
Virus culture of PBMC	Infective virus	95–100%	Subjects with undetectable viral load; virus genotyping/phenotyping	Expensive, labour-intensive
HIV RNA	Free plasma HIV RNA	90–95%	Therapeutic monitoring; prognostic significance	Sensitivity dependent on stage of HIV disease
HIV proviral DNA	Intracellular DNA	97–98%	Primary HIV-1 infection; neonatal infection; indeterminate serology	Not considered sufficiently accurate for HIV diagnosis without confirmatory serology
p24	Free viral core protein	8–32%	Primary HIV infection; prognostic significance	Usually detectable if plasma HIV RNA high; acid treatment increases sensitivity

The time from infection until the detection of antibodies has been described as the 'window period'. The estimation of the exact duration of this serological window is difficult. However, an average of 45 days, with 90% of patients having a window period of less than 141 days, has been calculated by mathematical modelling (Petersen et al., 1994). With the introduction of more sensitive assays the duration of the window period may be reduced by approximately 20 days (Busch et al., 1995). Currently available ELISA assays utilize highly immunogenic recombinant HIV antigens and may detect antibodies 1–2 weeks after onset of symptoms. IgM antibodies peak at 2–5 weeks and decline to undetectable levels after approximately 3 months (Cooper et al., 1987; Gaines et al., 1987b, 1988a; Lange et al., 1988). IgG antibodies appear 2–6 weeks after onset of illness (Cooper et al., 1987; Gaines et al., 1987b).

Immunoblotting is used for confirmation of a reactive ELISA test. The simultaneous detection of antibodies against several HIV (glyco)proteins such as gp41, gp120, gp160 (envelope), p18, p24, p55 (core) and p34, p53, p68 (structural proteins) significantly increases its specificity over an ELISA test. Serial immunoblotting during primary HIV infection may show typical patterns of development of different antibodies (Figure 1.3).

Several tests are available to detect HIV infection before seroconversion. The structural (core) p24 protein of HIV-1 may be detected in serum as early as 24 h after onset of the acute clinical illness (Gaines et al., 1987a; von Sydow et al., 1988; Mariotti et al., 1990). An enzyme immunoassay (EIA) for serum p24 antigen is a simple and inexpensive test. However, false-positive as well as false-negative p24 antigen tests do occur. In one series, p24 antigen was detected in only 75% of patients with acute HIV infection (Henrard et al., 1994). The level of serum p24 antigen also typically decreases as serum HIV-1 antibody titres increase and immune complexes develop (Goudsmit et al., 1986; von Sydow et al., 1988). False-positive tests can be detected by neutralization pre-treatment with p24 antibodies. Persistent antigenemia or the reappearance of antigenemia at a later time is a risk factor for a more rapid disease progression.

More recently, polymerase chain reaction (PCR) and branched DNA (bDNA) techniques have been introduced, permitting the detection of HIV RNA as well as integrated proviral HIV DNA. Those assays may test positive concomitantly with the p24 antigen EIA or even a few days earlier (Busch et al., 1995). They have a high sensitivity of 90–98%, which varies with the stage of the

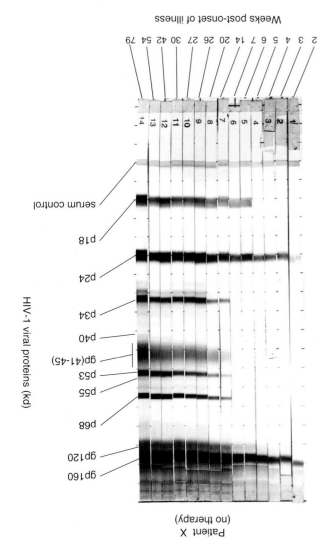

Figure 1.3 Immunoblotting (Western blot) of sequential samples obtained from a patient with primary HIV-1 infection. Courtesy of Philip Cunningham, Center for Immunology, St Vincent's Hospital, Sydney, Australia.

disease and the used technique (Owens et al., 1996). Specificity is about 97% for bDNA and closer to 100% for RT-PCR. These tests are particularly useful in patients with inconclusive or indeterminate serology and in newborns with maternal anti-HIV antibodies (Henrard et al., 1994).

Seronegative HIV-1 infection

Some studies have suggested that HIV-1 infection could persist for long periods without the development of HIV-1-specific antibodies (Ranki et al., 1987; Martin-Rico et al., 1995; Reimer et al., 1997). Early reports of seronegative HIV infection may be difficult to interpret because of relatively insensitive ELISA assays, which failed also to detect HIV-1 subtype O (Loussert-Ajaka et al., 1994; Schable et al., 1994). The small number of reports also suggests that a seronegative HIV-1 infection appears to be an extremely rare phenomenon.

Differential diagnosis

Several diseases may present with similar symptoms to primary HIV-1 infection and should be ruled out. They include cytomegalovirus (CMV) infection, Epstein–Barr virus (EBV) infection, toxoplasmosis, viral hepatitis, rubella, secondary syphilis, disseminated gonorrhoea, primary herpes simplex virus infection and allergic drug reactions. Although originally described as 'mononucleosis-like' (Cooper et al., 1985), and still described as such in much of the literature, symptomatic primary HIV-1 infection is a distinct and recognizable clinical syndrome. The diagnosis of primary HIV-1 infection should be considered in any person who presents with a febrile illness of acute onset and possible recent exposure to HIV-1. The major symptoms and signs that strengthen such a diagnosis include mucocutaneous ulceration, maculopapular rash, lymphadenopathy, and pharyngitis.

The skin rash associated with primary HIV-1 infection is a valuable diagnostic aid. Skin eruptions are rare in EBV infection (unless antibiotics have been given), toxoplasmosis or CMV infection and they do not affect the palms and soles in rubella. The rash of pityriasis rosea is typically scaly and may be pruritic. Both features are not typical of the rash in primary HIV-1 infection. Constitutional symptoms are generally mild or absent in persons with pityriasis rosea.

Mucocutaneous ulceration is another fairly distinctive finding, as it is unusual in most of the other diseases being considered in the differential diagnosis. Although serologic testing for HIV-1 and EBV will usually provide the definitive diagnosis, false-positive tests for heterophil antibodies have been reported during primary HIV-1 infection (Van Essen et al., 1988). The major differences between primary HIV-1 infection and EBV are summarized in Table 1.3.

Treatment

A placebo-controlled study evaluating the efficacy of zidovudine (ZDV) monotherapy in primary HIV-1 infection showed a modest benefit (Kinloch-de Loes et al., 1995). No significant changes of plasma viraemia and CD8 lymphocytes were noted and zidovudine did not shorten the dura-

Table 1.3 Clinical differences between primary HIV infection and Epstein–Barr virus (EBV) infection

Feature	Primary HIV infection	EBV infection
Onset	Acute	Insidious
Lymphadenopathy	39–52%	93–100%
Pharyngitis	36–70%	69–91%
exsudative	Uncommon	30%
Tonsillar hypertrophy	Mild	Prominent
Mucocutaneous ulcer	29–43%	None
Rash	24–68%	10%
Jaundice	<1%	8%
Elevated transaminases	Infrequent	90%
Splenomegaly	Rare	50%
Diarrhoea	10–46%	Absent
Neurological complications	17%	<1%
Cough	22–26%	5%

Adapted from Gaines et al. (1988b); Schacker et al. (1996); Kinloch-de Loes et al. (1995); Vanhems et al. (1997); Tindall et al. (1988). and Boufassa et al. (1995).

tion of the seroconversion illness. However, fewer minor opportunistic infections and a smaller CD4 lymphocyte decline were found during a follow-up of 18 months.

In a pilot study, which evaluated the combination of zidovudine and the NNRTI L-697,661, plasma HIV-1 RNA decreased rapidly in three of four individuals, in two patients to undetectable levels (Perrin et al., 1996). CD4 lymphocyte counts remained stable during the treatment period of 6 months.

In another pilot study, the combination of zidovudine, didanosine, and lamivudine was used in 10 patients (Lafeuillade et al., 1997). A rapid, sustained decline of plasma HIV-1 RNA levels was observed during the observation period of 10.7 months. Undetectable levels were reached at 108 days and CD4 T lymphocyte count increased by 243 cells/μl.

Studies evaluating combination therapies with PIs are under investigation. Preliminary results indicate that in most patients plasma viraemia can be reduced to undetectable levels (Conway et al., 1998; Hecht et al., 1998b).

Several theoretical considerations support starting antiretroviral treatment at the time of primary HIV-1 infection. First, it remains uncertain whether full immune reconstitution can ever be reached with the available therapeutic options (Kelleher et al., 1996; Autran et al., 1997). Therefore, the prevention of severe immunodeficiency by early therapeutic intervention may be crucial. Second, early treatment may prevent widespread viral dissemination and possibly the establishment of viral reservoirs, including the pool of latently infected cells. Conversely, the high cost of combination therapies and their side-effects are some of the reasons for delaying therapy. No studies are available yet to compare efficacy, durability and subsequent immunological benefits of an early and delayed therapy, which would justify the routine treatment of primary HIV-1 infection.

Counselling and prevention

The diagnosis of HIV-1 infection is often associated with profound psychosocial consequences. Specific factors that need to be considered in counselling individuals with primary HIV-1 infection include the acute physical distress that many people experience, the tentative nature of the diagnosis before seroconversion occurs, self-reproach due to recent risk behaviour and the potential development of mood disorders during primary HIV-1 infection (Carne et al., 1985; Tindall et al., 1988).

The identification of a patient with primary HIV-1 infection necessarily implies the existence of a source case of infection. Where possible, counselling for the source person is also indicated. Such persons may be unaware of their infection or of what constitutes safer sex or safer injecting practices, or may be in the process of seroconverting themselves. Counselling of such patients also needs to address their emotional reactions to having infected another individual.

Summary

A clinical syndrome commencing 2–4 weeks after inoculation with HIV-1 defines primary infection. Between 50 and 90% of patients experience symptoms, which last on average 2–3 weeks, but may persist for several months. The early diagnosis of primary HIV-1 infection is difficult and requires a high degree of suspicion. The most common symptoms include fever, headache, rash, sore throat, lymphadenopathy, myalgia and arthralgia. The duration and number of symptoms, as well as individual symptoms such as fever, rash, lethargy, odynophagy and oral candidiasis, have been associated with a poorer prognosis of the disease.

During the first weeks of the infection an extensive plasma viraemia is observed, with concomitant dramatic immunological disturbances including an expansion of CD8 lymphocytes and a decline of CD4 T lymphocytes. Not only the number of CD4 lymphocytes is reduced; the T and B lymphocyte-mediated immune response is also impaired. From peak plasma viraemia, HIV-1 RNA levels decline gradually, reaching stable values at 3–6 months. Cytotoxic T lymphocytes appear to be the most significant immune response reducing early plasma viraemia.

In a placebo-controlled study, ZDV reduced the decline of CD4 lymphocytes and the occurrence of minor opportunistic infections. Combination therapies including two or three reverse transcriptase inhibitors were tested only in small pilot studies and showed a more sustained reduction of viral load than a ZDV monotherapy. However, combination therapies of reverse transcriptase inhibitors with PIs are the therapy of choice in advanced HIV disease and may also prove beneficial in primary HIV-1 infection.

References

Alkhatib G, Combadiere C, Broder CC et al. (1996). CC CKR5: a RANTES, MIP-1α, MIP-1β receptor as a fusion cofactor for macrophage-tropic HIV-1. Science 272: 1955-8.

Autran B, Carcelain G, Li TS et al. (1997). Positive effects of combined antiretroviral therapy on CD4+ T cell homeostasis and function in advanced HIV disease. Science 277: 112-6.

Bailser E, Thomsen HK, Weismann K. (1990). Histopathology of acute human immunodeficiency virus exanthema. J Clin Pathol 43: 201-2.

Bartelsman JF, Lange JMA, van Leeuwen R et al. (1990). Acute primary HIV-esophagitis. Endoscopy 22: 184-5.

Bernard E, Dellamonica P, Michiels JF et al. (1990). Heparine-like anticoagulant vasculitis associated with severe primary infection by HIV. AIDS 4: 932-3.

Besnier JM, Barin F, Baillou A et al. (1990). Symptomatic HIV-2 primary infection. Lancet 335: 798.

Biggs B, Newton-John HF. (1986). Acute HTLV-III infection: a case followed from onset to seroconversion. Med J Aust 144: 545-7.

Boag FC, Dean R, Hawkins DA et al. (1992). Abnormalities of liver function during HIV seroconversion illness. Int J STD AIDS 3: 46-8.

Borrow P, Lewicki H, Hahn BH et al. (1994). Virus specific CD8+ cytotoxic T lymphocyte activity associated with control of viraemia in primary HIV-1 infection. J Virol 68: 6103-10.

Borrow P, Lewicki H, Wei XP et al. (1997). Antiviral pressure exerted by HIV-1-specific cytotoxic T lymphocytes (CTLs) during primary infection demonstrated by rapid selection of CTL escape virus. Nat Med 3: 205-11.

Boulassa F, Bachmeyer C, Carre N et al. (1995). Influence of neurologic manifestations of primary human immunodeficiency virus infection on disease progression. J Infect Dis 171: 1190-5.

Briones C, Perez-Olmeda M, Rodriguez C et al. (2001). Primary genotypic and phenotypic HIV-1 drug resistance in recent seroconverter in Madrid. J Acq Imm Dec Syndr 26: 145-50.

Brunnsgaard H, Pedersen C, Scheibel E et al. (1995). Increase in percentage of CD45RO+/CD8+ cells is associated with previous severe primary HIV infection. *J Acquir Immune Defic Syndr Hum Retrovirol* **10**: 107–14.

Busch MP, Lee LL, Satten GA *et al.* (1995). Time course of detection of viral and serologic markers preceding human immunodeficiency virus type 1 seroconversion: implications for screening of blood and tissue donors. *Transfusion* **35**: 91–7.

Carne CA, Tedder RS, Smith A *et al.* (1985). Acute encephalopathy coincident with seroconversion for anti HTLV-III. *Lancet.* **ii**: 1206–8.

Clark SJ, Saag MS, Decker WD *et al.* (1991). High titers of cytopathic virus in plasma of patients with symptomatic primary HIV-1 infection. *N Engl J Med* **324**: 954–60.

Cocchi F, DeVico AL, Garzino-Demo A *et al.* (1996). Identification of RANTES, MIP-1, and MIP-1 as the major HIV-suppressive factors produced by CD8+ T cells. *Science* **270**: 1811–5.

Connick E, Marr DG, Zhang XQ *et al.* (1996). HIV-specific cellular and humoral immune responses in primary HIV infection. *AIDS Res Hum Retrovir* **12**: 1129–40.

Conway B, Montessori J, Montaner J. (1998). Use of saquinavir-containing regimens for the treatment of primary HIV infection. In: *Book of abstracts, Fifth Conference on Retroviruses and Opportunistic Infections*, Chicago, IL, USA, 1998.

Cooper DA, Gold J, Maclean P *et al.* (1985). Acute AIDS retrovirus infection: definition of a clinical illness associated with seroconversion. *Lancet* **i**: 537–40.

Cooper DA, Imrie AA, Penny R. (1987). Antibody response to human immunodeficiency virus after primary infection. *J Infect Dis* **155**: 1113–8.

Cooper DA, Tindall B, Wilson EJ *et al.* (1988). Characterization of T lymphocyte responses during primary HIV infection. *J Infect Dis* **157**: 889–96.

Cossarizza A, Ortolani C, Mussini C *et al.* (1995). Massive activation of immune cells with an intact T cell repertoire in acute human immunodeficiency virus syndrome. *J Infect Dis* **172**: 105–12.

Daar ES, Moudgil T, Meyer RD *et al.* (1991). Transient high levels of viremia in patients with primary human immunodeficiency virus type 1 infection. *N Engl J Med* **324**: 961–4.

de Wolf F, Lange JMA, Bakker M *et al.* (1988). Influenza-like syndrome in homosexual men: a prospective diagnostic study. *J R Coll Gen Pract* **38**: 443–5.

del Rio C, Soffer O, Widell JL *et al.* (1990). Acute human immunodeficiency virus infection temporally associated with rhabdomyolysis, acute renal failure and nephrosis. *Rev Infect Dis* **12**: 282–5.

Deng H, Liu R, Ellmeier W *et al.* (1996). Identification of a major co-receptor for primary isolates of HIV-1. *Nature* **381**: 661–6.

Dorrucci M, Rezza G, Vlahov D *et al.* (1995). Clinical characteristics and prognostic value of acute retroviral syndrome among injecting drug users. *AIDS* **9**: 597–604.

Dragic T, Litwin V, Allaway GP *et al.* (1996). HIV-1 entry into CD4+ cells is mediated by the chemokine receptor CC-CKR-5. *Nature* **381**: 667–73.

Erice A, Mayers DL, Strike DG *et al.* (1993). Primary infection with zidovudine-resistant human immunodeficiency virus type 1. *N Engl J Med* **328**: 1163–5.

Ferbas J, Daar ES, Grovit-Ferbas K *et al.* (1996). Rapid evolution of human immunodeficiency virus strains with increased replicative capacity during the seronegative window of primary infection. *J Virol* **70**: 7285–9.

Fiore JR, Bjorndal A, Peipke KA *et al.* (1994). The biological phenotype of HIV-1 is usually retained during and after sexual transmission. *Virology* **204**: 297–303.

Fitzgibbon JE, Gaur S, Frenkel LD *et al.* (1993). Transmission from one child to another of human immunodeficiency virus type 1 with a zidovudine-resistant mutation. *N Engl J Med* **329**: 1835–41.

Fox R, Eldred LJ, Fuchs EJ *et al.* (1987). Clinical manifestations of acute infection with human immunodeficiency virus in a cohort of gay men. *AIDS* **1**: 35–8.

Gaines H, Albert J, von Sydow M *et al.* (1987a). HIV antigenaemia and virus isolation from plasma during primary HIV infection. *Lancet* **i**: 1317–8.

Gaines H, von Sydow M, Sonnerborg A *et al.* (1987b). Antibody response in primary human immunodeficiency virus infection. *Lancet* **i**: 1249–53.

Gaines H, von Sydow M, Parry JV *et al.* (1988a). Detection of immunoglobulin M antibody in primary human immunodeficiency virus infection. *AIDS* **2**: 11–5.

Gaines H, von Sydow M, Pehrson PO *et al.* (1988b). Clinical picture of primary HIV infection presenting as a glandular-fever-like illness. *Br Med J* **297**: 1363–8.

Gaines H, von Sydow M, von Stedingk LV *et al.* (1990). Immunological changes in primary HIV infection. *AIDS* **4**: 995–9.

Giorgi JV, Ho HN, Hirji K *et al.* (1994). CD8+ lymphocyte activation at human immunodeficiency virus seroconversion: development of HLA-DR+ CD38-CD8+ cells is associated with subsequent stable CD4+ cell levels. *J Infect Dis* **170**: 775–81.

Goudsmit J, de Wolf F, Paul DA *et al.* (1986). Expression of human immunodeficiency virus antigen in serum and cerebrospinal fluid during acute and chronic infection. *Lancet* **ii**: 177–80.

Graziosi C, Gantt KR, Vaccarezza M *et al.* (1996). Kinetics of cytokine expression during primary HIV-1 infection. *Proc Natl Acad Sci USA* **93**: 4386–91.

Hardy WD, Daar ES, Sokolov RT Jr, Ho DD. (1991). Acute neurologic deterioration in a young man. *Rev Infect Dis* **13**: 745–50.

Hecht FM, Grant RM, Petropoulos CJ *et al.* (1998a). Sexual transmission of an HIV-1 variant resistant to multiple reverse-transcriptase and protease inhibitors. *N Engl J Med* **339**: 307–11.

Hecht FM, Chesney MA, Busch MP *et al.* (1998b). Treatment of primary HIV with AZT, 3TC and Indinavir. In: *Book of abstracts, Fifth Conference on Retroviruses and Opportunistic Infections*, Chicago, IL, USA, 1998.

Henrard DR, Phillips J, Windsor I *et al.* (1994). Detection of human immunodeficiency virus type 1 p24 antigen and plasma RNA: relevance to indeterminate serologic tests. *Transfusion* **34**: 376–80.

Ho DD, Sarngadharan MG, Resnick L *et al.* (1985). Primary human T-lymphotropic virus type III infection. *Ann Intern Med* **103**: 880–3.

Ho DD, Moudgil T, Alam M. (1989). Quantitation of human immunodeficiency virus type 1 in the blood of infected persons. *N Engl J Med* **321**: 1621–5.

Imrie A, Carr A, Duncombe C *et al.* (1996). Primary infection with zidovudine-resistant HIV-1 does not adversely affect outcome at one year. *J Infect Dis* **174**: 195–8.

Imrie A, Beveridge A, Genn W *et al.* (1997). Transmission of human immunodeficiency virus resistant to nevirapine and zidovudine. *J Infect Dis* **176**: 1502–6.

Keet IP, Krijnen P, Koot M *et al.* (1993). Predictors of rapid progression to AIDS in HIV-1 seroconverters. *AIDS* **7**: 51–7.

Kelleher AD, Carr A, Zaunders J *et al.* (1996). Alterations in the immune response of human immunodeficiency virus (HIV) – infected subjects treated with an HIV-specific protease inhibitor, ritonavir. *J Infect Dis* **173**: 321–9.

Kieff ED, Johnson RP, Mark EJ. (1989). Case records of the Massachusetts General Hospital. Case 33-1989. N Engl J Med 321: 454-63.

Kinloch-de Loes S, de Saussure P, Saurat JH, Stalder H, Hirschel B, Perrin LH. (1994). Symptomatic primary infection due to human immunodeficiency virus type 1: review of 31 cases. Clin Infect Dis 17: 59-65.

Kinloch-de Loes S, Hirschel BJ, Hoen B et al. (1993). A controlled trial of zidovudine in primary HIV infection. N Engl J Med 333: 408-13.

Koup RA, Safrit JT, Cao YZ et al. (1994). Temporal association of cellular immune responses with the initial control of viremia in primary HIV-1 syndrome. J Virol 68: 4650-5.

Lafeuillade A, Poggi C, Tamalet C et al. (1997). Effects of a combination of zidovudine, didanosine, and lamivudine on primary human immunodeficiency virus type 1 infection. J Infect Dis 175: 1051-5.

Lange JM, Parry JV, de Wolf F et al. (1988). Diagnostic value of specific IgM antibodies in primary HIV infection. AIDS 2: 31-5.

Lapins J, Lindback S, Lidbrink P et al. (1996). Mucocutaneous manifestations in 22 consecutive cases of primary HIV-1 infection. Br J Dermatol 134: 257-61.

Lewis DA, Brook MG. (1992). Erythema multiforme as a presentation of human immunodeficiency virus seroconversion illness. Int J STD AIDS 3: 56-7.

Lindback S, Brostrom C, Karlsson A et al. (1994). Does symptomatic primary HIV-1 infection accelerate progression to CDC stage IV disease, CD4 count below 200 × 10 (6)/l, AIDS, and death from AIDS. Br Med J 309: 1535-7.

Loussert-Ajaka I, Ly TD, Chaix ML et al. (1994). HIV-1/HIV-2 seronegativity in HIV-1 subtype O infected patients. Lancet 343: 1393-4.

Mackewicz CE, Yang LC, Lifson JD et al. (1994). Non-cytolytic CD8 T-cell anti-HIV responses in primary infection. Lancet 344: 1671-3.

Mariotti M, Lefrere JJ, Noel B et al. (1990). DNA amplification of HIV-1 in seropositive individuals and in seronegative at-risk individuals. AIDS 4: 633-7.

Martin-Rico P, Pedersen C, Skinhoj P et al. (1995). Rapid development of AIDS in an HIV-1 antibody negative homosexual man. AIDS 9: 95-6.

Martinez-Escribano JA, Pedro F, Sabater V et al. (1996). Acute exanthem and pancreatic panniculitis in a patient with primary HIV infection and haemophagocytic syndrome. Br J Dermatol 134: 804-7.

McMillan A, Bishop PE, Aw D et al. (1989). Immunohistology of the skin rash associated with acute HIV infection. AIDS 3: 309-12.

Mellors JW, Kingsley LA, Rinaldo CR Jr et al. (1995). Quantitation of HIV-1 RNA plasma predicts outcome after seroconversion. Ann Intern Med 122: 573-9.

Mientjes GH, van Ameijden EJ, Weigel HM et al. (1993). Clinical symptoms associated with seroconversion for HIV-1 among misusers of intravenous drugs: comparison with homosexual men and intravenous and non-infected intravenous drug misusers. Br Med J 306: 371-3.

Moog C, Pellegrin I, Fleury HJ et al. (1997). Autologous and heterologous neutralizing antibody responses following initial seroconversion in human immunodeficiency virus type 1-infected individuals. J Virol 71: 3734-41.

Moore JP, Cao YZ, Ho DD et al. (1994). Development of the anti-gp120 antibody response during seroconversion to human immunodeficiency virus type 1. J Virol 68: 5142-55.

Musey L, Hughes J, Schacker T et al. (1997). Cytotoxic T-cell responses, viral load, and disease progression in early human immunodeficiency virus type 1 infection. N Engl J Med 337: 1267-74.

Nielsen C, Pedersen C, Lundgren JD et al. (1993). Biological properties of HIV isolates in primary HIV infection: Consequences for the subsequent course of infection. AIDS 7: 1035-40.

Ong EL, Mandal BK. (1991). Primary HIV-1 infection associated with pneumonitis. Postgrad Med J 67: 579-80.

Owens DK, Holodniy M, Garber AM et al. (1996). Polymerase chain reaction for the diagnosis of HIV infection in adults. A meta-analysis with recommendations for clinical practice and study design. Ann Intern Med 124: 803-15.

Pantaleo G, Graziosi C, Demarest JF et al. (1993). HIV infection is active and progressive in lymphoid tissue during the clinically latent stage of disease. Nature 362: 355-8.

Pantaleo G, Demarest JF, Schacker T et al. (1997a). The qualitative nature of the primary immune response to HIV infection is a prognosticator of disease progression independent of the initial level of plasma viremia. Proc Natl Acad Sci USA 94: 254-8.

Pantaleo G, Soudeyns H, Demarest JF et al. (1997b). Evidence for rapid disappearance of initially expanded HIV-specific CD8+ T cell clones during primary HIV infection. Proc Natl Acad Sci USA 94: 9848-53.

Pantaleo G, Cohen OJ, Schacker T et al. (1998). Evolutionary pattern of human immunodeficiency virus (HIV) replication and distribution in lymph nodes following primary infection: implications for antiviral therapy. Nature Med 4: 341-5.

Pedersen BK, Pedersen C. (1994). Epiglottitis as a manifestation of acute HIV infection. J Acquir Immune Defic Syndr 11: 1210-1.

Pedersen C, Lindhardt BO, Jensen BL et al. (1989). Clinical course of primary HIV infection: consequences for subsequent course of infection. Br Med J 299: 154-7.

Pedersen C, Dickmeiss E, Gaub J et al. (1990). T-cell subset alterations and lymphocyte responsiveness to mitogens and antigen during severe primary infection with HIV: a case series of seven consecutive HIV seroconverters. AIDS 4: 523-526.

Pellegrin I, Legrand E, Neau D et al. (1996). Kinetics of appearance of neutralizing antibodies in 12 patients with primary or recent HIV-1 infection and relationship with plasma and cellular viral loads. J Acquir Immune Defic Syndr 11: 438-47.

Peña JM, Martinez-Lopez MA, Arnalich F et al. (1991). Oesophageal candidiasis associated with acute infection due to human immunodeficiency virus: case report and review. Rev Infect Dis 13: 872-5.

Perrin L, Rakik A, Yerly S et al. (1996). Combined therapy with zidovudine and L-697,661 in primary HIV infection. AIDS 10: 1233-7.

Petersen LR, Satten GA, Dodd R et al. (1994). Duration of time from onset of human immunodeficiency virus type 1 infectiousness to development of detectable antibody. Transfusion 34: 283-9.

Phillips AN. (1996). Reduction of HIV concentration during acute infection: independence from a specific immune response. Science 271: 497-9.

Piatak M Jr, Saag MS, Yang LC et al. (1993). High levels of HIV-1 in plasma during all stages of infection determined by competitive PCR. Science 259: 1749-54.

Pilgrim AK, Pantaleo G, Cohen OJ et al. (1997). Neutralizing antibody responses to human immunodeficiency virus type 1 in primary infection and long-term nonprogressive infection. J Infect Dis 176: 924-32.

Price DA, Goulder PJR, Klenerman P et al. (1997). Positive selection of HIV-1 cytotoxic T lymphocyte escape variants during primary infection. Proc Natl Acad Sci USA 94: 1890-5.

Rabeneck L, Popovic M, Gartner S et al. (1990). Acute HIV infection presenting with painful swallowing and esophageal ulcers. JAMA 263: 2318–22.

Ranki A, Valle SL, Krohn M et al. (1987). Long latency precedes overt seroconversion in sexually transmitted human immunodeficiency virus infection. Lancet ii: 589–93.

Reimer L, Mottice S, Schable C et al. (1997). Absence of detectable antibody in a patient infected with human immunodeficiency virus. Clin Infect Dis 25: 98–100.

Ritter J, Chevallier P, Peyramond D et al. (1990). Serological markers during an acute HIV-2 infection. Vox Sang 59: 244–5.

Rizzardi GP, Barcellini W, Tambussi G et al. (1996). Plasma levels of soluble CD30, tumor necrosis factor (TNF)-α and TNF receptors during primary HIV-1 infection: correlation with HIV-1 RNA and the clinical outcome. AIDS 10: F45–50.

Roos MTL, Lange JMA, de Goede REY et al. (1992). Viral phenotype and immune response in primary human immunodeficiency virus type I infection. J Infect Dis 165: 427–32.

Samuel D, Castaing D, Adam R et al. (1988). Fatal acute HIV infection with aplastic anaemia, transmitted by liver graft. Lancet i: 1221–2.

Schable C, Zekeng L, Pau CP et al. (1994). Sensitivity of United States HIV antibody tests for detection of HIV-1 group O infections. Lancet 344: 1333–4.

Schacker T, Collier AC, Hughes J et al. (1996). Clinical and epidemiologic features of primary HIV infection. Ann Intern Med 125: 257–64.

Schacker T, Hughes J, Shea T et al. (1998). Biological and virologic characteristics of primary HIV infection. Ann Intern Med 125: 613–20.

Sinicco A, Biglino A, Sciandra M et al. (1993a). Cytokine network and acute primary HIV-1 infection. AIDS 7: 1167–72.

Sinicco A, Fora R, Sciandra M et al. (1993b). Risk of developing AIDS after primary acute HIV-1 infection. J Acquir Immune Defic Syndr 6: 575–81.

Sonnerborg AB, von Stedingk LV, Hansson LO et al. (1989). Elevated neopterin and beta2-microglobulin levels in blood and cerebrospinal fluid occur early in HIV-1 infection. AIDS 3: 277–83.

Strizki JM, Albright AV, Sheng H et al. (1996). Infection of primary human microglia and monocyte-derived macrophages with human immunodeficiency virus type 1 isolates: evidence of differential tropism. J Virol 70: 7654–62.

Terpstra FG, Al BJ, Roos MT et al. (1989). Longitudinal study of leukocyte functions in homosexual men seroconverted for HIV: rapid and persistent loss of B cell function after HIV infection. Eur J Immunol 19: 667–73.

Tindall B, Barker S, Donovan B et al. (1988). Characterization of the acute clinical illness associated with human immunodeficiency virus infection. Arch Intern Med 148: 945–9.

Tindall B, Hing M, Edwards P et al. (1989). Severe clinical manifestations of primary HIV infection. AIDS 3: 747–9.

Tindall B, Cooper DA. (1991). Primary HIV infection: Host responses and intervention strategies. AIDS 5: 1–14.

UK Collaborative Group on Monitoring the Transmission of HIV Drug Resistance (2001). Analysis of prevalence of HIV-1 drug resistance in primary infections in the UK. Br Med J 322: 1087–8.

Valle SL. (1987). Febrile pharyngitis as the primary sign of HIV infection in a cluster of cases linked by sexual contact. Scand J Infect Dis 19: 13–7.

Van Essen GG, Lieverse AG, Sprenger HG et al. (1988). False-positive Paul-Bunnell test in HIV seroconversion. Lancet ii: 747–8.

van Griensven GJP, de Vroome EMM, de Wolf F et al. (1990). Risk factors for progression of human immunodeficiency virus (HIV) infection among seroconverted and seropositive homosexual men. Am J Epidemiol 132: 203–10.

Vanhems P, Allard R, Cooper DA, et al. (1997). Acute HIV-1 disease as a mononucleosis-like illness: is the diagnosis too restrictive? Clin Infect Dis 24: 965–70.

Vanhems P, Lambert J, Cooper DA et al. (1998). Severity and prognosis of acute human immunodeficiency virus type 1 illness: a dose-response relationship. Clin Infect Dis 26: 323–9.

Vento S, Di Perri G, Garofano T et al. (1993). Pneumocystis carinii pneumonia during primary HIV-1 infection. Lancet 342: 24–5.

von Sydow M, Gaines H, Sonnerborg A et al. (1988). Antigen detection in primary HIV infection. Br Med J 296: 238–40.

von Sydow M, Sonnerborg A, Gaines H et al. (1991). Interferon-alpha and tumor necrosis factor alpha in serum of patients in varying stages of HIV-1 infection. AIDS Res Hum Retrovir 7: 375–80.

Ward JW, Bush TJ, Perkins HA et al. (1989). The natural history of transfusion-associated HIV infection: factors influencing progression to disease. N Engl J Med 321: 947–52.

Zaunders J, Carr A, McNally L et al. (1995). Effects of primary HIV-1 infection on subsets of CD4+ and CD8+ T lymphocytes. AIDS 9: 561–6.

Zhu TF, Mo H, Wang N et al. (1993). Genotypic and phenotypic characterization of HIV-1 in patients with primary HIV-1 infection. Science 261: 1179–81.

MARTYN FRENCH

The human immunodeficiency virus (HIV) exhibits tropism for cells of the immune system. Acute infection with HIV often gives rise to an illness with characteristics similar to those of the illness caused by other immunotropic viruses, such as cytomegalovirus (CMV) and Epstein–Barr virus (EBV). Following this acute infection, a chronic infection is established within various components of the immune system. The immunopathology arising in these sites as a consequence of the chronic infection gives rise, after a variable period of time, to diverse but characteristic disease manifestations, which reflect either viral replication itself, or the resulting immunodeficiency. These include constitutional symptoms, neurological disease, opportunistic tumours and opportunistic infections. Often, these disease manifestations occur together, but the degree to which each is expressed can vary. Thus, some patients have predominantly neurological disease with few if any complications of the immunodeficiency, while most have multiple infections and/or malignant disease without developing overt neurological disease. Furthermore, the rate at which these HIV disease manifestations develop varies from one individual to another and appears to be determined by genetic differences of the virus (Deacon et al., 1995), genetic factors in the host, especially polymorphism of major histocompatibility complex (MHC) genes (Keet et al., 1996; Hogan and Hammer, 2001) and chemokine or chemokine receptor genes (Hoffman and Doms, 1998), and the host immune response to HIV (Musey et al., 1997; Hogan and Hammer, 2001).

In developing strategies for the diagnosis and management of HIV-infected individuals, it is crucial to take into account this variability in the nature and time course of disease manifestations and use clinical assessments and laboratory investigations accordingly.

Presentation of HIV infection

Most people in developed countries, and many in developing countries, are aware of HIV infection and the activities that would place them at risk of acquiring infection. Consequently, many individuals discover that they are infected by HIV after they have sought diagnostic testing because of a belief that they are at risk of acquiring infection. As a result, HIV infection is often diagnosed prior to the onset of symptomatic disease. However, diagnosis of HIV infection at the time of presentation with an AIDS-defining illness continues to be a problem (Poznansky et al., 1995). Individuals presenting late with HIV infection are more likely to have Pneumocystis carinii pneumonia (PCP) than those who present earlier (and thus receive prophylaxis for PCP when their CD4 lymphocyte count places them at risk of reactivation). In these individuals, PCP is often severe and requires protracted hospitalization (Mallal et al., 1994). Because the occurrence of many HIV disease manifestations can be prevented or delayed by providing treatment for the HIV infection and prophylactic therapy for opportunistic infections, it is important to identify HIV-infected individuals as soon as possible and recruit them to treatment programmes. Furthermore, recruitment of patients to monitoring and treatment programmes will provide an opportunity to minimize transmission of HIV infection to other people.

The reasons for delaying medical assessment of HIV infection are not fully understood, but include a history of injecting drug use, lack of a supporting relative or partner, and not being aware of HIV risk (Samet et al., 1998). Education programmes promulgating the benefits of early diagnosis and treatment are therefore of paramount importance. Medical practitioners can also play a major role by actively searching for individuals with signs and symptoms of undiagnosed HIV infection, or evidence of behaviour patterns that would place that individual at risk of contracting the infection. Examples of the latter include signs of injecting drug use or anal sexually transmitted infections (e.g. warts) indicating anal intercourse. The routine questioning of patients about sexual behaviour and injecting drug use during the forming of a medical history will also increase the likelihood of detecting previously undiagnosed HIV infection.

Despite education programmes and active case detection, many HIV-infected individuals will still present with an HIV-related disease. It is therefore essential to consider HIV infection in the differential diagnosis of a wide range of medical problems. Disease caused by HIV infection presents in many ways, but some illnesses are particularly characteristic and should alert a medical or dental practitioner to the possibility of underlying HIV infection.

Acute HIV infection

Acute infection with HIV often presents as an infectious mononucleosis-like syndrome and may be confused with acute EBV or CMV infection. There are, however, a number of abnormalities characteristic or suggestive of acute HIV infection. These include neurological conditions such as meningoencephalitis, peripheral neuropathy, brachial neuritis, radiculopathy and Guillain–Barré syndrome; mucocutaneous manifestations such as oropharyngeal and genital ulceration, maculopapular skin rash, roseola-like rash, urticaria, desquamation and alopecia, and even the development of a transient cellular immunodeficiency syndrome (see Chapter 1). Acute HIV infection must therefore enter into the differential diagnosis of any acute febrile illness associated with diffuse lymphadenopathy, especially if there are additional clinical signs characteristic of HIV infection and particularly so if the patient has engaged in behaviour that would place him or her at risk of contracting the infection. Confirmation of acute HIV infection requires the use of laboratory investigations. Antibodies to HIV may be present within the first 2 weeks of the infection, especially IgM antibodies, but they often do not appear until 2–6 weeks after infection, and may take as long as 12 weeks. HIV RNA or p24 antigen may be detected in the patient's plasma before HIV antibodies are detected (Schacker et al., 1996) and, therefore, patients with suspected acute HIV infection should be tested for both HIV antibodies and HIV RNA or p24 antigen. However, it must be remembered that current

tests to quantify HIV RNA are not licensed for the detection of infection, and specificity is less than 100%. There is often a delay before a patient can be given a definitive diagnosis. An acutely infected individual is highly infectious because of the high plasma HIV viral load. A suspected case of acute HIV mononucleosis must therefore be managed as though it is HIV infection until proven otherwise. This management policy must include education of the patient about the importance of avoiding unprotected sexual intercourse and avoidance of organ and blood donation.

Lymphadenopathy

Much of the immunopathology that results from chronic HIV infection occurs within lymphoid tissue (Pantaleo et al., 1993). Consequently, lymphoid hyperplasia occurs in many individuals, especially early in the course of this chronic infection. Generalized lymphadenopathy occurs in 50–70% of HIV-infected individuals, and a smaller proportion have splenomegaly. HIV infection must therefore be considered in any person found to have generalized lymphadenopathy.

The enlarged nodes are not usually tender in chronic HIV infection. The degree of enlargement is not an indicator of the subsequent clinical course, though enlarged nodes often regress with the onset of severe immunodeficiency. Enlargement of a single node or group of nodes as the presenting manifestation of HIV infection, or as a new finding in patients with established immunodeficiency, should always raise the possibility of an abnormality other than HIV lymphadenitis, especially if the node is progressively increasing in size and is tender. Lymphoma, Kaposi's sarcoma (KS) and mycobacterial infections are the most common complications presenting in this way, particularly in the patient with severe immunodeficiency. Pathological examination of the enlarged node by fine-needle aspiration or surgical biopsy is indicated in this situation.

Mucocutaneous manifestations of HIV infection

Both infectious and neoplastic complications of cellular immunodeficiency can affect the skin and mucous membranes. In HIV-induced immunodeficiency, these may occur before the onset of severe opportunistic infections or constitutional symptoms and therefore may be the first manifestation of HIV infection.

Varicella zoster virus infection

Reactivation of varicella zoster virus (VZV) infection is common in individuals infected by HIV. This often occurs long before the onset of severe immunodeficiency and at a time when the CD4 lymphocyte count is relatively high. The development of shingles, including ophthalmic zoster, in a young person, should always alert the physician to the possibility of underlying HIV infection, particularly if there is a history of risk behaviour. The clinical course is usually similar to that seen in individuals not infected by HIV. However, more frequent, severe and prolonged illness has been described (see Chapter 32), though disease severity is not a good indicator of underlying HIV infection. Chronic relapsing dermatomal VZV infection and the presence of peripheral retinal perivasculitis and perivascular sheathing in patients with ophthalmic involvement (Karbassi *et al.*, 1992) are highly suggestive of HIV infection. Unlike many other opportunistic infections, the occurrence of herpes zoster infection in an HIV-infected patient does not portend a poor prognosis (McNulty *et al.*, 1997).

Dermatophyte infections

Fungal infections of the skin and nails are not uncommon in immunocompetent individuals, but extensive infections and infections that are recalcitrant to therapy may be an indicator of underlying HIV-induced cellular immunodeficiency. In this situation, infection of finger or toe nails often causes considerable onycholysis. Severe dermatophyte infections in HIV-infected individuals usually indicate advanced immunodeficiency.

Although eradication of dermatophyte infections is very difficult to achieve in HIV-infected patients, treatment may improve the condition and is worthwhile. Topical application of an imidazole cream to the skin is often successful, but oral administration of an imidazole may be necessary in severe cases. Nail infections usually require at least 6 months of oral griseofulvin, an imidazole or terbinafine (see Chapter 19).

Seborrhoeic dermatitis

Seborrhoeic dermatitis, although a relatively common problem in immunocompetent individuals, is a characteristic finding in HIV-infected individuals with moderate to severe immunodeficiency. Newly acquired seborrhoeic dermatitis, especially when severe or poorly responsive to therapy, could indicate underlying HIV infection. This is particularly so when it is associated with weight loss, fevers and oral candidiasis, a constellation of signs and symptoms that is characteristic of 'prodromal' PCP infection. *Pityrosporum* yeasts are probably implicated in the patho-

genesis of this condition and treatment with topical ketoconazole, in combination with topical hydrocortisone to reduce inflammation, is frequently effective. An alternative topical therapy is sulphur and salicylic acid cream (see Chapter 19).

Molluscum contagiosum

This poxvirus infection of the skin causes small nodular and often umbilicated lesions in immunocompetent individuals, occurs most commonly in children, mainly affects the trunk and often resolves spontaneously. In contrast, persistent progressively enlarging or giant lesions affecting the head and neck of adults are highly suggestive of underlying cellular immunodeficiency, especially HIV-induced immunodeficiency (see Chapter 19). Lesions may also occur elsewhere on the skin. Cryotherapy may be effective but recurrence is common. Recalcitrant lesions may respond to cidofovir therapy.

Herpes simplex virus infections

Mucocutaneous infections with herpes simplex virus (HSV) are relatively common in the general population, particularly sexually acquired ano-genital HSV infections. Patients presenting with recurrent HSV infections are rarely found to have immunodeficiency, but persistent, invasive and necrotic lesions, especially of the genitals and anus, are an indication for an evaluation of cellular immunity and testing for HIV infection.

Papillomavirus infections

Cutaneous and genital warts caused by infection with human papillomaviruses are not unduly common in patients with HIV infection. Indeed, genital warts would not be unexpected in a group of individuals who have another infection that is commonly acquired by sexual intercourse. However, persistent and large lesions and lesions recalcitrant to therapy can be the first indication of underlying HIV-induced immunodeficiency.

Kaposi's sarcoma

This proliferative tumour of vascular endothelial cells is endemic in some parts of Africa, Italy and Eastern Europe. Outside of these geographical areas, the occurrence of Kaposi's sarcoma (KS) indicates underlying immunodeficiency in the great majority of individuals. In the absence of therapeutic immunosuppression, this immunodeficiency is virtually always caused by HIV infection.

KS lesions can occur anywhere on the skin, as well as in the mucous membranes of the mouth and gastrointestinal tract. Cutaneous lesions have a characteristic reddish-brown colour and vary in size and shape from small macules to large bulbous lesions. Early KS lesions are sometimes difficult to differentiate from other skin lesions (particularly bacillary angiomatosis), and a skin biopsy may be necessary. They do not usually cause discomfort, but lesions on the feet can be very painful.

Mucosal candidiasis

Persistent infection of the mucosal surface of the mouth or oropharynx by Candida species in the absence of antibiotic therapy or an underlying illness is highly suggestive of immunodeficiency. Recurrent vaginal candidiasis is much less predictive of an immunodeficiency syndrome but abnormally severe and persistent vaginal candidiasis should alert the physician to the possibility of immuno-deficiency, including that caused by HIV infection.

Oral and oropharyngeal disease

In addition to candidiasis, there are several manifestations of HIV-induced immunodeficiency that affect the oral cavity and oropharynx (Greenspan and Greenspan, 1996; Weinart et al., 1996). While these are often first demon-strated in patients with established HIV infection, they may be the impetus for an individual with HIV infection to present to a dental or medical practitioner.

Hairy leukoplakia of the oral mucosa is a pathognomonic sign of cellular immunodeficiency that is nearly always sec-ondary to HIV infection. It most commonly affects the sides of the tongue as white plaques, which cannot be removed with a spatula or gauze. KS can take on many forms but commonly occurs as purplish-grey flat or protuberant lesions of the palate or gums. Severe gingivitis, especially necrotizing and associated with periodontal disease, also suggests immunodeficiency.

Laboratory test abnormalities

Chronic HIV infection commonly causes abnormalities of the immune and haemopoetic systems, which can be detected by laboratory testing. HIV infection may present with such abnormalities. Thrombocytopenia is usually immune mediated but may occasionally be a manifestation of thrombotic thrombocytopenic purpura (TTP) (see Chapter 17). HIV-associated immune thrombocytopenia (ITP) can be very pronounced and may occur long before the onset of immunodeficiency, when the affected indi-vidual is otherwise asymptomatic. Consequently, many clinicians now include investigations for HIV infection in protocols for the assessment of thrombocytopenia. In contrast, anaemia and neutropenia most commonly occur in the context of symptomatic HIV infection and related therapies. Lymphopenia is found almost universally in patients with severe immunodeficiency, and HIV infection should be a consideration in any patient who presents with unexplained lymphopenia. Likewise, hypergammaglobulin-aemia is a common occurrence, occurring in all stages of HIV infection. All isotypes of immunoglobulin can be affected, but increased serum concentrations of IgG and IgA are most characteristic (Fling et al., 1988).

Evaluation and management of the newly diagnosed patient

The patient with newly diagnosed HIV infection must be thoroughly evaluated to determine the severity of immuno-deficiency and whether or not complications of HIV infection are present. It is also important to evaluate the patient for latent infections that might reactivate if and when cellular immunodeficiency develops, and for conditions such as glucose-6-phosphate dehydrogenase (G6PD) deficiency, which may make the use of some drugs hazardous (Table 2.1). Thus, a full clinical examination,

Table 2.1 Investigations in the newly diagnosed patient

1. HIV antibodies to confirm the diagnosis (ELISA and Western Blot)
2. CD4 lymphocyte count (and percentage)
3. Plasma HIV RNA concentration
4. Mantoux test and measurement of DTH responses to antigens other than tuberculin
5. Serum antibodies to CMV, Toxoplasma gondii, Treponema pallidum, hepatitis A virus (HAV), hepatitis B virus (HBV) and hepatitis C virus (HCV)
6. Serum HBV surface antigen; plasma HCV RNA in HCV antibody-positive patients
7. Full blood count (especially a platelet count) and liver function tests
8. Measurement of red blood cell G6PD activity in males of black African or eastern Mediterranean descent (to detect those at risk of haemolysis from the use of anti-malarials or sulphonamides)

CMV: cytomegalovirus; DTH: delayed-type hypersensitivity.

including a neurological examination, and immunological and microbiological investigations, should be performed. The patient should also be assessed for other associated medical problems, especially other sexually transmissible infections and injecting drug use. Furthermore, many newly diagnosed patients experience difficulties in adjusting to the knowledge that they have HIV infection and will require counselling and occasionally referral to a clinical psychologist or psychiatrist.

Evaluation for latent infection by opportunistic pathogens

Assays for serum antibodies against CMV, hepatitis B virus (HBV), hepatitis C virus (HCV), *Toxoplasma gondii* and *Treponema pallidum* and for serum HBV surface antigen should be performed. If HCV antibodies are detected, plasma should be tested for HCV RNA to determine whether active HCV infection is present. Individuals with antibodies against *T. pallidum* who have not previously received adequate treatment for syphilis should have cerebrospinal fluid examined to determine whether asymptomatic neurosyphilis is present (Holtom *et al.*, 1992) and if so, appropriate treatment should be given.

A Mantoux test should also be performed, where possible in conjunction with skin testing of delayed-type hypersensitivity (DTH) to other antigens to exclude anergy and validate a negative Mantoux test. Induration from a Mantoux test of 5 mm or greater suggests latent infection with *Mycobacterium tuberculosis* (MTB) (Markowitz *et al.*, 1997) in individuals not previously immunized with BCG. However, intravenous drug users often have impaired DTH responses and a response of 2 mm or more may indicate latent MTB infection (Graham *et al.*, 1992). Mantoux test 'converters' and anergic patients with a CD4 lymphocyte count of less than 200 cells/μl and a high risk of acquiring MTB infection have a particularly high risk of developing tuberculosis (Markowitz *et al.*, 1997). Prophylactic isoniazid for 12 months or rifampin and pyrazinamide for 4 months (Halsey *et al.*, 1998) should be considered in patients with evidence of latent MTB infection and in patients who are anergic and at high risk of being infected by MTB (Perlman and Hanvanich, 1997) (see Chapter 23). Patients in whom it is difficult to test for MTB infection using a Mantoux test, because they may not return to have the test read, can be tested using a tuberculin interferon-gamma assay (Converse *et al.*, 1997).

Vaccination

The initial evaluation of an HIV-infected patient provides a valuable opportunity to determine whether or not vaccinations are necessary to increase the level of immunity against micro-organisms that might cause disease at a later date. Patients with HIV infection have a higher than normal risk of developing chronic HBV infection and homosexual men have a higher than normal risk of acquiring HAV infection. Patients should therefore be tested for HAV and HBV antibodies and vaccination offered if antibodies are not detected. However, antibody responses to both vaccines are often lower than in individuals without HIV infection and responsiveness progressively decreases with increasing levels of immunodeficiency (Hess *et al.*, 1995; Collier *et al.*, 1988). HIV-infected patients are also more susceptible to disease resulting from *Streptococcus pneumoniae* infection, particularly smokers, elderly patients and intravenous drug users (see Chapter 35). Routine vaccination with 23-valent pneumococcal polysaccharide vaccine is often recommended for all HIV-infected patients, but apart from patients with additional risk factors this practice may not be justified (Jain *et al.*, 1995). Vaccination with pneumococcal polysaccharides does not prevent pneumococcal disease (French *et al.*, 2000), and over 50% of patients with a CD4 lymphocyte count of less than 500 cells/μl respond poorly to vaccination, even when a second vaccination is given (Rodriguez-Barradas *et al.*, 1996; Dworkin *et al.*, 2001). Furthermore, vaccination with pneumococcal polysaccharides may increase HIV replication in some patients (Brichacek *et al.*, 1996). Although HIV-infected patients do not have an increased risk of influenza virus infection, secondary bacterial infections may be more severe and vaccination should be considered at presentation and when there is the possibility of a community outbreak. Immune responses to influenza virus antigens may be impaired in immunodeficient patients but vaccination appears not to increase HIV replication (Fowke *et al.*, 1997).

Patient education

The newly diagnosed HIV-infected patient should also be educated about HIV infection, its treatment and measures, which should be undertaken to prevent transmission of the infection to other people. Advice on safer sex practices should include information on sexual activities that do not involve transmission of bodily fluids and also information on the use of condoms. Oral sex without condoms should be strongly discouraged because there is good evidence that HIV infection can be transmitted by this means (Schacker et al., 1996). Injecting drug users should be provided with information on safe injecting techniques.

Clinical and laboratory monitoring of HIV-infected individuals

Given the panoply of HIV disease manifestations and their variable rate of progression, it is important to review HIV-infected individuals at regular intervals to detect clinical and laboratory indicators of disease progression and to monitor the effects of therapy in patients receiving antiretroviral therapy. Clinical and laboratory investigations used to monitor HIV-infected patients are shown in Table 2.2.

Clinical monitoring

Weight loss, night sweats, fevers and diarrhoea, for which there is no other cause, are common constitutional symptoms, which are part of the AIDS-related complex (ARC). Such symptoms may reflect the effects of excessive cytokine production and usually portend the onset of severe immunodeficiency. Regular inspection of the skin and mucous membranes will permit early detection of KS lesions, molluscum contagiosum, onycholysis caused by dermatophyte infections, candidiasis and oral hairy leukoplakia. Both oral candidiasis and hairy leukoplakia of the tongue predict the imminent progression to AIDS independently of CD4 lymphocyte counts (Katz et al., 1992) and presumably provide the clinical indication of a functional cellular immune defect. However, cigarette smokers

Table 2.2 Clinical and laboratory investigations used to monitor patients with HIV infection

Clinical	Laboratory
Weight	Blood CD4 lymphocyte count and percentage
Temperature	Plasma HIV RNA concentration
Examination of mouth for candidiasis and oral hairy leukoplakia	[a]Serum β_2-microglobulin, IgA or neopterin concentration
[a]Measurement of cutaneous DTH responses	

[a]Adjunctive investigations, not routinely done.

are more likely to develop oral candidiasis (Palacio et al., 1997), and the patient's smoking history should be taken into consideration when evaluating the significance of oral lesions.

Clinical monitoring in HIV-infected women should also include a cervical cytology examination every 6–12 months to detect cervical squamous intra-epithelial lesions (CSILs) of the cervix at an early stage (Palefsky, 1991). The place of routine anal cytology examination in HIV-infected males is yet to be established but it does appear to be indicated in patients with the highest risk of developing anal squamous intra-epithelial lesions (ASILs) (Palefsky et al., 1997). Such patients include those with anal warts or rectal discharge, a low CD4 lymphocyte count, anal human papilloma virus (HPV) infection and a high level of HPV DNA (Palefsky et al., 1998). Females with high-grade CSILs or cervical or vulval cancer also have a greater risk of developing ASILs and anal cancer (Hillemans et al., 1996) and should have a regular anal cytology examination performed. If abnormalities are detected by cytological examination, culposcopy or anoscopy should be performed to obtain biopsy material for histological examination.

Early signs of HIV encephalopathy are often detected by observing that the patient is becoming confused, forgetful, slow and less articulate. Such observations should prompt an evaluation of cognitive function and a neurological examination, to be followed, if indicated, by examination of cerebrospinal fluid and a cranial computerized tomography (CT) or magnetic resonance imaging (MRI) scan.

Laboratory monitoring

Serial measurement of the plasma HIV RNA concentration and CD4 lymphocyte count or percentage has the greatest clinical utility for monitoring HIV disease (Mellors et al., 1997), making decisions about therapy (Hughes et al., 1997), and determining the risk of developing opportunistic infections (Crowe et al., 1991). Measurements should be undertaken every 2–3 months, except when antiretroviral therapy is started or changed, when testing after 1 month will usually indicate whether therapy is effective or not.

CD4 lymphocyte counts can be used for clinical decision making, as outlined in Table 2.3. However, CD4 lymphocyte counts in patients treated with highly active antiretroviral therapy (HAART) may not have the same predictive value for opportunistic infections because clonal repletion of CD4 lymphocytes after HAART is often incomplete (Connors et al., 1997).

Table 2.3 CD4 lymphocyte counts in clinical decision making

CD4 lymphocyte count	Clinical decision
$<500/\mu l$	Consider starting antiretroviral therapy
$<200/\mu l$	Commence prophylaxis for *Pneumocystis carinii* and toxoplasma infection
$<100/\mu l$	Commence prophylaxis for MAC infection
$<50/\mu l$	Undertake regular examination of the fundi through dilated pupils to detect (CMV) retinitis

CMV: cytomegalovirus; MAC: *Mycobacterium avium* complex.

Opinion is divided on the use of HIV RNA assay results for clinical decision making. Some physicians argue that antiretroviral therapy should be commenced or changed if HIV RNA is detectable in any amount. Others accept the small risk of disease progression associated with low concentrations of HIV RNA in patients who are asymptomatic and have a CD4 lymphocyte count > 500 cells/μl, to avoid exposing the patient to drugs to which the virus might become resistant and to spare the patient from the rigours of taking antiretroviral therapy before it is essential to do so. However, antiretroviral therapy should be started or changed if the plasma HIV RNA concentration is > 30 000 copies/ml, irrespective of CD4 lymphocyte count, or > 5000 copies/ml if there is clinical or immunological evidence of disease progression (Saag *et al.*, 1996). Undetectable HIV RNA should be aimed for, but a value of < 5000 copies/ml may be acceptable if the patient or physician do not wish to change therapy.

A change in plasma HIV RNA concentration of less than threefold ($0.5 \log_{10}$) is not significant. Wherever possible, the same type of HIV RNA assay (either RT-PCR or bDNA) should be used for a particular patient. If HIV RNA is repeatedly undetectable or present in very low amounts using a RT-PCR assay in patients not treated with antiretroviral therapy, the possibility of infection with a subtype A, E or F strain of HIV should be considered, particularly if the infection may have been contracted in Africa or Asia. Plasma samples should be re-assayed using primers which will amplify reverse transcribed DNA from these strains of HIV (Dunne *et al.*, 1996).

Additional immunological investigations, including indicators of immune activation, such as the serum concentration of β_2-microglobulin, neopterin or IgA (Fahey

et al., 1990), and measurement of a functional cellular immune response, especially cutaneous DTH responses (Blatt *et al.*, 1993), provide information that supplements the measurement of CD4 lymphocyte counts. However, these investigations are probably only indicated when plasma HIV RNA concentrations cannot be measured.

Genotypical or phenotypical assays for demonstrating resistance of HIV isolates to antiretroviral drugs are now available but their role in managing patients being treated with combination antiretroviral therapy is still under investigation (Hirsch *et al.*, 2000). The demonstration of nucleotide substitutions associated with antiretroviral drug resistance in the reverse transcriptase and protease genes does appear to be of value in formulating a new drug regimen in patients failing antiretroviral therapy. In addition, testing of HIV isolates from all newly diagnosed cases of HIV infection may be indicated if transmission of drug-resistant strains of HIV is likely.

Evaluation of symptoms and signs in immunodeficient patients

Treatment of HIV-infected patients with highly active antiretroviral therapy (HAART) has resulted in a substantial reduction in the incidence of opportunistic infections and other HIV-related diseases (Palella *et al.*, 1998). However, patients who have progressively worsening HIV infection because they have not been treated with HAART for one reason or another, or because therapy has failed, will eventually develop symptoms and clinical signs of immunodeficiency and/or neurological disease. Many of these clinical problems present as characteristic manifestations of HIV-induced disease, the most common of which are described here by body system.

Treatment with HAART has increased the survival time of most patients, resulting in many patients having prolonged periods of antiretroviral therapy. Consequently, the adverse effect of drug therapy is now more of an issue than it was and must be taken into consideration when evaluating symptoms and signs (John *et al.*, 1998a).

Ear, nose and throat disease
Hearing impairment
Impairment of hearing is commonly caused by Eustachian tube dysfunction resulting from bacterial infection. It often accompanies bacterial infections of the nasal sinuses. Sensorineural deafness is uncommon but can be caused by

necrotic and bleed easily, especially when the gums are involved. Lymphoma may also present with nodular lesions but these are not as prone to bleed as KS lesions. Nodular lesions on the tongue must be differentiated from median rhomboid glossitis caused by *Candida* species infection.

Gingival and periodontal disease

Gingivitis and periodontitis are common and sometimes asymptomatic (Greenspan and Greenspan, 1996; Weinart et al., 1996). Consequently, regular dental assessments should be an essential component of a management plan for the immunodeficient patient. Gingivitis presents as diffuse erythematous lesions of the gums or linear marginal erythema. It is sometimes associated with petechiae and there is a tendency to spontaneous haemorrhage. Treatment comprises antibiotics active against Gram-positive cocci and anaerobes, together with antiseptic mouth washes. Necrotizing gingivitis results in extensive tissue loss, sometimes associated with ulceration, and is rapidly progressive. Some cases progress to periodontitis. Periodontal disease often causes deep pain in the gums and spontaneous bleeding. It can be a very aggressive disease and specialist assessment and management of this problem is strongly recommended. Acute necrotizing gingivitis and perio-dontitis are usually indicative of severe immunodeficiency and are poorly responsive to conventional therapy.

Dry mouth and disorders of taste and smell

These complaints may be very distressing and can result in a poor appetite and weight loss. A dry mouth is often an adverse effect of didanosine therapy, and may be so severe that the didanosine has to be ceased. Disorders of taste and smell are also usually attributable to drug therapies (Heald et al., 1998).

Respiratory tract disease

Chronic and subacute respiratory tract symptoms

The gradual onset of a non-productive cough associated with dyspnoea, weight loss and fever, in a person who has other evidence of immunodeficiency such as oral candidiasis or seborrhoeic dermatitis is highly suggestive of *Pneumocystis carinii* pneumonia (PCP). This is particularly so if the patient is not receiving adequate prophylactic therapy for PCP. Clinical signs and radiological changes of an interstitial pneumonitis are common in advanced disease but either may be absent, especially in early infection. Pneu-

cytotoxic drugs, including macrolide antibiotics and rarely by neurotoxic antiretroviral drugs such as zalcitabine (Martinez and French, 1993). It may also occur as a complication of severe meningitis, including cryptococcal meningitis. In rare circumstances, hearing loss may be due to disseminated pneumocystosis in a patient with advanced HIV infection.

Sinusitis

Infectious complications of both antibody- and cell-mediated immune defects are a cause of sinusitis in HIV-infected patients (Godofsky et al., 1992; Gradon et al., 1993). Patients usually present with nasal congestion and discharge associated with frontal headache or facial pain. Common bacterial causes of sinusitis, such as *Haemophilus influenzae* and *Streptococcus pneumoniae*, are often implicated and can be successfully treated with amoxycillin and clavulanic acid. Infection with *Pseudomonas aeruginosa* (O'Donnell et al., 1993) and a variety of opportunistic fungal infections occurs less commonly and mainly in severely immunodeficient patients. Initial investigations include sinus X-rays, or a CT scan of the sinuses, which is particularly useful in the diagnosis of sinusitis in this situation (Godofsky et al., 1992). Needle aspiration may be required for drainage and/or determining the microbial aetiology.

Oro-pharyngeal disease

Mucosal ulceration

Mucosal ulceration involving the mouth or oro-pharynx has a number of causes. Non-infective (aphthous) ulcers are most common and can be large, invasive and very painful. They are sometimes associated with oesophageal ulcers. Treatment with thalidomide (Jacobson et al., 1997a) or topical or systemic steroids is effective in many cases. Infective causes such as herpes simplex virus (HSV) must be excluded by culture of swabs from the lesions, particularly if topical or systemic steroids are to be used for treatment. Rarely, cytomegalovirus (CMV) can cause ulceration; diagnosis is based upon biopsy of a lesion. Single necrotic ulcers with raised edges must always raise the possibility of lymphoma, and biopsy of the lesion is again necessary to make the diagnosis. Mouth ulcers may also be an adverse effect of zalcitabine therapy.

Mass lesions

Nodular KS lesions are usually easy to recognize by their greyish-red colour. They can be large, and can become

monitis resulting from CMV infection may also present in a similar manner, but this is much less common than PCP and only occurs in severely immunodeficient patients.

Similar symptoms should also raise the possibility of tuberculosis in individuals from areas of the world in which this infection is endemic, as well as in injecting drug users and individuals from certain urban underprivileged groups. When tuberculosis is considered to be a possibility, it is strongly advisable to manage a patient with a productive cough as a case of 'open' tuberculosis until proven otherwise. This is particularly so when there is a possibility of infection with a multi-drug-resistant strain of MTB, which might infect other patients and hospital staff (Beck-Sague et al., 1992). Radiological changes can often help to differentiate tuberculosis from PCP. In patients with PCP, hilar lymphadenopathy and pleural effusions occur much less frequently than in patients with tuberculosis and the pleural effusions associated with tuberculosis are often much larger than in patients with PCP (Joseph et al., 1993). Furthermore, the probability of pulmonary tuberculosis (compared with other opportunistic infections of the lung) would be increased by demonstrating intact cutaneous DTH responses, including a tuberculin response (CDC, 1991), and a CD4 lymphocyte count of > 200 cells/μl. The latter occurs in approximately 25% of patients with tuberculosis (Dupon et al., 1992), compared with only 6% of patients with other pulmonary opportunistic infections (Masur et al., 1989).

Fungal infections of the lung are uncommon but may also present with fever and cough of insidious onset. Histoplasmosis, blastomycosis and coccidioidomycosis should be considered in a patient from an endemic area who presents with fever and respiratory symptoms. Pulmonary aspergillosis occurs in patients with severe immunodeficiency, particularly those with neutropenia or who are receiving corticosteroid therapy (Pursell et al., 1992). Most patients have invasive pulmonary disease but some have bronchial disease causing obstruction. Radiological changes are diverse and include cavities, nodules, pleural lesions and diffuse infiltrates. Cryptococcal pneumonia also causes interstitial infiltrates on chest X-ray, but does not commonly cause respiratory symptoms. Uncommon bacterial infections of the lower respiratory tract, such as those caused by Rhodococcus equi (Donisi et al., 1996), and Nocardia asteroides (Uttamchandani et al., 1994) should also be considered in patients with CD4 lymphocyte counts < 300 cells/μl and focal pulmonary lesions.

KS and lymphoma infrequently affect the lung. When there is pulmonary involvement, a chronic cough is common and may be accompanied by haemoptysis. Radiological abnormalities in the presence of extra-pulmonary KS or lymphoma lesions are often sufficient evidence to make a presumptive diagnosis of pulmonary involvement, but further investigation may be necessary. Bronchoscopy may demonstrate endobronchial lesions and sequential thallium and gallium scans can be used to discriminate between KS, lymphoma and infection. KS lesions take up thallium but not gallium, whereas opportunistic infections take up gallium but not thallium and lymphoma takes up both isotopes (Lee et al., 1991).

A chronic cough associated with purulent sputum production may indicate the presence of chronic suppurative bronchitis or bronchiectasis (Holmes et al., 1992). This is often complicated by acute infective exacerbations and may be associated with chronic sinusitis. The cause of the bronchial inflammation is usually unclear, but in some circumstances may be attributed to deficiency of IgG antibodies. Basal pulmonary rales are a very common clinical finding in these patients. A high resolution CT scan of the thorax during a phase without acute infection usually confirms the diagnosis.

Non-infective causes of dyspnoea are rare but must be considered in the dyspnoeic patient without a pulmonary infection (see Chapter 13). Pulmonary emphysema is usually associated with smoking cigarettes but there are features of this disease in HIV-infected patients that suggest that it is, at least in part, an HIV-associated disease (Diaz et al., 2000). Bronchiolitis obliterans, with or without organizing pneumonia, is an uncommon cause of severe dyspnoea and cough (Diaz et al., 1997). Dyspnoea may also be the presenting symptom of a dilated cardiomyopathy, particularly when there is involvement of the right side of the heart (Currie et al., 1994).

Acute respiratory tract symptoms

A cough of acute onset associated with fever suggests an acute bronchial or pulmonary infection. Bacterial infections usually result in the production of purulent sputum and are most often caused by Streptococcus pneumoniae (Dworkin et al., 2001) with Staphylococcus aureus, Haemophilus influenzae, Klebsiella pneumoniae and Pseudomonas aeruginosa being significant but less common pathogens (Hirschtick et al., 1995). S. pneumoniae infection often results in bacteraemia (Frankel et al., 1996). Bacterial pneumonia is particularly common in injecting drug users and older patients and may occur before the onset of severe cellular immuno-deficiency. Less common bacterial pathogens such as *Nocardia asteroides* should also be considered in the severely immunodeficient patient (Uttamchandani et al., 1994).

Gastrointestinal tract disease

Odynophagia and dysphagia

Infection of the oesophageal mucosa by *Candida species* and less commonly HSV or CMV usually causes odynophagia, which is sometimes accompanied by dysphagia. Odyno-phagia is also common in patients with non-infective (aphthous) mucosal ulceration and can occur with other less common ulcerative conditions, such as lymphoma. Substantial weight loss can occur because the patient is unable to eat normally. Dysphagia in a patient with KS or lymphoma may indicate involvement of the oesophagus, causing obstruction.

Odynophagia in the presence of oropharyngeal candidiasis is highly suggestive of oesophageal candidiasis and treatment with an azole antifungal agent is appropriate management. However, endoscopy should be performed when there is doubt about the cause of the odynophagia or if symptoms fail to improve after a course of therapy.

Abdominal pain

Abdominal pain may result from various infections and neoplastic complications of HIV-induced immunodefi-ciency, as well as from the adverse effects of drug therapy. The site and nature of the pain is often indicative of the cause, which can be established in most cases by under-taking biochemical, microbiological, imaging and gastro-enterological investigations (Thuluvath et al., 1991). Investigations that are valuable in the diagnosis of abdominal pain and the indications for their use are shown in Table 2.4. The investigations used and the order in which they are undertaken will be determined by the nature of the symptoms and the clinical findings.

Generalized abdominal pain is most commonly caused by enterocolitis resulting from an infection. Consequently, the pain is often associated with diarrhoea. Other causes of generalized abdominal pain include intestinal and/or nodal lymphoma and nodal *Mycobacterium avium* complex (MAC) infection. Abdominal lymphadenitis, resulting from restoration of an immune response against MAC

after commencing antiretroviral therapy (French et al., 1992; Race et al., 1998), can be extremely painful. Pain caused by intestinal lymphoma may be associated with intestinal obstruction. Causes of generalized abdom-inal pain that are unrelated to HIV infection must also be considered, especially inflammatory bowel disease and irritable bowel syndrome, both of which may cause diarrhoea.

Pain localized to the upper abdomen is most likely to be caused by gastric pathology such as KS, lymphoma or CMV infection; CMV duodenitis, or pancreatitis. Didanosine, zalcitabine and pentamidine may cause pancreatitis in HIV-infected patients but do so less often than previously because lower doses of drug are now used and monitoring for adverse drug effects is more effective. Hypertri-glyceridemia, as a complication associated with protease inhibitor (PI) therapy, may also contribute to pancreatitis (Carr et al., 1998).

The right upper quadrant of the abdomen is a common site of pain, which is caused by sclerosing cholangitis in the great majority of patients. When pain is associated with pronounced elevation of the serum alkaline phosphatase concentration and/or dilatation of the common bile duct on ultrasound examination, sclerosing cholangitis is present in virtually all cases. However, not all cases have these abnor-malities and endoscopic retrograde cholangiopancreatog-raphy (ERCP) may be necessary to establish the diagnosis. Specimens for microbiological examination can also be taken during this procedure. Infection by CMV, *Crypto-sporidium* or *microsporidia* is the most common cause. Other causes of right upper quadrant pain are much less common and include hepatic and/or nodal lymphoma, acalculous cholecystitis resulting from CMV or cryptosporidial infec-tion, hepatic steatosis associated with a nucleoside analogue-induced mitochondrial cytopathy (Lewis and Dalakas, 1995) or causes unrelated to HIV infection, such as cholelithiasis.

As is the case in immunocompetent individuals, pain in the right iliac fossa is commonly caused by acute appendicitis. However, in individuals with HIV-induced immunodeficiency, there may be histological changes in the appendix indicative of an opportunistic infection such as CMV. Pain in either flank or the lower back is suggestive of urinary tract stones or crystalluria in patients being treat-ed with indinavir (Kopp et al., 1997), particularly when the pain radiates to the lower abdomen or genitals and there is associated dysuria or haematuria.

Table 2.4 Investigation of abdominal pain

Investigation	Indications and interpretation
1. Biochemistry	
Liver function tests	Increased serum alkaline phosphatase in sclerosing cholangitis
Amylase	Acute pancreatitis
2. Microbiology	
Culture and microscopy of faeces for bacteria, mycobacteria and protozoa	Infectious enterocolitis
Blood cultures for bacteria and mycobacteria	Disseminated MAC infection involving the intestine and/or abdominal lymph nodes.
	Bacterial enterocolitis, e.g. *Salmonella* or *Campylobacter* species
Examination of urine	Haematuria, proteinuria in patients with indinavir-induced crystalluria
3. Imaging	
Plain abdominal radiograph	Sub-diaphragmatic air from a perforation of the gastrointestinal tract caused by CMV colitis, malignancy, etc.
	Toxic dilation of the colon, complicating colitis
	Intestinal obstruction caused by lymphoma
Abdominal ultrasound	Dilated bile ducts resulting from sclerosing cholangitis and/or papillary stenosis
	Gall bladder wall thickening resulting from acalculous cholecystitis
	Parenchymal liver disease caused by MAC infection, lymphoma or nucleoside analogue-induced hepatic steatosis
	Lymph node enlargement caused by MAC infection, KS or lymphoma
	Pancreatitis
ERCP	Sclerosing cholangitis
Abdominal CT scan	Parenchymal liver disease, pancreatitis, lymphadenopathy, intestinal infiltration
4. Endoscopy	
Gastroduodenoscopy	Inspection and biopsy of stomach or duodenum for KS, lymphoma, CMV infection
Colonoscopy	Infectious colitis (mainly CMV)

CMV: cytomegalovirus; CT: computerized tomography; ERCP: endoscopic retrograde cholangio-pancreatography; KS: Kaposi's sarcoma; MAC: *Mycobacterium avium* complex.

Diarrhoea

Diarrhoea is common in HIV-infected individuals and is often the presenting complaint. Between 30 and 60% of patients with AIDS in developed countries and up to 90% of patients in developing countries have diarrhoea during the course of their illness (Smith *et al.*, 1992). A number of enteric pathogens have been isolated from faeces, blood or biopsy material from HIV-infected patients with diarrhoea (Gordon *et al.*, 2001; Table 2.5). Most of these micro-organisms are clearly the cause of the diarrhoea, but for some, such as *Entamoeba histolytica*, the association is less clear. Infection with more than one microorganism is common. Diarrhoea in patients from the developing world may be caused by infections with pathogens that do not common-ly cause diarrhoea in the developed world, such as MTB or strongyloides (Lanjewar *et al.*, 1996).

HIV infection itself appears to cause an enteropathy, but the significance of this is unclear and with thorough clinical and laboratory investigation an enteric pathogen can be identified as the cause of diarrhoea in most patients (Sharpstone and Gazzard, 1996). However, HIV infection of the colon has been implicated in the pathogenesis of a chronic colitis in which diarrhoea is associated with rectal bleeding and stool leukocytosis (Hing *et al.*, 1992). Diarrhoea may also be an adverse effect of some anti-retroviral drugs, particularly didanosine and nelfinavir.

Involvement of the gastrointestinal tract by KS or lymphoma is an uncommon cause of diarrhoea, which is sometimes associated with lymphatic obstruction, bleeding, enteric protein loss, hypoalbuminemia and associated limb oedema.

The history is of limited value in diagnosing the cause of diarrhoea but abdominal cramps, bloating and nausea are suggestive of small intestinal infections, and bloody diarrhoea is indicative of colitis, most often caused by infection with Shigella, Campylobacter or CMV. Indicators of the cause of diarrhoea are also sometimes found during a general physical examination. For example, CMV retinitis may point to the presence of disseminated CMV infection and hepatomegaly may indicate disseminated MAC infection. The cause of diarrhoea will be demonstrated by a limited evaluation consisting of culture and microscopic examination of three stool specimens and a blood culture in about 80% of patients, and this is usually all the investigation that is needed in patients with mild to moderate immunodeficiency (CD4 lymphocyte count > 200/μl) (Sharpstone and Gazzard, 1996). A full evaluation (Table 2.6) can subsequently be undertaken if the initial investigations are uninformative and the diarrhoea fails to respond to antidiarrhoeal agents such as diphenoxylate hydrochloride, or relapses while the patient is being given therapy for any specific infection discovered. More intensive investigation is often necessary in severely immunodeficient patients and will demonstrate the cause of diarrhoea in

more than 90% of patients (Sharpstone and Gazzard, 1996). The CD4 lymphocyte count is of value in establishing the cause and predicting the outcome of diarrhoea. For example, CMV enterocolitis is very unlikely when the CD4 lymphocyte count is > 100 cells/μl and cryptosporidiosis will be fulminant only if the CD4 lymphocyte count is < 50 cells/μl (Blanchard et al., 1992).

Perianal and rectal disease

Diseases of the rectum and anus are often the medical complications of repeated anal intercourse, but the anus and rectum can be the site of primary complications of the immunodeficiency. Thus, inflammatory strictures and ulcers, warts and haemorrhoids may occur, in addition to the proctitis and malignancies that may complicate the immunodeficiency (Barrett et al., 1998).

Ano-rectal pain, sometimes associated with a muco-purulent discharge, diarrhoea or tenesmus, is a common presentation of proctitis. Chlamydia trachomatis or Neisseria gonorrhoea are sometimes identified as the cause of the proctitis, but an infectious agent is not demonstrated in many cases. Painful perianal ulceration, which may be associated with a proctitis, is most commonly caused by HSV infection, but can also result from CMV infection, in the severely immunodeficient patient. Chronic relapsing peri-

---

Table 2.5 Enteric pathogens causing diarrhoea in patients with HIV/AIDS

Bacteria	Protozoa
Salmonella sp.	Enterocytozoon bieneusi (microsporidia)
Shigella flexneri	Cryptosporidium parvum
Campylobacter jejuni	Isospora belli
Clostridium difficile	Giardia lamblia
	Septata intestinalis (microsporidia)

Mycobacteria	Viruses
MAC	CMV
	HIV
	Rotavirus[a]
	Adenovirus[a]

Fungi
Histoplasma capsulatum

[a] Associated with diarrhoea in some studies, but their significance as pathogens is uncertain.

CMV: cytomegalovirus; MAC: Mycobacterium avium complex.

Table 2.6 Comprehensive diagnostic evaluation of diarrhoea in patients with HIV/AIDS

1. History
2. Clinical examination
3. Collection of at least three specimens of faeces to culture for bacteria and mycobacteria, microscopically examine for ova and parasites, and assay for Clostridium difficile toxin
4. Culture of at least two blood specimens for bacterial or mycobacterial infection
5. CD4 lymphocyte count as an indication of the degree of immunodeficiency
6. Upper and lower gastrointestinal tract endoscopy
   – Histopathology on duodenal, rectal and colonic biopsies to detect infection with CMV, MAC and cryptosporidia, etc.
   – Electron microscopy of biopsies may be required to detect microsporidial infection
   – Microscopy and culture of duodenal aspirates
   Colonoscopy should include the ascending colon because CMV infection is sometimes localized to this site.

CMV: cytomegalovirus; MAC: Mycobacterium avium complex.

anal inflammation associated with ulceration and abscess formation, from which a particular pathogenic micro-organism cannot be isolated, occurs in some patients, and is a particularly difficult problem to manage.

External examination of the anus, followed by procto-scopy and sigmoidoscopy if necessary, will reveal the cause of perianal disease in most cases. Appropriate swabs should be taken for microbiological tests to demonstrate HSV, *Treponema pallidum*, *Neisseria gonorrhoea* and *Chlamydia trachomatis* and rectal biopsies can be obtained to culture for CMV and for histological examination. Infections should be treated with appropriate antimicrobial medication. Warts will regress with the use of topical podophyllin, or diathermy for anal canal lesions, but often recur. Haemorrhoids, fissures and chronic relapsing perianal inflammation of indeterminate cause frequently require surgical treatment.

Ocular disease

Apart from the ophthalmic complications of VZV infection, ocular disease is predominantly a complication of severe immunodeficiency. CMV retinitis is the most common ocular opportunistic infection, which occurs in up to 30% of patients with AIDS and is occasionally the presenting manifestation. Impaired visual acuity and 'floaters' are the most common presenting symptoms. Severe disease can cause retinal detachment. Because rapid treatment of early retinal lesions can arrest disease progression, it is important to undertake regular retinal examinations through dilated pupils in patients with a CD4 lymphocyte count of < 100 cells/μl to detect asymptomatic infection. Bilateral disease is common.

Established CMV retinitis appears as areas of retinal pallor associated with perivascular 'exudates' (actually areas of retinal necrosis) and haemorrhage. The diagnosis is essentially made by retinal examination and should be confirmed and disease extent evaluated by an ophthalmologist. Early CMV retinitis can sometimes be difficult to distinguish from the 'cotton-wool' lesions caused by HIV infection. These are discrete, fluffy, white lesions, which are not associated with exudates or haemorrhage, do not cause symptoms and spontaneously regress. Repeated retinal examination may be necessary to differentiate early CMV retinitis from 'cotton-wool' spots.

Other much less common causes of chorioretinitis include toxoplasmosis, tuberculosis, histoplasmosis, pneumocystosis and cryptococcosis. Candidal retinitis should be

a particular consideration in injecting drug users. It is often associated with an overlying vitreous reaction. Rapidly progressive herpetic retinal necrosis is an uncommon condition, caused by VZV infection in most cases, but it can be caused by HSV infection (Ormerod *et al.*, 1998). It results in an atrophic and necrotic retina, often complicated by retinal detachment, optic nerve involvement and loss of vision in most affected eyes. Prompt diagnosis is essential if therapy is to be of any value, as this condition responds very poorly to treatment.

The differential diagnosis of visual impairment in a patient with AIDS should also include an optic neuropathy and other lesions of the visual pathways. CMV infection, with or without retinitis, and VZV infection may cause optic neuritis, and cryptococcal meningitis is occasionally associated with total blindness of rapid onset by mechanisms that are unclear but might include an optic neuropathy (Rex *et al.*, 1993). Compressive lesions of the optic nerves such as lymphoma, and lesions in the intracerebral optic pathways including toxoplasmosis, cerebral lymphoma and progressive multifocal leucoencephalopathy (PML) may also present with visual impairment.

Neurological symptoms

Headache

Several intracranial and extracranial complications of HIV-induced immunodeficiency often present with headache. A generalized headache is the most common presenting feature of cryptococcal meningitis, which is often associated with fever. Neck stiffness and meningism are uncommon, though were reported to be present in 50–70% of patients in one study of African patients (Heyderman *et al.*, 1998). Less common causes of meningitis include *Mycobacterium tuberculosis* and *Listeria monocytogenes* (Jurado *et al.*, 1993) infections and occasionally HIV infection itself (Price, 1996). Intracerebral mass lesions, most commonly resulting from toxoplasmosis or lymphoma, may present with generalized or localized headaches, sometimes in association with fever and focal neurological signs. Frontal headaches may be caused by nasal sinusitis and, when unilateral, by early VZV infection of the ophthalmic division of the trigeminal nerve.

Careful history taking and clinical examination will often demonstrate the cause of headache due to extracranial lesions, but a CT or MRI scan of the head is sometimes necessary to demonstrate sinusitis (Godofsky *et al.*, 1992) and almost always necessary to demonstrate the presence of intracerebral space-occupying lesions (Table 2.7). Exami-nation of serum for cryptococcal antigen is a very valuable investigation because antigen is detected in virtually all patients with cryptococcal meningitis. Similarly, absence of toxoplasma antibodies from serum strongly suggests that cerebral mass lesions are not caused by toxoplasmosis, although antibody detection is assay dependent, with ELISA giving the most reliable results (Porter and Sande, 1992). If an intracerebral lesion is not demonstrated by neuroradiological investigations in a severely immunodefi-cient patient with a persistent headache, a lumbar puncture and CSF examination should be performed, especially in patients with fever or neck stiffness (Table 2.8). CSF exam-ination should include testing for viral DNA by a poly-merase chain reaction (PCR) method if infection by a herpes virus is suspected (Cinque et al., 1996).

Table 2.7 Causes of intracerebral space-occupying lesions in patients with AIDS

Infections	Neoplasms
Common	**Common**
Toxoplasma gondii	Primary cerebral lymphoma
Rare	**Rare**
Mycobacterium tuberculosis	Metastatic lymphoma
Cryptococcus neoformans	KS
Nocardia asteroides	
Histoplasma capsulatum	
CMV	

KS: Kaposi's sarcoma; CMV: cytomegalovirus.

Table 2.8 Cerebrospinal fluid examination in HIV-infected patients with headache

1. Cell count and differential, protein and glucose concen-trations
2. Microscopy for bacteria, mycobacteria and fungi (includ-ing an India ink preparation for cryptococci)
3. Culture for bacteria, mycobacteria and fungi
4. Assay for cryptococcal antigen
5. Antibody tests for Treponema pallidum infection
6. Cytology, especially in patients with imaging abnormali-ties compatible with lymphoma
7. Examination for viral DNA by a polymerase chain reac-tion (PCR) method in patients with a suspected herpes virus infection

Neuropsychiatric manifestations of HIV disease

Cognitive impairment is the most common manifestation of HIV encephalopathy (see Chapter 10). Neuropsycho-logical abnormalities can be demonstrated in many other-wise asymptomatic individuals and these become progressively worse as the severity of the HIV disease increases, eventually resulting in the development of the AIDS dementia complex (ADC) (Price, 1996). Less com-mon manifestations of HIV encephalopathy include motor abnormalities, seizures and psychiatric conditions, including acute psychoses and depression. Clinical, neuro-radiological and CSF examinations will often establish HIV encephalopathy as a cause of these problems, but other pos-sible causes resulting from the complications of HIV disease should be excluded. Thus, the apathy, social withdrawal and impaired concentration that are so common in ADC should be differentiated from reactive depression, frontal lobe cerebral mass lesions and indolent cryptococcal menin-gitis. Likewise, seizures should only be attributed to HIV encephalopathy following the exclusion of other causes, especially intracerebral mass lesions.

Neuromuscular symptoms in the lower limbs and bladder

Diseases of peripheral nerves or muscle may result from the effects of the HIV infection or from complications of the immunodeficiency (Price, 1996). A distal sensory neuro-pathy is common and causes pain, paresthesia, dysesthesia and hypoesthesia. The pathogenesis is unclear in most cases and, therefore, there is little value in undertaking extensive investigations to determine the cause. However, a rapidly progressive multi-focal sensorimotor neuropathy caused by CMV infection sometimes responds to ganciclovir therapy and a peripheral nerve biopsy and CSF examination may be indicated in patients with such symptoms (Said et al., 1991). Neuropathy may also be caused by some of the cancer chemotherapy agents and certain nucleoside analogues used to treat the HIV infection such as zalcitabine, didano-sine and stavudine. Acetyl-carnitine deficiency may con-tribute to nucleoside analogue-induced neurotoxicity (Famularo et al., 1997).

Discomfort in the upper legs associated with weakness and absent knee jerks may be the result of a radiculopathy or myeloradiculopathy, which is usually caused by CMV infection. Innervation of the bladder may also be affected, giving rise to bladder dysfunction and urinary retention. CSF examination characteristically demonstrates the presence of a neutrophil pleocytosis. Bladder dysfunction is also common in patients with HIV-related myelopathy but this is usually associated with increased leg reflexes and weakness of the legs, progressing to a spastic parapareisis (see Chapter 21).

Weakness may also be a manifestation of a myopathy, several types of which have been described in HIV-infected patients (Price, 1996). A mitochondrial myopathy caused by zidovudine (Peters *et al.*, 1993; Lewis and Dalakas, 1995) may cause muscle aching and wasting, which characteristically affects the gluteal muscles. It mainly occurs in patients over the age of 35 who have been taking zidovudine for a prolonged period of time. It is also most common in patients who have taken more than 600 mg of zidovudine daily and is therefore encountered less often than it was. The serum creatinine kinase concentration is usually increased and muscle biopsy, followed by electron microscopical examination of the tissue, usually confirms the diagnosis.

Constitutional symptoms

Fever

Fever commonly occurs as a consequence of the infectious or neoplastic complications of the immunodeficiency, or as a complication of the HIV infection itself. An infection is identified as the cause of fever in 80–90% of patients but the type of infection generally reflects the patient's HIV infection risk category (Barat *et al.*, 1996). Pneumonia and other bacterial infections are most common in intravenous drug users, whereas opportunistic infections are more common in homosexual men. Accompanying symptoms and clinical signs often point to the cause of the fever, but, when this is not the case, investigations are necessary to demonstrate its cause. Causes of fever of unknown origin that should be considered in HIV-infected patients are shown in Table 2.9.

Clinical examination should be thorough and focused, particularly on body sites at which occult infection or malignancy tend to occur. These sites include lymph nodes, sinuses, teeth and gums, heart valves (especially in injecting drug users), intravenous infusion sites and muscles, where a pyomyositis can remain undetected for some time. Routine microbiological and radiological investigations should be supplemented with blood cultures for bacteria, mycobacteria and fungi and assays for serum cryptococcal antigen. Lysis centrifugation blood cultures should also be undertaken in difficult cases because these can detect some

Table 2.9 Causes of fever of unknown origin in patients with HIV/AIDS

HIV infection
Infectious complications of HIV-induced immunodeficiency
• 'Prodromal' PCP
• Localized bacterial infections, e.g. sinusitis, dental abscess, pneumonia, endocarditis, pelvic inflammatory disease, pyomyositis
• Localized fungal infections, e.g. soft tissue infections, endocarditis
• Bacterial septicaemia
• Disseminated infections with MAC, CMV, fungi (such as cryptococci or histoplasma), toxoplasma, *Pneumocystis carinii* and other less common organisms, including *Bartonella henselae* and Leishmania
Neoplastic complications of HIV-induced immunodeficiency
• Lymphoma
• KS
Infected intravenous lines
Drug-induced fever

CMV: cytomegalovirus; KS: Kaposi's sarcoma; MAC: *Mycobacterium avium* complex.

infections that cannot be demonstrated by routine cultures, especially *Bartonella* spp. infections. Blood from indwelling central venous catheters should also be cultured, in addition to peripheral blood in those patients with a catheter. CMV disease is a very unlikely cause of fever unless the CD4 lymphocyte count is < 100 cells/μl and clinical examination will usually demonstrate the site of disease. In severely immunodeficient patients without clinical evidence of CMV, disease quantitation of CMV DNA in blood leucocytes or plasma by PCR is a better indicator of CMV disease than culture of blood or urine (Shinkai *et al.*, 1997; Boivin *et al.*, 1998).

Radionuclide scans using [67]Gallium and/or [111]Indium-labelled leucocytes may demonstrate the site of fever in patients without localizing signs, the latter investigation being much more sensitive (Rubin and Fischman, 1996). Microbiological or pathological investigations can then be undertaken on specimens obtained from involved areas. Culture of bone marrow in patients with pancytopenia, or a liver biopsy in patients with hepatomegaly or abnormal liver function tests, may also demonstrate infection, especially MAC infection. Bone marrow examination should include the use of stains for MAC and for *Histoplasma* and *Leishmania* in patients from endemic regions.

Drug-induced fevers may result from an immunological hypersensitivity reaction to the drug, often caused by sulphonamides or trimethoprim, a toxic effect of the drug itself, as seen with intravenous amphotericin B, or from the restoration of immunity to subclinical infections such as MAC following treatment of the HIV infection with antiretroviral therapy (French et al., 1992; Race et al., 1998).

Wasting

A wasting syndrome is a characteristic manifestation of advanced HIV infection that has become much less prevalent since the introduction of HAART. The pathogenesis of the wasting appears to be multi-factorial (see Chapter 18) but anorexia and reduced calorie intake associated with opportunistic infections, diarrhoea and malabsorption are the most important factors (Macallan et al., 1995). Regular measurement of body weight is a very important component of the monitoring of patients with HIV infection. A rapid change in weight (> 4 kg over 4 months) is most likely to indicate the presence of an opportunistic infection, whereas less rapid weight loss (< 4 kg over 4 months) is most often caused by diarrhoea and malabsorption (Macallan et al., 1993).

Weight loss in a patient with HIV infection should alert the physician to the possibility of an opportunistic infection, particularly infections of the upper and lower gastrointestinal tract, or to the possibility of malabsorption. Other causes of reduced calorie intake must also be considered, including depression, alcohol or drug abuse, AIDS-dementia complex and anorexia caused by drug therapy. Good nutrition is essential in the prevention and treatment of wasting and, therefore, dietetic advice should be available to all patients with HIV infection (American Dietetic Association, 1994).

Wasting may also be an adverse effect of some antiretroviral drugs. Zidovudine myopathy may present as muscle wasting, though this complication of zidovudine therapy is encountered much less commonly than it was now that the standard dose of zidovudine is 500–600 mg per day. Wasting of limbs and the face is a common presentation of the lipodystrophy, which is sometimes associated with hyperlipidaemia and very occasionally insulin-resistant diabetes in patients treated with combination antiretroviral therapy (Carr et al., 1998). The lipodystrophy is usually a manifestation of body fat redistribution which may include the development of abdominal obesity (Miller et al., 1998), 'buffalo humps' (Lo et al., 1998) and breast enlargement in women.

Opportunistic infections in patients treated with HAART

The presentation and natural history of many opportunistic infections have changed substantially since the introduction of HAART (Jacobson and French, 1998; Lee et al., 2001). The incidence of opportunistic infections such as PCP MAC disease and CMV retinitis has fallen progressively since 1995, due in part to the use of prophylactic antimicrobial therapy, but also attributable to the use of HAART (Palella et al., 1998). Suppression of HIV replication by HAART presumably maintains or restores pathogen-specific immune responses, which appears not only to prevent opportunistic infections but also to cause disease regression. Diseases such as progressive multifocal leucoencephalopathy (PML) and intestinal microsporidiosis or cryptosporidiosis, which were previously untreatable or very difficult to treat, may regress in patients treated with HAART. In addition, the presentation of disease related to infection by some opportunistic pathogens is significantly different in patients treated with HAART than in immunodeficient patients with uncontrolled HIV replication. This probably also reflects restoration of pathogen-specific immune responses by HAART and can therefore be considered to be 'immune restoration disease' (French et al., 2000).

MAC disease usually presents as a disseminated infection in immunodeficient patients and mycobacteremia is common. However, MAC disease, which presents following treatment with antiretroviral therapy is often limited to lymph nodes and occasionally to other organs, such as the liver (French et al., 1992; Race et al., 1998), and mycobacteraemia is unusual. Furthermore, MAC disease in such patients is characterized by a greater inflammatory response than in immunodeficient patients. Pronounced and protracted fever is common and there may be severe pain in affected lymph nodes or liver. Granulomatous inflammation may be present in affected tissues and there may be a cutaneous DTH response to mycobacterial antigens, suggesting that HAART is able to restore a specific immune response against mycobacteria. Steroid therapy is sometimes necessary, in addition to therapy for MAC to control tissue inflammation and pain.

A relapse of CMV retinitis in association with an increase of the CD4 lymphocyte count is also seen in some severely immunodeficient patients treated with HAART (Jacobson et al., 1997b). The retinitis in such patients differs from that in immunodeficient patients in that inflammatory changes such as a vitritis may also be present, and there is subsequent resolution of the retinitis without relapse when maintenance CMV therapy is ceased. Hepatitis associated with HBV or HCV infection after treatment with HAART may also be an 'immune restoration disease' (Carr and Cooper, 1997; John et al., 1998b).

Given that CD4 lymphocyte counts are increased and pathogen-specific immune responses appear to be restored after HAART, prophylactic antimicrobial therapy may not be necessary in patients treated with HAART. There are reports that prophylaxis for MAC or CMV infection have been ceased in patients responding to HAART. Data from observational studies of randomized trials suggest that primary prophylaxis for CMV or MAC disease may be ceased when the CD4 lymphocyte count is >100 cells/μl and that prophylaxis for PCP and toxoplasma cerebritis may be ceased when the CD4 lymphocyte count is >200 cell/μl (Kovacs and Masur, 2000). However, it is advisable to wait until the CD4 lymphocyte count has been above the suggested value for at least 6 months before ceasing prophylaxis, in order to ensure that the increased count is sustained and because CD4 lymphocyte clonal repletion may be incomplete immediately after commencing HAART (Connors et al., 1997). It is also advisable to cease prophylaxis only in patients with low levels of plasma HIV RNA.

References

American Dietetic Association. (1994). Position of the American Dietetic Association and the Canadian Dietetic Association: nutrition intervention in the care of persons with human immunodeficiency virus infection. J Am Dietetic Assoc **94**: 1042–5.

Barat LM, Gunn JE, Steger KA et al. (1996). Causes of fever in patients infected with human immunodeficiency virus who were admitted to Boston City Hospital. Clin Infect Dis **23**: 320–8.

Barrett WL, Callahan TD, Orkin BA. (1998). Perianal manifestations of human immunodeficiency virus infection. Dis Colon Rectum **41**: 606–12.

Beck-Sague C, Dooley SW, Hutton MD et al. (1992). Hospital outbreak of multidrug-resistant Mycobacterium tuberculosis infection. JAMA **268**: 1280–6.

Blanchard C, Jackson AM, Shanson DC et al. (1992). Cryptosporidiosis in HIV-seropositive patients. Q J Med **85**: 813–23.

Blatt SP, Hendrix CW, Butzin CA et al. (1993). Delayed-type hypersensitivity skin testing predicts progression to AIDS in HIV-infected patients. Ann Intern Med **119**: 177–84.

Boivin G, Handfield J, Toma E et al. (1998). Comparative evaluation of the cytomegalovirus DNA load in polymorphonuclear leukocytes and plasma of human immunodeficiency virus-infected subjects. J Infect Dis **177**: 355–60.

Brichacek B, Swindells S, Janoff EN et al. (1996). Increased plasma human immunodeficiency virus type 1 burden following anti-genic challenge with pneumococcal vaccine. J Infect Dis **174**: 1191–9.

Carr A, Cooper DA. (1997). Restoration of immunity to chronic hepatitis B infection in an HIV-infected patient on protease inhibitor. Lancet **349**: 996–7.

Carr A, Samsaras K, Chisholm D et al. (1998). A syndrome of peripheral lipodystrophy, hyperlipidaemia and insulin resistance in patients receiving HIV protease inhibitors. AIDS **12**: 51–8.

Centers for Disease Control and Prevention (1991). Purified protein derivative (PPD)-tuberculin allergy and HIV infection: guidelines for anergy testing and management of anergic persons at risk of tuberculosis. MMWR **40**: 27–33.

Cinque P, Vago L, Dahl H et al. (1996). Polymerase chain reaction on cerebrospinal fluid for diagnosis of virus-associated opportunistic diseases of the central nervous system in HIV-infected patients. AIDS **10**: 951–8.

Collier AC, Corey L, Murphy VL et al. (1988). Antibody to human immunodeficiency virus (HIV) and suboptimal response to hepatitis B vaccination. Ann Intern Med **109**: 101–5.

Connors M, Kovacs JA, Krevat S et al. (1997) HIV infection induces changes in CD4+ T-cell phenotype and depletions within the CD4+ T-cell repertoire that are not immediately restored by antiviral or immune-based therapies. Nat Med **3**: 533–40.

Converse PJ, Jones SL, Astemborski J et al. (1997). Comparison of a tuberculin interferon-gamma assay with the tuberculin skin test in high-risk adults: effect of human immunodeficiency virus infection. J Infect Dis **176**: 144–50.

Crowe SM, Carlin JB, Stewart KI et al. (1991). Predictive value of CD4 lymphocyte numbers for the development of opportunistic infections and malignancies in HIV-infected persons. J Acquir Immune Defic Syndr **4**: 770–6.

Currie PF, Jacob AJ, Foreman AR et al. (1994). Heart muscle disease related to HIV infection: prognostic implications. Br Med J **309**: 1605–7.

Deacon NJ, Tsykin A, Solomon A et al. (1995). Genomic structure of an attenuated quasi species of HIV-1 from a blood transfusion donor and recipients. Science **270**: 988–91.

Diaz F, Collazos J, Martinez E et al. (1997). Bronchiolitis obliterans in a patient with HIV infection. Respir Med **91**: 171–3.

Diaz F, King MA, Pacht Er et al. (2000). Increased susceptibility to pulmonary emphysema among HIV-seropositive smokers. Ann Intern Med **132**: 369–72.

Donisi A, Suardi MG, Casari S et al. (1996). Rhodococcus equi infection in HIV-infected patients. AIDS **10**: 359–62.

Dupon M, Ragnaud JM, and the Groupe des Infectiologues du Sud de la France. (1992). Tuberculosis in patients infected with human immunodeficiency virus 1. A retrospective multicentre study of 123 cases in France. Q J Med **85**: 719–30.

Dunne AL, Janky SE, Crowe SM. (1996). Comparison of branched DNA and RT-PCR for quantifying six different HIV-1 subtypes in plasma. AIDS **11**: 126–7.

Dworkin MS, Ward JW, Hanson DL et al. (2001) Pneumococcal disease among HIV-infected persons: incidence, risk factors and impact of vaccination. Clin Infect Dis **32**: 794–800.

Fahey JL, Taylor JMG, Detels R et al. (1990). The prognostic value of cellular and serologic markers in infection with human immunodeficiency virus type 1. New Engl J Med **322**: 166–72.

Famularo G, Moretti S, Marcellini S et al. (1997). Acetyl-carnitine deficiency in AIDS patients with neurotoxicity on treatment with antiretroviral nucleoside analogues. AIDS 11: 185-90.

Fling JA, Fischer JR, Baswell RN et al. (1988). The relationship of serum IgA concentration to human immunodeficiency virus (HIV) infection: a cross sectional study of HIV-seropositive individuals detected by screening in the United States Air Force. J Allergy Clin Immunol 82: 965-70.

Fowke KR, D'Amico R, Chernoff DN et al. (1997). Immunologic and virologic evaluation after influenza vaccination of HIV-1-infected patients. AIDS 11: 1013-21.

Frankel RE, Virata M, Hardalo C et al. (1996). Invasive pneumococcal disease: clinical features, serotypes, and antimicrobial resistance patterns in cases involving patients with and without human immunodeficiency virus infection. Clin Infect Dis 23: 577-84.

French MA, Lenzo N, John M et al. (2000). Immune restoration disease after the treatment of immunodeficient HIV-infected patients with highly active antiretroviral therapy. HIV Medicine 1: 107-15.

French MAH, Mallal SA, Dawkins RL. (1992). Zidovudine-induced restoration of cell-mediated immunity to mycobacteria in immuno-deficient HIV-infected patients. AIDS 6: 1293-7.

French N, Nakiyingi J, Carpenter LM et al. (2000). 23-Valent pneumococcal polysaccharide vaccine in HIV-1 infected Ugandan adults: double-blind, randomised and placebo-controlled trial. Lancet 355: 2106-11.

Godofsky MD, Zinreich J, Armstrong M et al. (1992). Sinusitis in HIV-infected patients: a clinical and radiographic review. Am J Med 93: 163-70.

Gordon MA, Walsh AL, Chaponda M et al. (2001). Bacteraemia and mortality among adult medical admissions in Malawi. J Infect Dis 42: 44-9.

Gradon JD, Timpone JG, Schnittman SM. (1993). Emergence of unusual opportunistic pathogens in AIDS: a review. Clin Infect Dis 15: 134-57.

Graham NMH, Nelson KE, Solomon L et al. (1992). Prevalence of tuberculin positivity and skin test anergy in HIV-1-seropositive and -seronegative intravenous drug users. JAMA 267: 369-73.

Greenspan D, Greenspan JS. (1996). HIV-related oral disease. Lancet 348: 729-33.

Halsey NA, Coberly JS, Desormeaux J et al. (1998). Randomised trial of isoniazid versus rifampicin and pyrazinamide for prevention of tuberculosis in HIV-1 infection. Lancet 351: 786-92.

Heald AE, Piper CF, Schiffman SS. (1998). Taste and smell complaints in HIV-1 infection. AIDS 12: 1667-74.

Hess G, Clemens R, Bienzle U et al. (1995). Immunogenicity and safety of an inactivated hepatitis A vaccine in anti-HIV positive and negative homosexual men. J Med Virol 46: 40-2.

Heyderman RS, Gangaidzo IT, Hakim JG et al. (1998). Cryptococcal meningitis in human immunodeficiency virus-infected patients in Harare, Zimbabwe. Clin Infect Dis 26: 284-9.

Hillemans P, Ellerbrock TV, McPhillips S et al. (1996). Prevalence of anal human papillomavirus infection and anal cytologic abnormalities in HIV-seropositive women. AIDS 10: 1641-7.

Hing MC, Goldschmidt C, Mathijs JM et al. (1992). Chronic colitis associated with human immunodeficiency virus infection. Med J Aust 156: 683-7.

Hirsch MS, Brun-Vézinet F, D'Aquila RT et al. (2000). Antiretroviral drug resistance testing in adult HIV-1 infection: recommendations of an international AIDS Society – USA panel. JAMA 283: 2417-26.

Hirschtick RE, Glassroth J, Jordan MC et al. (1995). Bacterial pneumonia in persons infected with the human immunodeficiency virus. N Engl J Med 333: 845-51.

Hoffman TL, Doms RW. (1998). Chemokines and co-receptors in HIV/SIV-host interactions. AIDS 12: S17-26.

Hogan CM and Hammer SM (2001). Host determinants in HIV infection. Part 2: genetic factors and implications for antiretroviral therapeutics. Ann Int Med 134: 978-96.

Holmes AH, Trotman-Dickenson B, Edwards A et al. (1992). Bronchiectasis in HIV disease. Q J Med 85: 875-82.

Holtom PD, Larsen RA, Leal ME et al. (1992). Prevalence of neurosyphilis in human immunodeficiency virus-infected patients with latent syphilis. Am J Med 93: 9-12.

Hughes MD, Johnson VA, Hirsch MS et al. (1997). Monitoring plasma HIV-1 RNA levels in addition to CD4+ lymphocyte count improves assessment of antiretroviral therapeutic response. Ann Intern Med 126: 929-38.

Jacobson JM, Greenspan JS, Spritzler J et al. (1997a). Thalidomide for the treatment of oral aphthous ulcers in patients with human immunodeficiency virus infection. New Engl J Med 336: 1487-93.

Jacobson MA, Zegans M, Pavan PR et al. (1997b). Cytomegalovirus retinitis after initiation of highly active antiretroviral therapy. Lancet 349: 1443-5.

Jacobson M, French M. (1998). Altered natural history of AIDS-related opportunistic infections in the era of potent combination antiretroviral therapy. AIDS – a year in review 12: S157-63.

Jain A, Jain S, Gant V. (1995). Should patients positive for HIV infection receive pneumococcal vaccine? BMJ 310: 1060-2.

John M, Mallal S, French M. (1998a). Emerging toxicity with long-term antiretroviral therapy. J HIV Ther 3: 58-62.

John M, Flexman J, French MA. (1998b). Hepatitis C virus – associated hepatitis following treatment of HIV-infected patients with HIV protease inhibitors: an immune restoration disease? AIDS 12: 2289-93.

Joseph J, Strange C, Sahn SA. (1993). Pleural effusions in hospitalized patients with AIDS. Ann Intern Med 118: 856-9.

Jurado RL, Farley MM, Pereira E et al. (1993). Increased risk of meningitis and bacteremia due to Listeria monocytogenes in patients with human immunodeficiency virus infection. Clin Infect Dis 17: 224-7.

Karbassi M, Raizman MB, Schuman JS. (1992). Herpes zoster ophthalmicus. Surv Ophthalmol 36: 395-410.

Katz MH, Greenspan D, Westenhouse J et al. (1992). Progression to AIDS in HIV-infected homosexual and bisexual men with hairy leukoplakia and oral candidiasis. AIDS 6: 95-100.

Keet IPM, Klein MR, Just JJ et al. (1996). The role of host genetics in the natural history of HIV-1 infection: the needles in the haystack. AIDS 10: S59-67.

Kopp JB, Miller KD, Mican JAM et al. (1997). Crystalluria and urinary tract abnormalities associated with indinavir. Ann Intern Med 127: 119-25.

Kovacs JA, Masur H. (2000). Prophylaxis against opportunistic infections in patients with human immunodeficiency virus infection. N Engl J Med 342: 1416-29.

Lanjewar DN, Anand BS, Genta R et al. (1996). Major differences in the spectrum of gastrointestinal infections associated with AIDS in India versus the West: an autopsy study. Clin Infect Dis 23: 482-5.

Lee LM, Karon JM, Selik R et al. (2001). Survival after AIDS diagnosis in adults and adolescents during the treatment era, US 1984-1997. JAMA 285: 1308-15.

Lee VW, Fuller JD, O'Brien MJ *et al.* (1991). Pulmonary Kaposi's sarcoma in patients with AIDS: scintigraphic diagnosis with sequential thallium and gallium scanning. *Radiology* **180**: 409–12.

Lewis W, Dalakas MC. (1995). Mitochondrial toxicity of antiviral drugs. *Nat Med* **1**: 417–21.

Lo JC, Mulligan K, Tai VW *et al.* (1998). 'Buffalo hump' in men with HIV-1 infection. *Lancet* **351**: 867–70.

Macallan DC, Noble C, Baldwin C *et al.* (1993). Prospective analysis of patterns of weight change in stage IV human immunodeficiency virus infection. *Am J Clin Nutr* **58**: 417–24.

Macallan DC, Noble C, Baldwin C *et al.* (1995). Energy expenditure and wasting in human immunodeficiency virus infection. *New Engl J Med* **333**: 83–8.

Mallal SA, Martinez OP, French MAH *et al.* (1994). Severity and outcome of *Pneumocystis carinii* pneumonia in patients of known and unknown HIV status. *J AIDS* **7**: 148–53.

Markowitz N, Hansen NI, Hopewell PC *et al.* (1997). Incidence of tuberculosis in the United States among HIV-infected persons. *Ann Intern Med* **126**: 123–32.

Martinez OP, French MAH. (1993). Acoustic neuropathy associated with Zalcitabine-induced peripheral neuropathy. *AIDS* **7**: 901–2.

Masur H, Ognibene FP, Yarchoan R *et al.* (1989). CD4 counts as predictors of opportunistic pneumonias in human immunodeficiency virus (HIV) infection. *Ann Intern Med* **111**: 223–31.

McNulty A, Li Y, Radtke U *et al.* (1997). Herpes zoster and the stage and prognosis of HIV-1 infection. *Genitourin Med* **73**: 467–70.

Mellors JW, Munoz A, Giorgi JV *et al.* (1997). Plasma viral load and CD4+ lymphocytes as prognostic markers of HIV-1 infection. *Ann Intern Med* **126**: 946–54.

Miller KD, Jones E, Yanovski JA *et al.* (1998). Visceral abdominal-fat accumulation associated with use of indinavir. *Lancet* **351**: 871–5.

Musey L, Hughes J, Schacker T *et al.* (1997). Cytotoxic T-cell responses, viral load, and disease progression in early human immunodeficiency virus type 1 infection. *New Engl J Med* **337**: 1267–72.

O'Donnell JG. Sorbello AF, Condoluci DV *et al.* (1993). Sinusitis due to *Pseudomonas aeruginosa* in patients with human immunodeficiency virus infection. *Clin Infect Dis* **16**: 404–6.

Ormerod DL, Larkin JA, Margo CA *et al.* (1998). Rapidly progressive herpetic retinal necrosis: a blinding disease characteristic of advanced AIDS. *Clin Infect Dis* **26**: 34–45.

Palacio H, Hilton JF, Canchola AJ *et al.* (1997). Effect of cigarette smoking on HIV-related oral lesions. *J Acquir Immune Defic Syndr Hum Retrovirol* **14**: 338–42.

Palefsky JM. (1991). Human papillomavirus infection among HIV-infected individuals. *Hematol Oncol Clin N Am* **5**: 357–70.

Palefsky JM, Holly EA, Hogeboom CJ *et al.* (1997). Anal cytology as a screening tool for anal squamous intraepithelial lesions. *J Acquir Immune Defic Syndr Hum Retrovirol* **14**: 415–22.

Palefsky JM, Holly EA, Ralston ML *et al.* (1998). Anal squamous intraepithelial lesions in HIV-positive and HIV-negative homosexual and bisexual men. *J Acquir Immune Defic Syndr Hum Retrovirol* **17**: 320–6.

Palella FJ, Delaney KM, Moorman AC *et al.* (1998). Declining morbidity and mortality among patients with advanced human immunodeficiency virus infection. *New Engl J Med* **338**: 853–60.

Pantaleo G, Graziosi C, Demarest JF *et al.* (1993). HIV infection is active and progressive in lymphoid tissue during the clinically latent stage of disease. *Nature* **362**: 355–8.

Perlman DC, Hanvanich M. (1997). Prophylaxis and treatment of HIV-related tuberculosis. *AIDS* **11**: S173–9.

Peters BS, Winer J, Landon DN *et al.* (1993). Mitochondrial myopathy associated with chronic zidovudine therapy in AIDS. *Q J Med* **86**: 5–15.

Porter SB, Sande MA. (1992). Toxoplasmosis of the central nervous system in the acquired immunodeficiency syndrome. *N Engl J Med* **327**: 1643–8.

Poznansky MC, Coke R, Skinner C *et al.* (1995). HIV positive patients first presenting with an AIDS defining illness: characteristics and survival. *Br Med J* **311**: 156–8.

Price RW (1996). Neurological complication of HIV infection. *Lancet* **348**: 445–52.

Pursell KJ, Telzak EE, Armstrong D. (1992). Aspergillus species colonization and invasive disease in patients with AIDS. *Clin Infect Dis* **14**: 141–8.

Race EM, Adelson-Mitty J, Kriegel GR *et al.* (1998). Focal mycobacterial lymphadenitis following initiation of protease-inhibitor therapy in patients with advanced HIV-1 disease. *Lancet* **351**: 252–5.

Rex JH, Larsen RA, Dismukes WE *et al.* (1993). Catastrophic visual loss due to *Cryptococcus neoformans* meningitis. *Medicine* **72**: 207–24.

Rodriguez-Barradas MC, Groover JE, Lacke CE *et al.* (1996). IgG antibody to pneumococcal capsular polysaccharide in human immunodeficiency virus-infected subjects: persistence of antibody in responders, revaccination in non-responders, and relationship of immunoglobulin allotype to response. *J Infect Dis* **173**: 1347–53.

Rubin RH, Fischman AJ. (1996). Radionuclide imaging of infection in the immunocompromised host. *Clin Infect Dis* **22**: 414–22.

Saag MS, Holodniy M, Kuritzkes DR *et al.* (1996). HIV viral load markers in clinical practice. *Nat Med* **2**: 625–9.

Said G, Lacroix C, Chemouilli P *et al.* (1991). Cytomegalovirus neuropathy in acquired immunodeficiency syndrome: a clinical and pathological study. *Ann Neurol* **29**: 138–46.

Samet JH, Freedberg KA, Stein MD *et al.* (1998). Trillion Virion Delay: time from testing positive for HIV to presentation for primary care. *Arch Intern Med* **158**: 734–40.

Schacker T, Collier AC, Hughes J *et al.* (1996). Clinical and epidemiologic features of primary HIV infection. *Ann Intern Med* **125**: 257–64.

Sharpstone D, Gazzard B. (1996). Gastrointestinal manifestations of HIV infection. *Lancet* **348**: 379–83.

Shinkai M, Bozzette SA, Powderly W *et al.* (1997). Utility of urine and leukocyte cultures and plasma DNA polymerase chain reaction for identification of AIDS patients at risk for developing human cytomegalovirus disease. *J Infect Dis* **175**: 302–8.

Smith PD, Quinn TC, Strober W *et al.* (1992). Gastrointestinal infections in AIDS. *Ann Intern Med* **116**: 63–74.

Thuluvath PJ, Connolly GM, Forbes A *et al.* (1991). Abdominal pain in HIV infection. *Q J Med* **287**: 275–85.

Uttamchandani RB, Daikos GL, Reyes RR *et al.* (1994). Nocardiosis in 30 patients with advanced human immunodeficiency virus infection: clinical features and outcome. *Clin Infect Dis* **18**: 348–53.

Weinart M, Grimes RM, Lynch DP. (1996). Oral manifestations of HIV infection. *Ann Intern Med* **125**: 485–96.

The pathogenesis of HIV infection

3

SHARON LEWIN AND DAVID HO

The human immunodeficiency virus type 1 (HIV-1) was identified as the causative agent of the acquired immuno-deficiency syndrome (AIDS) in 1983 (Barre-Sinoussi *et al.*, 1983; Gallo *et al.*, 1984). In the following years we have managed to acquire a significant understanding of the pathogenesis of HIV-1 infection so as to initiate treatments that have had a significant effect on patient prognosis (Palella *et al.*, 1998). HIV-1 primarily infects CD4 lympho-cytes and cells of the monocyte/macrophage lineage. Fol-lowing transmission, there are three clinical stages of infection. These stages include primary infection, a clini-cally latent asymptomatic period, followed by clinical pro-gression leading to AIDS. Each stage is characterized by a distinctive host immune response. However, throughout all stages of disease HIV-1 replicates at extremely high levels. The rate of disease progression is different among infected individuals and is dependent upon a complex interplay of viral and host factors (Hogan and Hammer, 2001).

HIV-1 entry

HIV-1 enters its target cells by interaction of the virion glycoproteins (gp120/41) with the CD4 molecule (Dalgleish *et al.*, 1984; Klatzmann *et al.*, 1984) and an additional receptor, now known to be a chemokine receptor. Chemokines are small proteins that serve as chemo-attractants in inflammation. The two most impor-tant chemoreceptors for HIV-1 are CXCR4 (also called fusin or LESTR [Feng *et al.*, 1996]) and CCR5 (Alkhatib *et al.*, 1996; Choe *et al.*, 1996; Deng *et al.*, 1996; Doranz *et al.*, 1996; Dragic *et al.*, 1996). CXCR4 is the receptor for the chemokine SDF-1 (Bleul *et al.*, 1996; Oberlin *et al.*, 1996). CCR5 serves as the receptor for the chemokines MIP-1 α and β, as well as RANTES (Alkhatib *et al.*, 1996). Although CCR5 and CXCR4 are believed to be the primary co-receptors for HIV-1, additional

chemokine receptors such as CCR2 and CCR3 have been shown by *in vitro* assays to serve as co-receptors for HIV-1 (reviewed by Cairns and D'Souza, 1998).

Macrophage-tropic (M-tropic) strains of HIV-1 replicate in macrophages and CD4 lymphocytes and use the chemokine receptor CCR5. T-tropic viruses replicate in primary CD4 lymphocytes, established CD4 lymphocyte cell lines, but not macrophages. T-tropic viruses use the chemokine receptor CXCR4 but can also use CCR5 (reviewed by Littman, 1998). The differences in tropism map to sequences in the gp120 subunit of the envelope gly-coprotein, particularly the V3 domain (Shioda *et al.*, 1991; Westervelt *et al.*, 1992).

Fusion of infected and uninfected cells leads to the for-mation of multinucleated giant cells, or syncytia. Not all primary isolates of HIV-1 induce syncytia *in vitro*. Most commonly, isolates derived early in the course of infection are non-syncytium inducing (NSI), while isolates from late-stage patients have a syncytium-inducing (SI) phenotype (Tersmette *et al.*, 1988; Connor *et al.*, 1993).

HIV-1 viruses are now classified on the basis of their co-receptor usage (Berger *et al.*, 1998) (Figure 3.1). The classification includes R5 (CCR5-tropic viruses or prev-iously M-tropic, NSI viruses), X4 (CXCR4-tropic viruses or previously T-tropic, SI viruses), and R5X4 (using both receptors with comparable efficiency or previously called dual tropic) (Malkevitch *et al.*, 2001).

Host range of cellular targets

The main targets for HIV-1 infection are CD4 lymphocytes (Dalgleish *et al.*, 1984; Klatzmann *et al.*, 1984; Schnittman *et al.*, 1989). HIV-1 also infects other CD4-expressing cells, including monocytes, macrophages and dendritic cells. Infection of CD4 lymphocytes and macrophages differs in several important ways.

HIV-1 infection of T lymphocytes

HIV-1 requires that CD4 lymphocytes are activated for optimal replication (McDougal et al., 1985; Zack et al., 1990). To understand HIV-1 replication in T cells, it is worthwhile to review the normal physiology of T-cell activation. Uninfected CD4 lymphocytes emerge from the thymus as naive cells and circulate until they encounter antigen. They then undergo blast transformation and begin to proliferate. Some cells survive and return to a resting state in which they persist as memory cells, able to respond to future encounters with the same antigen. X4 isolates can infect resting and activated CD4 lympho-cytes. R5 isolates only infect activated CD4 lymphocytes. This is likely to be related to the observation that CCR5 expression on the surface of CD4 lymphocytes increases with activation (Bleul et al., 1997). Furthermore, viral transcription is more efficient in activated cells due to an increase in important transcription factors (Nabel and Baltimore, 1987). Hence the major pathway to productive infection involves infection of activated CD4 lymphocytes. After producing virus, these cells die quickly due to viral cytolytic effect or host effector immune responses. A small fraction of cells may survive to revert back to a resting memory state, but now carrying an integrated copy of the HIV-1 genome (Folks et al., 1989; Pomerantz et al., 1990; Bagasra et al., 1992). Evidence suggests that in vivo only a fraction (< 0.1%) of infected CD4 lymphocytes carries a stably integrated provirus

capable of producing infectious virus following activation (Chun et al., 1997).

HIV-1 infection of monocytes/macrophages

Whereas HIV-1 infection of CD4 lymphocytes in vitro leads to extensive cell death, HIV-1 infection of monocyte/macrophages produces a sustained infection with limited cytopathicity in vitro (Crowe et al., 1987; Gendelman et al., 1988; Collman et al., 1989). This observation initially raised the suggestion that infected macrophages may represent a major reservoir for the virus in vivo, as observed for other lentiviruses (Haase, 1986). Tissue macrophage infection was first recognized in brains from individuals with HIV-1 associated neurological disease (Gartner et al., 1986; Koenig et al., 1986; Wiley et al., 1986). HIV-1 has subsequently been isolated from macrophages from the lung (Chayt et al., 1986; Salahuddin et al., 1986), lymph nodes (Embretson et al., 1993), bone marrow (McElrath et al., 1989), spleen (McIlroy et al., 1995) and liver (Cao et al., 1992). However, the contribution of HIV-1-infected macrophages in the untreated patient to overall viral load is low, estimated to be only 1–7% (Ho et al., 1995; Perelson et al., 1996).

Transmission

HIV-1 is transmitted by contact with infected body fluids, including blood or blood products (Ho et al., 1984), semen (Ho et al., 1984), vaginal and cervical secretions (Vogt et

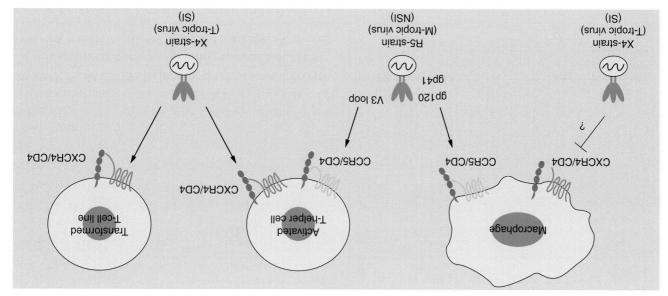

Figure 3.1 Basis of HIV-1 cellular tropism. Previous nomenclature for viral tropism is noted at the bottom. R5 strains were previously named macrophage-tropic or NSI (non-syncytium inducing in T-cell lines), whereas X4 isolates were known as T-cell-line tropic or SI (syncytium inducing) (adapted from Littman, 1998).

al., 1986); amniotic fluid (Mundy *et al.*, 1987) and breast milk (Thiry *et al.*, 1985). The precise mechanism of transmission of HIV-1 is not completely understood. Viruses must enter the body as either cell-free virions or infected cells. The R5 viruses are the strains most commonly transmitted and are present early in the disease. Analysis of HIV-1 isolates from donors and recipients following sexual transmission of HIV-1 shows that the transmitted virus is frequently only a minor variant in the blood of the transmitter (Zhu *et al.*, 1993). The transmitted virus is relatively homogenous in both sequence and phenotype (Zhang *et al.*, 1993; Zhu *et al.*, 1993). It is not yet clear what accounts for this sequence 'bottleneck' during transmission. However, the transmission of a restricted quasispecies occurs irrespective of the route of transmission: sexual (Zhu *et al.*, 1993), maternofetal (Wolinsky *et al.*, 1992); or parenteral (Wolfs *et al.*, 1992).

The most likely cellular target in the mucosa for initial viral infection is antigen-presenting cells, particularly macrophage-related cells of the dendritic-cell lineage. Dendritic cells residing in skin are called Langerhans cells (LCs), while those in the circulation are known as blood dendritic cells. Following intravaginal infection of rhesus macaques with simian immunodeficiency virus (SIV), the first cellular targets are tissue dendritic cells found in the lamina propria beneath the cervicovaginal epithelium (Spira *et al.*, 1996). Within two days of infection, SIV can be detected in the draining internal iliac lymph node (Spira *et al.*, 1996). A similar sequence of events probably occurs following HIV-1 infection (Figure 3.2). In fact, freshly isolated epidermal LCs from the skin (resembling resident mucosal LCs) express CCR5 but not CXCR4 (Zaitesva *et al.*, 1997). The presence of CCR5 would favour transmission of R5 viruses. Even though LCs are not highly permissive to HIV-1 infection, both blood dendritic cells and LCs are able to transmit HIV-1 to T cells very efficiently (Cameron *et al.*, 1992; Pope *et al.*, 1994). Breaks in the mucosal barrier, due to the presence of genital ulcer disease, urethritis or cervicitis, enhance viral transmission. Enhanced transmission occurs due not only to disruption of the integrity of the skin or mucosal lining but also due to the localization of activated lymphocytes at the site of the lesion (Greenblatt *et al.*, 1988; Stamm *et al.*, 1988). X4 strains are rarely, if ever, transmitted between individuals. If transmission of X4 viruses occurs, this is associated with more rapid disease progression (Nielsen *et al.*, 1993; Cornelissen *et al.*, 1995).

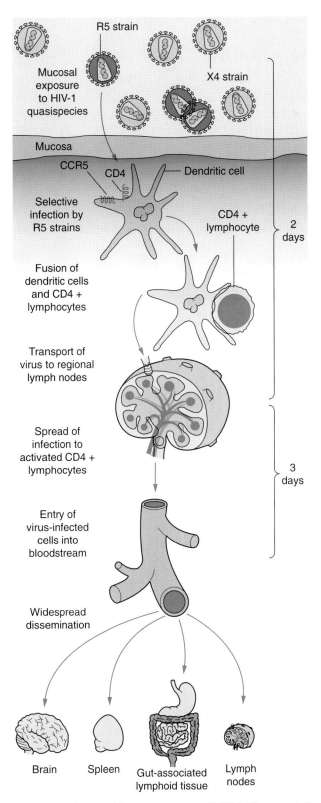

Figure 3.2 *Early events following transmission of HIV-1. The arrows indicate the path of the virus. Dendritic cells, which express the viral co-receptors CD4 and CCR5, are selectively infected by R5 strains. Within 2 days after mucosal exposure, virus can be detected in the lymph nodes. Within another 3 days, it can be cultured from the plasma (based on experiments with SIV) (reprinted with permission from Kahn and Walker, 1998).*

Clinical course of infection

Primary infection

Primary HIV-1 infection is associated with an acute mononucleosis-like clinical syndrome, which appears approximately 1 to a few weeks following infection (Tindall and Cooper, 1991; see Chapter 1). Although the majority of infected individuals do not report symptoms to their physicians, approximately 50–70% of individuals can recall symptoms appropriately associated with their estimated time of infection (Tindall and Cooper, 1991).

Acute infection is associated with a rapid rise in plasma viraemia, often to levels in excess of 1 million RNA molecules per ml (Clark et al., 1991; Daar et al., 1991; Piatak et al., 1993). This is followed by a marked reduction in plasma viraemia to a 'steady-state' level of viral replication (Clark et al., 1991; Daar et al., 1991; Piatak et al., 1993). The determinants of this so-called 'viral set-point' are complex and are dependent upon both viral and host factors (Mellors et al., 1996; Mellors et al., 1997) (see 'Factors determining disease progression' below). The peak in viral load is associated with a fall in the level of CD4 lymphocytes in the first 2–8 weeks following infection (Gaines et al., 1990). The level of CD4 lymphocytes usually rebounds toward normal but rarely returns to pre-infection levels (Figure 3.3).

The decrease in viral load following acute infection is largely due to virus-specific immune responses that limit viral replication (Cooper et al., 1987; Cooper et al., 1988). Multiple factors contribute to the decline in viraemia, including cellular and humoral immunity, the secretion of virus-suppressing cytokines (Cocchi et al., 1995) and the possible exhaustion of suitable lymphocyte target cells (Phillips, 1996). There is a strong temporal relationship between the appearance of HIV-1-specific cytotoxic T lymphocyte (CTL) responses and the striking fall in plasma viraemia (Koup et al., 1994; Musey et al., 1997). Similarly, studies in rhesus monkeys have shown that following infection with SIV, CTLs appear as early as 4–7 days after virus inoculation, and coincide with clearance of SIV from blood and lymph nodes (Letvin et al., 1993). Using limiting dilution analyses, the precursor frequency of HIV-specific CTL peaks at greater than 1% of peripheral blood CD8 lymphocytes (Koup et al., 1994; Borrow et al., 1997), but this is probably an underestimate (McMichael and O'Callaghan, 1998). Using newer assays, direct staining of antigen-specific CD8 lymphocytes is now possible (reviewed by McMichael and O'Callaghan, 1998). The assay uses tetrameric complexes of epitope peptide bound to the presenting class-I MHC molecule. Binding of the so-called 'tetramer' to cells displaying the appropriate T-cell receptor (TCR) can be detected by flow cytometry. The frequency of HIV-

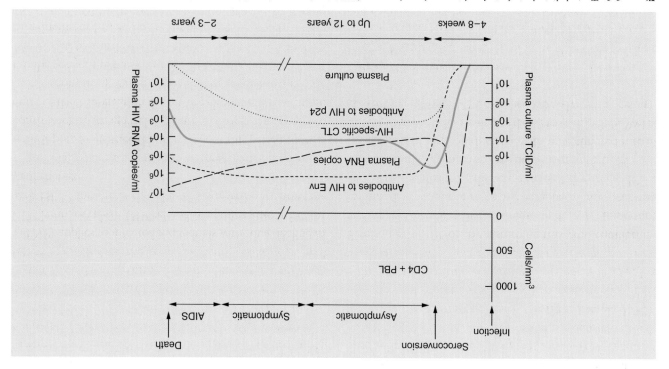

Figure 3.3 Typical clinical, virological and immunological course of HIV-1 infection (adapted from Pantaleo (1993a)).

1-specific CTL during acute infection using this method is thought to be closer to 5% (McMichael and O'Callaghan, 1998). The CTL responses peak as viraemia starts to fall and the expanded T-cell populations decrease secondary to apoptosis, while a small number of clones survive as memory cells. CTL responses then stabilize at a lower level, inversely correlated with viral load (Ogg et al., 1998).

All of this occurs prior to detection of neutralizing antibody (Koup et al., 1994; Musey et al., 1997). Neutralizing antibodies are defined by their ability to block, or neutralize, the infectivity of the virus. Although HIV-1 envelope-binding antibodies can be detected in the sera of HIV-1-infected individuals by 2–3 weeks following infection, most of these antibodies lack the ability to inhibit virus infection (Figure 3.3). Neutralizing antibodies become detectable in both humans and macaques several weeks after the initial high level of viraemia has subsided (Nara et al., 1987; Koup et al., 1994). These antibodies neutralize the infecting virus but often exhibit little or no activity against other strains. Therefore, it is generally considered that primary infection is predominantly contained by HIV-1-specific CTL responses.

Clinical latency

Following primary infection, there is usually a relatively long period that is characterized by few, if any, clinical manifestations. In adults, the average time between infection and development of AIDS is 10 years. However, a small number of individuals progress rapidly to AIDS within 5 years. At the other extreme, some infected individuals remain free of AIDS for more than 16 years (Buchbinder et al., 1994; Munoz et al., 1995). Although definitions differ among different investigators, the term 'long-term non-progressor' (LTNP) applies to infected individuals without a decline in CD4 lymphocytes or HIV-related symptoms after infection with HIV-1 for longer than 12–15 years without antiretroviral therapy.

Although there is a long-term asymptomatic phase, there is undisputed evidence that throughout this period there is continuous ongoing viral replication. Original attempts to detect HIV-1 replication during the clinically latent phase of infection, using culture techniques, suggested that the number of cells expressing viral RNA was in the range of 1 in 10 000 to 1 in 100 000. This was subsequently revised to estimates of 1 in 400 cells during the symptomatic phase and 1 in 50 000 cells infected during the asymptomatic phase (Ho et al., 1989).

Histological studies of lymph nodes using in situ hybridization have demonstrated high levels of viral RNA at all stages of HIV-1 infection (Tenner-Racz et al., 1989; Embretson et al., 1993; Pantaleo, 1993a). Most of the viruses produced within the lymph node are trapped on a specialized cell type known as a follicular dendritic cell (FDC) (Pantaleo, 1993a). FDCs are located in the germinal centres of the secondary lymphoid organs, where their function is to bind and present intact antigens to T lymphocytes. FDCs trap immune complexes, including viral particles that have reacted with antibodies. Although these cells are not directly infected with HIV-1, they may facilitate infection of associated CD4 lymphocytes. Within 3 months of acute infection, HIV-1 is mostly seen in individual virus-expressing cells with minimal or absent 'trapping'. Trapping of virions in the FDC network is most prominent in recent (4–20 months following primary infection) and long-term (> 2–3 years post primary infection) chronic infection (Pantaleo et al., 1998). However, in long-term chronic infection, the numbers of HIV-1 expressing cells in lymphoid tissue are significantly lower than in early disease (Pantaleo et al., 1998).

The development of sensitive and accurate methods for quantifying virus particles in the blood by branched DNA signal amplification (Cao et al., 1995a) and quantitative competitive RT-PCR (Piatak et al., 1993) has greatly facilitated the understanding of viral replication in vivo. Using these more sensitive methods of quantification, it became apparent that HIV-1 virions can be detected in cell-free plasma at all stages of infection (Piatak et al., 1993). The level of plasma HIV-1 RNA is reasonably stable, reflecting a 'quasi-steady state' in which virus production was predicted to equal viral clearance (Ho et al., 1995; Perelson et al., 1996). By disturbing this viral equilibrium with potent antiretroviral drugs, extremely important information about the rates of clearance of free virus and productively infected cells was obtained (Ho et al., 1995; Wei et al., 1995). These studies demonstrated an extremely high rate of viral production, with an estimated rate of > 10^{10} viral particles made per day (Ho et al., 1995; Wei et al., 1995; Perelson et al., 1996) (see 'Viral dynamics' below).

Clinically apparent disease

Eventually this steady state 'breaks down', leading to falling CD4 lymphocyte counts and increasing viral burdens characteristic of AIDS (Figure 3.3). The level of CD4 lymphocytes drops from a normal range of 600–1200 to below 500

CD4 lymphocytes/µl. Numerous HIV-related conditions, namely specific opportunistic infections and malignancies, occur. Their onset is associated with the level of CD4 lymphocytes (Crowe et al., 1991). On average, CD4 lympho-cytes decline at a yearly rate of 60 CD4 lymphocytes/µl (Lang et al., 1989). In the absence of antiretroviral therapy, the decline in CD4 lymphocytes continues until virtually all such cells are lost.

Determinants of disease progression

Overall, the most important correlate of progression to AIDS, prior to substantial immune destruction has occur-red, is the steady-state viral load, or 'set point' seen at the end of primary infection (Mellors et al., 1996; Mellors et al., 1997). Mellors et al. (1996, 1997) retrospectively studied a large cohort of infected individuals looking at the rela-tionship between CD4 lymphocyte counts, HIV-1 RNA levels and ultimate clinical outcomes. Baseline viral RNA levels provided an excellent indicator of time to AIDS and death. Plasma HIV-1 RNA levels of greater than 10^5 copies/ml after seroconversion were a strong predictor of progression to AIDS, while levels of HIV-1 RNA of less than 10^3 copies/ml were associated with a more stable clinical course. This was not the case with baseline CD4 lymphocyte counts. Furthermore, viral load change in response to antiretroviral therapy is also a stronger predic-tor of clinical progression than CD4 lymphocyte count changes (Hammer et al., 1996). However, the determinants of the viral load 'set-point' and consequently clinical prog-nosis, are complex and dependent upon the interplay of both viral and host factors (see Table 3.1).

Table 3.1 Factors associated with delayed disease progression

Viral	Attenuated strain, e.g. Δ nef
	R5 phenotype
Host	
Genetic	CCR5-Δ32 mutation
	Mutations in the CCR5 promoter
	CCR2-64 I mutation
	SDF-1 3' untranslated region (?)
HLA type	B13, B27, B51, B57
Immunology	High titre neutralizing antibody
	High level CD8+ HIV-1 specific T cells
	High level CD4+ HIV-1 specific proliferative responses
Age	Extremes of age (i.e. very old or very young) lead to a poorer prognosis

Viral factors

HIV-1 isolates from the infected individual change over time (Cheng-Mayer et al., 1988; Tersmette et al., 1989). Isolates from patients early in the course of HIV-1 infection are generally M-tropic, NSI, R5 viruses. The emergence of T-tropic, SI isolates correlates with increasing viral burden and increasing rate of CD4 lymphocyte decline (Connor et al., 1993; Koot et al., 1993). This change has also been shown to be associated with a switch in co-receptor use from CCR5 to CXCR4 (Connor et al., 1997). It is not clear whether disease progression is a direct result of cytopathic variants or whether declining immune competence allows the growth of variants with increased replicative capacity. In the rare instances of transmission of X4 virus (T-tropic, SI variant) a more rapid progression to AIDS is observed (Nielsen et al., 1993).

There are rare examples of genetic defects in the infect-ing virus playing a role in slow progression. A cohort of eight infected individuals from Sydney has been described (Learmont et al., 1992). The cohort comprises seven blood or blood-product recipients and the relevant donor. All CD4 lymphocyte counts have stable or very slowly declining CD4 lymphocyte counts 10–14 years after infection. Virus-es obtained from all the recipients and the donor had deletions in the viral nef gene with duplications and rearrangements within the long terminal repeat (LTR) (Deacon et al., 1995). Virus strains isolated from other non-progressing patients have also been found to have a defect in nef (Kirchhoff et al., 1995; Mariani et al., 1996). However, studies of other cohorts of LTNPs have not demonstrated genetic defects in nef (Huang et al., 1995). The possibility that alterations of nef might be responsible for long-term slow progression, at least in some cases, is consistent with observations in monkeys with SIV infec-tion. Infection of adult monkeys with cloned virus in which the nef gene was partially deleted became persistently infected but generally failed to develop clinical disease (Kestler et al., 1991).

Extensive genetic characterization of our own cohort of LTNPs demonstrated infrequent mutations within the LTR (Zhang et al., 1997a) and gag (Huang et al., 1998). Gene-tic analyses of pol (Huang et al., 1998) and the accessory genes vif, vpr and vpu (Zhang et al., 1997b) did not demon-strate any abnormality. In summary, it is generally consid-ered that the number of infected individuals with an attenuated form of HIV-1 is small and is a rare cause of non-progression.

Host factors

Chemokine receptors

Several reports have defined the role of chemokine receptors in HIV-1 disease progression (Figure 3.4). The 32-base-pair deletion in the CCR5 gene (CCR5-Δ32) confers resistance to HIV-1 infection in homozygotes (Dean et al., 1996; Liu et al., 1996; Samson et al., 1996). CCR5-Δ32 heterozygotes are not protected from HIV-1 infection but the onset of AIDS appears to be postponed by 2–4 years (Dean et al., 1996; Huang et al., 1996; Michael et al., 1997a). Approximately 10–15% of Caucasians are heterozygous for the CCR5-Δ32 allele. Levels of CCR5 expression on CD4 lymphocytes in these individuals are lower than in individuals homozygous for the wild type allele (Moore, 1997). This may influence the course of disease, but the mechanism of protection against progression remains to be further explored. Another much more rare mutation, CCR5-m303, with similar effects to CCR5-Δ32 has also been described (Quillent et al., 1998).

A valine to isoleucine switch at position 64 in the transmembrane domain of CCR2 (CCR2-64I) has also been associated with delayed disease progression (Smith et al., 1997; Kostrikis et al., 1998). There has been some debate over the effect of this mutation, but it appears that the effect is only apparent in seroconverters (Kostrikis et al., 1998; Rizzardi et al., 1998) and could be masked in studies of seroprevalent cohorts (Michael et al., 1997b), which are skewed against the inclusion of rapid progressors. A recent report describes finding the disease-retarding effects of the CCR2-64I allele only in African-Americans, not in Caucasians (Mummidi et al., 1998). It seems surprising that a single conservative amino acid substitution in the transmembrane (non-binding) region of a receptor, shown to be of minor importance in HIV-1 entry of target cells, should have an impact on disease progression. A potential mechanism explaining the mode of action of this mutation is related to strong linkage disequilibrium between CCR2-64I and mutations in the regulatory region of the closely linked CCR5 gene (Kostrikis et al., 1998; Mummidi et al., 1998 reviewed in Hogan and Hammer, 2001).

Another report of a mutation in the gene that codes for the chemokine stromal-derived factor 1 (SDF-1) has

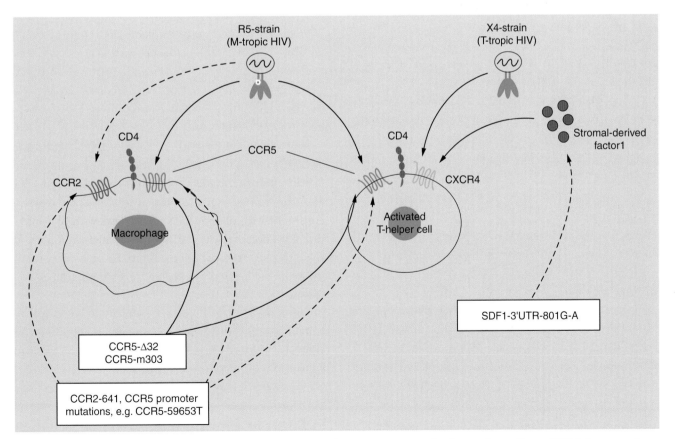

Figure 3.4 *Sites of action of mutations in the chemokine receptor network. Mutations associated with a significant effect on HIV-1 disease are shown in boxes (adapted from Stewart, 1998).*

been associated with delayed disease progression (Winkler et al., 1998), although this is controversial (Mummidi et al., 1998). SDF-1 is the principal ligand for CXCR4. Protection appears to be stronger than that conferred by the CCR5-Δ32 or CCR2-64I mutations (Winkler et al., 1998). The mechanism underlying protection is unclear but a possible explanation is that homozygotes for the mutant SDF-1, allele express higher levels of SDF-1, which delays the switch to T-tropic strains by competing with viruses for CXCR4. Alternatively, this allele may be in linkage disequilibrium with a truly protective gene. The mechanism underlying protection remains to be confirmed.

As expected, the frequency of these mutations is signif-icantly higher in cohorts of LTNPs. In fact, 25–30% of patients who remain AIDS-free for more than 16 years carry the CCR2-Δ35 or the CCR2-64I mutation (Smith et al., 1997 reviewed in Hogan and Hammer, 2001).

HLA type

Initial interest in the variability of host response to HIV-1 focused on HLA types (reviewed in Haynes et al., 1996). A number of major histocompatibility (MHC) alleles have been described, which may influence progression of disease. Certain alleles (e.g. A1, A24, C7, B8, DR3) (Cameron et al., 1990; Kaslow et al., 1990) have been asso-ciated with rapid progression, while others have been asso-ciated with protection from progression (B13, B27, B51, B57) (Kaslow and Mann, 1994). However, the HLA HIV-1 disease associations are not absolute. Combinations of particular MHC alleles may have a more significant impact (Kaslow et al., 1996). Several mechanisms have been pro-posed. For example, certain MHC alleles may serve as a restricting element for one or several immunodominant HIV T-helper or CTL epitopes promoting, or alternatively failing to generate, effective responses to HIV-1.

Immune response

Neutralizing antibody responses in LTNPs are improved in magnitude and breadth compared with other HIV-1 infected individuals (Cao et al., 1995b; Montefiori et al., 1996). It is unclear whether the broad neutralizing antibody response in LTNPs is a cause or effect of long-term non-pro-gression. A high and constantly changing complexity of viral quasispecies (Delwart et al., 1994) could possibly give rise to a wide range of neutralization epitopes for antigen presentation. In contrast, rapid progressors are character-

ized by lower levels of antibodies to HIV-1 proteins (Cao et al., 1995b; Pantaleo et al., 1995) and by low or absent anti-bodies that neutralize autologous HIV-1 variants (Cao et al., 1995b; Pantaleo et al., 1995).

HIV-1 specific CTL responses also play a significant role in determining disease progression. Many studies have shown that specific CTL responses deteriorate during dis-ease progression (Johnson et al., 1991; Klein et al., 1995; Rinaldo et al., 1995). Recent advances in the direct mea-surement of circulating HIV-1-specific CTL (effector CTL, CTLs, CTLe) using HLA-peptide tetramers have demon-strated an inverse correlation between HIV-1-specific CTL frequency and plasma RNA viral load (Ogg et al., 1998). Furthermore, when viral load was reduced following anti-retroviral therapy, CTLe decreased, suggesting that the virus did not have a significant inhibitory effect on CTLe and that generation of HIV-1-specific CTL responses required continued viral replication (Ogg et al., 1998). Studies of LTNPs show robust and persistent HIV-1-specific CTL responses (Cao et al., 1995b; Klein et al., 1995; Pantaleo et al., 1995). In fact, the initial immune response to HIV-1 may be responsible for distinct clinical outcomes. For exam-ple, a broadly directed CTL response during primary infec-tion appears to protect against rapid progression to AIDS (Pantaleo et al., 1997).

Despite seemingly potent CTL responses, HIV-1 is almost never eradicated from the body. There are many examples of HIV-1 evading CTL responses, either by muta-tional escape (Koenig et al., 1995; Borrow et al., 1997; Price et al., 1997) or non-mutational escape. Examples of non-mutational escape include sequestration, whereby HIV-1 exists in sites such as the central nervous system (CNS) or latent CD4 lymphocytes; down regulation of HLA expres-sion on infected cells (Collins et al., 1998); exhaustion of the responding CTL population (Borrow et al., 1997); or antagonism (Klenerman et al., 1994).

Finally, CD4 lymphocyte helper cells may also be a significant determinant of disease progression. CD4 lymphocyte helper function is central to an effective humoral and cell-mediated response to foreign antigens. However, as these very cells are the primary targets for HIV-1 infection, a state of T-helper cell tolerance to HIV-1 is readily induced. Rosenberg et al. (1997) showed that CD4 lymphocyte responses to an HIV-1 antigen, Gag, could be observed in a few long-term survivors and in patients treated very early after infection, suggesting that inhibition of virus replication by antiretroviral therapy rescued the

T-helper response. In chronic infection, T-helper proliferative responses were inversely correlated with viral load (Rosenberg *et al.*, 1997). The mechanisms whereby CD4 lymphocytes contribute to effective antiviral immunity are not known but may relate to enhanced CTL precursor activity, increased production of antiviral cytokines, or augmentation of humoral immune responses (McMichael, 1998).

Viral dynamics

The first phase of decay
Detailed analysis of the decline in plasma viraemia and the decline of HIV-1-infected peripheral blood mononuclear cells (PBMC) in patients undergoing antiretroviral therapy has given critical information about the dynamic processes that underlie HIV-1 infection (Ho *et al.*, 1995; Wei *et al.*, 1995). When potent inhibitors of HIV-1 protease (Ho *et al.*, 1995) or reverse transcriptase (Wei *et al.*, 1995) were administered to chronically infected patients, plasma levels of virus decreased approximately a hundred-fold in 2 weeks. In other words, plasma virus half-life was demonstrated to have a mean of about 2 days or less (Ho *et al.*, 1995; Wei *et al.*, 1995). From this it was deduced that a minimal estimate of the average rate of virus production and clearance was 10^9 virions per day (Ho *et al.*, 1995). This was a minimal estimate because monotherapy does not completely block viral replication and thus clearance must actually occur faster than what was observed to counterbalance the residual viral production.

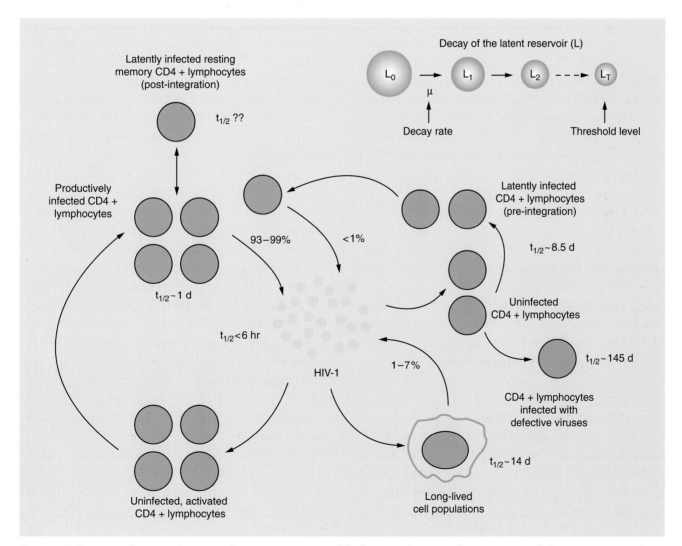

Figure 3.5 *Dynamics of HIV-1 infection. A schematic representation of the dynamics of HIV-1 replication in vivo. The latent reservoir L is shown at the top left, and its decay is hypothetically depicted in the insert.*

The rapid fall in plasma viraemia in fact reflects two processes: the clearance of free virions and the loss of the infected cells that produce most of the plasma virus (Perelson et al., 1996). The half-life of productively infected cells was 1.55 ± 0.57 days, while the half-life of HIV-1 RNA in plasma was at the most 6 h (Perelson et al., 1996) (Figure 3.5). Based on these new, higher estimates for the plasma virion clearance rate, the rate of production of virions was revised to 10^{10} virions/day (Perelson et al., 1996). If one assumes that about 100 virions are produced per productively infected cell (based on studies using in situ hybridization, ISH) (Haase et al., 1996), then on average there should be 10^8 new infections per day. Similar numbers have been obtained using ISH analysis of tonsillar biopsies from patients starting antiretroviral therapy (Cavert et al., 1997).

This high rate of virus production has significant implications for the generation of drug resistance and for the mechanism of CD4 lymphocyte depletion (see 'T cell dynamics'). The error rate of reverse transcriptase is estimated to be 3×10^{-5}/base/replication cycle (Mansky and Temin, 1995). One can predict that if 10^8 new cells are infected per day, then not only are all possible single-point mutations generated daily, but almost 1% of all possible two-point mutations are generated each day (Perelson et al., 1997b). Hence, the rapid emergence of drug-resistant virus

in plasma can be explained according to the dynamic processes maintaining the plasma viral load (Wei et al., 1995). Similarly, pressure for viral escape from immuno-protective mechanisms is strong.

The second phase of decay

After the rapid, initial decay of the virus during the first 1–2 weeks of treatment, plasma virus declines at a slower rate, reflecting the turnover of a longer-lived viral reservoir (Figure 3.6). This reservoir could be due to virus production from macrophages or dendritic cells, latently infected T cells or the release of trapped virions from lymphoid tissue (Coffin, 1995; Heath et al., 1995; Perelson et al., 1996; Perelson et al., 1997a) (Figure 3.6). This reservoir accounts for only a small portion of the total virus production in an untreated individual but becomes significant when cells that produce most of the plasma virus have largely decayed (Perelson et al., 1997a). The half-life of this second phase was calculated to be 1–4 weeks, with the loss of long-lived infected cells being a major contributor to this phase (Cavert et al., 1997; Perelson et al., 1997a). Mathematical projections suggested that these pools could be eliminated if fully effective treatment was continued for 2–3 years (Perelson et al., 1997a), raising the exciting possibility of virus eradication.

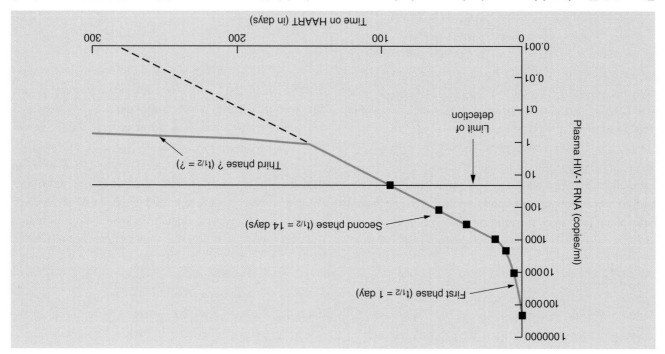

Figure 3.6 *Hypothetical decay curve for plasma virus levels in a patient treated with highly active antiretroviral therapy* (HAART) (reprinted with permission from Finzi and Siliciano, 1998).

The third phase of decay or the latent reservoir

Recent studies have demonstrated that infectious HIV-1 persists latently in resting CD4 memory lymphocytes in a post-integrated form despite 1–2 years of combination therapy (Chun *et al.*, 1997; Finzi *et al.*, 1997; Wong *et al.*, 1997). Even in patients who had undetectable virus in the periphery, HIV-1 could be isolated from resting CD4 lymphocytes using enhanced culture techniques (Finzi *et al.*, 1997). The so-called latent reservoir is small and estimated to be no larger than 10^7 cells (Chun *et al.*, 1997). Its decay rate has not been measured with any degree of accuracy, although one study reports no detectable decay of this pool during the first 2 years of treatment (Finzi *et al.*, 1997). However, it is known that memory CD4 lymphocytes have a mean half-life ($t_{1/2}$) of about 3–4 months (McLean and Michie, 1995). Although much of the pro-viral DNA harboured within memory CD4 lymphocytes of infected persons exists as defective forms (Chun *et al.*, 1997), the decay rate of this DNA may serve as a surrogate to assess the decay rate of the latent pool. An estimate of the half-life of the latent reservoir has been obtained by quantifying infectious virus isolated from resting CD4 T lymphocytes from patients receiving effective antiviral therapy. The half-life of the latent reservoir has been calculated to range from 6 months (Zhang, 1999a; Ramratnam, 2000) to 44 months (Finzi, 1999) depending on the degree of viral suppression (Ramratnam, 2000). Persistent viral replication despite undetectable virus in the plasma in individuals receiving effective antiviral therapy has been demonstrated by identifying evolution of *env* sequences (Zhang, 1999a) and by the detection of cell-associated HIV RNA using PCR (Lewin, 1999; Furado, 1999) and *in situ* hybridization (Zhang, 1999). Persistent viral replication will over-estimate the calculated half-life of the latent reservoir. A half life of 6 months is consistent with the previous estimates of the half life of memory lymphocytes (Mclean and Michie, 1995). Based on a decay rate of 6 months in order for the pool size to decay to less than 1, more than 10 years of continuous therapy would be required (Ho, 1998). However, it is conceivable that the residual pool need not be reduced to less than 1, but rather reduced to a threshold level (L_T; see Figure 3.5), while the spread of the virus could be controlled by the immune system without continuing antiretroviral therapy.

T-cell dynamics

The central immunopathogenic hallmark of HIV-1 disease is the progressive loss of CD4 lymphocytes. The exact mechanism of this is still incompletely understood. Numerous mechanisms have been proposed, including direct cell killing, syncytium formation, auto-immune destruction, impaired T-cell regeneration, or apoptosis (reviewed in Fauci and Desrosiers, 1997).

However, the central question remains whether T-cell decline is due to impaired regeneration, accelerated destruction, or both. Further light was shed on this issue when it was observed that following the administration of antiretroviral therapy to infected individuals, there was not only a rapid fall in plasma viraemia, but a rise in peripheral CD4 lymphocytes (Ho *et al.*, 1995; Wei *et al.*, 1995). These observations led to a hypothesis that high levels of virally induced T-cell destruction ($1–2 \times 10^9$ CD4 lymphocytes per day) placed considerable demand on CD4 lymphocyte proliferation, which resulted ultimately in collapse of the immune system. Alternative views suggested that the rise in CD4 lymphocytes following the introduction of effective therapy simply reflected 'redistribution'. A large number of T and B cells may be 'trapped' in peripheral sites (for example, by antigen, cytokine or chemokine signals). Following therapy, the amount of HIV-1 antigen declines and the immune response resolves and sequestered cells leave the inflamed lymph node and return to the circulation.

Other investigators have used different methods to quantify T-cell turnover in HIV-1-infected subjects. One approach is the measurement of telomere lengths as an indicator of replicative history. Basically, each time a cell divides the telomere length decreases. Greater telomere shortening correlates with greater cell division. Measurement of CD4 lymphocytes in HIV-1 infected patients using this method failed to detect shortening, suggesting normal or reduced CD4 lymphocyte turnover (Wolthers *et al.*, 1996). However, this method does not account for cells that have been destroyed and is biased towards non-dividing cells. Another technique of measuring T-cell turnover is the measurement of the nuclear antigen Ki-67, which is specific for cell proliferation. Using this technique, increased turnover of CD4 and CD8 lymphocytes was demonstrated in HIV-1 infected individuals compared with uninfected individuals (Sachsenberg *et al.*, 1998; Tenner-Racz *et al.*, 1998). Increased proliferation was demonstrated in both the periphery (Sachsenberg *et al.*, 1998; Tenner-Racz *et al.*, 1998) and within the germinal centres of lymph nodes (Tenner-Racz *et al.*, 1998).

By studying SIV-infected macaques following the ingestion of bromodeoxyuridine, a more direct measure of T cell proliferation *in vivo* has been obtained (Mohri *et al.*, 1998).

Bromodeoxyuridine is incorporated into the DNA of pro-liferating cells. This study demonstrated increased turnover of CD4 and CD8 lymphocytes, as well as NK cells, suggesting generalized immune activation in SIV infection. Studies using deuterated glucose found similar results in HIV-1 infected humans (Hellerstein et al., 1999). However, many questions regarding T-cell dynamics in HIV-1 infection remain unanswered. For example, even though increased proliferation of both CD4 and CD8 lymphocytes have been shown in both HIV-1 and SIV infection, it is unclear why only CD4 lymphocyte subsets are depleted and not CD8 lymphocyte subsets.

The role of the thymus in T-cell dynamics in HIV-1 infection remains controversial. Recent developments in the ability to quantify thymus function in vivo using a PCR-based assay that measures a byproduct of T-cell receptor synthesis, known as a T-cell receptor excision circle (TREC), have demonstrated that the thymus remains active throughout adult life (Douek, 1998; Zhang, 1999b). Although TREC is reduced in some HIV-infected individuals, it is certainly not reduced in all, suggesting that a defect in thymic function is unlikely to fully account for CD4 depletion in HIV infection (Zhang, 1999b).

However, HIV-1 disease is not characterized by a fall in CD4 lymphocyte alone. Other abnormalities in advanced disease include depletion of naive cells relative to memo-ry T-cell subsets, restricted diversity of the T-cell receptor repertoire, a greater proportion of CD8 lymphocytes com-pared with CD4 lymphocytes, and reduced functional com-petence of the T-lymphocyte system. Interestingly, following antiretroviral therapy there is an early rise in memory CD4 lymphocytes, followed by a reduction in T-cell activation, with an improved CD4 lymphocyte reac-tivity to recall antigens and finally a late rise in naive cells (Autran et al., 1997; Pakker et al., 1998). Other reports demonstrate reconstitution of the TCR repertoire (Goro-chov et al., 1998). These studies suggest that effective immune reconstitution may be achieved following effective antiretroviral therapy.

References

Alkhatib G, Combadiere C, Broder CC et al. (1996). CC CKR5: a RANTES, MIP-1alpha, MIP-1beta receptor as a fusion cofactor for macrophage-tropic HIV-1. Science 272: 1955-8.

Autran B, Carcelain G, Li T T et al. (1997). Positive effects of combined antiretroviral therapy on CD4+ T cell homeostasis and function in advanced HIV disease. Science 277: 112-6.

Bagasra O, Hauptman S, Lischner HW et al. (1992). Detection of human immunodeficiency virus type 1 provirus in mononuclear cells by in situ polymerase chain reaction. N Engl J Med 326: 1385-91.

Barre-Sinoussi P, Chermann J, Rey F et al. (1983). Isolation of a T-lym-photropic retrovirus from a patient at risk for acquired immune deficiency syndrome. Science 220: 868-71.

Berger EA, Doms RW, Fenyo EM et al. (1998). A new classification for HIV-1. Nature 391: 240.

Bleul CC, Farzan M, Choe H et al. (1996). The lymphocyte chemoat-tractant SDF-1 is a ligand for LESTR/fusin and blocks HIV-1 entry. Nature 382: 829-33.

Bleul CC, Wu L, Hoxie JA et al. (1997). The HIV coreceptors CXCR4 and CCR5 are differentially expressed and regulated on human T lymphocytes. Proc Natl Acad Sci USA 94: 1925-30.

Borrow P, Lewicki H, Wei X et al. (1997). Antiviral pressure exerted by HIV-1-specific cytotoxic T lymphocytes (CTLs) during primary infection demonstrated by rapid selection of CTL escape virus. Nat Med 3: 205-11.

Buchbinder SP, Katz MH, Hessol NA et al. (1994). Long-term HIV-1 infection without immunologic progression. AIDS 8: 1123-8.

Cairns J, D'Souza M. (1998). Chemokines and HIV-1 second receptors: the therapeutic connection. Nat Med 4: 563-8.

Cameron PU, Mallal SA, French MA et al. (1990). Major histocompat-ibility complex genes influence the outcome of HIV infection. Ances-tral haplotypes with C4 null alleles explain diverse HLA associations. Hum Immunol 29: 282-95.

Cameron P, Freudenthal P, Barker J et al. (1992). Dendritic cells exposed to human immunodeficiency virus type 1 transmit a vigorous cytopathic infection to CD4+ T cells. Science 257: 383-7.

Cao Y, Dieterich D, Thomas P et al. (1992). Identification and quantitation of HIV-1 in the liver of patients with AIDS. AIDS 6: 65-70.

Cao Y, Ho DD, Todd J et al. (1995a). Clinical evaluation of branched DNA signal amplification for quantifying HIV type 1 in human plas-ma. AIDS Res Hum Retrovir 11: 353-61.

Cao Y, Qin L, Zhang L et al. (1995b). Virologic and immunologic char-acterization of long-term survivors of human immunodeficiency virus type 1 infection. N Engl J Med 332: 201-8.

Cavert W, Notermans D, Staskus K et al. (1997). Kinetics of response in lymphoid tissues to antiretroviral therapy of HIV-1 infection. Science 276: 960-4.

Chayt KJ, Harper MA, Marselle LM et al. (1986). Detection of HTLV III RNA in lungs of patients with AIDS and pulmonary involvement. JAMA 256: 2356-9.

Cheng-Mayer C, Seto D, Tateno M et al. (1988). Biological features of HIV-1 that correlate with virulence in the host. Science 240: 80-2.

Choe H, Farzan M, Sun Y et al. (1996). The beta-chemokine receptors CCR3 and CCR5 facilitate infection by primary HIV-1 isolates. Cell 85: 1135-48.

Chun T-W, Carruth L, Finzi D et al. (1997). Quantification of latent tis-sue reservoirs and total body viral load in HIV-1 infection. Nature 387: 183-8.

Clark S, Saag MS, Decker D et al. (1991). High titers of cytopathic virus in plasma of patients with symptomatic primary HIV-1 infection. N Engl J Med 324: 954-60.

Cocchi F, DeVico A, Garzino-Demo A et al. (1995). Identification of RANTES, MIP-1α and MIP-1β as the major HIV-suppressive fac-tors produced by CD8+ T cells. Science 270: 1811-5.

Coffin J. (1995). HIV population dynamics in vivo: implications for genet-ic variation, pathogenesis and therapy. Science 267: 483-9.

Collins K, Chen B, Kalams S et al. (1998). HIV-1 Nef protein protects infected primary cells against killing by cytotoxic T lymphocytes. Nature 391: 397–401.

Collman R, Hassan N, Walker R et al. (1989). Infection of monocyte-derived macrophages with human immunodeficiency virus type 1 (HIV-1). J Exp Med 170: 1149–63.

Connor R, Mohri H, Cao Y et al. (1993). Increased viral burden and cytopathicity correlate temporally with CD4+ lymphocyte decline and clinical progression in human immunodeficiency virus type-1 infected individuals. J Virol 647: 1772–7.

Connor RI, Sheridan KE, Ceradini D et al. (1997). Change in co-receptor use coreceptor use: correlates with disease progression in HIV-1–infected individuals. J Exp Med 185: 621–8.

Cooper DA, Imrie AA, Penny R. (1987). Antibody response to human immunodeficiency virus after primary infection. J Infect Dis 155: 1113–8.

Cooper DA, Tindall B, Wilson EJ et al. (1988). Characterization of T lymphocyte responses during primary infection with human immunodeficiency virus. J Infect Dis 157: 889–96.

Cornelissen M, Mulder-Kampinga G, Veenstra J et al. (1995). Syncytium-inducing (SI) phenotype suppression at seroconversion after intramuscular inoculation of a non-syncytium-inducing/SI phenotypically mixed human immunodeficiency virus population. J Virol 69: 1810–8.

Crowe SM, Mills J, McGrath MS. (1987). HIV infection of monocyte/macrophages. Arch AIDS Res 1: 145–6.

Crowe SM, Carlin JB, Stewart KI et al. (1991). Predictive value of CD4 lymphocyte numbers for the development of opportunistic infections and malignancies in HIV-infected persons. J Acquir Immune Defic Syndr 4: 770–6.

Daar ES, Moudgil T, Meyer RD et al. (1991). Transient high levels of viraemia in patients with human immunodeficiency virus type 1 infection. N Engl J Med 324: 961–4.

Dalgleish G, Beverly P, Clapham P et al. (1984). The CD4 (T4) antigen is an essential component of the receptor for the AIDS retrovirus. Nature 312: 763–6.

Deacon NJ, Tsykin A, Solomon A et al. (1995). Genomic structure of an attenuated quasi species of HIV-1 from a blood transfusion donor and recipients. Science 270: 988–91.

Dean M, Carrington M, Winkler C et al. (1996). Genetic restriction of HIV-1 infection and progression to AIDS by a deletion allele of the CKR5 structural gene. Hemophilia Growth and Development Study, Multicenter AIDS Cohort Study, Multicenter Hemophilia Cohort Study, San Francisco City Cohort, ALIVE Study. Science 273: 1856–62.

Delwart EL, Sheppard HW, Walker BD et al. (1994). Human immunodeficiency virus type 1 evolution in vivo tracked by DNA heteroduplex mobility assays. J Virol 68: 6672–83.

Deng H, Liu R, Ellmeir W et al. (1996). Identification of a major co-receptor for primary isolates of HIV-1. Science 381: 661–6.

Doranz BJ, Rucker J, Yi Y et al. (1996). A dual-tropic primary HIV-1 isolate that uses fusin and the beta-chemokine receptors CKR-5, CKR-3, and CKR-2b as fusion cofactors. Cell 85: 1149–58.

Douek DC, McFarland RD, Keiser PH et al. (1998). Changes in thymic function with age and during the treatment of HIV infection. Nature 396: 690–5.

Dragic T, Litwin V, Allaway G et al. (1996). HIV-1 entry into CD4+ cells is mediated by the chemokine receptor CC-CKR-5. Science 381: 667–73.

Embretson M, Zupancic M, Ribas JL et al. (1993). Massive covert infection of helper T lymphocytes and macrophages by HIV during the incubation period of AIDS. Nature 362: 359–62.

Fauci A, Desrosiers R. (1997). Pathogenesis of HIV and SIV. In: J Coffin, S Hughes, H Varmus (eds.) Retroviruses. Plainview, NY: Cold Spring Harbor Laboratory Press, 587–636

Feng Y, Broder C, Kennedy P et al. (1996). HIV-1 entry cofactor: functional cDNA cloning of a seven-transmembrane, G protein-coupled receptor. Science 272: 872–7.

Finzi D, Silicano R. (1998). Viral dynamics in HIV-1 infection. Cell 93: 665–71.

Finzi D, Hermankova M, Pierson T et al. (1997). Identification of a reservoir for HIV-1 in patients on highly active antiretroviral therapy. Science 278: 1295–300.

Finzi D, Blankson J, Silicand JD et al. (1999). Latent infection of CD4+ T cells provides a mechanism for lifelong persistence of HIV-1, even in patients on effective combination therapy. Nat Med 5: 512–17.

Folks TM, Clouse KA, Justement J et al. (1989). Tumour necrosis factor alpha induces expression of human immunodeficiency virus in a chronically infected T-cell clone. Proc Natl Acad Sci USA 86: 2365–8.

Furtado MR, Callaway DS, Phair JP et al. (1999). Persistence of HIV-1 transcription in peripheral-blood mononuclear cells in patients receiving potent antiretroviral therapy. N Engl J Med 340: 1614–22.

Gaines H, von Sydow M, von Stedingk L et al. (1990). Immunological changes in primary HIV infection. AIDS 4: 995–9.

Gallo RC, Salahuddin SZ, Popovic M et al. (1984). Frequent detection and isolation of cytopathic retroviruses (HTLV-III) from patients with AIDS and at risk for AIDS. Science 224: 500–3.

Gartner S, Markovits P, Markovitz DM et al. (1986). The role of mononuclear phagocytes in HTLV-III/LAV infection. Science 233: 215–9.

Gendelman H, Orenstein J, Martin M et al. (1988). Efficient isolation and propagation of human immunodeficiency virus on recombinant colony-stimulating factor 1-treated monocytes. J Exp Med 167: 1428–41.

Gorochov G, Neumann A, Kereveur A et al. (1998). Pertubation of CD4+ and CD8+ T-cell repertoires during progression to AIDS and regulation of the CD4+ repertoire during antiviral therapy. Nat Med 4: 215–21.

Greenblatt RM, Lukehart SA, Plummer FA et al. (1988). Genital ulceration as a risk factor for human immunodeficiency virus infection. AIDS 2: 47–50.

Haase A. (1986). Pathogenesis of lentivirus infections. Nature 322: 130–6.

Haase A, Henry K, Zupancic M et al. (1996). Quantitative image analysis of HIV-1 infection in lymphoid tissue. Science 274: 985–9.

Hammer SM, Katzenstein DA, Hughes MD et al. (1996). A trial comparing nucleoside monotherapy with combination therapy in HIV-infected adults with CD4 cell counts from 200 to 500 per cubic millimeter. AIDS Clinical Trials Group Study 175 Study Team. N Engl J Med 335: 1081–90.

Haynes B, Pantaleo G, Fauci A. (1996). Toward an understanding of the correlates of protective immunity to HIV infection. Science 271: 324–8.

Heath SL, Tew JG, Tew JG et al. (1995). Follicular dendritic cells and human immunodeficiency virus infectivity. Nature 377: 740–4.

Hellerstein M, Hanley MB, Cesar D et al. (1999). Directly measured kinetics of circulating T lymphocytes in normal and HIV-1-infected humans. Nat Med 5: 83-9.

Ho DD. (1998). Toward HIV eradication or remission: the tasks ahead. Science 280: 1866-7.

Ho DD, Schooley R, Rota T. (1984). HTLV-III in the semen and blood of a healthy homosexual man. Science 226: 451.

Ho DD, Moudgil T, Alam M. (1989). Quantitation of human immunodeficiency virus type 1 in the blood of infected persons. N Engl J Med 321: 1621-5.

Ho DD, Neumann A, Perelson A et al. (1995). Rapid turnover of plasma virions and CD4 lymphocytes in HIV-1 infection. Nature 373: 123-6.

Hogan CM, Hammer SM (2001) Host determinants in HIV infection and disease. Part 2: genetic factors and implications for antiretroviral therapeutics. Ann Int Med 134: 978-96.

Huang Y, Zhang L, Ho DD. (1995). Characterization of nef sequences in long-term survivors of human immunodeficiency virus type 1 infection. J Virol 69: 93-100.

Huang Y, Paxton WA, Wolinsky SM et al. (1996). The role of a mutant CCR5 allele in HIV-1 transmission and disease progression. Nat Med 2: 1240-3.

Huang Y, Zhang L, Ho DD. (1998). Characterization of gag and pol sequences from long-term survivors of human immunodeficiency virus type 1 infection. Virology 240: 36-49.

Johnson RP, Trocha A, Yang L et al. (1991). HIV-1 gag-specific cytotoxic T lymphocytes recognize multiple highly conserved epitopes. Fine specificity of the gag-specific response defined by using unstimulated peripheral blood mononuclear cells and cloned effector cells. J Immunol 147: 1512-21.

Kahn J, Walker B. (1998). Current concepts: acute human immunodeficiency virus type 1 infection. N Engl J Med 339: 33-40.

Kaslow RA, Mann DL. (1994). The role of the major histocompatibility complex in human immunodeficiency virus infection – ever more complex? J Infect Dis 169: 1332-3.

Kaslow RA, VanRaden M et al. (1990). A1, Cw7, B8, DR3 HLA antigen combination associated with rapid decline of T-helper lymphocytes in HIV-1 infection. A report from the Multicenter AIDS Cohort Study. Lancet 335: 927-30.

Kaslow RA, Carrington M, Apple R et al. (1996). Influence of combinations of human major histocompatibility complex genes on the course of HIV-1 infection. Nat Med 2: 405-11.

Kestler HI, Ringler D, Mori K. (1991). Importance of the nef gene for maintenance of high virus loads and for development of AIDS. Cell 65: 651-2.

Kirchhoff F, Greenough TC, Brettler DB et al. (1995). Brief report: absence of intact nef sequences in a long-term survivor with nonprogressive HIV-1 infection. N Engl J Med 332: 228-32.

Klatzmann D, Champagne E, Chamaret S et al. (1984). T-lymphocyte T4 molecule behaves as receptor for human retrovirus LAV. Nature 312: 763-7.

Klein MR, van Baalen CA, Holwerda AM et al. (1995). Kinetics of Gag-specific cytotoxic T lymphocyte responses during the clinical course of HIV-1 infection: a longitudinal analysis of rapid progressors and long-term asymptomatics. J Exp Med 181: 1365-72.

Klenerman P, Rowland-Jones S, McAdam S et al. (1994). Cytotoxic T-cell activity antagonized by naturally occurring HIV-1 Gag variants. Nature 369: 403-7.

Koenig S, Gendelman H, Orenstein J et al. (1986). Detection of AIDS virus in macrophages in brain tissue from AIDS patients with encephalopathy. Science 233: 1089-93.

Koenig S, Conley AJ, Brewah YA et al. (1995). Transfer of HIV-1-specific cytotoxic T lymphocytes to an AIDS patient leads to selection for mutant HIV variants and subsequent disease progression. Nat Med 1: 330-6.

Koot M, Keet I, Vos A et al. (1993). Prognostic values of HIV-1 syncytium-inducing phenotype for rate of CD4+ cell depletion and progression to AIDS. Ann Intern Med 118: 681-8.

Kostrikis L, Huang Y, Moore J et al. (1998). A chemokine receptor CCR2 allele delays HIV-1 disease progression and is associated with a CCR5 promoter mutation. Nat Med 4: 350-3.

Koup R, Safrit J, Cao Y et al. (1994). Temporal association of cellular immune responses with the initial control of viremia in primary human immunodeficiency virus type 1 syndrome. J Virol 68: 4650-5.

Lang W, Perkins H, Anderson RE et al. (1989). Patterns of T lymphocyte changes with human immunodeficiency virus infection: from seroconversion to the development of AIDS. J Acquir Immune Defic Syndr 2: 63-9.

Learmont J, Tindall B, Evans L et al. (1992). Long-term symptomless HIV-1 infection in recipients of blood products from a single donor. Lancet 340: 863-7.

Levrin NL, Miller MD, Shen L et al. (1993). Simian immunodeficiency virus-specific cytotoxic T lymphocytes in rhesus monkeys: characterization and vaccine induction. Semin Immunol 5: 215-23.

Lewin SR, Vesanen M, Kostrikis L et al. (1999). The use of real-time PCR and molecular beacons to detect virus replication in HIV-1-infected individual on prolonged effective antiretroviral therapy. J Virol 73: 6099-103.

Littman D. (1998). Chemokine receptors: keys to AIDS pathogenesis? Cell 93: 677-80.

Liu R, Paxton WA, Choe S et al. (1996). Homozygous defect in HIV-1 co-receptor accounts for resistance of some multiply-exposed individuals to HIV-1 infection. Cell 86: 367-77.

Macallan DC, Fulleron CA, Neese RA et al. (1998). Measurement of cell proliferation by labeling of DNA with stable isotope-labeled glucose: studies in vitro, in animals, and in humans. Proc Natl Acad Sci USA 95: 708-13.

Malkevitch N, McDermott DH, Yi Y et al. (2001). Coreceptor choice and T cell depletion by R5, X4 and R5X4 HIV-1 variants in CCR5-deficient (CCR5 delta 32) and normal human lymphoid tissue. Virology 281: 239-47.

Mansky LM, Temin HM. (1995). Lower in vivo mutation rate of human immunodeficiency virus type 1 than that predicted from the fidelity of purified reverse transcriptase. J Virol 69: 5087-94.

Mariani R, Kirchhoff F, Greenough TC et al. (1996). High frequency of defective nef alleles in a long-term survivor with nonprogressive human immunodeficiency virus type 1 infection. J Virol 70: 7752-64.

McDougal J, Mawle A, Cort S. (1985). Cellular tropism of the human retrovirus HTLVIII/LAV: role of T cell activation and expression of the T4 antigen. J Immunol 135: 3151-62.

McElrath M, Pruett J, Cohn Z. (1989). Mononuclear phagocytes of blood and bone-marrow: comparative roles as viral reservoirs in human immunodeficiency virus type 1 infections. Proc Natl Acad Sci 86: 675-9.

McIlroy D, Autran B, Ceynier R et al. (1995). Infection frequency of dendritic cells and CD4+ T lymphocytes in spleens of human immunodeficiency virus-positive patients. *J Virol* **69**: 4737–45.

McLean A, Michie C. (1995). *In vivo* estimates of division and death rates of human T lymphocytes. *Proc Natl Acad Sci USA* **92**: 3707–11.

McMichael A. (1998). T cell responses and viral escape. *Cell* **93**: 673–6.

McMichael A, O'Callaghan C. (1998). A new look at T cells. *J Exp Med* **187**: 1367–71.

Mellors J, Rinaldo C, Gupta P *et al.* (1996). Prognosis in HIV-1 infection predicted by the quantity of virus in plasma. *Science* **272**: 1167–70.

Mellors JW, Munoz A, Giorgi JV *et al.* (1997). Plasma viral load and CD4+ lymphocytes as prognostic markers of HIV-1 infection. *Ann Intern Med* **126**: 946–54.

Michael N, Chang G, Louie L *et al.* (1997a). The role of viral phenotype and CCR-5 gene defects in HIV-1 transmission and disease progression. *Nat Med* **3**: 338–40.

Michael N, Louie L, Rohrbaugh A *et al.* (1997b). The role of CCR5 and CCR2 polymorphisms in HIV-1 transmission and disease progression. *Nat Med* **3**: 1160–2.

Mohri H, Bonhoeffer S, Monard S *et al.* (1998). Rapid turnover of T lymphocytes in SIV-infected rhesus macaques. *Science* **279**: 1223–7.

Montefiori DC, Pantaleo G, Fink LM *et al.* (1996). Neutralizing and infection-enhancing antibody responses to human immunodeficiency virus type 1 in long-term nonprogressors. *J Infect Dis* **173**: 60–7.

Moore J. (1997). Coreceptors: implications for HIV pathogenesis and therapy. *Science* **276**: 51–2.

Mummidi S, Ahuja S, Gonzalez E *et al.* (1998). Genealogy of the CCR5 locus and chemokine system gene variants with altered rates of HIV-1 disease progression. *Nat Med* **4**: 786–93.

Mundy D, Schinazi R, Gerber A. (1987). Human immunodeficiency virus isolated from amniotic fluid. *Lancet* **ii**: 891.

Munoz A, Kirby AJ, He YD *et al.* (1995). Long-term survivors with HIV-1 infection: incubation period and longitudinal patterns of CD4+ lymphocytes. *J Acquir Immune Defic Syndr Hum Retrovirol* **8**: 496–505.

Musey L, Hughes J, Schacker T *et al.* (1997). Cytotoxic-T-cell responses, viral load, and disease progression in early human immunodeficiency virus type 1 infection. *N Engl J Med* **337**: 1267–74.

Nabel G, Baltimore D. (1987). An inducible transcription factor activates expression of human immunodeficiency virus in T cells. *Nature* **326**: 711–3.

Nara PL, Robey WG, Arthur LO *et al.* (1987). Persistent infection of chimpanzees with human immunodeficiency virus: serological responses and properties of reisolated viruses. *J Virol* **61**: 3173–80.

Nielsen C, Pederson C, Lundgren J *et al.* (1993). Biological properties of HIV isolates in primary HIV infection: consequences for the subsequent course of infection. *AIDS* **7**: 1035–40.

Oberlin E, Amara A, Bachelerie F *et al.* (1996). The CXC chemokine SDF-1 is the ligand for LESTR/fusin and prevents infection by T-cell-line-adapted HIV-1. *Nature* **382**: 833–5.

Ogg G, Bonhoeffer S, Dunbar P *et al.* (1998). Quantification of HIV-1-specific cytotoxic T lymphocytes and plasma load of viral RNA. *Science* **279**: 2103–6.

Pakker N, Notermans D, de Boer R *et al.* (1998). Biphasic kinetics of peripheral blood T cells after triple combination therapy in HIV-1 infection: a composite of redistribution and proliferation. *Nat Med* **4**: 208–14.

Palella FJ, Jr, Delaney KM, Moorman AC *et al.* (1998). Declining morbidity and mortality among patients with advanced human immun-odeficiency virus infection. HIV Outpatient Study Investigators. *N Engl J Med* **338**: 853–60.

Pantaleo G, Graziosi C, Demarest JF *et al.* (1993a). HIV infection is active and progressive in lymphoid tissue during the clinically latent stage of disease. *Nature* **362**: 355–8.

Pantaleo G, Graziosi C, Fauci A. (1993b). The immunopathogenesis of human immunodeficiency virus infection. *N Engl J Med* **328**: 327.

Pantaleo G, Menzo S, Vaccarezza M *et al.* (1995). Studies in subjects with long-term nonprogressive human immunodeficiency virus infection. *N Engl J Med* **332**: 209–16.

Pantaleo G, Demarest JF, Schacker T *et al.* (1997). The qualitative nature of the primary immune response to HIV infection is a prognosticator of disease progression independent of the initial level of plasma viremia. *Proc Natl Acad Sci USA* **94**: 254–8.

Pantaleo G, Cohen OJ, Schacker T *et al.* (1998). Evolutionary pattern of human immunodeficiency virus (HIV) replication and distribution in lymph nodes following primary infection: implications for antiviral therapy. *Nat Med* **4**: 341–5.

Perelson A, Neumann A, Markowitz M *et al.* (1996). HIV-1 dynamics *in vivo*: virion clearance rate, infected cell life-span, and viral generation time. *Science* **271**: 1582–6.

Perelson A, Essunger P, Cao Y *et al.* (1997a). Decay characteristics of HIV-1-infected compartments during combination therapy. *Nature* **387**: 188–91.

Perelson A, Essunger P, Ho D. (1997b). Dynamics of HIV-1 and CD4+ lymphocytes *in vivo*. *AIDS* **11**: S17–24.

Phillips A. (1996). Reduction of HIV concentration during acute infection: independence from a specific immune response. *Science* **271**: 497–9.

Piatak Jr M, Saag M, Yang L *et al.* (1993). High levels of HIV-1 in plasma during all stages of infection determined by competitive PCR. *Science* **259**: 1749–54.

Pomerantz RJ, Trono D, Feinberg MB *et al.* (1990). Cells nonproductively infected with HIV-1 exhibit an aberrant pattern of viral RNA expression: a molecular model for latency. *Cell* **61**: 1271–6.

Pope M, Betjes MG, Romani N *et al.* (1994). Conjugates of dendritic cells and memory T lymphocytes from skin facilitate productive infection with HIV-1. *Cell* **78**: 389–98.

Price DA, Goulder PJ, Klenerman P *et al.* (1997). Positive selection of HIV-1 cytotoxic T lymphocyte escape variants during primary infection. *Proc Natl Acad Sci USA* **94**: 1890–5.

Quillent C, Oberlin E, Braun J *et al.* (1998). HIV-1-resistance phenotype conferred by combination of two separate inherited mutations of CCR5 gene. *Lancet* **351**: 14–8.

Ramaratnam B, Mitler JE, Zhang L *et al.* (2000). The decay of the latent reservoir of replication-competent HIV-1 is inversely correlated with the extent of residual viral replication during prolonged anti-retroviral therapy. *Nat Med* **6**: 82–5.

Rinaldo C, Huang XL, Fan ZF *et al.* (1995). High levels of anti-human immunodeficiency virus type 1 (HIV-1) memory cytotoxic T-lymphocyte activity and low viral load are associated with lack of disease in HIV-1-infected long-term nonprogressors. *J Virol* **69**: 5838–42.

Rizzardi G, Morawetz R, Vicenzi E *et al.* (1998). CCR2 polymorphism and HIV disease. *Nat Med* **3**: 252–3.

Rosenberg E, Billingsley J, Caliendo A *et al.* (1997). Vigorous HIV-1 specific CD4+ T cell responses associated with control of viremia. *Science* **278**: 1447–50.

Sachsenberg N, Perelson AS, Yerly S *et al.* (1998). Turnover of CD4+ and CD8+ T lymphocytes in HIV-1 infection as measured by Ki-67 antigen. *J Exp Med* **187**: 1295–303.

Salahuddin SZ, Rose RM, Groopman JE et al. (1986). Human T lymphotropic virus type III infection of alveolar macrophages. Blood 68: 281-4.

Samson M, Libert F, Doranz BJ et al. (1996). Resistance to HIV-1 infection in caucasian individuals bearing mutant alleles of the CCR-5 chemokine receptor gene. Nature 382: 722-5.

Schnittman S, Psallidopoulos M, Lan H et al. (1989). The reservoir for HIV-1 in human peripheral blood is a T cell that maintains expression of CD4. Science 245: 305-8.

Shioda T, Levy J, Cheng-Meyer C. (1991). Macrophage and T-cell line tropisms of HIV-1 are determined by specific regions of the envelope gp120 gene. Nature 349: 167-9.

Smith M, Dean M, Carrington M et al. (1997). Contrasting genetic influence of CCR2 and CCR5 variants on HIV-1 infection and disease progression. Science 277: 959-65.

Spira AI, Marx PA, Patterson BK et al. (1996). Cellular targets of infection and route of viral dissemination after an intravaginal inoculation of simian immunodeficiency virus into rhesus macaques. J Exp Med 183: 215-25.

Stamm W, Handsfield H, Rompalo A. (1988). The association between genital ulcer disease and acquisition of HIV infection in homosexual men. JAMA 260: 1429.

Stewart G. (1998). Chemokine genes-bearing the odds. Nat Med 4: 275-6.

Tenner-Racz K, Racz P, Gartner S et al. (1989). Ultrastructural analysis of germinal centers in lymph nodes of patients with HIV-1-induced persistent generalized lymphadenopathy: evidence for persistence of infection. Prog AIDS Pathol 1: 29-40.

Tenner-Racz K, Stellbrink HJ, van Lunzen J et al. (1998). The unenlarged lymph nodes of HIV-1-infected, asymptomatic patients with high CD4 T cell counts are sites for virus replication and CD4 T cell proliferation. The impact of highly active antiretroviral therapy. J Exp Med 187: 949-59.

Tersmette M, de Goede REY, Al BJM et al. (1988). Differential syncytium-inducing capacity of human immunodeficiency virus isolates: frequent detection of syncytium-inducing isolates in patients with acquired immunodeficiency syndrome (AIDS) and AIDS-related-complex. J Virol 62: 2026-32.

Tersmette M, Gruters RA, de Wolf F et al. (1989). Evidence for a role of virulent human immunodeficiency virus (HIV) variants in the pathogenesis of acquired immunodeficiency syndrome: studies on sequential HIV isolates. J Virol 63: 2118-25.

Thiry L, Sprecher-Goldberger S, Jonckheer T. (1985). Isolation of AIDS virus from cell-free breast milk of three healthy virus carriers. Lancet iii: 891.

Tindall B, Cooper D. (1991). Primary HIV infection: host responses and intervention strategies. AIDS 5: 1-14.

Vogt M, Witt D, Craven D. (1986). Isolation of HTLV-III/LAV from cervical secretions of women at risk for AIDS. Lancet i: 525.

Wei X, Ghosh S, Taylor M et al. (1995). Viral dynamics in human immunodeficiency virus type 1 infection. Nature 373: 117-22.

Westervelt P, Trowbridge DB, Epstein LG et al. (1992). Macrophage tropism determinants in human immunodeficiency virus type 1 in vivo. J Virol 66: 2577-82.

Wiley C, Schrier R, Nelson J et al. (1986). Cellular localization of human immunodeficiency virus infection within the brains of acquired immune deficiency syndrome patients. Proc Natl Acad Sci USA 83: 7089-93.

Winkler C, Modi W, Smith M et al. (1998). Genetic restriction of AIDS pathogenesis by an SDF-1 chemokine gene variant. Science 279: 389-93.

Wolfs T, Zwart G, Bakker M. (1992). HIV-1 genomic RNA diversification following sexual and parenteral virus transmission. Virology 189: 103-10.

Wolinsky S, Wike C, Korber B et al. (1992). Selective transmission of human immunodeficiency virus type-1 variants from mother to infant. Science 255: 1134-7.

Wolthers KC, Bea G, Wisman A et al. (1996). T cell telomere length in HIV-1 infection: no evidence for increased CD4+ T cell turnover. Science 274: 1543-7.

Wong J, Hezareh M, Gunthard H et al. (1997). Recovery of replication-competent HIV despite prolonged suppression of plasma viremia. Science 278: 1291-4.

Zack J, Arrigo S, Weisman S et al. (1990). HIV-1 entry into quiescent primary lymphocytes: molecular analysis reveals a labile, latent viral structure. Cell 61: 213-22.

Zaitseva M, Blauvelt A, Lee S et al. (1997). Expression and function of CCR5 and CXCR4 on human Langerhans cells and macrophages: implications for HIV primary infection. Nat Med 3: 1369-75.

Zhang L, MacKenzie P, Cleland A et al. (1993). Selection for specific sequences in the external envelope protein of HIV-1 upon primary infection. J Virol 67: 3345-56.

Zhang L, Huang Y, Yuan H et al. (1997a). Genotypic and phenotypic characterization of long terminal repeat sequences from long-term survivors of human immunodeficiency virus type 1 infection. J Virol 71: 5608-13.

Zhang L, Huang Y, Yuan H et al. (1997b). Genetic characterization of vif, vpr, and vpu sequences from long-term survivors of human immunodeficiency virus type 1 infection. Virology 228: 340-9.

Zhang L, Ramratnam B, Tenner-Racz K et al. (1999a). Quantifying residual HIV-1 replication and decay of he latent reservoir in patients on seemingly effective antiretroviral therapy. N Engl J Med 340: 1605-13.

Zhang L, Lewin SR, Markowitz M et al. (1999b). Measuring recent thymic emigrants is blood of normal persons and HIV-1 infected patients before and after effective therapy. J Exp Med 190: 725-32.

Zhu T, Mo H, Wang N et al. (1993). Genotypic and phenotypic characterization of HIV-1 in patients with primary infection. Science 261: 1179-81.

4

The use of the laboratory in the diagnosis and management of HIV

CHRIS BIRCH AND DOMINIC E. DWYER

Following the identification in 1983 of the virus responsible for AIDS (Barre-Sinoussi *et al.*, 1983), enormous effort has been expended in the development of tests capable of detecting HIV infection and characterizing the virus. A wide range of assay systems has become available, including those for HIV-specific antibody and antigen detection, virus isolation, molecular detection of RNA and DNA, quantitation of virus load, and assays that provide phenotypical and genotypical information about the virus. The range of HIV-specific assays available now allows clinicians to diagnose or confirm HIV infection, to assess prognosis for infected individuals and to monitor antiretroviral drug efficacy, and in addition provides insights into the pathogenesis of HIV infection. It is the latter areas that received the most attention during the last decade.

Current techniques used for the laboratory diagnosis of HIV infection

Enzyme-linked immunoassays and western blot

The first developments in diagnostic assays for HIV revolved around enzyme-linked immunoassays (EIA), the methods for which have been reviewed in depth elsewhere (Gurtler, 1996; Metcalf *et al.*, 1997). HIV-infected individuals develop an antibody response to most HIV proteins, usually within 3–4 weeks of exposure, and detection of these antibodies is the basis of screening assays. Inability to detect antibodies 3 months or more after infection is rare. First-generation EIAs were based on viral lysates derived from HIV cultures. Second-generation assays incorporated viral antigens produced by recombinant DNA technology, allowing the production of antigens with improved purity and in higher amounts than those obtained from viral lysates (although they may have a more limited repertoire of epitopes). Following the occasional detection of HIV-2 outside the geographical regions with the highest prevalence of HIV-2 (Western Africa and India), HIV-2 antigens have been incorporated into many commercial EIA systems. Assays that incorporate HIV-1 subtype O antigens (see below) are also now available following the failure of some EIA systems (particularly those using recombinant antigens) to diagnose subtype O infections (Benitez *et al.*, 1998).

EIA-based assays have a sensitivity of at least 99.5% and a specificity of over 99.8%. False positives are rare, although they are sometimes a problem when extensive testing of low-risk populations is undertaken. False positives may be due to procedural errors in handling samples, cross-reacting antibodies against some common human leucocyte antigens, autoreactive antibodies, heat inactivation of serum prior to testing, repetitive freeze–thaw cycles of samples, severe hepatic disease, passive immunoglobulin administration, recent exposure to some vaccine preparations and certain malignancies. False-negative results may arise because of procedural problems in assay performance, testing too early in the seroconversion period, hypogammaglobulinaemia, and unusual strains of HIV-1 (for example, subtype O). Whether other uncharacterized strains of HIV will react in current EIA systems is also unknown.

A positive reaction with an EIA test on a single serum sample is not sufficient to enable a diagnosis of HIV infection. The EIA should be repeated using a different commercial assay, whether on the same sample or a second sample. To exclude false-positive reactions (more likely to be seen in low-risk populations) or borderline reactivity with screening assays, confirmation with a more specific assay is required. The western blot (WB) assay is the most commonly used confirmatory test. Lysates of HIV-1 (or HIV-2) obtained from HIV-infected cell cultures are purified, separated by electrophoresis into individual proteins on the basis of molecular weight, and transferred onto nitrocellulose. Recombinant antigens can also be added. The nitrocellulose is cut into strips, which are then used as the basis of an antibody detection assay (Figure 4.1). A positive WB confirms the presence of HIV-specific antibodies, and enables identification of the specific viral components of that response qualitatively (and, in some cases, quantitatively). A positive WB generally reveals various degrees of antibody reactivity with the env, gag and pol gene products of HIV-1, although the correct interpretation of this reactivity has been an area of controversy. A negative WB is one in which no bands are present at any location, or where there are no bands corresponding to known HIV proteins. Detection of a protein or proteins from each of env (gp160, gp120 or gp41), Gag (p24) and pol (p66 or p51) is generally regarded as a positive result (Figure 4.1). WB results that cannot be classified as either positive or negative by these criteria are called indeterminate reactions (Figure 4.1).

In the absence of risk factors for HIV acquisition, most indeterminate WB results are usually not significant; in the presence of high-risk behaviour or possible recent HIV exposure, the finding of an indeterminate WB may indicate true HIV seroreactivity. In such cases, a further serum sample should be retested after 3–4 weeks. The high frequency of indeterminate WB reactivity makes the WB an inappropriate screening test, so its main use is as a confirmatory assay following a positive or indeterminate EIA or other screening test result. It is also likely to be a useful test for distinguishing between immune responses resulting from vaccination versus natural infection immune responses when vaccine trials become common.

HIV-2 infection shows cross-reactivity in about 80% of cases with WBs containing HIV-1 proteins, but is best confirmed by reactivity to HIV-2 recombinant antigens added to the HIV-1 WB strips, or with HIV-2-specific WBs. HIV-1 and HIV-2 WB, in conjunction with other HIV-1 or HIV-2-specific antibody assays and/or molecular assays, are needed to confirm dual infection with HIV-1 and HIV-2 and to exclude cross-reactivity between the two viruses.

Other diagnostic tests

Although EIA and WB are the most common antibody test systems worldwide, other assays are also available. The indirect immunofluorescence assay may be positive earlier in the course of acute infection than conventional EIA tests, and can be adapted for the detection of IgM antibody (Cooper et al., 1987). IgM testing is not always useful for the diagnosis of early infection as IgM reponses to HIV are not consistently produced. The immunofluorescence assay does not allow detection of specific antibody reactivity patterns and requires expert technical ability. The radio-immunoprecipitation (RIPA) assay is based on culturing HIV-infected cells in the presence of radiolabelled amino acids, allowing their incorporation into the viral proteins (Truillo et al., 1996). The requirement for HIV culture facilities, the use of radioactive reagents and the need for skilled

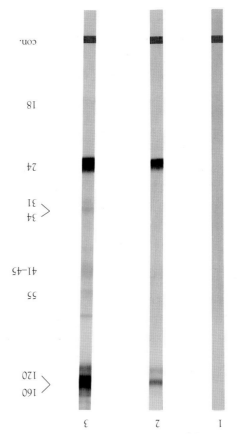

Figure 4.1 Western blot profiles of an individual undergoing HIV sero-conversion following infection due to a high-risk sexual exposure. The development of antibodies to HIV proteins is indicated. Lane 1, immediately after exposure; lane 2, 5 weeks after exposure; lane 3, 8 weeks after exposure. Only the profile in lane 3 satisfies the (current Australian) definition of an anti-HIV-positive western blot profile. Lane 2 is an indeterminate profile (courtesy of Dr Alan Breschkin, Victorian Infectious Diseases Reference Laboratory).

technical expertise means that this assay is now very rarely used by clinical laboratories. However, RIPA can be used for detecting low levels of antibody or evaluating individuals with indeterminate WB results.

Latex agglutination assays are a rapid antibody detection system based on the use of recombinant proteins, derived from highly conserved regions of the HIV-1 genome, that are chemically linked to polystyrene beads. Agglutination assays are used mainly for field testing in developing countries. They are generally easy to utilize, but their performance is variable (Malone et al., 1993; Windsor et al., 1997). A range of immunoblot assays are also available and are based on either viral antigens from lysates of HIV-infected cells or on recombinant antigens that are dotted onto a grid of absorbent nitrocellulose paper (Malone et al., 1993). Immunoblot assays have been developed that differentiate HIV-1 groups M and O and HIV-2 (Vallari et al., 1998). Other alternatives are the passive haemagglutination assays, an example of which is the autologous red cell agglutination assay (Kemp et al., 1988). This assay uses a non-agglutinating mouse monoclonal antibody reactive with human red blood cells chemically cross-linked to a synthetic gp41 peptide antigen. Addition of this antigen–antibody complex to small amounts of whole blood from an infected individual causes that person's red cells to become coated with the complex; HIV antibodies in the blood sample bind to the cell-bound antigen and cause agglutination of red cells into a visible mass. A result can be obtained in a few minutes, with the advantage that the test subject's own blood is used. In general, the more rapid assays, which may be used to test source patients following needlestick injury, or assays performed on body fluids other than blood, are slightly less sensitive and specific when compared to current EIA antibody assays on serum. Any positive result obtained with a rapid assay system requires confirmation with WB.

A number of assays can be adapted for use on body fluids other than serum, including saliva and urine. HIV antibody tests on saliva using EIA or WB techniques have proved sensitive and specific, although usually slightly less so than assays of serum (King et al., 1995; Luo et al., 1995; Martinez et al., 1995). Antibodies can also be detected in concentrated or unconcentrated urine using EIA, WB or other rapid antibody detection systems (Constantine et al., 1994; Berrios et al., 1995). These tests can be used for surveillance purposes or epidemiological studies, particularly where blood collection facilities are limited or health personnel insufficiently trained, or where phlebotomy is refused. Such assays can also be adapted to home testing for HIV infection. Testing cerebrospinal fluid (CSF) for HIV antibodies has demonstrated a relationship between intrathecal production of antibodies and isolation of HIV from the CSF (Sonnerborg et al., 1989), and has shown that high levels of antibodies to the HIV envelope protein are more common in patients with AIDS dementia complex than symptom-free, HIV-1 infected individuals (Trujillo et al., 1996). Any positive assay on body fluids other than serum should generally be confirmed using a standard test involving serum.

The serum HIV-1 p24 antigen solid-phase immunoassay has been used to provide a quantitative measure of the concentration of p24 antigen in serum or other body fluids, although this test has generally been replaced by viral load measurement. p24 antigen may be detected early after HIV exposure, often preceding the development of HIV-specific antibodies by several weeks. After seroconversion, p24 antigens usually become undetectable as p24 antibodies appear, although p24 antigens may reappear later as HIV infection progresses to AIDS. Because p24 antigens can only be detected in approximately 20–30% of individuals with asymptomatic infection (Lillo et al., 1997), it should not be used for diagnosis. It is sometimes used as a supplementary diagnostic test in patients with suspected HIV seroconversion illness or neonatal infection, and as a surrogate marker of antiviral efficacy in antiretroviral drug trials (Kappes et al., 1995). A positive p24 antigen result can be confirmed by repeating the test in the presence of a serum containing a known high concentration of HIV-1 antibody, thereby allowing neutralization of the positive result. The sensitivity of the p24 antigen assay has been increased using methods that disrupt immune complexes prior to performing the assay (Kappes et al., 1995). Despite these advances, the p24 antigen assay and other surrogate markers for HIV, including beta 2-microglobulin and neopterin, have been superseded by molecular methods of HIV quantitation (Dwyer et al., 1997).

Counselling, both pre- and post-testing, should accompany any decision to undertake screening for HIV antibodies and should be tailored to the behaviours, circumstances and special needs of the individual being tested. Counselling should be culturally and developmentally appropriate, sensitive to the needs of sexual identity, and linguistically specific. Pre-test discussion must include an individualized risk assessment, and should provide a plan for testing for risk reduction (MMWR, 1993a).

The role of widespread screening of low-risk patients, including admissions to emergency departments, routine surgery cases, antenatal screening, immigration and visa applications and home HIV testing needs to be discussed on a community by community basis. Factors such as the underlying HIV prevalence, availability, cost and perfor- mance of screening assays, and access to appropriate interventions should positive tests be found, will determine policies for widespread testing (MMWR, 1993b; Kelen et al., 1995; Phillips et al., 1995). Such issues are significantly more critical in developing countries, where high HIV prevalence and inadequate health budgets go hand-in- hand. Testing of HIV antibodies is becoming more accept- ed as a part of routine antenatal screening, particularly as antiretroviral treatment of infected mothers and their babies significantly reduces vertical transmission.

Detection of HIV subtypes

Following the publication of the first HIV-1 proviral sequences (Wain-Hobson et al., 1985; Alizon and Mon- tagnier, 1987), it became apparent that significant sequence variations occurred in HIV from different geo- graphical regions. As more phylogenetic analyses were undertaken globally, it was found that circulating HIV strains could be classified into three distinct groups: the main (M) group, containing at least 13 sequence subtypes and an outlier (O) group (including a number of recombi- nant forms) (Robertson et al., 2000) and a new (N) group. Approximately 30% intersubtype genetic divergence occurs in the env region of group M subtypes; the diver- gence is 14% in gag (Subbarao and Schochetman, 1996). Env amino acid variation ranges from 24% between differ- ent subtypes to 47% between the main groups.

The global dispersion of different subtypes is not uniform. The majority of published sequences from isolates from North America, Western Europe and Australasia are sub- type B. Subtype B also predominates in Brazil and other South American countries, with some subtype F and C also present. In sub-Saharan Africa, subtypes A and D predom- inate, although in some Central African countries many other subtypes cocirculate. In Southern Africa, the horn of Africa and Western India, subtype C is most common. Sub- type E is found predominantly in Thailand, and has spread to neighbouring countries, while subtype B is more fre-

quently found in other countries of East Asia. A variant of subtype B, with a different envelope V3 loop tip tetrapep- tide motif, has been described in injecting drug users in Bangkok, and has now spread to other injecting drug-using populations in Asia (Weniger et al., 1994; Myers et al., 1996). Dual infections with different subtypes may occur, and recombination between subtypes is common (Artenstein et al., 1995; Carr et al., 1996; Gao et al., 1998; Oelrichs et al., 1999). At least five genetic subtypes of HIV-2 exist, but widespread population studies of these (and possibly other) subtypes are yet to be performed (Gao et al., 1994).

Despite the enormous diversity of HIV group M sub- types, there do not appear to be significant biological dif- ferences between them with respect to their ability to replicate in different primary and continuous cell lines, co-receptor usage and antiretroviral drug susceptibility (Workshop Report, 1997). However, subtypes have rele- vance to diagnostic and monitoring assays. Comparisons of different commercially available viral load assays show vari- able sensitivity with respect to different subtypes present in plasma samples. All assays handle subtype B viruses satis- factorily, although it appears that the bDNA assay may be less sensitive to genotype variation than the current Amplicor Monitor and NASBA-QT assays (see below) (Dunne and Crowe, 1997; Chew et al., 1999a).

For clinical management, if an unusual subtype is sus- pected or the viral load results do not match other clinical and laboratory variables, discussion with the laboratory regarding testing for the presence of an unusual subtype, or the use of different viral load assays, is warranted. HIV sub- typing can be performed by sequencing and phylogenetic analysis of env, gag or other regions of the HIV genome, or alternatively, by the heteroduplex mobility assay (HMA). HIV-1 subtyping kits based on HMA have been developed in collaboration with the WHO Network on HIV Isolation and Characterization, and can be obtained from the National Institute of Health AIDS Research and Reference Reagent Program in the USA (Delwart et al., 1995). Sero- logical assays using subtype-specific peptides can also be used (Cheingsong-Popov et al., 1998; Devito et al., 1998), but are less sensitive and specific than molecularly based assays.

Molecular methods for diagnosis

As discussed above, infection with HIV is currently diag- nosed in the laboratory by detection of HIV antibodies using screening (e.g. EIA) and confirmatory or supplementary (e.g. WB) assays. However, there is a strong case for using other techniques for diagnosis, particularly when a seroconversion illness is suspected in an at-risk individual (Rutherford *et al.*, 2000). Many serum samples from individuals with early seroconversion syndrome are EIA and WB indeterminate, and these individuals may have to wait several weeks or months until their HIV antibody status is resolved. Early diagnosis of the HIV conversion syndrome is important to limit transmission to others and because early antiretroviral therapy may be beneficial. Several studies have shown that methods enabling detection of HIV RNA and/or DNA are specific and more rapid than existing serological diagnostic paradigms. One study used commercial and in-house assays to resolve indeterminate serology results in a group of patients subsequently shown to be uninfected with HIV (Sethoe *et al.*, 1995). Plasma HIV RNA has been shown to be useful for diagnosis of HIV infection in newborns, as it is detectable early and in a high proportion of infected infants born to HIV-positive mothers (Steketee *et al.*, 1997; Reisler *et al.*, 2001). In an Australian study of 13 patients with primary HIV-1 infection and indeterminate EIA and WB status, 12 had HIV RNA detected prior to EIA or WB becoming positive (Middleton *et al.*, 1997). In a second Australian investigation, a similar result was found by detecting proviral HIV DNA in infected cells (Cunningham *et al.*, 1997).

HIV isolation

HIV culture is rarely necessary for the diagnosis of HIV infection, although it may help to confirm infection in certain situations, including neonatal infection (Burgard *et al.*, 1992) or even early seroconversion. Assays to detect viral load have already largely replaced HIV isolation in the management of infection, although isolation may still have a role if drug resistance phenotypes are required (see below) or if some other property of the virus likely to affect prognosis is thought to be present (for example, syncytium-inducing phenotype).

When required, HIV is usually recovered by cocultivation of the infected individual's peripheral blood mononuclear cells (PBMCs) with those from an HIV-negative 'donor'. These cells are activated using phytohaemagglutinin, then incubated in a medium containing interleukin-2 to stimulate further cell replication (Neate *et al.*, 1987). Characteristic HIV-specific cytopathic effects, usually seen as production of syncytia and ballooning of individual cells

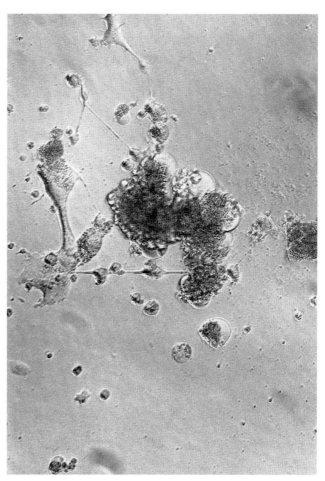

Figure 4.2 *Characteristic 'ballooning' and syncytial formation seen in T-lymphocytes (MT-2 cells) infected with a syncytial-inducing strain of HIV-1.*

(Figure 4.2), can be observed during isolation attempts, which may take up to 28 days. Cultures are confirmed as positive by detecting an HIV-specific marker (for example, p24 antigen using a commercial assay or exogenous reverse transcriptase (RT) activity using an in-house assay). The HIV strains obtained during isolation attempts are a reflection of the proviral DNA and replication-competent virions present in the patient's PBMCs. Isolation rates from PBMCs are directly proportional to the HIV RNA copy number per ml of plasma (Sebire *et al.*, 1998) (Figure 4.3). For copy numbers greater than 15 000/ml, isolation rates greater than 90% can be expected using the cocultivation method. This falls to 20% for plasma RNA levels of 0–500 copies/ml, unless highly specialized methods for recovering HIV are implemented. These include CD8 lymphocyte depletion to decrease the antiretroviral effects of chemokines, removal of contaminating macrophages and stimulation of donor cells with phytohaemagglutinin and interleukin-2 (Finzi et al., 1997; Wong et al., 1997).

HIV can also be isolated from the plasma of infected individuals, although less reliably than from cells. The likelihood of success is proportional to the viral load or stage of disease (Clarke et al., 1991; Daar et al., 1991; Shearer et al., 1997). HIV can also be cultured from biopsy and autopsy material, and other body fluids such as CSF but such testing is only necessary for investigating the pathogenesis of HIV infection (McGavin et al., 1996). Using dilution techniques, quantitative HIV isolation from PBMCs and plasma has been performed in the context of measuring antiretroviral drug efficacy in clinical trials (Ho et al., 1989), although this technique has been superseded by molecular viral load assays.

HIV viral load testing

Quantitation of HIV RNA in plasma (viral load) using commercial assays has become an essential tool for the management of infected individuals. Potential applications of HIV RNA measurement in diagnosis and management are given in Table 4.1. HIV RNA levels directly reflect the extent of virus replication at the site at which they are measured (Ho et al., 1995; Perelson et al., 1996), and have been shown to predict future disease progression in adults and children (Piatak et al., 1993; Mellors et al., 1995; Ho, 1996; Mellors et al., 1996; Shearer et al., 1997; Ariyoshi et al., 2000; Sterling et al., 2001). The peak HIV RNA level can also be used to predict clinical outcome early in infection (Katzenstein et al., 1996), and it helps indicate when antiretroviral drug therapy should be initiated in drug-naive patients. Transient increases in plasma HIV RNA levels may occur in the context of vaccination and intercurrent opportunistic infections. A significant increase in plasma HIV RNA levels subsequent to successful reduction in viral load following drug therapy indicates failure of that therapy, often as a result of developing drug resistance or due to poor compliance (Condra et al., 1996). The commercial assays currently available (see below) have been used to quantitate HIV RNA levels in the CSF (Brew et al., 1997). This is particularly relevant in the context of HIV establishing reservoirs of infection in sites relatively inaccessible to antiretroviral drugs. HIV RNA levels in the CSF give an (indirect) indication of the extent of replication in the CNS and the efficacy of drug therapy.

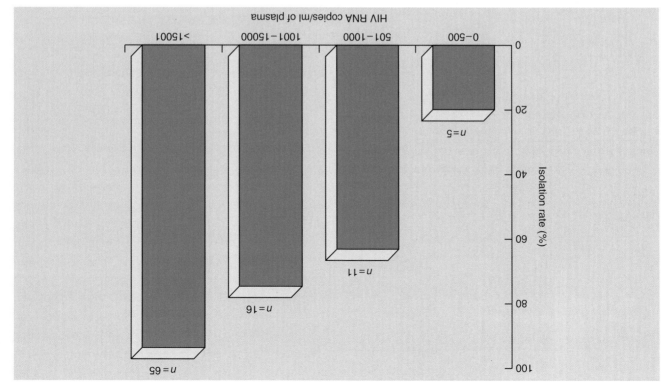

Figure 4.3 Relationship between HIV RNA copy number in plasma and ability to isolate HIV from PBMCs using coculture techniques (reproduced with permission from Sebire et al., 1998).

Table 4.1 Practical examples of molecular techniques used to detect and characterize HIV in clinical material

Method	Application
RNA detection, quantification and characterization	Diagnosis of primary infection (including neonatal transmission)
	Prognostic indicator in untreated patients (the virological set-point)
	Timing the initiation of HAART
	Response to HAART failure
	Detection of HIV in reservoirs (e.g. CSF)
	Determining drug resistance profiles
	Subtyping HIV strains
	Establishing epidemiology links in HIV transmission studies
DNA detection and characterization	Diagnosis of primary infection (including neonatal transmission)
	Detection of HIV in reservoirs (e.g. CSF, tissues)
	Studies of HIV pathogenesis
	Subtyping HIV strains
	Establishing epidemiological links in HIV transmission studies

HAART: highly active antiretroviral therapy; CSF: cerebrospinal fluid.

Accurate quantitation of HIV RNA levels is of considerable importance in the management of infected individuals. Several commercial quantitative assays are now available, and have largely usurped the use of in-house, polymerase chain reaction (PCR) based assays, which are often laborious, require considerable attention to quality control and may give results that are not directly comparable with those obtained by other laboratories. Examples of commercial assays for quantitation of HIV RNA in plasma include the Amplicor HIV-1 Monitor (Roche Diagnostic Systems), Quantiplex HIV RNA (Bayer) and NASBA-QT (Organon Teknika, amongst others). Guidelines outlining the appropriate use of these assays are available (MMWR, 1998).

The Amplicor HIV-1 assay involves the treatment of plasma with guanidium isothiocyanate and precipitation of HIV RNA by isopropanol. RT-PCR using the enzyme rTth (which has RT and polymerase activity) and biotinylated primers specific for *gag* (in association with a synthetic internal quantification standard) results in amplification of a 142 bp product (Revets *et al.*, 1996). Performance of the Quantiplex assay requires lysis of HIV virions that have

been pelleted from plasma by centifugation at 23 000g, and capture and immobilization of the viral RNA using multiple probes specific for the *pol* gene. bDNA amplifier molecules are then hybridized to the target-probe complexes. Multiple alkaline phosphatase-labelled probes are hybridized to the bDNA molecules, and following addition of a substrate (dioxetane), light emission is detected by chemiluminescence. The NASBA assay involves co-amplification of HIV RNA with three Q-RNA internal standards (QA, QB and QC) covering the *gag* region and part of *pol* in a reaction involving avian myeloblastosis virus RT, T7 RNA polymerase and RNase H. By using electrochemiluminescent (ECL)-labelled probes, individual detection and quantification of the RNA present can be derived from the ratio of the sample signal to the QA, QB and QC signals. In general, these assays are equally sensitive (Revets *et al.*, 1996), and yield relatively comparable results when they are directly compared (Schuurman *et al.*, 1996), although interassay differences may be more marked when viral loads are low (Chew *et al.*, 1999b). Clinicians should monitor individual patients using only one assay type, although this may cause a problem for laboratories wishing to change from one assay to another because of cost or technical reasons. Because of the primer design of existing commercial HIV RNA quantitation assays, they can only be used to measure HIV-1 RNA levels. Also, the quantitation of some strains of HIV-1 may be compromised because of the diversity (subtypes) of the HIV-1 genome. Manufacturers of assays previously facing this problem (for example, the Amplicor HIV Monitor) have responded by incorporating modified procedures (reduced sample volume and lower primer annealing temperatures) and altered primer sequences, with improved amplification efficiency across all group M subtypes as a result (Chew *et al.*, 1999a).

At present, the lower limit of detection of commercially available HIV RNA quantification assays varies from 400 (NASBA-QT and Amplicor) to 500 (Bayer) copies/ml of plasma. However, with an increased sample volume and incorporation of an ultracentrifugation step, second- and third-generation versions of these assays are now available and have lower limits of detection of approximately 50 RNA copies/ml of plasma. This increased sensitivity may be of prognostic value, since patients whose virus loads fall below 50 copies/ml following introduction of HAART maintain undetectable viral loads for longer than patients with levels between 50 and 500 copies/ml and patients with detectable virus loads below the normal quantitation range of commercial assays (less than 400 copies/ml) have a less durable virological response than patients with unde-tectable virus loads in the same assays (Pilcher et al., 1999). While intuition suggests that this will translate into improved clinical outcomes for those individuals in the former group, data supporting this assertion are not yet available.

Recently, the real-time TaqMan™ PR assay system has been developed for detection of either HIV RNA and DNA (Leutenegger et al., 2001; Desire et al., 2001). This assay sys-tem is fast and has a tremendous dynamic range ($\leq 10^{1.7}$ to 10^7 RNA or DNA copies per ml), and is likely to replace other systems for measuring HIV DNA and RNA in body fluids.

The effects of conditions often encountered during han-dling, transit and storage of blood specimens on the quan-tity of HIV RNA in plasma has been studied (Sébire et al., 1998). RNA copy numbers are maintained to within 0.5 $\log_{10}$ in blood and plasma samples held at room tempera-ture or 4°C for up to 3 days, and remain stable despite lim-ited freezing and thawing of the plasma. HIV RNA copy numbers are also maintained during long-term storage of plasma at -70°C.

HIV DNA PCR

HIV DNA can be detected qualitatively and quantitative-ly in PBMC (or other tissues including lymph node, tonsi-lar tissue, brain, an dried blood spots) using PCR. Detection of HIV DNA has been used for the early diag-nosis of neonatal infection and seroconversion illness (Palasanthiran et al., 1994; Steketee et al., 1997), for screen-ing of pooled blood from blood donors to exclude HIV-1 sero-negative but seroconverting individuals (Busch et al., 1991), to help interpret indeterminate serological screen-ing results (Perrin et al., 1990), and in situations where samples of blood or tissue are unsuitable for RNA mea-surements, virus isolation or serological analysis (Boriskin et al., 1995) (Table 4.1). It may also be used where DNA for sequence analysis is required for epidemiological purposes (Zhu et al., 1998), and to investigate the immunopatho-genesis of HIV infection (Pantaleo et al., 1991), including investigations of potential reservoirs of infection (for exam-ple, the lymph nodes) in individuals on antiretroviral drug therapy. Commercial qualitative proviral HIV-1 DNA PCR assays are now regarded as useful confirmatory assays in HIV diagnosis.

CD4 lymphocyte counts

Despite the current widespread use of HIV RNA quanti-tation in plasma as a means of monitoring the course of HIV infection, enumeration of CD4 lymphocytes remains an important method for evaluating the degree of immune dysfunction (and, indirectly, disease progression) in infected patients. The CD4 lymphocyte count helps to indicate when antiretroviral treatment should start, when prophylaxis for opportunistic infections should com-mence, and helps to indicate the likelihood of certain opportunistic infections in specific clinical situations. Nowadays few if any clinical trials rely exclusively on virus load measurements to assess the response to HAART, and an overall increase in CD4 lymphocytes during therapy still remains an important index of the response to treatment. Also, because of the cost of commercial HIV RNA quantification kits, CD4 lymphocyte enumeration is often the only available laboratory test in many geographical locations, including countries where the incidence of HIV infection is high.

To obtain a CD4 lymphocyte count, blood from the patient is mixed with a pool of monoclonal antibodies to cell surface markers (for example, CD3, CD4 and CD8). The antibodies are pre-conjugated to different dyes (PC5, RD1 and FITC for CD3, CD4 and CD8, respectively). Fol-lowing lysis of erythrocytes, stabilization of leucocytes and fixation of cellular membranes, the sample is analysed by flow cytometry to determine the relative proportions of CD3, CD4 and CD8 lymphocytes. From the total leucocyte count and lymphocyte percentage obtained from a full blood examination (FBE), the absolute number of CD4 lymphocytes per μL can then be calculated. The percentage of total lymphocytes expressing CD4 and the ratio between the number of CD4 lymphocytes and CD8 lym-phocytes can also be used for the same purpose, and may fluctuate less in individual patients. In advanced immune deficiency (CD4 lymphocytes less than 200/μL), a marked decline in the CD8 lymphocyte count indicates a poor prognosis.

Previous studies have shown that CD4 lymphocyte numbers are predictive for the development of certain opportunistic infections and malignancies in infected patients (Crowe et al., 1991). In this context, asymptomatic individuals tend to have counts greater than 500/μL. As counts decrease to between 250 and 500/μL, early opportunistic infections such as oropharyngeal candidiasis and tuberculosis are manifest. KS tends to occur in patients with CD4 lymphocyte counts between 150 and 200/ μl. AIDS-defining, life-threatening illnesses including *Pneumocystis carinii* pneumonia (PCP) and toxoplasmosis are common in individuals with approximately 100 cells/μl or less. Cytomegalovirus (CMV) retinitis and atypical mycobacterial infection, which occur in the terminal stages of disease, are associated with counts of 50–75/μl or below.

Sequencing HIV strains

Management of HIV infection may by influenced by knowledge of mutations in the HIV genome thought to be associated with long-term non-progression of disease. Studies of infected, clinically healthy individuals in the so-called 'Sydney Bloodbank Cohort' have revealed mutations in the *nef* and LTR regions of HIV DNA extracted from peripheral blood cells (Deacon *et al.*, 1995). Deletions of between 160 and 430 bp, along with a rearranged duplication of NFκB and SP1 transcription factor-binding regions within the U3 region of the LTR, appear to be responsible for the altered pathogenesis in these individuals. While unlikely to become a routine procedure, sequencing technique may be indicated for some individuals who are known to be infected yet do not progress, even in the absence of antiretroviral therapy.

Sequencing of HIV DNA derived from plasma virus has been used in a genetic evaluation of suspected cases of transient infection of infants (Frenkel *et al.*, 1998), a study that highlights the need for extreme care in handling specimens prior to PCR procedures. In 43 cases of suspected transient viraemia, repeat PCR failed to confirm the original result (20 cases), phylogenetic analysis of the env sequence from infant and maternal sources failed to identify the expected monophyletic relationship (17 cases), or typing of somatic loci demonstrated nonconcordance between HIV-positive and -negative specimens (six cases). These results suggest that sample mislabelling and laboratory contamination occur and should be avoided at all costs.

Investigations of cases of HIV infection involving uncommon or unusual routes of transmission have relied extensively on sequencing to identify epidemiological links. When coupled with phylogenetic analysis, sequencing is a powerful tool, which can show that a strain of HIV transmitted to one or more recipients derived from a single source. Conclusive demonstration of transmission of HIV from a dentist to several of his patients (Ou *et al.*, 1992), from a rapist to his victim (Albert *et al.*, 1994) and within the Scottish prison system (Yirrell *et al.*, 1997) have all relied on sequencing *env* and/or *gag* genes from the index case and recipients. Linkage between individuals associated with a legal case of knowing and reckless transmission of HIV has also been established using these techniques (Birch *et al.*, 2000)

Testing for antiretroviral drug resistance

At least 15 antiretroviral drugs are now available for the treatment of HIV infection (see Chapter 5). These drugs fall into the classes of reverse transcriptase (RT) or protease (PR) inhibitors. Current standard of care dictates that they be used in combinations containing at least three drugs, which may include examples from one or both classes. Because of the kinetics and nature of HIV replication, during which errors in the RT process may generate potentially resistant virus in patients who have never previously received antiretroviral therapy, strict adherence to the prescribed dosing of these drugs is necessary. Otherwise, selection of HIV strains with these existing resistance mutations may occur in the presence of suboptimal drug levels. Further mutations may then be selected, which increase the resistance or modify the replicative fitness of these strains.

The presence of drug resistance mutations impacts on virological and clinical responses to therapy. Several stages can be identified during HIV infection when knowledge of these mutations may impact on treatment. These include at the time of primary infection, when drug-resistant virus may have been transmitted (Boden *et al.*, 1999; Conlan *et al.*, 1994; Imrie *et al.*, 1997); during pregnancy, when treatment of the infected female with antiretroviral drugs may protect the fetus from infection; and at the time of virological failure in a previously treated patient, when a switch or intensification of therapy is considered. A growing number of prospectve studies have shown the potential clinical utility of drug resistance testing. In particular, the so-called VIRADAPT (Durant *et al.*, 1999) and GART (Baxter *et al.*, 1999) studies have demonstrated an improved virological response for periods of up to 12 months following laboratory-guided treatment alterations.

Currently, three methods have been described that fall into the category of antiretroviral drug resistance tests. These are genotyping, phenotyping and virtual phenotyping.

Genotyping

Determination of the nucleotide sequence (genotyping) of the RT and PR genes of HIV has enabled identification of specific amino acid mutations selected by antiretroviral therapy that result in drug resistance. A number of methods are available for assessing the HIV genotype, including direct sequencing, point mutation assays (Kay et al., 1992), the line probe assay and high density oligonucleotide array (gene chip) sequencing (Lipshutz, 1995) (see Table 4.2).

Direct sequencing involves extraction of HIV RNA from plasma with amplification by RT-PCR, or amplification of HIV DNA in PBMC by PCR, and sequencing of a region of the genome spanning the PR and RT genes. This procedure identifies the sequence of the major HIV species existing in plasma or PBMC at the time of blood collection. Cloning is required if the sequence of minor species is required (Condra et al., 1995). The presence of minor species may be important in predicting the likelihood of future resistance, particularly to PR inhibitors.

The process of translating the amino acid sequences derived from sequencing data into an antiretroviral drug susceptibility profile for HIV is not straightforward, although in general, the identification of specific mutations in the RT gene often predicts phenotypic resistance to certain nucleoside or nonnucleoside inhibitors. For example, M41-L and T215-Y mutations almost always indicate phenotypic resistance to zidovudine (ZDV) (Larder et al., 1989), and the M184-V mutation indicates resistance to lamivudine (3TC) (Tisdale et al., 1993) (and possibly a degree of cross-resistance to didanosine [ddI] and abacavir). Similarly, the presence of a K103N mutation in the RT suggests resistance to each of the nonnucleoside analogues available clinically (nevirapine, delavirdine and efavirenz) (Young et al., 1995). However, while the presence of both T215-Y and M184-V suggests pheno-typical resistance to ZDV and 3TC, the incompatibility of these mutations with respect to RT function may result in a virus that is phenotypically susceptible to ZDV but resistant to 3TC (Larder et al., 1995). Recently described polymorphisms at amino acid 333 in the RT (G333-Q or -D) are able to override this phenomenon, facilitating dual resistance to these agents (Kemp et al., 1998).

Extrapolating from genotypical data to the phenotype of HIV strains selected as a result of therapy with PIs can be especially problematic because of:

Table 4.2 Methods for the detection of drug-resistant HIV, and some of the technical advantages and disadvantages associated with each

Method	Advantages	Disadvantages
Phenotyping		
Primary isolate assay	Replication of clinical isolate assessed directly in presence of drug	Labour intensive; slow; virus may alter during passaging; Tests only single agents
Recombinant assay (RT and PR from clinical isolate in a laboratory backbone)	Replication of (recombinant) clinical isolate assessed in presence of drug; Assay can be automated	Does not assay for the effects of possible mutations at secondary sites; Restricted availability; Tests only single agents; May underestimate the role of the laboratory backbone
Genotyping		
Direct sequencing	General availability; Mutations may precede phenotypic resistance; Can provide entire sequence of region of interest	Is an indirect measure of phenotype; Expert interpretation of codon changes is required for many sequences
Gene chip assay	Can provide entire sequence of region of interest	May be insensitive to mixtures and low virus load; Needs to be updated when new mutations discovered
Line probe assay	Rapid; sensitive to mixtures; kit-based	Needs to be updated when new mutations discovered
Point mutation assay	Rapid; sensitive to mixtures	Insensitive to mixtures and low virus load
Virtual phenotyping	Requires only the sequence of interest; Subsequent virus replication not required	Depends on availability of phenotyped and genotyped strains in a database; Unable to analyse all mutations of potential importance

(1) the number of naturally occurring polymorphisms in the HIV protease (Kozal *et al.*, 1996);

(2) the variety and number of mutations that can be selected during therapy with PIs (at least 18 with indinavir);

(3) the presence of compensatory mutations, which improve protease function or alter cleavage sites in the gag-pol poly protein, and therefore contribute to improved virological fitness for the resistant strain; and

(4) the need for several mutations to be present before phenotypical resistance is measurable (a property particularly true of indinavir) (Condra *et al.*, 1996).

The gene chip assay provides sequence data on the HIV PR and RT genes through a system in which oligonucleotide probes distributed in an array on a silicon chip hybridize with fluorescein-labelled PCR products derived from the gene of interest (Lipshutz, 1995). Performance of the assay requires sophisticated hardware to enable data acquisition and analysis, but it is considered to be technically user-friendly.

A commercial genotyping assay for resistance to RT inhibitors has recently become available (Murex Innopa Lineprobe [LiPA]). RNA from plasma HIV virions is extracted and amplified by RT-PCR using biotinylated primers to create a DNA product that is then hybridized to oligonucleotides containing wild-type or resistant sequences on a nitrocellulose strip. Subsequent visual detection of hybridization involves interaction between alkaline phosphatase-labelled streptavidin and a chromagen. LiPA appears to have at least equivalent sensitivity and specificity to that of direct sequencing, and can often detect mixtures of wild-type and resistant strains. It will need to be constantly updated to incorporate newly discovered mutations of significance (for example, the G333-Q/D mutation conferring dual resistance to ZDV and 3TC (Kemp *et al.*, 1998) and E44A/D and V118I mutations that confer immediate level resistance of lamivudine (Herlogs *et al.*, 2000). An assay specific for the PR region has not yet been fully developed, possibly because of the interpretation difficulties outlined above.

Phenotyping

Difficulties in interpreting HIV drug resistance genotypes has stimulated somewhat of a renaissance in phenotyping assays. Traditionally, phenotyping assays have been time-consuming and cumbersome, and because of the time taken to obtain results (weeks to months) they had lost favour compared to genotyping. However, phenotyping assays that overcome most of these drawbacks have now been developed (Hertogs *et al.*, 1998). They involve amplification of a sequence encoding the entire PR and RT regions by RT-PCR from HIV virion RNA in the patient's plasma. This product is cotransfected into MT-4 cells with a plasmid containing the backbone of a laboratory-adapted, fully anti-retroviral-susceptible HIV-1 strain, but with a deletion corresponding to most of the PR and RT region. Homologous recombination results in production only of virus containing the introduced PR/RT sequence from the patient's virus in the background of a laboratory-adapted virus. This virus can be easily amplified in cell culture and tested for its susceptibility against any number of inhibitors using high-throughput, automated (robotic) technology, in which the end-point of the assay is measured as cell death (using an MTT-based assay) (Hertogs *et al.*, 1998). Such an assay represents an attempt both to increase the speed of phenotyping (by eliminating the need for primary culture of patient HIV strains) and to standardize the susceptibility testing procedure (by testing viruses having the same wild-type backbone). Factors such as the role of mutations external to the PR region on susceptibility to PIs (for example, at the p6/p1 and p1/p7 cleavage sites (Doyon *et al.*, 1996; Zhang *et al.*, 1997) require further evaluation.

Virtual phenotyping

A novel method to derive a drug susceptibility phenotype involves a comparison of locally generated PR and RT gene sequences from a virus with unknown phenotype with a similar or identical sequence derived from an HIV strain for which the phenotype is known. Such technology is available commercially from the Virco company. Its advantage is that it avoids the need to undertake phenotyping experiments with replication-component virus. However, further studies are required to determine the exact relationship between it and the actual phenotype.

Chemokine receptors: clinical use of polymorphism screening tests

The normal function of chemokines is to attract leucocytes to areas of inflammation during infection. Receptors for these soluble peptides are cell surface molecules, two of which have recently been identified as being the secondary receptors that permit the attachment and penetration of HIV into susceptible cells. In concert with the primary receptor CD4, the CCR-5 receptor enables infection of cells of the macrophage lineage by macrophage-tropic strains of HIV (Deng et al., 1996; Dragic et al., 1996). These strains predominate in the early stages of HIV infection. The CXCR-4 receptor enables infection of T-cell line-tropic strains, which emerge during disease progression (O'Brien and Dean, 1997).

A 32 base-pair deletion mutation (known as Δ32) in the gene for CCR-5 results in the production of a truncated protein that is not incorporated into the cell membrane. The Δ32 mutation can be detected by amplification of a 151 base-pair (bp) product of the CCR-5 gene compared to a 181 bp wild-type product (Biti et al., 1997). Although CD4 may be present on HIV-susceptible lymphocytes, the lack of the secondary receptor appears to be sufficient to prevent infection. Individuals homozygous for Δ32 appear to be markedly less susceptible to infection with HIV, although at least two such HIV-infected individuals have been reported (Balotta et al., 1997; Biti et al., 1997). While still fully vulnerable to infection, heterozygous individuals have a slower rate of disease progression than normals (Dean et al., 1996; Huang et al., 1996). The mutant allele is present at high frequency in Caucasians (10–20%), but occurs only at low frequency (< 1%) in black Africans and Asians (Huang et al., 1996; Samson et al., 1996).

While not likely to have a significant role in the area of HIV diagnosis, detection of the Δ32 mutation in infected, heterozygous individuals may indicate an improved prognosis because of delayed disease progression and the role of antiretroviral drug therapy. The relationships between the Δ32 mutation, viral load, disease progression and the role of antiretroviral therapy in heterozygotes are likely to come under more intense scrutiny in the future. The clinical significance of other mutations such as CCR2-64I, CCR5303, SDF1-3'A and CCR5-59653T is under study (Ometto et al., 2001); whether testing for these mutations offers value to the clinician managing HIV-infected patients is uncertain.

References

Albert J, Wahlberg J, Leitner J et al. (1994). Analysis of a rape case by direct sequencing of the human immunodeficiency virus type 1 pol and gag genes. J Virol 68: 5918-24.

Alizon M, Montagnier L. (1987). Genetic variability in human immunodeficiency viruses. Ann NY Acad Sci 511: 376-84.

Arriyoshi K, Jaffer S, Alabi AS et al. (2000). Plasma RNA viral load predicts the rate of CD4 T cell decline and death in HIV-2-infected patients in West Africa. AIDS 14: 339-44.

Arrernstein AW, VanCott TC, Mascola JR et al. (1995). Dual infections with human immunodeficiency virus type 1 of distinct envelope subtypes in humans. J Infect Dis 171: 805-10.

Balotta C, Bagnarelli P, Violin M et al. (1997). Homozygous Δ32 deletion of the CCR-5 chemokine receptor gene in an HIV-1 infected patient. AIDS 11: F67-71.

Barre-Sinoussi F, Chermann J-C, Rey F et al. (1983). Isolation of T-lymphotropic retrovirus from a patient at risk for the acquired immune deficiency syndrome (AIDS). Science 220: 868-71.

Baxter JD, Mayers DL, Wentworth DN et al. (2000). A randomized study of antiretroviral management based on plasma genotypic antiretroviral resistance testing in patients failing therapy. AIDS 14: F83-93.

Benitez J, Palenzuela D, Rivero J et al. (1998). A recombinant protein based immunoassay for the combined detection of antibodies to HIV-1, HIV-2 and HTLV-1. J Virol Methods 70: 85-91.

Berrios DC, Avins AL, Haynes-Sanstad K et al. (1995). Screening for human immunodeficiency virus antibody in urine. Arch Path Lab Med 119: 139-41.

Birch CJ, McCaw RF, Bulach DM et al. (2000). Molecular analysis of human immunodeficiency virus strains associated with a case of criminal transmission of the virus. J Infect Dis 182: 941-4.

Biti R, Ffrench R, Young J et al. (1997). HIV-1 infection in an individual homozygous for the CCR5 deletion allele. Nat Med 3: 252-3.

Boden D, Hurley A, Zhang L et al. (1999). HIV-1 drug resistance in newly infected individuals. JAMA 282: 1135-41.

Borskin YS, Booth JC, Fernando S et al. (1995). The detection of HIV-1 proviral DNA by PCR in clotted blood specimens. J Virol Methods 52: 87-94.

Brew B, Pemberton L, Cunningham P et al. (1997). Levels of human immunodeficiency virus type 1 RNA in cerebrospinal fluid correlate with AIDS dementia stage. J Infect Dis 175: 963-6.

Burgard M, Mayaux M-J, Blanche S et al. (1992). The use of viral culture and p24 antigen testing to diagnose human immunodeficiency virus infection in neonates. N Engl J Med 327: 1192-7.

Busch MP, Eble BE, Khayam-Bashi H et al. (1991). Evaluation of screened blood donations for human immunodeficiency virus type 1 infection by culture and DNA amplification of pooled cells. N Engl J Med 325: 1-5.

Carr JK, Salminen MO, Koch C et al. (1996). Full-length sequence and mosaic structure of a human immunodeficiency virus type 1 isolate from Thailand. J Virol 70: 5935-43.

Cheingsong-Popov R, Osmanov S, Pau CP et al. (1998). Serotyping of HIV type 1 infections: definition, relationship to viral genetic subtypes, and assay evaluation. UNAIDS Network for HIV-1 isolation and characterization. AIDS Res Hum Retrovir 14: 311-8.

Chew CB, Herring B, Zheng F et al. (1999a). Comparison of three commercial assays in the quantitation of HIV-1 RNA in plasma from individuals infected with different HIV-1 subtypes. J Clin Virol 14: 87-94.

Chew CB, Blyth K, Zheng F et al. (1999b). Comparison of three commercial assays for the quantitation of plasma HIV-1 RNA from individuals with low viral loads. AIDS 13: 1977-8.

Clarke SJ, Decker WD et al. (1991). High titers of cytopathic virus in plasma of patients with symptomatic primary HIV-1 infection. New Engl J Med 324: 954-60.

Condra JH, Schleif WA, Blahy OM et al. (1995). In vivo emergence of HIV-1 variants resistant to multiple protease inhibitors. Nature 374: 569-71.

Condra JH, Holder DJ, Schleif WA et al. (1996). Genetic correlates of in vivo viral resistance to indinavir, a human immunodeficiency virus type 1 protease inhibitor. J Virol **70**: 8270–6.

Conlan CP, Klenerman P, Edwards BA et al. (1994). Heterosexual transmission of human immunodeficiency virus type 1 variants associated with zidovudine resistance. J Infect Dis **169**: 411–5.

Cooper DA, Imrie AA, Penny R. (1987). Antibody response to human immunodeficiency virus after primary infection. J Infect Dis **155**: 1113.

Constantine NT, Zhang X, Li L et al. (1994). Application of a rapid assay for detection of antibodies to human immunodeficiency virus in urine. Am J Clin Path **101**: 157–61.

Crowe SM, Carlin JB, Stewart KI et al. (1991). Predictive value of CD4 lymphocyte numbers for the development of opportunistic infections and malignancies in HIV-infected persons. J Acquir Immune Def Syndr **4**: 770–6.

Cunningham P, Smith D, Temby C et al. (1997). Reduction of the HIV-1 pre-seroconversion window period with viral genomic detection assays. Abstract 26, Fourteenth National Reference Laboratory Workshop on Serology, September 26–27 1997, Adelaide University, Adelaide, South Australia.

Daar ES, Moudgil T, Meyer RD et al. (1991). Transient high levels of viremia in patients with primary human immunodeficiency virus type 1 infection. N Engl J Med **324**: 961–4.

Deacon NJ, Tsykin A, Solomon A et al. (1995). Genomic structure of an attenuated quasi species of HIV-1 from a blood transfusion donor and recipients. Science **270**: 988–91.

Dean M, Carrington M, Winkler C et al. (1996). Genetic restriction of HIV-1 infection and progression to AIDS by a detection allele of the CKR5 structural gene. Science **273**: 1856–62.

Delwart EL, Herring B, Rodrigo AG et al. (1995). Genetic subtyping of human immunodeficiency virus using a heteroduplex mobility assay. PCR Meth Appl **4**: S202–16.

Deng H, Liu R, Ellmeier W et al. (1996). Identification of a major co-receptor for primary isolates of HIV-1. Nature **381**: 661–6.

Desire N, Dehee A, Schneider V et al. (2001). Quantification of HIV-1 proviral load TaqMan real-time PCR assay. J Clin Microbiol **39**: 1303–10.

Devito C, Levi M, Hinkula J et al. (1998). Seroreactivity to HIV-1 V3 subtypes A to H peptides of Argentinian HIV-positive sera. J Acquir Immune Defic Syndr Hum Retrovirol **17**: 156–9.

Doyon L, Croteau G, Thibeault D et al. (1996). Second locus involved in human immunodeficiency virus type 1 resistance to protease inhibitors. J Virol **70**: 3763–9.

Dragic T, Litwin V, Allaway GP et al. (1996). HIV-1 entry into CD4+ cells is mediated by the chemokine receptor CC-CKR-5. Nature **381**: 667–73.

Dunne AL, Crowe SM. (1997). Comparison of branched DNA and reverse transcriptase polymerase chain reaction for quantifying six different HIV-1 subtypes in plasma. AIDS **11**: 126–7.

Durant J, Clevenbergh P, Halfon P et al. (1999). Durg-resistance genotyping in HIV-1 therapy: the VIRADAPT randomised contrlled trial. Lancet **353**: 2195–9.

Dwyer DE, Adelstein S, Cunningham AL et al. (1997). The laboratory in managing HIV infection. In: G Stewart (ed.) Managing HIV. 1st edition. Sydney: AMPCO, 59–61.

Finzi D, Hermankova M, Pierson T et al. (1997). Identification of a reservoir for HIV-1 in patients on highly active antiretroviral therapy. Science **278**: 1295–300.

Frenkel LM, Mullins JI, Learn GH et al. (1998). Genetic evaluation of suspected cases of transient HIV-1 infection of infants. Science **280**: 1073–7.

Gao F, Yue L, Robertson DL et al. (1994). Genetic diversity of human immunodeficiency virus type 2: evidence for distinct sequence subtypes with differences in virus biology. J. Virol **68**: 7433–47.

Gao F, Robertson DL, Carruther CD et al. (1998). A comprehensive panel of near-full-length clones and reference sequences for non-subtype B isolates of human immunodeficiency virus type 1. J Virol **72**: 5680–98.

Gurtler L. (1996). Difficulties and strategies of HIV diagnosis. Lancet **348**: 176–9.

Hertogs K, De Bethune M-P, Miller V et al. (1998). A rapid method for simultaneous detection of phenotypic resistance to inhibitors of protease and reverse transcriptase in recombinant human immunodeficiency virus type 1 isolates from patients treated with antiretroviral drugs. Antimicrob Agents Chemother **42**: 269–76.

Hertogs K, Bloor S, De Vroey V et al. (2000). A novel human immunodeficiency virus type 1 reverse transcriptase mutational pattern confers phenotypic lamivudine resistance in the absence of mutation M184V. Antimicrob Agents Chemother **44**: 568–73.

Ho DD. (1996). Viral counts in HIV infection. Science **272**: 1124–5.

Ho DD, Moudgil T, Alam M. (1989). Quantitation of the human immunodeficiency virus type 1 in the blood of infected persons. N Engl J Med **321**: 1621–5.

Ho DD, Neumann AU, Perelson AS et al. (1995). Rapid turnover of plasma virions and CD4 lymphocytes in HIV-1 infection. Nature **373**: 123–6.

Huang Y, Paxton WA, Wolinsky SM et al. (1996). The role of a mutant CCR5 allele in HIV-1 transmission and disease progression. Nat Med **2**: 1240–3.

Imrie A, Beveridge A, Genn W et al. (1997). Transmission of human immunodeficiency virus type 1 resistant to nevirapine and zidovudine. J Infect Dis **175**: 1502–6.

Kappes JC, Saag MS, Shaw GM et al. (1995). Assessment of antiretroviral therapy by plasma viral load testing: standard and ICD HIV-1 p24 antigen and viral RNA (QC-PCR) assays compared. J Acquir Immune Defic Syndr Hum Retrovirol **10**: 139–49.

Katzenstein TL, Pedersen C, Nielson C et al. (1996). Longitudinal serum HIV RNA quantification: correlation to viral phenotype at seroconversion and clinical outcome. AIDS **10**: 167–73.

Kay S, Loveday C, Tedder RS. (1992). A microtitre format point mutation assay: application to the detection of drug resistance in human immunodeficiency virus type 1 infected patients treated with zidovudine. J Med Virol **37**: 241.

Kelen GD, Hexter DA, Hansen KN et al. (1995). Trends in human immunodeficiency virus (HIV) infection among a patient population of an inner-city emergency department: Implications for emergency department-based screening programs for HIV infection. J Infect Dis **21**: 867–75.

Kemp BE, Rylatt DB, Bundesen PG et al. (1988). Autologous red cell agglutination assay for HIV-1 antibodies: simplified test with whole blood. Science **241**: 1352–4.

Kemp SD, Shi C, Bloor S et al. (1998). A novel polymorphism at codon 333 of human immunodeficiency virus type 1 reverse transcriptase can facilitate dual resistance to zidovudine and L-2′, 3′-dideoxy-3′-thiacytidine. J Virol **72**: 5093–8.

King A, Marion SA, Cook D et al. (1995). Accuracy of a saliva test for HIV antibody. J Acquir Immune Syndr Hum Retrovir 9: 172-5.

Kozal MJ, Shah N, Shen N et al. (1996). Extensive polymorphisms observed in HIV-1 clade B protease gene using high-density oligonucleotide arrays. Nat Med 2: 753-9.

Larder BA, Darby G, Richman DD. (1989). HIV with reduced sensitivity to zidovudine (AZT) isolated during prolonged therapy. Science 243: 1731-4.

Larder BA, Kemp SD, Harrigan PR et al. (1995). Potential mechanism for sustained antiretroviral efficacy of AZT-3TC combination therapy. Science 269: 696-9.

Learn GH, Korber BTM, Foley B et al. (1996). Maintaining the integrity of human immunodeficiency virus sequence databases. J Virol 70: 5720-30.

Leutenegger CM, Higgins J, Matthews TB et al. (2001). Real-time Tag-Man PCR as a specific and more sensitive alternative to the branched-chain DNA assay for quantitation of simian immunodeficiency virus RNA. AIDS Res Hum Retroviruses 17: 243-51.

Lillo FB, Maillard M, Saracco A et al. (1997). Monitoring antiretroviral activity using ICDp24 and CD4 counts in HIV infection. J Infect 35: 67-71.

Lipshutz RJ. (1995). Using oligonucleotide probe arrays to access genetic diversity. Bio Techniques 19: 442-7.

Luo N, Kasolo F, Ngwenya BK et al. (1995). Use of saliva as an alternative to serum for HIV screening in Africa. S Afr Med J 85: 156-7.

Malone JR, Smith ES, Sheffield J et al. (1993). Comparative evaluation of six rapid serological tests for HIV-1 antibody. J Acquir Immune Defic Syndr 6: 115-9.

Martinez P, de Lejarazu O, Eires JM et al. (1995). Comparison of two assays for detection of HIV antibodies in saliva. Eur J Clin Microbiol Infect Dis 14: 330-6.

McGavin CH, Land SA, Sebire KL et al. (1996). Syncytium-inducing phenotype and zidovudine susceptibility of HIV-1 isolated from post-mortem tissue. AIDS 10: 47-53.

Mellors JW, Kingsley LA, Rinaldo CR et al. (1995). Quantitation of HIV-1 RNA in plasma predicts outcome after seroconversion. Ann Intern Med 122: 573-9.

Mellors JW, Rinaldo CR, Gupta P et al. (1996). Prognosis in HIV-1 infection predicted by the quantity of virus in plasma. Science 272: 1167-70.

Metcalf JA, Davey RT, Lane CH. (1997). Acquired immunodeficiency syndrome: serologic and virologic tests. In: VT De Vita, S Hellman, SA Rosenberg (eds). AIDS. Etiology, diagnosis, treatment and prevention. 4th edition. Philadelphia, PA: Lippincott, Williams & Wilkins, 177-195.

Middleton T, Breschkin A, Land S et al. (1997). Detection and quantification of HIV-1 western blot indeterminate patients using commercially available assays. Fourteenth National Reference Laboratory Workshop on Serology, Adelaide University, Adelaide, South Australia.

MMWR (1993a). Technical guidance on HIV counseling. MMWR 42: 11-7.

MMWR (1995b). Recommendations for HIV testing services for in-patients and outpatients in acute-care hospital settings. MMWR 42: 1-6.

MMWR (1998). The Report of the NIH Panel to define principles of therapy of HIV infection and guidelines for the use of antiretroviral agents in HIV infected adults and adolescents. MMWR 47: 1-83.

Neate EV, Pringle RC, Jowett JBM et al. (1987). Isolation of HIV from Australian patients with AIDS, AIDS related conditions and healthy antibody positive individuals. Aust NZ J Med 17: 461-6.

O'Brien SJ, Dean M. (1997). In search of AIDS-resistance genes. Scientific American September: 28-35.

Oelrichs R, Dyer W, Downie J et al. (1999). Inaccurate HIV-1 viral load quantification by three major commercially available methods. AIDS 13: 727-8.

Ometto L, Bertorelle R, Mainardi M et al. (2001). Polymorphisms in the CCR5 promoter region influence disease progression in perinatally HIV type 1-infected children. J Infect Dis 183: 814-8.

Ou C-Y, Ciesielski CA, Myers G et al. (1992). Molecular epidemiology of HIV transmission in a dental practice. Science 256: 1165-71.

Palasanthiran P, Ziegler JB, Dwyer DE et al. (1994). Early detection of human immunodeficiency virus type 1 infection in Australian infants at risk of perinatal infection and factors affecting transmission. Pediatr Infect Dis J 13: 1083-90.

Pantaleo G, Graziosi C, Butini L et al. (1991). Lymphoid organs function as major reservoirs for human immunodeficiency virus. Proc Natl Acad Sci USA 88: 9838-42.

Perelson AS, Neumann AU, Markowitz M et al. (1996). HIV-1 dynamics in vivo: virion clearance rate, infected cell life span and viral generation time. Science 271: 1582-6.

Perrin LH, Yerly S, Adami N et al. (1990). Human immunodeficiency virus DNA amplification and serology in blood donors. Blood 76: 641-5.

Phillips KA, Flatt SJ, Morrison KR et al. (1995). Potential use of home HIV testing. N Engl J Med 332: 1308-10.

Piatak M, Saag MS, Yang LC et al. (1993). High levels of HIV-1 in plasma during all stages of infection determined by competitive PCR. Science 259: 1749-54.

Pilcher CD, Miller WC, Beatty ZA et al. (1999). Detectable HIV-1 RNA levels below quantifiable limits by Amplicor HIV-1 Monitor is associated with virologic relapse on antiretroviral therapy. AIDS 13: 1337-42.

Reisler RB, Thea DM, Pliner V et al. (2001). Early detection of reverse transcriptase activity in plasma of neonates infected with HIV-1: a comparative analysis with RNA-based and DNA-based testing using PCR. J Acquir Immune Defic Syndr 26: 93-102.

Revets H, Marissens D, De Wit S et al. (1996). Comparative evaluation of NASBA HIV-1 RNA QT, AMPLICOR-HIV Monitor, and QUANTIPLEX HIV RNA assay, three methods for quantification of human immunodeficiency virus type 1 RNA in plasma. J Clin Microbiol 34: 1058-64.

Robertson DL, Anderson JP, Brodac JA et al. (2000). HIV-1 nomenclature proposal. Science 288: 55-6.

Rutherford GW, Schwarcz SK, McFarland W. (2000). Surveillance for incident HIV infection: new technology and new opportunities. J Acquir Immune Defic Syndr 25: S115-19.

Samson M, Libert F, Doranz BJ et al. (1996). Resistance to HIV-1 infection in Caucasian individuals bearing mutant alleles of the CCR-5 chemokine receptor gene. Nature 382: 722-5.

Schuurman R, Descamps D, Weverling GJ et al. (1996). Multicenter comparison of three commercial methods for quantification of human immunodeficiency virus type 1 RNA in plasma. J Clin Microbiol 34: 3016-22.

Sebire K, McGavin K, Land S et al. (1998). Stability of human immunodeficiency virus RNA in blood specimens as measured by a commercial PCR-based assay. J Clin Microbiol 36: 493-8.

Sethoe SY, Ling AE, Sug EH et al. (1995). PCR as a confirmatory test for human immunodeficiency virus type 1 infection in individuals with indeterminate western blot (immunoblot) profile. J Clin Microbiol 33: 3034–6.

Shearer WT, Quinn TC, LaRussa P et al. (1997). Viral load and disease progression in infants infected with human immunodeficiency virus type 1. Women and Infants Transmission Study Group. N Engl J Med 336: 1337–42.

Sonnerborg AB, von Sydow MA, Forsgren M et al. (1989). Association between intrathecal anti-HIV-1 immunoglobulin G synthesis and occurrence of HIV-1 in cerebrospinal fluid. AIDS 3: 701–5.

Steketee RW, Abrams EJ, Thea DM et al. (1997). Early detection of perinatal human immunodeficiency virus (HIV) type 1 infection using HIV RNA amplification and detection. J Infect Dis 175: 707–11.

Sterling TR, Vlahov D, Astemborski J et al. (2001). Initial HIV-1 RNA levels and progression to AIDS in women and men. N Engl J Med 344: 720–5.

Subbarao S and Schochetman G. (1996). Genetic variability of HIV-1. AIDS 10: S13–23.

Tisdale M, Kemp SD, Parry NR et al. (1993). Rapid in-vitro selection of human immunodeficiency virus type 1 resistant to 3'-thiacytidine inhibitors due to a mutation in the YMDD region of reverse transcriptase. Proc Natl Acad Sci USA 90: 5653–6.

Trujillo JR, Navia BA, Worth J et al. (1996). High levels of anti-HIV-1 envelope antibodies in cerebrospinal fluid as compared to serum from patients with AIDS dementia complex. J Acquir Immune Defic Hum Retrovirol 12: 19–25.

Vallari AS, Hickman RK, Hackett JR Jr et al. (1998). Rapid assay for simultaneous detection and differentiation of immunoglobulin G antibodies to human immunodeficiency virus type 1 (HIV-1) group M, HIV-1 group O, and HIV-2. J Clin Microbiol 36: 3657–61.

Wain-Hobson S, Sonigo P, Danos O et al. (1985). Nucleotide sequence of the AIDS virus, LAV. Cell 40: 9–17.

Weniger BG, Takebe Y, Ou Cy et al. (1994). The molecular epidemiology of HIV in Asia. AIDS 8: 13–28.

Windsor IM, Gomes dos Santos ML, de la Hunt LI et al. (1997). An evaluation of the capillus HIV-1/HIV-2 latex agglutination test using serum and whole blood. Int J STD AIDS 8: 192–5.

Wong JK, Hezareh M, Gunthard HF et al. (1997). Recovery of replication-competent HIV despite prolonged suppression of plasma viremia. Science 278: 1291–5.

Workshop Report from the European Commission and the Joint United Nations Program on HIV/AIDS. (1997). HIV and subtypes: implications for epidemiology, pathogenicity, vaccines and diagnostics. AIDS 11: 17–36.

Yirrell DL, Robertson P, Goldberg DJ et al. (1997). Molecular investigation into outbreak of HIV in a Scottish prison. Brit Med J 314: 1146–50.

Young SD, Britcher SF, Tran LO et al. (1995). L-743,726 (DMP-266): a novel, highly potent nonnucleoside inhibitor of the human immunodeficiency virus type 1 reverse transcriptase. Antimicrob Agents Chemother 39: 2602–5.

Zhang YM, Imamichi H, Imamichi T et al. (1997). Drug resistance during indinavir therapy is caused by mutations in the protease gene and its gag substrate cleavage sites. J Virol 71: 6662–70.

Zhu T, Korber BT, Nahmias AJ et al. (1998). An African HIV-1 sequence from 1959 and implications for the origin of the epidemic. Nature. 391: 594–7.

Antiretroviral drugs

5

SUZANNE CROWE

Three classes of antiretroviral drugs are currently available to treat HIV infection: nucleoside analogue reverse transcriptase inhibitors ('nucleosides', NRTIs), non-nucleoside analogue reverse transcriptase inhibitors (NNRTIs), and protease inhibitors (PIs) (Table 5.1). A fourth class, known as 'entry inhibitors' (e.g. T-20, CCR5 and CXCR4 chemokine receptor inhibitors), is undergoing clinical trial.

Table 5.1 Classes of antiretroviral drugs

Nucleoside analogue reverse transcriptase inhibitors	
	Trade name
Zidovudine	Retrovir
Didanosine	Videx
Zalcitabine	Hivid
Lamivudine	3TC
Stavudine	Zerit
Abacavir	Ziagen
Non-nucleoside analogue reverse transcriptase inhibitors	
Nevirapine	Viramune
Delavirdine	Rescriptor
Efavirenz	Sustiva
Protease inhibitors	
Saquinavir (soft gel)	Fortovase
Ritonavir	Norvir
Nelfinavir	Viracept
Indinavir	Crixivan
Amprenavir	Agenerase
Lopinavir	Kaletra

Nucleoside analogue reverse transcriptase inhibitors (NRTIs)

These antiretroviral drugs were the first class of drugs discovered and used for the treatment of HIV infection. They are all potent inhibitors of HIV-1 replication and are also active against HIV-2. They require intracellular phosphorylation to the triphosphate derivative for activity against HIV reverse transcriptase, and as such inhibit reverse transcriptase and terminate DNA chain synthesis (reviewed in detail in Kucers et al., 1997).

Zidovudine
Zidovudine is the nucleoside analogue of the pyrimidine thymidine. It is marketed by GlaxoWellcome (Research Triangle Park, NC, USA) under the trade name Retrovir®.

In vitro *activity*
Zidovudine has activity against HIV-1 subtypes M (A–H) and O groups (Descamps et al., 1995). The IC_{90} value of 0.002–0.2 μM (Mohri et al., 1993; Shafer et al., 1993) of zidovudine in vitro is easily achieved in vivo, with plasma levels after an oral dose of 5–10 mg/kg being greater than 4–6 μM (Yarchoan et al., 1986). Zidovudine administered at a dose of 5–10 mg/kg achieves plasma levels greater than 4–6 μM, which is well above the IC_{90} of 0.002–0.2 μM for zidovudine in vitro (Yarchoan et al., 1986).

Zidovudine is additive or synergistic, with most other NRTIs against zidovudine-sensitive and zidovudine-resistant strains of HIV-1 (Dornsife et al., 1991; St Clair et al., 1995) with the exception of stavudine (Merrill et al., 1996). NNRTIs (Richman et al., 1991a). PIs (Craig et al., 1990) also demonstrate synergism with zidovudine. Ribavirin and stavudine antagonize zidovudine's action by inhibiting its phosphorylation (Vogt et al., 1987).

Resistance
HIV-1 strains resistant to zidovudine have developed after the passage of HIV-1 in cell culture in the presence of zidovudine (Larder et al., 1991) and in patients treated with zidovudine (Larder et al., 1989; Land et al., 1990). Resistance to zidovudine monotherapy develops relatively slowly (usually after months or years), compared to patients treated with NNRTI monotherapy (in whom

resistance may develop within weeks) (Medina et al., 1995). The time to development of resistance has been predicted in the past by the CD4 lymphocyte number and disease stage (probably relating to higher viral load levels in more advanced disease) but has not been conclusively linked to dose (Richman et al., 1990).

Mutations in the reverse transcriptase gene mediating resistance to zidovudine are detected earlier in plasma HIV RNA than in HIV DNA, and thus HIV strains isolated from plasma and cells may differ in susceptibility to zidovudine (Kozal et al., 1993). A number of mutations have been described in HIV-1 strains with reduced susceptibility to zidovudine (Larder et al., 1991; Larder, 1994) (Table 5.2). These mutations generally appear in chronological order (Figure 5.1) and various combinations of mutations confer differing degrees of resistance. The mutation in codon 215 has been reported to correlate with disease progression (Boucher et al., 1990). Zidovudine-resistant strains of HIV generally remain susceptible to other NRTIs, although some reports of cross-resistance have emerged (Rooke et al., 1991; Mayers et al., 1994). Resistant strains may slowly revert to being zidovudine susceptible following cessation of drug therapy, with these mutations reported as persisting from 8 to 22 months (Boucher et al., 1993a; Gurusinghe et al., 1995). Transmission of zidovudine-resistant strains of HIV is well documented (Conlon et al., 1994; Kuritzkes et al., 1994).

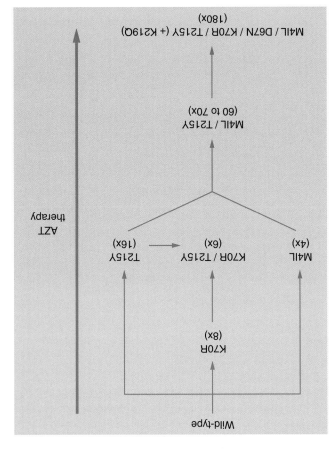

Figure 5.1 *Cumulative development of mutations within HIV reverse transcriptase conferring resistance to zidovudine during treatment (fold decrease in susceptibility is shown in parentheses) (reproduced with permission from Larder, 1994).*

Table 5.2 Major mutations within reverse transcriptase gene codons associated with resistance to NRTIs

Zidovudine	Didanosine	Zalcitabine	Stavudine	Lamivudine	Abacavir
M41L					M41L
				E44D*	
	K65R	K65R			K65R[a]
D67N					
		T69D[a]			
K70R					
	L74V[a]	L74V[a]			L74V[a]
			V75T[a]		
					Y115F
				V118I[a]	
	M184V/I	M184V/I[a]		M184V/I[a]	M184V/I[a]
L210W					
T215Y/F[a]					
K219Q					

[a]Mutations, which are often the first selected during viral evolution under drug pressure. These primary mutations cause resistance due to reduced binding of the inhibitor. All other mutations are secondary, and contribute to resistance. This list is not complete, and requires regular updating (data from Hirsch et al., 2000, O'Brien, 2000, Schinazi et al., 2000).

Clinically relevant pharmacokinetics

Dosage and administration. Zidovudine is available as capsules (100 mg and 250 mg) and as syrup containing 50 mg of zidovudine in 5 ml (Table 5.3). The adult dose of zidovudine is 250 mg administered orally twice daily or 200 mg three times daily. Higher doses are used if the primary intention is to treat AIDS dementia (see Chapter 10). The recommended oral dose for children aged over 3 months is 180 mg/m^2 administered 6 hourly (Table 5.4) (see also Chapter 9). Zidovudine is also available in combination with lamivudine (Combivir®, Glaxo Wellcome), and in combination with both lamivudine and abacavir (Trizivir®).

Absorption. There is good oral bioavailability (46–69%; Yarchoan *et al.*, 1989) and the drug can be taken without regard for food.

Distribution. Zidovudine crosses the placenta by simple diffusion and is found in cerebrospinal fluid (CSF; CSF:plasma ratio of about 0.6) (Yarchoan *et al.*, 1986, 1989). It has a plasma half-life of about 1 h and, of greater clinical importance, an intracellular half-life of 3–4 h (Furman *et al.*, 1986).

Metabolism and excretion. Zidovudine is metabolized mainly by glucuronidation in the liver, and the inactive glucuronide is rapidly cleared from plasma. Less than 20% of zidovudine is present unchanged in the urine. Zidovudine and its metabolites are eliminated by glomerular filtration and tubular secretion.

Important drug interactions

As zidovudine is myelotoxic, severe neutropenia may result from co-administration with ganciclovir (Hochster *et al.*, 1990). Co-administration of zidovudine and chemotherapeutic agents or high-dose co-trimoxazole should also be avoided. Drugs that are metabolized by hepatic glucuronidation, such as zidovudine, may inhibit metabolism of zidovudine and thus prolong its half-life. These drugs include probenecid, non-steroidal anti-inflammatory agents, narcotic analgesics, and sulfonamide antibiotics (Yarchoan *et al.*, 1989).

Major or frequent adverse reactions

During the first 6 weeks of therapy, zidovudine may cause nausea in up to 50% of patients, with anorexia, lethargy and headaches being less frequently described (see Chapter 6 for details of toxicity). Zidovudine may be associated with the development of anaemia, neutropenia, or leukopenia (reviewed in Kucers *et al.*, 1997). Zidovudine-induced myopathy, presenting with proximal weakness and wasting, occurs in about 20% of patients treated for more than 12 months with the drug, is not dose related, resolves with cessation of therapy and recurs with rechallenge (Gertner *et al.*, 1989; Dalakas *et al.*, 1990). There are rare reports of zidovudine causing acute hepatitis, with markedly increased transaminase levels and variable elevation of alkaline phosphatase (Gradon *et al.*, 1992). A syndrome of fatal lactic acidosis, massive hepatomegaly and steatosis is also a rare complication of zidovudine therapy (Chattha *et al.*, 1993).

Major clinical use

Although zidovudine was initially used as monotherapy (Yarchoan *et al.*, 1986; Fischl *et al.*, 1987, 1990; Volberding *et al.*, 1990; Hamilton, 1992; Cooper, 1993a; Concorde Co-ordinating Committee, 1994; reviewed in Kucers *et al.*, 1997), and then as part of dual NRTI therapy (Meng *et al.*, 1992; Collier et al, 1993; Eron *et al.*, 1995; Fischl *et al.*, 1995; Delta Co-ordinating Committee, 1996; Hammer *et al.*, 1996; Katlama *et al.*, 1996; reviewed in Kucers *et al.*, 1997), it is now used only as one component of triple- or quadruple-combination regimens in countries where resources are not constrained (see Chapter 7). Zidovudine is also commonly used to treat paediatric HIV infection, again usually as part of a combination regimen (see Chapter 9).

Zidovudine is often specifically included in antiretroviral regimens to treat HIV-related dementia (Yarchoan *et al.*, 1987) and other neurological disease, as it has a relatively high CSF:plasma ratio (see Chapter 10). Recent studies have demonstrated that zidovudine administered to HIV-infected pregnant women during pregnancy (and in some studies during parturition and then to the neonate for the first 6 weeks) can reduce transmission to the infant (Connor *et al.*, 1994) (see Chapter 8). Zidovudine has also been shown to be of benefit to health-care workers who have significant occupational exposure to HIV, with a case–control study demonstrating a reduction in risk of HIV transmission by 80% (Anon., 1995) (see Chapter 34). Marked clinical improvement has been observed in patients with HIV-related thrombocytopenia (Swiss Group, 1988; Chow *et al.*, 1993) and HIV-related psoriasis (Kaplan et al., 1989) who are treated with zidovudine. The mechanism by which zidovudine exerts these latter effects is not clear; zidovudine may improve platelet survival by decreasing plasma glycocalicin levels (Panzer et al., 1989).

Didanosine

Didanosine is the nucleoside analogue of the purine inosine. The drug is marketed by Bristol-Myers-Squibb (Princeton, NJ, USA) under the trade name Videx®.

In vitro activity

Didanosine is a less potent inhibitor of HIV-1 replication than zidovudine in vitro (Hitchcock, 1993). It is active against both group M and O strains of HIV-1 (Descamps et al., 1997). Plasma levels of approximately 30 μM (when didanosine is taken in the fasted state) are significantly higher than the IC_{50} of 2.5–10 μM (Shelton et al., 1992) and IC_{99} of 20 μM (Hayashi et al., 1990). Didanosine is more potent in inhibiting HIV replication in resting cells such as macrophages than in activated T lymphocytes (Gao et al., 1994).

When zidovudine, didanosine and lamivudine are used together in vitro, there is greater synergism than in double combinations of these drugs or monotherapy (St Clair et al., 1995). Additive to synergistic interactions occur between PIs and didanosine (Kageyama et al., 1992).

Resistance

Didanosine resistance develops less readily than zido-vudine resistance. The main mutation within the reverse transcriptase gene that is associated with the develop-ment of resistance is Leu74Val, which is associated with cross-resistance to zalcitabine but not to zidovudine (St Clair et al., 1991). Other reported mutations that confer resistance to didanosine are Lys 65 Arg, Met 184 Val, which is associated with cross-resistance to lamivudine and zalcitabine and Val 75 Thr, associated with cross-resistance to stavudine and zalcitabine (reviewed in Kucers et al., 1997; Table 5.2). Mutations in codons 62, 75, 77, 116 and 151 have been reported in association with multiple drug resistance (Shirasaka et al., 1995).

Clinically relevant pharmacokinetics

Dosage and administration. Didanosine is available as chewable buffered tablets containing 25 mg or 100 mg of didanosine or as paediatric powder for oral solution (Table 5.3). These formulations of didanosine include antacid, as the drug is destroyed by exposure to low pH. Didanosine has recently also become available in 400 mg enteric coated capsules, which do not require buffer and also remove the need to take tablets in the fasted state (see below).

The recommended dosage is dependent on weight: for adult patients greater than 60 kg the dose is 200 mg twice daily; for those less than 60 kg the dose is 125 mg twice daily. The dose for children is again weight dependent; for body surface areas of 1.5–2m², 1.0–1.4m², 0.5–0.9m² the doses are 200 mg twice daily, 150 mg twice daily and 50 mg twice daily, respectively.

Recent data suggest that didanosine can be taken once daily in a dose of 400 mg, although studies suggest that the durability of efficacy is shortened by taking the drug once daily and twice-daily administration is recommended.

Absorption. As the mean bioavailability of didanosine is only 35% and this decreases with food, didanosine must be taken on an empty stomach (4 h or more after the last meal, at least 30 min before a meal) (Table 5.4).

Distribution. Didanosine crosses the placenta by simple diffusion, but less than 50% reaches the placental cir-culation due to placental metabolism of the drug (Dancis et al., 1993). The CSF:plasma ratio of didanosine is only about 0.2, less than that of zidovudine (0.6) and similar to that of zalcitabine (0.1–0.2).

Metabolism and excretion. Similar to zidovudine, the intracellular half-life of didanosine (8–24 h) greatly exceeds the plasma half-life (0.6–2.7 h), providing the rationale for once or twice daily dosing. Didanosine is metabolized to hypoxanthine, the major metabolite, with small amounts of uric acid being formed through the action of xanthine oxidase (Back et al., 1992). Up to 50% of administered didanosine is cleared by renal mechanisms, via both tubular secretion and glomerular filtration.

Important drug interactions

The buffer within didanosine preparations may interfere with the absorption of dapsone, ketoconazole and ciprofloxacin; these drugs should be administered 2 h prior to or 6 h after didanosine (Sahai et al., 1993). The

Table 5.3 Dosing of antiretroviral therapies

Zidovudine	2 × 100 mg capsules	Three times daily
	1 × 250 mg capsule	Twice daily
Didanosine	2 × 100 mg tablets	Twice daily (if ≥60 kg)[a]
Zalcitabine	1 × 0.75 mg tablet	Three times daily
Stavudine	1 × 40 mg capsule	Twice daily (if ≥60 kg)
	1 × 30 mg capsule	Twice daily (if ≥60 kg)
Lamivudine	1 × 150 mg tablet	Twice daily
Combivir (lamivudine/zidovudine)	1 × 150 mg/300 mg capsule	Twice daily
Abacavir	1 × 300 mg tablet	Twice daily
Nevirapine	1 × 200 mg tablet	Twice daily[b]
Delavirdine	4 × 100 mg tablets	Three times daily[c]
Efavirenz	3 × 200 mg capsules	Once daily[d]
Indinavir	2 × 400 mg capsules	Three times daily[e]
	2 × 400 mg capsules	Twice daily with ritonavir 100 mg twice daily[f]
Saquinavir soft gel	6 × 200 mg capsules	Three times daily[g]
	2 × 200 mg capsules	Twice daily with ritonavir 400 mg twice daily
Ritanovir	7.5 ml[h] or 600 mg soft elastic capsule[i]	Twice daily
Nelfinavir	3 × 250 mg tablets	Three times daily[j]
	5 × 250 mg tablets	Twice daily
	3 × 250 mg tablets	Twice daily with ritonavir 400 mg twice daily
Amprenavir	4 × 200 mg capsules	Three times daily

[a]Take 1 or 2 h after a meal.
[b]For first 14 days of therapy, 1 × 200 mg tablet, once daily.
[c]Take 1 h or more away from didanosine and antacid.
[d]Take at night to minimize noticeable side-effects.
[e]Take 1 h before or 2 h after meal, or; take 1 h or more away from didanosine and antacids (drink 2 litres of liquid daily).
[f]Can be taken without regard to food (reviewed in Swanstrom et al., 2000).
[g]Take immediately after a meal.
[h]For first 4 days, 4 ml twice daily; for next 4 days, 4 ml twice daily; for next 4 days, 6 ml twice daily, then full dose. Take with meals.
[i]300 mg twice daily initially, increasing to 600 mg twice daily over 2 weeks.
[j]Take with meal or snack.

buffer contains aluminum and therefore tetracyclines should not be co-administered with didanosine. Drugs that are causally linked with pancreatitis (e.g. pentamidine) or those that cause peripheral neuropathy (e.g. zalcitabine, vincristine) should not be co-administered with didanosine (Lelacheur and Simon, 1991).

Major adverse reactions

Peripheral neuropathy and pancreatitis are the most important adverse reactions to didanosine therapy (see Chapter 6 for details of toxicity). The most frequent toxicity is a peripheral neuropathy, which is dose related, predominantly sensory, bilateral, symmetrical, and generally reversible within 3–5 weeks of cessation of therapy (Cooley et al., 1990). Pancreatitis may be fatal, is dose related, and occurs in up to 2% of patients, particularly those with advanced HIV disease (Yarchoan et al., 1990; Schindzielorz et al., 1994). Elevations in serum amylase, lipase or triglycerides may precede symptoms of pancreatitis (Seidlin et al., 1992) and patients receiving didanosine should have serum amylase and triglyceride levels monitored routinely. Hyperglycaemia and diabetes mellitus have been reported in patients receiving didanosine (Munshi et al., 1994). Haematological toxicity is generally not a concern in patients treated with didanosine (Connolly et al., 1991). Diarrhoea is common, but rarely requires discontinuing the drug.

Major clinical use

Didanosine has been used in the past as monotherapy (Cooley et al., 1990; Hartman et al., 1990; Lambert et al., 1990; Valentine et al., 1990; Connolly et al., 1991; Kahn et al., 1992), and in combination with zidovudine (Ragni et al., 1995; Delta Co-ordinating Committee, 1996; Hammer et al., 1996). Didanosine is now only used in combination with another NRTI and either one or more PIs or an NNRTI (see Chapter 7).

Zalcitabine

Zalcitabine is the nucleoside analogue of the pyrimidine cytidine. The drug is marketed by Roche (Roche Laboratories, Nutley, NJ, USA) under the trade name Hivid®.

In vitro activity

Zalcitabine is more potent *in vitro* than didanosine on a molar basis and inhibits HIV replication about as well as zidovudine (Jeffries, 1989). The IC_{99} of zalcitabine is 0.5–1 μM, and the IC_{50} is in the range of 0.03–0.5 μM, with the reported maximal plasma concentrations being 0.25–0.6 μM (Klecker et al., 1988). Zalcitabine has activity against other HIV subtypes, including group O, which is resistant to certain NNRTIs (Descamps et al., 1995).

With zidovudine, zalcitabine has synergistic activity against zidovudine-sensitive and zidovudine-resistant strains of HIV-1 *in vitro* (Eron et al., 1992). Saquinavir and certain NNRTIs also have additive to synergistic effects with zalcitabine (Craig et al., 1990; Chong et al., 1994). GM-CSF has been reported to slightly reduce the inhibitory effect of both zalcitabine and didanosine (Perno et al., 1992), but the clinical significance of this observation is unclear.

Resistance

Zalcitabine resistance arises more slowly than resistance to zidovudine during *in vitro* passage of HIV (Shirasaka et al., 1993). A single mutation within the reverse transcriptase gene is sufficient to cause resistance. The following mutations have been reported to confer reduced susceptibility to zalcitabine: Lys 65 Arg/Asn; Thr 69 Asp; Leu 74 Val; Val 75 Thr and Met 184 Val (this last mutation is also associated with resistance to didanosine, lamivudine and abacavir). Zalcitabine-resistant strains are infrequently recovered from patients receiving prolonged zalcitabine monotherapy; resistant strains were not found in a study of patients receiving zidovudine and zalcitabine combination therapy (Richman et al., 1994b).

In general, zalcitabine-resistant strains remain sensitive to zidovudine but become resistant to didanosine (mutations in codons 65, 74, 75 and 184). The resistant strain may also be cross-resistant to lamivudine (mutations in codons 65, 184) and stavudine (mutation in codon 75).

Clinically relevant pharmacokinetics

Dosage and administration. Zalcitabine is available as tablets containing 0.375 and 0.75 mg. The dose of zalcitabine for adults is 0.75 mg administered every 8 h (Table 5.3). Children may be given a dose of 0.01 mg/kg every 8 h (Spector, 1994). Zalcitabine has excellent oral bioavailability (70–88%) in persons with HIV infection), with a modest reduction in absorption if taken with food (Table 5.4), resulting in a lower maximal concentration (C_{max}) reduced by 35%) and slower time (T_{max}) to achieve this concentration (Gustavson et al., 1990). Zalcitabine has a low CSF:plasma ratio (0.1:0.2), which is similar to that of didanosine but lower than zidovudine. Zalcitabine crosses the placenta by simple diffusion. Glomerular filtration and tubular secretion are the major mechanisms involved in the clearance of zalcitabine (Klecker et al., 1988). There is minimal first-pass metabolism of zalcitabine.

Important drug interactions

Zalcitabine should not be co-administered with drugs that cause pancreatitis and should be used with extreme caution with drugs that cause peripheral neuropathy (see Chapter 6).

Major adverse reactions

The major toxicity of zalcitabine is development of a dose-related peripheral neuropathy that occurs in up to 30% of patients taking 2.25 mg of zalcitabine daily (see

Table 5.4 Major pharmacokinetic features of antiretroviral drugs

	Absorption in humans	Effect of food	CSF:plasma ratio	Cytochrome p450 metabolism	Excretion
Didanosine	35%	↓	0.2	No	Renal(50%)
Zidovudine	46–69%	↔	0.6	No	Renal
Zalcitabine	70–88%	Mild↓	0.1–0.2	No	Renal
Lamivudine	80%	↔	0.05–0.3	No	Renal (70%)
Stavudine	70–90%	↔	0.3–0.5	No	Renal (33%)
Abacavir	80%	↔	0.3	No	Renal (80%)
Nevirapine	>90%	↔	0.45	Yes	Renal
Delavirdine	85%	↓	0.04	Yes	Renal (50%)
Efavirenz	16% (in rats)	↔	0.6	Yes	Renal hepatobiliary (<1%)
Saquinavir	4% (hard gel) 12% (soft gel)	↑	0.01–0.06	Yes	Renal hepatobiliary (<4%) Hepatobiliary (96%)
Indinavir	60%	↓(high fat) ↔(low-fat snack)	0.02–0.76	Yes	Renal (20%)
Ritonavir	60–80%	↑	0.01	Yes	Renal (11%) Hepatobiliary (86%)
Nelfinavir	78%	↑	a	Yes	Renal (2%) Hepatobiliary (98%)
Amprenavir	>70%	↔	0.01	Yes	Hepatobiliary

aNo data currently available.

Chapter 6) (Shelton *et al.*, 1993). Similar to other NRTI-induced peripheral neuropathies, the cause is inhibition of mitochondrial function by zalcitabine (Werth *et al.*, 1994). Zalcitabine also causes pancreatitis in about 1% of recipients. Haematological toxicity is not a prominent feature of zalcitabine therapy. Apthous ulceration is not uncommon in zalcitabine recipients (McNeely *et al.*, 1989), but it may resolve with continuing treatment in some patients (Adkins *et al.*, 1997).

Major clinical use

In the past, zalcitabine has been used as monotherapy, based on clinical trials (Merigan *et al.*, 1989; Fischl *et al.*, 1993; Abrams *et al.*, 1994) but was generally less commonly used in this manner than zidovudine and didanosine. It was also demonstrated to have efficacy in combination with zidovudine (Meng *et al.*, 1990; Fischl *et al.*, 1995; Schooley *et al.*, 1996) and saquinavir (Collier *et al.*, 1996). Currently the place of zalcitabine is in combination therapy with another NRTI and one or two PIs or an NNRTI.

Lamivudine

Lamivudine is the dideoxynucleoside analogue of the pyrimidine cytidine. The drug is marketed by Glaxo Wellcome under the trade names 3TC® and Epivir® and in combination with zidovudine as Combivir®.

In vitro *activity*

The IC_{90} of lamivudine against HIV replication in T lymphocytes is approximately 0.1 μM (Gray *et al.*, 1995), well below the C_{max} of lamivudine (about 7 μM) and the trough plasma concentrations (about 0.7 μM) (St Clair *et al.*, 1995). Lamivudine also inhibits hepatitis B virus replication. Lamivudine is additive to synergistic against HIV replication *in vitro* with zidovudine, zalcitabine, didanosine, stavudine, nevirapine and saquinavir (Merrill *et al.*, 1996). Ganciclovir and ciprofloxacin have been found to reduce the activity of lamivudine by two- to threefold *in vitro* (Glaxo Wellcome, unpubl. data).

Resistance

Passage of HIV-infected cells in increasing concentrations of lamivudine results in the rapid emergence of high-level resistance to the drug (Tisdale *et al.*, 1993). Similarly, patients treated with lamivudine monotherapy developed evidence of resistant strains within weeks of starting therapy (as early as 1 week in some patients) (Schuurman *et al.*, 1995). Mutations in codons 44 and 118 have been associated with ~tenfold reduction in susceptibility to lamivudine in the absence of the 184 mutation (Hertogs *et al.*, 2000). High-level resistance (greater than a hundredfold reduction in susceptibility) can develop following a single mutation (Met 184 Val)

lama et al., 1996; CAESAR Co-ordinating Committee, 1997). Due to its low toxicity, good bioavailability and recognized clinical efficacy in combination, therapy lamivudine is a common component of combination regimens (see Chapter 7).

Stavudine

Stavudine (d4T) is a nucleoside analogue of the pyrimidine thymidine. The drug is marketed by Bristol-Myers-Squibb under the trade name of Zerit®.

In vitro activity

Stavudine and zidovudine inhibit HIV-1 replication in vitro at equivalent concentrations, with the stavudine IC_{50} being about 0.2 μM (Friedland et al., 1996) and a C_{max} of 3 μM (Seifert et al., 1994). Stavudine is additive to synergistic with zalcitabine, didanosine, lamivudine, saquinavir, and nevirapine. Although data remain controversial, it is generally accepted that stavudine is antagonistic with zidovudine by inhibiting the intracellular phosphorylation of zidovudine (Ho and Hitchcock, 1989) and this combination should be avoided in patients (Carpenter et al., 1998).

Resistance

Resistance has been reported to stavudine both in vitro and in treated patients, with at least two mutations conferring resistance (Val 75 Thr and Ile 50 Thr). In patients treated with stavudine the development of resistance is associated only with the appearance of Val 75 Thr (Lacey and Larder, 1994) (Table 5.2). Resistance to stavudine develops slowly and in a minority of treated patients (20%) after 18–22 months of therapy in one study) (reviewed in Moyle 1995). The codon 75 mutation also results in cross-resistance to didanosine and zalcitabine (Lacey and Larder, 1994). Zidovudine-associated resistance mutations are now known to confer reduced susceptibility to stavudine.

Clinically relevant pharmacokinetics

Stavudine is available as capsules containing 15 mg, 20 mg, 30 mg and 40 mg of stavudine and has recently also become available as a powder for oral solution containing 1 mg/ml. The dose of stavudine is 40 mg twice daily in adult patients who weigh 60 kg or more, and 30 mg twice daily in those less than 60 kg (Table 5.3). The dose should be modified in patients with renal

(Boucher et al., 1993b, Table 5.2). Another mutation in this codon (Met 184 Ile) also results in resistance to zidovudine, but if it occurs in a zidovudine-resistant strain of HIV that has mutations in codons 41 and 215, the strain reverts to zidovudine-susceptible (Boucher et al., 1995b). A mutation in codon 333 causes resistance to both zidovudine and lamivudine (Kemp et al., 1998).

Clinically relevant pharmacokinetics

Lamivudine is available as 150 mg tablets. Combivir® is available as a tablet containing 150 mg lamivudine and 300 mg zidovudine. The dose of lamivudine for adults is 150 mg administered twice daily (Table 5.3). In children aged 3 months to 12 years, the dose is 8 mg/kg daily in two divided doses. The oral bioavailability of lamivudine is 80% (65%) in children; hence the higher dose in this group). The drug can be taken without regard to food (Table 5.3). The penetration of lamivudine into CSF is poor, with CSF:plasma ratios ranging from 0.05 to 0.3. There are no data published regarding placental transfer of lamivudine. Most (about 70%) of an oral dose of lamivudine is excreted unchanged in the urine (van Leeuwen et al., 1992).

Important drug interactions

There are no known major drug interactions with lamivudine. Co-trimoxazole results in an increase in plasma concentrations of lamivudine (45% increase in the area-under-the-curve [AUC]) and reduces its clearance. There are no significant interactions when zidovudine is co-administrated with lamivudine, although the C_{max} and AUC for zidovudine increase modestly.

Major adverse reactions

Virtually no major toxicities of lamivudine have been reported in adults. However, up to 15% of children in two studies developed pancreatitis and thus lamivudine should be avoided in patients with a history of, or with risk factors for pancreatitis.

Major clinical use

It was quickly recognized that lamivudine was unsuitable for use as monotherapy due to the rapid emergence of resistance (Schuurman et al., 1995; van Leeuwen et al., 1995). However, when used in combination with zidovudine, reductions in viral load and improvement in CD4 lymphocyte counts were sustained in participants in clinical trials (Eron et al., 1995; Staszewski, 1995; Kat-

impairment. The optimal paediatric dose of stavudine has not been established. Stavudine has good bioavailability (in the range of 70–90%) (Dudley et al., 1992). The drug may be taken without regard for food (Table 4.4). Stavudine crosses the placenta by simple diffusion (Bawdon et al., 1994). The CSF:plasma ratio of stavudine ranges from 0.3 to 0.5 (Bristol-Myers Squibb, unpubl. data). About one-third of the administered dose of stavudine is excreted unchanged in the urine (Dudley et al., 1992), via glomerular filtration and tubular secretion. The rest of the dose of stavudine is probably cleaved to form thymidine (Dudley, 1995).

Important drug interactions

There are no significant drug interactions with stavudine, apart from that described with zidovudine. Didanosine and stavudine may cause peripheral neuropathy, and this combination is now recommended for use with caution.

Major adverse reactions

Like didanosine and zalcitabine, stavudine causes a dose-related, predominantly sensory peripheral neuropathy, which is more common in patients with a prior history of neuropathy and generally resolves on cessation of therapy (Skowron, 1995). This is predominantly due to mitochondrial toxicity, which may also be responsible for lipoatrophy. Serum lactate levels should be monitored in patients receiving stavudine therapy. Serum stavudine is more potent in causing inhibition of mitochondrial metabolism than didanosine and zidovudine but less so than zalcitabine; abacavir has least effect of the NRTIs on mitochondria (Chen et al., 1991).

Major clinical use

Stavudine was used initially as monotherapy, based on efficacy demonstrated in clinical trials (Browne et al., 1993; Anderson et al., 1995; Kline et al., 1995; Murray et al., 1995; Petersen et al., 1995; Skowron, 1995). It is currently a common component of combination therapy (see Chapter 7). A comparison of lamivudine in combination with either stavudine or zidovudine found both regimens to be equally efficacious (Foudraine et al., 1998).

Abacavir

Abacavir (1592U89) is a synthetic carbocyclic nucleoside analogue of guanine. It exerts its activity after intracellular phosphorylation to carbovir triphosphate (Faletto et al., 1997). The drug is marketed by Glaxo Wellcome under the trade name of Ziagen®.

In vitro activity

Abacavir has similar potency in vitro to zidovudine (Foster and Faulds, 1998). The IC_{50} of abacavir is in the range of 0.26 μM for clinical isolates of HIV-1 (Daluge et al., 1997) with a C_{max} of about 10 μM. (1 μM = 0.28 μg/ml). Abacavir has been reported to have synergistic activity against HIV-1 with amprenavir, nevirapine and zidovudine, and additive activity with didanosine, lamivudine, stavudine and zalcitabine (Daluge et al., 1997; Drusano et al., 1998).

Resistance

Resistance to abacavir develops relatively slowly when compared to certain other NRTIs (Foster and Faulds, 1998). Resistant strains of HIV-1 have been isolated from patients treated with abacavir; these strains have had Leu 74 Val and Met 184 Val mutations, with the Lys 65 Arg and Tyr 115 Phe mutations also occurring. The codon 184 mutation alone (which may arise from lamivudine therapy) results in only low-level resistance (less than fivefold reduction in susceptibility) and at least one additional mutation is required for high-level resistance (Tisdale et al., 1997; Miller et al., 1998; Hirsch et al., 2000; Table 5.2). Some abacavir-resistant strains of HIV-1 are cross-resistant to didanosine, zalcitabine and lamivudine but not to zidovudine or stavudine (Tisdale et al., 1997).

Clinically relevant pharmacokinetics

Abacavir is available as tablets containing 300 mg of abacavir and as an oral solution (20 mg/ml). The dose of abacavir for adults is 300 mg twice daily (Table 5.3). The paediatric dose is 8 mg/kg up to a maximum of 300 mg twice daily. Abacavir is rapidly absorbed after oral administration, with bioavailability assessed as being about 80%. It may be taken without regard for food (Table 5.4). The CSF:plasma ratio of abacavir is 0.27–0.33. Abacavir is metabolized via glucuronyl transferase and alcohol dehydrogenase to form inactive metabolites and is not metabolized by the cytochrome p450 pathway. The drug is excreted predominantly in urine, largely as these metabolites (5′ carboxylic acid derivative and 5′ glucuronide derivative), with less than 1% being abacavir itself.

Major clinical use

Abacavir is used only in combination with other antiretroviral agents, usually one or two other RIs, and one or two PIs (see Chapter 7) (Kadama et al., 2000; Khanna et al., 2000).

Major adverse reactions

Hypersensitivity reactions (manifest as maculopapular or urticarial skin rash, fever, gastrointestinal symptoms, which may rarely progress to multiorgan failure) have been associated with abacavir therapy in about 5% of patients. In all patients with hypersensitivity, the drug should be ceased immediately as symptoms worsen with continued therapy or with rechallenge (see Chapter 6). Abacavir has been associated with nausea and vomiting in up to one-third of patients taking this drug in combination with zidovudine and lamivudine. Mild elevation of blood glucose and serum triglyceride levels has been reported with infrequent elevation of liver enzymes and pancreatitis. Lactic acidosis, in association with steatosis and severe hepatomegaly, has been reported in patients receiving abacavir in combination with other antiretroviral drugs. Obesity and prolonged exposure to nucleoside analogues may increase the risk.

Important drug interactions

Moderately heavy alcohol consumption (e.g. five standard drinks per day) increases the AUC of abacavir by about 40%, without altering the pharmacokinetics of the alcohol.

Non-nucleoside analogue reverse transcriptase inhibitors (NNRTIs)

These compounds are unrelated chemically. They only inhibit HIV-1 replication and have no activity against the reverse transcriptase of HIV-2. They are also generally inactive against group O strains of HIV-1 (Descamps et al., 1997). They do not require intra-cellular phosphorylation for their activity. Their mode of action is solely through inhibition of reverse transcriptase and they do not cause DNA chain termination (reviewed in Kucers et al., 1997; Moyle, 2001).

Nevirapine

Nevirapine is a dipyridodiazepinone derivative. It is marketed by Boehringer-Ingelheim (Sydney, Australia) under the trade name of Viramune®.

In vitro activity

Nevirapine potently inhibits HIV-1 with an IC_{50} value ranging from 0.015 to 0.04 µM, far less than the plasma trough levels of 16 µM (Havlir et al., 1995a). Additive to synergistic interactions occur in vitro between nevirapine and zidovudine, lamivudine, didanosine, stavudine and saquinavir (Richman et al., 1991a; Gu et al., 1995; Merrill et al., 1996). Delavirdine has been reported to be antagonistic with nevirapine in vitro (Gu et al., 1995).

Resistance

Resistance to nevirapine appears very rapidly in vitro (Table 5.5) due to the rapid development of reverse transcriptase gene mutations in codons 180-188 and 100-110. These mutations affect the binding pocket of NNRTIs, which is adjacent to the catalytic site of the enzyme (Nunberg et al., 1991; Larder, 1992; Larder, 1995). The Tyr 181 Cys mutation is found in all nevirapine-resistant strains of HIV-1 (Mellors et al., 1992) and results in a hundredfold or greater decrease in susceptibility to nevirapine (Richman et al., 1991b). A codon 188 mutation is also of major importance in the development of nevirapine resistance (Richman et al., 1991b). HIV-1 isolated from patients receiving nevirapine monotherapy was found to accumulate mutations in codon 181 (80% of patients by week 8 of therapy) and in codon 188, 103, 106, 108 and 190 (Dueweke et al., 1993a; Richman et al., 1994a; Hirsch et al., 2000; Table 5.5). Co-administration of zidovudine with nevirapine suppresses the 181 mutation but other mutations still emerge (Richman et al., 1994a). Sustained virological suppression may be maintained in some patients, despite the acquisition of mutations that confer resistance to nevirapine.

Clinically relevant pharmacokinetics

Dosage and administration. Nevirapine is available as 200 mg tablets and in adults the dose is 200 mg daily for the first 14 days and 200 mg twice daily thereafter (Table 5.3). This sequence is important because for the first 2 weeks of therapy nevirapine induces cytochrome p450 enzymes (metabolic autoinduction) that are necessary for its metabolism (reviewed in Carr and Cooper, 1996). If the lower dose is not given initially, the incidence of rash due to nevirapine is greatly increased.

In children aged 2 months to 8 years the recommended dose is 4 mg/kg once daily for the first 14 days and then 7 mg/kg given twice daily thereafter. For older chil-

Table 5.5 Mutations in reverse transcriptase gene codons that confer resistance to NNRTIs

Nevirapine	Delavirdine	Efavirenz
L100I		L100I
K103N[a]	K103N[a]	K103I/N/A[a]
V106[a]		
V108I[a]		Y188L*
Y181C/I[a]	Y181C[a]	
Y188CL/H[a]		
G190A[a]		G190S/A[a]
		P225H
	P236L	

[a]Mutations, which are often the first selected during viral evolution under drug pressure. These primary mutations cause resistance due to reduced binding of the inhibitor. All other mutations are secondary, and contribute to resistance. This list is not complete, and requires regular updating (data from Hirsch et al., 2000; O'Brien, 2000; Schinazi et al., 2000).

dren, the initial starting dose is 4 mg/kg per day for the first 14 days, followed by 4 mg/kg twice daily thereafter.

Absorption. The oral bioavailability of nevirapine is greater than 90% (reviewed in Carr and Cooper, 1996). The drug can be taken without regard for food (Table 5.4).

Distribution. The CSF:plasma ratio is approximately 0.45. In an *in vitro* model, the order of permeability of the blood–brain barrier to antiretroviral drugs was nevirapine ≫ didanosine, stavudine, zalcitabine, zidovudine > indinavir > saquinavir (Glynn and Yazdanian, 1998). Nevirapine also crosses the placenta and is present in breast milk.

Metabolism. Nevirapine is metabolized predominantly by the hepatic cytochrome p450 pathway, followed by glucuronidation. During the first 14 days of nevirapine therapy there is metabolic autoinduction of cytochrome p450 enzymes, resulting in a decrease in the plasma half-life from 43 to 23 h. About 80% of an oral dose of nevirapine is excreted via the kidneys.

Important drug interactions

As nevirapine induces cytochrome p450 enzymes, the plasma level of any other drug metabolized by this system may be decreased in patients receiving nevirapine. Alternatively, inducers of cytochrome p450 such as rifabutin and rifampicin may alter plasma concentrations of nevirapine (see Chapter 6).

Major adverse reactions

The most common and most important adverse reaction is the development of a rash, which occurs in up to 50% of patients if they commence with a dose of 200 mg twice daily, but in only 20% when the dose is halved for the first 14 days (Havlir et al., 1995a). Stevens-Johnson syndrome may occur rarely (reviewed in Moyle, 2001).

Major clinical use

Nevirapine monotherapy is associated with rapid development of resistance (Grob et al., 1992; De-Jong et al., 1994; Havlir et al., 1995a, b; Carr and Cooper, 1996; D'Aquila et al., 1996), and the drug is only used in combination with other antiretroviral drugs, usually with two NRTIs, with or without one PI (Montaner et al., 1998a) (see Chapter 7).

Delavirdine

Delavirdine mesylate is a bisheteroarylpiperazine (BHAP) derivative that is active against the reverse transcriptase of HIV-1. It is marketed by Pharmacia and Upjohn (Kelamazoon, MI, USA) under the trade name of Rescriptor®.

In vitro *activity*

Although delavirdine is active against HIV-1, most work relates solely to subtype B strains. Group O HIV-1 may not be inhibited by delavirdine. The IC_{50} and IC_{90} of delavirdine against clinical isolates of HIV-1 are 0.001–0.7 μM and 0.1 μM, respectively (Dueweke et al., 1993b; Nottet et al., 1994), which is significantly less than the steady-state C_{max} of 35 μM and trough levels of 10 μM. However, plasma concentrations of delavirdine vary greatly between individuals, ranging from 1 to 60 μM (reviewed in Havlir and Lange, 1998). Additive to synergistic interactions exist between delavirdine and zidovudine, didanosine, zalcitabine (Campbell et al., 1993; Chong et al., 1994). Delavirdine and nevirapine are antagonistic *in vitro* (Gu et al., 1995).

Resistance

Delavirdine monotherapy results in high-level resistance (between fifty- and five-hundredfold reduction in susceptibility within 8 weeks of starting therapy). Resistance is due primarily to the Lys 103 Asn mutation and secondarily to Tyr 181 Lys and Pro 236 Leu mutations in the reverse transcriptase gene (Fan et al., 1995; Freimuth, 1996).

Delavirdine is available as 100 mg tablets. The oral dose of delavirdine for adults is 400 mg three times daily (Table 5.3). The oral bioavailability of delavirdine is about 85%. Although delavirdine may be taken without regard for food, food slightly reduces the peak plasma concentration (by about 20%). A high-fat meal reduces the C_{max} by about 60%. The CSF:plasma ratio of delavirdine is low – about 0.04. Delavirdine is metabolized primarily by cytochrome p450 isoenzyme and particularly CYP3A4 (probably CYP2D6) in hepatic microsomes. Delavirdine inhibits CYP3A4 and thus inhibits its own metabolism. Half of the drug is excreted in the faeces and half in the urine (less than 5% unchanged).

Major clinical use

Delavirdine is less commonly used than nevirapine or efavirenz. It is useful only in combination with other antiretroviral agents and is most often used in combination with two NRTIs (reviewed in Freimuth, 1996; also in Havlir and Lange, 1998) and is not used in combination with another NNRTI (see Chapter 7).

Major adverse reactions

Skin rash (macular, often pruritic) is a common adverse reaction, being reported in up to 20% of patients receiving delavirdine in combination with other antiretrovirals (see Chapter 6). In most cases patients can continue therapy and the rash disappears in less than 2 weeks (Freimuth, 1996). Other common side-effects include nausea and vomiting.

Important drug interactions

Inducers of cytochrome p450, including rifampicin, rifabutin and phenytoin, reduce the plasma concentrations of delavirdine (see Chapter 6). As delavirdine inhibits CYP3A4, it may inhibit the metabolism of drugs, including terfenadine, midazolam and cisapride (and the PI). Serum levels of coumadin (warfarin) may be prolonged.

Clinically relevant pharmacokinetics

Efavirenz

Efavirenz (DMP 266) is a benzoxazinone derivative NNRTI with activity against HIV-1 reverse transcriptase (Young et al., 1995). It is marketed by DuPont Merck (Wilmington, DE, USA) under the trade name of Sustiva® (reviewed in Moyle, 2001).

In vitro activity in relation to plasma levels

The IC_{90} to IC_{95} of efavirenz ranges from 1.7 to 25 μM for both laboratory-adapted strains and clinical isolates of HIV-1. This is well below the steady-state C_{max} of about 13 μM and trough level of 5.6 μM in patients receiving 600 mg daily. Efavirenz is synergistic in vitro with zidovudine, didanosine and indinavir.

Resistance

In direct comparison to nevirapine and delavirdine, selection of resistant mutants of HIV to efavirenz requires multiple passages in vitro (Winslow et al., 1996). The Val 179 Asp, Leu 100 Ile and Tyr 181 Cys reverse transcriptor mutations have been reported to reduce efavirenz susceptibility of HIV strains by up to a thousand fold (Winslow et al., 1996). In patients receiving efavirenz in combination with one or more NRTIs or indinavir, the Lys 103 Arg mutation was most commonly seen at the time of virological rebound, often followed by the development of mutations codons 108, 188 and 225, and less frequently in 100, 101 and 190 (Bacheler et al., 1998; Hirsch et al., 2000; Schinazi et al., 2000, Table 5.5). Efavirenz-resistant strains of HIV-1 are cross-resistant to nevirapine and delavirdine.

Clinically relevant pharmacokinetics

Dosage and administration. Efavirenz is available as capsules containing 50 mg, 100 mg or 200 mg. The adult dose of efavirenz is 600 mg daily (usually taken at night to minimize side-effects) (Table 5.3). Paediatric dosing is according to weight for children over 3 years of age (see Table 5.6). Once daily dosing is possible because of the very long (40-53 h) half-life of efavirenz (Ruiz and DuPont Merck Study Group, 1997). The oral bioavailability of efavirenz is 16% in rats (Young et al., 1995) but has not been reported in humans. High-fat meals may increase the absorption of efavirenz, but otherwise the drug may be taken with or without food (Table 5.4). Efavirenz is 99% protein bound (Bacheler et al., 1997) and has a CSF:plasma ratio of about 0.6 (Tashima et al., 1998), with wide patient-to-patient variability (range 0.26-1.19) in patients receiving a daily dose of 200-600 mg. Efavirenz is mainly metabolized by the hepatic cytochrome p450 pathway (isoenzymes 3A4 and 2B6) to hydroxylated metabolites, followed by glucuronidation. Efavirenz induces these enzymes (metabolic auto-induction). The drug has a long plasma half-life of 40-55 h, allowing once daily dosing. Less than 1% of an oral dose of efavirenz is excreted in urine.

Important drug interactions

As efavirenz is metabolized via cytochrome p450 pathways, interactions may be expected with other drugs metabolized via this route (see Chapter 6). Efavirenz induces cytochrome p450 isoenzymes, including CYP3A4; it may hasten the metabolism of drugs that use this pathway, such as saquinavir and indinavir plasma concentrations of these PI are significantly reduced when administered with efavirenz. The level by which ritonavir inhibits cytochrome CYP3A4 is similar to the level at which efavirenz inhibits ritonavir's metabolism; thus, the effects of the two drugs on each other's metabolism cancel one another out (Fiske *et al.*, 1998). Drugs that induce CYP3A4 (e.g. rifampin, rifabutin) would be expected to accelerate clearance of efavirenz and thus to lower its plasma concentrations (Benedek *et al.*, 1998).

Major adverse reactions

The major side-effects of efavirenz, seen in over 50% of patients, involve the central nervous system: dizziness, impairment of concentration, drowsiness, insomnia, abnormally vivid dreams, and rarely delusions and severe depression. Symptoms tend to occur within the first few days of therapy and resolve within 2–4 weeks. Rash (rarely Stevens-Johnson syndrome and erythema multiforme) occurs in up to one-quarter of recipients, again being most frequent during the first few weeks of therapy and requiring cessation of treatment in about 1% of patients. Increases in fasting serum cholesterol levels have been observed in a minority of recipients.

Major clinical use

Efavirenz is used clinically only in combination with other antiretroviral drugs, as monotherapy rapidly induces resistance. It is most commonly used in combination with two NRTIs with or without a PI (Mayers *et al.*, 1997; Riddler

Table 5.6 Recommended dosing of efavirenz for children over the age of 3 years, based on weight

Child's weight	Dosing
10–15 kg	200 mg
15–20 kg	250 mg
20–25 kg	300 mg
25–32.5 kg	350 mg
32.5–40 kg	400 mg
Over 40 kg	600 mg

et al., 1997; Staszewski *et al.*, 1998). It is not used in combination with other NNRTIs (see Chapter 7).

Other non-nucleoside reverse transcriptase inhibitors

MKC-442 (Triangle Pharmaceuticals) is now in phase III clinical trials (Pederson *et al.*, 2000). DPC 083 and 961 are second-generation NNRTIs (Dupont Merck), which are undergoing evaluation.

Protease inhibitors

The HIV aspartyl protease is encoded by the *gag* gene and expressed as part of the Gag-Pol polyprotein. The protease is responsible for cleavage of the Gag polyprotein, a process that occurs soon after the virion buds from the cell membrane and which is necessary for maturation of the virion. HIV PIs prevent cleavage of these proteins, resulting in the production of immature, non-infectious virions (reviewed in Kucers *et al.*, 1997). PIs inhibit acute HIV infection of cells as well as chronically-infected cells, although the activity is up to twentyfold lower than in acutely-infected cells (Perno *et al.*, 1998).

All the HIV PIs described below are metabolized via cytochrome p450 enzymes, predominantly CYP3A4 (Fitzsimmons and Collins, 1997; Kumar *et al.*, 1997). These drugs can also inhibit or induce cytochrome p450 enzymes; ritonavir is the most potent inhibitor of cytochrome p450, while saquinavir is the weakest (Fitzsimmons and Collins, 1997). Toxicities and drug interactions are detailed in Chapter 5, and the clinical use of these antiretroviral drugs is detailed in the Chapter 7.

In general (for all PIs), a single mutation within the protease results in only a modest reduction in susceptibility, with further mutations needing to accumulate before high-level resistance occurs (reviewed in Flexner, 1998).

Saquinavir

Saquinavir mesylate is a potent inhibitor of HIV protease, with virtually no activity against human aspartic proteases. It is marketed under the brand names of Invirase® (hard-gel capsule) and Fortovase® (soft-gel capsule, both by Roche Laboratories).

In vitro activity

The IC_{90} of saquinavir against HIV-1 is 6–30 nM (Craig *et al.*, 1991; Eberle *et al.*, 1995), which is markedly less than the steady-state plasma C_{max} of approximately 2500 nM (Flexner, 1998). Saquinavir shows additive to synergistic activity with zidovudine, zalcitabine, lamivudine, stavudine, and some NRTIs (Craig et al., 1990; Johnson et al., 1992; Craig et al., 1994; Merrill et al., 1996). Saquinavir and indinavir are antagonistic in action (Merrill et al., 1997).

Resistance

Resistance to saquinavir develops fairly slowly *in vitro* and to a modest degree when compared with NRTIs such as lamivudine and NNRTIs such as efavirenz.

The mutations leading to saquinavir resistance develop in stepwise fashion, starting with Gly 48 Val, with Leu 90 Met and/or Ile 54 Val appearing later (Turriziani et al., 1994; Tisdale et al., 1995) (Table 5.7). Together these mutations result in a fiftyfold increase in the IC_{90} (Eberle et al., 1995). In patients who develop resistance to saquinavir, the codon 90 mutation is most frequently detected; codon 48 mutation is uncommon and the double mutation is rare (Boucher, 1996; Jacobsen et al., 1996). Other mutations have been reported (in codons 36, 71, 82, 84) (Ives et al., 1997). There is cross-resistance of varying degrees between saquinavir and other PIs.

Clinically relevant pharmacokinetics

Dosage and administration. Saquinavir is available in hard-gelatin (200 mg) and soft-gelatin (200 mg) capsules and in powder and liquid paediatric formulations. The adult dose is 600 mg three times daily for the hard-gel capsule and 1200 mg three times daily for the soft-gel capsule (Table 5.3). The dose of saquinavir should be decreased if saquinavir is used with ritonavir (Merry et al., 1997). Saquinavir at a dose of 400 mg twice daily can be administered with ritonavir 400 mg twice daily (Buss, 2000).

Absorption. A high-fat meal increases the bioavailability of saquinavir (Flexner, 1998) and the drug should be taken with meals (Table 5.4). Saquinavir hard-gel has low oral bioavailability (less than 4%) (Noble and Faulds, 1996); unrefined grapefruit juice improves absorption of saquinavir. The soft-gel formulation of saquinavir is absorbed about three times better than the hard-gel capsules (Buss et al., 1998), and the steady-state AUC for the soft-gel is eightfold higher than that of the hard-gel formulation (reviewed in Perry and Noble, 1998).

Distribution. Saquinavir is highly protein bound. Due to high protein binding, the CSF:plasma ratio of saquinavir is low, in the range of 0.01–0.06 (Flexner, 1998).

Metabolism. Saquinavir is predominantly metabolized in the liver by cytochrome p450 isoenzyme CYP3A4 to inactive derivatives (Farrar et al., 1994; Fitzsimmons and Collins, 1997). Renal excretion accounts for only 4% of the drug; the remainder is found in the faeces.

Important drug interactions

As saquinavir is metabolized via cytochrome p450, any drug that is a substrate, inducer or inhibitor of the enzymes should be used with caution (see Chapter 6). Inhibitors of cytochrome p450 such as ketoconazole significantly increase the plasma concentration of saquinavir (reviewed in Flexner, 1998). Inducers of cytochrome p450, such as rifampin, increase the metabolism of saquinavir and significantly reduce the plasma concentration of saquinavir (Anon., 1996); saquinavir and rifampin cotherapy is contraindicated (reviewed in Vella and Floridia, 1998). Saquinavir is not an inducer or significant inhibitor of cytochrome p450 (reviewed in Flexner, 1998). However, it is recommended that saquinavir should not be co-administered with terfenadine, midazolam cisapride or astemizole. Indinavir, nelfinavir and ritonavir increase the plasma concentrations of saquinavir by up to fivefold, fivefold and thirtyfold, respectively (Cohen et al., 1996; Merry et al., 1997; McCrea et al., 1997).

Major adverse reactions

Saquinavir is well tolerated. The major adverse effects are elevation of serum aminotransferase levels (although hepatitis rarely develops) (Brau et al., 1997), increased serum cholesterol and triglyceride levels in association with lipodystrophy and glucose intolerance (Carr et al., 1998), and gastrointestinal symptoms, particularly with the soft-gel formulation.

Major clinical use

Saquinavir is generally used in combination with two NRTIs (Collier et al., 1996). In some patients a NNRTI will be included in the regimen (Chapter 7).

Indinavir

Indinavir sulfate is an inhibitor of HIV-1 and HIV-2 protease of the hydroxyaminopentane amide class. It is marketed by Merck Sharpe and Dohme (Merck & Co., Inc.) under the trade name of Crixivan®.

In vitro activity

Indinavir has an IC_{95} of 50–100 nM against laboratory strains of HIV-1 and 20–50 μM against clinical isolates (Dorsey et al., 1994), well below the plasma C_{max} of 4.9 μM and trough levels of 0.3 μM (Stein et al., 1996). The drug is also highly active against strains of HIV-2. Indinavir is synergistic with NRTIs such as zidovudine and didanosine and several NNRTIs (Vacca et al., 1994). Antagonism between saquinavir and indinavir has been reported (Merrill et al., 1997).

Resistance

Multiple mutations are required for the development of resistance to indinavir (Tisdale et al., 1995). A Val 82 Ala/Phe mutation in the binding cleft region of the protease, in addition to other mutations, is required for phenotypic resistance in vitro (Emini et al., 1996). A Met 46 Ile/Leu mutation within the flap region is also critical for the development of resistance to indinavir (Hirsch et al., 2000; Schinazi et al., 2000; Table 5.7).

Numerous other mutations, which vary in their order of appearance, have been described in patients failing indinavir therapy, including mutations within codons 8, 10, 15, 32, 34, 36, 47, 48, 54, 57, 63, 71, 84, 90 and 93 (Condra et al., 1995a, b; Ridky and Leis, 1995; Schmit et al., 1996; Eastman et al., 1998). A number of these 'accessory' mutations have been detected in strains of HIV isolated from patients who are naïve to PI therapy and may be polymorphisms unrelated to the development of resistance (Moyle, 1998).

Cross-resistance to other PIs may result from a minimum of four mutations involving codons 46, 63, 82 and 84, with the Ile 84 Val mutation being specifically required for development of resistance to saquinavir and amprenavir (reviewed in Moyle, 1998). Changing therapy prior to emergence of important mutations such as these may preserve susceptibility to other PIs.

Table 5.7 Major mutations within HIV protease gene codons associated with resistance to protease inhibitors

Indinavir	Ritonair	Saqinavir	Nelfinavir	Amprenavir	Lopinavir	Tipranavir
L10I/R/V		L10I/R/V	L10/F/I	L10F/I/R/V	L10F	
K20/M/R	K20M/R					
L24I						
			D30N[a]			
V32I/L	V32I			V32I	V32I	
	L33F					
M36I	M36I		M36I			
M46I[a]	M46I/L		M46I/L	M46I	M46I	
				I47V	I47V	
					V47A	
		G48V[a]				
				I50V[a]		
I54V	I54V/L	I54V		I54V		
A71V/T	A71V/T	A71V/T	A71V/T			
G73S/A		G73S				
V77I	V77I	V77I	V77I			
V82A/F/T/S[a]	V82A/F/T/S[a]	V82A	V82A/F/T/S			V82T
I84V	I84V		I84V	I84A/F/T/Sa	I84V	I84V
			N88D			
L90M	L90M	L90M[a]	L90M[a]			L90M
					T91S	

[a]Mutations, which are often the first selected during viral evolution under drug pressure. These primary mutations cause resistance due to reduced binding of the inhibitor. All other mutations are secondary, and contribute to resistance. This list is not complete, and requires regular updating (data 2000 from Hirsch et al., 2000; O'Brien, 2000; Schinazi et al., 2000).

Clinically relevant pharmacokinetics

Dosage and administration. Indinavir is available as capsules containing 200 mg and 400 mg. For adults the usual dose is 800 mg every 8 h (Table 5.3). Co-administration of ritonavir with indinavir significantly increases the blood levels of the latter and allows indinavir to be dosed twice daily without food restrictions (indinavir 800 mg twice daily, plus ritonavir 100–200 mg twice daily). Indinavir 400 mg twice daily co-administered with ritonavir 400 mg twice daily is also an accepted alternative dosing schedule, although ritonavir-induced gastrointestinal side-effects may limit its use.

Absorption. Indinavir is absorbed rapidly in the fasted state, with an oral bioavailability of about 60% (Yeh et al., 1998). A high-fat meal decreases the bioavailability of indinavir; a light meal does not alter the plasma AUC. Thus, it is recommended that indinavir be taken when fasting or with a light, low-fat snack (Flexner, 1998) (Table 5.4). Preliminary data suggest that lower doses of indinavir (800 mg or 400 mg twice daily) in combination with ritonavir (100 mg or 400 mg) appear to extend the half-life of both drugs and to allow indinavir to be administered without regard for food (Hsu et al., 1998a).

Distribution. The CSF:plasma ratio of indinavir is highly variable, being reported to range from 0.02 to 0.76 (Flexner, 1998).

Metabolism. Indinavir is metabolized similarly to other PIs, via cytochrome p450 enzymes, predominantly CYP3A4. The major excretory route of indinavir is in faeces (Balani et al., 1996). Urinary excretion of indinavir is by both glomerular filtration and tubular secretion and accounts for about 20% of the oral dose, with varying but often high levels of the drug are excreted unchanged (Balani et al., 1995).

Important drug interactions. As indinavir is metabolized via cytochrome p450, any drug that is a substrate, inducer or inhibitor of the cytochrome p450 enzymes should be used with caution in patients being treated with indinavir (see Chapter 6). The dose of indinavir will need to be increased if it is used in combination with efavirenz or nevirapine.

Ketoconazole, which inhibits CYP3A4, increases the plasma concentration of indinavir (reviewed in Flexner, 1998). Rifabutin, an inducer of cytochrome p450, decreases the plasma concentration of indinavir, while that of rifabutin is increased due to inhibition of the metabolism of rifabutin by ritonavir with co-administration of these drugs (Cato et al., 1998). Drugs metabolized by the cytochrome p450 pathway, including midazolam, terfenadine and astemizole, should be avoided or used with extreme caution in indinavir-treated patients as competitive inhibition of their metabolism by indinavir may lead to high plasma levels and life-threatening reactions.

Major adverse reactions

Nephrolithiasis is probably the most serious adverse effect of indinavir, occurring in about 4% of patients receiving the drug and resulting from deposition of indinavir crystals within the kidney. Patients generally present with symptomatic renal colic associated with microscopic or macroscopic haematuria; urinary tract obstruction may occur (Gentle et al., 1997). Encouraging the patient to drink at least 2 litres of water each day helps to minimize this risk. Elevated unconjugated bilirubin levels occurred in about 10% of patients receiving indinavir in early clinical trials and hepatitis has been reported (Vergis et al., 1998). Hyperlipidaemia associated with elevated blood glucose levels and lipodystrophy have been reported with indinavir use (Carr et al., 1998), and premature coronary artery disease has been associated with PI therapy in general (see Chapters 15 and 18). Breast hypertrophy (Lui et al., 1998) and paronychia have also been associated with indinavir therapy (Bouscarat et al., 1998).

Major clinical use

Indinavir in combination with two NRTIs has been found to be very effective in reducing viral load and increasing CD4 lymphocyte counts in patients at all stages of HIV infection, including patients with prior antiretroviral therapy (Gulick et al., 1997; Hammer et al., 1997; Gulick et al., 1998) (see Chapter 7).

Ritonavir

Ritonavir is a peptidomimetic inhibitor of HIV-1 and HIV-2 protease (reviewed in Kucers et al., 1997). It is marketed by Abbott (Abbott Laboratories, Abbott Park, IL, USA) under the brand name of Norvir®.

In vitro *activity*

The IC_{90} of ritonavir is approximately 100 nM, with steady-state plasma C_{max} of about 16 μM and trough levels of about 5 μM with doses of 600 mg administered twice daily (Danner *et al.*, 1995; Kempf *et al.*, 1995). Ritonavir is less active against group O strains of HIV-1 than group M subtype B strains (Descamps *et al.*, 1997); there is no significant difference in susceptibility between group M subtypes A, B, C, D and E of HIV-1 (Palmer *et al.*, 1998).

Resistance

Similar to indinavir, resistance to ritonavir is associated with the accumulation of mutations within the HIV protease enzyme. A key mutation conferring resistance is Val 82 Ala/Phe (reviewed in Hirsch *et al.*, 2000; Schinazi *et al.*, 2000), although Ile 36 Leu, Ile 52 Val, Ile 54 Val, Ala 71 Val and Ile 84 Val also contribute (Markowitz *et al.*, 1995a; Molla *et al.*, 1995; Norbeck *et al.*, 1995). The codon 82 mutation is necessary for the development of phenotypic resistance, although other mutations are usually also required (reviewed in Hirsch *et al.*, 2000; Schinazi *et al.*, 2000; Table 5.7). Ritonavir-resistant strains of HIV-1 are almost invariably cross-resistant to indinavir and nelfinavir (Molla *et al.*, 1996), while ritonavir-resistant strains often remain susceptible to saquinavir and amprenavir (Moyle, 1998).

Clinically relevant pharmacokinetics

Dosage and administration. Ritonavir is available in soft-elastic capsules containing 100 mg ritonavir and also as a liquid containing 80 mg/ml (Table 5.3). (As crystallization was detected within the early capsule formulation, patients were switched to liquid formulation). The dose of ritonavir for adults is 600 mg twice daily. Due to metabolic autoinduction, therapy is initiated with low dose, which is gradually increased (300 mg twice daily for 4 days, then 400 mg twice daily for 4 days, then 500 mg twice daily for 4 days, then routine dose of 600 mg twice daily). If ritonavir is administered with other PIs the dose may change due to interactions according to the involved metabolic pathway. (For example, ritonavir is given in a dose of 100 mg twice daily when co-administered with indinavir).

Absorption. The oral bioavailability of ritonavir is high but it is still recommended that the drug be taken with meals to improve absorption (Table 5.4).

Distribution. Ritonavir is highly protein bound (Lazdins *et al.*, 1997) and the CSF:plasma ratio is low, approximately 0.01 (Flexner, 1998). Ritonavir does not cross the placenta into fetal tissue and does not accumulate in the placenta (Casey and Bawdon, 1998).

Metabolism. Ritonavir is metabolized by cytochrome p450 enzymes and autoinduces the enzymes required for its metabolism. Thus the dose of ritonavir is increased during the first 2 weeks of therapy from 300 mg twice daily to 600 mg twice daily (Flexner, 1998). The drug is cleared primarily by the hepatobiliary tract (Denissen *et al.*, 1997). Only 11% of an oral dose of ritonavir is excreted in urine (3% unchanged), while 86% is eliminated in faeces (33% unchanged) (Hsu *et al.*, 1997).

Important drug interactions

As ritonavir is metabolized via cytochrome p450 pathways, any drug that is a substrate, inducer or inhibitor of cytochrome enzymes of this system should be used with caution in ritonavir-treated patients (see Chapter 6).

Cytochrome p450 enzyme inducers such as rifampin will accelerate the clearance of ritonavir and lower the plasma level of the protease inhibitor. In contrast, co-administration of ritonavir with rifabutin increases the plasma concentration of rifabutin by more than three-fold, and the risk of rifabutin-associated uveitis is increased by ritonavir co-administration (Sun *et al.*, 1996). Ritonavir is a potent inhibitor of cytochrome p450 CYP3A4 isoenzyme, and thus may increase the plasma levels of drugs that are metabolized by this route, including terfenadine, midazolam and PIs (von Moltke *et al.*, 1998). Ritonavir potently inhibits cytochrome p450-mediated metabolism of saquinavir, nelfinavir, indinavir and amprenavir, increasing plasma concentrations of these drugs (Kempf *et al.*, 1997; Hsu *et al.*, 1998b), a finding that has been exploited clinically in combination regimens (Lorenzi *et al.*, 1997; Rhone *et al.*, 1998).

Major adverse reactions

Gastrointestinal symptoms are frequently reported by patients receiving ritonavir (see Chapter 6). Elevations of serum bilirubin and aminotransferase levels are found in up to 15% of patients and are generally reversible on cessation of therapy. Similar to the other PIs, a syndrome comprising glucose intolerance, elevation of serum cholesterol and triglyceride levels and lipodystrophy has been described with ritonavir therapy (Sullivan and Nelson, 1997; Carr et al., 1998). A maculopapular rash associated with fever has also been described in patients receiving ritonavir (Bachmeyer et al., 1997).

Major clinical use

Although effective in the short-term as monotherapy (Ho et al., 1994; Danner et al., 1995, Markowitz et al., 1995b; Cameron et al., 1997), ritonavir is used only as a component of combination therapy. Ritonavir is less pop- ular with patients than other PIs due to gastrointestinal side-effects. Increasingly, however, low doses of ritonavir are being used with a second PI to increase the plasma concentrations of the second drug; these combinations achieve excellent antiretroviral activity while reducing adverse reactions, especially those due to ritonavir (see Chapter 7).

Nelfinavir

Nelfinavir mesylate is a non-peptidic inhibitor of HIV-1 and HIV-2 protease (Kaldor et al., 1997 reviewed in Bardsley-Eliot et al., 2000). It is marketed by Agouron (Pharmaceuticals Inc, La Jolla, CA, USA) under the trade name of Viracept®.

In vitro activity

Nelfinavir has an IC_{50} ranging from 9 to 60 nM and an IC_{90} of 7–196 nM against laboratory strains and clinical isolates of HIV-1, with steady-state plasma C_{max} levels of approximately 5000 nM and trough levels of 1700–3300 nM. Nelfinavir is additive to synergistic against HIV-1 with zidovudine, didanosine, lamivudine, zalcitabine, stavudine, ritonavir and saquinavir; nelfinavir is slightly antagonistic with indinavir (Patick et al., 1997).

Resistance

A unique Asp 30 Asn mutation confers low-level resis- tance to nelfinavir without cross-resistance to other PIs (Markowitz et al., 1998). The Leu 90 Met mutation results in a fivefold reduction in susceptibility but is rare in vivo (Schinazi et al., 2000). Additional mutations Met 46 Ile and Ile 84 Val/Ala result in a thirtyfold reduction in susceptibility to nelfinavir (Patick et al., 1996); muta- tions have also been detected in codons 36, 63, 71 and 90 (Moyle, 1995; Hirsch et al., 2000; Schinazi et al., 2000; Table 5.7). Clinically significant

levels of resistance require the development of multiple mutations. Mutations commonly associated with resis- tance to other PIs (within codons 48, 82 and 84) have not generally been detected in patients receiving nelfinavir therapy, although patients failing nelfinavir may not respond to other PIs (Sampson et al., 1997)

Clinically relevant pharmacokinetics

Nelfinavir is available as film-coated tablets containing 250 mg nelfinavir and as a powder formulation for paediatric use. The adult dose is 750 mg taken three times daily or 1250 mg taken twice daily (Bardsley-Elliot et al., 2000; Table 5.3). An alternative regimen of 1250 mg administered twice daily may be as effective (Jarvis and Faulds, 1998). The oral bioavailability of nelfinavir is greater than 78% and it is increased by a high-fat meal (Flexner, 1998). The drug should be taken with meals, as the plasma AUC is increased by up to 50% when taken with food compared to fasted volun- teers (reviewed in Bardsley-Elliot et al., 2000). There are no published data currently available regarding distri- bution of the drug in tissues. Nelfinavir is metabolized by cytochrome p450 enzymes, similar to other PIs (reviewed in Bardsley-Elliot et al., 2000). Protein binding exceeds 98%. The drug is both an inducer and an inhibitor of cytochrome p450 enzymes.

Important drug interactions

As nelfinavir is metabolized via cytochrome p450, any drug that is a substrate, inducer or inhibitor of this enzyme system should be used with caution in patients receiving nelfinavir (see Chapter 6).

Ketoconazole increases plasma nelfinavir levels through inhibition of the cytochrome p450 enzymes required for metabolism of the PI. Inducers of this enzyme system, such as rifampin, and nevirapine, decrease the AUC of nelfinavir, resulting in subtherapeutic levels by accele- rating its clearance (reviewed in Flexner, 1998). As an inhibitor of cytochrome p450, nelfinavir can reduce the metabolism of other drugs, thus increasing their plasma concentrations; these include other PIs, terfenadine, and other drugs of its class, including cisapride and mida- zolam. The plasma level of rifabutin increases approxi- mately twofold with nelfinavir cotherapy, requiring a reduction in its dose to 150 mg daily (Anon, 1996). Nelfinavir plasma levels are reduced by about 50% with nevirapine co-administration (Merry et al., 1998).

Major adverse reactions

Nelfinavir can cause mild to moderate diarrhoea, elevation of serum aminotransferase levels, rash, nausea, headache and asthenia (reviewed in Jarvis and Faulds, 1998). As with other PIs, a syndrome comprising lipodystrophy in association with hyperlipidaemia and hyperglycaemia has been described in nelfinavir recipients (reviewed in Jarvis and Faulds, 1998; see also Chapter 6).

Major clinical use

Nelfinavir is highly potent in reducing HIV-1 viral load and increasing CD4 lymphocyte counts. It is used in combination with NRTIs and NNRTIs (reviewed in Havlir and Lange, 1998; see also Chapter 7). A European study evaluating nelfinavir in combination with saquinavir (SPICE study) found that quadruple therapy provided a more durable response than triple therapy with a single PI (Moyle *et al.*, 2000).

Amprenavir

Amprenavir (141W94) is an inhibitor of HIV-1 and HIV-2 protease. It was synthesized by Vertex Pharmaceuticals (Chicago, IL, USA) and is marketed by Glaxo Wellcome under the trade name Agenerase®.

In vitro *activity*

Amprenavir has an IC_{50} of 0.01–0.41 µM against HIV-1 (St Clair *et al.*, 1996). Amprenavir is additive to synergistic in action with zidovudine, abacavir, didanosine, saquinavir, indinavir and ritonavir (St Clair *et al.*, 1996; Drusano *et al.*, 1998).

Resistance

The resistance pattern of amprenavir differs to that of saquinavir and indinavir (Adkins and Faulds, 1998). *In vitro*, significant resistance to amprenavir required the development of at least two or three mutations within codons 10, 46, 47 and 50 (Ile → Val) of the HIV-1 protease (Pazhanisamy *et al.*, 1996) (Table 5.7). The codon 50 mutation is thought to be critical to the development of resistance (Parteledis *et al.*, 1995). Mutations within codon 184 are considered to be important contributors to resistance. Amprenavir-resistant strains are cross-resistant to ritonavir, but may actually increase the susceptibility of HIV to saquinavir, indinavir and nelfinavir (reviewed in Moyle, 1998). This will be assessed more effectively as widespread use of amprenavir occurs.

Clinically relevant pharmacokinetics

Dosage and administration. Amprenavir is available in 150 and 200 mg soft-gelatin capsules. The adult dose is 800 mg three times daily or 1200 mg twice daily (Haubrich *et al.*, 1999; Sadler *et al.*, 2001) (Table 5.3). Amprenavir can be taken without regard for food (Table 5.4). The CSF:plasma ratio of amprenavir is low (<0.01), a finding that is not surprising as the drug is highly protein bound. Amprenavir is metabolized via cytochrome p450 enzymes. Amprenavir inhibits certain isoforms including CYP2E1, 2C19 and 3A4; inhibition of CYP3A4 is greater than that by saquinavir, similar to that by indinavir and nelfinavir, and less than that by ritonavir (Decker *et al.*, 1998).

Important drug interactions

As amprenavir is metabolized via cytochrome p450, any drug that is a substrate, inducer or inhibitor of the cytochrome enzymes should be used with caution as described above for other PIs (see Chapter 6).

Major adverse reactions

The most common adverse effects of amprenavir are headache, nausea and diarrhoea, rash, and circumoral paresthesia. Mild increases in levels of serum triglycerides have been frequently reported (see Chapter 6).

Major clinical use

Amprenavir is used to treat patients at all stages of HIV infection in combination regimens with NRTIs, and in some cases also with an NNRTI (see Chapter 7).

Lopinavir

Lopinavir [ABT-378] is a second-generation PI synthesized by Abbott Laboratories. Lopinavir and ritonavir are co-formulated into a single capsule, with ritonavir acting as a pharmacokinetic enhancer, by blocking metabolism of lopinavir by the cytochrome p450 isoform CYP3A.

In vitro *activity*

Lopinavir is significantly more active against HIV-1 in cell culture than ritonavir (Carillo *et al.*, 1998). The IC_{50} of lopinavir ranges from 0.006 to 0.17 µM, when tested against both laboratory-adapted and clinical strains of HIV-1. The drug is also active against ritonavir-resistant strains of HIV-1 with a mutation in codon 82 (IC_{50} of 0.06 µM) (Sham *et al.*, 1998).

Resistance

Lopinavir-resistant strains of HIV-1 can be detected by serial passage *in vitro*, with sequential appearance of mutations in the protease gene Ile 84 Val, Leu 10 Phe, Thr 91 Ser, Val 32 Ile, Ile 47 Val, Val 47 Ala. Other mutations have also been detected within p1/p6 and p7/p1 gag proteolytic processing sites, which appear to be necessary for replication of highly-resistant strains of HIV-1 (Carillo et al., 1998).

Clinically relevant pharmacokinetics

The metabolism of lopinavir is inhibited by ritonavir, resulting in higher plasma concentrations of lopinavir, exceeding the *in vitro* IC_{50} by fiftyfold and the AUC by seventy-sevenfold (Sham et al., 1998). The dose of lopinavir is 400 mg lopinavir/100 mg ritonavir, three co-formulated capsules administered twice daily, best taken with food.

Important drug interactions

No dosage adjustment is required when lopinavir is co-administered with nevirapine or efavirenz. Alternatives to oestrogen-based oral contraceptives should be used in female patients receiving lopinavir. Similar precautions would be used as with other PIs regarding drugs that are metabolized by CYP3A.

Major adverse reactions

The most commonly reported side-effects are loose stools and nausea. Rash has occurred in fewer than 3% of clinical trial participants. Elevations in cholesterol and asymptomatic elevations in hepatic transaminases (particularly in patients with baseline abnormalities in these enzymes) have been observed (Investigator's brochure, Abbott Laboratories (Murphy et al., 2001; reviewed in Hurst and Faulds, 2000)).

Major clinical use

Lopinavir is currently in phase III clinical trial. As with other PIs, lopinavir is used as a component of combination regimens. Clinical trials suggest that lopinavir is useful for the treatment of patients with PI-resistant strains of HIV.

Tipranavir

Tipranavir, a non-peptidic PI, is active against strains of HIV-1 that are resistant to other PIs (Poppe et al., 1997;

Larder et al., 1999; Swanstrom et al., 2000). In a dose-ranging study, 1500 mg (10 capsules) administered three times daily had potent antiviral activity. Ritonavir co-administration significantly improves the pharmacokinetics of tipranavir.

HIV entry inhibitors

T-20

T-20 (DP178) is a 36-amino acid synthetic peptide derived from the transmembrane glycoprotein gp41 (amino acid residues 643–678) of HIV-1. It inhibits fusion between the virus and the cell membrane (Pine et al., 1998), and is manufactured by Trimeris.

In vitro activity

T-20 inhibits HIV-1 infectivity *in vitro* in a cell fusion assay with an IC_{90} of 2–30 ng/ml without evidence of cytotoxicity (Wild et al., 1993; Lawless et al., 1996). It appears to be more active *in vitro* against syncytium-inducing strains of HIV-1 than non-syncytium-inducing strains. It is about 5000-fold less active against HIV-2 (Investigator's brochure, Trimeris).

Resistance

Serial passage of HIV-1 in increasing concentrations of T-20 results in emergence of resistant strains of virus. Resistance has been mapped to a three-amino-acid motif at positions 552–554 within gp41, close to the leucine zipper region (residues 558–595), which comprises the binding region of T-20 to gp41 (Su et al., 1999; Kliger et al., 2000; Investigator's brochure, Trimeris).

Clinically relevant pharmacokinetics

Animal studies suggest that microgram levels of the drug are available following intravenous administration. In humans, subcutaneous administration of T-20 results in >70% bioavailability.

Major adverse reactions

During a 14-day clinical trial of intravenous T-20 given twice daily by infusion, fevers and headaches were reported in about 25% of recipients (Investigator's brochure, Trimeris).

Major clinical use

T-20 is in clinical trial. Early studies showed that intravenous administration by twice-daily infusion for 14 days resulted in a 1–2 $\log_{10}$ decrease in plasma HIV RNA (Kilby *et al.*, 1998).

Other antiretroviral drugs

Hydroxyurea

Hydroxyurea, used in the treatment of cancer and sickle cell anaemia, is an inhibitor of the cellular enzyme ribonucleotide reductase (the rate-limiting enzyme of DNA synthesis), and as such prevents HIV DNA synthesis by inhibiting deoxynucleotide triphosphate (particularly dATP) generation within cells (Lori *et al.*, 1994; Gao *et al.*, 1995; Gao *et al.*, 1998). In addition, drugs of this class have been reported to stimulate uptake and phosphorylation of extracellular deoxynucleosides such as zidovudine (Giacca *et al.*, 1996a) and to reduce cellular activation and thus also decrease HIV-1 replication. The drug is marketed by Bristol-Myers Squibb under the brand name Hydrea®.

In vitro *activity and resistance*

Hydroxyurea is synergistic *in vitro* with didanosine (Gao *et al.*, 1998) and modestly enhances the activity of zidovudine, and zalcitabine (Gao *et al.*, 1995). Since hydroxyurea inhibits cellular proteins, which are less prone to mutations than viral proteins, resistance is not expected to occur. Hydroxyurea has been reported to reverse HIV resistance to didanosine (Lori *et al.*, 1997).

Clinically relevant pharmacokinetics

Hydroxyurea is available as 500 mg capsules. A frequently used dose of hydroxyurea in a 70 kg person is 500 mg twice daily orally (approximately 15 mg/kg per day). However, dosing regimens are still under evaluation. As the plasma half-life is short (2.5 h) and bone marrow toxicity may be related to peak concentration, it may be more effective and less toxic when administered three or four times daily; there are currently no data to support this hypothesis. Hydroxyurea is well absorbed following oral administration (Gwilt and Tracewell, 1998), with peak serum levels within 2 h. Hydroxyurea is present in breast milk and is predominantly excreted in urine.

Important drug interactions

Hydroxyurea should not be used in combination with myelosuppressive drugs.

Major adverse reactions

Hydroxyurea causes dose-related bone marrow suppression, with anaemia, neutropenia and thrombocytopenia being common effects. The development of neutropenia is more likely if patients have low neutrophil levels at start of therapy (Galpin *et al.*, 1998). Lymphopenia is seen in most patients, including reduction in CD4 lymphocyte subsets (Lucht *et al.*, 1998). Nausea and vomiting, rash, and alopecia occur less frequently. Alopecia is more common in patients with advanced HIV infection and lymphopenia (Rutschmann *et al.*, 1998).

Major clinical use

There is a paucity of large, randomized controlled clinical trials assessing the activity of hydroxyurea in patients with HIV infection. The drug is currently being evaluated in AIDS Clinical Trials Group (ACTG) Study No. 307. Meanwhile, based largely on small studies and anecdotal reports, hydroxyurea is used by some clinicians in combination with other NRTIs (usually didanosine) to potentiate the antiviral activity of the latter class of drugs. Hydroxyurea is most commonly used as part of a salvage regimen in patients with virological failure following multiple antiretroviral regimens (Montaner *et al.*, 1998b). However, as it causes lymphopenia it is not generally used in patients with advanced HIV infection and CD4 lymphocyte counts below 50 lymphocytes/μl.

In the randomized, double-blinded prospective Swiss HIV Cohort Study of 144 patients, hydroxyurea was found to modestly improve the antiviral activity of didanosine and stavudine for up to 12 weeks, with only a small improvement in terms of CD4 lymphocyte numbers (Rutschmann *et al.*, 1998). These data, showing modest benefit, support the results of a pilot study of hydroxyurea in patients on long-term didanosine therapy and CD4 lymphocyte counts of between 100 and 350 cells/μl treated with didanosine and hydroxyurea or didanosine alone (Montaner *et al.*, 1997), but not results from other small trials with this drug in combination with didanosine (Simonelli *et al.*, 1997) or as monotherapy (Giacca *et al.*, 1996b), where hydroxyurea appeared to have no effect.

Adefovir dipivoxil (Bis-Pom PMEA)

This drug is an acyclic monophosphorylated nucleoside (nucleotide) analogue, the orally bioavailable prodrug of adefovir. It is marketed by Gilead (CA, USA), under the trade name Preveon®. It is converted to adefovir within cells prior to being phosphorylated by mitochondria to the active form. It is an inhibitor of HIV reverse transcriptase.

In vitro activity and resistance

Adefovir dipivoxil has activity against a number of viruses including HIV, herpes viruses including cyto-megalovirus, hepadnaviruses including hepatitis B virus, and a number of other retroviruses (De Clercq, 1997). It inhibits HIV with an IC_{50} of 1.6–2 μM. The drug is synergistic in vitro against HIV with zidovudine, stavudine, zalcitabine, (De Clercq et al., 1986) dida-nosine, nelfinavir, ritonavir and saquinavir (Mulato and Cherrington, 1997). Within 12 months of treatment with adefovir dipivoxil, mutations develop within the HIV reverse transcriptase (Lys 65 Arg and Lys 70 Glu), resulting in sixteen- and ninefold decreases in suscepti-bility to adefovir, respectively (Foli et al., 1996; Mulato et al., 1998; Miller et al., 1999).

Clinically relevant pharmacokinetics

In humans the oral bioavailability of adefovir is less than 12% (Cundy et al., 1995); the oral bioavailability of the dipivoxil derivative is significantly higher. About 90% of an intravenous dose of adefovir is recovered unchanged in urine, with active tubular secretion accounting for about 60% of the clearance of adefovir (Cundy et al., 1995).

Major adverse reactions

The drug is well tolerated in doses of 125 and 250 mg daily over 12 weeks (Deeks et al., 1997). Gastrointestinal complaints and reversible elevation of hepatic transa-minase levels and decreases in serum free carnitine levels are the most frequently noted adverse events (Barditch Crovo et al., 1997). Supplementation with oral L-carnitine 500 mg daily is recommended.

Major clinical use

Patients receiving adefovir dipivoxil monotherapy in a dose of 125 mg daily orally for 12 weeks experienced a median decrease in HIV RNA levels of 0.5 $\log_{10}$ copies/ml (Mulato et al., 1998). As monotherapy, adefovir dipivoxil reduces plasma HIV RNA levels by 0.4–0.6 $\log_{10}$ copies/ml (Barditch Crovo et al., 1997).

Tenofovir disoproxil fumarate (bis-POC PMPA)

This second-generation nucleotide analogue, marketed by Gilead Sciences Inc. (Foster City, CA, USA), is now in phase III clinical trials.

The drug is in phase II and phase III studies for treatment of hepatitis B and HIV infections. As for other antiretroviral therapies this drug will be used as part of a combination therapy regimen. Gilead has terminated the development of Adefovir within the USA as an anti-HIV agent, resulting from US FDA requests for longer-term placebo-controlled studies of the drug.

Current guidelines for the treatment of HIV infection

http://hivatis.org/trtgdlns.html

References

Abrams DI, Goldman AI, Launer C et al. (1994). A comparative trial of didanosine or zalcitabine after treatment with zidovudine in patients with human immunodeficiency virus infection. The Terry Beirn Community Programs for Clinical Research on AIDS. N Engl J Med 330: 657.

Adkins JC, Faulds D. (1998). Amprenavir. Drugs 55: 837–42.

Adkins JC, Peters DH, Faulds D. (1997). Zalcitabine. An update of its pharmacodynamic and pharmacokinetic properties and clinical efficacy in the management of HIV infection. Drugs 53: 1054–80.

Anderson RE, Dunkle LM, Smaldone L et al. (1995). Design and implementation of the stavudine parallel track program. J Infect Dis 171: S118.

Anon. (1995). Case control study of HIV seroconversion in health care workers after percutaneous exposure to HIV-infected blood – France, United Kingdom and United States, Jan 1988–Aug 1994. MMWR 44: 929.

Anon. (1996). Impact of HIV protease inhibitors on the treatment of HIV-infected tuberculosis patients with rifampin. MMWR 45: 921–5.

Bachelez LT, Anton E, Baker D et al. (1997). Impact of mutation, plasma protein binding and pharmacokinetics on clinical efficacy of the HIV-1 non-nucleoside reverse transcriptase inhibitor, DMP 266. Thirty-seventh Interscience Conference on Antimicrobial Agents and Chemotherapy, Toronto, Ontario, Canada.

Bachelet L, Weislow O, Snyder S et al. (1998). Virologic resistance to stavudine. Twelfth World AIDS Conference Geneva, Switzerland (abstract).

Bachmeyer C, Blum L, Cordier F et al. (1997). Early ritonavir induced maculopapular eruption. Dermatology 195: 301–2.

Back DJ, Ormesher S, Tjia JP et al. (1992). Metabolism of 2',3'-dideoxyinosine (ddI) in human blood. Br J Clin Pharmacol 33: 319.

Balani SK, Arison BH, Mathai L et al. (1995). Metabolites of L-735,524 a potent HIV-1 protease inhibitor in human urine. Drug Metabol Disposit 23: 266.

Balani SK, Woolf EJ, Hoagland VL et al. (1996). Disposition of indinavir, a potent HIV-1 protease inhibitor, after an oral dose in humans. *Drug Metab Disposit* **24**: 1389–94.

Barditch Crovo P, Toole J, Hendrix CW et al. (1997). Anti-human immunodeficiency virus (HIV) activity, safety, and pharma-cokinetics of adefovir dipivoxil (9-[2-(bis-pivaloyloxymethyl)-phosphonylmethoxyethyl]adenine) in HIV-infected patients. *J Infect Dis* **176**: 406–13.

Bardsley-Eliot A, Plosker GL. (2000). Nelfinavir. An update on its use in HIV infection. *Drugs* **89**: 581–620.

Bawdon RE, Kaul S, Sobhi S. (1994). The *ex vivo* transfer of the anti HIV nucleoside compound d4T in the human placenta. *Gynecol Obstet Invest* **38**: 1.

Benedek IH, Joshi A, Fiske WD et al. (1998). *Pharmacokinetic inter-action between efavirenz (EFV) and rifampin (RIF) in healthy volun-teers*. Twelfth World AIDS Conference, Geneva, Switzerland.

Boucher CA, Tersmette M, Lange JM et al. (1990). Zidovudine sensitivity of human immunodeficiency viruses from high-risk, symptom-free individuals during therapy. *Lancet* **336**: 585.

Boucher CA, Leeuwen RB, Kellam P et al. (1993a). Effects of discontinuation of zidovudine treatment on zidovudine sensitivity of human immunodeficiency virus type 1 isolates. *Antimicrob Agents Chemother* **37**: 1525.

Boucher CA, Cammack N, Schipper P et al. (1993b). High-level resistance to (–) enantiomeric 2′-deoxy-3′-thiacytidine *in vitro* is due to one amino acid substitution in the catalytic site of human immunodeficiency virus type 1 reverse transcriptase. *Antimicrob Agents Chemother* **37**: 2231.

Boucher C. (1996). Rational approaches to resistance; using saquinavir. *AIDS* **10**: S15–19.

Bouscarat F, Bouchard C, Bouchour D. (1998). Paronychia and pyogenic granuloma of the great toes in patients treated with indinavir. *N Engl J Med* **338**: 1176–7.

Brau N, Leaf HL, Wieczorek RL et al. (1997). Severe hepatitis in three AIDS patients treated with indinavir. *Lancet* **349**: 924–5.

Browne MJ, Mayer KH, Chafee SB et al. (1993). 2′, 3′-didehydro 3′-deoxythymidine (d4T) in patients with AIDS or AIDS related complex, a phase I trial. *J Infect Dis* **167**: 21.

Buss N (on behalf of the Fortovase Study Group). (1998). *Saquinavir soft gel capsules (Fortovase) pharmacokinetics and drug interactions*. Fifth Conference on Retroviruses and Opportunistic Infections, Chicago, IL, USA.

Buss N. (2000). Effect of ritonavir on saquinavir metabolism. *JAMA* **283**: 2936–7.

CAESAR Co-ordinating Committee. (1997). Randomized trial of addition of lamivudine or lamivudine plus loviride to zidovudine-containing regimens for patients with HIV-1 infection; the CAESAR trial. *Lancet* **349**: 1413–21.

Cameron DW, Heath-Chiozzi M, Danner S et al. (1997). Randomized placebo-controlled trial of ritonavir in advanced HIV-1 disease. The advanced HIV disease ritonavir study group. *Lancet* **351**: 543–9.

Campbell TB, Young RK, Eron JJ et al. (1993). Inhibition of human immunodeficiency virus type 1 replication *in vitro* by the bisheteroaryl-piperazine atevirdine (U-87201E) in combination with zidovudine or didanosine. *J Infect Dis* **168**: 318.

Carillo A, Stewart KD, Sham HL et al. (1998). *In vitro* selection and characterization of human immunodeficiency virus type 1 variants with increased resistance to ABT-378, a novel protease inhibitor. *J Virol* **72**: 7532–41.

Carpenter CJ, Fischl MA, Hammer SM et al. (1998). Antiretroviral therapy for HIV infection in 1998. *JAMA* **280**: 78–86.

Carr A, Cooper DA. (1996). Current clinical experience with nevirapine for HIV infection. In: J Mills, P Volberding, L Corey (eds.) *Antiviral chemotherapy, new directions for clinical applications and research*. Volume 4. 299.

Carr A, Samaras K, Burton S et al. (1998). A syndrome of peripheral lipodystrophy, hyperlipidaemia and insulin resistance in patients receiving HIV protease inhibitors. *AIDS* **12**: F51–8.

Casey BM, Bawdon RE. (1998). Placental transfer of ritonavir with zidovudine in the *ex vivo* placental perfusion model. *Am J Obstet Gynecol* **179**: 758–61.

Cato A, Cavanaugh J, Shi H et al. (1998). The effect of multiple doses of ritonavir on the pharmacokinetics of rifabutin. *Clin Pharmacol Ther* **63**: 414–21.

Chattha G, Arieff AI, Cummings C et al. (1993). Lactic acidosis complicating the acquired immunodeficiency syndrome. *Ann Intern Med* **118**: 37.

Chen CH, Vazquez Padua M, Chang YC. (1991). Effect of anti-human immunodeficiency virus nucleoside analogs on mitochondrial DNA and its implication for delayed toxicity. *Mol Pharmacol* **39**: 625.

Chong KT, Pagano PJ, Hinshaw RR. (1994). Bisheteroarylpiperazine reverse transcriptase inhibitor in combination with 3′-azido-3′-deoxythymidine or 2,3′-dideoxycytidine synergistically inhibits human immunodeficiency virus type 1 replication *in vitro*. *Antimicrob Agents Chemother* **38**: 288.

Chow FP, Chen RB, Hamburger AW. (1993). Sustained elevation of platelet counts by long term azidothymidine treatment of immunosuppressed mice. *J Lab Clin Med* **121**: 562.

Cohen C, Sun E, Cameron W et al. (1996). Ritonavir-saquinavir combination treatment in HIV-infected patients. In: *Addendum to program and abstracts of the Thirty-sixth Interscience Conference on Antimicrobial Agents and Chemotherapy*, New Orleans, Washington, DC. New York: American Society for Microbiology.

Collier AC, Coombs RW, Fischl MA. (1993). Combination therapy with zidovudine and didanosine compared with zidovudine alone in HIV-1 infection. *Ann Intern Med* **119**: 786.

Collier AC, Coombs RW, Schoenfeld DA. (1996). Treatment of human immunodeficiency virus infection with saquinavir, zidovudine and zalcitabine. *N Engl J Med* **334**: 1011.

Concorde Co-ordinating Committee. (1994). MRC/ANRS randomiz-ed double blind controlled trial of immediate and deferred zidovudine in symptom free HIV infection. *Lancet* **343**: 871.

Condra JH, Schleif WA, Blahy OM et al. (1995a). *In vivo* emergence of HIV-1 variants resistant to multiple protease inhibitors. *Nature* **374**: 569.

Condra JH, Schleif WA, Blahy OM et al. (1995b). Dynamics of acquired HIV-1 clinical resistance to the protease inhibitor MK-639. *J AIDS Hum Retrovir* **10**: S35.

Conlon CP, Klenerman P, Edwards A et al. (1994). Heterosexual transmission of human immunodeficiency virus type 1 variants associated with zidovudine resistance. *J Infect Dis* **169**: 411.

Connolly KJ, Allan JD, Fitch H et al. (1991). Phase I study of 2′-3′-dideoxyinosine administered orally twice daily to patients with AIDS or AIDS-related complex and hematologic intolerance to zidovudine. *Am J Med* **91**: 471.

Connor EM, Sperling RS, Gelber R et al. (1994). Reduction of maternal infant transmission of human immunodeficiency virus type 1 with zidovudine treatment. Pediatric AIDS Clinical Trials Group Protocol 076 Study Group. *N Engl J Med* **331**: 1173.

Cooley TP, Kinches LM, Saunders CA et al. (1990). Once daily administration of 2',3'-dideoxyinosine (ddI) in patients with the acquired immunodeficiency syndrome or AIDS-related complex. Results of a Phase I trial. N Engl J Med 322: 1340.

Cooper DA, Gatell JM, Kroon S et al. (1993) Zidovudine in persons with asymptomatic HIV infection and CD4+ cell counts greater than 400 per cubic millimeter. NEJM 329: 297–303.

Craig JC, Duncan IB, Whittaker L et al. (1990). Antiviral synergy between inhibitors of HIV proteinase and reverse transcriptase. Antiviral Chem Chemother 4: 161.

Craig JC, Duncan IB, Hockley D et al. (1991). Antiviral properties of Ro 31-8959, an inhibitor of human immunodeficiency virus (HIV) proteinase. Antiviral Res 16: 295.

Craig JC, Whittaker L, Duncan IB et al. (1994). In vitro anti-HIV and cytotoxicological evaluation of the triple combination, ACT and ddC with HIV proteinase inhibitor saquinavir (Ro 31-8959). Antiviral Chem Chemother 5: 380.

Cundy KC, Barditch-Crovo P, Walker RE et al. (1995). Clinical pharmacokinetics of adefovir in human immunodeficiency virus type 1-infected patients. Antimicrob Agents Chemother 39: 2401–5.

D'Aquila RT, Hughes MD, Johnson VA et al. (1996). Nevirapine, zidovudine and didanosine compared with zidovudine and didanosine in patients with HIV-1 infection. Ann Intern Med 124: 1019.

Dalakas MC, Illa I, Pezeshkpour GH et al. (1990). Mitochondrial myopathy caused by long term zidovudine therapy. N Engl J Med 322: 1098.

Daluge SM, Faletto MB, Good SS et al. (1997). 1592U89, a novel carbocyclic nucleoside analog with potent, selective anti-human immunodeficiency virus activity. Antimicrob Agents Chemother 41: 1082–93.

Dancis J, Lee JD, Mendoza S et al. (1993). Transfer and metabolism of dideoxyinosine by the perfused human placenta. J AIDS 6: 2.

Danner SA, Carr A, Leonard JM et al. (1995). A short term study of the safety, pharmacokinetics and efficacy of ritonavir an inhibitor of HIV-1 protease. European Australian Collaborative Ritonavir Study Group. N Engl J Med 333: 1528–33.

De-Clercq E. (1997). Acyclic nucleoside phosphonates in the chemotherapy of DNA virus and retrovirus infections. Intervirology 40: 295–303.

De Clercq E, Holy A, Rosenberg I, et al. (1986). A novel selective broad-spectrum anti-DNA virus agent. Nature 323: 464–7.

De Jong MD, Loewenthal M, Boucher CA et al. (1994). Alternating nevirapine and zidovudine treatment of human immunodeficiency virus type 1-infected persons does not prolong nevirapine activity. J Infect Dis 169: 1346.

Decker CJ, Laitinen LM, Bridson GW et al. (1998). Metabolism of amprenavir in liver microsomes: role of CYP3A4 inhibition for drug interactions. J Pharm Sci 87: 803–7.

Deeks SG, Collier A, Lalezari J et al. (1997). The safety and efficacy of adefovir dipivoxil, a novel anti-human immunodeficiency virus (HIV) therapy, in HIV-infected adults; a randomized, double-blind placebo-controlled trial. J Infect Dis 176: 1517–23.

Delta Co-ordinating Committee. (1996). Delta: a randomized double blind controlled trial comparing combinations of zidovudine plus didanosine or zalcitabine with zidovudine alone in HIV-infected individuals. Lancet 348: 283.

Denissen JF, Grabowski BA, Johnson MK et al. (1997). Metabolism and disposition of the HIV-1 protease inhibitor ritonavir (ABT-538) in rats, dogs and humans. Drug Metab Dispos 25: 489–501.

Descamps D, Collin G, Loussert-Ajaka I et al. (1995). HIV-1 group O sensitivity to antiretroviral drugs. AIDS 9: 977.

Descamps D, Collin G, Letourneur F et al. (1997). Susceptibility of human immunodeficiency virus type 1 group O isolates to antiretroviral agents; in vitro phenotypic and genotypic analyses. J Virol 71: 8893–8.

Dornsife RE, St Clair MH, Huang AT et al. (1991). Anti-human immunodeficiency virus synergism by zidovudine (c'-azidothymidine) and didanosine (dideoxyinosine) contrasts with their additive inhibition of normal human marrow progenitor cells. Antimicrob Agents Chemother 35: 322.

Dorsey BD, Levin RB, McDaniel SL et al. (1994). L-735,524 the design of a potent and orally bioavailable HIV protease inhibitor. J Med Chem 37: 3443.

Drusano GL, D'Argenio DZ, Symonds W et al. (1998). Nucleoside analog 1592U89 and human immunodeficiency virus protease inhibitor 141W94 are synergistic in vitro. Antimicrob Agents Chemother 42: 2153–9.

Dueweke TJ, Pushkarskaya T, Poppe SM et al. (1993a). A mutation in reverse transcriptase of bis(heteroaryl)piperazine-resistant human immunodeficiency virus type 1 that confers increased sensitivity to other non-nucleoside inhibitors. Proc Natl Acad Sci USA 90: 4713.

Dueweke TJ, Poppe SM, Romero DL et al. (1993b). U-90152S, a potent inhibitor of human deficiency virus type 1 replication. Antimicrob Agents Chemother 37: 1127.

Dudley MW, Graham KK, Kaul S et al. (1992). Pharmacokinetics of stavudine in patients with AIDS or AIDS related complex. J Infect Dis 166: 480.

Dudley MN. (1995). Clinical pharmacokinetics of nucleoside antiretroviral agents. J Infect Dis 171: S99.

Eastman PS, Mitler J, Kelso R et al. (1998). Genotypic changes in human immunodeficiency virus type 1 associated with loss of suppression of plasma viral RNA levels in subjects treated with ritonavir (Norvir) monotherapy. J Virol 72: 5154–64.

Eberle J, Bechowsky B, Rose D et al. (1995). Resistance of HIV type 1 to proteinase inhibitor Ro 31-8959. AIDS Res Hum Retrovir 11: 671.

Emini EA, Schleif WA, Deutsch P et al. (1996). In vitro selection of HIV-1 variants with reduced susceptibility to the protease inhibitor L-735,524 and related compounds. In: J Mills, P Volberding, L Corey (eds). Antiviral chemotherapy, new directions for clinical application and research. Volume 4. New York: Plenum Press, 327.

Eron JJ, Johnson VA, Merrill DP et al. (1992). Synergistic inhibition of replication of human immunodeficiency virus type 1, including that of a zidovudine-resistant isolate, by zidovudine and 2',3'-dideoxycytidine in vitro. Antimicrob Agents Chemother 36: 1559.

Eron JJ, Benoit SL, Jemsek J et al. (1995). Treatment with lamivudine, zidovudine or both in HIV positive patients with 200 to 500 CD4+ cells per cubic millimeter. North American HIV Working Party. N Engl J Med 333: 1662.

Faletto MB, Miller WH, Garvey EP et al. (1997). Unique intracellular activation of the potent anti-human immunodeficiency virus agent 1592U89. Antimicrob Agents Chemother 41: 1099–107.

Fan N, Rank KB, Evans DT et al. (1995). Simultaneous mutations of Tyr-181 and Tyr-188 in HIV-1 reverse transcriptase prevents inhibition of RNA dependent DNA polymerase activity by the bisheteroarylpiperazine (BHAP) U-90152S. FEBS Lett 370: 59.

Farrar G, Mitchell AM, Hopper H et al. (1994). Prediction of potential drug interactions of saquinavir (Ro 31-8959) from in vitro data. Br J Clin Pharmacol 38: 162.

Fischl MA, Richman DD, Grieco MH et al. (1987). The efficacy of azidothymidine (AZT) in the treatment of patients with AIDS and AIDS-related complex. N Engl J Med 317: 185.

Fischl MA, Richman DD, Hansen N et al. (1990). The safety and efficacy of zidovudine (AZT) in the treatment of subjects with mildly symptomatic human immunodeficiency virus type 1 (HIV) infection: a double-blind, placebo controlled trial. Ann Intern Med 112: 727.

Fischl MA, Olson RM, Follansbee SE et al. (1993). Zalcitabine compared with zidovudine in patients with advanced HIV-1 infection who received previous zidovudine therapy. Ann Intern Med 118: 762.

Fischl MA, Stanley K, Collier AC et al. (1995). Combination and monotherapy with zidovudine and zalcitabine in patients with advanced HIV disease. The NIAID AIDS Clinical Trials Group. Ann Intern Med 122: 24.

Fiske WD, Benedek IH, Joseph JL et al. (1998). Pharmacokinetics of efavirenz (EFV) and ritonavir (RIT) after multiple oral doses in health volunteers. Twelflth World AIDS Conference, Geneva, Switzerland.

Fitzsimmons ME, Collins JM. (1997). Selective biotransformation of the human immunodeficiency virus protease inhibitor saquinavir by human small intestinal cytochrome P4503A4: potential contribution to high first pass metabolism. Drug Metab Dispos 25: 256–66.

Flexner C. (1998). HIV-protease inhibitors. N Engl J Med 338: 1281–92.

Foli A, Sogocio KM, Anderson B et al. (1996). In vitro selection and molecular characterization of human immunodeficiency virus type 1 with reduced sensitivity to 9-2-(phosphonomethoxy) ethyl]adenine (PMEA). Antiviral Res 32: 91–8.

Foster RH, Faulds D. (1998). Abacavir. Drugs 55: 729–36.

Foudraine NA, de-Jong JJ, Jan-Weverling G et al, (1998). An open randomized controlled trial of zidovudine plus lamivudine versus stavudine plus lamivudine. AIDS 12: 1513–19.

Freimuth W. (1996). Delavirdine mesylate, a potent non nucleoside HIV-1 reverse transcriptase inhibitor. In: J Mills, P Volberding, L Corey (eds.) Antiviral chemotherapy, new directions for clinical application and research. New York: Plenum Press, 279.

Friedland G, Dunkle LW, Cross AP. (1996). Stavudine (D4T, Zerit). Antiviral Chemother 4: 271.

Furman PA, Fyfe JA, St. Clair MH et al. (1986). Phosphorylation of 3′-azido-3′-deoxythymidine and selective interaction of the 5′-triphosphate with human immunodeficiency virus reverse transcriptase. Proc Natl Acad Sci USA 83: 8333.

Galpin JE, Lori F, Globe DR et al. (1998). Safety, sheltering and synergy of hydroxyurea (HU) with ddl or ddl plus d4T in HIV-infected patients. Fifth Conference of Retroviruses and Opportunistic Infections, Chicago, IL, USA.

Gao WY, Agbaria R, Driscoll JS et al. (1994). Divergent anti-human immunodeficiency virus activity and anabolic phosphorylation of 2′,3′-dideoxynucleoside analogs in testing and activated human cells. J Biol Chem 269: 12633.

Gao WY, Johns DG, Chokekuchyai S et al. (1995). Disparate actions of hydroxyurea in potentiation of purine and pyrimidine 2′,3-dideoxynucleoside activities against replication of human immunodeficiency virus. Proc Natl Acad Sci USA 92: 8333–7.

Gao WY, Zhou BS, Johns DG et al. (1998). Role of the M2 subunit of ribonucleotide reductase in regulation by hydroxyurea of the activity of the anti-HIV-1 agent 2′,3′-dideoxyinosine. Biochem Pharmacol 56: 105–12.

Gentle DL, Stoller ML, Jarrett TW et al. (1997). Protease inhibitor induced urolithiasis. Urology 50: 508–11.

Gertner E, Thurn JR, Williams DN. (1989). Zidovudine associated myopathy. Am J Med 86: 814.

Giacca M, Borella S, Calderazzo F et al. (1996a). Synergistic antiviral action of ribonucleotide reductase inhibitors and 3′-azido-3′-deoxythymidine on HIV type 1 infection in vitro. AIDS Res Hum Retrovir 12: 677–82.

Giacca M, Zanussi S, Comar M et al. (1996b). Treatment of human immunodeficiency virus infection with hydroxyurea; virologic and clinical evaluation. J Infect Dis 174: 204–9.

Glynn SL, Yazdanian M. (1998). In vitro blood brain barrier permeability of nevirapine compared to other HIV antiretroviral agents. J Pharm Sci 87: 306–10.

Gradon JD, Chapnick EK, Sepkowitz DV. (1992). Zidovudine induced hepatitis. J Intern Med 231: 317.

Gray NM, Marr CL, Penn CR et al. (1995). The intracellular phosphorylation of (-)-2′-deoxy-3′-thiacytidine (3TC) and the incorporation of 3TC 5′-monophosphate into DNA by HIV-1 reverse transcriptase and human DNA polymerase gamma. Biochem Pharmacol 50: 1043.

Grob PM, Wu JC, Cohen KA et al. (1992). Non-nucleoside inhibitors of HIV-1 reverse transcriptase; nevirapine as a prototype drug. AIDS Res Hum Retrovir 8: 145.

Gu Z, Quan Y, Li Z et al. (1995). Effects of non-nucleoside inhibitors of human immunodeficiency virus type 1 in cell free recombinant reverse transcriptase assays. J Biol Chem 270: 31046.

Gulick RM, Mellors JW, Havlir D et al. (1997). Treatment with indinavir, zidovudine, and lamivudine in adults with human immunodeficiency virus infection and prior antiretroviral therapy. N Engl J Med 337: 734–9.

Gulick RM, Mellors JW, Havlir D et al. (1998). Simultaneous vs sequential initiation of therapy with indinavir, zidovudine, and lamivudine for HIV-1 infection. JAMA 280: 35–41.

Gurusinghe AD, Land SA, Birch C et al. (1995). Reverse transcriptase mutations in sequential HIV-1 isolates in a patient with AIDS. J Med Virol 46: 238.

Gustavson LE, Pukuda EK, Rubio FA et al. (1990). A pilot study of the bioavailability and pharmacokinetics of 2′,3′-dideoxycytidine in patients with AIDS or AIDS-related complex. J AIDS 3: 28.

Gwilt PR, Tracewell WG. (1998). Pharmacokinetics and pharmacodynamics of hydroxyurea. Clin Pharmacokinetics 34: 347–58.

Hamilton JD. (1992). Late treatment of HIV infection – is it better? Infect Agents Dis 1: 156–62.

Hammer SM, Katzenstein DA, Hughes MD et al. (1996). A trial comparing nucleoside monotherapy with combination therapy in HIV-infected adults with CD4 cell counts from 200 to 500 per cubic millimeter. N Engl J Med 335: 1081.

Hammer SM, Squires KE, Hughes MD et al. (1997). A controlled trial of two nucleoside analogues plus indinavir in persons with human immunodeficiency virus infection and CD4 cell counts of 200 per cubic millimeter or less. AIDS Clinical Trials Group 320 Study Team. N Engl J Med 337: 725–33.

Hartman NR, Yarchoan R, Pluda JM et al. (1990). Pharmacokinetics of 2′,3′-dideoxyadenosine and 2′,3′-dideoxyinosine in patients with severe human immunodeficiency virus infection. *Clin Pharmacol Ther* **47**: 647.

Haubrich R, Thompson M, Schooley R *et al.* (1999). A phase II safety and efficacy study of amprenavir in combination with zidovudine and lamivudine in HIV-infected patients with limited antiretroviral experience. *AIDS* **13**: 2411–20.

Havlir DV, Lange JMA. (1998). New antiretrovirals and new combinations. *AIDS* **12**: S165–74.

Havlir DE, Cheeseman SH, McLaughlin M *et al.* (1995a). High dose nevirapine; safety, pharmacokinetics and antiviral effect in patients with human immunodeficiency virus infection. *J Infect Dis* **171**: 537.

Havlir D, McLaughlin MM, Richman DD. (1995b). A pilot study to evaluate the development of resistance to nevirapine in asymptomatic human immunodeficiency virus infected patients with CD4 cell counts of >500/mm³; AIDS Clinical Trials Group Protocol 208. *J Infect Dis* **171**: 537.

Hayashi S, Fine RL, Chou JC *et al.* (1990). In vitro inhibition of the infectivity and replication of human immunodeficiency virus type 1 by combination of antiretroviral 2',3'-dideoxynucleosides and virus binding inhibitors. *Antimicrob Agents Chemother* **34**: 82.

Hertogs K, Bloor S, De Vroey V *et al.* (2000). A novel human immunodeficiency virus type 1 reverse transcriptase mutational pattern confers phenotypic lamivudine resistance in the absence of mutation 184V. *Antimicrob Agents Chemother* **44**: 568–73.

Hirsch MS, Brun Vezinet F, D'Aquila RT *et al.* (2000). Antiretroviral drug resistance testing in adult HIV-1 infection: recommendations of an International AIDS Society – USA panel. *JAMA* **283**: 2417–26.

Hitchcock MJ. (1993). In vitro antiviral activity of didanosine compared with that of other dideoxynucleoside analogs against laboratory strains and clinical isolates of human immunodeficiency virus. *Clin Infect Dis* **1**: S16.

Ho DD, Hitchcock MJM. (1989). Cellular pharmacology of 2',3'-didehydrothymidine, a nucleoside analog active against human immunodeficiency virus. *Antimicrob Agents Chemother* **33**: 844.

Ho DD, Toyoshima T, Mo H *et al.* (1994). Characterization of human immunodeficiency virus type 1 variants with increased resistance to a C2-symmetric protease inhibitor. *J Virol* **68**: 2016–20.

Hochster H, Dieterich D, Bozzette S *et al.* (1990). Toxicity of combined ganciclovir and zidovudine for cytomegalovirus disease associated with AIDS. An AIDS Clinical Trials Group Study. *Ann Intern Med* **113**: 111.

Hsu A, Granneman GR, Witt G *et al.* (1997). Multiple dose pharmacokinetics of ritonavir in human immunodeficiency virus infected subjects. *Antimicrob Agents Chemother* **41**: 898–905.

Hsu A, Granneman R, Heath-Chiozzi M et al. (1998a). Indinavir can be taken with regular meals when administered with ritonavir. Twelfth World AIDS Conference, Geneva, Switzerland.

Hsu A, Granneman GR, Cao G *et al.* (1998b). Pharmacokinetic interactions between two human immunodeficiency virus protease inhibitors, ritonavir and saquinavir. *Clin Pharmacol Ther* **63**: 453–64.

Hurst M and Faulds D (2000). Lopinavir *Drugs* **60**: 1371–9.

Ives KJ, Jacobsen H, Galpin SA et al. (1997). Emergence of resistant variants of HIV in vivo during monotherapy with the proteinase inhibitor saquinavir. *J Antimicrob Chemother* **39**: 771–9.

Jacobsen H, Hanggi M, Ou M *et al.* (1996). In vivo resistance to a human immunodeficiency virus type 1 proteinase inhibitor; mutations, kinetics and frequencies. *J Infect Dis* **173**: 1379.

Jarvis B, Faulds D. (1998). Nelfinavir. A review of its therapeutic efficacy in HIV infection. *Drugs* **56**: 147–67.

Jeffries DJ. (1989). The antiviral activity of dideoxycytidine. *J Antimicrob Chemother* **23**: 29.

Johnson VA, Merrill DP, Chou TC *et al.* (1992). Human immunodeficiency virus type 1 (HIV-1) inhibitory interactions between protease inhibitor Ro 31-8959 and zidovudine, 2'3'-dideoxycytidine, or recombinant interferon-alpha A against zidovudine sensitive or resistant HIV-1 in vitro. *J Infect Dis* **166**: 1143.

Kageyama S, Weinstein JN, Shirasaka T *et al.* (1992). In vitro inhibition of human immunodeficiency virus (HIV) type 1 replication by C2 symmetry-based HIV protease inhibitors as single agents or in combinations. *Antimicrob Agents Chemother* **36**: 926.

Kahn JO, Lagakos SW, Richman DD *et al.* (1992). A controlled trial comparing continued zidovudine with didanosine in human immunodeficiency virus infection. *N Engl J Med* **327**: 581.

Kaldor SW, Kalish VJ, Davies JF *et al.* (1997). Viracept (nelfinavir mesylate, AG1343), a potent, orally bioavailable inhibitor of HIV-1 protease. *J Med Chem* **40**: 3979–85.

Kaplan MH, Sadick NS, Wieder J *et al.* (1989). Antipsoriatic effects of zidovudine in human immunodeficiency virus associated psoriasis. *J Am Acad Dermatol* **20**: 76.

Katlama C, Ingrand D, Loveday C *et al.* (1996). Safety and efficacy of lamivudine-zidovudine combination therapy in antiretroviral naive patients. A randomized controlled comparison with zidovudine monotherapy. *JAMA* **276**: 118.

Katlama C, Clotet B, Plettenberg A *et al.* (2000). The role of abacavir (ABC, 1592) in antiretroviral therapy-experienced patients: results from a randomized, double-blind trial. *AIDS* **14**: 781–9.

Kemp SD, Shi C, Bloor S, et al. (1998). A novel polymorphism at codon 333 of human immunodeficiency virus type 1 reverse transcriptase can facilitate dual resistance to zidovudine and L-2',3'-dideoxy-3'-thiacytidine. *J Virol* **72**: 5093–8.

Kempf DJ, Marsh KC, Denissen JF *et al.* (1995). ABT-538 is a potent inhibitor of human immunodeficiency virus protease and has high oral bioavailability in humans. *Proc Natl Acad Sci USA* **92**: 2484.

Kempf DJ, Marsh KC, Kumar G *et al.* (1997). Pharmacokinetic enhancement of inhibitors of the human immunodeficiency virus protease by co-administration with ritonavir. *Antimicrob Agents Chemother* **41**: 654–60.

Khanna N, Klimkait T, Schiffer V *et al.* (2000). Salvage therapy with abacavir plus a non-nucleoside reverse transcriptase inhibitor and a protease inhibitor in heavily pre-treated HIV-1 infected patients. *AIDS* **14**: 791–9.

Kilby JM, Hopkins S, Venetta TM *et al.* (1998). Potent suppression of HIV-1 replication in humans by T-20, a peptide inhibitor of gp41-mediated virus entry. *Nat Med* **4**: 1302–7.

Klecker RW, Collins JM, Yarchoan RC *et al.* (1988). Pharmacokinetics of 2',3'-dideoxycytidine in patients with AIDS and related disorders. *J Clin Pharmacol* **28**: 837.

Kliger Y, Shai Y. (2000). Inhibition of HIV-1 entry before gp41 folds into its fusion-active conformation. *J Mol Biol* **295**: 163–8.

Kline MW, Dunkle LM, Church JA *et al.* (1995). A phase I/II evaluation of stavudine (D4T) in children with human immunodeficiency virus infection. *Pediatrics* **96**: 247.

Kozal MJ, Shafer RW, Winters MA *et al.* (1993). A mutation in human immunodeficiency virus reverse transcriptase and decline in CD4 lymphocyte numbers in long term zidovudine recipients. *J Infect Dis* **167**: 526.

Kucers A, Crowe SM, Grayson L et al. (1997). Ritonavir. In: The use of antibiotics: a clinical review of antibacterial antifungal and antiviral drugs. 5th edition. New York: Butterworth Heinemann, 1795–9.

Kumar GN, Rodrigues AD, Buko AM et al. (1997). Cytochrome P450-mediated metabolism of the HIV-1 protease inhibitor ritonavir (ABT-538) in human liver microsomes. J Pharmacol Exp Ther 281: 1506.

Kuritzkes DR, Bell S, Bakhtiari M. (1994). Rapid CD4+ cell decline after sexual transmission of a zidovudine resistant syncytium inducing isolate of HIV-1. AIDS 8: 1017.

Lacey SF, Larder BA. (1994). Novel mutation (V75T) in human immunodeficiency virus type 1 reverse transcriptase confers resistance to 2',3'-dideoxythymidine in cell culture. Antimicrob Agents Chemother 38: 1428.

Lambert JS, Seidlin M, Reichman RC et al. (1990). 2',3' dideoxyinosine (ddI) in patients with the acquired immunodeficiency syndrome or AIDS-related complex A phase I trial. N Engl J Med 322: 1333.

Land S, Treloar G, McPhee D et al. (1990). Decreased in vitro susceptibility to zidovudine of HIV isolate obtained from patients with AIDS. J Infect Dis 161: 326.

Larder BA. (1992). 3'-azido-3'-deoxythymidine resistance suppressed by a mutation conferring human immunodeficiency virus type 1 resistance to non-nucleoside reverse transcriptase inhibitors. Antimicrob Agents Chemother 36: 2664.

Larder BA. (1994). Interactions between drug resistance mutations in human immunodeficiency virus type 1 reverse transcriptase. J Gen Virol 75: 951.

Larder BA. (1995). Viral resistance and the selection of antiretroviral combinations. J AIDS Hum Retrovirol 10: S28.

Larder BA, Darby G, Richman DD. (1989). HIV with reduced sensitivity to zidovudine (AZT) isolated during prolonged therapy. Science 243: 1731.

Larder BA, Coates KE, Kemp SD. (1991). Zidovudine resistant human immunodeficiency virus selected by passage in cell culture. J Virol 65: 5232.

Larder BA, Bloor S, Hertogs K et al. (1999). Tipranavir is active against a large selection of highly protease inhibitor-resistant HIV-1 clinical samples. In: Abstracts of the third International Workshop on HIV Drug Resistance and Treatment Strategies. San Diego, CA: 5.

Lawless MK, Barney S, Guthrie KI et al. (1996). HIV-1 membrane fusion mechanism: structural studies of the interactions between biologically active peptides from gp41. Biochemistry 35: 13697–708.

Lazdins JK, Mestan J, Goutte G et al. (1997). In vitro effect of alpha 1 acid glycoprotein on the anti-human immunodeficiency virus (HIV) activity of the protease inhibitor CGP 61755, a comparative study with other relevant HIV protease inhibitors. J Infect Dis 175: 1063–70.

LeLacheur SF, Simon GL. (1991). Exacerbation of dideoxycytidine induced neuropathy with dideoxyinosine. J AIDS 4: 538.

Lorenzi P, Yerly S, Abderrakim K et al. (1997). Toxicity, efficacy, plasma drug concentrations and protease mutations in patients with advanced HIV infection treated with ritonavir plus saquinavir. Swiss HIV Cohort Study. AIDS 11: F95–9.

Lori F, Malykh A, Cara A et al. (1994). Hydroxyurea as an inhibitor of human immunodeficiency virus-type 1 replication. Science 266: 801–805.

Lori F, Malykh AG, Foli A et al. (1997). Combination of a drug targeting the cell with a drug targeting the virus controls human immunodeficiency virus type 1 resistance. AIDS Res Hum Retroviruses 13: 1403–9.

Lucht F, Charreau I, Biron F et al. (1998). A randomized phase II trial comparing two different doses of hydroxyurea plus didanosine, ddI alone or ddI plus zidovudine in HIV-1 infected naive patients with CD4(+) lymphocytes between 250 and 500/mm³. Thirty-eighth Interscience Conference on Antimicrobial Agents and Chemotherapy, San Diego, CA, USA.

Lui A, Karter D, Turett G. (1998). Another case of breast hypertrophy in a patient treated with indinavir. Clin Infect Dis 26: 1482.

Markowitz M, Mo H, Kempf DJ et al. (1995a). Selection and analysis of human immunodeficiency virus type 1 variants with increased resistance to ABT-538, a novel protease inhibitor. J Virol 69: 701–6.

Markowitz M, Saag M, Powderly WG et al. (1995b). A preliminary study of ritonavir, an inhibitor of HIV-1 protease, to treat HIV-1 infection. N Engl J Med 333:1534–9.

Markowitz M, Conant M, Hurley A, et al. (1998). A preliminary evaluation of nelfinavir mesylate, an inhibitor of human immunodeficiency virus (HIV)-1 protease to treat HIV infection. J Infect Dis 177: 1533–40.

Mayers DL, Japour AJ, Arduino JM et al. (1994). Dideoxynucleoside resistance emerges with prolonged zidovudine monotherapy. Antimicrob Agents Chemother 38: 307.

Mayers D, Riddler S, Bach M et al. (1997). Durable clinical anti-HIV-1 activity and tolerability for DMP 266 in combination with indinavir (IDV) at 24 weeks. Thirty-Seventh Interscience Conference on Antimicrobial Agents and Chemotherapy. Toronto, Ontario, Canada.

McCrea J, Buss N, Stone J et al. (1997). Indinavir-saquinavir single dose pharmacokinetic study. In: Program and abstracts of the Fourth Conference on Retroviruses and Opportunistic Infections, Washington DC, USA.

McNeely MC, Yarchoan R, Broder S et al. (1989). Dermatologic complications associated with administration of 2',3'-dideoxycytidine in patients with human immunodeficiency virus infection. J Am Acad Dermatol 21: 1213.

Medina DJ, Tung PP, Lerner-Tung MB et al. (1995). Sanctuary growth of human immunodeficiency virus in the presence of 3'-azido-3'-deoxythymidine. J Virol 69: 1606.

Mellors JW, Dutschman GE, Im GJ et al. (1992). In vitro selection and molecular characterization of human immunodeficiency virus 1 resistant to non-nucleoside inhibitors of reverse transcriptase. Mol Pharmacol 41: 446.

Meng TC, Fischl MA, Richman DD. (1990). AIDS Clinical Trials Group; phase I/II study of combination 2',3'-dideoxycytidine and zidovudine in patients with acquired immunodeficiency syndrome (AIDS) and advanced AIDS-related complex. Am J Med 88: 27.

Meng TC, Fischl MA, Boota AM et al. (1992). Combination therapy with zidovudine and dideoxycytidine in patients with advanced human immunodeficiency virus infection. A phase I/II study. Ann Intern Med 116: 13.

Merigan TC, Skowron G, Bozzette SA et al. (1989). Circulating p24 antigen levels and responses to dideoxycytidine in human immunodeficiency virus (HIV) infection. A phase I and II study. Ann Intern Med 110: 189.

Merrill DP, Moonis M, Chou TC et al. (1996). Lamivudine or stavudine in two and three drug combinations against human immunodeficiency virus type 1 replication in vitro. J Infect Dis 173: 355.

Merrill DP, Manion DJ, Chou TC et al. (1997). Antagonism between human immunodeficiency virus type 1 protease inhibitors indinavir and saquinavir in vitro. J Infect Dis 176: 265–8.

Merry C, Barry MG, Mulcahy F et al. (1998). The pharmacokinetics of combination therapy with nelfinavir plus nevirapine. AIDS **12**: 1163–7.

Merry C, Barry MG, Mulcahy F et al. (1997). Saquinavir pharmacokinetics alone and in combination with nelfinavir in HIV-infected patients. AIDS **11**: F29–33.

Miller V, Sturmer M, Staszewski et al. (1998). The M184V mutation in HIV-1 reverse transcriptase (RT) conferring lamivudine resistance does not result in broad cross resistance to nucleoside analogue RT inhibitors. AIDS **12**: 705–12.

Miller MD, Anton KE, Mulato AS et al. (1999). Human immunodeficiency virus type 1 expressing the lamivudine associated M184V mutation in reverse transcriptase shows increased susceptibility to adefovir and decreased replication capability in vitro. J Infect Dis **179**: 92–100.

Mohri H, Singh MK, Ching WT et al. (1993). Quantitation of zidovudine-resistant human immunodeficiency virus type 1 in the blood of treated and untreated patients. Proc Natl Acad Sci USA **90**: 25.

Molla A, Boucher C, Korneyeva M et al. (1995). Evolution of resistance to protease inhibitor ritonavir (ABT-538) in HIV-infected patients. J AIDS Hum Retrovirol **10**: S34.

Molla A, Korneyeva M, Gao Q et al. (1996). Ordered accumulation of mutations in HIV protease confers resistance to ritonavir. Nature Med **2**: 760–6.

Montaner JS, Zala C, Conway B et al. (1997). A pilot study of hydroxyurea among patients with advanced human immunodeficiency virus (HIV) disease receiving chronic didanosine therapy; Canadian HIV trials network protocol 080. J Infect Dis **175**: 801–6.

Montaner JSG, Reiss P, Cooper D et al. (1998a). A randomized, double-blind trial comparing combinations of nevirapine, didanosine and zidovudine for HIV-infected patients; the INCAS trial. JAMA **279**: 930–7.

Montaner JSG, Jahnke N, Hogg R et al. (1998b). Multi drug rescue therapy (MDRT) for HIV-infected individuals with prior virologic failure to multiple regimens; preliminary results. Thirty-eighth Interscience Conference on Antimicrobial Agents and Chemotherapy, San Diego, CA, USA.

Moyle G. (1995). Resistance to antiretroviral compound for clinical management of HIV infection. Immunol Infect Dis **5**: 170.

Moyle G. (1998). The role of combinations of HIV protease inhibitors in the management of persons with HIV infection. Exp Opin Invest Drugs **7**: 413–26.

Moyle G. (2001). The emerging roles of non-nucleoside reverse transcriptase inhibitors in antiretroviral therapy. Drugs **61**: 19–26.

Moyle G, Pozniak A, Opravil M et al. (2000). The SPICE study: 48 week activity of combinations of saquinavir and nelfinavir with and without nucleoside analogues. J Acquir Immune Defic Synd **23**: 128–37.

Mulato AS, Cherrington JM. (1997). Anti-HIV activity of adefovir (PMEA) and PMPA in combination with antiretroviral compounds: in vitro analyses. Antiviral Res **36**: 91–7.

Mulato AS, Lamy PD, Miller MD et al. (1998). Genotypic and phenotypic characterization of human immunodeficiency virus type 1 variants isolated from AIDS patients after prolonged adefovir dipivoxil therapy. Antimicrob Agents Chemother **42**: 1620–8.

Munshi NM, Martin RL, Fonseca VA. (1994). Hyperosmolar nonketotic diabetic syndrome following treatment of human immunodeficiency virus infection with didanosine. Diabetes Care **17**: 316.

Murray HW, Squires KE, Weiss W et al. (1995). Stavudine in patients with AIDS and AIDS-related complex; AIDS Clinical Trials Group 089. J Infect Dis **171**: S123.

Murphy RL, Bruns, Hicks C et al. (2001). ABT-378/ritonavir plus stavudine and lamivudine for the treatment of antiretroviral-naive adults with HIV infection: 48 week results. AIDS **15**: F1–F9.

Noble S, Faulds D. (1996). Saquinavir: a review of its pharmacology and clinical potential in the management of HIV infection. Drugs **52**: 93.

Norbeck D, Hsu A, Granneman R et al. (1995). Virologic and immunologic response to ritonavir (ABT 538) an inhibitor of HIV protease. J AIDS Hum Retrovir **10**: S34.

Notermans DW, Jurriaans S, de Wolf F et al. (1998). Decrease of HIV-1 RNA levels in lymphoid tissue and peripheral blood during treatment with ritonavir, lamivudine and zidovudine. AIDS **12**: 167–73.

Nottet H, Oteman M, Visser MR et al. (1994). Anti HIV-1 activities of novel non-nucleoside reverse transcriptase inhibitors. J Antimicrob Agents Chemother **33**: 366.

Nunberg JH, Schleif WA, Boots EJ et al. (1991). Viral resistance to human immunodeficiency virus type 1 specific pyridinone reverse transcriptase inhibitors. J Virol **65**: 4887.

O'Brien WA. (2000). Resistance against reverse transcriptase inhibitors. Clin Infect Dis **30**(2): S185–92.

Palmer S, Alaeus A, Albert J et al. (1998). Drug susceptibility of subtypes A, B, C. D and E human immunodeficiency virus type 1 primary isolates. AIDS Res Hum Retrovir **14**: 157–62.

Panzer S, Stain C, Benda H et al. (1989). Effects of 3-azidothymidine on platelet counts, indium-iii-labeled platelet kinetics, and antiplatelet antibodies. Vox Sang **57**: 120.

Parteledis JA, Yamaguchi K, Tisdale M et al. (1995). In vitro selection and characterization of human immunodeficiency virus type 1 (HIV-1) isolate with reduced sensitivity to hydroxy-ethylamino sulfonamide inhibitors of HIV-1 aspatyl protease. J Virol **69**: 5228–35.

Patick AK, Mo H, Markowitz M et al. (1996). Antiviral and resistance studies of AG1343, an orally bioavailable inhibitor of human immunodeficiency virus protease. Antimicrob Agents Chemother **40**: 292–7.

Patick AK, Boritzki TJ, Bloom LA. (1997). Activities of the human immunodeficiency virus type 1 (HIV-1) protease inhibitor nelfinavir mesylate in combination with reverse transcriptase and protease inhibitors against acute HIV-1 infection in vitro. Antimicrob Agents Chemother **41**: 2159–64.

Pazhanisamy S, Stuver CM, Cullinan AB et al. (1996). Kinetic characterization of human immunodeficiency virus type 1 protease-resistant variants. J Biol Chem **271**: 17979–85.

Pederson OS, Pedersen EB. (2000). Non-nucleoside reverse transcriptase inhibitors: the NNRTI boom. Antiviral Chem Chemother **10**: 285–314.

Perno CF, Cooney DA, Gao WY et al. (1992). Effects of bone marrow stimulatory cytokines on human immunodeficiency virus replication and the antiviral activity of dideoxynucleosides in cultures of monocytes macrophages. Blood **80**: 995.

Perno CF, Newcomb FM, Davis DA et al. (1998). Relative potency of protease inhibitors in monocytes/macrophages acutely and chronically infected with human immunodeficiency virus. J Infect Dis **178**: 413–22.

Perry CM, Benfield P. (1997). Nelfinavir. Drugs **54**: 81–7.

Perry CM, Noble S. (1998). Saquinavir soft gel capsule formulation. A review of its use in patients with HIV infection. *Drugs* **55**: 461–86.

Petersen EA, Ramirez Ronda CH, Hardy WD. (1995). Dose related activity of stavudine in patients infected with human immunodeficiency virus. *J Infect Dis* **171**: S131.

Pine PS, Weaver JL, Oravecz T et al. (1998). A semiautomated fluorescence-based cell-to-cell fusion assay for gp120–gp41 and CD4 expressing cells. *Exp Cell Res* **240**: 49–57.

Poppe SM, Slade DE, Chong KT et al. (1997). Antiviral activity of the dihydropyrone PNU-140690, a new nonpiptidic human immunodeficiency virus protease inhibitor. *Antimicrob Agents Chemother* **41**: 1058–63.

Ragni MV, Amato DA, LoFaro ML et al. (1995). Randomized study of didanosine monotherapy and combination therapy with zidovudine in hemophilic and nonhemophilic subjects with asymptomatic human immunodeficiency virus-1 infection. AIDS Clinical Trial Groups. *Blood* **85**: 2337.

Rhone SA, Hogg RS, Yip B et al. (1998). The antiviral effect of ritonavir and saquinavir in combination amongst HIV-infected adults; results from a community-based study. *AIDS* **12**: 619–24.

Richman DD, Grimes JM, Lagakos SW. (1990). Effect of stage of disease and drug dose on zidovudine susceptibilities of isolates of human immunodeficiency virus. *J AIDS* **3**: 743.

Richman DD, Rosenthal AS, Skoog M et al. (1991a). BI RG 587 is active against zidovudine resistant human immunodeficiency virus type 1 and synergistic with zidovudine. *Antimicrob Agents Chemother* **35**: 305.

Richman DD, Shih CK, Lowy I et al. (1991b). Human immunodeficiency virus type 1 mutants resistant to non-nucleoside inhibitors of reverse transcriptase arise in tissue culture. *Proc Natl Acad Sci USA* **88**: 11241.

Richman DD, Havlir D, Corbeil J et al. (1994a). Nevirapine resistance mutations of human immunodeficiency virus type 1 selected during therapy. *J Virol* **68**: 1660.

Richman DD, Meng TC, Spector SA et al. (1994b). Resistance to AZT and ddC during long term combination therapy in patients with advanced infection with human immunodeficiency virus. *J AIDS* **7**: 135.

Riddler S, Stein D, Mayers D et al. (1997). *Durable clinical anti-HIV-1 activity (48 weeks) and tolerability (24 weeks) for DMP 266 in combination with indinavir (IDV) (DMP 266-003, Cohort IV).* Thirty-fifth Annual Meeting of the Infectious Diseases Society of America, San Francisco, CA, USA, 770.

Ridky T. Leis J. (1995). Development of drug resistance to HIV-1 protease inhibitors. *J Biol Chem* **270**: 29621.

Rooke R, Parniak MA, Tremblay M et al. (1991). Biological comparison of wild type and zidovudine resistant isolates of human immunodeficiency virus type 1 from the same subjects; susceptibility and resistance to other drugs. *Antimicrob Agents Chemother* **35**: 988.

Ruiz N, DuPont Merck Study Group. (1997). *A double blind pilot study to evaluate the antiretroviral activity, tolerability of DMP 266 in combination with indinavir (Cohort III).* Fourth Conference on Retroviruses and Opportunistic Infections, Washington DC, USA.

Rutschmann OT, Opravil M, Iten A et al. (1998). A placebo-controlled trial of didanosine plus stavudine, with and without hydroxyurea, for HIV infection. The Swiss HIV Cohort Study. *AIDS* **12**: F71–7.

Sadler BM, Gillotin C, Lou Y et al. (2001). Pharmacokinetic and pharmacodynamic study of the human immunodeficiency virus protease imhibitor amprenavir after multiple oral dosing. *Antimicrob Agents Chemother* **45**: 30–7.

Sahai J, Gallicano K, Oliveras L et al. (1993). Cations in the didanosine tablet reduce ciprofloxacin bioavailability. *Clin Pharmacol* **53**: 292.

Sampson MS, Barr MR, Torres RA et al. (1997). *Viral load changes in nelfinavir treated patients switched to a second protease inhibitor after loss of viral suppression.* Thirty-Seventh Interscience Conference on Antimicrobial Agents and Chemotherapy, Toronto, Ontario, Canada.

Schinazi RF, Larder BA, Mellors JW. (2000). Mutations in retroviral genes associated with drug resistance: 2000–2001 update. *Int Antiretrovir News* **8**: 65–91.

Schindzielorz A, Pike I, Daniels M et al. (1994). Rates and risk factors for adverse events associated with didanosine in the expanded access program. *Clin Infect Dis* **19**: 1076.

Schmit JC, Ruiz L, Clotet B et al. (1996). Resistance related mutations in the HIV-1 protease gene of patients treated for 1 year with the protease inhibitor ritonavir (ABT-538). *AIDS* **10**: 995–9.

Schooley RT, Ramirez-Ronda C, Lange JM et al. (1996). Virologic and immunologic benefits of initial combination therapy with zidovudine and zalcitabine or didanosine compared with zidovudine monotherapy. Wellcome Resistance Study Collaborative Group. *J Infect Dis* **173**: 1354.

Schuurman R, Nijhuis M, van Leeuwen R et al. (1995). Rapid changes in human immunodeficiency virus type 1 RNA load and appearance of drug resistant virus populations in persons treated with lamivudine (3TC). *J Infect Dis* **171**: 1411.

Seidlin M, Lambert JS, Dolin R et al. (1992). Pancreatitis and pancreatic dysfunction in patients taking dideoxyinosine. *AIDS* **6**: 831.

Seifert RD, Stewart MB, Sramek JJ et al. (1994). Pharmacokinetics of co-administered didanosine and stavudine in HIV seropositive male patients. *Br J Clin Pharmacol* **38**: 405.

Shafer RW, Kozal MJ, Katzenstein DA et al. (1993). Zidovudine susceptibility testing of human immunodeficiency virus type 1 (HIV) clinical isolates. *J Virol Meth* **41**: 297.

Sham HL, Kempf DJ, Molla A et al. (1998). ABT-378, a highly potent inhibitor of the human immunodeficiency virus protease. *Antimicrob Agents Chemother* **42**: 3218–24.

Shelton MJ, O'Donnell AM, Morse GD et al. (1992). Didanosine. *Ann Pharmacother* **26**: 660.

Shelton MJ, O'Donnell AM, Morse GD. (1993). Zalcitabine. *Ann Pharmacother* **27**: 480.

Shirasaka T, Yarchoan R, O'Brien MC et al. (1993). Changes in drug sensitivity of human immunodeficiency virus type 1 during therapy with azidothymidine, dideoxycytidine and dideoxyinosine, an *in vitro* comparative study. *Proc Natl Acad Sci USA* **90**: 562.

Shirasaka T, Kavlick MF, Ueno T et al. (1995). Emergence of human immunodeficiency virus type 1 variants with resistance to multiple dideoxynucleosides in patients receiving therapy with dideoxynucleosides. *Proc Natl Acad Sci USA* **92**: 2398.

Simonelli C, Comar M, Zanussi S et al. (1997). No therapeutic advantage from didanosine (ddI) and hydroxyurea versus ddI alone in patients with HIV infection. *AIDS* **11**: 1299–300.

Skowron G. (1995). Biologic effects and safety of stavudine; overview of phase I and II clinical trials. *J Infect Dis* **171**: S113.

Spector SA. (1994). Pediatric antiretroviral choices. *AIDS* **8**: S15.

St Clair MH, Martin JL, Tudor-Williams G et al. (1991). Resistance to ddI and sensitivity to AZT induced by a mutation in HIV-1 reverse transcriptase. *Science* **253**: 1557.

St Clair MH, Pennington KN, Rooney J et al. (1995). In vitro comparison of selected triple drug combinations for suppression of HIV-1 replication. The Inter Company Collaboration Protocol. J AIDS Hum Retrovir 10: S83.

St Clair MH, Millard J Rooney J, et al. (1996). In vitro antiviral activity of 141W94 (VX–478) in combination with other antiretroviral agents. Antiviral Res 29: 53–6.

Staszewski S. (1995). Zidovudine and lamivudine; results of phase III studies. J AIDS Hum Retrovir. 10: S57.

Staszewski S, Morales-Ramirez J, Tashima K et al. (1998). A phase III, multicenter, randomized, open-label study to compare the antiretroviral activity and tolerability of efavirenz (EFV) + indinavir (IDV), versus EFV + zidovudine (ZDV) + lamivudine (3TC) versus IDV + ZDV + 3TC at 24 weeks [study DMP 266-006]. Twelfth World AIDS Conference, Geneva, Switzerland.

Stein DS, Fish DG, Bilello JA et al. (1996). A 24-week open label phase I/II evaluation of the HIV protease inhibitor MK 639 (indinavir). AIDS 10: 485.

Su SB, Gong WH, Gao JL et al. (1999). 120/DP178, an ectodomain peptide of human immunodeficiency virus type 1 gp41, is an activator of human phagocyte N-formyl peptide receptor. Blood 93: 3885–92.

Sullivan AK, Nelson MR. (1997). Marked hyperlipidaemia on ritonavir therapy. AIDS 11: 938–9.

Sun E, Heath-Chiozzi M, Cameron DW et al. (1996). Concurrent ritonavir and rifabutin increases risk of rifabutin associated adverse events. In: Program and abstracts of the Eleventh International Conference on AIDS, Vancouver, Canada.

Swanstrom R, Erona J. (2000). Human immunodeficiency virus type-1 protease inhibitors: therapeutic successes and failures, suppression and resistance. Pharmacol Ther 86: 145–70.

Swiss Group for Clinical Studies on the Acquired Immunodeficiency Syndrome (AIDS) (1988). Zidovudine for the treatment of thrombocytopenia associated with human immunodeficiency virus (HIV). A prospective study. Ann Intern Med 109: 718.

Tashima KT, Caliendo AMC, Ahmad MA. (1998). Cerebrospinal Fluid HIV-1 RNA levels and efavirenz concentrations in patients enrolled in clinical trials. Twelfth World AIDS Conference, Geneva, Switzerland.

Tisdale M, Kemp SD, Parry NR et al. (1993). Rapid in vitro selection of human immunodeficiency virus type 1 resistant to 3'-thiacytidine inhibitors due to a mutation in the YMDD region of reverse transcriptase. Proc Natl Acad Sci USA 90: 5653.

Tisdale M, Myers RE, Maschera B et al. (1995). Cross resistance analysis of human immunodeficiency virus type 1 variants individually selected for resistance to five different protease inhibitors. Antimicrob Agents Chemother 39: 1704.

Tisdale M, Alnadaf T, Cousens D. (1997). Combination of mutations in human immunodeficiency virus type 1 reverse transcriptase required for resistance to the carbocyclic nucleoside 1592U89. Antimicrob Agents Chemother 41: 1094–8.

Turriziani O, Antonelli G. Jacobsen H et al. (1994). Identification of an amino acid substitution involved in the reduction of sensitivity of HIV-1 to an inhibitor of viral proteinase. Acta Virologica 38: 297.

Vacca JP, Dorsey BD, Schleif WA et al. (1994). L-735,524 an orally bioavailable human immunodeficiency virus type-1 protease inhibitor. Proc Natl Acad Sci USA 91: 4096.

Valentine FT, Seidlin M, Hochster H et al. (1990). Phase I study of 2',3'-dideoxyinosine; experience with 19 patients at New York University Medical Center. Rev Infect Dis 5: S534.

Van Leeuwen R, Lange JM, Hussey EK et al. (1992). The safety and pharmacokinetics of a reverse transcriptase inhibitor, 3TC in patients with HIV infection; a phase 1 study. AIDS 6: 1471.

Van Leeuwen R, Katlama C, Kitchen V et al. (1995). Evaluation of safety and efficacy of 3TC (lamivudine) in patients with asymptomatic or mildly symptomatic human immunodeficiency virus infection; a phase I/II study. J Infect Dis 171: 1166.

Vella S, Floridia M. (1998). Saquinavir. Clinical pharmacology and efficacy. Clin Pharmacokinet 34: 189–201.

Vergis E, Paterson DL, Singh N. (1998). Indinavir associated hepatitis in patients with advanced HIV infection. Int J STD AIDS 9: 53.

Vogt MW, Hartshorn KL, Furman PA et al. (1987). Ribavirin antagonizes the effect of azidothymidine on HIV replication. Science 235: 1376.

Volberding PA, Lagakos SW, Koch MA et al. (1990). Zidovudine in asymptomatic human immunodeficiency virus infection. A controlled trial in persons with fewer than 500 CD4 positive cells per cubic millimeter. The AIDS Clinical Trials Group of the National Institute of Allergy and Infectious Diseases. N Engl J Med 322: 941.

von Moltke LL, Greenblatt DJ, Grassi JM et al. (1998). Protease inhibitors as inhibitors of human cytochromes P450: high risk associated with ritonavir. J Clin Pharmacol 38: 106–11.

Werth JL, Zhou B, Nutter LM et al. (1994). 2',3'-dideoxycytidine alters calcium buffering in cultured dorsal root ganglion neurons. Mol Pharmacol 45: 1119.

Wild C, Greenwell T, Matthews T. (1993). A synthetic peptide from HIV-1 gp41 is a potent inhibitor of virus-mediated cell–cell fusion. AIDS Res Hum Retrovir 9: 1051–3.

Winslow DL, Garber S, Reid C et al. (1996). Selection conditions affect the evolution of specific mutations in the reverse transcriptase gene associated with resistance to DMP 266. AIDS 10: 1205–9.

Yarchoan R, Klecker RW, Weinbold KJ et al. (1986). Administration of 3'-azido-3'-deoxythymidine, an inhibitor of HTLV-III/LAV replication, to patients with AIDS or AIDS-related complex. Lancet i: 575.

Yarchoan R, Berg G, Brouwers P et al. (1987). Response of human immunodeficiency virus associated neurological disease to 3'-azido 3'-deoxythymidine. Lancet i: 132.

Yarchoan R, Mitsuya H, Myers CE et al. (1989). Clinical pharmacology of 3'-azido-2'-3'-dideoxythymidine (zidovudine) and related dideoxynucleosides. N Engl J Med 321: 726.

Yarchoan R, Mitsuya H, Pluda JM et al. (1990). The National Cancer Institute phase I study of 2',3'-dideoxyinosine administration in adults with AIDS or AIDS-related complex; analysis of activity and toxicity profiles. Rev Infect Dis 12: S522–33.

Yeh KC, Deutsch PJ, Haddix H et al. (1998). Single dose pharmacokinetics of indinavir and the effect of food. Antimicrob Agents Chemother 42: 332–8.

Young SD, Britcher SF, Tran LO et al. (1995). L-743-726 (DMP-266); a novel, highly potent non-nucleoside inhibitor of the human immunodeficiency virus type 1 reverse transcriptase. Antimicrob Agents Chemother 39: 2602–5.

Antiretroviral therapy: adverse effects and drug interactions

S. ERALP BELLIBAS, MASATO HOMMA AND FRANCESCA AWEEKA

Antiretroviral therapy for HIV has changed dramatically over the past few years. With the introduction of the protease inhibitors, the potency of antiretroviral regimens has profoundly improved the clinical and virological responses in HIV-infected patients. This has resulted in a longer life span and dramatically reduced susceptibility to the complications of HIV disease. Life-threatening opportunistic infections such as *Pneumocystis carinii* pneumonia, cytomegalovirus and toxoplasmosis rarely occur, so that 'complications of HIV' are now in essence the complications of the therapy itself.

The antiretroviral drugs that are the focus of this chapter include the reverse transcriptase inhibitors (both nucleoside analogue and non-nucleoside reverse transcriptase inhibitors) and the protease inhibitors. The primary toxicities of each of the currently approved agents will be reviewed and their drug interactions summarized.

Reverse transcriptase inhibitors

The reverse transcriptase inhibitors (RTIs) specifically inhibit the transcription of viral RNA into DNA. Currently six nucleoside analogues (NRTIs) are approved for clinical use: zidovudine, didanosine, zalcitabine, lamivudine, stavudine and, most recently, abacavir. Three non-nucleoside reverse transcriptase inhibitors (NNRTIs) are available: nevirapine, delavirdine and efavirenz. All of these drugs are commonly used as part of combination antiretroviral regimens with or without the potent anti-HIV protease inhibitors (PIs). Although both classes of drugs target HIV similarly, the NRTIs and NNRTIs are largely distinct pharmacologically (reviewed in Kucers *et al.*, 1997).

Nucleoside (purine or pyrimidine) analogue RTIs enter the target cells and are phosphorylated by host cellular kinases to their active 5'-triphosphates. The active triphosphates competitively inhibit the binding of endogenous nucleoside triphosphates to the viral RT (Peter and Gambertoglio, 1998), assuring the required antiviral effect. Unfortunately, these NRTIs also inhibit mammalian DNA polymerase, including gamma polymerase, an enzyme essential for mitochondrial DNA replication. It is proposed that mitochondrial toxicity contributes to the occurrence of multiple adverse effects, including bone marrow suppression, neuropathy, and myopathy.

In contrast, the NNRTIs bind directly to RT without prior intracellular phosphorylation and block DNA polymerase by disrupting the catalytic site of viral RT. Unlike the NRTIs, the NNRTIs do not inhibit gamma polymerase. Such differentiation at least partially explains the lack of concordance for adverse events attributed to these two drug classes.

Zidovudine (AZT, ZDV)

Zidovudine is a thymidine analogue, approved by the US Food and Drug Administration (FDA) for treatment of patients with HIV infection in 1987. Zidovudine is also a primary agent used in pregnancy to reduce transmission of HIV from mother to fetus and has received additional approval for this specific indication.

Adverse effects

The major adverse reactions of zidovudine are anaemia and neutropenia, with a wide range of frequency (2–37%), depending on the stage of HIV disease (Retrovir® package insert, GlaxoWellcome, Research Triangle Park, NC, USA, 1998). These haematological toxicities are dose (and therefore exposure) dependent and often dose limiting. Haematological toxicity is more likely to occur in patients with advanced disease, low CD4 lymphocyte counts, vitamin B_{12} and folate deficiency, and baseline anaemia and neutropenia (McLeod and Hammer, 1992).

The proposed mechanism is inhibition of haem synthesis by zidovudine and has been associated with the ZDV metabolite, 3'-amino-3'-deoxythymidine (Cretton et al., 1991). Management of anaemia and neutropenia has included the use of packed red blood cell transfusions, recombinant erythropoietin, granulocyte-colony-stimulating factor (G-CSF), and granulocyte-macrophage-colony-stimulating factor (GM-CSF) (Miles et al., 1991).

Nausea, anorexia, myalgia, malaise, fatigue, and insomnia may also occur in zidovudine-treated patients, particularly during the first 6 weeks or so of therapy (Table 6.1). Other reported adverse effects include seizures, macular oedema, and the Stevens-Johnson syndrome, although the causal relationship remains uncertain (McLeod and Hammer, 1992).

Long-term studies have documented liver and muscle abnormalities (myopathy) from zidovudine therapy. Increases in liver function tests were seen in a large population of patients receiving long-term zidovudine (>10 months), although dose adjustment was required in less than 3.3% of patients (Fischl et al., 1989). The incidence of zidovudine-related myopathy likely to develop remains unclear as it is difficult to differentiate zidovudine-related myopathy from a similar phenomenon caused directly by HIV infection. Biochemical or immunochemical differences may exist between the two entities (Gherardi et al., 1994). Clinical improvement of myopathy may occur following cessation of zidovudine (Peters et al., 1993).

Occasional cases of severe liver damage including hepatitis (Gradon et al., 1992), fulminant hepatic failure (Shintaku et al., 1993), and hepatomegaly with steatosis (Freiman et al., 1993), and lactic acidosis (Chattha et al., 1993) with or without liver damage (Olano et al., 1995) have been reported. Lactic acidosis should be considered when zidovudine-treated patients develop unexplained tachypnoea, dyspnoea, or a fall in serum bicarbonate level (Retrovir® product information, Glaxo Wellcome, Research Triangle Park, NC, USA, 1998).

Drug interactions

Haematological toxicity of zidovudine can be exacerbated via concomitant renal disease (resulting in decreased erythropoietin production) or indirectly by drugs that are highly nephrotoxic, such as amphotericin. Cytotoxic compounds that may worsen anaemia or neutropenia include flucytosine, vincristine, doxorubicin, and alpha-interferon-α and those that interfere with erythro-

cyte/leucocyte number or function include aciclovir, ganciclovir, pentamidine and dapsone. The combination of zidovudine and ganciclovir is poorly tolerated in patients with AIDS and cytomegalovirus disease (Hochester et al., 1990). The toxicity results from the combined myelosuppressive effect of the two drugs. Concurrent administration of these two agents should therefore be undertaken with extreme caution. For other drugs, such as high doses of co-trimoxazole (trimethoprim-sulfamethoxazole), dapsone, flucytosine, amphotericin B and pyrimethamine, careful monitoring of haematological parameters is required when co-administered with zidovudine (Burger et al., 1993).

Several drugs affect zidovudine pharmacokinetics by inhibiting its metabolism by glucuronidation or its excretion (acetaminophen, cimetidine, indomethacin, lorazepam, probenecid, aspirin, valproic acid, and trimethoprim). For example, probenecid and methadone both inhibit hepatic glucuronidation, resulting in increased serum concentrations of zidovudine and a prolonged elimination half-life (De Miranda et al., 1989; McCance-Katz et al., 1989). Thus, ZDV dose modification may be required in patients receiving either of these drugs concurrently with ZDV (Kornhauser et al., 1989; McCance-Katz et al., 1989). Not all the potential drug interactions are of clinical importance, as shown in Table 6.2 (Taburet and Singlas, 1996).

Administration with a fatty meal decreases both the ZDV plasma area-under-the-curve (AUC) and peak plasma concentration (C_{max}). However, these food effects are not of major importance and have not resulted in specific recommendations regarding the timing of meals in relation to drug intake for patients receiving this therapy.

Ribavirin, recently approved for the treatment of hepatitis C, was initially shown in vitro to antagonize the anti-HIV activity of zidovudine by inhibiting intracellular phosphorylation of zidovudine (Burger et al., 1993). Therefore, concomitant use of these drugs was initially avoided. However, recent clinical findings indicate no antagonistic change in viral load when ribaviron is coadministered with ZDV (Dieterich et al., 2000). Additionally, zidovudine alters the phosphorylation of stavudine (d4T), a mechanism explaining the poor clinical response observed when this combination was evaluated in AIDS Clinical Trials Group protocol 290 (Sommadossi et al., 1998). There is no significant pharmacokinetic interaction between zidovudine and the NNRTIs or PIs.

Table 6.1 Adverse effects of NRTIs and NNRTIs

Zidovudine (ZDV, AZT)*
CNS	Headache (>10%), insomnia (>10%)
GIS	Nausea, anorexia, vomiting (1–10%)
NMS	Myopathy
Dermatological	Rash, nail discoloration (1–10%)
Haematological	Anaemia (>10%), granulocytopenia (1–10%), bone marrow depression (<1%)
Hepatic	Hepatotoxicity (<1%)
General	Myalgia (>10%), malaise (1–10%)

Didanosine (ddI)*
CNS	Headache (>10%), depression (1–10%)
GIS	Diarrhoea, nausea, vomiting, abdominal pain (10%), pancreatitis (1–10%)
NMS	Neuropathy (>10%)
Dermatological	Rash, pruritis (1–10%)
Haematological	Leukopenia (>10%), anaemia, granulocytopenia, thrombocytopenia (1–10%)
Hepatic	Elevated AST/ALT, alkaline phosphatase, biluribin (1–10%)

Zalcitabine (ddc)*
CNS	Headache, dizziness, myalgia, fatigue (1–10%), neuropathy (17–31%)
GIS	Diarrhoea (1–10%), nausea, vomiting, oral ulcers (>10%), dysphagia, anorexia, pharyngitis
Dermatological	Rash, pruritis (1–10%)
CVS	Chest pain (1–10%), atrial fibrillation, tachycardia (<1%)
Haematological	Granulocytopenia (1–10%), epistaxis, anaemia

Stavudine (d4T)*
CNS	Headache, anxiety, insomnia, depression
GIS	Diarrhoea, nausea, vomiting, abdominal pain (1–10%), pancreatitis
NMS	Peripheral neuropathy (>10%), myalgia, back pain (1–10%)
Hepatic	Elevated AST/ALT
General	Asthenia, malaise, chills/fever

Lamivudine (3TC)*
CNS	Headache, insomnia, depression, dizziness
GIS	Nausea, anorexia, vomiting (>10%), diarrhoea, abdominal pain, dyspepsia, elevated amylase
NMS	Peripheral neuropathy, paresthesia (>10%), myalgia, artralgia (1–10%)
Dermatological	Rash (1–10%)
Haematological	Anaemia (1–10%), thrombocytopenia (<1%), neutropenia
Hepatic	Elevated AST, ALT (1–10%)
Respiratory	Cough (>10%), nasal sign and symptoms
General	Malaise, fatigue, chills (1–10%), fever

Abacavir*
CNS	Headache (35%), insomnia (17%)
GIS	Diarrhoea (21%), nausea (44%), vomiting (13%), abdominal pain, anorexia
Dermatological	Rash
Respiratory	Sore throat, cough
General	Hypersensitivity reaction (2–5%), fever, fatigue and malaise (29%)

Nevirapine
CNS	Headache
GIS	Nausea, diarrhoea
Dermatological	Rash, Stevens-Johnson syndrome
Hepatic	Elevated ALT and AST and/or GGT
General	Fatigue, fever

Delavirdine
CNS	Headache
GIS	Nausea, vomiting, diarrhoea, dyspepsia
Dermatological	Rash
Hepatic	Elevated AST, ALT
General	Fatigue

Efavirenz
CNS	Headache, dizziness, insomnia, light-headedness, anxiety, dysphoria, ataxia, tremor
GIS	Diarrhoea, nausea, vomiting, dyspepsia
Dermatological	Rash (27%), erythema multiforme and Stevens-Johnson syndrome (3.5% in children)
General	Influenza-like symptoms, sinusitis, fatigue, elevated AST/ALT

ALT: alanine aminotransferase; AST: aspartate aminotransferase; CNS: central nervous system; CVS: cardiovascular system; GGT: gamma glutamyl transferase; GIS: gastrointestinal system; NMS: neuromuscular system.

*Lactic acidosis with hepatic steatosis is a rare but potentially life-threatening toxicity with the use of NRTIs.

Table 6.2 Pharmacokinetic drug interactions with NRTIs and NNRTIs

	Effect	Comments
Zidovudine (ZDV)		
Atovaquone	Increases ZDV AUC (33%)	Inhibition of ZDV glucuronidation
Fluconazole	Increases ZDV AUC (74%)	Inhibition of ZDV glucuronidation
Methadone	Increases ZDV AUC (41%)	Inhibition of ZDV glucuronidation and/or reducing excretion
Valproic acid	Increases ZDV AUC (80%)	Inhibition of ZDV glucuronidation
Probenecid	Increases ZDV AUC (80%)	Inhibition of ZDV glucuronidation
Rifampicin (rifampin)	Decreases ZDV AUC (36–75%)	Induction of ZDV glucuronidation
Cotrimoxazole	Decreases ZDV CLr (48–58%)	No effect on total CL and AUC
Cimetidine	Decreases ZDV CLr	No effect on total CL (Ranitidine no effect)
Paracetamol	Decreases ZDV AUC (10–30%)	Not clinically relevant
Rifabutin	Decreases ZDV AUC and C_{max}	Not clinically relevant
Stavudine	Antiviral antagonism	Inhibition of phosphorylation (*avoid*)
Ribavirin	Inhibits phosphorylation of ZDV	Avoid if possible
Didanosine (ddI)		
Ciprofloxacin	Decrease ciprofloxacin absorption	Ciprofloxacin should be given >1 h before or 6 h after ddI
Tetracycline	Decrease tetracycline absorption	Tetracycline should be administered 2 h before or after ddI
Itraconazole	Decrease itraconazole absorption	Itraconazole should be administered >1 h before or 2 h after ddI
Ketoconazole	Decrease ketoconazole absorption	Ketoconazole should be administered >1 h before or 2 h after ddI
Dapsone	Decrease dapsone absorption	Dapsone should be administered >1 h before or 2 h after ddI
Ranitidine	Increase ddI absorption	Ranitidine should be administered 2 h before or after ddI
Zidovudine	Increase ZDV AUC (35%)	Decrease in ZDV oral clearance
Ganciclovir	Increase ddI AUC	Close monitoring for adverse effects required
Delavirdine	Decrease delavirdine absorption	Separate administration by at least 1 h
Protease inhibitors	Decrease PI absorption	Separate administration by at least 1 h
Methadone	Decrease in ddI levels (41%)	Consider ddI dose increase
Zalcitabine (ddC)		
Didanosine	Additive toxicity	Close monitoring for adverse effects required
Stavudine	Additive toxicity	Close monitoring for adverse effects required
Lamivudine	Additive toxicity	Close monitoring for adverse effects required
Cimetidine	Increases ddC AUC (36%)	Inhibition ddC renal CL
Trimethoprim	Increases ddC AUC (37%)	Inhibition ddC renal CL
Al and Mg hydroxide	Decreases ddC bioavailability (25%)	Antacid drug is administered 2 hours apart
Dapsone	Slightly increase dapsone C_{max}	Not clinically relevant
Stavudine (d4T)		
Zidovudine	Antiviral antagonism	Inhibition of phosphorylation (*avoid*)
Didanosine	Additive toxicity	Close monitoring for adverse effects required
Zalcitabine	Additive toxicity	Close monitoring for adverse effects required
Methadone	Decrease in d4T levels (27%)	No dose adjustment
Lamivudine (3TC)		
Zidovudine	Increases ZDV C_{max} (40%)	No significant change in AUC
Cotrimoxazole	Increases lamivudine AUC (44%)	30% decrease in 3TC CL
Abacavir		
Ethanol	Increases abacavir AUC (40%)	Common metabolic pathway (alcohol dehydrogenase)
Nevirapine		
Zidovudine	Decreases ZDV AUC (32%)	Induction of P450; no data regarding dose adjustment
Indinavir	Decreases indinavir AUC (28%)	Induction of P450; increase indinavir dosage 1000 mg every 8 h
Saquinavir	Decreases saquinavir AUC (25%)	Induction of P450; no data regarding dose adjustment
Rifampin	Decreases nevirapine AUC (68%)	Induction of P450; increase nevirapine dose (50%)
Ketoconazole	Decreases ketoconazole AUC (63%)	Induction of P450; alternative antifungal should be used
Clarithromycin	Decreases clarithromycin levels (30%)	No dose adjustment
Oral contraceptives	Decreases ethinyl estradiol levels (20%)	Use alternative or additional methods
Methadone	Decreases methadone levels significantly	Titrate methadone dose to effect

Continued.

Table 6.2 *Continued.*

Delavirdine (DLV)

Rifampicin	Decreases delavirdine level	Induction of CYP3A4 (*avoid*)
Rifabutin	Decreases delavirdine level	Induction of CYP3A4 (*avoid*)
Indinavir	Increases indinavir AUC (50%)	Inhibition of CYP3A4; Indinavir dose 600 mg every 8 h
Saquinavir	Increases saquinavir AUC (500%)	Inhibition of CYP3A4; standard dose
Ritonavir	Increases ritonavir AUC (60%)	Inhibition of CYP3A4; no recommendations regarding dose adjustment
Nelfinavir	Increases nelfinavir AUC (92%)	Decreases nelfinavir metabolite AUC (50%)
Clarithromycin	Increases delavirdine AUC (44%)	Increases clarithromycin AUC (100%)
Fluoxetine	Increases delavirdine trough levels (50%)	Inhibition of CYP2C6
Fluconazole	Increases delavirdine AUC (30%)	Inhibition of CYP3A4
Ketoconazole	Increases delavirdine trough levels (50%)	Inhibition of CYP3A4
Terfenadine	Predict plasma levels increased	Serious cardiac arrhythmias (*avoid*)
Astemizole	Predict plasma levels increased	Serious cardiac arrhythmias (*avoid*)
Cisapride	Predict plasma levels increased	Serious cardiac arrhythmias (*avoid*)
Warfarin	Predict plasma levels increased	Serious bleeding problems; close monitoring of PT
Midazolam	Predict plasma levels increased	Excessive sedation (*avoid*)

Efavirenz

Indinavir	Decreases indinavir AUC (31%)	Increases indinavir dose to 1000 mg every 8 h
Ritonavir	Increases ritonavir and efavirenz AUC (20%)	No dosage adjustment necessary
Amprenavir	Decreases amprenavir AUC (36%)	Dosage adjustment should be considered
Nelfinavir	Increases nelfinavir plasma levels (20%)	No dose adjustment necessary
Saquinavir	Decreases saquinavir AUC (62%)	Co-administration, as a sole PI is not recommended
Ethinyl estradiol	Increases ethinyl estradiol levels (37%)	Clinical significance unknown
Clarithromycin	Decreases clarithromycin levels (39%)	Alternative agent should be considered
Rifampin	Decreases efavirenz AUC (33%)	Efavirenz dose should be increased to 800 mg daily
Terfenadin	Predict plasma levels increased	Serious cardiac arrhythmias (*avoid*)
Astemizole	Predict plasma levels increased	Serious cardiac arrhythmias (*avoid*)
Midazolam	Predict plasma levels increased	Excessive sedation (*avoid*)
Methadone	Decreases methadone levels significantly	Titrate methadone dose to effect
Nevirapine	Decreases efavirenz AUC (22%)	
Cisaprid	Predict plasma levels increased	Serious cardiac arrhythmias (*avoid*)
Methadone	Decreases methadone levels significantly	Titrate methadone dose to effect
Nevirapine	Decreases efavirenz AUC (22%)	

AL: aluminium; AUC: area-under-the-curve; CL: clearance; Clr: renal clearance; Mg: magnesium; PT: prothrombin time.

Didanosine (ddI)

Didanosine is an inosine analogue, approved by the FDA since 1991 for the treatment of HIV infection. Didanosine is phosphorylated intracellularly to its active metabolite, dideoxyadenosine triphosphate (ddATP).

Adverse effects

Dose-limiting adverse reactions associated with didanosine therapy are peripheral neuropathy occurring in 13–34% of patients and pancreatitis in 5% (Table 6.1) (Perry and Balfour, 1996). These reactions may be exposure related and reversible. Peripheral neuropathy is more likely to be observed in patients with a history of peripheral neuropathy or previous neurotoxic drug therapy. Due to increasing concern over didanosine-associated pancreatitis, pancreatic function (serum amylase and lipase levels) should be carefully monitored to avoid subsequent development of diabetes and serious pancreatitis. Glucose intolerance during didanosine therapy is an early sign of pancreatitis (Albrecht *et al.*, 1993). Predisposing factors to the development of this disorder include prior history of pancreatic disease and advanced HIV disease coupled with a low CD4 lymphocyte count (<50 cells/μl).

Other adverse events include diarrhoea, nausea, vomiting, headache, depression and liver function abnormalities resembling hepatitis. Diarrhoea is relatively frequent and is generally attributed to the citrate/phosphate buffer used in the preparation of this drug.

The incidence of gastrointestinal adverse reactions (diarrhoea, nausea, and vomiting) with didanosine therapy is significantly greater than with zidovudine (Saravolatz et al., 1996). Myelosuppression, however, is generally minimal with didanosine. Zidovudine-associated bone marrow suppression may be reversed when patients are switched from zidovudine to didanosine (Spruance et al., 1994).

Retinal changes and optic neuritis have been reported in several paediatric patients who received didanosine at or above the recommended dose (Videx® product information, Bristol-Myers Squibb, Princeton, NJ, USA, 1996) and a couple of cases of fulminant hepatitis have also been reported (Lai et al., 1991; Bissuel et al., 1994).

Drug interactions

Concurrent administration of ganciclovir increases the didanosine plasma AUC by 72%, possibly due to competition for active tubular secretion in the kidneys (Trapnell et al., 1994). Therefore, lower doses of didanosine are warranted during co-administration of these drugs. Concomitant administration of other drugs (dapsone, metronidazole, pentamidine, phenytoin, ribavirin and vincristine), which have the potential to cause peripheral neuropathy or pancreatitis, may increase the risk of these toxicities (Taburet and Singlas, 1996).

Didanosine impacts on the pharmacokinetic disposition of several AIDS-related compounds. Didanosine is available as a chewable/dispersible tablet, which is buffered with sodium citrate and the antacids calcium carbonate and magnesium hydroxide, and also as a powder for oral solution buffered with citrate/phosphate (Perry and Balfour, 1996). These formulations, which acutely alkalinize the gastric environment to prevent didanosine degradation in the stomach, contribute to drug interactions at the absorption stage. For example, didanosine decreases the absorption of ketoconazole, itraconazole, and dapsone, which require gastric acid for absorption as well as ciprofloxacin and tetracycline, which form chelate complexes with magnesium and aluminum. These agents should be administered at least 2 h prior to didanosine. The new enteric-coated formulation of didanosine is unlikely to interact in the same way as the buffered formulation.

Ranitidine slightly increases didanosine bioavailability, whereas food reduces it by twofold (Shyu et al., 1991). Therefore, didanosine should be given while fasting and at least 30 min before a meal (Videx® product information, Bristol-Myers Squibb).

Zalcitabine (ddC)

Zalcitabine is a cytosine analogue, also phosphorylated intracellularly, which was approved by the FDA for the treatment of HIV infection in 1992. It is currently less commonly used than other NRTIs, owing to its relatively lower potency and higher toxicity profile.

Adverse effects

The most common adverse effect reported with zalcitabine is a dose-dependent peripheral neuropathy (17–31%) (Table 6.1) (Adkins et al., 1997). Although the range of reported frequencies of this toxicity varies widely and is thus similar for didanosine and zalcitabine, peripheral neuropathy is considered more common with zalcitabine than didanosine (Abrams et al., 1994). The symptoms are predominantly sensory with distal dyesthesia, pain and numbness, any of which may necessitate treatment termination. Risk factors include diabetes, low serum cobalamin, history of nerve dysfunction or peripheral neuropathy, and CD4 lymphocyte count of less than 50 cells/μl (Blum et al., 1996).

Another untoward effect of zalcitabine therapy is oral stomatitis. In a comparative trial of zalcitabine versus didanosine (following zidovudine therapy), stomatitis was observed only in those receiving zalcitabine. Conversely as expected, diarrhoea and pancreatitis were more commonly linked to didanosine treatment (Styrt et al., 1996).

Other potential adverse effects of zalcitabine include granulocytopenia, leukopenia, anaemia, diarrhoea, abnormal liver function tests, rash and pancreatitis (Adkins et al., 1997). Haematological changes are less frequently observed with zalcitabine than zidovudine. Pancreatitis appears to be rare (<1%), but appropriate laboratory studies including monitoring amylase and lipase levels should be carried out.

Drug interactions

The primary route for zalcitabine elimination is renal excretion of unchanged drug. Trimethoprim significantly increases the zalcitabine AUC (37%) by inhibiting renal tubular secretion (Lee et al., 1995). In addition, cimetidine reduces the renal clearance of zalcitabine (owing to competition for renal tubular secretion), increasing the AUC

(36%), whereas C_{max} remains unchanged (Taburet and Singlas, 1996). Nephrotoxic agents (amphotericin, foscarnet, and aminoglycosides) may potentiate the risk of zalcitabine toxicities if renal function deteriorates, resulting in zalcitabine accumulation (Taburet and Singlas, 1996). Guidelines for definitive dosage adjustments are not available. However, when used together zalcitabine toxicity must be monitored carefully.

Co-administration of 'Maalox' results in a significant reduction in zalcitabine bioavailability with decreases in C_{max} and AUC (Massarella et al., 1994). Therefore, it is recommended that zalcitabine and antacid drugs are administered 2 h apart to minimize this interaction. Although dapsone does not substantially alter the disposition of zalcitabine, the AUC of dapsone is slightly increased by zalcitabine.

Considering that peripheral neuropathy is the most common adverse effect of zalcitabine, concomitant administration with drugs (chloramphenicol, cisplatin, dapsone, disulfiram, ethionamide, glutethimide, gold hydralazine, iodoquinol, isoniazid, metronidazole, nitrofurantoin, phenytoin, ribavirin, and vincristine) that cause peripheral neuropathy should be avoided (Adkins et al., 1997). Co-administration of zalcitabine and didanosine is also not recommended, owing to reports of severe left ventricular hypokinesis (MacGregor et al., 1995), in addition to an increased risk of peripheral neuropathy. The concomitant use of pentamidine and zalcitabine should be avoided because of increased risk of severe pancreatitis.

Stavudine (d4T)

Stavudine is a nucleoside thymidine analogue, which was approved for the treatment of HIV infection in the USA in 1994. Its active metabolite stavudine-5′-triphosphate inhibits HIV replication, by competing with thymidine-5′-triphosphate for inclusion into proviral DNA and/or by causing DNA chain termination.

Adverse effects

An important dose-limiting adverse effect caused by stavudine is peripheral neuropathy, which is reversible in the majority of cases on cessation of treatment (Lea and Faulds, 1996; Styrt et al., 1996). Compared to didanosine and zalcitabine, peripheral neuropathy is less frequent with stavudine. Other reported adverse effects are hepatotoxicity (mild to moderate increase in transaminases) and haematological abnormalities (anaemia,

leukopenia, myelosuppression and neutropenia). Compared to zidovudine, haematological effects are less frequent; however, asymptomatic elevations of transaminases are more common. Further, a lower incidence of nausea and vomiting have been reported, but flu-like syndrome and fungal dermatitis are more common than with zidovudine (Mellors et al., 1995).

Pancreatitis was noted in 1% of stavudine recipients in clinical trials carried out prior to FDA approval. Occasional cases of cardiomyopathy and diabetes mellitus have also been reported (Styrt et al., 1996).

Drug interactions

Stavudine has relatively few drug interactions. Like other NRTIs, stavudine is converted to its active triphosphate form by intracellular phosphorylation. Zidovudine inhibits the phosphorylation of stavudine resulting in antiviral antagonism, but stavudine has no effect on zidovudine phosphorylation (Sommadossi et al., 1998). Concomitant administration of stavudine and zidovudine must be avoided.

The absorption rate of stavudine is affected by food intake (C_{max} decreases by 50% and T_{max} delays 1 h); however, the overall AUC is unchanged. Stavudine, therefore, can be taken with or without food.

Lamivudine

Lamivudine is the (−)enantiomer of a dideoxy analogue of cytidine, which was approved for use in the treatment of HIV infection in the USA in 1995. Intracellularly, lamivudine is phosphorylated to its active metabolite, lamivudine triphosphate.

Adverse effects

In contrast to other NRTIs, lamivudine is not incorporated into mitochondrial DNA and shows relatively little inhibition of mitochondrial DNA synthesis (Hart et al., 1992; Swartz, 1995). Therefore, lamivudine has relatively little severe toxicity. Haematological adverse effects are rare and an absence of all lamivudine-related toxicity was reported in asymptomatic HIV-infected patients (van Leeuwen et al., 1992). In one dose-escalation study of lamivudine monotherapy, the most commonly reported adverse events were headache, insomnia, nausea and diarrhoea (van Leeuwen et al., 1995). In addition, a trend toward decreased neutrophil counts was noted at high doses (Perry and Balfour, 1996).

Lamivudine has also been approved for use in combination with zidovudine and is available both as the drug alone and in a combined formulation. It is also now available with both abacavir and zidovudine in a combined formulation (Trizivir®). Generally, adverse events associated with combination therapy are no different to those of zidovudine monotherapy. Dizziness, depression, nasal symptoms and cough are reported at a slightly higher percentage with combination therapy than with zidovudine alone. The incidence of myelosuppression was no different when both drugs are used together (Combivir® prescription information, Glaxo Wellcome, 1998). One potential benefit of the combination is the delayed appearance of zidovudine-resistant mutations.

Pancreatitis and paresthesia or neuropathy associated with lamivudine have been reported only in children (Perry and Faulds, 1997), but there is no evidence that these events are directly attributable to lamivudine treatment.

Drug interactions

Lamivudine increases zidovudine concentrations in plasma significantly (approximately 39%) (Horton et al., 1994). Co-trimoxazole (trimethoprim/sulfamethoxazole) decreases the renal clearance of lamivudine (29%) and alters bioavailability, resulting in an AUC increase of 44% (Taburet and Singlas, 1996). As observed for zalcitabine, trimethoprim competes with the tubular secretion of lamivudine and therefore lower doses of lamivudine may be warranted. Food results in slowed lamivudine absorption and a diminished C_{max} (40%), but no change in AUC. Thus, as is true for most NRTIs, recommendations stand that lamivudine may be administered without regard for the timing of meals.

Abacavir

Abacavir is a carbocyclic NRTI approved by the FDA in 1998 for the treatment of HIV infection. Intracellularly, abacavir is converted to the active metabolite carbovir triphosphate, which in turn inhibits the activity of HIV-1 reverse transcriptase.

The most common side-effects reported during therapy with abacavir (300 mg, bid) plus lamivudine and zidovudine include nausea (47%), nausea and vomiting (16%), diarrhoea (12%), loss of appetite and anorexia (11%), insomnia and other sleep disorders (7%). The most important safety issue with abacavir is a hypersensitivity reaction (2–5%) that occurs several days to 4 weeks after initiating therapy. The reaction is characterized by flu-like symptoms, possibly followed by a measles-like rash, however a rash does not always occur. Other signs and symptoms include fever, fatigue, gastrointestinal symptoms, malaise, lethargy, myalgia, myolysis, arthralgia, oedema, pharyngitis, cough, dyspnoea, headache and paresthesia. When a reaction occurs, abacavir therapy must cease and should not resume as rechallenge may be life-threatening (Frissen et al., 2001).

To date, no important drug interactions have been observed with abacavir (Sadler et al., 1998), although multiple antiretroviral combination regimens involving abacavir are currently being evaluated for pharmacokinetic changes. Due to their metabolic pathways via alcohol dehydrogenase, co-administration of ethanol and abacavir resulted in a 41% increase in abacavir AUC in HIV-infected male patients (Ziagen® product information, Glaxo Wellcome, 2000).

Non-nucleoside reverse transcriptase inhibitors

Nevirapine

Nevirapine is an NNRTI of HIV-1. It binds directly to reverse transcriptase and blocks the RNA-dependent and DNA-dependent DNA polymerase activities by causing a disruption of the catalytic site of the enzyme.

Adverse effects

The most frequently reported adverse events are rash, fever, nausea, headache and liver function abnormalities. Rash, which is usually mild and self-limited, typically develops within the first 6 weeks of initiation of therapy. Severe rashes including Stevens-Johnson syndrome, have been reported in 6–7% of patients (Metry et al., 2001). If a rash develops, the dosage of nevirapine should not be escalated until it abates. If the rash is extensive, moist, involves the mucous membranes, or is associated with fever, nevirapine must be discontinued.

Abnormal liver function tests have been observed particularly in the first few weeks of nevirapine therapy (Viramune® prescription information, Roxane Laboratories, Columbus, OH, USA, 1996). Hepatitis occurs as an uncommon adverse event associated with nevirapine use. Therefore, monitoring of liver function tests is recommended.

Drug interactions

Nevirapine is an inducer of CYP3A4 and CYP2B6, two metabolic isoenzymes located mainly in the liver (Lamson et al., 1999). Therefore, nevirapine therapy may result in lower plasma concentrations or other drugs that are CYP3A4 and also CYP2B6 substrates (see protease inhibitors). A completed drug interaction study on 24 HIV-infected subjects revealed that co-administration of nevirapine with indinavir resulted in a 28% decrease in indinavir AUC. However, some authors argue that dosage adjustments may not be necessary, since indinavir plasma levels remain above an effective antiviral threshold (Murphy et al., 1999). Others recommend an indinavir dose adjustment to 1000 mg/8 h. Nevirapine has no significant effect on ritonavir AUC (Murphy et al., 1997), but saquinavir AUC decreased 25% with nevirapine co-administration (Buss et al., 1998). Nevirapine co-administration with clarithromycin (Robinson et al., 1999) and lamivudine (Leitz et al., 1998) resulted in an interaction. However, no dosage adjustment is necessary for either drug. When nevirapine was administered in combination with zidovudine, a statistically significant decline in zidovudine AUC (32%) was observed. However, nevirapine levels were not affected (MacGregor et al., 1995). No dosage adjustment is recommended.

Rifampin, a CYP3A4 inducer caused a 68% reduction in nevirapine concentrations. Therefore, the nevirapine dose should be increased by 50% when given concomitantly with this drug (Robinson et al., 1998). Alternatively, co-administration of nevirapine with ketoconazole, a CYP3A4 inhibitor, resulted in increased nevirapine levels (15–20%) and a significantly decreased ketoconazole AUC of 63%, suggesting that an alternative antifungal agent should be considered (Lamson et al., 1998).

Delavirdine

Delavirdine is a NNRTI of HIV-1. It binds directly to reverse transcriptase and blocks RNA-dependent and DNA-dependent DNA polymerase.

Adverse effects

The most common adverse reaction associated with delavirdine is rash and the risk appears to be higher in those with lower CD4 lymphocyte counts (of less than 300 cells/μl). Delavirdine produced a rash in 16% of subjects participating in phase II and III clinical trials

(Rescriptor® prescription information, Pharmacia & Upjohn, Kalamazoo, MI, USA, 1998). The rash usually presents between 1 and 3 weeks after initiating treatment. In clinical trials, participants were allowed to continue delavirdine in the presence of the rash, unless it was severe or associated with accompanying systemic symptoms, such as fever or myalgia. Rash typically resolves within 3–14 days after onset and may be treated symptomatically. Severe rash was reported in 3.6% of patients receiving delavirdine (Murphy, 1997). Other adverse effects included nausea, diarrhoea, headache, fatigue, and increases in alanine aminotransferase (ALT) and aspartate aminotransferase (AST) levels.

Drug interactions

Since delavirdine is metabolized by cytochrome P450 enzymes (CYP3A4, 2D6, and 2C9), co-administration of drugs that act as enzyme inducers such as rifabutin (Borin et al., 1997a) and rifampicin (Borin et al., 1997b), result in a decreased delavirdine AUC by fivefold and twenty-sevenfold, respectively. In turn, delavirdine inhibits drug metabolism (especially of drugs metabolized by CYP3A4), and results in an increase in plasma concentrations of clarithromycin (Freimuth, 1996), indinavir AUC by 40% (Ferry et al., 1997), ritonavir AUC by 60% (Morse et al., 1998), and saquinavir AUC by fivefold (Cox et al., 1997). Co-administration of delavirdine with nelfinavir in healthy volunteers resulted in an increased nelfinavir AUC of 92%, but a decreased AUC of 50% for the active metabolite of nelfinavir (Cox et al., 1998). Although not every potential interaction has been definitively evaluated, known CYP3A4 substrates such as astemizole, terfenadine, cisapride, midazolam and warfarin must be avoided when delavirdine is co-administered.

Efavirenz

Efavirenz is a new NNRTI compound, which was approved by the FDA for the treatment of HIV infection in 1998. Efavirenz activity is mediated predominantly by non-competitive inhibition of HIV-1 reverse transcriptase. A major advantage of this NNRTI compared with the others is its once-daily dosing schedule.

Adverse effects

Most significant adverse events associated with efavirenz therapy are nervous system symptoms (52%) (including headache, dizziness, insomnia) and skin rash (27%). Rash is more common in children (40%) and more severe. Erythema multiforme and Stevens-Johnson syndrome have been reported. Efavirenz should be discontinued in patients developing severe rash associated with blistering, desquamation, mucosal involvement or fever. A moderate increase in total cholesterol has been observed in some healthy volunteers and patients receiving efavirenz. Other major adverse events are nausea, vomiting, diarrhoea and serious psychiatric symptoms, including severe depression, suicide attempts, delusions, paranoia, aggressive behaviour and psychosis-like symptoms (Sustiva™ prescription information, DuPont Pharmaceuticals, Wilmington, DE, USA, 2000; Marzolini et al., 2001).

Drug interactions

In vitro, efavirenz is both an inducer and inhibitor of the CYP3A4 isoenzyme. Clinically, efavirenz has been shown to decrease the AUC of indinavir and saquinavir by 31% and 62%, respectively and to increase nelfinavir AUC by 20%. Neither indinavir nor nelfinavir altered efavirenz exposure, but saquinavir decreased efavirenz AUC by 12%.

Co-administration of efavirenz with ritonavir in healthy volunteers resulted in an AUC increase of 20% for each drug. While no dosage adjustment is necessary when nelfinavir and ritonavir are administered in combination with efavirenz, co-administration of efavirenz with saquinavir as the sole protease inhibitor is not recommended, and the indinavir dose should be increased to 1000 mg every 8 h when it is administered with efavirenz. Efavirenz also increases the plasma AUC of ethinyl estradiol by 37% and decreases clarithromycin AUC by 39%. Co-administration of efavirenz with certain antihistamines (terfenadine and astemizole) and cisapride may result in potentially serious and/or life-threatening adverse events. These drugs should not be used with efavirenz (Sustiva™ prescription information, DuPont Pharmaceuticals, 1998). A recent study revealed that co-administration of efavirenz with rifampin results in significantly lower C_{max} and AUC values of efavirenz than those obtained alone (Benedek et al., 1998). The pharmacokinetic interaction between efavirenz and rifabutin has not been evaluated to date. However, a similar interaction is expected.

Protease inhibitors

The PIs inhibit the protease enzyme, an enzyme essential for viral replication and maturation. Treatment of HIV has been revolutionized with the availability of these novel compounds. Currently there are six approved drugs (saquinavir, ritonavir, indinavir, nelfinavir, amprenavir and lopinavir/ritonavir) in clinical practice. Although the PIs are highly efficacious for HIV, they are associated with pronounced adverse effects, including metabolic complications with altered fat distribution. This has compromised their use and resulted in suboptimal compliance for those patients experiencing such untoward effects (see Chapter 18).

Protease inhibitor-associated altered body fat syndrome

Protease inhibitor-associated altered body fat syndrome (PIABFS) was previously called lipodystrophy (reviewed in Strawford and Hellerstein, 2001). However, since lipodystrophy refers to the regional or generalized absence of subcutaneous adipose tissue (Senior and Gellis, 1964), body shape changes in HIV-infected patients on PI therapy are not always consistent with this description. PI-associated body shape changes have reportedly variable prevalences, from 16% (Dong et al., 1998) to 64% (Carr et al., 1998a). A predominant feature in most patients has been fat accumulation, rather than subcutaneous fat loss (Lo et al., 1998a). Recently, a uniform case definition has been proposed (Lo et al., 1998b). In this chapter, we use the term PIABFS to describe body shape changes and metabolic disorders observed in HIV-infected patients treated with PIs as part of their antiretroviral regimen.

The principal features of PIABFS are peripheral lipodystrophy, central-truncal obesity (protease paunch), dorsal fat pad (buffalo hump), ectodermal dysplasia, diabetes mellitus and hyperlipidemia. In the case of the latter, high blood lipids secondary to PI therapy was deemed the cause in two cases of premature coronary artery disease in men (Henry et al., 1998). Although this syndrome resembles Cushing's syndrome, consistent with the description mentioned above, endocrinological evaluation, including 24-h urine cortisol measurements (Roth et al., 1998) and use of the dexamethasone suppression test (Lo et al., 1998a), show that the two syndromes are distinct.

A proposed mechanism for this syndrome is suggested by the observation of a 60–70% homology between the active site of PIs and several key proteins controlling lipid metabolism (Carr et al., 1998b). These include cytoplasmic retinoic-acid binding protein type-1 (CRABP-1) and LDL-receptor-related protein (LRP). It has been postulated that PIs bind to CRABP-1 and inhibit binding to retinoic acid resulting in hyperlipidemia. The factors linked to the pathogenesis of PIABFS are under intense investigation. Interestingly, some of these clinical manifestations occur in the absence of PI therapy. Lo and colleagues (1998a) reported that four of eight patients with buffalo hump were receiving antiretrovirals other than PIs. Additionally, a study presented recently revealed that more than 100 patients with HIV infection who were not exposed to PIs had developed some alterations in body fat distribution (Kotler et al., 1998), calling into question the influence of hormonal and metabolic changes of HIV infection itself, rather than a specific class of drugs on the pathogenesis of this syndrome.

CYP450 enzyme system

The cytochrome P450 (CYP450) isoenzymes are a family of enzymes localized mainly in the lipid bilayer of hepatocytes. These enzymes play an important role in the metabolism of a large number of drugs, as well as streoid hormones, fatty acids and prostaglandins via oxidative reactions. Major isoenzymes responsible for drug metabolism are CYP3A4, CYP2D6, CYP2C, CYP1A2 and CYP2E1 subfamilies. The CYP3A4 isoenzymes account for 60% of all cytochrome enzymes in the liver. Numerous drug interactions observed in clinical practice are based on the inhibition or induction of CYP450 isoenzymes by concomitantly administered drugs (Michalets, 1998).

Saquinavir

Saquinavir was the first PI licensed in the USA by the FDA (December 1995) for the treatment of HIV infection. The original formulation was characterized by a very low absolute bioavailability (approximately 4%) owing to high first-pass metabolism and incomplete absorption. The newer soft-gelatin formulation of saquinavir has minimized this problem, with bioavailability enhanced threefold when compared to the original product (Fortovase® product information, Roche Laboratories, Nutley, NJ, USA, 1997).

Saquinavir is 98% protein bound and metabolized by hepatic and gastrointestinal isozymes (especially cytochrome P450 3A4). Its half-life ranges from 1 to 2 h, with nearly 90% eliminated in the faeces (Invirase® product information, Roche Laboratories, 1997).

Adverse effects

Saquinavir is generally well tolerated. The majority of adverse reactions attributed to saquinavir are associated with the gastrointestinal system (Table 6.3). In one large trial involving 940 patients receiving either saquinavir, zalcitabine or a combination of both drugs, the most frequently reported adverse event with saquinavir monotherapy was diarrhoea (5%). Other reported side-effects included nausea (2%), peripheral neuropathy (3%), rash (2%), abdominal discomfort/pain, headache (2%), elevation of serum transaminase levels (2%) and fever (Haubrich et al., 1996).

An increased incidence of adverse effects has been reported with the soft-gel formulation (presumably due to increased drug exposure). Reported adverse events are diarrhoea (20%), nausea (11%), abdominal discomfort (9%), dyspepsia (8%), flatulence (6%), vomiting (3%), fatigue (5%), headache (5%) and depression (3%). Laboratory abnormalities are also higher with the improved formulation (Gill et al., 1998).

Drug interactions

As is true for all the PIs, clinically significant drug interactions are very common with saquinavir. This is due to the affinity of PIs for cytochrome P450 isozymes (especially cytochrome P450 3A4 [CYP3A4]), contained in the liver and gastrointestinal tract. PIs are both metabolized by these enzymes, as well as being inhibitors (and potential inducers) of these enzymes. Therefore, they are susceptible to the effects of concomitant medications that alter P450 metabolism and/or are capable of altering drug metabolism themselves (Table 6.4). Regarding the latter, saquinavir is a less potent inhibitor than ritonavir, nelfinavir or indinavir in inhibiting CYP3A4. The Ki for the inhibition of terfenadine metabolism is 0.017 μM for ritonavir and 0.7 μM for saquinavir, a fortyfold difference in potency (Flexner, 1998). Despite lower potency, saquinavir can alter the metabolism of multiple compounds, including other antiretroviral agents dependent on CYP3A4. Further, saquinavir inhibits the metabolism of antihistamines such as astemizole and terfenadine causing prolonged QT interval and potentially fatal arrhythmias. Similarly, excessive sedation can occur when co-administered with midazolam, a sedative benzodiazepine (Merry et al., 1997).

Other AIDS-related therapies alter saquinavir disposition. It has been reported that rifampicin, rifabutin

Table 6.3 Adverse effects of protease inhibitors*

Saquinavir

CNS	Headache (2%), paresthesia, dizziness
GIS	Diarrhoea (5%), nausea (2%), abdominal discomfort/pain, buccal mucosa ulceration, dyspepsia, acid reflux, intestinal gas, mucosal damage
NMS	Peripheral neuropathy (3%), pain, myalgia
Dermatological	Rash (2%), pruritis
Endocrinological	Altered body fat syndrome
Haematological	Neutropenia, thrombocytopenia
Hepatic	Elevated AST/ALT (2%), total biluribin
General	Asthenia, fatigue, appetite disturbances
Other lab abnormalities	Elevated CPK, triglycerides, elevated or decreased blood sugar, K, P

Ritonavir

CNS	Headache (6%), dizziness (3%)
GIS	Diarrhoea (18%), nausea (26%), vomiting (15%), abdominal pain (7%), taste perversion (5%), pancreatitis
NMS	Peripheral and circumoral paresthesia (5–6%)
Dermatological	Rash, urticaria, Stevens-Johnson syndrome
Endocrinological	Altered body fat syndrome
Haematological	Anaemia, thrombocytopenia
Hepatic	Elevated AST/ALT, GGT, total bilirubin, hepatitis
General	Asthenia (14%), anorexia (6%), bronchospasm, angioedema, anaphylaxis, insomnia/somnolence, fever, sweating
Other lab abnormalities	Elevated CPK, LDH, triglycerides, blood sugar, AP, K, uric acid

Indinavir

CNS	Headache (6%), blurred vision, dizziness
GIS	Diarrhoea (5%), nausea (12%), abdominal pain (9%), vomiting, acid reflux, taste perversion
Dermatological	Hypertrophic paronychia of the great toe (4%), dry skin, rash, alopecia
Endocrinological	Altered body fat syndrome, gynaecomastia
Haematological	Anaemia, thrombocytopenia, neutropenia
Hepatic	Elevated ALT (5.5%), AST (4%), bilirubin (12.5%)
GUS	Nephrolithiais (9%), back pain, nephropathy (?)
General	Fever (4%), asthenia, fatigue, anorexia, insomnia/somnolence, allergic reaction, respiratory failure (?)
Other lab abnormalities	Elevated amylase, triglycerides, blood sugar, ketoacidosis

Nelfinavir

CNS	Headache
GIS	Diarrhoea (25%), nausea (5%), abdominal pain, flatulence (3.3%)
Dermatological	Rash (3%)
Endocrinological	Altered body fat syndrome, gynaecomastia
Hepatic	Elevated ALT/AST
General	Asthenia
Other lab abnormalities	Elevated creatine kinase, triglycerides, blood sugar

Amprenavir

CNS	Headache
GIS	Nausea, diarrhoea, loose stools, vomiting, taste disorders
NMS	Oral/perioral/peripheral paresthesia
Dermatological	Rashes, Stevens-Johnson syndrome
Endocrinological	Altered body fat syndrome
Hepatic	Elevated AST/ALT, bilirubin
General	Mood disorders
Other lab abnormalities	Elevated amylase, hyperglycaemia, hypertriglyceridaemia, hypercholestererolaemia

Lopinavir/ritonavir

CNS	Headache
GIS	Nausea, vomiting, diarrhoea, abnormal stools, abdominal pain, pancreatitis
Endocrinological	Altered body fat syndrome
Hepatic	Abnormal liver function
General	Fatigue
Other lab abnormalities	Hypertriglyceridaemia, hypercholesterolaemia, elevated ALT/AST, hyperglycemia

ALT: alanine aminotransferase; AP: alkaline phosphatase; AST: aspartate aminotransferase; CNS: central nervous system; CPK: creatinine phosphokinase; GGT: gamma glutamyl transferase; GIS: gastrointestinal system; K: potassium; LDH: lactic dehydrogenase; NMS: neuromuscular system; P: phosphate; (?): effect not proven.
*All protease inhibitors may cause increased bleeding in patients with hemophilia.

and nevirapine increase saquinavir drug clearance, resulting in diminished AUCs. Further, antiretroviral drugs such as ritonavir, nelfinavir, delavirdine, the anti-fungal agent ketoconazole and grapefruit juice inhibit saquinavir metabolism, resulting in between a threefold and thirtyfold increase in saquinavir AUCs (Invirase™ prescribing information, Roche Laboratories, 1997). When co-administered with nelfinavir 750 mg every 8 h, suggested saquinavir soft-gel capsule (SGC) dosage is 800 mg (Kravcik *et al.*, 1998). No dosage adjustment is necessary when co-administered with ketoconazole. Contraindicated medications when managing patients with saquinavir include rifampin, ergot alkaloids, astemizole, terfenadine, cisapride, midazolam and triazolam.

Ritonavir

Ritonavir was the second PI approved by the FDA (February 1996). In contrast to saquinavir, it has a relatively high bioavailability (approximately 60–75%). For optimal absorption ritonavir should be administered with food. Like saquinavir, it is highly bound to plasma proteins at 98–99%. It is also metabolized via hepatic and gastrointestinal CYP3A4 isozymes (and partially via CYP2D6), with an elimination half-life of 3–5 h.

Adverse effects

The most common adverse events associated with ritonavir are gastrointestinal disturbances such as nausea (26%), diarrhoea (18%), vomiting (15%), abdominal pain (7%) and taste perversion (5%); neurological disturbances such as peripheral and circumoral paresthesia (5–6%), headache (6%), dizziness (3%) and additional general side-effects such as asthenia (14%), anorexia (6%) and abnormal laboratory values (elevation in serum AST, ALT, GGT, CPK, LDH and triglyceride levels). Ritonavir use is associated with a sixfold higher risk of severe hepatotoxicity compared to other antiretrovirals (Sulkowski *et al.*, 1998). Allergic reactions including urticaria, skin eruptions, bronchospasm, angioedema and rare cases of anaphylaxis and Stevens-Johnson syndrome have also been reported (Norvir®, Abbott Laboratories, 1997). Severe renal impairment in patients managed with combination saquinavir and ritonavir has been reported (Witzke *et al.*, 1997). While saquinavir alone is not known to be nephrotoxic, this adverse event may be associated with elevated saquinavir exposure due to the interactive effects of ritonavir. Myasthenia gravis has also

been reported during ritonavir treatment (Saadat and Kaminski, 1998).

Drug interactions

Due to the high affinity of ritonavir for several metabolic isozymes including CYP3A4, CYP2D6 and CYP2C9, it is the most potent interacting drug of all antiretrovirals. Its metabolic characteristics are highly complex. Ritonavir is metabolized primarily via CYP3A4 but partially by CYP2D6. Ritonavir in turn inhibits CYP3A4, 2D6 and 2C9/19 (Kumar *et al.*, 1996). Additional data indicate that ritonavir induces 1A2 and 2C9/19 as well as its own metabolism (Hsu *et al.*, 1997a). In the context of inhibition, large dose reductions (>50%) and careful therapeutic drug monitoring is often recommended when susceptible drugs are used concomitantly with ritonavir (Table 6.4). In addition, co-administration of ritonavir with certain analgesics, antihistamines, sedative hypnotics, anti-arrhythymics, ergot alkaloids and cisapride may result in potentially serious and/or life-threatening adverse events. These drugs should not be used with ritonavir (Table 6.5).

Indinavir

The third PI approved by the FDA in March 1996 (only 1 month after ritonavir), for treatment of HIV infection was indinavir. For optimal absorption, indinavir should be administered without food but with water, 1 h before or 2 h after a meal. It is also metabolized via CYP3A4. Less than 20% of unchanged drug is found in the urine (Balani *et al.*, 1996). The half-life of indinavir is 2 h and its protein binding is 60%.

Adverse effects

The most frequent adverse events observed with indinavir are abdominal pain (9%), nausea (12%), diarrhoea (5%), vomiting (4%), headache (6%), fever (4%) and nephrolithiasis (including renal colic and flank pain with and without haematuria, in 9%). To prevent nephrolithiasis, patients should consume large quantities of water (>3 litres) daily. Indinavir nephropathy may be associated with normal glomeruli and interstitial inflammation with fibrosis (Sarcletti *et al.*, 1998). Indinavir nephropathy has also been diagnosed in a paediatric haemophiliac HIV patient (Ascher and Lucy, 1997). The patient's nephritis resolved and serum creatinine decreased to 1.1 mg/dl (1.3–1.7 mg/dl) within 1 month of

Table 6.4 Pharmacokinetic drug interactions between protease inhibitors and other drugs

Effects of other drugs on protease inhibitors[a]

	Saquinavir	Ritonavir	Indinavir	Nelfinavir	Amprenavir	Lopinavir
Increase in AUC (%)	Ritonavir (1600) Delavirdine (500) Indinavir (620) Nelfinavir (400) Ketoconazole (300) Clarithromycin (180)	Fluoxetine (19) Fluconazole (12) Clarithromycin (12) Nelfinavir (9) Efavirenz (18)	Delavirdine (40) Ritonavir (500) Ketoconazole (68) Nelfinavir (50) Clarithromycin (30) Zidovudine (13)	Amprenavir (15) Delavirdine (92) Ritonavir (152) Indinavir (83) Ketoconazole (35) Saquinavir (18) Efavirenz (20)	Ketoconazole (31) Clarithromycin (18) Indinavir (33) Abacavir (29)	Ritonavir (46) Delavirdine (92)
Decrease in AUC (%)	Amprenavir (18) Rifampin (80) (*avoid*) Rifabutin (40) Nevirapine (27) Efavirenz (60)	Rifampin (35) (*avoid*) Tobacco (18) Nevirapine (11)	Amprenavir (38) Rifampin (92) (*avoid*) Rifabutin (32) Nevirapine (28) Efavirenz (31)	Rifampin (82) (*avoid*) Rifabutin (32)	Rifampin (82) (*avoid*) Efavirenz (36) Saquinavir (32)	Ketoconazole (13) Rifampin (75) (*avoid*) Efavirenz (40)

Effects of protease inhibitors on other drugs

	Saquinavir	Ritonavir	Indinavir	Nelfinavir	Amprenavir	Lopinavir
Increase in AUC (%)	Nelfinavir (18) Sildenafil (300)	Amprenavir (250) Saquinavir (1600) Indinavir (500) Rifabutin (350) Nelfinavir (150) Drobinol (>300) Desipramine (145) Efavirenz (20) Clarithromycin (77) Trimethoprim (20) Sildenafil (1100)	Saquinavir (620) Rifabutin (204) Ketoconazole (68) Nelfinavir (83) Clarithromycin (53) Stavudine (25) Zidovudine (17–36) Norethindrone (26) Ethinyl estradiol (24) Trimethoprim (19) Isoniazid (13) Sildenafil (200)	Saquinavir (400) Rifabutin (207) Indinavir (50) Lamivudine (10)	Sildenafil (200) Ketoconazole (44) Rifabutin (193) Zidovudine (31)	Ketoconazole (300) Rifabutin (300) Atorvastatin (600) Pravastatin (33) Sildenafil (*probable*) Saquinavir* Indinavir* Amprenavir*
Decrease in AUC (%)	Amprenavir (36)	Theophylline (43) Ethinyl estradiol (40) Zidovudine (25) Didanosine (13) Methadone (37)	Lamivudine (6)	Ethinyl estradiol (47) Zidovudine (35) Norethindrone (18)		Ethinyl estradiol (42) Methadone (53)

[a]Affected drugs are protease inhibitors, provided as column headings.

AUC: area-under-the-curve.

*Similar AUC, lower C_{max} (no information for SQV) and higher C_{min}.

discontinuing indinavir therapy. Further, indinavir use in two perinatally acquired HIV-infected children was associated with interstitial nephritis (Rutstein *et al.*, 1997).

Additional adverse effects associated with indinavir include some laboratory abnormalities of severe or life-threatening intensity, such as increased serum bilirubin (12.5%), increased ALT (5.5%) and AST (4%) (Crixivan® prescribing information, Merck & Co., Inc., West Point, PA, USA, 1998). Recently, paronychia and pyogenic granuloma of the great toes has been reported in 4% of patients treated with indinavir (Bouscarat and Bouhour, 1998). Of greatest severity are recent reports of rare cases of acute respiratory failure (Dieleman *et al.*, 1998), fatal acute haemolysis (Prazuck *et al.*, 1998), severe allergic reaction (Rijnders and Kooman, 1998), severe coronary artery disease (Karmochkine and Raguin, 1998) and ketoacidosis (Besson *et al.*, 1998). Inhibition of the cellular protease that converts pro-insulin to insulin has been postulated as the mechanism underlying development of ketoacidosis. This is likely to occur also with other PIs. Breast hypertrophy has been noted in a couple of patients treated with indinavir (Herry *et al.*, 1997; Lui *et al.*, 1998).

Drug interactions

Similar to the other PIs, drugs that induce the activity of CYP3A4 (such as rifabutin) decrease the plasma AUC of indinavir, whereas other drugs that inhibit the enzyme (such as ketoconazole and clarithromycin) increase indinavir AUC (Chiba *et al.*, 1996; Ferry *et al.*, 1998; Crixivan® prescription information, Merck & Co., Inc., 1998). Due to a fivefold increase in indinavir AUC when co-administered with ritonavir, indinavir should be administered at a reduced dosage (Hsu *et al.*, 1997b). A dose reduction of rifabutin to half the standard dose and a dose increase of indinavir to 1000 mg every 8 h is recommended when rifabutin and indinavir are co-administered. Also dose reduction of indinavir to 600 mg every 8 h should be considered when administering ketoconazole concurrently (Crixivan® product information, Merck & Co., Inc., 1998). Conversely, indinavir inhibits CYP3A4, resulting in significant increases in the plasma levels of co-administered drugs, such as cisapride, terfenadine, astemizole, midazolam, and triazolam. Such combinations should be avoided in clinical practice due to the high incidence of serious adverse reactions (Table 6.5).

Table 6.5 Drugs that should not be used with protease inhibitors

Analgesics	Meperidine[a]
	Piroxicam[a]
	Propoxyphene[a]
Anti-arrhythmic	Amiodarone[a]
	Encainide[a]
	Flecainide[c]
	Propafenone[c]
	Quinidine[a]
Cardiac drugs	Bepridil[b]
Lipid lowering agents	Simvastatin
	Lovastatin
Antimicrobials	Rifampin
	Rifabutin[a]
Antihistamine	Astemizole
	Terfenadine
Ergot alkaloids	Dihydroergotamine[a]
	Ergotamine[a]
Gastrointestinal drugs	Cisapride
Psychotropics	Bupropion[a]
	Clozapine[a]
	Pimozide[c]
Sedative/hypnotics	Alprazolam[a]
	Clorazepate[a]
	Diazepam[a]
	Estazolam[a]
	Flurozepam[a]
	Midazolam
	Triazolam
	Zolpidem[a]
Herbs	St. John's Wort

[a]With ritonavir only.
[b]With ritonavir or amprenavir.
[c]With ritonavir or lopinavir/ritonavir.

Nelfinavir

Nelfinavir is the fourth PI to be approved by the FDA. It is well absorbed following oral administration, particularly when taken with food. It is more than 98% protein bound and is also metabolized mainly in the liver by CYP3A4 and 2C19 (primarily to a potentially active M8 metabolite). Its elimination half-life ranges from 3 to 5 h. Only 2% of the dose is recovered in the urine (Viracept® product information, Agouron Pharmaceuticals Inc., La Jolla, CA, USA, 1997).

Adverse effects

The most commonly adverse reaction reported is diarrhoea (25%), followed by nausea (5%), flatulence (3.3%) and rash (3%). Less common side-effects include asthenia, headache, abdominal pain, elevated creatinine kinase and transaminases and haematological changes such as neutrophil and lymphocyte count abnormalities. One case of gynaecomastia attributed to nelfinavir treatment has been reported (Schurmann et al., 1998).

Drug interactions

Agents that affect CYP3A4 or 2C19 are expected to alter the plasma concentrations of nelfinavir. Co-administration of ketoconazole, a potent inhibitor of CYP3A4, results in a 35% increase in the nelfinavir plasma AUC; however, dosage adjustment might not be necessary. In addition, other PIs (indinavir and ritonavir) increase nelfinavir concentrations. On the other hand, inducers of this isozyme including rifampin, rifabutin, carbamazepine, phenobarbital and phenytoin, decrease nelfinavir levels. Nelfinavir AUC decreased by 32%, accompanied by a twofold increase in rifabutin plasma AUC when these drugs were co-administered. Thus, a dose reduction of rifabutin to half the standard dose is recommended when co-administered with nelfinavir. The co-administration of rifampicin and nelfinavir should be avoided (Viracept® prescription information, Agouron Pharmaceuticals, Inc., 1997).

Nelfinavir itself inhibits CYP3A4, resulting in a decrease in the metabolism of saquinavir, indinavir, terfenadine, rifabutin and lamivudine (Viracept® product information, Agouron Pharmaceuticals Inc., 1997; Table 6.4). Merry and colleagues (1998) reported that there was a 50% reduction in the plasma AUC of nelfinavir when co-administered with nevirapine in seven HIV-infected patients. Given the autoinduction of nelfinavir, the validity of these results was argued (Skowron et al., 1998) and a well-designed pharmacokinetic study is necessary to conclude on a nelfinavir–nevirapine interaction. While nelfinavir did not affect efavirenz plasma AUC, nelfinavir AUC has been increased by 20% with efavirenz co-administration (Sustiva™ prescription information, DuPont Pharmaceuticals, 1998).

Amprenavir

Amprenavir is the fifth member of PI antiretroviral drugs which was approved by FDA in February 1999. It is well absorbed after oral administration with a time to peak concentration (t_{max}) between 1 to 2 hours after a single oral dose. Large amounts of vitamin E are included in the formulation to enhance the bioavailability. It may be taken with or without food, but should not be taken with a high-fat meal. Amprenavir is metabolized in the liver by the cytochrome P450 enzyme system and also inhibits CYP3A4.

Adverse effects

The most common reported adverse events associated with amprenavir include nausea, diarrhoea and loose stools, vomiting, taste disorders, rashes, headache, oral/perioral and peripheral paresthesia and some mood disorders. The rash occurs in 28% of patients, of whom 4% have severe or life-threatening rash, including Stevens–Johnson syndrome. Amprenavir therapy should be discontinued for severe rashes and for moderate rashes accompanied by systemic symptoms. Rash due to cross-sensitivity with sulfa drugs may also occur.

Laboratory abnormalities reported include hyperglycaemia, hypertriglyceridaemia, hypercholesterolaemia and elevations of AST, ALT, amylase and bilirubin levels. (Agenerase, product information, GlaxoWellcome, 2000).

Drug interactions

Sadler and colleagues (1998) reported results for the interactive effects of amprenavir with zidovudine, lamivudine, indinavir, saquinavir, nelfinavir, ketoconazole and clarithromycin. However, most of these interactions do not require dosage adjustment. In contrast, efavirenz caused a 36% decrease in AUC of amprenavir, suggesting the need for dosage adjustment. Additionally, the AUC of amprenavir decreased by 82% with rifampin. Therefore, these drugs should not be co-administered. Rifabutin doses should be reduced when used concomitantly with amprenavir, due to a twofold increase in its AUC (Sadler et al., 1998).

Lopinavir/ritonavir (ABT-378/r)

Lopinavir is the latest PI to be approved by FDA in September 2000. It is a peptidomimetic substrate analogue that inhibits the activity of HIV protease. Lopinavir's antiviral properties are combined with a low dose of ritonavir that inhibits lopinavir's metabolism and increases its blood levels (Kaletra, Abbott Laboratories, Abbott Park, IL, USA, 2000).

Adverse effects

The most commonly reported adverse effects are: abdominal pain, abnormal stools, diarrhoea, fatigue, headache, nausea and vomiting. Lopinavir/ritonavir also produces increases in triglycerides and cholesterol levels. Pancreatitis and abnormal liver function have been reported in patients receiving lopinavir/ritonavir. As observed with other PIs, it may also be associated with other significant adverse effects including increases in blood glucose, altered body fat distribution and life-threatening drug interactions.

Drug interactions

Lopinavir is metabolized primarily by CYP3A4 system. Thus, there is a potential for pharmacokinetic interaction between lopinavir and other drugs metabolized by the same pathway. Co-formulation with ritonavir will likely complicate the drug interaction profile of lopinavir.

Acknowledgment

S. Eralp Bellibas MD was supported by a Merck Sharp and Dohme International Fellowship in Clinical Pharmacology Award from the Merck Co. Foundation.

References

Abrams DI, Goldman AI, Launer C et al. (1994). A comparative trial of didanosine or zalcitabine after treatment with zidovudine in patients with human immunodeficiency virus infection. *N Engl J Med* **330**: 657–62.

Adkins JC, Peters DH, Faulds D. (1997). Zalcitabine: an update on its pharmacodynamic and pharmacokinetic properties and clinical efficacy in the management of HIV infection. *Drugs* **53**: 1054–80.

Albrecht H, Stellbrink HJ, Arasteh K. (1993). Didanosine-induced disorders of glucose tolerance [letter]. *Ann Intern Med* **119**: 1050.

Ascher DP, Lucy MD. (1997). indinavir sulfate renal toxicity in a pediatric hemophiliac with HIV infection. *Ann Pharmacother* **31**: 1146–9.

Balani SK, Woolf EJ, Hoagland VL et al. (1996). Disposition of indinavir, a potent HIV-1 protease inhibitor, after an oral dose in humans. *Drug Met Disposition* **24**: 1389–94.

Benedek I, Joshi A, Fiske WD et al. (1998). *Pharmacokinetic interaction between efavirenz (EFV) and rifampin (RIF) in healthy volunteers.* Twelfth World AIDS Conference, Geneva, Switzerland.

Besson C, Jubault V, Viard JP et al. (1998). Ketoacidosis associated with protease inhibitor therapy. *AIDS* **12**: 1399–400.

Bissuel F, Bruneel F, Habersetzer F et al. (1994). Fulminant hepatitis with severe lactate acidosis in HIV-infected patients in didanosine therapy. *J Intern Med* **253**: 367–71.

Blum AS, Dal PGJ, Feinberg J et al. (1996). Low-dose zalcitabine-related toxic neuropathy: frequency, natural history, and risk factors. *Neurology* **46**: 999–1003.

Borin MT, Chambers JH, Carel BJ et al. (1997a). Pharmacokinetic study of the interaction between rifabutin and delavirdine mesylate in HIV-1 infected patients. *Antivir Res* **35**: 53–63.

Borin MT, Chambers JH, Carel BJ et al. (1997b). Pharmacokinetic study of the interaction between rifampin and delavirdine mesylate. *Clin Pharmacol Ther* **61**: 544–53.

Bouscarat F, Bouhour D. (1998). Paronychia and pyogenic granuloma of the great toes in patients treated with indinavir. *N Engl J Med* **338**: 1776–7.

Burger DM, Meenhost PL, Koks CHW et al. (1993). Drug interaction with zidovudine. *AIDS* **7**: 111–17.

Buss N, and the Fortovase® Study Group. (1998). *Saquinavir soft gel capsule (Fortovase®) pharmacokinetics and drug interactions.* Fifth Conference on Retroviruses and Opportunistic Infections, Chicago, IL, USA.

Carr A, Samaras K, Burton S et al. (1998a). A syndrome of peripheral lipodystrophy, hyperlipidemia and insulin resistence in patients receiving HIV protease inhibitors. *AIDS* **12**: F51–8.

Carr A, Samaras K, Chisholm DJ et al. (1998b). Pathogenesis of HIV-1-protease inhibitor-associated peripheral lipodystrophy, hyperlipidemia, and insulin resistence. *Lancet* **351**: 1881–3.

Chattha G, Arieff AI, Cummings C et al. (1993). Lactic acidosis complicating the acquired immunodeficiency syndrome. *Ann Intern Med* **118**: 37–9.

Chiba M, Hensleigh M, Nishime JA et al. (1996). Role of cytochrome P4503A4 in human metabolism of MK-639, a potent human immunodeficiency virus protease inhibitor. *Drug Met Disposition* **24**: 307–14.

Cox SR, Batts DH, Stewart F et al. (1997). *Evaluation of pharmacokinetic interaction between saquinavir and delavirdine in healthy volunteers.* Fourth Conference on Retroviruses and Opportunistic Infections, Washington, DC, USA.

Cox SR, Schneck DW, Herman BD et al. (1998). *Delavirdine and nelfinavir. A pharmacokinetic drug–drug interaction study in healthy adult volunteers.* Fifth Conference on Retroviruses and Opportunistic Infections. Chicago, IL, USA.

Cretton EM, Xie MY, Bevan RJ et al. (1991). Catabolism of 3-azido-3-deoxythymidine in hepatocytes and liver microsomes, with evidence of formation of 3-amino-3-deoxythymidine, a highly toxic catabolite for human bone marrow cells. *Mol Pharmacol* **39**: 258–66.

De Miranda P, Good SS, Yarchoan R et al. (1989). Alteration of zidovudine pharmacokinetics by probenecid in patients with AIDS or AIDS-related complex. *Clin Pharmacol Ther* **46**: 494–9.

Dieleman JP, Veld B, Borleffs JC et al. (1998). Acute respiratory failure associated with the human immunodeficiency virus (HIV) peotease inhibitor indinavir in an HIV-infected patient. *Clin Infect Dis* **26**: 1012–13.

Dieterich D et al. (2000). *Sustained virologic response (SVR) following interferon and ribavirin therapy for hepatitis C patients who are connected with HIV.* Thirty-eighth Annual Meeting of the Infectious Diseases Society of America, New Orleans, LA, USA, 17.

Dong K, Flynn MM, Dickinson BP et al. (1998). Changes in body habitus in HIV(+) women after initiation of protease inhibitor therapy. Twelfth World AIDS Conference, Geneva, Switzerland, Abs. No. 12373.

Ferry JJ, Herman BD, Cox SR et al. (1997). Delavirdine and indinavir: a pharmacokinetic drug–drug interaction study in healthy adult volunteers. Fourth Conference on Retroviruses and Opportunistic Infections, Washington, DC, USA.

Ferry JJ, Herman BD, Carel BJ et al. (1998). Pharmacokinetic drug interaction study of delavirdine and indinavir in healthy volunteers. J AIDS Hum Retrovir 18: 252–9.

Fischl MA, Richman DD, Causey DM et al. (1989). Prolonged zidovudine therapy in patients with AIDS and advanced AIDS-related complex. JAMA 262: 2405–10.

Flexner C. (1998). HIV-protease inhibitors. N Engl J Med 338: 1281–92.

Freiman JP, Helfert KE, Hamrell MR et al. (1993). Hepatomegaly with severe steatosis in HIV-seropositive patients. AIDS 7: 379–85.

Freimuth WW. (1996). Delavirdine mesylate, a potent non-nucleoside HIV-1 reverse transcriptase inhibitor. Adv Exp Med Biol 394: 279–89.

Frissen PH, de Vries J, Weigal HM et al. (2001). Severe anaphylactic shock after re-challenge with abacavir without preceding hypersensitivity. AIDS 15: 289.

Gherardi RK, Florea-Strat A, Fromont G et al. (1994). Cytokine expression in the muscle of HIV-infected patients: evidence for interleukin-1-alfa accumulation in mitochondria AZT fibers. Ann Neurol 30: 752–8.

Gill M (NV15182 Study Team). (1998). Safety profile of soft gelatin formulation of saquinavir in combination with nucleosides in a broad patient population. AIDS 12: 1400–3.

Gradon JD, Chapnick EK, Sepkowitz DV. (1992). Zidovudine induced hepatitis. J Intern Med 231: 317–18.

Hart GJ, Orr DC, Penn CR et al. (1992). Effects of (−)-2′-deoxy-3′-thiacytidine (3TC) 5′-triphosphate on human immunodeficiency virus reverse transcriptase and mammalian DNA polymerases alpha, beta, and gamma. Antimicrob Agents Chemother 36: 1688–94.

Haubrich R, Burger HU, Beattie D et al. (1996). Saquinavir + zalcitabine vs saquinavir or zalcitabine monotherapy in HIV-infected patients discontinuing or intolerant to zidovudine: results of randomized, double blind trial. AIDS 10: S17.

Henry K, Melroe H, Huebsch J et al. (1998). Severe premature coronary artery disease with protease inhibitors. Lancet 351: 1328.

Herry I, Bernard L, de Truchis P et al. (1997). Hypertrophy of the breasts in a patient treated with indinavir. Clin Infect Dis 25: 937–8.

Hochester H, Dieterich D, Bozzette S et al. (1990). Toxicity of combined ganciclovir and zidovudine for cytomegalovirus disease associated with AIDS. Ann Intern Med 113: 111–17.

Horton CM, Yuen G, Mikolich DM et al. (1994). Pharmacokinetics of oral lamivudine administered alone and with oral zidovudine in asymptomatic patients with human immunodeficiency virus infection. Clin Pharmacol Ther 55: 198.

Hsu A, Granneman GR, Witt G et al. (1997a). Multiple-dose pharmacokinetics of ritonavir in human immunodeficiency virus-infected subjects. Antimicrob Agents Chemother 41: 898–905.

Hsu A, Granneman GR, Japour A et al. (1997b). Evaluation of potential ritonavir and indinavir combination bid regimens. Thirty-seventh Interscience Conference on Antimicrobial Agents and Chemotherapy, Toronto, Ontario, Canada.

Karmochkine M, Raguin G. (1998). Severe coronary artery disease in a young HIV-infected man with no cardiovascular risk factor who was treated with indinavir. AIDS 12: 2499–514.

Kornhauser DM, Petty BG, Hendrix CW et al. (1989). Probenecid and zidovudine metabolism. Lancet ii: 473–5.

Kotler DP, Rosenbaum KB, Wang J et al. (1998). Alterations in body fat distribution in HIV-infected men and women. Twelfth World AIDS Conference, Geneva, Switzerland, Abs. No. 32173.

Kravcik S, Farnsworth A, Patick A et al. (1998). Long-term follow-up of combination protease inhibitor therapy with nelfinavir and saquinavir (soft gel) in HIV infection. Fifth Conference on Retroviruses and Opportunistic Infections, Chicago, IL, USA.

Kucers A, Crowe SM, Grayson L et al. (1997). Use of antibiotics, a clinical review of antibacterial, antifungal and antiviral drugs. 5th edition. London: Butterworth-Heinmann.

Kumar GN, Rodrigues AD, Buko AM et al. (1996). Cytochrome P450 mediated metabolism of the HIV-1 protease inhibitor ritonavir (ABT-538) in human liver microsomes. J Pharmacol Exp Ther 277: 423–32.

Lai KK, Gang DL, Zawacki JK et al. (1991). Fulminant hepatic failure associated with 2′,3′-dideoxyinosine (ddI). Ann Intern Med 115: 283–4.

Lamson M, Robinson P, Gigliotti M et al. (1998). Pharmacokinetic interaction between nevirapine and ketoconazole. Twelfth World AIDS Conference, Geneva, Switzerland.

Lamson M, MacGregor T, Riska P et al. (1999). Nevirapine induces both CYP3A4 and CYP2B6 metabolic pathways. Hundredth Annual Meeting of American Society for Clinical Pharmacology and Therapeutics. San Antonia, TX, USA.

Lea AP, Faulds D. (1996) Stavudine a review of its pharmacodynamic and pharmacokinetic properties and clinical potential in HIV infection. Drugs 51: 846–64.

Lee BL, Tauber MG, Chambers HF et al. (1995) The effect of trimethoprim on the pharmacokinetics of zalcitabine in HIV-infected patients [abstract]. Thirty-fifth Interscience Conference on Antimicrobial Agents and Chemotherapy, San Francisco. Antimicrob Agents Chemother 35: 6.

Leitz G, Lamson M, Lionetti D et al. (1998). Nevirapine/lamivudine drug–drug interaction study in HIV infected patients. Twelfth World AIDS Conference, Geneva, Switzerland.

Lo JC, Mulligan K, Tai VW et al. (1998a). 'Buffalo hump' in men with HIV-1 infection. Lancet 351: 867–70.

Lo JC, Mulligan K, Tai VW et al. (1998b). Body shape changes in HIV-infected patients. J AIDS Hum Retrovir 19: 307–8.

Lui A, Karter D, Turett G. (1998). Another case of breast hyper trophy in a patient treated with indinavir. Clin Infect Dis 26: 1482.

MacGregor TR, Lamson MJ, Cort S et al. (1995). Steady state pharmacokinetics of nevirapine, didanosine, zalcitabine, and zidovudine combination therapy in HIV-1 positive patients. Pharm Res 12: S101.

Marzolini C, Telenti A, Decosterd LA et al. (2001). Efavirenz plasma levels can predict treatment failure and central nervous system side effects in HIV-1 infected patients. AIDS 15: 71–5.

Massarella JW, Holazo AA, Koss-Twardy S et al. (1994). The effects of cimetidine and maalox on the pharmacokinetics of zalcitabine in HIV-positive patients. Pharm Res 11: 415.

McCance-Katz EF, Rainey PM, Jatlow P et al. (1989). Methadone effects on zidovudine disposition (AIDS Clinical Trials Group 262). J AIDS Hum Retrovir 18: 435–43.

McLeod GX, Hammer SM. (1992). Zidovudine: five years later. *Ann Intern Med* **117**: 487–501.

Mellors J, Stool E, Connaughton E *et al.* (1995). *Safety and tolerability of ZERIT (Stavudine, d4T) versus retrovir (zidovudine, ZDV) in HIV-infected adults with <500 CD4 cells/mm³ after at least 6 months of ZDV treatment.* Thirty-fifth Interscience Conference on Antimicrobial Agents and Chemotherapy, San Francisco, CA, USA, 235.

Merry C, Mulcahy F, Barry M *et al.* (1997). Saquinavir interaction with midazolam: pharmacokinetic considerations when prescribing protease inhibitors for patients with HIV disease. *AIDS* **11**: 268–9.

Merry C, Barry MG, Mulcahy F *et al.* (1998). The pharmacokinetics of combination therapy with nelfinavir plus nevirapine. *AIDS* **12**: 1163–7.

Metry DW, Lahart CJ, Farmer KL *et al.* (2001). Stevens-Johnson syndrome caused by the antiretroviral drug nevirapine. *J Am Acad Dermatol* **44**: 354–7.

Michalets EL. (1998). Update: clinically significant cytochrome P450 drug interactions. *Pharmacother* **18**: 84–112.

Miles SA, Mitsuyasu RT, Moreno J *et al.* (1991) Combined therapy with recombinant granulocyte colony-stimulating factor and erythropoietine decreases hematologic toxicity from zidovudine. *Blood* **77**: 2109–17.

Morse GD, Shelton MJ, Hewitt RG *et al.* (1998). *Ritonavir pharmacokinetics during combination therapy with delavirdine.* Fifth Conference on Retroviruses and Opportunistic Infections, Chicago, IL, USA.

Murphy R. (1997). Non-nucleoside reverse transcriptase inhibitors. *AIDS Clin Care* **9**: 75–9.

Murphy R, Gagnier P, Lamson M *et al.* (1997). *Effect of nevirapine on pharmacokinetics of indinavir and ritonavir in HIV-1 patients.* Fourth Conference on Retroviruses and Opportunistic Infections, January, Washington, DC, USA.

Murphy R, Sommadossi JP, Lamson M *et al.* (1999) Antiviral effect and pharmacokinetic interaction between nevirapine and indinavir correlation with antiviral activity. *J Infect Dis* **179**: 1116–23.

Olano JP, Borucki MJ, Wen JW *et al.* (1995). Massive hepatic steatosis and lactic acidosis in a patient with AIDS who was receiving zidovudine. *Clin Infect Dis* **21**: 973–6.

Perry CM, Balfour JA. (1996). Didanosine, an update on its antiviral activity, Pharmacokinetics properties and therapeutic efficacy in the management of HIV disease. *Drugs* **52**: 928–62.

Perry CM, Faulds D. (1997). Lamivudine, a review of its antiviral activity, pharmacokinetic properties and therapeutic efficacy in the management of HIV infection. *Drugs* **53**: 657–80.

Peter K, Gambertoglio JG. (1998). Intracellular phosphorylation of zidovudine (ZDV) and other nucleoside reverse transcriptase inhibitors (RTI) used for human immunodeficiency virus (HIV) infection. *Pharm Res* **15**: 821–7.

Peters BS, Winter J, Landon DN *et al.* (1993) Mitochondrial myopathy associated with chronic zidovudine therapy in AIDS. *Q J Med* **86**: 5–15.

Prazuck T, Semaille C, Roques S. (1998). Fatal acute haemolysis in an AIDS patient treated with indinavir. *AIDS* **12**: 531–3.

Rijnders B, Kooman J. (1998). Severe allergic reaction after repeated exposure to indinavir. *Clin Infect Dis* **26**: 523–4.

Robinson P, Lamson M, Cigliotti M *et al.* (1998). *Pharmacokinetic interaction between nevirapine and rifampin.* Twelfth World AIDS Conference, Geneva, Switzerland.

Robinson P, Gigliotti M, Lamson M *et al.* (1999). *Effect of reverse transcriptase inhibitor, nevirapine, on steady state pharmacokinetics of clarithromycin in HIV-positive patients.* Sixth Conference on Retroviruses and Opportunistic Infections, Chicago, IL, USA.

Roth VR, Angel JB, Kravcik S. (1998). *Development of a cervical fat pad following treatment with HIV-1 protease inhibitors.* Fifth Conference on Retrovirus and Opportunistic Infections, Chicago, IL, USA, 411.

Russ N, and the Fortovase® Study Group. (1998). *Saquinavir soft gel capsule (Fortovase®) pharmacokinetics and drug interactions.* Fifth Conference on Retroviruses and Opportunistic Infections, Chicago, IL, USA.

Rutstein RM, Feingold A, Meislich D *et al.* (1997). Protease inhibitor therapy in children with perinatally acquired HIV infection. *AIDS* **11**: F107–11.

Saadat K, Kaminski HJ. (1998). Ritonavir-associated myasthenia gravis. *Muscle Nerve* **21**: 680–1.

Sadler BM, Gillotin C, Chittick GE *et al.* (1998). *Pharmacokinetic drug interactions with Amprenavir.* Twelfth World AIDS Conference, Geneva, Switzerland, Abs. No. 12389.

Saravolatz LD, Winslow DL, Collins G *et al.* (1996) Zidovudine alone or in combination with didanosine or zalcitabine in HIV-infected patients with the acquired immunodeficiency syndrome or fewer than 200 CD4 cells per cubic millimeter. *N Engl J Med* **335**: 1099–106.

Sarcletti M, Petter A, Lhotta K *et al.* (1998). *Increased risk of indinavir nephropathy in women.* Fifth Conference on Retrovirus and Opportunistic Infections, Chicago, IL, USA, 418.

Schurmann D, Bergmann F, Ehrenstein T *et al.* (1998). Gynaecomastia in a male patient during protease inhibitor treatment for acute HIV disease. *AIDS* **12**: 2232–3.

Senior B, Gellis SS. (1964) The syndromes of total lipodystrophy and of partial lipodystrophy. *Pediatrics* **33**: 593–612.

Shintaku M, Nasu K, Shimizu T. (1993). Fulminant hepatic failure in an AIDS patient; possible zidovudine-induced hepatotoxicity. *Am J Gasteoenterol* **88**: 464–6.

Shyu WC, Knupp CA, Pittman KA *et al.* (1991). Food-induced reduction in bioavailability of didanosine. *Clin Pharmacol Ther* **50**: 503–7.

Skowron G, Leoung G, Kerr B *et al.* (1998). Lack of pharmacokinetic interaction between nelfinavir and nevirapine. *AIDS* **12**: 1243–4.

Sommadossi JP, Zhou XJ, Moore J *et al.* (1998). *Impairment of stavudine (d4T) phosphorylation in patients receiving a combination of zidovudine (ZDV) and d4T (ACTG 290).* Fifth Conference on Retrovirus and Opportunistic Infections, Chicago, IL, USA, 3.

Spruance SL, Pavia AT, Peterson D *et al.* (1994). Didanosine compared with continuation of zidovudine in HIV-infected patients with single of clinical deterioration while receiving zidovudine. A randomized, double-blind clinical trial. *Ann Intern Med* **120**: 360–8.

Strawford A, Hellerstein MK. (2001). Metabolic complications of HIV and AIDS. *Curr Infect Dis Rep* **3**: 183–92.

Styrt BA, Piazza-Hepp TD, Chikami GK. (1996). Clinical toxicity of antiretroviral nucleoside analogs. *Antiviral Res* **31**: 121–35.

Sulkowski MS, Thomas DL, Chaisson RD *et al.* (1998). *Hepatotoxicity with antiretroviral therapy among HIV-infected adults: The role of protease inhibitors and hepatitis C infection.* Thirty-eighth Interscience Conference on Antimicrobial Agents and Chemotherapy, San Diego, CA, USA, 116.

Swartz MN. (1995). Mitochondrial toxicity – new adverse drug effects. *N Engl J Med* **333**: 1146–8.

Taburet AM, Singlas E. (1996). Drug interaction with antiviral drugs. *Clin Pharmacokinet* **30**: 385–401.

Trapnell CB, Cimoch P, Games K *et al.* (1994). Altered didanosine pharmacokinetics with concomitant oral ganciclovir. *Clin Pharmacol Ther* **55**: 93.

van Leeuwen R, Lange JM, Hussey EK *et al.* (1992). The safety and pharmacokinetics of a reverse transcriptase inhibitor, 3TC, in patients with HIV infection: a phase I study. *AIDS* **6**: 1471–5.

van Leeuwen R, Katlama C, Kitchen V *et al.* (1995). Evaluation of safety and efficacy of 3TC (lamivudine) in patients with asymptomatic or mildly symptomatic human immunodeficiency virus infection; a phase I/II study. *J Infect Dis* **171**: 1166–71.

Wainberg MA, Salomon H, Gu Z *et al.* (1995). Development of HIV-1 resistance to (-)2′-deoxy-3′-thiacytidine in patients with AIDS or advanced AIDS-related complex. *AIDS* **9**: 351–7.

Witzke O, Plentz A, Schafers RF *et al.* (1997). Side-effects of ritonavir and its combination with saquinavir with special regard to renal function. *AIDS* **11**: 836–8.

Treatment of HIV infection

7

ROBERT MURPHY

Significant advances have been made in the treatment of HIV-infected individuals during the past 5 years, primarily because of a better understanding of HIV dynamics and more aggressive antiretroviral treatment approaches (Ho et al., 1995; Perelson et al., 1996). Clinically, this has dramatically translated into fewer hospital admissions, lower rates of opportunistic infection and decreased mortality (Mouton et al., 1997; Hogg et al., 1998; Palella et al., 1998). Prior to the use of potent antiretroviral regimens, often referred to as 'highly active antiretroviral therapy' or HAART, significant treatment benefits were relatively short-lived and limited to people with more advanced disease. By 1996, treatment with double combinations of nucleoside analogues was found to improve survival in asymptomatic patients (Hammer et al., 1996; CAESAR Co-ordinating Committee, 1997). By 1997, the impact of protease inhibitor-based triple drug therapy had been demonstrated to improve morbidity and mortality even further (Hammer et al., 1997), quickly becoming the standard of care in developed countries.

In 1996, fewer than half the estimated number of HIV-infected patients in the USA was receiving treatment for HIV infection. Treated patients were more likely to have advanced disease, to be male, working and to have private medical insurance. The annual cost of patient care was roughly US$20 000 per patient year; a considerable amount, but accounting for less than 1% of the total amount spent on personal health care in the USA in 1996. This proportion is not excessive, considering that HIV infection accounted for about 7% of the total potential years of life lost in the USA (Bozzette et al., 1998). The bulk of the monies spent on HIV patient care was related to hospitalization costs. Since that time, overall costs have dropped, due to the effects of improved treatment on hospitalization rates, despite the increase in pharmacy charges. The effect of improved therapies has also indirectly attracted more patients with less advanced HIV infection into initiating antiretroviral therapy and is expected to extend the potential life span of those with all stages of infection considerably.

There are several published guidelines regarding the management of the HIV-infected patient (Carpenter et al., 2000; Department of Health and Human Services, 2000). Practically, these guidelines offer a foundation from which the patient and clinician can begin to contemplate and design an appropriate treatment strategy. There are currently 15 antiretroviral drugs available to patients in the developed world. Unfortunately, these 15 agents must be used in combinations of at least three drugs. Many have overlapping toxicities, similar resistance profiles, incompatible dosing administration properties, and/or long-term potential toxicities. Suboptimal treatment regimens or improper monitoring and management can have disastrous consequences for the patient. Clinicians unfamiliar with the most up-to-date treatment of HIV infection should defer to colleagues who have such expertise. This has been vividly demonstrated in one study, where patients cared for by the most experienced physicians had a 31% lower risk of death than patients cared for by physicians with the least experience ($p < 0.02$) (Kitahara et al., 1996).

The current treatment guidelines for the USA can be found on http://hivatis.org/trtgdlns.html.

Which patients with HIV infection should be offered antiretroviral therapy?

Almost all patients with documented HIV infection will benefit from antiretroviral therapy at some point in their disease, as fewer than 2% of infected people seem able to contain viral replication and to maintain adequate CD4 lymphocyte counts in the absence of antiretroviral therapy for prolonged periods of time (Haynes *et al.*, 1996). The question is really when to initiate therapy. Treatment is complex, costly, and not tolerated by many. Non-adherence to a prescribed treatment regimen can have severe negative consequences for the individual patient, as resistance can readily develop to most of the prescribed agents and related class compounds. If the patient is reluctant to begin therapy, treatment should not be initiated until the person is 'ready'. This may take a considerable amount of time and education on the clinician's part.

There is universal agreement that therapy should be offered to people who have symptomatic HIV disease, regardless of the plasma HIV RNA concentration or CD4 lymphocyte count. Further evidence strongly supports the use of antiretroviral therapy if the CD4 lymphocyte count falls below 500 cells/ml or the plasma HIV RNA is greater than 10 000 copies/ml, as measured by RT PCR or the bDNA. Controversy exists as to the recommendation for treatment in persons with CD4 lymphocyte counts greater than 500 cells/ml and plasma HIV RNA less than 10 000 copies/ml (Carpenter, 1998; Department of Health and Human Services, 1998). Controversy also exists as to whether or not patients with acute HIV infection should be offered therapy. While a short-term treatment benefit has been noted for patients with recently acquired HIV infection, long-term data regarding outcome do not exist (Lafeuillade *et al.*, 1997). Table 7.1 outlines the current consensus on whom should be offered therapy.

Monitoring the effect of therapy

Monitoring the effect of therapy is critical to patient management and has been considerably improved by the widespread availability of measuring plasma concentrations of HIV RNA, frequently referred to as 'viral load', in addition to circulating CD4 lymphocyte counts (Saag *et al.*, 1996; Mellors *et al.*, 1997; Marschner *et al.*, 1998; Lepri *et al.*, 2001). The viral load is a direct measurement of HIV in the plasma. This circulating level of virus actually represents less than 1% of all HIV in the body. However, plasma levels proportionally represent total body virus, and a decrease in the measurement of the plasma compartment generally corresponds to decreases in the lymph tissue compartment, where the bulk of virus resides. Prior to the initiation of therapy, both viral load and CD4 lymphocyte count should be performed. The immediate goal of therapy is to decrease the viral load to the lowest level possible for as long as possible. With the currently available assays, this means a decrease to less than 50 copies of HIV RNA/ml. This magnitude of reduction in viral load takes 16–24 weeks, and even longer if the baseline viral load is very high (i.e. >100 000 copies/ml). With a sustained and significant reduction in viral load, the CD4 lymphocyte count should increase by 100–200 cells/µl (although the rise in absolute numbers of CD4 lymphocytes varies considerably from patient to patient) and the incidence of clinical events, including death, will be markedly decreased. Following the initiation of therapy, the viral load should be repeated after 1 month. If possible, the patient should have the viral load, CD4

Table 7.1 Indications for initiating antiretroviral therapy

Clinical category	CD4 lymphocyte count (cells/mm^3)	Viral load MIV RNA (copies/ml)	Recommendation
Acute infection	Any	Any	Strong consideration
Symptomatic	Any	Any	Treat
Asymptomatic	<350	Any	Treat
Asymptomatic	350–500	>5000	Treat
Asymptomatic	350–500	<5000	Consider treatment
Asymptomatic	>500	>30 000	Treat
Asymptomatic	>500	5000–30 000	Consider treatment
Asymptomatic	>500	<5000	Deter therapy

Adapted from Carpenter *et al.* (2000); Department of Health and Human Services (2000).

lymphocyte count, full blood count and chemistries done prior to the first follow-up visit in order that the clinician can review these results with the patient at the time of the visit. At a minimum, the viral load should be reduced at that time by 0.5 log_{10} copies/ml (threefold) from the baseline level. If it is not, it is important to assess why this has not occurred. A drug resistance test should be performed (Lepri *et al.*, 2001). Common reasons for initial failure to achieve an appropriate virological response include suboptimal treatment regimen, community-acquired drug resistance, inadequate absorption, and non-adherence.

If the initial response is adequate, the viral load should be repeated no later than 12 weeks after initiating therapy and then quarterly or when the clinical condition suggests disease progression. Within 24 weeks most patients will have maximally reduced their viral load to the lowest level measurable (Lepri *et al.*, 2001). Following maximal suppression of virus, an occasional small increase in measurable viral load may be observed, usually to levels less than 1000 copies/ml. This will typically return to an 'undetectable' level if the patient continues to take the treatment regimen as prescribed. Intercurrent illness, immunizations and some therapies, such as IL-2, are known to increase viral load transiently; however, viral load levels usually fall back towards baseline within 1 month. If a small rise in viral load is noted, this value should be repeated before the next visit (typically within 1 month).

Antiretroviral therapy

There are currently three available classes of antiretroviral drugs: nucleoside analogue reverse transcriptase inhibitors, non-nucleoside reverse transcriptase inhibitors, and protease inhibitors (see Chapters 5 and 6). The currently available drugs, their recommended dosages and expected side-effects are listed in Table 7.2. Typically, potent regimens include at least three antiretroviral drugs, two of them being nucleoside analogues that inhibit reverse transcriptase. While inhibitors of HIV protease were originally considered as an essential third component of a potent regimen, protease inhibitor-sparing regimens that substitute a non-nucleoside reverse transcriptase inhibitor for the protease inhibitor are also highly effective, and are now included as a first-line option in formal treatment guidelines

(Carpenter *et al.*, 1998; Department of Health and Human Services, 1998).

Nucleoside reverse transcriptase inhibitor 'backbone'

It is recommended that double nucleoside reverse transcriptase inhibitor (NRTI) therapy be included as a component of every initial, as well as most subsequent, treatment regimens. Various combinations of NRTIs have been shown to be synergistic, additive or antagonistic *in vitro*, depending on the combination studied. By the mid-1990s, specific double NRTI therapy was shown to be superior to NRTI monotherapy (Delta Co-ordinating Committee, 1996; Hammer *et al.*, 1996; Saravolatz *et al.*, 1996). Within a very short period of time, double NRTI therapy with one of five recommended combinations had become the standard treatment recommendation. While there are five recommended double nucleoside combinations, three are preferred because of proven or perceived antiviral and/or clinical benefit. These include:

(1) stavudine/lamivudine (Katlama *et al.*, 1998);
(2) zidovudine/lamivudine (Eron *et al.*, 1995; Bartlett *et al.*, 1996; Katlama *et al.*, 1996; Staszewski *et al.*, 1996); and
(3) didanosine/stavudine (Fisher, 1998; Molina *et al.*, 1998).

They are outlined in Table 7.3. Two other combinations have been extensively studied (Delta Co-ordinating Committee, 1996; Hammer *et al.*, 1996; Saravolatz *et al.*, 1996), but are rarely used in clinical practice because of intolerance (zidovudine/didanosine) or suboptimal efficacy (zalcitabine/zidovudine). Other combinations are generally not used because of significant overlapping toxicity (stavudine/zalcitabine) or antagonism (stavudine/zidovudine).

Initial treatment approaches

Current guidelines recommend initiation of antiretroviral therapy using at least three drugs. Included in the treatment options are one of the NRTI combinations noted in Table 7.3, plus the addition of a protease inhibitor or a non-nucleoside reverse transcriptase inhibitor (NNRTI) noted in Table 7.2. In 2000, the most common initial treatment regimens included one of the dual NRTI combinations plus either the protease

Table 7.2 Available antiretroviral agents, commonly used dosages and side-effects

Name	Other names	Dosage	Side-effects	Comments
Nucleoside (or nucleotide) reverse transcriptase inhibitors[a]				
Abacavir	Ziagen™	300 mg twice daily	Fever, malaise, rash, 'hypersensitivity reaction' (2–5%)	The hypersensitivity reaction can be lethal; if suspected, patients should discontinue drug immediately and never be rechallenged
Didanosine	ddI; Videx™; Videx EC	200 mg twice daily or 400 mg once daily, EC dosage is 400 mg daily (250 mg if less than 60 kg)	Peripheral neuropathy, pancreatitis, gastrointestinal symptoms	No food must be taken within 1 h of dosing; pills are large Videx EC is a capsule and much better tolerated than the tablets
Lamivudine	3TC; Epivir™	150 mg twice daily	Minimal toxicities have been reported	Very well tolerated; resistance can develop rapidly
Stavudine	d4T; Zerit™	40 mg twice daily (30 mg if less than 60 kg)	Peripheral neuropathy	Resistance profile favourable
Zalcitabine	ddC; Hivid™	0.75 mg every 8 h	Peripheral neuropathy, stomatitis	Relatively weak potency limits usefulness
Zidovudine	ZDV; AZT; Retrovir™	250–300 mg twice daily	Anaemia, neutropenia, myopathy, gastrointestinal symptoms, headache	Resistance to this drug may limit usefulness for entire drug class
Non-nucleoside reverse transcriptase inhibitors				
Delavirdine	Rescriptor™	400 mg three times daily	Rash	Pill burden high; inhibits hepatic P450 and may increase levels of drugs metabolized by this pathway
Efavirenz	Sustiva™	600 mg once daily	Central nervous system effects common (50%) but self-limited; rash	Induces hepatic P450 and may lower levels of drugs metabolized by this pathway; teratogenic in animals, avoid in pregnancy; false-positive cannabinoid test
Nevirapine	Viramune™	200 mg once daily for 14 days, then 400 mg once daily, or 200 mg twice daily	Rash (may be severe); hepatitis	Induces hepatic P450 and may lower levels of drugs metabolized by this pathway
Hepatitis and Stevens–Johnson syndrome potentially fatal but rare; should not be used in post-exposure prophylaxis regimens if possible
Protease inhibitors[b]				
Amprenavir	Agenerase™	1200 mg twice daily	Rash, gastrointestinal symptoms	No food restrictions; high-fat meals should be avoided; high pill burden
Indinavir	Crixivan™	800 mg three times daily	Nephrolithiasis, gastrointestinal symptoms	Must be taken with no food or low-protein, low-fat meal
Lopinavir/ritonavir	Kaletra™, ABT-378lr	400/100 mg twice daily with food. Increase to 533/133 mg if taken with nevirapine/efavirenz	Gastrointestinal symptoms; hyperlipidaemia	In subjects co-infected with hepatitis B and C, transaminase levels may rise significantly
Nelfinavir	Viracept™	1250 mg twice daily	Diarrhoea and other gastrointestinal symptoms	Must be taken with a fatty snack; high pill burden
Ritonavir	Norvir™	600 mg twice daily	Gastrointestinal symptoms very common; circumoral paresthesias	Current liquid formulation has foul taste; gel caps (when available) need refrigeration; no food restrictions; very potent inhibitor of hepatic P450; used in combination with other protease inhibitors, the dose is usually lowered to 100–400 mg twice daily
Saquinavir	Fortovase™ (Invirase™, the old hard gel formulation should not be used)	1200 mg three times daily	Gastrointestinal symptoms	Must be taken with a snack or meal; high pill burden
Lopinavir/ritonavir	Kaletra™	400/100 mg twice daily	Gastrointestinal symptoms	May cause hyperlipidemia and increased lepatic transquivers levels in patients co-infected with hepatitis C

[a]Lactic acidosis with hepatic steatosis is a rare but potentially life threatening toxicity with the use of all nucleoside reverse transcriptase inhibitors.

[b]All protease inhibitors inhibit (or affect) the hepatic cytochrome P450 enzymes and may significantly alter the levels of drugs metabolized by that pathway; lipodystrophy and other metabolic complications may be a late complication, hyperlipidaemia may be an early adverse occurrence.

Table 7.3 The three most commonly used NRTI backbone combinations

Nucleoside combination	Advantages	Disadvantages
Stavudine plus lamivudine	Best tolerated; no food restrictions; stavudine resistance profile favourable	Stavudine may cause peripheral neuropathy. Lactic acidosis (rare and lipodystrophy)
Zidovudine plus lamivudine	Convenient dosing as one pill twice daily (Combivir®); no food restrictions	Gastrointestinal intolerance, anaemia, and/or leucopenia occur in less than 5%; zidovudine may cause myopathy; zidovudine resistance may affect activity against other antiretrovirals; lipoatrophy possible
Didanosine plus stavudine	Didanosine may cause pancreatitis and gastrointestinal symptoms, both drugs may cause peripheral neuropathy, hepatic steatosis and should be used together with extreme caution if at all during pregnancy	Didanosine must not be given within 1 h of eating; both drugs may cause peripheral neuropathy; didanosine may cause pancreatitis and gastrointestinal symptoms

inhibitor nelfinavir or indinavir, or the NNRTI efavirenz or nevirapine (Table 7.4). A new approach involves initiating therapy with three NRTIs (Staszewski et al., 2001; Saez-Llorens et al., 2001). Combination tablets (lamivudine/zidovudine and abacavir/lamivudine/zidovudine) are now in clinical use (cremieux et al., 2001)

Protease inhibitor-based approach

Most data exist on initiating therapy with two NRTIs and the protease inhibitor (PI) indinavir. It was this regimen that first clearly demonstrated the sustained benefit of potent antiretroviral therapy in individuals who were treatment-naïve to lamivudine and PIs. In these studies, sustained antiviral responses with indinavir, lamivudine and zidovudine occurred in 60–78% of recipients; more importantly, patients survived longer than if treated with only two NRTIs (Gulick et al., 1997; Hammer et al., 1997; Gulick et al., 1998). Similar sustained antiviral responses have been observed with the other licensed PIs when used in triple drug

Table 7.4 Common treatment approaches in 2000

NRTI backbone	Third agent	Comments
Stavudine plus lamivudine or Zidovudine plus lamivudine or Stavudine plus didanosine	Nelfinavir	Pill burden high; diarrhoea and GI side-effects common; long-term PI effects a concern
	Indinavir	Every 8 h dosing and food restrictions for indinavir complicate regimen; well studied; kidney stones, long-term PI effects a concern; when given with ritonavir 100–400 mg can be dosed twice daily, 40 mg, cause dorsal bid
	Efavirenz	Dosing regimen easy; pill burden low; 50% CNS side-effects (generally self-limited); efavirenz is a potent P450 inducer and many drug levels may be affected; teratogenicity in animals prohibits use in women who are pregnant or considering pregnancy; rash frequency low
	Nevirapine	Less well studied in patients with advanced disease; rash problematic and may be severe (3–5%); nevirapine is a modest P450 inducer and may affect other drug levels; has been safely used in pregnant women to date; hepatitis rare, but can be fatal. Should not be used for post-exposure prophylaxis if possible
	Lopinavir/ritonavir	Minor GI side-effects; hyperlipidaemia; otherwise potent as well tolerated should be used for post-exposure prophylaxis

GI: gastrointestinal; NRTI: nucleoside analogue reverse transcriptase inhibitor; PI: protease inhibitor.

combinations, such as nelfinavir (Clendennin *et al.*, 1998), ritonavir (Connick *et al.*, 1998), amprenavir (Murphy *et al.*, 1999), the soft-gel formulation of saquinavir (Mitsuyasu *et al.*, 1998) and 10 prenavir/ritonavir (Murphy *et al.*, 2001). Likewise, treatment comparisons have been made with a variety of dual NRTI combinations and the same PI. To date, no difference has been observed in patients treated with stavudine plus lamivudine, stavudine plus didanosine or zidovudine plus lamivudine in addition to indinavir (Gulick, 1998).

Initiating therapy with two PIs, such as ritonavir and saquinavir, both given in a dose of 400 mg twice daily, has also been studied in combination with dual NRTI therapy. From an antiviral perspective, results have been encouraging (Cameron *et al.*, 1999). In one study, the proportion of patients with plasma HIV RNA levels of less than 200 copies/ml after 24 weeks of treatment was significantly better for the dual PI treatment than in those commencing treatment with a single PI in combination with dual NRTI therapy. Of 119 treatment-naïve patients enrolled in this trial, 89% of those with a ritonavir plus saquinavir-based treatment compared to 63% and 57% for those with indinavir alone – or ritonavir alone in combination with dual NRTIs (p < 0.01) (Kirk *et al.*, 1999). Typically, these dual PI combinations are not used in an initial therapy regimen, but are reserved for subsequent treatment regimens following virological or clinical failure.

Initial therapy with protease-sparing regimens has recently become more common, due to the difficulty individuals have in taking any of the available PIs, coupled with additional concerns regarding the metabolic complications that have been associated with PI-based treatment (see Chapter 6). These complications include diabetes and clinical lipodystrophy, or fat redistribution syndrome, and are only now being fully explored (Dube *et al.*, 1997; Eastone and Decker, 1997; Visnegarwala *et al.*, 1997; Carr *et al.* 1998a, b; Lo *et al.*, 1998; Miller *et al.*, 1998a, b; Roth *et al.*, 1998). While no agreed definition of lipodystrophy exists, the syndrome can be characterized by any of the following physical changes:

(1) development of a dorsocervical fat pad (buffalo hump);
(2) perinasal fat pad wasting;

(3) decreased subcutaneous fat in the extremities (veins often become prominent); and
(4) central obesity, including breast enlargement in women.

Regardless of the absence of a formal definition, it is a condition that is becoming more and more commonly observed. In addition to the physical changes, elevations in cholesterol and triglyceride levels are often observed early after the initiation of PI-based therapy. The clinical relevance of these plasma lipid abnormalities remains an issue of concern.

Protease inhibitor-sparing approaches

The problems relating to toxicity due to the PIs have accelerated the push to find PI-sparing treatment approaches, particularly for those individuals with only early or moderately advanced disease. It was first noted in 1996 that patients treated with the non-nucleoside nevirapine plus didanosine and zidovudine (the INCAS study) had a durable antiviral response, similar to that observed with the PI-based regimens (Montaner *et al.*, 1998a). This study has been criticized because the baseline plasma HIV RNA level for the group was relatively low (17 732 HIV RNA copies/ml), and there was no direct comparison with a PI-containing regimen. There are now two trials that have directly compared a non-nucleoside-based regimen with a PI-based regimen. Preliminary results suggest that the treatment approaches are equivalent (Katlama *et al.*, 1999; Staszewski *et al.*, 1999).

In the first head-on comparison to be reported, the NNRTI efavirenz was compared to indinavir; both treatment regimens included zidovudine and lamivudine. Additionally, a treatment arm containing indinavir and efavirenz together was included in the trial design. The results after 48 weeks demonstrated that 70% of patients enrolled in the efavirenz arm had plasma HIV RNA of less than 400 copies/ml, compared to 48% of patients in the indinavir arm (p < 0.001). While these results are encouraging, it is unlikely that the indinavir arm is truly performing as poorly as suggested from the intent-to-treat analysis described above. The drop-out rate in this study was extremely high, being 27% in the efavirenz arm and 43% in the indinavir arm (p = 6.005). This difference in treatment effect is more probably explained by the relative difficulty patients had in taking indinavir three times daily compared to the once daily dosing of efavirenz with no food restrictions (Staszewski et al., 1999).

The other trial (the Atlantic study) compared the non-nucleoside nevirapine with indinavir in a regimen that also included didanosine and stavudine. This trial also had an arm containing three nucleosides alone. Another novel feature of this study was that the didanosine was administered in a dose of 400 mg once daily. Similarly, the nevirapine was also administered in a dose of 400 mg once daily. The preliminary on-treatment analysis of this study after 24 weeks of treatment revealed that the proportion of subjects with HIV RNA of less than 50 copies/ml was 81% for both the indinavir and nevirapine groups. The intent-to-treat analysis was also similar, but the results were not given due to their preliminary nature. All treatment groups tolerated their regimens well (Katlama et al., 1999).

A new approach to initiating therapy is with three nucleoside reverse transcriptase inhibitors, without a PI or an NNRTI. This approach is considered novel and experimental at present, but preliminary results from two clinical trials suggest that triple NRTI combinations may become a viable option for some patients. The two regimens that have been formally studied are stavudine plus didanosine, plus lamivudine (the Atlantic study) and zidovudine plus lamivudine plus abacavir, all administered at the full recommended dosage. To date, the virological responses of both of these regimens after 48 weeks of treatment are comparable to regimens that contain a PI or NNRTI. In the Atlantic study the as-treated analysis demonstrated that 76% of subjects receiving stavudine plus didanosine plus lamivudine had HIV RNA levels of less than 50 copies/ml after 24 weeks (Katlama et al., 1999). This regimen was well tolerated, without any unusual side-effects reported thus far. The other triple NRTI regimen studied is zidovudine plus lamivudine plus abacavir. In the CNA3005 study, this combination was compared to zidovudine plus lamivudine plus indinavir in a blinded manner. After 24 weeks, both arms showed equivalent results. At 16 weeks, 45% of the abacavir-treated patients and 42% of the indinavir-treated patients had HIV RNA levels of less than 50 copies/ml. It was noted that cholesterol levels were 15–20 mg/dl higher in the indinavir arm. Toxicity was also observed among abacavir recipients, with 5%

experiencing hypersensitivity reactions, including one death (Staszewski et al., 1999).

These two triple NRTI trials open the door to a new treatment strategy option. Advantages of this approach are that other NRTIs could potentially be used following treatment failure and the sparing of two other potent classes of antiretroviral agents. It is important to keep in mind that the data on these studies are preliminary.

Treatment of patients experiencing clinical or virological failure

The reasons for treatment failure are multiple and include resistance to one or more of the chosen anti-retroviral drugs (Montaner et al., 2001), non-adherence to the prescribed treatment regimen, drug–drug interactions resulting in subtherapeutic levels of the antiretroviral agents, and postulated intracellular mechanisms. The reasons for treatment failure and the subsequent choice of treatment must be individualized.

Despite our best efforts, the likelihood of achieving a sustained antiretroviral response in patients treated with any of the triple therapy regimens presumed to be effective approximates 50% (Montaner et al., 1998). While antiviral rebound or failure does not necessarily translate to immediate clinical failure, it certainly predicts a poorer outcome than if the replication of the virus could be controlled. The development of clinical disease while receiving antiretroviral therapy constitutes clinical failure. Long before this happens, the viral load typically increases, indicating that viral replication is taking place in the presence of the therapy being prescribed. Persistent viral replication during anti-retroviral therapy places the patient at great risk for the development of resistance to the exposed treatment regimen. This should be avoided if at all possible, as many of the currently available drugs are cross-resistant to other members of their class (Moyle, 1996). For example, drugs within the non-nucleoside class (efavirenz, nevirapine, and delavirdine) all select for the single K103N reverse transcriptase mutation and are completely cross-resistant. While the protease resistance profile shows some variability and specificity, there is a risk of cross-resistance following acquisition of three or more codon mutations (Condra et al., 1995). The NRTIs have different resistance profiles. However, following treatment failure, subsequent response to supposedly susceptible nucleosides may be significantly blunted. It has been postulated that this may be due to an alteration in intracellular kinetics of nucleoside phosphorylation (Sommadossi, 1998). Resistance testing, either by genotype or phenotype, is commercially available, but its exact utility has yet to be fully characterized. It is likely that resistance testing will become a useful management tool when treatment changes based on these types of test results are proved beneficial and the assays receive formal regulatory approval.

The numerical threshold for defining virological failure has not been determined. A rise in viral load of at least 0.5 $\log_{10}$ copies/ml (threefold) is known to be significant. A rise to greater than, or equal to, the pretherapy level is generally agreed to constitute treatment failure. However, the significance in rises in the viral load to levels less than 500, 1000, 5000, or 10000 copies/ml is not completely understood. Current guidelines recommend that when a change of antiretroviral treatment is considered, two new NRTIs are chosen plus a different PI to which the virus is likely to be sensitive (Carpenter et al., 2000; Department of Health and Human Services, 2000). In practice, what occurs is that the patient is placed on double PI therapy with or without a non-nucleoside RTI, in addition to NRTIs if possible. Response rates to these approaches vary and are dependent upon how long the patient has been receiving the failing regimen, how many prior drugs have already been administered, and genotypical and/or phenotypical resistance to the various drugs. Virological success rates with subsequent therapy range from 28 to 80%. The cohorts of patients that have fared best are those where therapy was changed very quickly after the viral load rebounded to greater than 500 copies/ml (Murphy et al., 1998) and those where combination PI therapy was employed (Deeks et al., 1998; Kaufmann et al., 1998; Tebas et al., 1999). The use of resistance testing to assist in the choice of subsequent antiretroviral therapy has been used with a favourable response in several clinical trials (Baxter et al., 2000; Durant et al., 1999). While not widely available at present, these assays are now coming into broader clinical use (Montaner et al., 2001).

Treatment intensification

While not formally recommended, one experimental approach taken in a limited number of clinical studies is the addition of a single active agent described as 'treatment intensification', to a regimen in a patient experiencing a rebound in plasma viraemia. The potential advantage of such an approach is preservation of more aggressive treatment strategies for a later time. The results from one of the first treatment intensification strategies was first reported in a group of patients with a history of extensive pre-treatment with NRTIs who were then switched to ritonavir plus saquinavir therapy. In several patients who experienced virological rebound following many months of optimal suppression with ritonavir plus saquinavir, the addition of lamivudine and stavudine, two NRTIs that the patients had never previously received, resulted in a renewed and sustained antiretroviral suppression (Cameron et al., 1999).

'Treatment intensification' has also been successfully observed when the antimetabolite hydroxyurea was added to the regimen of patients with measurable viraemia following therapy with didanosine and stavudine (Rutschmann et al., 1998) (see Chapter 5). In this study, patients naïve to therapy were treated with didanosine plus stavudine plus either hydroxyurea or placebo. After 12 weeks, the virological non-responders assigned to placebo were given open-label hydroxyurea. By 24 weeks, the antiviral response in the patients originally treated with hydroxyurea and in those who added it after 12 weeks was equivalent, with approximately 79% achieving optimal suppression. However, these results were not sustained over time

The only placebo controlled trial of 'treatment intensification' is a study of patients receiving their first antiretroviral regimen with plasma HIV RNA levels up to 50 000 copies/ml. Intensification of their regimen had undetectable plasma HIV RNA levels (of less than 400 copies/ml) in abacavir (or placebo). After 24 weeks, 39% in the abacavir group versus 8% receiving placebo demonstrated that a significant proportion of those treated were able to achieve an effective antiretroviral response by intensifying their regimen (Katlama et al., 1998).

While 'treatment intensification' is an attractive alternative to the standard approach of changing the entire therapeutic regimen, it must be approached with caution. In patients with extensive treatment histories, this approach is likely to fail, due to significant baseline resistance at the time of intensification.

Drugs with low thresholds for the development of resistance, such as the non-nucleoside RTIs and lamivudine, should be avoided because of the likelihood of the development of further resistance. Patients with relatively high plasma viral loads should also not be considered candidates for intensification, as the power of any single available agent may not be sufficient. Clinicians considering this approach should consider utilizing a commercial resistance assay to determine the viral genotype prior to making the switch (Baxter et al., 2000). Blood samples for resistance testing should be drawn while patients are receiving their treatment regimens.

Switching regimens

Current guidelines recommend that patients experiencing virological failure or rebound, should change their entire regimen (Carpenter et al., 2000; Department of Health and Human Services, 2000). For purely virological reasons, this makes sense. However, if a patient has difficulty with adherence, changing medications, often to an even more complicated regimen, is not going to be very helpful. There have been no controlled studies comparing different strategies in patients who have failed an active three-drug antiretroviral regimen, although there have been multiple studies describing results in patients who have failed dual NRTI regimens.

There have been two reports of trials describing results of patients who experienced virological rebound during their first three-drug, PI-based therapy. In one study, 24 patients treated with nelfinavir in combination with NRTIs for at least 48 weeks and having detectable viral load (median viral load of 46 674 copies/ml), were treated with a ritonavir plus saquinavir-based regimen. In 22 of the 24 patients, viral load decreased to less than 500 copies/ml on at least one occasion and 14 of 24 (58.3%) had sustained antiviral suppression. In this trial, a higher baseline viral load predicted subsequent treatment failure. Interestingly, the D30N mutation, unique to nelfinavir, did not predict the treatment response, suggesting that subsequent PI-based approaches may be successful (Tebas et al., 1999). In the second study, 55 patients who had failed an amprenavir-based regimen were treated with indinavir, nevirapine, stavudine and lamivudine. In this group, 79% experienced a sustained antiretroviral response for 48 weeks (Murphy et al., 1998). Many of the

Table 7.5 Pharmacologically enhanced protease inhibitors

Prior regimen	Enhanced regimen
Indinavir 800 mg POBID	Indinavir/ritonavir 400/400 mg POBID 800/200 mg POBID 800/100 mg POBID
Ampranavir 1200 mg POBID	Amprenavir/ritonavir 600/100 mg POBID 900/100 mg POBID
Saquinavir (Fortrase®) 1200 mg POBID	Saquinavir (Fortrase®)/ritonavir 400/400 mg BID 1600/100 mg QD
None	Lopinavir/ritonavir (Kaletra®) 400/100 mg BID

GI: gastrointestinal; IDV: indinavir; NNRTI: non-nucleoside analogue reverse transcriptase inhibitor; NRTI: nucleoside analogue reverse transcriptase inhibitor; PI: protease inhibitor; RTV: ritonavir.

patients in this study did not have demonstrable PI mutations, suggesting that early treatment changes when there are fewer mutations may present a response to other PIs useful in salvage regimens.

The key to successful salvage regimens lies in (1) improved adherence, (2) use of drugs that the virus is susceptible, and (3) to maximize potency inhibitors (Table 7.5).

'MegaHAART' for patients with extensive prior antiretroviral treatment

A novel treatment approach has more recently received serious attention in a very advanced group of patients who have failed multiple drug treatments. In one such cohort, the administration of six or more drugs, many of them having been used in the past, has been attempted and has been termed 'MegaHAART'. In one such group of patients treated with at least six antiretroviral drugs, 10 of 24 (who were followed for at least 8 months) were shown to have decreased their viral load to less than 500 copies/ml. Prior drug 'holidays' and drug-sensitive virus based on the resistance assays were associated with a successful antiviral response. Long-term therapy with this amount of drugs was not feasible for the majority of the patients because of intolerance (Miller et al., 1999). This study, among others, highlights important points such as drug holidays, resistance testing, and recycling of drugs, all topics worthy of further, more definitive, study.

Table 7.6 Examples of common treatment strategies

Treatment course	Protease inhibitor based	Non-nucleoside based	Double protease inhibitor based	Triple nucleoside based
Initial regimen	Indinavir or nelfinavir plus NRTI[1] plus NRTI[2]	Efavirenz or nevirapine plus NRTI[1] plus NRTI[2]	Ritonavir (400 mg twice daily) plus saquinavir (400 mg twice daily) or indinavir (400 mg every 12 h) plus NRT[1] plus NRTI[2]	Stavudine plus didanosine plus lamivudine or abacavir plus zidovudine plus lamivudine
Second regimen line	Double protease inhibitors (see above) plus NRTI[3] plus NRTI[4] (optional to add efavirenz or nevirapine)	Indinavir or nelfinavir plus NRTI[3] plus NRTI[4]	Efavirenz or nevirapine plus NRTI[3] plus NRTI[4] (optional to add to fifth NRTI and/or hydroxyurea)	Indinavir or nelfinavir plus NRTI[4] plus nevirapine or efavirenz
Third regimen line	No recommendation	Double protease inhibitor (see above) plus NRTI[5] plus NRTI[6]	No recommendation	Double protease inhibitor (see above) plus NRTI[5] plus NRT[1]

NRTI: nucleoside reverse transcriptase inhibitor.

Structured treatment interruption

Structured treatment interruptions (STI) of HAART are being tested in clinical trials to examine virologic and immunologic consequences. Studies in macaques suggest such regimens may be an effective alternative to continuous treatment (Lori et al., 2000). However, in clinical trials to date (which have generally been uncontrolled and involving small numbers of patients) no clear benefit has been demonstrated. The risks of STI include induction of drug resistance and increasing the viral reservoir (Bonhoeffer et al., 2000; Miller, 2001; Deeks et al., 2001).

Formulating a strategy

Initiating therapy and following published guidelines superficially appears quite easy. However, if a miscalculation is made, the results can be quite unfavourable for the patient, as subsequent options are limited. It is necessary to strategize a sequence of therapeutic interventions. A realistic goal at the present time is to attempt to control the replication of the virus as much as possible, but at least for the next 1–2 years. The reason for this is that the antiretroviral drugs currently in development coupled with the potential for immune interventions look promising and are likely to provide further significant benefit to our patients. Table 7.6 outlines several strategic approaches currently available to HIV-infected patients in the developed world.

References

Department of Health and Human Services and the Henry J. Kaiser Family Foundation. (2000). *Guidelines for the use of antiretroviral agents in the HIV-infected adult and adolescent.* January 28.

Bartlett JA, Benoit SL, Johnson VA et al. (1996). Lamivudine plus zidovudine compared with zalcitabine plus zidovudine in patients with HIV infection. A randomized, double-blind, placebo-controlled trial. *Ann Intern Med* **125**: 161–72.

Baxter JD, Mayers DL, Wentworth DN et al. (2000). A randomized study of antiretroviral management based on plasma genotypic antiretroviral resistance testing in patients failing therapy. *AIDS* **14**: F83–F93.

Bozzette SA, Berry SH, Duan N et al. (1998). The care of HIV-infected adults in the United States. *N Engl J Med* **339**: 1897–904.

Bonhoeffer S, Rembiszewski M, Ortiz GM et al. (2000). Risks and benefits of structured treatement interruptions in HIV-1 infection. *AIDS* **14**: 2313–22.

CAESAR Coordinating Committee. (1997). Randomized trial of addition of lamivudine or lamivudine plus loviride to zidovudine-containing regimens for patients with HIV-1 infection. *Lancet* **349**: 1413–21.

Cameron DW, Japour AJ, Xu Y et al. (1999). Ritonavir and saquinavir combination therapy for the treatment of HIV infection. *AIDS* **13**: 213–24.

Carpenter CJ, Cooper DAFischl MA et al. (1998). Antiretroviral therapy in adults: updated recommendations of the International AIDS Society – USA Panel. *JAMA* **280**: 78–86.

Carr A, Samaras K, Burton S et al. (1998a). A syndrome of peripheral lipodystrophy, hyperlipidaemia and insulin resistance in patients receiving HIV protease inhibitors. *AIDS* **12**: F51–8.

Carr A, Samaras K, Chisholm DJ et al. (1998b). Pathogenesis of HIV-1 protease inhibitor-associated peripheral lipodystrophy, hyperlipidaemia, and insulin resistance. Lancet 351: 1881–3.

Clendennin N, Quart B, Anderson R et al. (1998). Analysis of long-term virologic data from the Viracept (nelfinavir, NFV) 511 protocol using 3 HIV-RNA assays. In: Program and abstracts of the Fifth Conference on Retroviruses and Opportunistic Infections, Chicago, IL, USA.

Condra JH, Schleif WA, Blahy OM et al. (1995). In vivo emergence of HIV-1 variants resistant to multiple protease inhibitors. Nature 374: 569–71.

Connick E, Lederman M, Kotzin B et al. (1998). Immunologic effects of 48 weeks of AZT/3TC/ritonavir. In: Program and abstracts of the Fifth Conference on Retroviruses and Opportunistic Infections, Chicago, IL, USA.

Cremieux AC, Katlama C, Gillotin C et al. (2001). A comparison of the steady-state pharmacokinetics and safety of abacavir, lamivudine and zidovudine taken as a triple combination tablet and as abacavir plus a lamivudine-zidovudine double combination tablet by HIV-infected adults. Pharmacother 21: 424–30.

Deeks SG, Grant RM, Beatty GW (1998). Activity of a ritonavir plus saquinavir-containing regimen in patients with virologic evidence of indinavir or ritonavir failure. AIDS 12: F97–102.

Deeks SG, Wrin T, Liegler et al. (2001). Virologic and immunologic consequences of discontinuing combination antiretroviral therapy in HIV-infected patients with detectable viremia. N Engl J Med 344: 472–80.

Delta Coordinating Committee. (1996). Delta: a randomised double-blind controlled trial comparing combinations of zidovudine plus didanosine or zalcitabine with zidovudine alone in HIV-infected individuals. Lancet 348: 283–91.

Dube M, Johnson D, Currier J et al. (1997). Protease inhibitor-associated hyperglycemia. Lancet 350: 713–14.

Durant J, Clevenbergh P, Halfon P et al. (1999) Drug-resistance genotyping in HIV-1 therapy: the VIRADAPT randomized, controlled trial. JAMA 353: 2195–2199

Eastone J, Decker C. (1997). New-onset diabetes mellitus associated with use of protease inhibitors. Ann Intern Med 127: 948.

Eron JJ, Benoit Sl, Jemsek J et al. (1995). Treatment with lamivudine, zidovudine, or both in HIV-positive patients with 200 to 500 CD4+ cells per cubic millimeter. N Engl J Med 333: 1662–9.

Fisher M. (1998). Nucleoside combinations for antiretroviral therapy: efficacy of stavudine in combination with either didanosine or lamivudine. AIDS 12: S9–16.

Gulick RM. (1998). Combination therapy for patients with HIV-1 infection: the use of dual nucleoside analogues with protease inhibitors and other agents. AIDS 12: S17–22.

Gulick RM, Mellors JW, Havlir D et al. (1997). Treatment with indinavir, zidovudine, and lamivudine in adults with human immunodeficiency virus infection and prior antiretroviral therapy. N Engl J Med 337: 734–9.

Gulick RM, Mellors JW, Havlir D et al. (1998). Simultaneous vs. sequential initiation of therapy with indinavir, zidovudine, and lamivudine for HIV-1 infection: 100-week follow-up. JAMA 280: 35–41.

Hammer SM, Katzenstein DA, Hughes MD et al. (1996). A trial comparing nucleoside monotherapy with combination therapy in HIV-infected adults with CD4 cell counts from 200 to 500 per cubic millimeter. N Engl J Med 335: 1081–90.

Hammer SM, Squires KE, Hughes MD et al. (1997). A controlled trial of two nucleoside analogues plus indinavir in persons with human immunodeficiency virus infection and CD4 cell counts of 200 per cubic millimeter or less. N Engl J Med 337: 725–33.

Haynes BF, Panteleo G, Fauce AS. (1996). Toward an understanding of the correlates of protective immunity to HIV infection. Science 271: 324–8.

Ho DD, Neumann AU, Perelson AS et al. (1995). Rapid turnover of plasma virions and CD4+ lymphocytes in HIV-1 infection. Nature 373: 123–6.

Hogg RS, Heath KV, Yip B et al. (1998). Improved survival among HIV-infected individuals following initiation of antiretroviral therapy. JAMA 279: 450–4.

Katlama C, Ingrand D, Loveday C et al. (1996). Safety and efficacy of lamivudine–zidovudine combination therapy in antiretroviral-naïve patients. A randomized controlled comparison with zidovudine monotherapy. JAMA 276: 118–25.

Katlama C, Valantin M-A, Matheron S et al. (1998). Efficacy and tolerability of stavudine plus lamivudine in treatment-naïve and treatment-experienced patients with HIV-1 infection. Ann Intern Med 129: 525–31.

Katlama C, Murphy R, Johnson V et al. (1999). The Atlantic Study: a randomized, open-label study comparing two protease inhibitor (PI)-sparing antiretroviral strategies versus a standard PI-containing regimen. In: Program and abstracts of the Sixth Conference on Retroviruses and Opportunistic Infections, Chicago, IL, USA.

Kaufmann GR, Duncombe C, Cunningham P et al. (1998). Treatment response and durability of a double protease inhibitor therapy with saquinavir and ritonavir in an observational cohort of HIV-1 infected individuals. AIDS 12: 1625–30.

Kirk Ole, Katzenstein TL, Gerstoft, et al. (1999). Combination therapy containing ritonavir plus saquinavir has superior short-term antiretroviral efficacy: a randomized trial. AIDS 13: F9–16.

Kitahara MM, Koepsell TD, Deyo RA, (1996). Physicians' experience with the acquired immunodeficiency syndrome as a factor in patients' survival. N Engl J Med 334: 701–6.

Lafeuillade A, Poggi C, Tamalet C et al. (1997). Effects of a combination of zidovudine, didanosine, and lamivudine on primary human immunodeficiency virus type 1 infection. J Infect Dis 175: 1051–5.

Lepri AC, Miller V, Phillips AN et al. (2001). The virological response to highly active antiretroviral therapy over the first 24 weeks of therapy according to pre-therapy viral load and week 4–8 viral load. AIDS 15: 47–54.

Lo JC, Mulligan K, Tai VW. (1998). 'Buffalo hump' in men with HIV-1 infection. Lancet 351: 867–70.

Lori F, Lewis MG, Xu J et al. (2000). Control of SIV rebound through structured treatment interruptions during early infection. Science 290: 1591–3.

Marschner IC, Collier AC, Coombs RW et al. (1998). Use of changes in plasma levels of human immunodeficiency virus type RNA to assess clinical benefit of antiretroviral therapy. J Infect Dis 177: 40–7.

Mellors JW, Munoz AM, Giorgi JV et al. (1997). Plasma viral load and CD4+ lymphocytes as prognostic markers of HIV-1 infection. Ann Intern Med 126: 946–54.

Miller KD, Jones E, Yanovski JA. (1998a). Visceral abdominal-fat accumulation associated with the use of indinavir. Lancet 351: 871–5.

Miller KK, Daly PA, Sentochnik D et al. (1998b). Pseudo-Cushing's syndrome in human immunodeficiency virus-infected patients. Clin Infect Dis 27: 68–72.

Miller V. (2001). Structured treatment interruptions in antiretroviral management of HIV-1. Curr Opin Infect Dis 14: 29–37.

Miller V, Mocroft A, Reiss P et al. (1999). Relations among CD4 lymphocyte count nadir, antiretroviral therapy, and HIV-1 disease progression: results from the EuroSIDA study. Ann Intern Med 130: 570–7.

Mitsuyasu RT, Skolnik PR, Cohen SR et al. (1998). Activity of the soft gelatin formulation of saquinavir in combination therapy in antiretroviral-naïve patients. AIDS 12: F103–9.

Molina J-M, Journot V, Ferchal F et al. (1998). ALBI (ANRS 070): a randomized, controlled trial to evaluate the efficacy and safety of AZT/3TC vs alternating d4T/ddI and AZT/3TC vs. d4T/ddI. In: Programs and abstracts of the Twelfth World AIDS Conference, Geneva, Switzerland.

Montaner JSG, Hogg R, Raboud J. (1998a). Antiretroviral treatment in 1998. Lancet 352: 1919–22.

Montaner JSG, Reiss P, Cooper D et al. (1998b). A randomized, double-blind trial comparing combinations of nevirapine, didanosine, and zidovudine for HIV-infected patients: the INCAS Trial. JAMA 279: 930–7.

Montaner JS, Harrigan PR, Jahnke N et al. (2001). Multiple drug rescue therapy for HIV infected individuals with prior virologic failure to multiple regimens. AIDS 15: 117–9.

Mouton Y, Alfandare S, Valette M et al. (1997). Impact of protease inhibitors on AIDS-defining events hospitalizations in 10 French AIDS reference centers. AIDS 11: F101–5.

Moyle G. (1996). Use of viral resistance patterns to antiretroviral drugs in optimizing selection of drug combinations and sequences. Drugs 52: 168–85.

Murphy RL, Brun S, Hicks C et al. (2001). ABT378/ritonavir plus stavudine and lamivudine for the treatment of antiretroviral-naive adults with HIV-1 infection: 48 week results. AIDS 15: F1–F9.

Murphy RL, Gulick R, Smeaton L et al. (1998). Long-term evaluation of subjects following therapy with an amprenavir-containing regimen: ACTG 373. Antivir Ther 3: 97.

Murphy RL, Gulick RM, DeGruttola V et al. (1999). Treatment with amprenavir alone or with zidovudine and lamivudine in adults with human immunodeficiency virus infection. J Infect Dis 179: 808–16.

Murphy RL, Brun S, Hicks C et al. (2000). ABT378/ritonavir plus stavudine and lamivudine for the treatment of antiretroviral-naive adults with HIV-1 infection: 48 week results. AIDS 15: F1–F9.

Palella FJ, Delaney KM, Moorman AC et al. (1998). Declining morbidity and mortality among patients with advance human immunodeficiency virus infection. N Engl J Med 338: 853–60.

Perelson AS, Neumann AU, Markowitz M et al. (1996). HIV-1 dynamics in vivo: virion clearance rate, infected cell life-span, and viral generation time. Science 271: 1582–6.

Roth VR, Kravcik S, Angel JB. (1998). Development of cervical fat pads following therapy with human immunodeficiency virus type 1 protease inhibitors. Clin Infect Dis 27: 65–7.

Rutschmann OT, Opravil M, Iten A et al. (1998). A placebo-controlled trial of didanosine plus stavudine, with and without hydroxyurea, for HIV infection. The Swiss HIV Cohort Study. AIDS 12: F71–7.

Saag MS, Holodniy M, Kuritzkes DR et al. (1996). HIV viral load markers in clinical practice. Nature Med 2: 627–9.

Saez-Llorens X, Nelson RP, Emmanuel P et al. (2001). A randomized, double-blind study of triple nucleoside therapy of abacavir, lamivudine and zidovudine versus lamivudine and zidovudine in previously treated HIV-1 infected children. Pediatrics 107: E4.

Saravolatz LD, Winslow DL, Collins G et al. (1996). Zidovudine alone or in combination with didanosine or zalcitabine in HIV-infected patients with the acquired immunodeficiency syndrome or fewer than 200 CD4 cells per cubic millimeter. N Engl J Med 335: 1099–106.

Sommadossi J-P. (1998). Cellular nucleoside pharmacokinetics and pharmacology: a potentially important determinant of antiretroviral efficacy. AIDS 12: S1–8.

Staszewski S, Loveday C, Picazo JJ et al. (1996). Safety and efficacy of lamivudine-zidovudine combination therapy in zidovudine-experienced patients. A randomized, controlled comparison with zidovudine monotherapy. JAMA 276: 111–17.

Staszewski S, Keisser P, Gathe J et al. (1999). Ziagen/Combivir is equivalent to indinavir/Combivir in antiretroviral therapy (ART) naïve adults at 24 weeks (CNA3005). In: Program and abstracts of the Sixth Conference on Retroviruses and Opportunistic Infections, Chicago, IL, USA.

Staszewski S, Keiser P, Montaner J et al. (2001). Abacavir-lamivudine-zidovudine in antiretroviral – naive HIV-infected adults: a randomized equivalence trial. JAMA 285: 1155–63

Staszewski S, Morales–Ramirez J, Tashima K et al. (1999). Efavirenz plus zidovudine and lamivudine, efavirenz plus indinavir, and indinavir plus zidovudine and lamivudine in the treatment of HIV infection in adults. N Engl J Med 341: 1865–73

Tebas P, Patick AK, Kane EM et al. (1999). Virologic responses to a ritonavir–saquinavir-containing regimen in patients who had previously failed nelfinavir. AIDS 13: F23–8.

Visnegarwala F, Krause K, Musher D. (1997). Severe diabetes associated with protease inhibitor therapy. Ann Intern Med 127: 947.

The HIV-infected woman

8

ALISON KESSON AND KATE CLEZY

Women are now estimated to comprise almost half of all newly human immunodeficiency virus (HIV) infected adults and most new infections occur in those aged between 15 and 24, the beginning of the childbearing years. This leads to complex issues surrounding fertility, pregnancy and childbirth. In addition, women experience a number of gender-specific medical problems. This was recognized by the Centres for Disease Control and Prevention (CDC) in 1993, when invasive cervical cancer was added to the list of AIDS-defining conditions. In addition, three gynaecologic conditions were included in the revised classification system for HIV infection as conditions for which course or management are affected by HIV infection. These are persistent, frequent, or poorly responsive Candida vulvovaginitis, moderate to severe cervical dysplasia/carcinoma *in situ*, and pelvic inflammatory disease (see Table 8.1).

In societies where women are disadvantaged socially, financially and politically, their access to preventative health care may be limited and the ability to negotiate safe sex may be significantly compromised. Worldwide, many women rely on prostitution, or sex work, for economic survival. In countries where poor economy and high levels of unemployment exist, these factors are seen as an important component of the spread of HIV.

The advent of the female condom may assist women in negotiating safe sex and in 1997, four million female condoms were sold in the developing world as a direct result of a UNAIDS initiative encouraging their use. In a study in Thailand, the female condom has been shown to decrease the sexually transmitted diseases in female sex workers by 34%.

Although there have been significant advances in the knowledge about and treatment of HIV infection, most natural history studies and clinical trials have consisted largely of men. Recently, the National Institutes of Health (NIH) promulgated and implemented new guidelines concerning participation of women and minorities in all clinical trials. This will increase the body of knowledge about HIV and women. Currently, in the USA women comprise 12% of study participants in government-sponsored trials (compared with 18% of AIDS notifications). In addition, the NIH is funding two large studies, the Women's Interagency HIV Study (WIHS) and the HIV Epidemiology Research Study (HERS), which will help to determine the medical, gynaecological, virological, immunological and psychosocial parameters of HIV infection in women.

Epidemiology, risk factors for HIV infection and pathogenesis

On a global basis, women comprise about 40% of those infected. However, this proportion varies significantly between countries (WHO, 1998). In general, where HIV has largely been transmitted by heterosexual contact (such as in southern Africa), rates in women almost equal those of men. Where HIV is predominantly transmitted through men having sex with men (in Australia, for example) HIV rates in women remain low. In Botswana, in 1997,

Table 8.1 Clinical categories of HIV infection specific to women – 1993 revision of the CDC criteria

Category B
Vulvovaginal candidiasis that is persistent, frequent, or poorly responsive to therapy
Cervical dysplasia that is moderate or severe; cervical carcinoma *in situ*
Pelvic inflammatory disease, particularly if complicated by tubo-ovarian abscess

Category C (AIDS)
Invasive cervical cancer

43% of pregnant women tested HIV-positive in the major urban centre of Francistown. In Harare, 32% of pregnant women were already infected in 1995 (UNAIDS, WHO, 1998). In contrast, in Australia the rate of HIV infection and proportion of women infected remain low, with women comprising 5.5% of the total infected population and rates in women between 17 and 176 infections per 100 000 population. In some countries, HIV transmission and AIDS cases are falling in homosexual men and are either stable or increasing in women. In Australia, the number of men diagnosed with HIV infection declined significantly between the years 1989 and 1997 (from 2512 to 734); however, the number of women infected each year has remained stable. In the USA in 1996, new AIDS cases among African-Americans rose by 19% in heterosexual men and 12% in heterosexual women. In contrast, there was an 11% drop in AIDS cases in homosexual men.

Transmission of HIV through unprotected vaginal intercourse is the most common route of acquisition of HIV for women. HIV has been demonstrated to readily pass through cervical epithelium, infecting mononuclear cells in the lamina propria (Fantini et al., 1998). The recently described HIV coreceptors, CCR5 and CXCR4, are found more commonly on cells in the cervix than in the vagina and this may facilitate cellular viral entry (Zhang et al., 1998).

There is epidemiological evidence that some sexually transmitted diseases (STDs) increase the risk of HIV transmission to women. The STDs for which there is evidence of increased HIV transmission are chancroid, syphilis and herpes, as well as trichomonas, chlamydia and gonorrhoea (Laga et al., 1993; Sorvillo and Kerndt, 1998). Laga and coworkers (1993) found that the adjusted odds ratios for HIV seroconversion were 4.8 for gonorrhoea, 3.6 for chlamydial infection and 1.9 for trichomonas. Therefore, the treatment of STDs may reduce the risk of HIV transmission. This was shown in a study in Tanzania, where the treatment of STDs decreased the rate of HIV transmission by 40% (Grosskurth et al., 1995).

There have been a number of studies assessing the role of hormonal contraceptives in HIV transmission and, to date, the data are inconclusive. With recent attention on the viral load in various body compartments, it appears that the risk of HIV transmission increases with higher viral loads in semen and vaginal fluids. As there is an association with plasma viral load and the viral load in cervical secre-

tions or semen, it follows that the risk of HIV transmission may be reduced by the use of potent antiretroviral agents (Uvin and Caliendo, 1997; Vernazza et al., 1997).

Clinical aspects of HIV infection in women

The natural history of HIV infection is similar in men and women with comparable complications and similar survival times after an AIDS diagnosis, although viral load tends to be lower in women than in men (Sterling et al., 2001). Some early studies suggested that women have a poorer outcome than men; however, this may reflect socioeconomic factors, different access to medical care and rates of treatment with antiretroviral agents. In a number of recent studies, there have been no gender or race differences in disease progression or survival after an AIDS diagnosis (Chaisson et al., 1995; Palella et al., 1998).

In the HERS study, less than half of HIV-infected women with CD4 lymphocyte counts of less than $200/\mu l$ reported current use of antiretroviral therapy, and only 58% reported current use of Pneumocystis carinii pneumonia (PCP) prophylaxis (Solomon et al., 1998). In a similar study from the UK, only 40% of women with an AIDS diagnosis were taking antiretroviral drugs (Mercey et al., 1996). The use of highly active antiretroviral therapy (HAART) has been associated with a significant reduction in mortality in patients with low CD4 lymphocyte counts, regardless of sex, race, age, and risk factors for transmission of HIV. The use of HAART has also been associated with a reduction in the incidence opportunistic infections (in particular PCP, Mycobacterium avium complex disease [MAC], and cytomegalovirus [CMV] retinitis). Combination antiretroviral therapy with the inclusion of protease inhibitors (PIs) in treatment regimens was associated with the most benefit (Palella et al., 1998).

The AIDS-defining opportunistic infections occur at similar rates in men and women, although some studies have suggested that oesophageal candidiasis and bacterial pneumonia are more common in women. Although AIDS-related-lymphoma occurs equally in men and women, Kaposi's sarcoma (KS) is much less common in women. In one serological study of women with HIV infection (WIHS), the prevalence of serological reactivity to human herpes virus 8 (HHV-8) antigens was 4.0% in the 301 HIV-infected participants and 1.2% in the 84 HIV-uninfected participants. Two of the HIV-infected women had KS and both were sero-positive (Kedes *et al.*, 1997). This contrasts with high levels of HHV-8 serological reactivity and rates of clinical KS in homosexual males, with HIV infection higher than those seen in women. The clinical manifestations of the opportunistic infections and the response to treatment have not been formally evaluated in women compared to men. Apart from the problems of access to medical care and consequent delayed diagnosis, there is no suggestion that women behave differently to men.

Gynaecological disease

Women with advanced HIV disease have frequent gynaecological comorbidity (Korn and Landers, 1995). In one study of women admitted to an AIDS inpatient unit, 83% had gynaecologic disease detected on examination, although only 9% of women had been admitted for primary gynaecological or genito-urinary diagnoses. Vaginitis was the most common diagnosis, occurring in 51%. Cervical dysplasia was found in 45%; genital condylomata, genital herpes, and pelvic inflammatory disease were found in 23%, 20%, and 5%, respectively. The absence of symptoms in these patients was a poor predictor of the absence of disease (Frankel *et al.*, 1997). Women may also have infrequent gynaecological examinations as part of their routine care and therefore these conditions may remain undiagnosed (Thackway *et al.*, 1998).

Vulvovaginal candidiasis

Several studies report that vaginal candidiasis, usually due to *C. albicans*, occurs frequently in HIV-infected women and that it may be the earliest opportunistic infection in these women (Rhoads *et al.*, 1987). Although candida and other yeasts are commonly isolated from the female genital tract of HIV-infected women, they are also isolated in approximately 25% of HIV-uninfected women. However, women infected with HIV are at higher risk of symptomatic vulvovaginitis. The risks for colonization and symptomatic vulvovaginitis appear to be related to the degree of immunodeficiency. In women with CD4 lymphocyte counts of less than 200/μl, the risk for symptomatic vaginitis is three or four times higher than for women with a CD4 lymphocyte count of more than 500/μl, or HIV-uninfected women. In immunocompetent HIV-infected women, there may be no significant difference in the prevalence of candidiasis compared with HIV-uninfected women (Duerr *et al.*, 1997). Vulvovaginal candidiasis that is persistent or recurrent

should suggest the possibility of underlying HIV infection.

Vulvovaginitis causes morbidity with pruritus, persistent vaginal discharge, chronic vaginal soreness and dyspareunia. Topical antifungal therapy is usually curative, although application may need to be repeated. If there is significant immunodeficiency (CD4 lymphocyte counts of less than 100/μl), oral antifungal agents may be required. Both fluconazole and ketoconazole are effective antifungal agents; however, as ketoconazole is associated with more drug interactions, fluconazole is recommended for systemic therapy. In women with recurrent candidiasis, fluconazole at a dose of 200 mg weekly reduces the risk of recurrent disease by about 40%. In this study of 323 women, the incidence of fluconazole-resistant isolates was less than 5% after treatment for 29 months (Schuman *et al.*, 1997). It has been established that advanced immunodeficiency and exposure to oral azoles are risk factors for the development of fluconazole resistance in candida isolates (Maenza *et al.*, 1996). Suggested treatment regimens are outlined in Table 8.2.

Pelvic inflammatory disease (PID)

Pelvic inflammatory disease (PID) was included in the CDC category B classification of HIV infection, based on a study of women hospitalized in New York City with PID (Hoesgberg *et al.*, 1990). In this study, women with HIV infection were more likely to have normal leucocyte counts and to require surgical intervention than HIV-uninfected women. In a recent study of 423 women with PID presenting to a New York hospital, HIV-infected women had higher body temperatures at admission and lower leucocyte counts than HIV-uninfected women. They were more likely to have persistent fever 2–4 days after starting antibiotic therapy and were four times more likely to require a change of antibiotics and to have longer hospital stays. However, in this study, HIV-infected women did not undergo more surgery, or have a higher incidence of tubo-ovarian abscesses than HIV-uninfected women (Barbosa *et al.*, 1997).

The diagnostic features of PID have been based on studies in HIV-uninfected women and include the clinical findings of lower abdominal pain, adnexal tenderness, cervicitis, fever and adnexal mass, elevated erythrocyte sedimentation rate (ESR) or C-reactive protein. In addition, PID may be diagnosed by the aspiration of purulent material from the peritoneal cavity by laparoscopy. However, many women with PID have minimal or no symptoms.

Table 8.2 Treatment of vulvovaginal candidiasis

	Topical		Systemic
Indication	Initial treatment		Inadequate response to topical therapy Recurrent disease Fluconazole 200 mg daily
Formulations/dose	Clotrimazole	1% cream 2% cream	
	Econazole	100 mg pessary	
	Miconazole	1.5% cream	
	Nystatin cream	2% cream	
Treatment duration	10–14 days		10–14 days
Maintenance therapy	Not required		Fluconazole 150 mg weekly or 50–100 mg daily

The usual associated organisms are of endogenous genital origin such as *Bacteroides fragilis*, anaerobic streptococci, *Escherichia coli*, group B streptococci and *Gardnerella vaginalis*. *Neisseria gonorrhoea* and *Chlamydia trachomatis* may also cause PID.

Although the optimal antibiotic regimen has not been determined by clinical trials, there are several regimens that are effective. Third-generation cephalosporins such as cefotaxime or ceftriaxone can be used in combination with metronidazole. In patients allergic to β-lactam drugs, clindamycin plus an aminogylcoside is a suitable alternative

Table 8.3 Suggested antimicrobial regimens for pelvic inflammatory disease

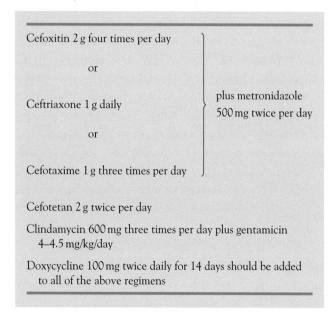

Cefoxitin 2 g four times per day

or

Ceftriaxone 1 g daily

or

Cefotaxime 1 g three times per day

plus metronidazole 500 mg twice per day

Cefotetan 2 g twice per day

Clindamycin 600 mg three times per day plus gentamicin 4–4.5 mg/kg/day

Doxycycline 100 mg twice daily for 14 days should be added to all of the above regimens

regimen. All patients should be given doxycycline 100 mg twice daily for 14 days for presumed concurrent chlamydial infection (see Table 8.3).

PID in HIV-infected women appears to have a more complicated course than in HIV-uninfected women and further studies with longer follow-up periods are required to assess long-term outcomes. The current CDC recommendations are that women with PID should be offered HIV counselling and testing, and that known HIV-infected women with PID should be hospitalized for treatment.

Human papilloma virus infection and cervical neoplasia

Human papilloma virus (HPV) is considered the aetiological agent of most dysplastic and neoplastic lesions of the lower female genital tract (Robinson and Morris, 1996). Alteration of the immune system (for example, in pregnancy) and in patients treated with immunosuppressive therapy for organ transplants is known to be associated with aggressive disease. Several studies have shown that HIV infection, and in particular, worsening immunodeficiency, increase the risk of HPV infection and the development of cervical neoplasia (Boccalon *et al.*, 1996; Melbye *et al.*, 1996; Wright *et al.*, 1996). About one-third of HIV-infected women will have abnormal cervical cytology on routine screening, which is four to five times more common than HIV-uninfected women. Independent risk factors for abnormal cervical cytology are immunodeficiency (odds ratio, [OR], of 8–17) and HPV infection (OR of 5) (Maiman *et al.*, 1998). The prevalence of HPV co-infection increases with more profound immunodeficiency, with approximately 50% of HIV-infected women being positive for HPV (using PCR technology). In women with symptomatic HIV infection, the prevalence may reach 80%. HIV-infected women with persistent HPV infection are more likely to be infected with serotypes of HPV that are most often associated with carcinoma (Sun *et al.*, 1997).

In comparison with HIV-uninfected women, HIV-infected women are more likely to have co-existent cervical intra-epithelial neoplasia (CIN) when mild cervical atypia is detected in smear, have faster rates of progression of CIN and are more likely to relapse after standard therapy. In a longitudinal study of 127 HIV-infected women and 193 HIV-uninfected women treated for CIN, after 3 years of follow-up, recurrent CIN was found in 62% of the HIV-infected women, compared with 18% of the HIV-uninfected women. If there was co-existent immunodeficiency (CD4 lymphocyte counts of less than 200/μl), the recurrence rate was 87%. In those who had recurrent CIN, the median CD4 lymphocyte count was 193/μl, compared to 316/μl for the whole cohort (Fruchter *et al.*, 1996). Once cervical cancer occurs, it usually has an aggressive course (Holcomb *et al.*, 1998). However, currently there are no data that indicate increasing incidence of cervical invasive carcinoma in HIV-infected women.

Therefore, HIV-infected women should undergo regular cervical smear tests (every 6–12 months), with colposcopy if cytology is abnormal or if inflammation is present. Treatment of dysplasia or neoplasia should be as for HIV-uninfected women and careful long-term follow-up is essential.

Pregnancy and HIV

In vitro fertilization and sperm washing

Some HIV sero-discordant heterosexual couples wish to conceive and have children. Unprotected intercourse may result in pregnancy, but there is a significant risk that the HIV-uninfected woman may acquire HIV and that her fetus may also become infected with the virus. Seroconversion has also been well documented after artificial insemination with infected donor semen (Chiasson *et al.*, 1990). One option for assisted reproduction in such couples is insemination of washed semen from the male HIV-infected partner. Semen washing using a percoll gradient, which allows sperm to swim to an upper layer, has been shown in a small number of samples to reduce extracellular RNA to below detectable limits. Cellular pro-viral DNA can be reduced

to below detectable limits in one-third of samples (Lasheeb *et al.*, 1997). This technique is not widely available, as there is ongoing concern about the potential infectivity of sperm. About one-third of the licensed fertility units in the UK offer intrauterine insemination after sperm washing to sero-discordant couples if the male partner is HIV-infected and the couple is offered *in vitro* fertilization (IVF). If the woman is HIV-infected, occasional centres offer intrauterine insemination or IVF (Balet *et al.*, 1998). In Italy, semen washing and insemination have been practised since 1989. Up until 1996, there had been more than 1000 insemination attempts in 350 couples, resulting in 200 pregnancies with no maternal or paediatric infection (Semprini *et al.*, 1998). In this centre, couples are counselled that the risk of HIV infection after insemination with washed sperm cannot be completely excluded.

Clinical approach to HIV infection in pregnancy

Most pregnant women with HIV infection are asymptomatic and many have learned of their HIV status for the first time during pregnancy. As in the non-pregnant woman, counselling, education about the disease and infection control, contact tracing and medical and laboratory assessment are all required. Consideration of treatment in pregnant woman has two major goals: the optimal management of the woman's HIV infection and the prevention of perinatal transmission to her infant.

Vertical transmission

The interruption of vertical transmission may be the most important and effective therapeutic intervention applied to control the spread of HIV infection (see also Chapter 9). The rates of transmission of HIV from mother to infant ranges from 13 to 40%. These differences in transmission rates are unexplained, being 13% in Europe, 30% in USA and Australia and 40% in Africa. The reasons for this variation in transmission may be related to geographical variation in the prevalence of cofactors associated with transmission, such as the incidence of sexually transmitted diseases, chorioamnionitis, maternal disease, nutritional deficiencies, breast feeding and the HIV subtype in the mother.

Vertical transmission rates vary among different populations. It has been shown that maternal CD4 lymphocyte counts are an independent predictor of transmission, with increased rates of vertical transmission in women with lower CD4 lymphocyte counts (European Collaborative Study Group, 1992; Mayaux et al., 1995; European Collaborative Study Group, 1996). Other factors influencing vertical transmission have not been clearly defined, though there is evidence that specific neutralizing antibodies of maternal origin may offer some protection (Rossi et al., 1989; Devash et al., 1990; Bryson et al., 1993; Scarlatti et al., 1993; Mofenson, 1994). Transmitting mothers only rarely had neutralizing antibodies against their child's HIV isolate. These observations have not been supported by other studies, where the presence of maternal neutralizing antibodies had no influence on the rate of vertical transmission (Husson et al., 1995). Adoptive transfer of neutralizing antibodies has been shown to be protective against a subsequent lethal challenge of homologous virus in several animal models of viral infections. A study comparing the effect of zidovudine (ZDV) and HIV-hyperimmune globulin with ZDV and intravenous immunoglobulin without HIV antibodies was inconclusive because of the significant reduction in vertical transmission due to ZDV alone (Steihm et al., 1999). Whether passive immunization of the mother with neutralizing antibody or other materials (e.g. recombinant CD4-immunoglobulin) or active immunization with recombinant gp160 or gp120 will be protective against vertical transmission of HIV has yet to be determined.

Another factor influencing the risk of vertical transmission is the quantity of infectious virus to which the infant is exposed. In several studies, high maternal viral burden (determined by quantitative plasma or cell cultures, and more recently by high plasma HIV RNA plasma copy number) has been associated with increased transmission risk (Borkowsky et al., 1994; Weiser et al., 1994; Fang et al., 1995; Dickover et al., 1996; Shaffer et al., 1999). Some investigators have suggested that there is a threshold plasma HIV viral level below which transmission does not occur (Dickover et al., 1996; Shaffer et al., 1999), but this is not supported by larger studies and transmission may occur at all levels, even in those whose plasma HIV RNA is below the limits of detection of the test used (Sperling et al., 1996).

The timing of vertical transmission may be antepartum, peripartum or postpartum (Table 8.4). It is not yet possible to predict which exposed infants will contract HIV infection, and there are few prospective data about the predominant mechanism. Current data suggest that more than 50% of infections may be acquired in late pregnancy or at

Table 8.4 Mechanisms of vertical transmission

- Antepartum: presumably by transplacental transmission
- Peripartum: as a result of contact with contaminated blood or body fluid during delivery
- Postpartum: via breast milk

the time of proposed delivery (Bryson et al., 1992). Definitions for *in utero* and intrapartum transmission can be found in Table 8.5. It is important to differentiate between *in utero* and intrapartum transmission in order to establish the efficacy of therapeutic strategies aimed at preventing or decreasing vertical transmission.

In utero transmission of HIV infection

There is good evidence supporting transmission of HIV *in utero* from mother to infant. Intrauterine transmission has been detected by recovery of HIV from fetal tissues or infant blood within 48 hours of birth, either by cell culture (Specter et al., 1986; DiMaria et al., 1986), or detection of HIV genome by molecular techniques such as polymerase chain reaction (PCR) (Laure et al., 1988; Wolinsky et al., 1988), or *in situ* hybridization (Harnish et al., 1987).

Recent studies suggest that the rate of vertical transmission during the mid trimester is approximately 5% (Phuapradit et al., 1999).

Table 8.5 Timing of vertical transmission

Early (*in utero*)[a]	Late (intrapartum)[b]
HIV-1 isolated from blood	HIV-1 isolated from blood
HIV-1 genome detected by polymerase chain reaction	HIV-1 genome detected by polymerase chain reaction
p24 antigen detected in blood	

[a]An infant is considered to have early infection if HIV-1 is isolated from the blood within 48 h of birth. This must be confirmed with a second specimen by culture or polymerase chain reaction. Ideally, both cord and peripheral blood should give concordant results. Results from a cord blood sample must be confirmed with a peripheral blood sample.

Detection of p24 antigen in the blood within the first 7 days of life is not diagnostic of HIV-1 infection due to the possibility of passive transfer of p24 antigen across the placenta without infection.

[b]HIV detected on two occasions during the period from day 7 to day 90 in an infant who has not been breast fed. One test must be a positive HIV-1 culture. The tests must be negative on blood specimens in the first week of life.

Intrapartum transmission of HIV infection

There is considerable debate about the major route of HIV transmission to infants born to HIV-infected mothers, with few conclusive data. Although fetal placental villi are bathed with infectious maternal blood throughout pregnancy, the majority of infants escape infection *in utero*. Significant and extensive mucous membrane exposure to blood and secretions occurs during birth. It is probable that a significant proportion of infants are infected during labour and delivery but there is no actual proof of intrapartum infection (Rouzioux *et al.*, 1995). However, there are a number of observations that support the role of intrapartum transmission. HIV-1 has been isolated from vaginal and cervical secretions from approximately 50% of HIV-infected women (Wolfsy *et al.*, 1986; Vogt *et al.*, 1987). In addition, some infants with HIV viraemia or p24 antigenaemia have had negative results when these assays were performed shortly after birth (Krivine *et al.*, 1992). This, coupled with the fact that HIV-specific IgM antibody has not been found in the first months of life in some infants subsequently shown to be infected, suggests that infection has occurred during delivery (Gaetano *et al.*, 1987; Pyun *et al.*, 1987). The observation that there is a much higher incidence of perinatally acquired HIV infection in first-born twins (Duliege *et al.*, 1995) and the observation that rupture of the membranes for greater than 4 hours (Minkoff *et al.*, 1995; Landesman *et al.*, 1996) is also associated with an increased rate of transmission both lend support to the theory that infant exposure to infected maternal secretions during labour and delivery are a significant risk factor in transmission. Furthermore, intrapartum transmission is the principal mechanism by which infants are infected with some other blood-borne viruses, such as hepatitis B.

Establishing the rate of intrapartum infection and its contribution to the overall rate of vertical transmission is important because intrapartum transmission is probably more amenable to preventive strategies than is *in utero* transmission. Diagnosis and treatment of genital infections, which may lead to premature rupture of the membranes, may be advisable and virucidal cleansing of the vagina may also be effective in reducing transmission, although there is no evidence to date that this intervention is efficacious (Biggar *et al.*, 1996).

Role of Caesarean section

The role of Caesarean section in the prevention of vertical transmission of HIV has been quite contentious. Many studies have shown there there is some protective effect, but the level of protection has never reached statistical significance.

A French prospective study, which distinguished between elective and non-elective Caesarean sections, did not reveal any relationship between mode of delivery and risk of vertical transmission (Mandelbrot *et al.*, 1996). However, in a more recent study elective Caesarean section was associated with a lower rate of vertical transmission, when the mother also received ZDV (Mandelbrot *et al.*, 1998).

A recent meta-analysis of 15 prospective studies has clearly demonstrated that the risk of vertical transmission was significantly lower among HIV-infected women who underwent elective Caesarean section before the onset of labour, compared with other modes of delivery. Elective Caesarean section reduced the risk of vertical transmission by approximately 50% (adjusted odds ratio 0.43; 95% confidence intervals 0.33–0.56). This protective effect was present even after adjustment for the covariates, non-receipt of antiretroviral therapy, advanced maternal stage of disease and low infant birth weight, each of which is independently associated with an increased risk of transmission (The International Perinatal HIV Group, 1999). Postpartum morbidity was not examined in these studies, but HIV-infected women have an increased risk of peripartum and postpartum complications and an increased risk of post-operative complications (Semprini *et al.*, 1995). In less developed countries, the risk of elective Caesarean section to the mother and infant may outweigh the potential benefits and the relative risks of various modes of delivery should be discussed with all pregnant HIV-infected woman. During labour and delivery, every attempt should be made to assess fetal welfare by non-invasive methods, as invasive procedures such as fetal scalp electrode monitoring and fetal sampling of scalp blood may increase the risk of transmission of HIV to the child.

Postpartum transmission of HIV infection

There is now a considerable evidence that breast milk is a vehicle for vertical transmission of HIV. The evidence includes case reports describing HIV infection in breast-fed infants whose mothers became sero-positive postpartum (Ziegler *et al.*, 1985), and studies reporting isolation of HIV from samples of breast milk (Thirty *et al.*, 1985). A retrospective study of women infected postpartum showed a risk of 27% for breast feeding during primary HIV infection (95% confidence interval 6–61%) (Palasanthiran *et al.*, 1993). In addition, vertical transmission of other retroviruses via breast milk in humans (HTLV-1) (Tsuji *et al.*, 1990) and other species is well described (Marrack *et al.*, 1991). Although prospective studies have shown a twofold increase in HIV infection in breast-fed infants compared with bottle-fed infants, the numbers are too small to define the risk accurately.

Although HIV has been isolated from breast milk, the rates of detection and titre of HIV in breast milk during varying clinical stages of HIV in the mother is unknown and the risk of vertical transmission may be considerably lower during the asymptomatic stage of HIV infection than during HIV seroconversion or in late stage infection, when plasma and peripheral blood mononuclear cell viral titres are highest. In most of the described cases and in the retrospective study of Palasanthiran and colleagues, the women were studied during primary infection, when the HIV titres in serum can be expected to be relatively high (Palasanthiran *et al.*, 1993). During this transient high viraemia, HIV may readily enter breast milk at a time when HIV-specific antibody levels would be low. The role of specific antibody in breast milk in protecting infants from HIV has yet to be determined. In the case of HTLV-1 and CMV, both of which can be transmitted in breast milk, antibody is not protective.

Prevention of transmission of HIV via breast milk is easily achieved by avoidance of breast feeding. This strategy is appropriate for the developed world where infant formula is affordable and not contaminated with pathogenic organisms, and the marginal protection from infection afforded to the infant by breast feeding is of little consequence. However, in many parts of the world where HIV is endemic, breast feeding is closely linked with infant survival. Breast-fed infants have a lower incidence of respiratory and diarrhoeal diseases of infection. Currently, WHO recommends that mothers in developing countries should breast feed their infants regardless of maternal HIV-1 status (WHO, 1987). However, breast feeding is not recommended in the developed world, as the risk of HIV-1 infection far outweighs the marginal benefit derived from breast feeding.

Screening for HIV infection in pregnant women

There are three compelling reasons to screen for HIV infection in pregnant women: to influence the medical consequences of HIV infection in the women; to help prevent horizontal transmission to sexual and other contacts at risk, and to try to reduce the risk, of vertical transmission. Initial

recommendations for antenatal screening were made with the assumptions that 'at risk' women could be identified and would be available for screening. In fact, testing only women who admit to being at risk for HIV infection may fail to identify as many as 43–86% of infected women in populations with a seroprevalence of around 2% (MacDonald *et al.*, 1991). Many studies have shown that HIV-infected women have rates of pregnancy, terminations and second pregnancies concordant with women of similar backgrounds. HIV-infected women, like all other women, are influenced by issues relating to their desire to have children, self-image and cultural roles, when making reproductive decisions. Furthermore, it has been incorrectly assumed that women infected with HIV would choose not to bear children because of their risk of transmitting HIV to their offspring.

From a public health perspective, the decision to offer routine antenatal screening to women should be based on the prevalence of HIV infection in the population – it has been suggested that screening is appropriate if greater than 1:1000 of women in the community are infected (Minkoff and Landesman, 1988). With the high sensitivity and specificity of current screening tests, false-positive test results occur at a frequency of about 1:1000. Thus, 50% of positive screening tests will be incorrect in populations with a seroprevalence of 1:1000 or less. Confirmation of results is expensive and time consuming, resulting in a period of great anxiety for the woman and her partner. At present, in low prevalence populations, it is appropriate to screen only women at risk of HIV infection; however, in areas with a prevalence of 1:1000 or above, screening for HIV should be incorporated into the routine battery of antenatal tests. Determination of serum HIV antibody status should be repeated at 36 weeks gestation in sero-negative women, especially those at risk (MacDonald *et al.*, 1991). With an increasing seroprevalence in many populations and improved confirmatory tests for HIV, it is likely that routine antenatal screening will eventually be recommended in all countries.

Prevention of HIV infection – counselling issues

Prevention of horizontal transmission of HIV requires that the woman and her partner are educated about safe sex practices and the dangers of needle sharing in a non-judgmental way. The consistent use of condoms during sexual intercourse will reduce but not eliminate the risk of viral transmission. The need for behavioural change should be presented logically, then sympathetically and continually reinforced. Behaviour modification is difficult, particularly as women are often in unequal power relationships with their male partners, and within society. Women should be encouraged and assisted in their efforts to make sexual choice an option socially, culturally and economically. Counselling directed solely at the women and not including the partner may at best be ineffective or at worst lead to abuse.

Condoms are an effective means of preventing transmission of HIV, but are an inferior means of contraception and thus should be used in conjunction with alternative contraception when prevention of pregnancy is desired. Hormonal contraceptives have not been proven to affect the course of HIV infection, but may influence the pharmacokinetics of other drugs through their effect on protein-binding and hepatic metabolism. Rifampicin, tricyclic antidepressants and benzodiazepines all interact with oral contraceptive hormones in this way. No interactions have been reported with ZDV; however, there are variable effects when used in conjunction with PIs or non-nucleoside reverse transcriptase inhibitors (NNRTIs).

Caution should be exercised in recommending the use of intrauterine contraceptive devices, as they may render the woman more susceptible to ascending infections and PID. These devices are also associated with increased menstrual blood loss and hence potentially increased infectivity of genital secretions. Surgical sterilization should be recommended only when indicated for reasons other than HIV serological status.

If a woman is to make an informed choice about pregnancy several issues need to be discussed. These include the risk of vertical transmission, the prognosis of HIV infection in the woman, the future of her partner and her unborn child (depending on the HIV status), the sequelae of termination of pregnancy, loss of opportunity of parenting, relinquishing the role of care-giver during illness, effect on the family and orphaned children, social isolation, the financial cost of health care and potential loss of income. Women should be helped to assess the resources available to them. They should also involve their partners, or alternatively others who may be significant to them, in the counselling and decision-making process. It is appropriate to consider the role of the woman in the society of which she is part. In some cultures, a woman is not complete until she is a mother, and children strengthen a woman's role in the culture. For example, in areas of high unemployment and low socio-economic status, child bearing and child rearing may be the most fulfilling role for a woman. The wishes of the male partner can be very influential in the decision a woman makes, or she may face physical or emotional abuse if she does not follow her partner's wishes. A woman may not be able to dictate the use of contraceptives should she wish to avoid pregnancy or HIV transmission.

Counselling is not straightforward because the line between clinical recommendations and value judgements is ambiguous. The counsellor should be aware of the woman's expectations and cultural background and help her to fully explore all available options. The woman's decision should be respected and imposition of unwanted advice or opinions by the counsellor may simply trigger rejection in women who may otherwise consider their reproductive options more thoughtfully.

Approach to HIV infection in pregnancy

There is no convincing data to suggest that pregnancy accelerates HIV disease progression. In one study, which followed the HIV RNA plasma viral load in pregnant women, an increase in viral load was seen in a proportion of women 6 months postpartum when compared with their antepartum levels. The increase in HIV load was independent of whether the woman had received zidovudine (AZT, ZDV) during pregnancy (Cao et al., 1997).

The 1994 interim analysis of data from Paediatric AIDS Clinical Trials Group (PACTG) Protocol 076 demonstrated that zidovudine chemoprophylaxis could significantly reduce the vertical transmission of HIV from mother to infant (Connor et al., 1994).

There have been significant advances in the understanding of the pathogenesis of HIV, in particular the kinetics of HIV replication and CD4 lymphocyte turnover. This and the availability of more potent combination antiretroviral drug regimens has resulted in marked changes to standard antiretroviral therapy for HIV-infected adults. Combination therapy with two nucleoside analogues and a PI will suppress viral replication in the majority of patients with subsequent increases in CD4 lymphocyte numbers and improvement in clinical outcome and survival.

There are unique considerations for use of antiretrovirals in pregnancy, including alterations in pharmacokinetics due to physiological changes in pregnancy, the effective reduction in the risk of vertical transmission to the infant and the theoretical potential for short-term and long-term side-effects on the fetus and newborn infant. Therefore

Table 8.6 USA animal and human data relevant to use of antiretrovirals in pregnancy

Antiretroviral agent	FDA pregnancy category	Placental passage- newborn: material ratio	Long-term animal carcinogenicity studies
Zidovudine	C	0.85 (human)	Rodents: non-invasive Vaginal epithelial tumours
Didanosine	B	0.30–0.50	Rhesus: no tumours; lifetime rodent study
Zalcitabine	C	0.5 (human)	Rodents: thymic lymphoma
Stavudine	C	0.76	Rhesus: not completed
Lamivudine	C	1.0 (human)	No tumours; lifetime rodent study
Nevirapine	C	1.0 (human)	Not completed
Delavirdine	C	Unknown	Not completed
Indinavir	C	Unknown	Not completed
Ritonavir	B	Mid-term 1.15 Late-term 0.15–0.64	Not completed
Saquinavir	B	Unknown	Not completed
Nelfinavir	B	Unknown	Not completed

A: adequate and well-controlled studies of pregnant women fail to demonstrate a risk to the foetus during the first trimester of pregnancy (and there is no evidence of risk during later trimesters); B: animal reproduction studies fail to demonstrate a risk to the fetus and adequate but well-controlled studies of pregnant women have not been conducted; C: safety in human pregnancy has not been determined, animal studies are either positive for foetal risk or have not been conducted, and the drug should not be used unless the potential benefit outweighs the potential risk to the fetus; D: positive evidence of human fetal risk based on adverse reaction data from investigational or marketing experiences, but the potential benefits from the use of the drug in pregnant women may be acceptable despite its potential risks.

(Courtesy of US Public Health Service, 1997.)

when considering antiretroviral therapy in a pregnant woman, the physician has to balance the advantages of therapy to the maternal HIV disease, and the reduction of vertical transmission with the short- and long-term benefits and risks of such therapy for her and her infant (Perinatal HIV Guidelines Working Group, 2001).

Management of the HIV-infected pregnant woman

Treatment of HIV-infected pregnant women is based on the principle that therapies beneficial for a woman should not be withheld during pregnancy unless the adverse effects on either the mother or fetus outweigh the benefits to the woman. ZDV alone has been demonstrated to significantly reduce the risk of perinatal transmission; however, monotherapy is now considered suboptimal for treatment of HIV infection, and combination therapy is considered the standard of care. Care of an HIV-infected pregnant woman should involve collaboration between the HIV specialist, the obstetrician and the woman herself. The decision to use antiretroviral therapy in pregnancy should be made by the woman after discussion of the known and unknown benefits and risks of therapy with her health-care providers.

The choice of antiretroviral therapy in a pregnant woman has some unique considerations, including altered pharmacokinetics and potential toxic effects on the fetus. Physiological changes that occur during pregnancy may affect the kinetics of drug absorption, distribution, metabolism and elimination, thereby affecting drug dosing requirements. In addition, placental transport of drugs and compartmentalization in metabolism by either the fetus or placenta may affect the pharmacokinetics of antiretroviral drugs in a pregnant woman.

Another major concern of drug use in pregnancy is the potential for teratogenic, mutagenic or carcinogenic effects on the fetus and newborn. Information about drug safety in pregnancy is very limited and comes from animal toxicity data, anecdotal reports, registry data and clinical trials.

Table 8.7 Recommended regimen of zidovudine in pregnancy (PACTG 076 regimen)

Pregnancy	500 mg orally per day from 14 to 34 weeks gestation, continued throughout pregnancy
Labour	Intravenous administration 2 mg/kg over 1 h, then continuous infusion at 1 mg/kg body weight until delivery
Newborn	Zidovudine syrup, 2 mg/kg body weight oral administration every 6 h for 6 weeks, starting 8–12 h after delivery

The pharmacokinetics of only two nucleoside analogues, ZDV and lamivudine, have been evaluated in human pregnancies and both drugs are well tolerated in pregnancy. ZDV was evaluated in the PACTG 076 study and is tolerated well from 14 weeks gestation. Lamivudine has had only limited evaluation from 38 weeks gestation. The pharmacokinetics of 3TC at a dose of 150 mg twice daily were similar to those seen in non-pregnant adults.

Carcinogenicity has been demonstrated for some agents in animal studies and the relative risks of these agents is summarized in Table 8.6. These drugs have been classified by the Federal Drug Administration (FDA) on available animal carcinogenesis studies; however, the relevance of these data to humans is unknown. The proven effect of ZDV in reducing the risk of vertical transmission of HIV to the infant far outweighs the theoretical risk of carcinogenesis derived from these animal studies. The theoretical risk of carcinogenesis should be discussed with the woman in the course of counselling on the relative benefits and risks of antiretroviral therapy during pregnancy and emphasis should be placed on the need for long-term follow-up of the infant exposed to these agents *in utero*, even if they are uninfected, to monitor them for untoward effects.

Table 8.8 Short-course ZDV regimen to reduce mother-to-child transmission – possible schedule

Respond to symptoms	First visit – 16 weeks	Second visit – 24–28 weeks	Third visit – 34–36 weeks	Fourth visit – antenatal care	Delivery postnatal
Screen for risk factors	History, observe scar, etc.		Assess obvious multiple pregnancy	Assess obvious multiple pregnancy	
Screen and treat as needed	Anaemia, blood pressure, rapid plasma reagin	Anaemia, blood pressure	Anaemia, blood pressure	Anaemia, blood pressure	
HIV-testing	HIV pre-test, counselling/ testing	HIV testing[a]			
Prophylaxis	Mebendazole, iron plus folate	Antimalaria prophylaxis[a], iron plus folate	Antimalaria prophylaxis[b], iron plus folate	Antimalaria prophylaxis, iron plus folate	
	Check/give tetanus, toxoid immunizations	Check/give tetanus, toxoid immunization	Oral zidovudine 300 mg twice a day from 36 weeks until delivery	Oral zidovudine 300 mg twice a day from 36 weeks until delivery	Intensive treatment with oral zidovudine, 300 mg every 3 h of labour–delivery
Counsel individually	Where to give birth, results rapid plasma reagin Benefits of VCT	Post-test counselling and test results, refer to support groups	Infant feeding counselling If positive – ARV therapy (consent)	Birth plan Decision of infant feeding Adherence issues	Support decision on infant feeding, breast feeding technique cup feeding
Inform	Obtain clean delivery kit, when to seek care	How to prepare for birth, plan for emergency	If home delivery planned, safe steps	Check if clean delivery kit obtained	Refer HIV-positive women for care and social support
Plan for follow-up	Next visit – routine Bring partner	Next visit – routine	Follow-up after birth (child immunization)		Family planning, possible partner/ family counselling

[a]In malaria-endemic areas according to national guidelines.
VCT: voluntary counselling and testing; ARV: antiretroviral.

A randomized, double-blind, placebo-controlled trial of the safety and efficacy of ZDV in reducing the risk of maternal–infant HIV transmission, PACTG 076, was commenced in 1991. In this study, women with CD4 lymphocyte counts of greater than 200/μl who had not received antiretroviral therapy were enrolled between 14 and 34 weeks gestation (Connor et al., 1994). The final results of protocol PACTG 076 showed in 402 infant mother pairs a rate of vertical transmission of HIV of 7.6% (95% confidence intervals, 4.3–12.3%) with ZDV treatment and a rate of 22.6% (95% confidence intervals, 17.0–29.0%) with placebo ($p < 0.001$) (Sperling et al., 1996).

Follow-up of infants exposed to ZDV in utero demonstrated only a short-term toxic effect of a lower haemoglobin, with a difference of < 1 g/dl, in the ZDV-exposed group, compared with the placebo-treated group. This difference had no discernible clinical effects. There have been no increase in congenital abnormalities, delayed growth or development or incidence of malignancies in the follow-up of these exposed infants to date (Culnane et al., 1999). However, in a recent study by Blanche et al. (1999), eight of 1754 HIV-negative children exposed to ZDV and/or lamivudine have developed a possible mitochodrial dysfunction, which is well in excess of the number expected. While these findings are of concern, it must be remembered that ZDV prophylaxis to prevent vertical transmission of HIV has significantly reduced transmission and prevented thousands of paediatric infections and subsequent deaths.

The efficacy of ZDV in reducing vertical transmission of HIV is not totally explained by the reduction of maternal HIV RNA copy number that was observed in PACTG 076. If the pre-exposure prophylaxis of the infant has a significant effect in reducing the rate of perinatal transmission, then it is possible that any antiretroviral therapy that has significant transplacental transfer to the fetus would be efficacious. If antiretroviral activity in placental tissues is an important arm of protection, ZDV may be unique among the nucleoside analogue antiretroviral agents as it is phosphorylated to an active form in placental tissue. While HAART is highly advantageous to the woman's own therapy and management, it is unknown whether there is an additional advantage to HAART for reducing perinatal transmission. However, combination therapy is used commonly in the developed world, and a safe option might include ZDV, lamivudine and nevirapine.

In the developing world a short course of ZDV is currently recommended for prevention of mother-to-child transmission of HIV (WHO, 1998) (Table 8.7). More recently, in a study comparing the safety and efficacy of short-course nevirapine or ZDV during labour and the first week of life, nevirapine lowered the risk of HIV-1 transmission during the first 14–16 weeks of life by almost 50% in a breastfeeding population. This simple and inexpensive regime may have a significant impact on the rate of vertical transmission in less developed, poorer countries (Guay et al., 1999).

In summary, all HIV-infected pregnant women should be offered antiretroviral therapy and AZT should be included in any therapeutic regimen, as outlined in Table 8.8.

Current guidelines for management of HIV-infected women can be found at: www.hab.hrsa.gov/womencare.htm.

References

Balet R, Lower AM, Wilson C et al. (1998). Attitudes towards routine human immunodeficiency virus (HIV) screening and fertility treatment in HIV positive patients-a UK survey. Hum Reprod 13: 1085–7.

Barbosa C, Macasaet M, Brockmann S et al. (1997). Pelvic inflammatory disease and human immunodeficiency virus infection. Obstet Gynecol 89: 65–70.

Biggar RJ, Miotti PG, Taha TE et al. (1996). Perinatal intervention trial in Africa: effect of a birth canal cleansing intervention to prevent HIV transmission. Lancet 347: 1647–50.

Blanche S, Tardieu M, Rurlin P et al. (1999). Persistent mitochondrial dysfunction and perinatal exposure to antiretroviral nucleoside analogues. Lancet 354: 1084–9.

Boccalon M, Tirelli U, Sopracordevole F et al. (1996). Intra-epithelial and invasive cervical neoplasia during HIV infection. Eur J Cancer 32: 2212–7.

Borkowsky W, Krasiniski K, Cao Y et al. (1994). Correlation of perinatal transmission of human immunodeficiency virus type 1 with maternal viraemia and lymphocyte phenotypes. J Pediatr 125: 345–51.

Bryson Y, Luzuriaga K, Sullivan J et al. (1992). Proposed definition for in utero verses intrapartum transmission of HIV-1. N Engl J Med 327: 1246–7.

Bryson Y, Lehman D, Garraty E. (1993). The role of maternal autologous neutralising antibody in prevention of maternal to foetal HIV-1 transmission. In: Proceedings of UCLA Symposia, 1993.

Cao Y, Krogstad P, Korber BT et al. (1997). Maternal HIV-1 viral load and vertical transmission of infection: the Ariel project for the prevention of HIV transmission from mother to infant. Nat Med 3: 549–52.

Chiasson MA, Stoneburner RL, Joseph SC. (1990). Human immunodeficiency virus transmission through artificial insemination. J Acquir Immune Defic Syndr 3: 69–72.

Chaisson RF, Keruly JC, Moore RD. (1995). Race, sex, drug use, and progression of human immunodeficiency virus disease. N Engl J Med 333: 751–6.

Connor E, Sperling R, Gelber B et al. (1994). Reduction in maternal–infant transmission of human immunodeficiency virus type 1 with zidovudine treatment. N Engl J Med 331: 1174–80.

Culnane M, Fowler M, Lee SS et al. (1999). Lack of long-term effects of in utero exposure to zidovudine among uninfected children born to HIV-infected women. Pediatric AIDS Clinical Trial Group Protocol 219/076 Teams. JAMA 281: 151–7.

Devash Y, Cavelli T, Wood D et al. (1990). Vertical transmission of human immunodeficiency virus is correlated with the absence of high affinity/avidity maternal antibodies to the gp120 principal neutralizing domain. Proc Natl Acad Sci 87: 3445–9.

Dickover RE, Garraty E, Horman SA. (1996). Identification of levels of maternal HIV-1 RNA associated with risk of perinatal transmission. JAMA 275: 599–605.

DiMaria H, Courotin C, Rouzioux C. (1996). Transplacental transmission of human immunodeficiency virus. Lancet 2: 215–6.

Duerr A, Sierra MF, Feldman J et al. (1997). Immune compromise and prevalence of Candida vulvovaginitis in human immunodeficiency virus-infected women. Obstet Gynecol 90: 252–6.

Duliege AM, Amos CI, Felton S et al. (1995). Birth order, delivery route, and concordance in the transmission of the human immunodeficiency virus type 1 from mothers to twins. J Pediatr 126: 625–32.

European Collaborative Study Group. (1992). Risk factors for mother-to-child transmission of HIV-1. Lancet 339: 1007–12.

European Collaborative Study Group. (1996). Vertical transmission of HIV-1: maternal immune status and obstetric factors. AIDS 10: 1675–81.

Fang G, Burger H, Grimson R. (1995). Maternal plasma human immunodeficiency virus type 1 RNA level: a determinant and projected threshold for mother-to-child transmission. Proc Natl Acad Sci 92: 12100–4.

Fantini J, Yahi N, Tourres C et al. (1997). HIV-1 transmission across the vaginal epithelium. AIDS 11: 1663–4.

Frankel RE, Selwyn PA, Mezger J et al. (1997). High prevalence of gynecologic disease among hospitalized women with human immunodeficiency virus infection. Clin Infect Dis 5: 706–12.

Fruchter R, Maiman M, Sedlis A et al. (1996). Multiple recurrences of cervical intraepithelial neoplasia in women with the human immunodeficiency virus. Obstet Gynecol 87: 338–44.

Gaetano C, Scano G, Carbonari T et al. (1987). Delayed and defective anti-IgM response in infants. Lancet i: 631.

Grosskurth H, Mosha F, Todd J et al. (1995). Impact of improved treatment of sexually transmitted diseases on HIV infection in rural Tanzania: randomised controlled trial. Lancet 346: 530–6.

Guay LA, Musoke P, Fleming T et al. (1999). Intrapartum and neonatal single-dose nevirapine compared with zidovodine for prevention of mother-to-child transmission of HIV-1 in Kampala, Uganda: HIVET 012 randomised trial. Lancet 354: 795–802.

Harnish D, Hammberg O, Walker I et al. (1987). Early detection of HIV in a newborn. N Engl J Med 316: 272–3.

Hoegsberg B, Abulafia O, Sedlis A et al. (1990). Sexually transmitted diseases and human immunodeficiency virus infection among women with pelvic inflammatory disease. Am J Obstet Gynecol 163: 1135–9.

Holcomb K, Maiman M, Dimaio T et al. (1998). Rapid progression to invasive cervix cancer in a woman infected with the human immunodeficiency virus. Obstet Gynecol 91: 848–50.

Husson R, Lan Y, Kojima E et al. (1995). Vertical transmission of human immunodeficiency virus type 1: autologous neutralising antibody, virus load, and virus phenotype. J Pediatr 126: 865–71.

The International Perinatal HIV Group (1999). The mode of delivery and the risk of vertical transmission of human immunodeficiency virus type 1. N Engl J Med 340: 977–87.

Kedes DH, Ganem D, Ameli N et al. (1997). The prevalence of serum antibody to human herpesvirus 8 (Kaposi sarcoma-associated herpesvirus) among HIV-seropositive and high-risk HIV-seronegative women. JAMA 277: 478–81.

Korn AP, Landers DV. (1995). Gynecologic disease in women infected with human immunodeficiency virus type 1. J Acquir Immune Defic Syndr Hum Retrovirol 9: 361–70.

Krivine A, Firtion G, Cao L et al. (1992). HIV replication during the first weeks of life. Lancet 339: 1187–9.

Laga M, Manoka A, Kivuvu M et al. (1993). Non-ulcerative sexually transmitted diseases as risk factors for HIV-1 transmission in women: results from a cohort study. AIDS 7: 95–102.

Landesman SH, Kalish L, Burns DN et al. (1996). Obstetrical factors in the transmission of human immunodeficiency virus from mother to child. N Engl J Med 334: 1617–23.

Lasheeb AS, King J, Ball JK et al. (1997). Semen characteristics in HIV-1 positive men and the effect of semen washing. Genitourin Med 73: 303–5.

Laure F, Courgnaud V, Rouzioux C et al. (1988). Detection of HIV-1 DNA in infants and children by means of polymerase chain reaction. Lancet 339: 538–41.

MacDonald MG, Ginzburg HM, Bolan JC et al. (1991). HIV infection in pregnancy: epidemiology and clinical management. J AIDS 4: 100–8.

Maenza JR, Keruly JC, Moore RD et al. (1996). Risk factors for fluconazole-resistant candidiasis in human immunodeficiency virus-infected patients. J Infect Dis 173: 219–25.

Maiman M, Fruchter RG, Sedlis A et al. (1998). Prevalence, risk factors, and accuracy of cytologic screening for cervical intraepithelial neoplasia in women with the human immunodeficiency virus. Gynecol Oncol 68: 233–9.

Mandelbrot L, Mayaux MJ, Bougain A et al. (1996). Obstetric factors in mother to child transmission of human immunodeficiency virus type 1: the French perinatal cohorts. Am J Obstet Gynaecol 175: 611–7.

Mandelbrot L, Le Chenadec J, Berrebi A et al. (1998). Perinatal HIV transmission. Interaction between zidovudine prophylaxis and mode of delivery in the French perinatal cohort. JAMA 280: 55–60.

Marrack P, Kushnir E, Kappler J. (1991). A maternally inherited superantigen encoded by mouse mammary tumour virus. Nature 349: 524–6.

Mayaux MJ, Blanche C, Riozioux P et al. (1995). Maternal factors associated with perinatal HIV 1 transmission: the French Cohort Study: 7 years follow-up observation. The French Pediatric HIV Infection Study Group. J Acquir Immune Defic Syndr Hum Retrovirol 8: 188–94.

Melbye M, Smith E, Wohlfahrt J et al. (1996). Anal and cervical abnormality in women–prediction by human papillomavirus tests. Int J Cancer 68: 559–64.

Mercey D, Griffioen A, Woronowski H et al. (1996). Uptake of medical interventions in women with HIV infection in Britain and Ireland. Genitourin Med 72: 281–2.

Minkoff H, Landesman S. (1988). The case for routinely offering prenatal testing for human immunodeficiency virus. Am J Obstet Gynaecol 159: 793–6.

Minkoff H, Burns DN, Landesman S et al. (1995). The relationship of ruptured membranes to the vertical transmission of human immunodeficiency virus. Am J Obstet Gynaecol 173: 585–9.

Mofenson LM. (1994). Epidemiology and determinants of vertical HIV transmission. Sem Ped Infect Dis 5: 252–65.

Palasanthiran P, Ziegler J, Stewart GJ et al. (1993). Breast-feeding during primary maternal human immunodeficiency virus infection and risk of transmission from mother to infant. J Ped Infect Dis 167: 441–4.

Palella FJ, Delaney KM, Moorman AC et al. (1998). Declining morbidity and mortality among patients with advanced human immunodeficiency virus infection. HIV Outpatient Study Investigators. N Engl J Med 338: 853–60.

Perinatal HIV Guidelines Working Group. (2001). Public Health Service Task Force recommendations for use of antiretroviral drugs in pregnant HIV-1 infected women for Maternal Health and Interventions to Reduce Perinatal HIV-1 Transmission in the United States. http://www.hivatis.org.

Phuapradit W, Panburana P, Jaovisidha A et al. (1999). Maternal viral load and vertical transmission of HIV-1 in mid-trimester gestation. AIDS 13: 1927–31.

Pyun K, Ochs H, Dufford T et al. (1987). Perinatal infection with human immunodeficiency virus: specific antibody responses by the neonate. N Engl J Med 317: 611–4.

Rhoads JL, Wright DC, Redfield RR et al. (1987). Chronic vaginal candidiasis in women with human immunodeficiency virus infection. JAMA 257: 3105–7.

Robinson W, Morris C. (1996). Cervical neoplasia. Pathogenesis, diagnosis and management. Hematol Oncol Clin N Am 10: 1163–76.

Rossi P, Moschese V, Broliden PA et al. (1989). Presence of maternal antibodies to human immunodeficiency virus type 1 envelope glycoprotein gp120 epitopes correlates with the uninfected status of children born to seropositive mothers. Proc Natl Acad Sci 86: 8055–8.

Rouzioux C, Costagliola D, Burgard M et al. (1995). Estimated timing of mother-to-child human immunodeficiency virus type-1 (HIV-1) transmission by use of a Markov model: the HIV Infections in Newborns Collaborative Study Group. Am J Epidemiol 142: 1330–7.

Scarlatti G, Albert J, Rossi P. (1993). Mother to child transmission of human immunodeficiency virus type 1: correlation with neutralising antibodies against primary isolates. J Infect Dis 168: 207–10.

Schuman P, Capps L, Peng G et al. (1997). Weekly fluconazole for the prevention of mucosal candidiasis in women with HIV infection. A randomized, double-blind, placebo-controlled trial. Terry Beirn Community Programs for Clinical Research on AIDS. Ann Intern Med 126: 689–96.

Semprini AE, Castagna C, Ravizza M et al. (1995). The incidence of complications from caesarean section in 156 HIV-positive women. AIDS 9: 913–7.

Semprini AE, Fiore S, Savasi V et al. (1998). Assisted conception to reduce the risk of male-to-female sexual transfer of HIV in serodiscordant couples: and update. Proceedings of the Annual Meeting of the American Society for Reproductive Medicine, Boston, MA, USA.

Shaffer N, Roongpisuthipong A, Siriwasin W et al. (1999). Maternal virus load and perinatal human immunodeficiency virus type 1 subtype E transmission, Thailand. J Infect Dis 179: 590–9.

Solomon L, Stein M, Flynn C et al. (1998). Health services use by urban women with or at risk for HIV-1 infection: the HIV Epidemiology Research Study (HERS). J Acquir Immune Defic Syndr Hum Retrovirol 17: 253–61.

Sorvillo F, Kerndt P. (1998). Trichomonas vaginalis and amplification of HIV-1 transmission. Lancet 351: 213–4.

Specter S, Soumenkoff G, Puissant F et al. (1986). Vertical transmission of HIV in a 15 week foetus. Lancet ii: 288–9.

Sperling RS, Shapiro DE, Coombs RW et al. (1996). Maternal viral load, zidovudine treatment and the risk of transmission of human immunodeficiency virus type 1 from mother to infant. N Engl J Med 335: 1621–9.

Steihm ER, Lambert JS, Mofenson LM et al. (1999). Efficacy of zidovudine and human immunodeficiency virus (HIV) hyperimmune immunoglobulin for reducing perinatal transmission from HIV-infected women with advanced disease: results of pediatric AIDS clinical trials group protocol 185. J Infect Dis 179: 567–75.

Sterling TR, Vlahov D, Astemborski J et al. (2001) Initial plasma HIV-1 RNA levels and progression to AIDS in women and men. N Engl J Med 344: 720–5.

Sun XW, Kuhn L, Ellerbrock TV et al. (1997). Human papillomavirus infection in women infected with the human immunodeficiency virus. N Engl J Med 337: 1343–9.

Thackway S, Furner V, Mijch A et al. (1998). HIV Infection in women in the Asia-Pacific: the Australian experience. J HIV Therapy 3: 9–12.

Thirty L, Specher-Goldberger S, Jonckheer T et al. (1985). Isolation of AIDS virus from cell-free breast milk of three healthy virus carriers. Lancet 2: 891.

Tsuji Y, Doi H, Yamabe T et al. (1990). Prevention of mother to child transmission of human T-lymphotropic virus type-1. Pediatrics 86: 11–7.

Uvin SC, Caliendo AM. (1997). Cervicovaginal human immunodeficiency virus secretion and plasma viral load in human immunodeficiency virus-seropositive women. Obstet Gynecol 90: 739–43.

Vernazza PL, Gilliam BL, Dyer J et al. (1997). Quantification of HIV in semen: correlation with antiviral treatment and immune status. AIDS 11: 987–93.

Vogt MW, Witt DJ, Craven DE et al. (1987). Isolation patterns of human immunodeficiency virus from cervical secretions during the menstrual cycle of women at risk of the acquired immunodeficiency syndrome. Ann Intern Med 106: 380–2.

Weiser B, Nachman S, Tropper P et al. (1994). Quantitation of human immunodeficiency virus type 1 during pregnancy: relationship of viral titre to mother-to-child transmission and stability of viral load. Proc Nat Acad Sci 91: 8031–41.

World Health Organization. (1987). Breast-feeding/breast milk and human immunodeficiency virus. Weekly Epidemiol Record 62: 245.

WHO (1998). Recommendations on the safe and effective use of short-course ZDV for prevention of mother-to-child transmission of HIV. Weekly Epidemiol Record 73: 41.

Wolfsy CB, Cohen JB, Hayer LB et al. (1986). Isolation of AIDS–associated retrovirus from genital secretions of women with antibody to the virus. Lancet 1: 527–9.

Wolinsky S, Mack D, Yogev R. (1988). Detection of HIV – infection in pediatric patients and their mothers by polymerase chain reaction (PCR). In: Proceedings of the Fourth International AIDS Conference, Stockholm, Sweden.

Wright T, Moscarelli R, Dole P et al. (1996). Significance of mild cytologic atypia in women infected with Human Immunodeficiency Virus. Obstet Gynecol 87: 515–9.

Zhang L, He T, Talal A et al. (1998). In vivo distribution of the human immunodeficiency virus/simian immunodeficiency virus co-receptors: CXCR4, CCR3, and CCR5. J Virol 72: 5035–45.

Ziegler JB, Johnson RO, Gold J. (1985). Postnatal transmission of AIDS-associated retrovirus from mother to infant. Lancet 1: 896–7.

ROSS McKINNEY AND RUSSELL VAN DYKE

Biology of HIV infection in infants

Although the course of paediatric HIV disease is analogous to that in adults, there are certain characteristics of HIV infection in children that make it distinct. These unique aspects are the result of the mode of transmission, the timing of transmission, and immaturity of the infant's immune system. Further, there are aspects of the diagnosis, staging and management of HIV-infected infants that differ significantly from those of adults.

The time at which HIV is transmitted from mother to infant can be defined fairly tightly for most pregnancies. Transmission can occur before birth (*in utero*), during the delivery process (peripartum), or via breast feeding postpartum. Although infection through breast feeding is common in much of the world, it is an uncommon means of transmission in developed countries, largely because relatively few HIV-infected women breast feed.

The standard means used to determine the timing of an infant's infection is an HIV culture or DNA polymerase chain reaction (PCR) test within the first week of life (Bryson *et al.*, 1992). In the case of an infant infected peripartum (as opposed to *in utero*), the amount of virus present in the first days after infection is small, and as a result HIV cannot be detected using standard PCR or culture techniques. In contrast, if the newborn was infected *in utero*, viral replication will have proceeded for a period of time, producing a high level of HIV in plasma, which is easily detected. Integrated (proviral) HIV DNA has been found in a subset of abortuses, suggesting fetal infection (Soeiro *et al.*, 1992).

Current estimates are that in the absence of breast feeding, less than half of infants who acquire HIV infection do so while *in utero*. Most *in utero* transmissions are thought to occur late in gestation (Kalish *et al.*, 1997). Breast feeding probably adds an additional 10–15% risk of transmitting HIV infection, although this rate is related to the length of breast feeding and is increased to about 30% if the mother acquires primary HIV infection postpartum (Dunn *et al.*, 1992; Miotti *et al.*, 1999). The risk factors for transmission of HIV from mother to infant are summarized in Table 9.1.

The fact that infection of infants occurs at a well-defined time offers an unusual opportunity to intervene therapeutically. Studies in adults have shown that shortly after infection HIV disseminates rapidly to multiple organs, particularly lymph nodes (Fauci, 1993). A relatively high-level viraemia follows, as evidenced by high concentrations of viral RNA in plasma. The adult immune response usually controls this viraemia within a matter of weeks, and a period of relatively low viral replication (the 'viral load set-point') ensues, which is associated with generally good health (the clinical latent period), which may last years or even decades (Daar *et al.*, 1991). Infants rapidly develop elevated virus loads, which are higher than adults and which decline more slowly (Shearer *et al.*, 1997) (Figure 9.1). The immune system of children does not appear to

Table 9.1 Maternal risk factors for vertical transmission

- Failure to receive zidovudine preventive therapy
- Breast feeding
- Advanced HIV infection in the mother (decreased CD4 lymphocyte count, high plasma viral load)
- Prolonged rupture of membranes
- Vaginal delivery (versus Caesarian section)
- Prematurity or low birth weight
- Placental inflammation or chorio-amnionitis
- First-born of twins
- Maternal injecting drug use
- Bloody amniotic fluid
- Placental levels of leukemia inhibitory factor

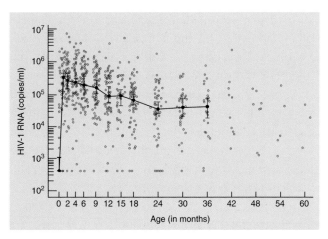

Figure 9.1 *Plasma HIV-1 RNA concentrations in multiple samples from 106 infants with HIV infection. The solid line connects the median values of the individual data points. The vertical bars represent the 95% confidence intervals (from Shearer et al., 1997).*

control virus replication as well as that of adults (Rosenberg *et al.*, 1997), in that few or no cytotoxic T cells are generated (Pikora *et al.*, 1997) and viral load does not fall to the same degree as that in adults (Palumbo *et al.*, 1995; Shearer *et al.*, 1997). Thus, there may be a particular niche for early antiviral therapy in children in an attempt to limit viral dissemination while the immune response matures.

Epidemiology of paediatric HIV infection

Most paediatric HIV disease has been the result of vertical (maternal–fetal) transmission (John and Kreiss, 1996). There are some instances of horizontal transmission, such as males with haemophilia prior to full protection of the blood supply and the Romanian neonates either transfused with infected blood products or given injections using HIV-contaminated equipment, but they are the exception to the global rule. The prevalence of paediatric HIV infection is thus directly related to the prevalence of HIV infection among women.

As of late 1999, the UN AIDS Programme estimated that 34.3 million people were HIV infected, of whom 15.7 million were women and 1.3 million were children under 15 years of age. Regional infection rates vary tremendously, from a country like Australia, where only 900 women and less than 150 children are thought to be HIV infected (approximately 0.003% of the population), to KwaZulu Natal Province in South Africa, where nearly 30% of pregnant women are HIV infected (UNAIDS, 1998; Report on the

global HIV/AIDS epidemic: www.us.unaids.org). The highest prevalence rates among women are currently in Central and Southern Africa, but there are other problem areas within South east Asia and in countries like India, where the epidemic is growing at an explosive rate.

In addition to geographical variations in the prevalence of HIV infection, there are also variations in vertical transmission rates. These rates reflect many factors, most importantly the availability of antiretroviral therapy to use as perinatal prophylaxis. Transmission rates in Africa, where antiretroviral prophylaxis is largely unavailable, are in the range of 25–40%, while in the USA and Europe, where prophylaxis is widely used, rates as low as 2–4% have been reported. These differences reflect disparities in the ability to recognize infected women, as well as the availability of prophylactic antiviral regimens.

The state of the epidemic in women of child-bearing age is an important predictor of the degree to which vertical transmission of HIV is a problem. Countries such as the USA and European nations have a low prevalence in women – less than 3 per 1000. Unfortunately, women have been one of the groups experiencing a rapid rise in the HIV infection rate, especially in the southeastern USA (Centers for Disease Control and Prevention, 1995). In many developing countries, nearly half the infections are in women.

Injecting drug use is also a major cause of HIV infection in women and children, primarily because of sexual transmission (including commercial sex) from HIV-infected male contacts who are injecting drug users, and less frequently because of injecting drug use by the women themselves.

Natural history

Paediatric HIV disease

HIV infection is more aggressive in children than in adults. The median life expectancy of a child born in the USA with vertically-acquired HIV infection is about 8 years. Children are more likely to have central nervous system disease, to have lethal *Pneumocystis carinii* pneumonia (PCP), and to have impaired growth (Oxtoby, 1994).

Untreated HIV infection acquired in infancy has a rate of progression that is bimodally distributed (Auger *et al.*, 1988). Roughly one-quarter of children will develop AIDS within the first year of life, while the other three-quarters have a slower progression, with a median time to AIDS of greater than 5 years, similar to the incubation period of adults with HIV infection (European Collaborative Study,

1991). The 'rapid progressor' group typically has a high viral load in plasma and a high proportion of infected CD4 lymphocytes, experiences rapid depletion of CD4 lymphocytes, has a high risk for encephalopathy, and has more numerous opportunistic infections. Rapid progressors are likely to have been infected *in utero*, while the slow progressors are thought to have been infected peripartum. There is, however, considerable overlap in plasma HIV RNA concentrations between children with rapid and slow progression when early viral loads are evaluated.

The rapid progression seen in some HIV-infected infants may thus reflect an inadequate immune response, rather than *in utero* infections. Luzuriaga and Sullivan, while investigating the early T-cell response to HIV infection, showed that HIV-infected infants had almost no detectable HIV-specific T cells. In contrast, in adults an early cytolytic response to HIV infection is easily demonstrable (Luzuriaga and Sullivan, 1998). There is thus a need in children for interventions that can either contain the virus or boost the child's immune response.

It has been suggested that some perinatally infected infants will spontaneously clear their infection (e.g. Bryson *et al.*, 1995). However, in at least some of the cases reported, comparison of maternal and infant viral sequences has shown them to be unrelated, suggesting a laboratory error or mixing of blood samples (Frenkel *et al.*, 1998). Thus, spontaneous resolution of neonatal infection must be an extremely rare event, if it occurs at all.

The most typical early manifestations of HIV in infants are oral candidiasis, hepatomegaly, splenomegaly, generalized lymphadenopathy, and a subtle growth delay (McKinney and Robertson, 1993; Moye *et al.*, 1996). In the typical growth pattern, HIV-infected infants gain weight and length more slowly than uninfected infants born to HIV-infected women. The HIV effects are seen equally with height and weight growth, so the infected children are smaller than normal but have normal body proportions, a pattern consistent with growth delay (Figure 9.2). This is in contrast to the adult wasting syndrome, wherein patients become lean (attaining a low weight-for-height). While some children do become lean late in their disease, loss of lean body mass is rarely an early manifestation of HIV disease in children. Unless extreme, growth problems in early HIV disease are almost impossible to diagnose in the individual child, and are better seen in aggregate data from groups of children who are infected, compared to those who are simply exposed and not infected.

The most common AIDS defining opportunistic infection in North America and Europe is PCP. In comparison to adult PCP, the onset in children is more abrupt, the progression to severe hypoxaemia more rapid, and the disease can occur when CD4 counts are still within the normal range. PCP is also associated with a higher mortality in children than in adults. As prevention of PCP is more effective than treatment, most HIV-infected children are given co-trimoxazole prophylaxis for their first year of life, regardless of their CD4 count (Figure 9.3).

Fungal infections are relatively common in HIV-infected children. The most frequent problem infections are *Candida albicans*, dermatophytes, and histoplasmosis.

Bacterial infections are also frequent in HIV-infected children. The most severe problems are with polysaccharide-encapsulated bacteria (*Streptococcus pneumoniae*, *Neisseria meningitidis*), and infected children can have unusually frequent bouts of acute otitis media and sinusitis. Invasive bacterial diseases such as meningitis and pneumonia are also more common in HIV-infected children than in their uninfected peers.

Mycobacterial infections have likewise been a major problem for both adult and paediatric patients with end-stage HIV infection. The most common disease is disseminated infection with *Mycobacterium avium* complex (MAC), which typically affects children with fewer than 100 CD4 lymphocytes/μl. As in adults, disseminated MAC in children manifests itself with fevers, weight loss, anaemia (or pancytopenia), and fatigue. The disease is severe enough for prophylaxis with one of the macrolides (most frequently azithromycin) to be warranted once a child's CD4 lymphocyte counts fall to below 75–100 cells/μl.

In parts of the world where BCG vaccine is used to prevent severe tuberculosis, infants with HIV and disseminated BCG infection have been reported (Raton *et al.*, 1997). Knowing a child's HIV status prior to BCG vaccination would be useful, although in many countries where BCG is routinely employed, the relative risk of BCG vaccine is felt to be lower than the risk from exposure to wild-type tuberculosis.

Viral infections controlled by cell-mediated immune responses are also a significant problem for HIV-infected children, although to a lesser degree than might be expected. Primary infections with herpes simplex and varicella-zoster virus (VZV) are generally well controlled (Gershon *et al.*, 1997). However, recurrent zoster (shingles) is

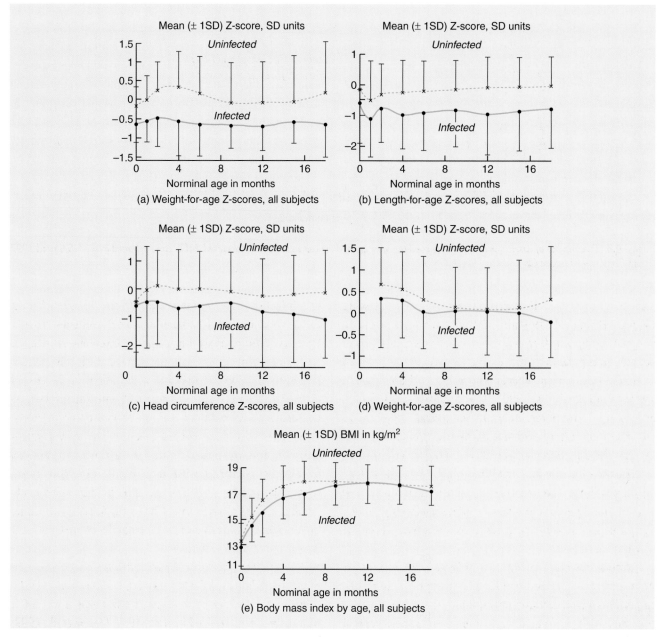

Figure 9.2 *Growth characteristics of infants born to HIV-1 infected women and then prospectively followed from birth. The groups are divided into HIV-1 infected and uninfected patients (from Moye et al., 1996).*

common in children with falling CD4 lymphocyte numbers. Some children with end-stage HIV disease develop a chronic form of VZV disease, with painful, thick, lichenified lesions in multiple sites.

Mechanisms of perinatal transmission

HIV infection among infants and pre-adolescent children results almost exclusively from the transmission of HIV from an infected mother to her child (see also Chapter 8). Consequently, in most countries over 90% of HIV-infect-

ed children have an infected mother. Children can be infected through the receipt of blood or blood products if blood is not tested for the presence of HIV, although this is a rare event in developed countries, where donor deferral and rigorous HIV testing protect the blood supply. Rare cases of infection in children result from sexual abuse, or from close contact with another infected individual through exchange of blood or bloody secretions.

Transmission from mother to child occurs not only *in utero* but also *intrapartum* by exposure to maternal blood

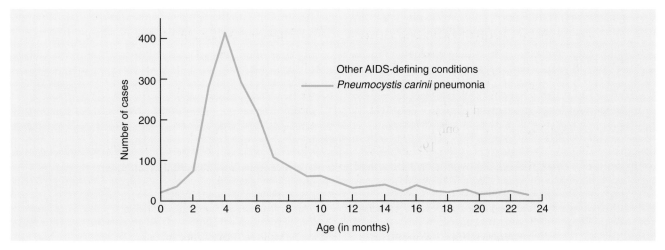

Figure 9.3 *The number of cases of AIDS-defining conditions by age of diagnosis in perinatally-acquired AIDS cases reported in the USA until 1997 (From Centers for Disease Control and Prevention, 1997).*

and secretions, as well as postpartum via breast feeding (Van De Perre *et al.*, 1991; Bryson, 1996). However, in the absence of breast feeding, most transmission probably occurs during labour and delivery, with a minority of infections occurring *in utero* late in gestation (Bertolli *et al.*, 1996; John and Kreiss, 1996). This conclusion is supported by a number of observations. Infected infants rarely have clinical or laboratory evidence of disease at birth, suggesting that the infection was recently acquired. In addition, in at least two-thirds of infants ultimately shown to be infected, HIV will not be detectable in blood during the first few days of life. These infants develop detectable viraemia by 4–8 weeks of age, suggesting that transmission occurs in the peripartum period.

Intrapartum HIV infection of infants probably results from exposure to blood or bloody secretions in the birth canal. This would account for the substantially higher infection rate with prolonged rupture of membranes, vaginal delivery (versus Caesarian section) and in the first born of twins (Duliege *et al.*, 1995; Landesman *et al.*, 1996; The International Perinatal HIV Group, 1999). Alternatively, small amounts of maternal blood may enter the child's circulation through the placenta during labour. Infants with detectable virus in the peripheral blood in the first 48 h of life are presumed to have *in utero* acquisition of infection (Bryson *et al.*, 1992).

Risk factors for maternal–child transmission

In the absence of preventive therapy with zidovudine, the risk of infection for a non-breast-fed infant born to an infected mother is approximately 25%. However,

the infection rate varies widely (from 15 to 50%) in different studies and geographical regions. Transmission by breast feeding is well documented and the additional risk of infection to the infant posed by breast feeding is estimated to be from 3.2% (Leroy *et al.*, 1998). In developed countries, it is recommended that HIV-infected mothers do not breast feed. However, the risk of breast feeding needs to be balanced with its marked benefit in preventing gastroenteritis and malnutrition in young infants. Thus, in developing countries with high infant mortality rates, recommendations regarding breast feeding must be made locally, and most authorities have suggested continuing breast feeding. Strategies are being developed to limit infection via this mechanism.

A number of risk factors for maternal–child transmission have been identified (Table 9.1) (Gabiano *et al.*, 1992; St Louis *et al.*, 1993; Dickover *et al.*, 1996; Leroy *et al.*, 2001; Mandelbrot *et al.*, 1996; Pitt *et al.*, 1997; Garcia *et al.*, 1999; Mofenson *et al.*, 1999; Patterson *et al.*, 2001). It is likely that variability in these factors accounts for the broad range of transmission rates seen in different studies. Maternal–fetal transmission rates are high in women with advanced HIV infection, as defined by high viral loads and low CD4 lymphocyte counts. However, women with all levels of viral load can transmit HIV to their child, and there is no threshold level of viral load below which transmission does not occur (Cao *et al.*, 1997; Ioannidis *et al.*, 2001). Thus, for an individual woman, the viral load (or CD4 lymphocyte count) has little ability to predict her risk of transmission.

Most studies that defined risk factors for mother–child transmission of HIV were performed prior to the routine use of antiretroviral chemoprophylaxis to prevent transmission. In the context of preventative therapy, most risk factors lose their importance, including maternal viral load and CD4 lymphocyte count (Sperling *et al.*, 1996). In a recent study of a non-breast-feeding population in which most women and infants received preventive zidovudine, histological chorioamnionitis was the only independent risk factor for transmission (Van Dyke *et al.*, 1999). However, other studies of maternal–fetal transmission with zidovudine-treated mothers have continued to identify elevated maternal plasma HIV RNA concentration (viral load) as the major factor predicting transmission (Garcia *et al.*, 1999; Mofenson *et al.*, 1999).

Prevention of maternal–child transmission

In 1994, the Paediatric AIDS Clinical Trials Group (PACTG) Study 076 demonstrated that zidovudine (ZDV) can dramatically reduce the rate of maternal–child transmission of HIV (Connor *et al.*, 1994; Sperling *et al.*, 1996). In this placebo-controlled study, ZDV was administered orally to HIV-infected women during the second and third trimesters of pregnancy, by intravenous infusion during labour, and orally to the infant for 6 weeks following birth. This regimen decreased the transmission rate by two-thirds, from 22.6% to 7.6% (Connor *et al.*, 1994; Sperling *et al.*, 1996).

As a result of this study, in April 1994, the US Public Health Service recommended the administration of ZDV to all HIV-infected pregnant women and their infants (Table 9.2) (Centers for Disease Control and Prevention, 1994a; Centers for Disease Control and Prevention, 1994b). All pregnant HIV-infected women should receive zidovudine during the second and third trimester, with an intravenous infusion during active labour until delivery.

The infant should receive 6 weeks of oral therapy. Although the PACTG 076 study administered 200 mg of ZDV five times a day to the mother and four times a day to the infant, many authorities now recommend zidovudine 200 mg po three times daily or 300 mg twice daily for the mother and 2.6 mg/kg po three times daily for the infant.

In order for this intervention to be successful, HIV-infected pregnant women must be identified prior to the second trimester of pregnancy. It is recommended that HIV antibody testing is routinely performed early in pregnancy, albeit only voluntarily (Stoto *et al.*, 1998). Women who have participated in high-risk behaviour during pregnancy should be re-tested during the third trimester.

The 'PACTG 076 prevention protocol' has been well accepted in the USA and other developed countries. Indeed, in the USA it is estimated that 87% of HIV-infected pregnant women are now identified during pregnancy and more than 65% receive preventative treatment with ZDV (Centers for Disease Control and Prevention, 1998c). This has resulted in a dramatic reduction in the number of HIV-infected children born in the USA; between 1992 and 1996, there was a 43% reduction in the estimated number of perinatally infected children (Centers for Disease Control and Prevention, 1997).

However, in much of the developing world, the 'PACTG 076 protocol' cannot be routinely implemented. Women often do not receive pre-natal care until late in pregnancy and many deliver outside of the hospital, making the intrapartum infusion of ZDV impossible. In addition, the cost of ZDV is prohibitive for most developing countries. In an attempt to define a more practical intervention, short-course ZDV was recently evaluated in Thailand. Pregnant women received oral ZDV (300 mg twice daily), starting at 36 weeks gestation, with oral ZDV (300 mg every

Table 9.2 Prevention of maternal–fetal transmission of HIV: *The United States Public Health Service Guidelines*, 1994

Subject	Timing	Dose of zidovudine
Mother	*Begin* in late second trimester (or as soon as possible if this date is missed); *continue* until onset of labour, delivery	200 mg three times daily, or 250–300 mg twice daily
	Begin at onset of labour, end of delivery	2 mg/kg intravenous loading dose, followed by 1 mg/kg/hour
Newborn	*Begin* at 8–12 h after birth; *end* at age 6 weeks[a]	2 mg/kg orally every 6 h, or 2.6 mg/kg orally three times per day

(Courtesy of Centers for Disease Control and Prevention, 1994.)
[a]Should be continued, adding full antiretroviral therapy, if there is evidence that the infant has become infected despite antiretroviral prophylaxis. See also http://hivatis.org/trtgdlns.html.

3 h) continued during labour. No ZDV was given to the infants and the women did not breast feed. In this placebo-controlled study, there was a 50% reduction in the rate of transmission, from 18.9 to 9.4% (Centers for Disease Control and Prevention, 1998a; Shaffer et al., 1999; Chot-pitayasunondh et al., 2001). Similar results have been seen in two studies of very similar dosing regimens in Burkina Faso and Coté d'Ivoire, Africa (Dabis et al., 1999; Wiktor et al., 1999). Short-course ZDV intervention is safe and inexpensive and is likely to become the standard of care in many developing countries. The results also support the belief that most transmission occurs late in pregnancy or at delivery. Zidovudine combined with lamivudine may be more effective than zidovudine alone, but was also more toxic (Mandelbrot et al., 2001).

Because of its long half-life nevirapine (see section on treatments, below) was evaluated as part of a regimen for perinatal prophylaxis in Uganda in the US NIH HIVNET 012 study (Gray et al., 1999). One dose administered orally to the mother followed by one dose given to the infant appeared to reduce maternal–fetal transmission by about 50%, approximately the same as a longer course of zido-vudine. This is also a practical and inexpensive alternative to PACTG 076 zidovudine prophylaxis for developing countries.

A meta-analysis of 15 prospective cohort (uncontrolled) studies suggests that Caesarian section, when performed prior to the rupture of membranes, results in a 50% reduction in infection rate of the infant after adjustment for antiretroviral therapy, maternal stage of disease and infant birth weight (The International Perinatal HIV Group, 1999). Preliminary results from a randomized prospective study conducted in Europe show a 71% reduction in the transmission rate with elective Caesarian section (from 10.3 to 3.0%) (Semprini, 1998). However, the morbidity of Caesarian section in HIV-infected women remains to be adequately defined. At the present time, Caesarian section is not routinely recommended in the USA to prevent trans-mission of HIV, because of the low transmission rates cur-rently observed with the use of ZDV therapy (possibly less than 5%) (Pediatric ACTG Protocol 185 Executive Sum-mary, 1997). Interventions at delivery that limit exposure of the infant to maternal blood, such as cleansing of the birth canal, do not appear to reduce the transmission rate (Bigger et al., 1996).

Up-to-date guidelines for the prevention of mothers-to-child transmission of HIV can be found at: http://hivatis.org/trtgdlns.html.

Of course, the easiest, cheapest and most effective means of reducing HIV infection in children is by reducing the incidence and prevalence of HIV infection among women of child-bearing age. As a consequence, public policies and attention need to be focused on women in order to reduce the number of infected infants. Interventional efforts have focused on education, improving access to condoms, and empowering women to refuse intercourse when condoms are not going to be used. Sexually transmitted disease (STD) prevention and treatment are important (e.g. because ulcerative STDs facilitate transmission of HIV), but the same steps that prevent heterosexual HIV trans-mission will also prevent most STDs.

Management of the HIV-exposed infant

HIV-infected infants rarely have clinical evidence of disease at birth and their lymphocyte subset values are usually nor-mal for age. In addition, virtually all infants born to HIV-infected mothers will be HIV-seropositive themselves, due to placental transfer of maternal IgG antibody. Thus, HIV infection in the infant is diagnosed by detecting virus or viral RNA or DNA in peripheral blood (see below). HIV-exposed infants should have virological testing performed on peripheral blood (not cord blood) prior to discharge from the nursery and at 1–2 months and 4 months of age (Table 9.3). A positive test should be repeated as soon as possible. HIV infection is confirmed if a child has positive virologi-cal tests on two separate occasions. A child who is not breast fed can be considered free of infection with two neg-ative virological tests if one was obtained after 1 month of age and the second after 4 months of age. Absence of infec-tion can be confirmed by a negative HIV antibody test, reflecting loss of maternal antibody; this frequently does not occur until after 12 months of age (Van Dyke et al., 1999). Since anaemia and neutropenia are the major toxicities seen with ZDV and trimethoprim-sulfamethoxazole, the infant should be evaluated with regular complete blood counts, as suggested in Table 9.3.

All HIV-exposed infants should receive 6 weeks of ZDV, according to the 'ACTG 076 protocol', as noted above. In developed countries, infants of HIV-infected mothers should not breast feed. In developing countries, the risks and benefits of breast feeding should be considered local-ly. At 6 weeks of age, prophylaxis for PCP with trimetho-prim-sulfamethoxazole is started and discontinued once the child is shown to be HIV-uninfected (see section on chemo-prophylaxis of opportunistic infections).

Table 9.3 Schema for evaluating children at risk of HIV infection

Age at initial Presentation	HIV status	Test on infant	Schedule (months)	Comments
< 2 weeks	1) Maternal HIV status unknown	HIV serology (mother and infant)	Immediate	If either mother or infant is positive, warrants further evaluation per outline below
	2) Mother HIV infected	HIV peripheral blood cDNA[a] and/or culture	Birth 1–2 months, 4–6 months	cDNA and culture are roughly equal in sensitivity. Two negative tests for HIV cDNA at 2 months and 4–6 months are good evidence that the child is not infected. Consider doing two early cDNA assays or HIV cultures (1 and 2 months), as well as at 6 months
2 weeks–6 months	1) Maternal HIV status unknown	HIV serology (mother and infant)	Immediate	If positive, proceed to next step to determine whether the child is infected in addition to being at risk for HIV
	2) Mother HIV-infected	HIV cDNA and/or culture	Initial visit, 4–6 months old	Consider doing two cDNA tests 4 weeks apart, then one at more than 6 months of age
6–15 months	1) Maternal HIV status unknown	HIV serology[b] (mother and infant)	Immediate	If HIV serology on mother or infant is positive, proceed to next step
	2) Mother HIV infected	HIV serology and HIV cDNA or culture	Once immediately; repeat every 3 months until negative	Children whose HIV serology is going to revert to negative will do so at a median of 10 months old. Perform cDNA testing or culture initially to identify the child who might need PCP prophylaxis or antiretroviral treatment. If HIV serology does not revert to negative by 15–18 months old, the child is HIV infected
> 15 months	All at-risk children	HIV serology	Once as a screen; twice if confirmation needed	HIV serology will suffice at more than 15 months old, because a positive assay means that the child is HIV infected. To avoid lab. errors, in a high-risk child a repeat assay may be worthwhile, regardless of first assay's result

[a]cDNA: complementary DNA; detection of HIV cDNA in the infant following polymerase chain reaction amplification from peripheral blood mononuclear cells.
[b]Combination screening and confirmatory testing (e.g. ELISA followed by western blot).

Diagnosis of HIV infection in infants

The detection of HIV infection in an individual older than 15 months is a straightforward process, since antibody detection by combined enzyme-linked immunosorbent assay (ELISA) and western blot is both sensitive and specific (see also Chapter 4) (Rogers *et al.*, 1994). Unfortunately, in younger children the utility of antibody-based diagnostic tests is vitiated by the presence of transplacentally acquired maternal antibodies. Antibody assays can determine whether an infant was exposed to HIV *in utero*, but cannot separate the 'at risk' infant from the infected one. Whether newborns are infected or not is determined using one of several strategies; detection of virus-specific proteins in serum (generally the major capsid protein, p24), or finding virus-specific genetic sequences (in RNA or

DNA) in plasma or peripheral blood mononuclear cells. These techniques vary in their cost, their sensitivity, and in the time it takes to obtain a result (see Chapter 4).

Because infants exposed to HIV *in utero* are HIV sero-positive but have indeterminate HIV infection status, they have been given a specific CDC classification, category 'E' (for exposed) (Centers for Disease Control, 1994c). In the previous terminology, indeterminate children were category 'P–0', as opposed to the 'P–1' children, who had mild symptoms of HIV disease and 'P–2' children with more serious manifestations.

Tests for HIV infection
Detection of HIV antibodies
The validity of antibody-based HIV assays depends on the fact that an adult or child will make specific anti-HIV antibodies only when they are HIV infected. However, as IgG antibodies are transferred across the placenta from mother to fetus during pregnancy, a newborn child will have most of the IgG antibody types his mother possessed at the time of birth. Unfortunately, it is generally not possible to know whether the antibodies found in an infant less than 15 months old were endogenously produced in response to HIV infection or were transplacentally acquired.

The most widely used antibody detection technique is the ELISA. ELISA assays are very sensitive (> 99%), and rarely yield false-positive tests after the first 15 months of life (Rogers *et al.*, 1994), although repeatedly positive ELISA tests are always confirmed using a second category of antibody detection assays, most commonly a western blot (see Chapter 4). A few children will have a negative ELISA and persistently indeterminate western blot results, with one or more bands that which do not meet the diagnostic criteria for positive. If at low risk, these patients are almost certainly not infected (Jackson *et al.*, 1990). If the child has clinical symptoms suggesting a high risk of HIV infection, an indeterminate western blot may be a stage in transition to positive.

Antigen detection
HIV antigen detection is a relatively inexpensive and rapid test, but unfortunately insensitive. The antigen most commonly assayed is p24 antigen, one of the structural protein components of the virus capsid, which is also found in serum (see Chapter 4). HIV p24 antigen is detected and quantified using an antibody-capture ELISA (see Chapter 4). The sensitivity of the assay has been increased by breaking up p24 immune complexes, the 'immune-complex dis-

sociated' p24 assay (ICD-p24) (Miles *et al.*, 1993). As the overall sensitivity of ICD-p24 detection is 81% in children aged 6 weeks to 13 years (Miles *et al.*, 1993), less sensitive than detection of HIV RNA or DNA, the ICD-p24 is generally considered a second-line diagnostic assay.

HIV culture
The traditional gold standard for the determination of HIV infection status was culture (see Chapter 4). HIV culture has excellent sensitivity in newborns (equivalent to DNA or RNA detection) and also excellent specificity (Bryson *et al.*, 1991; Frenkel *et al.*, 1998). Both HIV culture and nucleic acid detection tests are negative in about 50% of infected newborns (less than 7 days old), probably because virus transmission often occurs perinatally at this time, when virus concentrations are below the level of detection (Borkowsky *et al.*, 1992). The virtues of HIV culture include the ability to perform quantitative assays, to determine certain *in vitro* properties of the virus that correlate with prognosis, and the ability to obtain large amounts of virus for molecular and antiviral resistance studies. The greatest drawbacks of HIV culture are the need for a biohazard containment laboratory (to protect laboratory staff), the length of time until culture becomes positive (as long as 3–4 weeks), and the expense of the technicians and reagents. For these reasons, and because excellent assays to detect and quantitate HIV RNA and DNA are now commercially available, HIV culture is used primarily as a research tool.

Detection of HIV-specific DNA or RNA
HIV genomic RNA and complementary DNA (cDNA, either unintegrated or integrated [proviral] DNA) can be detected and quantitated by several different techniques (see Chapter 4). To detect whether or not an infant is infected, probing for HIV cDNA in peripheral blood mononuclear cells using PCR amplification appears to be the most sensitive test (Rogers *et al.*, 1989). This test has a sensitivity greater than or equal to HIV culture, and is positive in virtually 100% of HIV-infected children after the first month of life (Rogers *et al.*, 1994). The major concern with PCR is false-positive results from contaminating HIV cDNA (Borkowsky *et al.*, 1992), which should not occur if proper laboratory procedures are followed. The tests used to quantitate HIV RNA in plasma may be more sensitive than detection of HIV cDNA, especially in the first 2 weeks after birth, but they are not licenced for diagnosis of HIV infection and false-positive tests do occur (Reisler *et al.*, 2001).

Strategies for diagnosis of HIV infection of infants

When HIV infection in an infant less than 18 months old is being considered, the first step is to determine whether the child is at risk of infection by performing an HIV ELISA and confirmatory western blot on the mother or infant. If either mother or child is seropositive, further evaluations should be performed, as determining whether infants are HIV-infected or not can only be established serologically after they are more than 18 months old or if they have had an AIDS-defining clinical event. At-risk infants should therefore have a test for the presence of HIV cDNA or an HIV culture (see Chapter 4).

While there are no absolute guidelines for diagnostic strategies, most HIV-exposed children should have a culture and/or a test for HIV cDNA performed as soon as possible after birth (Table 9.3). A positive test on a sample obtained within the first 7 days of life is felt to be a poor prognostic sign because it appears to indicate *in utero* infection, and perhaps a larger virus inoculum. Given the poor sensitivity of assays in the first weeks of life, an initial negative test should be repeated at 2–4 weeks of age. Most authorities recommend further re-testing at 2–4 months, and again at 4–5 months or older if negative tests persist. Three negative HIV cultures or tests for HIV cDNA, including at least one at age 4 months or older, is considered adequate evidence that a child is uninfected.

For those children who present at age 18 months or older, the diagnosis of HIV can be made using standard serological testing, by HIV ELISA and western blot. If the child has symptoms consistent with HIV and a negative ELISA, quantitative immunoglobulin concentrations should be obtained to be certain that the child is not hypogammaglobulinaemic, and in this instance testing for HIV cDNA or HIV culture is also warranted. A small proportion of HIV-infected children, particularly those severely affected by the virus, may be ELISA positive but western blot negative (Walter *et al.*, 1990); in this instance, the child should also be tested for the presence of HIV cDNA.

Treatment of HIV infection in children

Paediatric HIV infection is a difficult condition to manage. The disease is complex, manifests itself as more than simple immunosuppression, and often occurs in families ill-equipped to administer medications according to complex schedules. The best approach for patient care is to use a multidisciplinary team able to optimize medical management, minimize psychosocial problems, improve nutrition, and monitor developmental progress. The medical issues are the most straightforward aspect of paediatric HIV care; the psychosocial problems, which have enormous effect, are

Table 9.4 Suggested management of the infant born to an HIV-infected mother

Age	Management
Birth	Complete blood count
	Test for HIV cDNA in peripheral blood (not cord blood)
	Start oral zidovudine (2 mg/kg every 6 h or 2.6 mg/kg every 8 h) within 6–12 h of birth. If the child cannot take medications orally within 24 h, give intravenous zidovudine (1.5 mg/kg intravenously every 6 h) until oral medications are tolerated
2–3 weeks	Complete blood count; repeat HIV cDNA in peripheral blood (particularly if not done at birth)
6 weeks	Complete blood count; discontinue zidovudine if testing fails to detect HIV cDNA
	Start oral trimethoprim-sulfamethoxazole, 75 mg/kg twice daily, three times a week (e.g. on Monday, Wednesday and Friday)[a]
3 months	Complete blood count
4 months	Complete blood count and lymphocyte subset analysis; repeat HIV cDNA in peripheral blood (particularly if not done at birth)[b]
9–12 months	HIV antibody testing if uninfected or of indeterminate HIV status[c]
18 months	HIV antibody testing if uninfected or of indeterminate HIV status

[a]Continue trimethoprim-sulfamethoxazole until 12 months of age if the child is infected or remains of indeterminate status; discontinue if uninfected.

[b]If two HIV cDNA tests are negative (one at more than 1 month and one at more than 4 months of age), lymphocyte subsets are normal for age, and the child has no clinical signs/symptoms of HIV infection, the child is considered uninfected. Trimethoprim-sulfamethoxazole prophylaxis can be discontinued and no further CD4 lymphocyte enumeration is necessary. HIV antibody testing should be performed at 9–12 months and repeated as necessary to document loss of passive maternal antibody, confirming absence of HIV infection.

[c]Two positive HIV cDNA tests (or cultures positive) constitute proof of HIV infection. Trimethoprim-sulfamethoxazole prophylaxis should be continued through the first year of life, and then managed according to the Centres for Disease Control guidelines, based upon the child's CD4 lymphocyte count.

beyond the scope of this text. An approach to the overall management of an infant born to an HIV-infected mother is outlined in Table 9.4.

Up-to-date guidelines for treating HIV-infected children can be found at: http://hivatis.org/trtgdlns.html.

Antiretroviral therapy

The range of drugs available for children is smaller than the spectrum of agents from which physicians for adults can choose (see Chapters 5, 6 and 7). In some cases the compounds are difficult to prepare as liquids or in other formulations suitable for use in infants and children. In other cases, toxicities make it difficult to use the compounds in this age group. For example, it is very difficult to diagnose either peripheral neuropathy or the early symptoms of pancreatitis in a pre-verbal child, both of which are known adverse events with some antiretroviral drugs.

Reverse transcriptase inhibitors

Reverse transcriptase inhibitors (RTIs) can be divided into two broad categories the nucleoside analogue reverse transcriptase inhibitors (NRTIs) and the non-nucleoside reverse transcriptase inhibitors (NNRTIs). The NRTIs are modified nucleosides that take advantage of a relatively high affinity of the virus reverse transcriptase (RT) for certain types of nucleotide modifications. Two of the commonly used NRTIs are derived from thymidine, ZDV and stavudine (SVD). One or the other is used as a foundation for most therapeutic regimens; however, since ZDV inhibits stavudine phosphorylation and thus activation, they should not be used simultaneously (see Chapter 5).

Both ZDV and stavudine are available in liquid and solid preparations and clinical trials support their use in children (McKinney et al., 1991; Kline et al., 1998). They are comparable in their virological effect, typically lowering viral load by 0.5–1.0 $\log_{10}$ RNA when used alone (McKinney, 1996a).

The most common adverse events with ZDV in children are anaemia and neutropenia. Rarely, children may have a ZDV-related myopathy (Morgello et al., 1995), and some children appear to develop a drug-related attention deficit disorder. Nausea, headaches, and fatigue often occur shortly after initiation of ZDV, but usually improve with time. SVD is well tolerated by most children (Kline et al., 1998). There are rare instances of peripheral neuropathy, but this seems less common than in adults. Pancreatitis also occurs rarely.

In a pattern similar to the thymidine analogs, non-thymidine NRTIs such as didanosine (ddI), lamivudine (3TC), and zalcitabine (ddC), are generally not given in combination with each other. The non-thymidine NRTIs are typically combined with ZDV or SVD.

3TC is available as a liquid or tablet. While lamivudine is moderately potent as monotherapy, high-level resistance develops with a single-point mutation at RT codon 184 (Kuritzkes et al., 1996). When combined with ZDV in HIV-infected children, 3TC therapy accelerates normal growth and prevents disease progression (McKinney et al., 1998). 3TC is generally very well tolerated, with few adverse events. Pancreatitis, suggested by some early case reports, has not proved to be a significant problem.

ddI is acid labile and thus must be given in combination with antacids. The absorption of ddI may also be improved if it is taken with the stomach empty (at least 2 h after the last meal), although the marginal increase in absorption should be weighed against the effect of avoiding mealtimes on compliance. The paediatric suspension is usually dissolved in a liquid antacid like Maalox®, although tablets that can be dissolved in water are also available. The suspension must be kept refrigerated, and the shelf life is relatively short (approximately 4 weeks).

ddI has proved to be a potent nucleoside, with virological and clinical effects comparable to combination nucleosides (for example, Paediatric ACTG Study 152; Englund et al., 1997). ddI is generally well tolerated, although adverse events such as peripheral neuropathy and pancreatitis can occur. The pancreatitis is typically symptomatic, with elevations in both serum amylase and lipase. It should be noted that many HIV-infected children also have elevated serum amylase concentrations related to salivary gland inflammation, so that increased amylase concentrations should be further evaluated with a fractionated amylase (to separate pancreatic and salivary isoenzymes), or by confirming the presence or absence of pancreatitis with a serum lipase determination. Salivary inflammation does not generally lead to an increased serum lipase, while pancreatic inflammation does.

ddC is only commercially available in capsules. Its virological effects are similar to ddI, and there is a high degree of cross-resistance between the two compounds. ddC monotherapy in antiretroviral-experienced children led to improved weight gain (Spector et al., 1997). ddC has also been studied in combination with ZDV producing a modest rise in CD4 lymphocyte counts (Bakshi et al., 1997).

The most common adverse events of zalcitabine are peripheral neuropathy and oral ulcers.

The most recently developed nucleoside has been abacavir (ABC). This drug appears to be very potent as first-line therapy of HIV infection in children, but is less effective as secondary therapy (Kline et al., 1999). The primary side-effect has been a hypersensitivity reaction, usually seen in the first few weeks of ABC use. The reaction presents with manifestations including fever, abdominal pain, headache, hepatitis, and rash. If a child has these symptoms, the drug should be stopped and not restarted. Serious reactions, including hypotension and death, have occurred on re-challenging patients who had symptoms of ABC hypersensitivity. Rarely, patients have hypersensitivity after stopping and restarting ABC, even without an antecedent hypersensitivity. However, this appears to be quite rare. ABC is available as a capsule or a liquid.

Non-nucleoside reverse transcriptase inhibitors

Two NNRTIs, nevirapine and efavirenz, are licensed for paediatric use (see Chapters 5, 6 and 7). Only nevirapine is available as a liquid preparation. As NNRTI resistance develops very quickly when the drugs are used as monotherapy (Richman et al., 1994), they must always be used in combinations. In addition, as there appears to be extensive cross-resistance among NNRTIs, switching from one NNRTI to another will seldom be useful if antiretroviral failure was due to drug resistance.

Nevirapine has been evaluated in combination with NRTIs in children and has shown beneficial effects (Luzuriaga et al., 1996). Although it may be less potent than protease inhibitors (PIs), comparative studies have not been performed.

The two major problems with nevirapine are rash and hepatitis. Patients who develop a severe macular rash, especially if it is associated with fever, should generally stop nevirapine, as this early rash can progress into a life-threatening Stevens–Johnson syndrome. The incidence of rash appears to be the same in children and adults. Hepatitis occurs most frequently early during nevirapine administration, but can appear at any point during therapy.

Clinical experience with efavirenz in children is relatively limited. However, it appears to be an effective alternative to PIs, and has also been used effectively in combination with them (Kahn et al., 1998). The drug has a very long half-life and can be administered once daily. The major side-effect of efavirenz has been rash, which is probably more common in children than adults. In most cases, the efavirenz rash will fade if the drug is continued. Some children have sleep disturbances and behavioural problems during efavirenz administration (Teglas et al., 2001).

Protease inhibitors

PIs have been developed relatively slowly for children. They are difficult to formulate into palatable liquid preparations, and the pharmacokinetics of PIs in children appear to be disadvantageous when compared to adults. The capsule forms of several agents are large, soft-gel preparations, which exceed the size (and dose) a child can swallow.

Nelfinavir is the most widely used PI in children, as it is available as both capsules and as a granular powder, which allows size-adjusted dosing in children. The initial pharmacokinetic studies of nelfinavir suggested a dosage range of 25–30 mg/kg/dose every 8 h. However, more recent studies indicate that a higher dose should be used, especially in young children, and some physicians are using doses in the range 40–55 mg/kg/dose every 12 h.

Although nelfinavir-containing combination antiretroviral regimens reduce viral load to undetectable levels in some children, the proportion achieving this goal is less than in adults. The relatively poor success in children is probably related to low compliance with complex dosing regimens, unfavourable pharmacology, and the higher viral loads with which most children begin (Martel et al., 1998). The major side-effect of nelfinavir is diarrhoea, which is generally manageable using symptomatic therapy with anti-diarrhoeal agents. The powder is somewhat difficult to use, and many children dislike its gritty taste.

Ritonavir is approved for children in the USA, and has proved to be clinically effective (Mueller et al., 1998). Unfortunately, ritonavir is a difficult drug to use, with a vile-tasting liquid preparation and numerous side-effects. The liquid is 43% ethanol, which in and of itself makes it difficult for children (or their parents) to tolerate. Side-effects include nausea, chemical hepatitis, elevated serum lipid concentrations, peri-oral paresthesias, and numerous drug interactions. All these problems are similar to those seen in ritonavir-treated adults. Ritonavir soft-gel capsules are relatively large and difficult for a child to swallow.

Indinavir is also difficult to use in children because there is no liquid preparation. Older children can be treated with capsules, although it appears that clearance of the drug may be more rapid in children than in adults. The side-effect profile is similar to that in adults: nephrolithiasis, elevated liver function tests, occasional hyperbilirubinaemia, and numerous drug interactions.

There is little experience with saquinavir in children, since the introduction of the relatively large but well-absorbed soft-gel capsules.

Amprenavir has unique resistance pattern, which gives it some limited utility when other PIs have failed (Church *et al.*, 2000). However, the capsules are large and and liquid somewhat unpalatable. The liquid is also only suitable for children 3 years and older.

Lopinavir is available as a combination with ritoavir. It has the advantage of a unique resistance pattern and a liquid preparation. The gel cap preparation for older children and adults is quite large and difficult to swallow. There is little published to date on lopinavir use in children.

Antiretroviral treatment strategies in children

Considerable controversy exists about when to start antiretroviral drugs in children (McKinney, 1996b), although consensus guidelines have been published (Centers for Disease Control and Prevention, 1998b). Most of the controlled data comes from adult studies, which cannot be confidently extrapolated to paediatric patients. There are several important differences between paediatric and adult HIV disease that make such extrapolation tenuous. Children are more likely than adults to have central nervous system (CNS) involvement and HIV has different effects on a growing immune system than a mature one. Finally, perinatally transmitted paediatric disease appears to be more aggressive than adult HIV disease (Scott *et al.*, 1989; Shearer *et al.*, 1997).

Treatment of adults during 'primary infection', the time immediately after HIV inoculation, appears to be beneficial (Rosenberg *et al.*, 1997). However, adults are rarely aware of their disease in time for early therapy. In contrast, infants infected with HIV have only been infected for a few months and thus can be treated at a time when virus dissemination is less well established. Consequently, many specialists believe all infected infants should be started on antiviral therapy as soon as they are identified. While this hypothesis has not yet been clinically verified, there is supporting animal model data. The difficulty comes in trying to persuade a family to treat their infant, who appears perfectly healthy, with a complex and rigid regimen, including several poorly tolerated medications.

There are thus two approaches most often used in the decision about whether to treat an HIV-infected child with antiretroviral therapy. If a child is known to be HIV-infected in the first few months of life, early treatment is justified. The infected child is at high risk of progression, and laboratory tests are of little prognostic value (because all HIV-infected newborns have a high viral load). If the child is more than 3–6 months old at the time that HIV infection is first diagnosed, there are no data on which to base a recommendation about when to start treatment. However, all children should be treated before they reach the threshold where pneumocystis prophylaxis is warranted, and most paediatric infectious disease specialists will begin therapy as soon as Centres for Disease Control and Prevention immunological category 2 or CDC clinical category B or C is reached (Centers for Disease Control and Prevention, 1994c, 1998b).

When antiretroviral therapy is started, combinations of drugs must be given, as it is no longer appropriate to initiate monotherapy (see Chapter 7). While there are only limited data, as a nucleoside base for a regimen, ZDV/ddI appears to be similar to ZDV/zalcitabine. ZDV/lamivudine is probably equal to ZDV/didanosine (and is less toxic) (McKinney *et al.*, 1998) and combinations of either ddI or 3TC with stavudine are probably comparable to ZDV-containing regimens. Most paediatricians begin children on a three-drug regimen containing two NRTIs and either a PI or NNRTI, as is currently the practice in adults. Some practitioners believe that a four-drug regimen will be more effective than one containing three drugs, particularly in young infants with their high initial viral loads. However, compliance is a serious problem for most families, especially those with infants, and if the family is non-compliant with a four-drug regimen, future therapeutic options will be severely limited. We therefore do not recommend initiating therapy with four-drug antiretroviral regimens except in very unusual circumstances, as defined by a multi-disciplinary team. Thus, selection of children suitable for treatment with a complex antiretroviral regimen is difficult and should usually involve a multi-disciplinary team.

Immunoprophylaxis of opportunistic infections

HIV-infected children are predisposed to recurrent bacterial infections. In order to reduce the number of infections, some clinicians use monthly infusions of intravenous immunoglobulin (IVIG). Two controlled studies address the utility of this therapy, which is very expensive in many countries (Mofenson *et al.*, 1992; Spector *et al.*, 1994). The first trial began at a time when neither antiretroviral therapy nor PCP prophylaxis were routinely provided. During the study many children were started on ZDV and trimethoprim-sulfamethoxazole. Although children with CD4 lymphocyte counts above 200 cells/μl who received IVIG had fewer bacterial infections and fewer recurrences of certain viral infections than the control group, there was no effect on survival. In order to address the additive effect of ZDV and trimethoprim-sulfamethoxazole on bacterial infections, another study of IVIG (AIDS Clinical Trials Group Protocol 051) was performed (Spector et al., 1994). While there were fewer bacterial infections in the IVIG group, the benefit was not large, and there was no beneficial effect of IVIG in children who received trimethoprim-sulfamethoxazole. Given its considerable cost in the USA (more than US$1000/month) and limited benefit, IVIG should probably be reserved for children with a history of recurrent bacterial infections in spite of trimethoprim-sulfamethoxazole prophylaxis.

Chemoprophylaxis of opportunistic infections

Probably the single most effective therapeutic intervention for HIV-infected children has been the introduction of prophylaxis for PCP. Since PCP is most common in children less than 8 months old, prophylaxis needs to be started early in infancy. Guidelines regarding the timing and method of PCP prophylaxis have been published (Grubman and Simonds, 1996).

All HIV-infected infants should be started on trimethoprim-sulfamethoxazole when they are 4–6 weeks old and their peripartum ZDV prophylaxis has ended. They should remain on PCP prophylaxis until the child is proved not to be infected by HIV. If the child is infected, they should remain on prophylaxis for at least 1 year. The original Centers for Disease Control and Prevention PCP guidelines waited to start prophylaxis until the CD4 lymphocyte count in an infant was less than 1500 cells/μl or less than 20%; however, several children were reported to have PCP at CD4 lymphocyte counts above those levels, making the broader use of PCP prophylaxis desirable. Trimethoprim-sulfamethoxazole is inexpensive, easy to administer and has a low rate of toxicity at the doses used for prophylaxis.

HIV-infected children between 1 and 5 years old with a CD4 lymphocyte count of less than 500 cells/μl or with CD4 lymphocytes less than 15% of total lymphocytes should receive PCP prophylaxis, as should children older than 6 years with lymphocyte counts of less than

200 cells/μl, proportions of less than 15%. Any child who has had PCP, regardless of their CD4 lymphocyte count, should remain on lifelong PCP prophylaxis (see Chapter 25).

If a child does not tolerate trimethoprim-sulfamethoxazole, the alternatives are much less appealing (see Chapter 25). In young children (less than 4 years of age), the most useful option is dapsone (1–2 mg/kg/day administered once daily [not to exceed 100 mg]). There is little doubt that dapsone is less effective than trimethoprim-sulfamethoxazole, and that breakthrough PCP is more common. A second alternative is pentamidine, which can be given as an aerosol to those children who are old enough to breathe deeply on command (300 mg via nebulizer), or as an intravenous infusion (4 mg/kg every 3–4 weeks). There is no proof that the latter approach works in children, although it is been effective in adults (see Chapter 25), and it is virtually the only option available for those children who have allergies to both trimethoprim-sulfamethoxazole and dapsone (unfortunately, a common overlap). Atovaqone also has potential, but at present there are no completed clinical studies of prophylactic atovoquone.

Children with HIV infection have an increased rate of bacterial infections, both serious and minor. Antiretroviral prophylaxis may have a role in limiting the number and severity of such infections. The most commonly used antimicrobial for prophylaxis in HIV-infected patients is trimethoprim-sulfamethoxazole, since it is already being administered for PCP prevention. While no controlled studies have specifically addressed the efficacy of trimethoprim-sulfamethoxazole for this purpose in children, the large ACTG trial of PCP prophylaxis in adults showed a reduction in bacterial infections in the trimethoprim-sulfonamide-treated group (see Chapter 25). In children, the ACTG trial of IVIG and ZDV (ACTG 051) gave indirect evidence of benefit (Spector et al., 1997). IVIG prophylaxis produced no reduction in the rate of bacterial infections in children who were on trimethoprim-sulfamethoxazole at the beginning of the study, while it did reduce the infection rate in those who were not initially on trimethoprim-sulfamethoxazole (Spector et al., 1997).

Another bacterial infection which may warrant antimicrobial prophylaxis in children is Mycobacterium avium complex (MAC). This infection occurs only in the late stages of HIV infection, and can produce fever, fatigue, weight loss, anaemia and neutropenia (see also Chapter 24). Studies in adults have demonstrated that prophylaxis with rifabutin, azithromycin or clarithromycin decreases the rate of symptomatic MAC disease by 50% (see Chapter 25 and Mofenson, 1998). However, rifabutin has many adverse reactions including uveitis, hepatitis, anorexia, and neutropenia, and alters metabolism of many other medicines including PIs (see Chapters 5 and 24). Azithromycin is more popular for prophylaxis as there are fewer drug interactions and adverse reactions and it can be given once weekly (see Chapter 25). The experience with prophylaxis in children is very limited, and no rigorous trials have been conducted.

Supportive therapies

Anaemia and neutropenia are commonly observed in HIV-infected children (see Chapter 17). These haematological findings may be produced by HIV infection itself, as an adverse outcome of drug therapy (e.g. with ZDV), or as a consequence of superinfections by bone marrow-tropic agents such as parvovirus B-19 and MAC. Although chronic anaemia can be treated with transfusions such therapy carries the risk of blood-borne infections, especially hepatitis C virus.

Chronic anaemia is best treated with recombinant erythropoietin. Although erythopoietin is safe, it is also very expensive, and 25–50% of patients still require periodic transfusions. Erythopoietin must be given subcutaneously several days each week. It is a reasonable option for patients with chronic anaemia, particularly those who have ZDV-related anaemia and for whom other NRTIs are not an option. ZDV-related anaemia may also respond to decreasing the ZDV dose, typically by increments of 30%, changing PCP prophylaxis to a drug other than trimethoprim-sulfamethoxazole or dapsone, or treatment of superinfections (parvovirus with IVIG, MAC with a combination of antimycobacterial drugs).

Neutropenia is also a common problem in HIV-infected children and it often responds to granulocyte colony stimulating factor (G-CSF) (see Chapter 17). The usual dose is 1–20 μg/kg/day as a single subcutaneous injection. Therapy should begin at the low end of the dosage range, with increases as needed. As G-CSF is expensive, it is worth first lowering ZDV or trimethoprim-sulfamethoxazole doses (or substituting equivalent drugs without bone marrow toxicity), to determine whether they may be the cause of the neutropenia.

Nutrition

HIV-infected children do not grow at a normal rate (McKinney et al., 1993; Moye et al., 1996). HIV infection produces a growth delay that affects both height and weight within a few months of birth. However, because the effect is comparable for both height and weight, these children generally have an appropriate weight for height. Only in the late stages of HIV disease do children become lean (i.e. have a low weight-for-height).

Early in the course of HIV infection, all that is usually required to ensure adequate nutrition and weight gain is a reasonable emphasis on an appropriate, balanced diet. There is no point in constructing rigid dietary plans, since children are unlikely to comply.

The issue of dietary supplements for HIV-infected children is unresolved. While there are advocates for formulas containing 24 calories/30 ml, (instead of the standard 20 calories/ml), no evidence yet exists for their benefit. Children in the late stages of HIV disease are often given nutritional supplements such as Ensure® and Sustacal® (see Chapter 18). While these can help to provide a balanced diet, their main advantage is the ease with which they can be swallowed. Some children are fed via a nasogastric or gastrostomy tube, but this drastic step has its cost, particularly in quality of life for the child. Intravenous nutrition is primarily indicated as temporary support for a child with an acute gastrointestinal problem, as chronic total parenteral nutrition (TPN) is very expensive, and requires placement of a central venous access line with its attendant complications. Appetite stimulants such as Megace® (megestrol acelate) and Periactin® may increase oral intake and produce some growth. Unfortunately, in late-stage HIV disease almost all interventions increase body fat rather than lean body mass, making their utility marginal.

Effective antiretroviral therapy and aggressive treatment of opportunistic infections are probably the single most important determinants of optimal growth. In the future, recombinant growth hormone may prove to have a role. Preliminary studies in adults have shown improved lean body mass and few side-effects. Since the growth pattern in HIV-infected children appears to be a growth delay, growth hormone may be particularly useful in small, HIV-infected children.

Management of HIV cardiomyopathy

Cardiomyopathy is a frequent complication of HIV in children, which often manifests itself as an acute deterioration in cardiac function (see Chapter 15). While some children ultimately recover completely, most are left with some residual cardiac dysfunction. No single therapeutic strategy can be used, but most patients will respond to a combination of digoxin, an after load-reduction agent such as enalopril, and diuretics.

Summary

The management of paediatric HIV infection is complex because of the nature of the disease. Effective antiretroviral therapy must be combined with a holistic approach, which considers the overall picture, especially the global functioning and quality of life of the child and their family. The next few years will almost certainly show improvements in the range of antiretroviral drugs available, a better understanding of how to use these agents, and more options for the prophylaxis of opportunistic infections.

References

Auger I, Thomas P, DeGruttola V et al. (1998). Incubation periods for paediatric AIDS patients. Nature 336: 575–7.

Bakshi SS, Britto P, Capparelli E et al. (1997). Evaluation of pharmacokinetics, safety, tolerance and activity of combination of zalcitabine and zidovudine in stable, zidovudine-treated paediatric patients with human immunodeficiency virus infection. J Infect Dis 175: 1039–50.

Bertolli J, St Louis ME, Simonds RJ et al. (1996). Estimating the timing of mother-to-child transmission of human immunodeficiency virus in the breast feeding population in Kinshasa, Zaire. J Infect Dis 174: 722–6.

Bigger RJ, Miotti PG, Taha TE et al. (1996). Perinatal intervention trial in Africa; effect of birth canal cleansing intervention to prevent HIV transmission. Lancet 347: 1647–50.

Borkowsky W, Krasinski K, Pollack H et al. (1992). Early diagnosis of human immunodeficiency virus infection in children less than 6 months of age. Comparison of polymerase chain reaction, culture, and plasma antigen capture techniques. J Infect Dis 166: 616–9.

Bryson YJ (1996). Perinatal HIV-1 transmission. Recent advances and therapeutic interventions. AIDS 3: S33–42.

Bryson Y, Chen I, Miles S et al. (1991). A prospective evaluation of HIV co-culture for early diagnosis of perinatal HIV infection. In: Proceedings and abstracts. VII International Conference on AIDS, Florence, Italy.

Bryson YJ, Luzuriaga K, Sullivan JL et al. (1992). Proposed definitions for in utero versus intrapartum transmission of HIV-1. N Engl J Med 327: 1246–7.

Bryson YJ, Pang S, Wei LS et al. (1995). Clearance of HIV infection in a perinatally infected infant. N Engl J Med 332: 833–8.

Cao Y, Krogstad P, Korber TB et al. (1997). Maternal HIV-1 viral load and vertical transmission. Nat Med 3: 549–52.

Centers for Disease Control and Prevention. (1994a). Recommendations of the US Public Health Service Task Force on the use of zidovudine to reduce perinatal transmission of human immunodeficiency virus. MMWR 43: 1–20.

Centers for Disease Control and Prevention. (1994b). Zidovudine for the prevention of HIV transmission from mother to infant. MMWR 43: 285–7.

Centers for Disease Control and Prevention. (1994c). Revised classification system for HIV infection in children less than 13 years of age. MMWR 43: 1–10.

Centers for Disease Control and Prevention. (1995). Update. AIDS among women – United States, MMWR 44: 81–4.

Centers for Disease Control and Prevention. (1997). Update. Perinatally acquired HIV/AIDS – United States. MMWR 46: 1086–92.

Centers for Disease Control and Prevention. (1998a). Administration of zidovudine during late pregnancy and delivery to prevent perinatal HIV transmission – Thailand, 1995–1998. MMWR 47: 151–4.

Centers for Disease Control and Prevention. (1998b). Guidelines for the use of antiretroviral agents in paediatric HIV infection. MMWR 47: 1–43.

Centers for Disease Control and Prevention. (1998c). Success in implementing public health service guidelines to reduce perinatal transmission of HIV. MMWR 47: 688–91.

Chotpitayasunondh T, Vanprar N, Simonds RJ et al. (2001). Safety of in utero exposure to zidovudine in infants born to HIV-infected mothers: Bangkok. Pediatrics 107: E5.

Church J, Rathore M, Rubio R et al. (2000). A phase III study of amprenavir (APV, Agenerase™) in protease-inhibitor-naïve and -experienced HIV-infected children and adolescents. In: Program and abstracts of the seventh conference on retroviruses and opportunistic infections, San Francisco, January–February 2000.

Connor EM, Sperling RS, Gelber R et al. (1994). Reduction of maternal infant transmission of human immunodeficiency virus type 1 with zidovudine treatment. Results of AIDS clinical trials group protocol 076. N Engl J Med 331: 1173–80.

Daar ES, Moudgil T, Meyer RD et al. (1991). Transient high levels of viraemia in patients with primary human immunodeficiency virus type 1 infection. N Engl J Med 324: 961–4.

Dabis F, Msellati P, Meda N et al. (1999). Six month efficacy, tolerance, and acceptability of a short regimen or oral zidovudine to reduce vertical transmission of HIV in breast fed children in Cote di Voire and Burkina Faso: a double blind placebo-controlled multicentre trial. Lancet 353: 786–92.

Dickover RE, Garratty EM, Herman SA et al. (1996). Identification of levels of maternal HIV-1 RNA associated with risk of perinatal transmission. Effect of maternal zidovudine treatment on viral load. JAMA 275: 599–605.

Duliege AM, Amos CI, Felton S et al. (1995). Birth order, delivery route, and concordance in the transmission of human immunodeficiency virus type 1 from mothers to twins. J Pediatr 126: 625–32.

Dunn DT, Newell ML, Ades ME et al. (1992). Risk of HIV-1 transmission through breast feeding. Lancet 340: 585–8.

Englund JA, Baker CJ, Raskino C et al. (1997). Zidovudine, didanosine or both as the initial treatment for symptomatic HIV-infected children. N Engl J Med 336: 1704–12.

European Collaborative Study. (1991). Children born to women with HIV-1 infection. Natural history and risk of transmission. Lancet 337: 253–60.

Fauci AS. (1993). Multifactorial nature of human immunodeficiency virus disease. Implications for therapy. *Science* **262**: 1011–8.

Frenkel LM, Mullins JI, Learn GH *et al.* (1998). Genetic evaluation of suspected cases of transient HIV-1 infection of infants. *Science* **280**: 1073–7.

Gabiano C, Tovo PA, deMartino M *et al.* (1992). Mother to child transmission of human immunodeficiency virus type 1. Risk of infection and correlates of transmission. *Pediatrics* **90**: 369–74.

Garcia PM, Kalish LA, Pitt J *et al.* (1999). Maternal levels of plasma human immunodeficiency virus type 1 RNA and the risk of perinatal transmission. *N Engl J Med* **341**: 394.

Gershon AA, Mervish N, LaRussa P *et al.* (1997). Varicella-zoster virus infection in children with underlying human immunodeficiency virus infection. *J Infect Dis* **176**: 1496–500.

Gray LA, Musoke P, Fleming T *et al.* (1999). Intrapartum and neonatal single dose nevirapine compared with zidovudine for prevention of mother-to-child transmission of HIV-1 in Kampala, Uganda; HIVNET 012 randomised trial. *Lancet* **354**: 795–802.

Grubman S, Simonds RJ. (1996). Preventing *Pneumocystis carinii* pneumonia in human immunodeficiency virus infected children, new guidelines for prophylaxis. *Ped Infect Dis* **15**: 165–8.

Ionnidis JP, Abrams EJ, Ammann A *et al.* (2001). Perinatal transmission of HIV-1 by pregnant women with RNA virus loads <1000 copies/ml. *J Infect Dis* **183**: 539.

International Perinatal HIV Group. (1999). The mode of delivery and the risk of vertical transmission of human immunodeficiency virus type 1. A meta-analysis of 15 prospective cohort studies. *N Engl J Med* **340**: 877–89.

Jackson JB, MacDonald KL, Caldwell J *et al.* (1990). Absence of HIV infection in blood donors with indeterminate western blot tests for antibody to HIV-1. *N Engl J Med* **322**: 217.

John GC, Kreiss J. (1996). Mother to child transmission of human immunodeficiency virus type 1. *Epidemiol. Rev* **18**: 149–57.

Kahn J, Mayers D, Riddler S *et al.* (1998). Durable clinical anti-HIV-1 activity (60 weeks) and tolerability for efavirenz (DMP 266) in combination with indinavir (IDV) suppression to 'less 1 copy/ml' (OD = background) by Amplicor as a predictor of virologic treatment response [DMP 266-003, cohort IV]. In: *Program and abstracts of the Fifth Conference on Retroviruses and Opportunistic Infections*, Chicago, IL, USA.

Kalish LA, Pitt J, Lew J *et al.* (1997). Defining the time of fetal or perinatal acquisition of human immunodeficiency virus type 1 infection on the basis of age at first positive culture. *J Infect Dis* **175**: 712–5.

Kline MW, Van Dyke RB, Lindsey JC *et al.* (1998). A randomized comparative trial of stavudine (d4T) versus zidovudine (ZDV, AZT) in children with human immunodeficiency virus infection. *Pediatrics* **101**: 214–20.

Kline MW, Blanchard S, Fletcher CV *et al.* (1999). AIDS Clinical Trials Group 330 Team. *Pediatrics* **103**: URL: http://www.pediatrics.org/cgi/content/full/103/4/e47.

Kuritzkes DR, Quinn JB, Benoit SL *et al.* (1996). Drug resistance and virologic response in NUCA 3001, a randomized trial of lamivudine (3TC) versus zidovudine (ZDV) versus ZDV plus 3TC in previously untreated patients. *AIDS* **10**: 975–81.

Landesman SH, Kalish LA, Burns DN *et al.* (1996). Obstetrical factors and the transmission of human immunodeficiency virus type 1 from mother to child. *N Engl J Med* **334**: 1617–23.

Leroy V, Newell ML, Dabis F *et al.* (1998). Late postnatal mother-to-child transmission of HIV-1: international multicentre pooled analysis. *The Twelfth World AIDS Conference*, Geneva, Switzerland.

Leroy V, Montcho L, Manigart O *et al.* (2001). Maternal viral load, zidovudine and mother-to-child transmission of HIV-1 in Africa. *AIDS* **15**: 517–22.

Luzuriaga K, Sullivan JL. (1998). Prevention and treatment of paediatric HIV infection. *JAMA* **280**: 17–8.

Luzuriaga K, Bryson Y, McSherry G *et al.* (1996). Pharmacokinetics, safety and activity of nevirapine in human immunodeficiency virus type 1 infected children. *J Infect Dis* **174**: 713–21.

Mandelbrot L, Landreau-Mascaro A, Rekacewicz C *et al.* (2001). Lamivudine-zidovudine combination for prevention of maternal–infant transmission of HIV-1. *JAMA* **285**: 2083–93.

Mandelbrot L, Mayaux MJ, Bongain A *et al.* (1996). Obstetric factors and mother-to-child transmission of human immunodeficiency virus type 1. The French perinatal cohorts. *Am J Obstet Gynecol* **175**: 661–7.

Martel L, Valentine M, Ferguson L *et al.* (1998). Virologic and CD4 response to treatment with nelfinavir in therapy experienced but protease inhibitor naive HIV-infected children. In: *Program and abstracts of the Fifth Conference on Retroviruses and Opportunistic Infections*, Chicago, IL, USA.

McKinney RE. (1996a). Antiretroviral therapy. Evaluating the new era in HIV treatment. *Adv Pediatr Infect Dis* **12**: 297–323.

McKinney RE. (1996b). Use of antiretroviral therapy in children and pregnant women. *Adv Exp Med Biol* **394**: 345–54.

McKinney RE, Maha MA, Connor EM *et al.* (1991). A multicenter trial of oral zidovudine in children with advanced human immunodeficiency virus disease. *N Engl J Med* **324**: 1018–25.

McKinney RE, Robertson JWR, Duke Pediatric AIDS Clinical Trials Unit. (1993). The effect of human immunodeficiency virus infection on the growth of young children. *J Pediatr* **123**: 579–82.

McKinney RE, Johnson GM, Stanley K *et al.* (1998). A randomized study of combined zidovudine-lamivudine versus didanosine monotherapy in children with symptomatic therapy-naive HIV-1 infection. *J Pediatr* **133**: 500–8.

Miles SA, Balden E, Magpantay L *et al.* (1993). Rapid serologic testing with immune complex-dissociated HIV p24 antigen for early detection of HIV infection in neonates. *N Engl J Med* **328**: 297.

Miotti PG, Taha ET, Kumwenda NJ *et al.* (1999). HIV transmission through breast feeding. *JAMA* **282**: 744–9.

Mofenson LM. (1998). Rifabutin. *Ped Infect Dis J* **17**: 71–2.

Mofenson LM, Moye J, Bethel J *et al.* (1992). Prophylactic intravenous immunoglobulin in HIV-infected children with CD4+ counts of 0.20 × 10⁹/L or more. Effect on viral, opportunistic and bacterial infections. *JAMA* **268**: 483–8.

Mofenson LM, Lambert JS, Stiehm ER *et al.* (1999). Risk factors for perinatal transmission of human immunodeficiencyvirus type 1 in women treated with zidovudine. *N Engl J Med* **341**: 385.

Morgello S, Wolfe D, Godfrey E *et al.* (1995). Mitochondrial abnormalities in human immunodeficiency virus associated myopathy. *Acta Neuropathologica* **90**: 366–74.

Moye J, Rich KC, Kalish LA *et al.* (1996). Natural history of somatic growth in infants born to women infected by human immunodeficiency virus. *J Pediatr* **128**: 58–69.

Mueller BU, Nelson RP, Sleasman J et al. (1998). A phase I/II study of the protease inhibitor ritonavir in children with human immunodeficiency virus infection. *Pediatrics* **101**: 335–43.

Oxtoby MJ. (1994). Vertically acquired HIV infection in the United States. In: PA Pizzo, CM Wilfert (eds.). *Pediatric AIDS. The challenge of HIV infection in infants, children and adolescents.* 2nd edition. Baltimore, MD: Williams and Wilkins, 3–20.

Palumbo PE, Kwok S, Waters S et al. (1995). Viral measurement by polymerase chain reaction-based assays in human immunodeficiency virus-infected infants. *J Pediatr* **126**: 592–5.

Patterson BK, Bebbahani H, Kabat WJ et al. (2001). Leukemia inhibits HIV-1 replication and is upregulated in placentae from non-transmitting women. *J Clin Invest* **107**: 287–94.

Pediatric ACTG *Protocol 185 executive summary.* (1997). Bethesda, MD: National Institute of Child Health and Human Development, NIH.

Pikora CA, Sullivan JL, Panicali D et al. (1997). Early HIV-1 envelope-specific cytotoxic T lymphocyte responses in vertically infected infants. *J Exp Med* **185**: 1153–61.

Pitt J, Brambilla D, Reichelderfer P et al. (1997). Maternal immunologic and virologic risk factors for infant human immunodeficiency virus type 1 infection. Findings from the Woman and Infants Transmission Study. *J Infect Dis* **175**: 567–75.

Raton JA, Pocheville I, Vicente JM et al. (1997). Disseminated Bacillus Calmette-Guerin infection in an HIV-infected child; a case with cutaneous lesion. *Pediatr Dermatol* **14**: 365–8.

Reisler RB, Thea DM, Pliner V et al. (2001). Early detection of reverse transcriptase activity in plasma of neonates infected with HIV-1: a comparative analysis of RNA-based and DNA-based testing using PCR. *J Acquir Immune Defic Syndr* **26**: 93–102.

Richman DD, Havlir D, Corbeil J et al. (1994). Nevirapine resistance mutations of human immunodeficiency virus type 1 selected during therapy. *J Virol* **68**: 1660–6.

Rogers MF, Ou CY, Rayfield M et al. (1989). Use of the polymerase chain reaction for early detection of the proviral sequences of human immunodeficiency virus in infants born to seropositive mothers. *N Engl J Med* **320**: 1649.

Rogers MF, Schochetman G, Hoff R. (1994). Advances in diagnosis of HIV infection in infants. In: PA Pizzo, CM Wilfert. *The Challenge of HIV infection in infants, children and adolescents.* 2nd edition. Baltimore, MD: Williams and Wilkins.

Rosenberg ES, Billingsley JM, Caliendo AM et al. (1997). Vigorous HIV-1-specific CD4+ T cell responses associated with control of viraemia. *Science* **278**: 1447–50.

Scott GB, Hutto C, Makuch RW et al. (1989). Survival in children with perinatally acquired human immunodeficiency virus type 1 infection. *N Engl J Med* **321**: 1791

Semprini AE. (1998). An international randomized trial of mode of delivery in HIV infected women. *The Twelfth World AIDS Conference,* Geneva, Switzerland.

Shaffer N, Chuachoowong R, Mock RA et al. (1999). Short-course zidovudine for perinatal HIV-1 transmission in Bangkok, Thailand: a randomized controlled trial. *Lancet* **353**: 773–80.

Shearer WT, Quinn TC, LaRussa P et al. (1997). Viral load and disease progression in infants infected with human immunodeficiency virus type 1. *N Engl J Med* **336**: 1337–42.

Soeiro R, Rubinstein A, Rashbaum WK et al. (1992). Maternofetal transmission of AIDS: frequency of human immunodeficiency virus type 1 nucleic acid sequences in human fetal DNA. *J Infect Dis* **166**: 699–703.

Stoto MA, Almario DA, McCornick MC. (1998). *Reducing the odds. Preventing perinatal transmission of HIV in the United States (Summary).* Washington, DC: National Academy Press [available at: www.nap.edu/readingroom].

Spector SA, Gelber RD, McGrath N et al. (1994). A controlled trial of intravenous immune globulin for the prevention of serious bacterial infections in children receiving zidovudine for advanced human immunodeficiency virus infection. *N Engl J Med* **331**: 1181–7.

Spector SA, Blanchard S, Wara DW et al. (1997). Comparative trial of two dosages of zalcitabine in zidovudine-experienced children with advanced human immunodeficiency virus disease. *Ped Infect Dis J* **16**: 623–6.

Sperling RS, Shapiro DE, Coombs RW et al. (1996). Maternal viral load, zidovudine treatment, and the risk of transmission of human immunodeficiency virus type 1 from mother to infant. *N Engl J Med* **335**: 1621–9.

St Louis ME, Kamenga M, Brown C et al. (1993). Risk for perinatal HIV-1 transmission according to maternal immunologic, virologic and placental factors. *JAMA* **269**: 2853–9.

Teglas JP, Quartier P, Treluyer JM et al. (2001). Tolerance of efavirenz in children. *AIDS* **15**: 241–3.

Van de Perre P, Simonon A, Msellati P et al. (1991). Postnatal transmission of human immunodeficiency virus type 1 from mother to infant. A prospective cohort study in Kigali, Rwanda. *N Engl J Med* **325**: 593–8.

Van Dyke RB, Korber BT, Popek E et al. (1999). A prospective cohort study of risk factors for maternal child transmission of HIV in the era of maternal zidovudine therapy. The Ariel Project. *J Infect Dis* **179**: 319–28.

Walter EB, McKinney RE, Lane BA et al. (1990). Interpretation of western blots in HIV-1 infected children. Implications for prognosis and diagnosis. *J Pediatr* **117**: 255.

Wiktor SZ, Ekpini E, Karon JM et al. (1999). Short course oral zidovudine for prevention of mother to child transmission of HIV-1 in Abidjan, Cote d'Ivoire; a randomized trial. *Lancet* **353**: 781–5.

BRUCE JAMES BREW

Involvement of the nervous system frequently occurs during the course of human immunodeficiency virus (HIV) infection, and results in disease affecting the brain, spinal cord, peripheral nerve and muscle (Brew 1992). Within each of these components of the neuraxis, a multiplicity of pathological processes may occur, which are often layered upon each other and which may simultaneously involve different parts of the neuraxis. To assist the clinician confronted with a patient in whom HIV-related neurological disease is suspected, this review will first categorize the disorders according to the anatomical level of the neurological involvement and focus largely upon those disorders that are directly related to HIV infection. In addition, as explained later in this chapter, the probability of a particular neurological complication of HIV disease occurring is determined by the degree of advancement of HIV disease, the best measure of which is the CD4 lymphocyte count; the three categories for CD4 lymphocyte count of 500 or more cells/μl, 200–500 cells/μl, and less than 200 cells/μl have been chosen to concur with the Center for Diseases Control and Prevention revised definition of HIV infection. In this era of highly active antiretroviral therapy (HAART), CD4 lymphocyte counts may fluctuate widely, with some patients experiencing dramatic increases. While it is not known whether a patient's risk of a particular neurological complication is related to their current CD4 lymphocyte count or their lowest count, it seems prudent to place more emphasis on the nadir count, as there is evidence that the increase in CD4 lymphocytes that occurs in some patients may not represent fully functional CD4 lymphocytes.

Central nervous system: brain involvement

AIDS dementia complex

Direct involvement by HIV has been known under a variety of terms, such as HIV encephalopathy, subacute encephalitis, AIDS-related dementia, and AIDS dementia complex. More recently, HIV-1-associated minor cognitive/motor deficit and HIV-1-associated dementia have been chosen in order to differentiate mild cognitive impairment that does not meet the usual criteria for dementia because activities of daily living have not been disturbed (Working Group of the American Academy of Neurology AIDS Task Force, 1991). In the past there has been doubt as to whether the mild cognitive deficit related to HIV has the same causation and natural history as the more severe HIV-1-associated dementia. Recent data suggest that this is not the case (Stern et al., 1998). For this reason, this review will continue to use the term AIDS dementia complex (ADC).

Clinical features

The clinical features of ADC have been well described over the past few years (Navia et al., 1986a). The disorder is a subcortical dementia, in that the usual cortical features of aphasia, alexia and agraphia that characterize dementias such as Alzheimer's disease are absent and there is a prominent motor disturbance. The recent pathological demonstration of cortical neuronal loss (Ketzler et al., 1990; Everall et al., 1991), does not alter the fact that the clinical presentation is predominantly that of a subcortical process with complaints of poor concentration, disturbed short-term memory, slowing of thought processes, motor inco-ordination and unsteadiness of gait. Behavioural symptoms such as social apathy and withdrawal are less common. Cortical symptoms occur when the dementia is advanced and the deficit has become more global.

Most investigators agree that the symptoms and signs of ADC can be grouped into three spheres of abnormality: cognition, motor function and behaviour. Dysfunction often occurs in each of these, but the cognitive and motor disturbances are most closely linked. Patients complain of decreased concentration, manifest as losing track of the conversation while speaking to people and having to reread a paragraph or page to fully understand it. Forgetfulness, especially for day-to-day events and slowing of thought processes, are also prominent. In addition to these cognitive symptoms, patients frequently have motor complaints of clumsiness, sloppy handwriting, tremor and poor balance, especially with rapid head turns. Less commonly, patients may be socially withdrawn and apathetic. Indeed, patients may be mistakenly diagnosed as suffering from depression, but careful clinical assessment reveals that while they may have the outer mask of depression, they do not have the inner feelings of depression. Insight is preserved until late in the illness, so that patients often accurately report these difficulties.

The neurological examination of patients with ADC is often characterized by few abnormalities, especially in the early stage of the disorder. The mini-mental state examination is usually normal, although responses are delayed. Subtle signs, such as slowing and inaccuracy of saccadic and pursuit eye movements and fine finger movements are common. Deep tendon reflexes are frequently brisker in the lower limbs but the ankle jerks may be depressed or absent as a consequence of an associated peripheral neuropathy, which may lead to a sensory disturbance. Tandem gait is commonly abnormal. As the disorder progresses, patients become globally demented, mute, paraparetic and incontinent of urine and faeces.

In order to stage ADC, a scheme has been developed that stratifies patients from 0 through to 4 (Price and Brew, 1988). This has now been modified to include only cognitive changes, as the motor disturbance in an individual patient may be related either to brain disease or spinal cord dysfunction (Table 10.1). In essence, the staging scheme is similar to a neurologically based Karnofsky assessment. In addition to this scheme, the World Health Organization and the American Academy of Neurology have developed a similar classification (Working Group of the American Academy of Neurology AIDS Task Force, 1991) although they only recognize dementia at stage 2.

ADC occurs at a moderately advanced stage of immunosuppression in HIV disease. In a personally examined group of ADC patients, the mean CD4 lymphocyte count was $94 \pm 139/\mu l$ (unpubl. data). Portegies *et al.* (1993) found a similar mean of $109/\mu l$. The finding of Sidtis *et al.* (1993), where the mean CD4 lymphocyte count for

Table 10.1 Modified staging scheme for AIDS dementia complex

Stage	Category	Clinical features
0	Normal	Normal mental and motor function
0.5	Subclinical	Minimal or equivocal symptoms without impairment of work or activities of daily living (ADL) 'background' neurological signs, such as slowed fine finger movements or primitive reflexes may be present
1	Mild	Cognitive deficit that compromises the performance of the more demanding aspects of work or ADL
2	Moderate	Cognitive deficit makes the patient unable to perform work or the more demanding aspects of ADL; the patient may require assistance with walking
3	Severe	Cognitive deficit makes it possible for the patient to perform only the most rudimentary tasks; for example, the patient cannot follow news or sustain a conversation of any complexity; the patient often requires some support for walking
4	End-stage	Cognitive deficit has reached the point where the patient has virtually no understanding of his surroundings and is virtually mute; the patient is paraparetic or paraplegic, often with double incontinence

patients with ADC was $535/\mu l$, probably reflects a selection bias as the zidovudine (ZDV) trial was designed for patients presenting with ADC who had no previous antiretroviral drug exposure.

Prevalence and natural history

The prevalence of ADC has been variably estimated, with groups reporting rates ranging from 7 to 90% (Brew 1992). It is now agreed that approximately 20% of patients with advanced HIV disease have the disorder (McArthur *et al.*, 1993; Portegies *et al.*, 1993). The risk of developing ADC in patients with advanced HIV disease is approximately 7% per year (McArthur *et al.*, 1993). The discrepancies in previous estimates probably relate to several factors. First, ADC prevalence varies according to the degree of HIV-associated immunodeficiency, with the disorder being uncommon in patients with a CD4 lymphocyte count of between 200 and 500 cells/μl and rare in patients with counts above 500 cells/μl. Second, some studies did not adequately exclude the confounding effects of fatigue, anxiety and depression on ADC assessment. Third, variation in the clinical 'cut-off' that is used to diagnose dementia will influence prevalence figures: if mild or stage 1 ADC is included, then approximately 25–30% of patients with advanced HIV disease will have the disorder, whereas if mild disease is excluded then the figure is reduced to around 12% (Brew et al., 1992a). Finally, the prevalence of ADC will be influenced by the proportion of patients taking ZDV (Portegies et al., 1989) as well as newer antiretroviral drugs in combination (Fernando et al., 1998; Foudraine et al., 1998, Sacktor et al., 2001).

The natural history of ADC is difficult to evaluate, as patients often develop other AIDS-related complications and antiretroviral drugs may alter the course of ADC. The mean time to death for patients with varying degrees of severity of ADC is 6 months, although those with milder disease (stage 1 and some stage 2 patients) may remain stable for a year or more. Occasional patients are rapid progressors, but the early identification of these patients is not currently possible (McArthur et al., 1993).

Investigations

At the present time, there is no investigation that is diagnostic of ADC. Nonetheless, investigations have two major roles: exclusion and confirmation. Potentially treatable complications should be excluded as they may exacerbate existing ADC or previously subclinical HIV brain disease to the point where the clinical manifestations of ADC overshadow those of the precipitant infection. Moreover, the results of certain investigations can show changes that are suggestive of ADC, and indeed their absence may render the possibility of ADC less likely.

Computed tomographic (CT) scanning of the brain usually demonstrates cerebral atrophy, and magnetic resonance imaging (MRI) may reveal T2 weighted periventricular abnormalities that are either patchy or diffuse (Jarvik et al., 1988). However, both of these neuroradiological abnormalities may occur in patients who are not demented (McArthur et al., 1989). The MRI changes probably relate to the breakdown of the blood–brain barrier and excess water content of the brain, rather than true white matter damage (Smith et al., 1990; Power et al., 1993).

More refined use of magnetic scanning with employment of functional imaging and magnetic resonance spectroscopy may assist in diagnosis, though their precise utility is still unclear. Functional imaging studies have shown that abnor-

malities may first occur in subcortical structures. These changes may be found in neurologically asymptomatic patients (Navia et al., 1997). Magnetic resonance spectroscopy has revealed a significant reduction in N-acetyl aspartate (NAA), a marker of mature neurons, in cortical areas. The reduction in NAA correlates to some extent with the severity of cognitive impairment in ADC (Barker et al., 1995). Significant elevations in choline and myoinositol have been described in the white matter of patients with mild ADC. However, this has also been observed in those who are neurologically asymptomatic (McConnell et al., 1994; Tracey et al., 1996).

Similar problems beset other neuro-imaging modalities, such as single photon emission computed tomography (SPECT), where multifocal cortical and subcortical areas of hypoperfusion are often found (Masdeu et al., 1991). SPECT is more sensitive than the other imaging techniques but at the expense of decreased specificity (Schielke et al., 1990). SPECT may have a role in measuring response to therapy (Brew et al., 1996a; Szeto et al., 1998). Positron emission tomography (PET) studies have consistently shown relative basal ganglia hypermetabolism early in ADC, with more diffuse defects occurring with disease progression (Rottenberg et al., 1987; Van Gorp et al., 1992; Hinken et al., 1995).

For practical purposes, patients with suspected ADC should have a CT brain scan with and without contrast to exclude a concomitant opportunistic infection or neoplasm. If the scan does not show any changes, then it is probably unnecessary to consider other neuro-imaging. However, if the clinical features of a patient with suspected ADC are atypical, or the CT brain scan shows an area of hypodensity, then an MRI of the brain should be performed with gadolinium to address the possibility of progressive multifocal leukoencephalopathy.

Analysis of cerebrospinal fluid (CSF) may reveal non-specific abnormalities such as a minor mononuclear pleocytosis, raised CSF protein, intrathecal IgG synthesis and oligoclonal bands, which also occur in non-demented HIV-infected patients (Marshall et al., 1988). A modest mononuclear pleocytosis of up to several hundred mononuclear cells is occasionally seen (Navia et al., 1986a), though in general CSF mononuclear cell counts correlate with the degree of immunodeficiency, with higher cell counts occurring in individuals with less advanced HIV disease. There are several virological indices in the CSF that may be useful in the diagnosis of ADC. The most important of these is the number of HIV RNA copies in the CSF (CSF viral load). Of all the markers for ADC, CSF viral load best correlates with severity of ADC (Brew *et al.*, 1997a; Ellis *et al.*, 1997; McArthur *et al.*, 1997). Presently, it is not known whether there is a critical 'cut off' level of CSF viral load that can be used to diagnose the presence of ADC, though this seems unlikely. On a population basis there is no correlation between CSF and plasma viral loads. In individual cases it is recommended that some measure of the integrity of the blood–brain barrier, such as the CSF/serum albumin ratio, is included. The clinician should be aware of other caveats in the interpretation of CSF viral load. CNS infections such as cryptococcal meningitis and toxoplasmosis can lead to significant elevations in CSF viral load in the absence of ADC, and when these infections are successfully treated the CSF viral load falls. There are four sources of viral load in the CSF:

(1) 'leak' from the plasma through a disturbed blood brain barrier;
(2) 'spill over' from brain infection;
(3) 'shedding' from productive infection of the meningeal compartment (meningeal macrophages); and
(4) 'shedding' of HIV from trafficking of activated CD4 lymphocytes through the CNS as part of their normal regulatory immune function.

These aspects should be evaluated when interpreting the significance of CSF viral load. The precise role of measurement of CSF viral load in clinical practice is beginning to be clarified. It has a role as an ancillary tool to support the diagnosis of ADC. Whether it can be used to predict ADC or its response to therapy is under assessment.

Other virological markers are less useful. The core protein of HIV-1, p24 antigen, is infrequently found in the CSF of ADC patients, but when present it may be a useful confirmatory adjunct to ADC assessment. Approximately 50% of severely demented patients will have detectable p24 antigen in the CSF (Portegies *et al.*, 1989; Brew *et al.*, 1994) while the detection of CSF p24 antigen in a non-demented patient is rare. Conversely, caution should be exercised, as CSF p24 antigen will be negative in up to 50% of patients with severe ADC (Brew *et al.*, 1994). The detection of HIV-1 antibodies in CSF (Resnick *et al.*, 1988) and culture of CSF for HIV-1 (Chiodi *et al.*, 1988) are less useful, as HIV-1 antibodies are not found in the CSF of every ADC patient and viruses can be cultured from the CSF of only 30% of ADC patients.

Measures of immune activation within the CSF may be useful as adjuncts to the diagnosis of ADC. Elevated CSF concentrations of β_2 microglobulin (Brew *et al.*, 1992), the invariant light chain of the major histocompatibility complex class I, neopterin (Brew *et al.*, 1990) (a product of activated macrophages) and quinolinic acid (Heyes *et al.*, 1991) are related to both the presence and severity of ADC in patients without confounding neurological illnesses. Other markers of immune activation such as tumor necrosis factor concentrations (Gallo *et al.*, 1989; Grimaldi *et al.*, 1991) remain controversial. Interleukins 1β and 6 have been associated with the presence but not the severity of ADC (Gallo *et al.*, 1989). The significance of antimyelin basic protein antibodies in the CSF requires confirmation (Mastroianni *et al.*, 1991).

Which CSF variables should be considered in the day-to-day assessment of the patient suspected of having ADC? It is suggested that routine CSF parameters such as cell count and protein should be assessed, with emphasis placed on the differential of the white cell count: a mononuclear pleocytosis would be consistent with ADC but the finding of a polymorphonuclear pleocytosis would strongly favour an alternative diagnosis such as cytomegalovirus (CMV) encephalitis (see below). CSF cryptococcal antigen should be performed to exclude cryptococcal meningitis, and syphilis serology should also be performed. Markers of immune activation such as β_2 microglobulin and/or neopterin would be useful adjuncts to the diagnosis if other infections have been excluded.

The clinical utility of neurophysiological investigations in the assessment of a patient with ADC is limited, and in most instances no extra information can be gained from performance of these tests.

Neurophysiological investigations are frequently abnormal in patients with ADC, but these abnormalities are also often found in asymptomatic patients. Disturbances in pursuit and saccadic eye movements become increasingly common with increasing severity of HIV disease and with the presence of ADC (Currie *et al.*, 1988; Merrill *et al.*, 1991; Sweeney *et al.*, 1991). Abnormal brainstem auditory evoked potentials (Koralnik *et al.*, 1990) and long latency event-related potentials (Goodin *et al.*, 1990) have similarly been found. The significance of electroencephalographic (EEG) abnormalities is less clear. Two studies have described an increased frequency of EEG abnormalities in asymptomatic patients (Parisi *et al.*, 1989; Koralnik *et al.*, 1990), but a larger and more rigorously controlled study has not supported the earlier findings (Nuwer *et al.*, 1992). Whether one or a combination of these investigations will predict the subsequent development of ADC is unclear. One group has claimed prognostic significance of EEG abnormalities in asymptomatic patients (Parisi *et al.*, 1989), but their data have not been confirmed.

Neuropsychology

Neuropsychological testing can be used to confirm the diagnosis in a patient suspected of having ADC. The essential features of ADC in neuropsychological terms are impaired attention and slowing of intellectual processes (Tross *et al.*, 1988; Dunbar and Brew, 1996) but this pattern is not pathognomonic of ADC. A number of testing strategies has been suggested by various authors. Presently, the AIDS Clinical Trials Group in the USA uses timed gait, trail-making tests A and B, finger tapping (dominant and non-dominant), grooved pegboard (dominant and non-dominant), and digit symbol tests. An impairment score is then derived by allotting a value of 1 for each standard deviation from the mean of each test; these are then added to arrive at the impairment score. Scores with values greater than or equal to 4 are consistent with ADC (Price and Sidtis, 1990). Reaction time is one of the most sensitive parameters of ADC (Perdices and Cooper, 1989) and has the additional advantage that it can be computerized for ease of administration.

Neuropsychological assessment has several limitations. First, the evaluation must be linked to a clinical neurological examination and confounding illnesses such as opportunistic infections or tumours must be excluded. Second, impaired test performance does not translate directly into ADC as patients may perform poorly because of fatigue, anxiety and depression. The latter illnesses can be assessed with further tests, such as the profile of mood states. Patients with a high premorbid intellect may not have impairment adequately assessed with the currently used measures unless more sophisticated testing strategies are used. Third, agreement has not been reached on the precise definition of what is abnormal in neuropsychological terms. Nonetheless, neuropsychological assessment provides a useful quantitative assessment of the patient with ADC and can be of assistance in the evaluation of response to treatment.

Given the limitations and usefulness of neuropsychological testing, what is its role in the practical management of a patient with ADC? Neuropsychological evaluation should be employed as an ancillary investigation. The results should be combined with the clinical assessment and results of investigations. The diagnosis of ADC is ultimately clinical. It should not be made on the basis of one abnormal test, regardless of whether that test is a CT brain scan, CSF viral load or a neuropsychological evaluation.

Neuropathology

The neuropathology of ADC has recently been revised (Budka *et al.*, 1991). It may be divided into five categories, which frequently overlap with each other (Table 10.1). HIV leukoencephalopathy, diffuse poliodystrophy, HIV encephalitis, vacuolar leukoencephalopathy and cerebral vasculitis (Table 10.2). HIV leukoencephalopathy consists of diffuse, especially subcortical, damage to the white matter, reactive astrocytosis and the presence of macrophages and multinucleated giant cells with minimal or no inflammatory infiltrate. It is the most common disorder in this classification. A similar leukoencephalopathy where evidence of HIV infection in the brain tissue is absent is not addressed by this classification because of the lack of

Table 10.2 Neuropathology of AIDS dementia complex

Pathological classification	Principal neutropathological features	Comments
HIV leukoencephalopathy	Diffuse subcortical white matter damage, reactive astrocytosis; macrophages, multinucleated giant cells; minimal or no inflammatory infiltrate	Most common
Diffuse poliodystrophy	Diffuse reactive astrogliosis and microgial activation in cerebral gray matter	Common
HIV encephalitis	Perivascular inflammatory infiltrates of multinucleated giant cells, predominantly subcortical involvement	Less frequent
Vacuolar leukoencephalopathy	Vacuolation throughout white matter	Rare
Cerebral vasculitis		Rare

definite association with HIV infection, although the disorder occurs frequently in patients with ADC (Navia et al., 1986b). Diffuse poliodystrophy is also a reasonably common finding where there is diffuse reactive astrogliosis and microglial activation involving the cerebral grey matter. Less frequent is HIV encephalitis, where there are perivascular inflammatory infiltrates of multinucleated giant cells again in a predominantly subcortical distribution. Rarely, the pathology may be characterized by vacuolation throughout the white matter, which has been termed vacuolar leukoencephalopathy. Finally, cerebral vasculitis has been described but it would appear to be distinctly uncommon (Mizusawa et al., 1989). Cortical atrophy with neuronal loss is most likely associated with HIV diffuse poliodystrophy and HIV encephalitis (Everall et al., 1991). The precise relationship between the latter abnormalities is unknown. Some investigators have suggested that leukoencephalopathy forms a base, upon which are added the changes of diffuse poliodystrophy and HIV encephalitis in moderate to severe cases of ADC. Others have suggested that the leukoencephalopathy and poliodystrophy are separate but parallel processes. The overriding principles, however, are that the neuropathological changes are predominantly subcortical and that within these subcortical areas there appear to be certain structures that are more commonly involved, for example the basal ganglia, especially the globus pallidus (Kure et al., 1990; Brew et al., 1995a).

Neurovirology

Productive HIV infection occurs mainly in subcortical rather than cortical structures and even within subcortical structures there is topographic localization to certain parts of the basal ganglia, for example the globus pallidus (Budka, 1990). The only intrinsic neural cell that consistently supports HIV replication is the microglial cell (Michaels et al., 1988; Brew et al., 1995a). There is some evidence that endothelial cells can be productively infected, but the data need to be carefully evaluated to exclude actual infection of the microglial component of the perivascular glial barrier (Budka, 1990). Previous reports of infection of oligodendroglial cells were controversial (Gyorkey et al., 1987; Sharer and Prineas, 1988), although recently Esiri et al. (1991) have raised the possibility again, albeit as a distinctly uncommon event. The issue of astrocyte infection is more complex in that these cells support restricted infection with the production of regulatory proteins only and not whole

virions. How commonly this occurs is the subject of debate (Takahaski et al., 1996; Wiley, 1996), but it appears to be more common in children (Wiley, 1996). Latent infection may occur in astrocytes and two groups have shown that it may be found infrequently in neurons (Nuovo et al., 1994; Bagasra et al., 1996).

Pathogenesis

Understanding of the pathogenesis of ADC has progressed considerably over the past few years. Before approaching a hypothetical model, it is useful to emphasize certain pivotal aspects of ADC. Subclinical involvement of the nervous system is common throughout the course of HIV-1 infection. Various brain imaging studies have demonstrated abnormalities in asymptomatic HIV-infected patients. The CSF of asymptomatic patients is frequently abnormal, with a mild mononuclear pleocytosis, an elevated protein and recovery of HIV-1 from the CSF, as well as a detectable HIV RNA in a small percentage of patients. Evidence of neurophysiological dysfunction has also been defined by demonstration of EEG abnormalities, long latency potentials and eye movement disturbances. Minor neuropsychological disturbance in the absence of any symptoms has been described but larger studies have not shown any significant deficit at a population level (McArthur et al., 1989). Abnormalities have even been found at a neuropathological level. Astrogliosis, vasculitis and a lymphocytic meningitis have been described in the brains of patients who had been asymptomatically infected and who had died accidental deaths (Gray et al., 1992). Thus, at every level there is overwhelming evidence of CNS abnormalities, although they are not clinically evident.

While there is subclinical involvement of the CNS, its clinical expression, namely ADC, is usually a feature of advanced HIV disease when there is significant immunodeficiency with a CD4 lymphocyte cell count of less than 200/µl.

Despite significant immunodeficiency, ADC develops only in some patients. As previously mentioned, the prevalence of ADC is approximately 20% and even with the inclusion of milder deficits it increases to approximately 33%. Despite the fact that patients are living longer because of more potent antiretroviral therapy, there has been no major change in ADC prevalence over the past few years (Bacellar et al., 1994). The effect of HAART or ADC incidence and prevalence has not yet been fully defined.

The presence and severity of ADC are linked to immune activation within the CSF and brain parenchyma, as demonstrated by elevated CSF concentrations of β_2 microglobulin, neopterin, quinolinic acid, interleukins 1 and 6 (Gallo et al., 1989) and increased expression of MHC class I and II molecules on cells in the brains of patients with ADC (Tyor et al., 1992).

The neuropathological and neurovirological features are predominantly subcortical and perivascular in location, with a specific predisposition for the subcortical structures, especially the globus pallidus. Additionally, there is cortical neuronal loss, mainly affecting the frontal lobes. From a pathogenetic viewpoint, there are two important observations: the absence of productive infection of the choroid plexus (Kure et al., 1990) arguing against simple spread of infection from the choroid plexus, and the lack of a uniformly centrifugal distribution of neuropathological changes that makes dissemination of infection from the meninges to various subcortical structures unlikely (Kure et al., 1990; Brew et al., 1995a). Productive infection of the brain is confined to cells of the monocyte/macrophage lineage, including the microglial cell. Restricted infection appears to occur in astrocytes (Wiley, 1996).

Purely virological factors seem unlikely as causative agents for ADC. This hypothesis is supported by the clinical–virological dissociation observed, both when the clinical severity of ADC is often greater than the amount of productive HIV-1 infection found at autopsy (Brew et al., 1995a; Glass et al., 1995), and in some paediatric patients with ADC in whom there is no evidence of productive infection despite severe dementia (Vazeux et al., 1992). Moreover, there is viral–pathological dissociation when the pathological changes are more extensive than the amount of productive infection (Brew et al., 1995a). Thus, productive brain infection appears to be sufficient, but not necessary, for the development of ADC.

In summary, ADC is restricted in time (the degree of advancement of HIV disease), place (both the anatomical site and supportive cell), and person. Moreover, there are three paradoxes in ADC: the disorder is related to immune activation at a time of immunodeficiency; the clinical deficit exceeds the amount of virus in the brain; and like other lentiviral infections, the neural cells capable of supporting infection are not the ones that die.

A hypothetical model of the pathogenesis of ADC is proposed. HIV enters the CNS early in the course of the disease, probably at the time of seroconversion. Entry is by way of blood-borne infection and to a lesser extent by 'spread' from chronic meningeal infection, which is related to low-level infection of the choroid plexus (Harouse et al., 1989) and perhaps infection of meningeal macrophages (Perry et al., 1994). Productive infection of the choroid plexus cannot be demonstrated in the brains of patients with ADC, and this is probably the result of the death of the original cells capable of supporting infection by the time the patient died. Low-level infection is kept in check by a relatively intact immune system, and the variety of subclinical nervous system abnormalities is related to the production of toxins, both locally and systemically. As HIV disease progresses, both brain and systemic infection are no longer controlled, resulting in the production of cytokines that can cause CNS dysfunction. Additionally, the low-level brain and meningeal compartment infection may be amplified by the similarly uncontrolled systemic disease, thereby accounting for the perivascular distribution of the pathology of ADC.

There are probably three mechanisms by which HIV enters the brain, namely through trafficking of activated T cells and monocytes, the so-called 'Trojan horse' mechanism, since these cells can cross the intact blood–brain barrier, and through the passage of cell-free virus across a disrupted blood–brain barrier, which occurs in advanced HIV-1 disease (Petito and Cash, 1992). The third mechanism is by spread of infection from the meningeal compartment.

At the cellular level, HIV enters cells of macrophage lineage by binding to the CD4 molecule; entry is facilitated by CCR5, CCR3 and possibly other chemokine co-receptors (Cairns and D'Souza, 1998). Once in the cell, HIV may replicate, thereby producing further viruses and a variety of viral products that are injurious to other cells (virus-coded toxins). If the cell is incapable of fully supporting replication, restricted infection may occur, for example in the astrocyte, with disruption of normal astrocyte function and secondary neuronal death. Uninfected, but activated immune cells produce a variety of toxins aimed at the death of cells supporting HIV infection, but in the process lead to the death of normal neural cells (host-coded toxins). The precise mechanism of neuronal damage is by activation of the N-methyl D-aspartate (NMDA) receptor, with consequent influx into the cell of calcium and secondary production of nitric oxide in those neurons containing nitric oxide synthetase (Dawson et al., 1993). Other virus-coded toxins are the regulatory proteins Tat and Nef, but again these mediate their toxicity at least in part by way of host-determined toxins. Host-coded toxins (some of which are as yet undefined) are largely produced by cells of macrophage lineage, while others are nitric oxide, arachidonic acid metabolites, Ntox, tumor necrosis factor (TNF) and platelet activating factor, that require cell-to-cell interactions for toxicity (Brenneman *et al.*, 1988; Epstein and Gendelman, 1993). Our group has also shown that the excitotoxin quinolinic acid, an NMDA receptor agonist, is elevated in the CSF of ADC patients (Heyes *et al.*, 1991) and that macrophages infected with HIV-1 *in vitro* can produce large quantities of quinolinic acid, with this production being dependent upon the degree of macrophage tropism of HIV and certain cytokines (Brew *et al.*, 1995b, 1996b; Pemberton *et al.*, 1997). Further support for the role of quinolinic acid is provided by the fact that it is both acutely (Kerr *et al.*, 1995) and chronically (Kerr *et al.*, 1998) toxic to human neurons in concentrations that are clinically relevant and that inhibition of its production results in a significant amelioration in the neurotoxicity of supernatants from HIV-infected macrophage cultures (Kerr *et al.*, 1997).

The pathogenesis of HIV leukoencephalopathy probably follows the same model. White matter abnormalities caused by virus-coded toxins were not thought to be as important as those caused by toxins until recently. The demonstration that gp120 may bind the galactosyl ceramide receptor and possibly other glycolipid receptors suggests that it may be implicated in leukoencephalopathy by binding to oligodendrocytes, with resultant dysfunction (Harouse *et al.*, 1991; Kimura-Kuroda *et al.*, 1993). Host-coded toxins also play an important role, with cytokines released by cells of macrophage lineage in an attempt to control infection. Similar leukoencephalopathic changes have been observed in patients receiving high doses of various cytokines, particularly the interleukins, as part of cancer chemotherapy. Another possible host-coded toxin effect is the documented methylation defect (Keating *et al.*, 1991) in infected individuals that may lead to changes similar to cyanocobalamin deficiency. The actual toxin, however, has not been precisely identified.

Treatment

Currently, the treatment of ADC is limited. There is only one antiretroviral medication that has been proven to be efficacious for ADC. ZDV efficacy has been documented by several anecdotal case reports, open-label observational studies (Portegies *et al.*, 1993; Tozzi *et al.*, 1993) and a place-bo-controlled trial (Sidtis *et al.*, 1993). The latter study only showed significant improvement with regard to neuropsychological scores in the group that was treated with high-dose ZDV (2000 mg/day). Brain and CSF ZDV concentrations are 30–50% of serum ZDV levels; thus, it is reasonable to expect that doses higher than those used for systemic infection would be necessary. However, the use of high-dose ZDV is impractical due to haematological intolerance. As a consequence, it is usually recommended that the highest tolerable dose of ZDV is given. The average time taken to respond to ZDV is approximately 8 weeks and the limited data that exist suggest that approximately 50% will respond (Portegies *et al.*, 1993; Tozzi *et al.*, 1993). The clinical response is mirrored in the CSF by a decline in markers of immune activation, β_2 microglobulin, neopterin, quinolinic acid, and viral load (Brew *et al.*, 1990, 1992; Heyes *et al.*, 1991; Foudraine *et al.*, 1998).

The efficacy of other nucleoside analogue reverse transcriptase inhibitors (NRTIs) in the treatment of ADC is uncertain. Didanosine (ddI) has been found effective in improving the neuropsychological deficits of HIV-1-infected children (Butler *et al.*, 1991), but data from the Alpha study of the efficacy of ddI in advanced ZDV-intolerant patients suggests that ddI may not be effective in adults (Portegies, 1995). This is further supported by the poor CSF penetration of ddI and lack of viral load reduction in the CSF with its use (Gisslen *et al.*, 1997). While there are no data on the efficacy of zalcitabine (ddC) in ADC, it has poor CSF penetration and thus is not an optimal agent for ADC treatment. Stavudine (d4T) has been shown to penetrate into the CSF in efficacious concentrations and decrease CSF viral load to below detection in a small number of patients (Foudraine *et al.*, 1998). Similarly, lamivudine (3TC) can reach efficacious steady-state concentrations in the CSF and may have a role in the treatment of ADC as part of a combination of antiviral drugs (Foudraine *et al.*, 1998). Abacavir is a new, potent NRTI with good CSF penetration. In a large, randomized double-blind placebo-controlled trial of its efficacy in ADC, the drug failed to show benefit over continuation of existing combination therapy, which included the protease inhibitor (PI) indinavir in most patients. In subgroup analyses the drug was found to be efficacious in those patients not on PIs, especially those with more severe ADC (Brew *et al.*, 1998).

Of the currently available non-nucleoside reverse transcriptase inhibitors (NNRTIs), (nevirapine, efavirenz and delavirdine) the first two may be effective. Nevirapine can reach efficacious steady-state CSF concentrations (Yazdanian *et al.*, 1997), while a small study failed to show any efficacy for delavirdine in ADC (Brew *et al.*, unpubl. data). Recent data have shown that efavirenz may reach efficacious CSF concentrations and reduce CSF viral load in combination therapy (Tashima *et al.*, 1998).

Of the four PIs available (saquinavir, ritonavir, indinavir and nelfinavir, data for potential ADC efficacy exist only for indinavir and consist only of favourable CSF steady-state concentrations (Collier *et al.*, 1997).

In clinical practice, the ADC patient should be treated with a combination of drugs, but it is not clear how many and which drugs should be used, with the caveat that ZDV and d4T should not be used together. This author recommends ZDV or d4T with abacavir plus indinavir plus 3TC and nevirapine or efavirenz; however, data to support this recommendation are not yet available. 3TC would perhaps be best used with ZDV to 'reverse' ZDV resistance. Preliminary data suggest that appropriate combination therapy may be chosen by the pattern of genotypic mutations in the CSF (Cunningham *et al.*, 1998). It is now apparent that resistance patterns may be different between CSF and blood compartments, with individual patients having sensitive virus in the blood but resistant virus in the CSF, and vice versa.

In the future, other non-antiviral agents may be available as adjunctive therapy to block the cascade of immune activation-related damage or to block the NMDA receptor, the probable final common pathway for neuronal damage in ADC. Memantine, an open channel NMDA antagonist, is currently being trialed for ADC.

Symptomatic treatment of patients with ADC is also an important aspect of management. It should be appreciated, however, that ADC patients are very susceptible to the extrapyramidal effects of neuroleptics, so that low doses should be used, and preference given to those that have a low propensity for extrapyrmidal side-effects, such as clozapine and olanzapine. Similarly, patients are prone to the development of confusion with other psychoactive drugs, such as the antidepressants, and low doses should be used cautiously.

Major psychosocial and medicolegal issues abound in the management of patients with ADC. Not only do healthcare professionals have to address the problems of an incompetent, and often insightful patient, but there are aspects of ADC that make it more taxing to manage than other dementing disorders. First, the dominant apathy and amotivational aspects of ADC make caring for the patient difficult. Such patients have to be encouraged to maintain personal hygiene and to take their medications. Second, response to treatment often takes several weeks to 2 months. During this period it is important to support the carers of the patient and not to 'give up' because the patient has not improved after several days or weeks.

Medicolegally, patients with ADC stage 2 or greater should not be allowed to drive and should be supervised at home. Decisions as to when a patient should stop work and relinquish power of attorney have to be individualized, but in general once the patient has reached stage 2 the issues should be seriously considered.

Prediction of and prophylaxis against ADC

Currently, there are three investigations that can assess the risk of the subsequent development of ADC in asymptomatic patients (Brew, 1997). The first relates to the level of haemoglobin: the lower the level, the higher the risk. These data pertain to HIV-infected patients in general. The risk may be further increased in patients with advanced HIV disease, as judged by CD4 lymphocyte counts below 200 cells/μl (McArthur *et al.*, 1993). Risk assessment for ADC can also be ascertained by neuropsychological evaluation. Provided that other confounding factors, for example previous head injury, have been excluded, a pattern of psychomotor slowing carries a risk of approximately fourfold. These data are relevant to patients with a CD4 lymphocyte count of less than 200 cells/μl (Sacktor *et al.*, 1996). The third investigation is measurement of CSF β_2 microglobulin; there is a graded risk with concentrations above 5 mg/l, carrying a seventeenfold risk in the subsequent 6 months (Brew *et al.*, 1996c).

Prophylaxis against ADC is a difficult issue. Epidemiological data and neurovirological studies suggest that ADC is not an inevitable consequence of HIV disease. It is much more likely that it only occurs in small number of patients (20% of those with advanced HIV disease). In the near future, there may be tools that can be used to assess risk more precisely, such as; delineation of certain genetic factors akin to the CCR5 gene polymorphism, and certain virological characteristics, such as dementia-associated envelope mutations. At present, patients with advanced HIV disease should have at least two neurologically active drugs in their combination regimen, to reduce the risk of development of ADC.

Other central nervous system manifestations

Sequelae of primary infection

There are several disorders less common than ADC that appear directly related to HIV. Patients may develop an aseptic meningitis, encephalitis or cerebellar syndrome, shortly after the glandular fever-like illness that is associated with initial infection by HIV (Brew et al., 1989a; Brew and Tindall, 1997). These are almost always mild, usually with complete resolution occurring over several weeks. The diagnosis is made by exclusion of other causes with appropriate investigations. Although numbers are small, the patients do not appear to be at greater risk of subsequent neurological involvement when significant immunodeficiency develops. The pathogenesis of these complications is unknown (see Table 10.3).

Multiple sclerosis-like illness

Several years after initial infection with HIV, rare patients with only mild immunodeficiency may develop a syndrome very similar to multiple sclerosis (Berger et al., 1989). Although it is still not clear whether this represents the concurrence of two disorders in the one patient, it is conceivable that it is related to HIV and that it has an auto-immune pathogenesis (see Table 10.3).

Aseptic meningitis and HIV-1 headache

An aseptic meningitis may occur following the development of mild to moderate immunodeficiency, sometimes in combination with cranial neuropathies, especially of nerves V, VII and VIII (Brew, 1992) (see Table 10.3). Patients may have the acute onset of a non-specific headache over several days or an indolent illness in which headaches have been present for months. Brew & Miller (1993) have described both acute and chronic non-specific headaches occurring without a raised CSF cell count. Because a CSF pleocytosis may occur in asymptomatic HIV-infected patients, it is probable that headaches occurring with and without CSF pleocytosis are in fact the same disorder, with the CSF pleocytosis being unrelated. Nonetheless, the relationship between headaches and HIV disease is still debated. The recent paper by Singer et al., (1996) showing no increased frequency of headaches in HIV-infected patients, included patients with headaches of varying types and severity. Other groups have observed a relationship between HIV disease and headache (Kapoor et al., 1998; Mirsattari et al., 1998). Low doses of amitriptylline or other tricyclic antidepressant drugs are effective in managing the headaches.

Seizures

Seizures in the HIV-infected patient may result from an underlying opportunistic complication, electrolyte imbal-

Table 10.3 The central nervous system complications[a] of HIV infection as a function of advancement of HIV-1 infection by CD4 lymphocyte count

	CD4 lymphocyte count/μl		
	>500	200–500	<200
AIDS dementia complex			<---------->
Primary infection sequelae	<---->		
Multiple sclerosis-like illness		<---->	
Aseptic meningitis	<-->		
HIV headache		<----------------------------------->	
Seizures		<--------------------->	
Transient neurological disorders		<--------------------->	
Opportunistic infection			<--->
Meningovascular syphilis	<--->		
Primary CNS lymphoma			<---------->
Metastatic systemic lymphoma			<---------->
Vacuolar myelopathy			<--->
Multinucleated cell myelitis			<--->

[a]Complications have been placed in the CD4 lymphocyte count category, where the disorder is most common, not where it may occur.

ance or HIV infection itself (Holtzman *et al.*, 1989; Dore *et al.*, 1996). In patients in whom there is no cause apart from HIV infection, there is a relationship with ADC: approximately 10% of patients with ADC have seizures, whereas an unknown proportion of patients with seizures have ADC (see Table 10.3). Seizures occurring in the absence of an identifiable cause seem to indicate subclinical HIV involvement of the brain and place the patient at a higher risk of subsequent development of ADC. The investigation of the HIV-infected patient with a seizure should be directed towards the exclusion of an underlying treatable condition: electrolytes, particularly calcium and magnesium, should be measured and a CT brain scan and CSF analysis performed. As there is a high relapse rate, indefinite anticonvulsant therapy should be initiated after the first seizure. Because approximately 14% of patients will develop a rash with phenytoin and probably carbamazepine, a useful alternative drug is valproic acid. This has the added advantage that it does not use the cytochrome P450 system for its metabolism and so will not interact with the PI antiretroviral medications. Some of the newer anticonvalescent drugs such as lamotrigene and gabapentin also do not require the cytochrome P450 system, for metabolism, but there is probably a greater propensity for the development of a rash with lamotrigene.

Transient neurological deficits and strokes

Cerebrovascular complications occur in HIV infection, often as the result of an underlying opportunistic infection, lymphoma, marantic endocarditis or occasionally meningovascular syphilis. However, some patients may develop transient neurological deficits without an underlying condition (Engstrom *et al.*, 1989; Brew and Miller, 1996) (see Table 10.3). At autopsy, 20% of patients have evidence of small areas of infarction in the basal ganglia, but few had clinically apparent strokes (Mizusawa *et al.*, 1989). The pathogenesis of these vascular events is unknown. Some patients have significantly elevated titres of anticardiolipin antibodies and low levels of protein S, which may be contributory (Brew and Miller, 1996). There seems to be an association with active HIV disease and these patients seem more likely to have ADC, so that intensification of antiretroviral drugs may be useful (Brew and Miller, 1996).

Some patients with transient ischaemic attacks and stroke may have a cerebral vasculitis due to varicella zoster virus (Gray *et al.*, 1994). How such a diagnosis should be made is unclear; cerebral angiography may play a role and

amplification of the varicella zoster virus (VZV) genome in the CSF by polymerase chain reaction (PCR) may also be helpful. Treatment is the same as that employed in the HIV-uninfected patient; namely, consideration is given to anticoagulation and, when appropriate, to aciclovir.

Uncommon central nervous system opportunistic complications of the brain

For the most part these conditions will be discussed elsewhere in this book, but mention will be made here of those complications that have either distinct neurological complications or that have neurological involvement as their major or sole clinical expression.

Cytomegalovirus encephalitis

CMV affecting the CNS is a feature of advanced immunodeficiency; usually when the CD4 lymphocyte count is less than 50 cells/μl (see Chapter 21). CMV may cause a poorly defined encephalitis that can develop over days to several weeks (Brew, 1992), with a clinical picture consisting of progressive obtundation, fevers and seizures. In addition, some patients may have a focal encephalitis, sometimes with mass lesions (Dyer *et al.*, 1995) or a brainstem encephalitis, often involving the third, fourth and sixth nerves with nystagmus (Fuller *et al.*, 1989; Holland *et al.*, 1994). There may not be clinical evidence of CMV organ involvement elsewhere. Infrequently, patients have a preexisting CMV retinopathy or CMV colitis controlled on maintenance antiviral therapy (Berman and Kim, 1994). CT brain scan often shows the background abnormality of cerebral atrophy, and occasionally may show periventricular contrast enhancement, reflecting the associated ventriculitis that is found pathologically. Analysis of the CSF may demonstrate a polymorphonuclear pleocytosis, a finding highly suggestive of CMV infection of the CNS, after exclusion of bacterial and tuberculous meningitis. Amplification of CMV DNA from the CSF by the PCR is useful diagnostically (Cinque *et al.*, 1997). Ganciclovir may be beneficial, but objective data on its efficacy are unavailable. Some clinicians utilize combination therapy with ganciclovir and foscarnet.

Progressive multifocal leukoencephalopathy

Progressive multifocal leukoencephalopathy (PML) is another uncommon disorder found in approximately 4% of AIDS patients, usually at an advanced stage of HIV infection (Major *et al.*, 1992). The clinical picture is that of a multifocal deficit with preservation of consciousness that develops gradually, over several weeks. Patients are afebrile unless there is a complicating illness. The CT brain scan often reveals areas of hypodensity without mass effect and usually without contrast enhancement. Occasionally, the CT brain scan will be unremarkable, while an MRI brain scan reveals multiple lesions confined to the white matter with sparing of the cortex. Although these radiological appearances are highly suggestive of PML, VZV infection may rarely produce similar changes. At present, the only definitive method of diagnosis is by brain biopsy, but amplification of the genome of the causative agent, the JC virus, by PCR from the CSF can be very useful, with a 60–90% sensitivity and almost 100% specificity (Cinque *et al.*, 1997). There is no proven therapy for this disorder. There have been several anecdotal reports of the efficacy of cytosine arabinoside but in a large, randomized trial there was no evidence of efficacy using either systemic or intrathecal administration (Hall *et al.*, 1998). There are also anecdotal reports of resolution with HAART (Mileno *et al.*, 1997) and with interferon alpha (Huang *et al.*, 1998).

Syphilis

There is some evidence that syphilis may behave more aggressively in HIV-infected patients with earlier neurological complications and atypical presentations (Katz and Berger, 1989). Patients have presented with meningovascular syphilis after adequate treatment for primary syphilis. There have been no reports of general paresis of the insane or tabes dorsalis. Meningovascular syphilis may lead to transient ischaemic attacks and strokes. The diagnosis of neurosyphilis in HIV-infected patients may be exceptionally difficult (Davis, 1990), as infection with both pathogens may have similar clinical manifestations and both frequently lead to CSF abnormalities. Certainly neurosyphilis may occur with a negative CSF Venereal Disease Research Laboratories (VDRL) test and rarely a negative fluorescent treponemal antibody test (FTA). For practical purposes, however, negative syphilis serology makes the diagnosis of neurosyphilis very unlikely. The treatment course and dose of intravenous penicillin are no different to those employed in the HIV-uninfected patient with neurosyphilis, except that benzathine penicillin should be avoided as it has poor CSF penetration (see Chapter 22).

Central nervous system: spinal cord involvement

Vacuolar myelopathy and multinucleated cell myelitis

Approximately one-third of AIDS patients at autopsy have a condition that has been termed vacuolar myelopathy (Petito *et al.*, 1985), although only the more severely affected have a clinically apparent spastic paraparesis, usually without a definite sensory level (Dal Pan *et al.*, 1994) (see Table 10.3). Posterior column sensory loss of diminished proprioception and vibration sense is common and dominant over pinprick or light-touch abnormalities. The clinical picture is similar to subacute combined degeneration of the spinal cord but serum vitamin B_{12} levels are normal. The deficits are largely confined to the lower limbs, and the onset is usually over weeks to months. The disorder is uncommon in HIV-infected children. Although the features of this myelopathy may exist alone, it often co-exists with ADC and sometimes with a peripheral neuropathy.

Some HIV-infected patients develop multinucleated cell myelitis or HIV myelitis. The prevalence and clinical features are less precisely known, but the myelitis appears to cause a myelopathy that is not necessarily confined to the posterior and lateral columns of the spinal cord, as compared with vacuolar myelopathy. The major difficulty is that the two conditions may occur in the same patient. The main differential diagnosis of these two conditions is the myelopathy that may occur after exposure to nitrous oxide, which causes a clinical picture similar to vacuolar myelopathy. Inquiry into any recreational use of nitrous oxide should clarify the diagnosis.

Neuropathology

Vacuolar myelopathy is pathologically similar to subacute combined degeneration of the cord, with multiple vacuoles in the white matter of the posterior and lateral columns of the spinal cord, infrequent lipid-laden macrophages and separation of the myelin lamellae on electron microscopy. Importantly, the changes are not confined to a particular tract. The thoracic cord is most often involved but changes can extend into the brainstem.

Multinucleated cell myelitis is characterized by multinucleated cell infiltrates that do not seem to have a predilection for any particular part of the cord. There are parenchymal and perivascular infiltrates of microglial cells, macrophages and multinucleated giant cells involving both the grey and white matter of the cord. This is probably the spinal cord equivalent of HIV encephalitis.

Pathogenesis

The pathogenesis of vacuolar myelopathy is unknown. HIV itself is unlikely because vacuolar myelopathy has been described in immunocompromised non-HIV-infected patients (Kamin and Petito, 1991). Similarly, although other retroviruses such as human T-lymphotropic virus type 1 have been associated with a myelopathy, the possibility that vacuolar myelopathy might be related to dual infection with HTLV-1 has been excluded (Brew *et al.*, 1989b). The observation that vacuolar myelopathy is uncommon in children (Sharer *et al.*, 1990) supports the hypothesis that it is in fact another opportunistic infection and not a consequence of a metabolic disturbance. Children have a low prevalence of opportunistic infections as they have not lived long enough to be primarily infected with the usual opportunistic pathogens that are later reactivated. A metabolic disturbance such as a methylation defect of cobalamin has been identified in HIV infection (Keating *et al.*, 1991), but as this has been described in HIV-infected children (Surtees *et al.*, 1990), the very group where vacuolar myelopathy is rare, it would seem unlikely to play a causative role.

Multinucleated cell myelitis is related, in part at least, to productive infection of the infiltrating cells because immunohistochemical evaluation has demonstrated various HIV antigens. The precise mechanisms of spinal cord damage are likely to be similar to those that operate in ADC.

Investigations

Presently, there is no clinically useful diagnostic investigation. Myelography and CSF analysis are employed only for the exclusion of other diseases. MRI scanning of the cord has not proved helpful, although one group have identified MRI changes in autopsy tissue that are said to be suggestive of the presence of vacuolar myelopathy (Santosh *et al.*, 1993).

Treatment

Anecdotal experience suggests that vacuolar myelopathy does not respond to antiretroviral therapy, while multinucleated cell myelitis does. However, further data are required. A trial using S-adenosyl methionine to correct a possible cobalamin metabolic defect is currently underway.

Peripheral nervous system: peripheral nerve and root

HIV-related peripheral neuropathy
Classification

HIV-related peripheral neuropathy may take the form of distal symmetrical predominantly sensory neuropathy, autonomic neuropathy, mononeuritis multiplex, inflammatory demyelinating polyneuropathy, mononeuropathy and diffuse infiltrative lymphocytosis syndrome-associated neuropathy (Simpson and Wolfe, 1991; Moulignier *et al.*, 1997; Gherardi *et al.*, 1998). The American Academy of Neurology Working Group has defined two conditions: HIV-associated acute inflammatory demyelinating polyneuropathy and HIV-associated predominantly sensory neuropathy (Working Group of the American Academy of Neurology AIDS Task Force, 1991). An important cause of neuropathy is that which is secondary to the use of certain nucleoside analogues. As this is very similar to distal symmetrical neuropathy, it will be discussed in that section.

General principles. There are certain general principles that are relevant to neuropathies. First, as with other neurological complications, the type of neuropathy is related to the degree of advancement of HIV disease, as measured by the CD4 lymphocyte count (see Table 10.4). Treatment of these neuropathies varies according to the type, and includes optimization of nutrition and minimization of exposure to potential neuropathical insults (e.g. neurotoxic nucleosides). There are certain risk factors for the development of HIV-related neuropathy:

(1) advanced HIV disease, especially CD4 lymphocyte below 50 cells/μl;
(2) pre-existing neuropathy, including subclinical distal predominantly sensory neuropathy; and
(3) presence of predisposing factors, such as nutritional disturbance or exposure to vincristine.

HIV-associated distal predominantly sensory neuropathy (including nucleoside and painful neuropathy). This is the most common and probably the most important of the HIV-related neuropathies. It is a feature of advanced HIV disease and is estimated to occur in approximately 45% of AIDS patients (Simpson and Wolfe, 1991). Nucleoside neuropathy occurs in approximately 15% of patients taking one or more of ddI (didanosine), ddC (zalcitabine) or d4T

Table 10.4 The peripheral neurological complications[a] of HIV infection as a function of advancement of HIV-1 infection by CD4 lymphocyte count

	CD4 lymphocyte count/μl		
	>500	200–500	<200
Predominantly sensory neuropathy		<------------------>	
Distal painful sensory neuropathy			<--->
Autonomic neuropathy			<--------->
Mononeuritis multiplex	<-------------------->		
Acute demyelinating neuropathy	<------------------------>		
Chronic demyelinating neuropathy		<----->	
Mononeuropathies	<--->		<--->
Opportunistic infection			<--->
Syphilitic polyradiculopathy		<-------------------->	
Non-inflammatory myopathies	<--->		
Polymyositis	<--->		

[a]Complications have been placed in the CD4 lymphocyte count category, where the disorder is most common, not where it may occur.

(stavudine). It is also more common in patients with advanced HIV disease. Painful neuropathy may occur as a result of either of the above neuropathies.

The clinical manifestations of these neuropathies are essentially the same. Initially, there is mildly diminished temperature perception in the legs, with absent or depressed ankle jerks and minimal or no symptoms. With time, the patients develop tingling or numbness in the feet, which gradually spreads to the knees. The hands are involved less frequently. Significant limb weakness is uncommon. In a small proportion of patients a painful distal sensory neuropathy develops, which progresses to the point where it is difficult for the patient to walk. This peripheral neuropathy is uncommon in HIV-infected children. Recognition of the neuropathy, even in its early stages, is important as it may worsen dramatically with administration of ddI, ddC, d4T or the vinca alkaloids. Infection with *Mycobacterium avium* complex (MAC) may precipitate or exacerbate the neuropathy (Norton *et al.*, 1996).

The pathogenesis of distal predominantly sensory neuropathy is unknown. Productive HIV infection of the nerve has not been convincingly demonstrated (Grafe and Wiley, 1989). Similarly, CMV infection is unlikely, as the neuropathy may occur at a CD4 lymphocyte count not usually associated with CMV disease. The reason for the rarity of peripheral neuropathy in HIV-infected children is unknown, but as with vacuolar myelopathy it may point to an indirect pathogenesis, such as another opportunistic infection. Macrophages have been found to be prominent in the peripheral nerves of HIV-infected patients, arguing against a purely metabolic disturbance (Griffin *et al.*, 1998).

Treatment is mainly symptomatic. When pain is prominent, capsaicin cream may be useful in single, double or even triple strength. In those patients who do not benefit from capsaicin, low doses of amitriptylline, starting at 10 mg each night and slowly increasing to approximately 50 mg, may be beneficial. If the side-effect of drowsiness is problematic, then desipramine may be useful. Topical lidocaine also appears effective in some patients (Khan *et al.*, 1998) and valproic acid may also be useful. A recent controlled trial demonstrated that lamotrigene is effective, although doses did not exceed 300 mg each day, and there did not appear to be any efficacy in those patients with nucleoside-related painful neuropathy (Simpson *et al.*, 1998). Nerve growth factor appears to have modest benefit in this disorder (McArthur *et al.*, 1998). Some patients who do not respond to any of the above measures require narcotic analgesic medication.

HIV-associated autonomic neuropathy. In the more advanced phase of HIV-1 infection, a small number of patients develop an autonomic neuropathy that is clinically significant (Freeman *et al.*, 1990), with postural hypotension, diarrhoea and sudden arrhythmias. A subclinical autonomic neuropathy has been found in approximately 50% of patients with advanced HIV disease. The autonomic neuropathy usually occurs in conjunction with the predominantly sensory neuropathy. Treatment is symptomatic, with the use of agents such as fludrocortisone acetate for stabilization of blood pressure.

HIV-associated mononeuritis multiplex. Mononeuritis multiplex was first described by Lipkin *et al.* (1985) and seems to occur when the CD4 lymphocyte count is subnormal but not below 250 cells/μl. The disorder is rare and may require corticosteroids and immunosuppressant therapy for control, as is required with other vasculitic neuropathies. HAART may have a role (Markus and Brew, 1998).

Demyelinating neuropathies. A demyelinating neuropathy may occur acutely at seroconversion or chronically at a later stage of HIV disease when there is only mild immunodeficiency (Simpson and Wolfe, 1991). The clinical presentation is identical to that seen in the non-HIV-infected population, except that investigations reveal a mild CSF mononuclear pleocytosis in contrast to the classic 'albumino-cytologique dissociation' of Guillain-Barré syndrome. It is likely that the CSF pleocytosis represents the subclinical aseptic meningitis common in HIV-1 infected individuals; that is, the pleocytosis is an asymptomatic background abnormality brought to clinical attention by the chance occurrence of the neuropathy. Treatment with plasmapheresis and response is no different from that seen in non-HIV-infected patients.

Mononeuropathy. In the context of primary HIV infection or the early stage of HIV disease, patients may develop a variety of mononeuropathies, usually cranial and most often involving the seventh nerve. These are often short-lived and infrequently related to herpes zoster or lymphoma. In advanced HIV disease, mononeuropathies may also occur, usually related to pressure in the context of debility and wasting. When pressure is deemed an unlikely cause, CMV should be considered (Said *et al.*, 1991) and treated where appropriate.

Diffuse infiltrative lymphocytosis syndrome associated neuropathy. This newly described entity has been defined as a neuropathy that occurs in a subgroup of patients with marked increases in CD8 lymphocytes and a consequent Sjogren-like syndrome with multivisceral infiltration (Moulignier *et al.*, 1997; Gherardi *et al.*, 1998). It usually occurs in patients with CD4 lymphocyte counts above 200 cells/μl. The clinical features include the development of a

usually symmetrical, often painful sensorimotor neuropathy. The neuropathy often co-exists with parotidomegaly and a sicca syndrome (Moulignier *et al.*, 1997). The pathological features are those of an axonal neuropathy with CD8 lymphocyte infiltrates. There is no proven treatment, but some patients respond to HAART and others require corticosteroid treatment.

Uncommon central nervous system opportunistic complications of the peripheral nervous system

Cytomegalovirus radiculomyelopathy
Clinical features
In approximately 2% of AIDS patients, CMV infection may lead to a polyradiculopathy mainly affecting the legs, with some spinal cord involvement (de Gans *et al.*, 1990). Usually, patients complain of an ascending numbness in both lower limbs associated with leg weakness, back pain and sometimes saddle anaesthesia, with the later development of urinary dysfunction. Onset is gradual over a few days to weeks. Deep tendon reflexes are lost in the legs and there is evidence of distal sensory loss with leg weakness. Rarely, there is involvement of the hands. Antecedent or co-existent CMV organ involvement occurs in approximately half of patients.

Investigations. Analysis of CSF reveals a polymorphonuclear pleocytosis in the absence of any other identifiable organism in the majority of patients and is very suggestive of the diagnosis. Amplification of CMV DNA from the CSF by the PCR is the definitive investigation.

Treatment. Intravenous ganciclovir at a dose of 5 mg/kg twice daily for 3 weeks is effective in some patients (de Gans *et al.*, 1990). However, as this disorder is rare, there have been no controlled studies to determine optimal dose and duration of induction therapy. Patients should be placed on indefinite maintenance therapy. If there is no response to ganciclovir after 2–3 weeks, or if there is suspicion of resistance to ganciclovir, foscarnet should be used.

Cytomegalovirus mononeuritis multiplex
In a small number of patients with advanced HIV disease, a mononeuritis multiplex caused by CMV may develop (Said *et al.*, 1991). The presentation is similar to HIV-associated mononeuritis multiplex, except that the patient has

more advanced HIV disease with a CD4 lymphocyte count of less than 50 cells/μl. The diagnosis is usually made on clinical grounds, as the CSF may show no abnormalities and nerve biopsy may not reveal CMV because of the patchy nature of involvement. Treatment is the same as that used for CMV disease elsewhere.

Syphilitic polyradiculopathy

Rarely, patients may develop a polyradiculopathy related to syphilis (Lanska et al., 1988). This may occur without any other syphilitic complications. The symptoms and signs resemble a lumbosacral radiculopathy, and the CSF is abnormal, with a low glucose and markedly raised white cell count and protein. Treatment with intravenous penicillin is effective.

Peripheral nervous system: muscle

HIV myopathy

HIV-associated myopathies are poorly defined (Simpson and Wolfe, 1991). The myopathies may be grouped into inflammatory and non-inflammatory conditions. The inflammatory myopathy is similar to polymyositis and seems to occur in patients with mild to moderate immunodeficiency. Diagnosis is made by muscle biopsy. The management of patients with this type of myopathy is difficult because they often need corticosteroid therapy to control the myopathy. This places them at greater risk of opportunistic infections and they should be monitored closely when the CD4 lymphocyte count is less than 100 cells/μl. When patients reach this level of immunodeficiency it may be prudent to consider alternative therapy such as intravenous gamma globulin. When patients are commenced on corticosteroids, appropriate prophylaxis should be instituted; namely, cotrimoxazole for Pneumocystis carinii and toxoplasmosis prevention.

Rarely, patients may develop a non-inflammatory myopathy that usually affects all limbs, although the development of severe weakness has not been reported. The disorder does not seem to be linked to the stage of HIV disease and there is no known treatment for this complication.

Very uncommonly, patients may develop a myopathy secondary to opportunistic conditions such as toxoplasmosis, microsporidial infection, cryptococcosis and MAC infection. These myopathies are characterized by their acute development, sometimes with systemic involvement.

Zidovudine myopathy

Currently, the most important myopathy in HIV-infected individuals is that related to ZDV therapy. It generally develops after 1 year on therapy, in less than 20% of patients, and is manifest as wasting of the buttock muscles, with associated leg weakness (Dalakas et al. 1990). The risk of myopathy increases with daily dose and duration of ZDV treatment. The disorder is a mitochondrial myopathy with inhibition of gamma DNA polymerase by ZDV (Dalakas et al., 1990). Definitive diagnosis requires a biopsy, but there is some evidence that affected patients have raised blood lactate/pyruvate ratios, as seen in a mitochondrial myopathy. In practical terms, patients who have been on ZDV for longer than several months should have their creatinine kinase (CK) monitored regularly, perhaps every month to 6 weeks, so that the ZDV dose can be decreased or ceased when serum CK increases. If the CK does not fall within several days to weeks, an alternate diagnosis should be considered. When the complication is recognized early, improvement and in some cases resolution should occur.

Approach to diagnosis of neurological symptoms and signs

In an individual patient, the diagnosis of the nature of the neurological disturbance can be approached in the following way. First, the anatomical site of the lesion should be determined and then consideration should be given to the likely pathology. In HIV-related neurological disease, the differential diagnosis of the pathology is largely determined by the stage of HIV disease, as illustrated in Tables 10.3 and 10.4. The best measure of stage of HIV disease is the CD4 lymphocyte count, with the nadir count being taken as a guide at the present time. In the future, the CD4 lymphocyte count elevation that occurs with potent antiretroviral therapy may be found to represent fully functioning CD4 cells, and the risk of a particular neurological complication may change with the CD4 lymphocyte count. It is also not apparent at the moment whether the degree of elevation of plasma viral load determines the occurrence of certain complications, such as, peripheral neuropathy.

In HIV-related brain involvement, it is also useful to consider whether the clinical presentation is predominantly focal or non-focal (Table 10.5). While there are some patients where such a distinction is difficult, most will be one or the other.

Table 10.5 HIV-related complications of the brain according to clinical presentation

Focal	Non-focal
Toxoplasmosis	AIDS dementia complex
Primary brain lymphoma	Cytomegalovirus (CMV)
Progressive multifocal	encephalitis
leukoencephalopathy	Cryptococcal meningitis
Cryptococcoma	Tuberculous meningitis
Varicella zoster virus	Lymphomatous meningitis
Meningovascular syphilis	HIV headache
Metastatic lymphoma	
Transient neurological	
disorders	
Miscellaneous (tuberculosis,	
aspergillosis,	
histoplasmosis, etc.)	

Two disorders are rarely if ever associated with neurological disease: Kaposi's sarcoma (KS) and *Mycobacterium avium* complex (MAC). While there have been occasional reports of metastatic KS to the nervous system, it is exceptionally rare. Similarly, MAC may involve the meninges or brain, but it is uncommon. It is now evident that toxoplasmosis is very unlikely if the patient is taking cotrimoxazole and cryptococcal disease is unlikely if the patient is taking either ketoconazole or fluconazole.

The physician should also consider that within each part of the nervous system there may be several complications 'layered' upon each other. For example, a patient may have background abnormalities of the CSF, consisting of a mild mononuclear pleocytosis and raised protein, added to the characteristic CSF findings of CMV radiculomyelopathy (a polymorphonuclear pleocytosis). Another example is the patient with an HIV-associated predominantly sensory neuropathy, who develops a superimposed vincristine neuropathy as part of treatment for KS and later develops a painful neuropathy secondary to ddI. At a particular time point the diagnosis of the most recent complication may therefore be confounded by the pre-existing pathologies. This has special relevance to ADC where a previously compensated subclinical deficit may be unmasked by another complication, such as toxoplasmosis. Similarly, a number of pathological processes may be occurring at different parts of the nervous system, at the same time further complicating accurate diagnosis; a concept that has been termed 'parallel tracking'. As an example, it is not uncommon for a patient to have varying combinations of ADC, a myelopathy, sensory and autonomic neuropathies. If the patient then develops urinary incontinence, is it related to progression of ADC with involvement of the micturition centre or is it progression of the myelopathy or the autonomic neuropathy, or a combination of all three? Despite these complexities, it is usually possible to arrive at an accurate diagnosis by using the latter principles and thereby to institute appropriate treatment.

References

Bacellar H, Munoz A, Miller EN et al. (1994). Temporal trends in the incidence of HIV-1 related neurologic diseases: multicentre AIDS cohort study 1985–1992. *Neurology* **44**: 1892–900.

Bagasra O, Lavi E, Bobroski L et al. (1996). Cellular reservoirs of HIV-1 in the central nervous system of infected individuals: identification by the combination of *in situ* polymerase chain reaction and immunochemistry. *AIDS* **10**: 573–86.

Barker PB, Lee RR, McArthur JC. (1995). AIDS dementia complex: evaluation with proton MR spectroscopic imaging. *Radiology* **195**: 58–4.

Berger JR, Sheremata WA, Resnick L et al. (1989). Multiple sclerosis-like illness occurring with human immunodeficiency virus infection. *Neurology* **39**: 324–9.

Berman SM, Kim RC. (1994). The development of cytomegalovirus encephalitis in AIDS patients receiving ganciclovir. *Am J Med* **96**: 415–9.

Brenneman DE, Westbrook GL, Fitzgerald SP et al. (1988). Neuronal cell killing by the envelope protein of HIV and its prevention by vasoactive intestinal peptide. *Nature* **335**: 639–42.

Brew BJ. (1992). Central and peripheral nervous system abnormalities in HIV-1 infection. In: White DA, Gold JWM (eds.) *Medical management of AIDS patients. Medical clinics of North America*. Volume 76. Philadelphia, PA: WB Saunders, 63–81.

Brew BJ. (1997). AIDS dementia complex and its prevention. *Antiviral Ther* **2**: 69–73.

Brew BJ, Miller J. (1993). Human immunodeficiency related headache. *Neurology* **43**: 1098–100.

Brew BJ, Miller J. (1996). Human immunodeficiency virus type 1 related transient neurologic deficits. *Am J Med* **101**: 257–61.

Brew BJ, Tindall B. (1997). Neurologic manifestations of primary HIV-1 infection. In: J Berger, R Levy (eds.) *AIDS and the nervous system*. 2nd edition. Philadelphia, PA: Raven Press, 517–26.

Brew BJ, Perdices M, Darveniza P et al. (1989a). The neurological features of early and 'latent' human immunodeficiency virus infection. *Aust NZ J Med* **19**: 700–5.

Brew BJ, Hardy W, Zuckerman E et al. (1989b). AIDS-related vacuolar myelopathy is not associated with co-infection by HTLV-1. *Ann Neurol* **26**: 679–81.

Brew BJ, Bhalla RB, Paul M et al. (1990). CSF neopterin in HIV-1 infection. *Ann Neurol* **28**: 556–60.

Brew BJ, Bhalla RB, Paul M et al. (1992). Cerebrospinal fluid β_2 microglobulin in patients with AIDS dementia complex: an expanded series including response to zidovudine treatment. *AIDS* **6**: 461–5.

Brew BJ, Paul M, Nakajima G et al. (1994). Cerebrospinal fluid HIV-1 p24 antigen and culture: sensitivity and specificity for AIDS dementia complex. *J Neurol Neurosurg Psychiatr* **57**: 784–9.

Brew BJ, Rosenblum M, Cronin K et al. (1995a). The AIDS dementia complex and human immunodeficiency virus type 1 brain infection: clinical-virological correlations. Ann Neurol **38**: 563–70.

Brew BJ, Corbeil J, Pemberton L et al. (1995b). Quinolinic acid production by macrophages infected with HIV-1 isolates from patients with and without AIDS dementia complex. J Neurovirol **6**: 369–74.

Brew BJ, Dunbar N, Druett J et al. (1996a). Pilot study of the efficacy of atevirdine in the treatment of AIDS dementia complex. AIDS **10**: 1357–60.

Brew BJ, Evans L, Byrne C et al. (1996b). The relationship between AIDS dementia complex and the presence of macrophage tropic and non syncytium inducing isolates of human immunodeficiency virus type 1 in the cerebrospinal fluid. J Neurovirol **2**: 152–7.

Brew BJ, Dunbar N, Pemberton L et al. (1996c). Cerebrospinal fluid concentrations of β_2 microglobulin and neopterin predict the development of AIDS dementia Complex. J Infect Dis **174**: 294–8.

Brew BJ, Pemberton L, Cunningham P et al. (1997). Levels of HIV-1 RNA correlate with AIDS dementia. J Infect Dis **175**: 963–6.

Brew BJ, Brown SJ, Catalan J et al. (1998). Safety and efficacy of Abacavir (ABC, 1592) in AIDS Twelfth dementia complex (Study CNAB 3001), Twelfth World AIDS Conference, Geneva, Switzerland.

Budka H. (1990). Human immunodeficiency virus (HIV) envelope and core proteins in CNS tissues of patients with the acquired immune deficiency syndrome (AIDS). Acta Neuropathol **79**: 611–9.

Budka H, Wiley CA, Kleihues P et al. (1991). HIV associated disease of the nervous system: review of nomenclature and proposal for neuropathology based terminology. Brain Pathol **1**: 143–52.

Butler KM, Husson RN, Balis FM et al. (1991). Dideoxyinosine in children with symptomatic human immunodeficiency virus infection. N Engl J Med **324**: 137–44.

Cairns JS, D'Souza MP. (1998). Chemokines and HIV-1 second receptors: the therapeutic connection. Nat Med **4**: 563–8.

Chiodi F, Albert J, Olausson E et al. (1988). Isolation frequency of Human Immunodeficiency Virus from cerebrospinal fluid and blood of patients with varying severity of HIV infection. AIDS Res Hum Retrovir **4**: 351–8.

Cinque P, Scarpellini P, Vago L et al. (1997). Diagnosis of central nervous system complications in HIV-infected patients: cerebrospinal fluid analysis by the polymerase chain reaction. AIDS **11**: 1–17.

Collier AC, Marra C, Coombs et al. (1997). Cerebrospinal fluid indinavir and HIV RNA levels in patients on chronic indinavir therapy. In: Program and abstracts of the Infectious Diseases Society of America Thirty-fifth Annual Meeting, San Francisco, CA, USA.

Cunningham P, Smith D, Satchell C et al. (1998). Evidence for independent development of RT inhibitor resistance patterns in cerebrospinal fluid compartment. Twelfth World AIDS Conference, Geneva, Switzerland.

Currie J, Benson E, Ramsden B et al. (1988). Eye movement abnormalities as a predictor of the acquired immunodeficiency syndrome dementia complex. Arch Neurol **45**: 949–53.

Dalakas MC, Illa I, Pezeshkpour GH et al. (1990). Mitochondrial myopathy caused by long term zidovudine therapy. N Engl J Med **322**: 1098–105.

Dal Pan GJ, Glass JD, McArthur JC. (1994). Clinicopathologic correlations of HIV-1 associated myelopathy: an autopsy-based case control study. Neurology **44**: 2159–64.

Davis LE. (1990). Neurosyphilis in the patient infected with human immunodeficiency virus. Ann Neurol **27**: 211–2.

Dawson VL, Dawson TM, Uhl GR et al. (1993). Human immunodeficiency virus type 1 coat protein neurotoxicity mediated by nitric oxide in primary cortical cultures. Proc Natl Acad Sci USA **90**: 3256–9.

de Gans J, Portegies P, Tiessens G et al. (1990). Therapy for cytomegalovirus polyradiculomyelitis in patients with AIDS: treatment with ganciclovir. AIDS **4**: 421–5.

Dore GJ, Law M, Brew BJ. (1996). Prospective analysis of seizures occurring in human immunodeficiency virus type 1 infection. J Neurol AIDS **1**: 59–70.

Dunbar N, Brew BJ. (1996). Neuropsychological dysfunction in HIV infection: a review. J Neuro-AIDS **1**: 73–102.

Dyer JR, French MAH, Mallal SM. (1995). Cerebral mass lesions due to cytomegalovirus in patients with AIDS: report of two cases. J Infect Dis **30**: 147–51.

Ellis R, Hsia K, Spector SA et al. (1997). Cerebrospinal fluid human immunodeficiency virus type 1 RNA levels are elevated in neurocognitively impaired individuals with acquired immunodeficiency syndrome. Ann Neurol **42**: 679–88.

Engstrom JW, Lowenstein DH, Bredesen DE. (1989). Cerebral infarctions and transient neurologic deficits associated with acquired immunodeficiency syndrome. Am J Med **86**: 528–32.

Epstein LG, Gendelman HE (1993). Human immunodeficiency virus type 1 infection of the nervous system: pathogenetic mechanisms. Ann Neurol **33**: 429–36.

Esiri M, Morris CS, Millard PR. (1991). Fate of oligodendrocytes in HIV-1 infection. AIDS **5**: 1081–8.

Everall IP, Luthert PJ, Lantos PL. (1991). Neuronal loss in the frontal cortex in HIV infection. Lancet **337**: 1119–21.

Fernando S, van Gorp W, McElhiney M et al. (1998). Highly active antiretroviral treatment in HIV infection: benefits for neuropsychological function. AIDS **12**: F65–70.

Foudraine NA, Hetelmans RMW, Lange JA et al. (1998). Cerebrospinal fluid HIV-1 RNA and drug concentrations after treatment with lamivudine plus zidovudine or stavudine. Lancet **351**: 1547–51.

Freeman R, Roberts MS, Friedman LS et al. (1990). Autonomic function and human immunodeficiency virus infection. Neurology **40**: 575–80.

Fuller GN, Guiloff RJ, Scaravilli F et al. (1989). Combined HIV-CMV encephalitis presenting with brainstem signs. J Neurol Neurosurg Psychiatry **52**: 975–9.

Gallo P, Frei K, Rordorf C et al. (1989). Human immunodeficiency virus type 1 (HIV-1) infection of the central nervous system: an evaluation of cytokines in cerebrospinal fluid. J Neuroimmunol **23**: 109–16.

Gherardi RK, Chretien F, Delfau-Larue M-H et al. (1998). Neuropathy in diffuse infiltrative lymphocytosis syndrome: an HIV neuropathy, not a lymphoma. Neurology **50**: 1041–5.

Gisslen M, Norkrans G, Svennerholm L et al. (1997). The effect on cerebrospinal fluid HIV RNA levels after initiation of zidovudine or didanosine. J Infect Dis **175**: 434–7.

Glass JD, Fedor H, Wesselingh SL et al. (1995). Immunocytochemical quantitation of human immunodeficiency virus in the brain: correlations with dementia. Ann Neurol **38**: 755–62.

Goodin DS, Aminoff MJ, Chernoff DN et al. (1990). Long latency event-related potentials in patients infected with human immunodeficiency virus. Ann Neurol **27**: 414–9.

Grafe MR, Wiley CA. (1989). Spinal cord and peripheral nerve pathology in AIDS: the roles of cytomegalovirus and human immunodeficiency virus. *Ann Neurol* **25**: 561–6.

Gray F, Lescs MC, Keohane C *et al.* (1992). Early brain changes in HIV infection: neuropathological study of 11 HIV seropositive, non-AIDS cases. *J Neuropathol Exp Neurol* **51**: 177–85.

Gray F, Belec L, Lescs MC *et al.* (1994). Varicella zoster virus infection of the central nervous system in AIDS. *Brain* **117**: 987–99.

Griffin JW, Thomas O, Crawford MO, McArthur JC. (1998). Peripheral neuropathies associated with infection. In: HE Gendelman, SA Lipton, L Epstein, S Swindells (eds.). *The neurology of AIDS*. New York: Chapman and Hall, 275–91.

Grimaldi LM, Martino GV, Franciotta DM *et al.* (1991). Elevated alpha tumor necrosis factor levels in spinal fluid from HIV-1 infected patients with central nervous system involvement. *Ann Neurol* **29**: 21–5.

Gyorkey F, Melnick JL, Gyorkey P. (1987). Human immunodeficiency virus in brain biopsies of patients with AIDS and progressive encephalopathy. *J Infect Dis* **155**: 870–6.

Hall CD, Dafni U, Simpson D *et al.* (1998). Failure of cytarabine in progressive multifocal leukoencephalopathy associated with human immunodeficiency virus infection. *N Engl J Med* **338**: 1345–51.

Harouse JM, Wroblewska Z, Laughlin MA *et al.* (1989). Human choroid plexus cells can be latently infected with human immunodeficiency virus. *Ann Neurol* **25**: 406–11.

Harouse JM, Bhat S, Spitalnik SL *et al.* (1991). Inhibition of entry of HIV-1 in neural cell lines by antibodies against galactosyl-ceramide. *Science* **253**: 320–3.

Heyes MP, Brew BJ, Martin A *et al.* (1991). Increased cerebrospinal fluid concentrations of the excitotoxin quinolinic acid in human immunodeficiency virus infection and AIDS dementia complex. *Ann Neurol* **29**: 202–9.

Hinken CH, Van Gorp WG, Mandelkern MA *et al.* (1995). Cerebral metabolic change in patients with AIDS: report of a six-month follow-up positron emission tomography. *J Neuropsychiatry Clin Neurosci* **7**: 180–7.

Holland NR, Power C, Matthews VP *et al.* (1994). Cytomegalovirus encephalitis in acquired immunodeficiency syndrome (AIDS). *Neurology* **44**: 507–14

Holtzman DM, Kaku DA, So YT. (1989). New onset seizures associated with human immunodeficiency virus infection: causation and clinical features in 100 cases. *Am J Med* **87**: 173–7.

Huang SS, Skolansky RL, Dal Pan G *et al.* (1998). Survival prolongation in HIV-associated progressive multifocal leukoencephalopathy treated with alpha-interferon: an observational study. *J Neurovirol* **4**: 324–32.

Jarvik JG, Hesselink JR, Kennedy C *et al.* (1988). Acquired immunodeficiency syndrome: magnetic resonance patterns of brain involvement with pathologic correlation. *Arch Neurol* **45**: 731–6.

Kamin SS, Petito CK. (1991). Idiopathic myelopathies with white matter vacuolation in non-acquired immunodeficiency syndrome patients. *Hum Pathol* **22**: 816–24.

Kapoor C, Robertson K, Vaughn B *et al.* (1998). Headache in HIV infection. *J Neurovirol* **4**: 354.

Katz DA, Berger JR. (1989). Neurosyphilis in acquired immunodeficiency syndrome. *Arch Neurol* **46**: 895–8.

Keating JN, Trimble KC, Mulcahy F *et al.* (1991). Evidence of brain methyltransferase inhibition and early brain involvement in HIV positive patients. *Lancet* **337**: 935–9.

Kerr SJ, Armati PJ, Brew BJ. (1995). Neurocytotoxicity of quinolinic acid in human brain cultures. *J Neurovirol* **1**: 375–80.

Kerr SJ, Armati PJ, Pemberton LA *et al.* (1997). Kynurenine pathway inhibition with 6-chloro-D-tryptohan reduces neurotoxicity of HIV-1 infected macrophage supernatants. *Neurology* **49**: 1671–81.

Kerr SJ, Armati PJ, Brew BJ. (1998). Chronic exposure of human neurons to quinolinic acid results in neuronal changes consistent with AIDS dementia complex. *AIDS* **12**: 357–65.

Ketzler S *et al.* (1990). Loss of neurons in the frontal cortex in AIDS brains. *Acta Neuropathological* **80**: 92–4.

Khan A, Dorfman D, Dalton A *et al.* (1998). Treatment of painful neuropathy in HIV infection with a topical agent: results of an open label study using 5% lidocaine. *J Neurovirol* **4**: 355.

Kimura-Kuroda J, Nagashima K, Yasui K. (1993). HIV-1 gp120 causes demyelination in a primary culture of rat cerebral cortex. *Clin Neuropathol* **12**: S3.

Koralnik IJ, Beaumanoir A, Hausler R *et al.* (1990). A controlled study of of neurologic abnormalities in men with asymptomatic immunodeficiency virus infection. *N Engl J Med* **323**: 864–70.

Kure K, Lyman WD, Weidenheim KM *et al.* (1990). Cellular localization of an HIV-1 antigen in subacute AIDS encephalitis using an improved double-labeling immunohistochemical method. *Am J Pathol* **136**: 1085–92.

Lanska M, Lanska DJ, Schmidley JW. (1988). Syphilitic polyradiculopathy in an HIV-positive man. *Neurology* **38**: 1297–301.

Lipkin W, Parry G, Kiprov D *et al.* (1985). Inflammatory neuropathy in homosexual men with lymphadenopathy. *Neurology* **35**: 1479.

Major EO, Amemiya K, Tornatore CS *et al.* (1992). Pathogenesis and molecular biology of progressive multifocal leukoencephalopathy, the JC virus-induced demyelinating disease of the human brain. *Clin Microbiol Rev* **5**: 49–73.

Markus R, Brew BJ. (1998). HIV-1 peripheral neuropathy: response to combination antiretroviral therapy. *Lancet* **352**: 1906–7.

Marshall DW, Brey RL, Cahill WT *et al.* (1988). Spectrum of cerebrospinal fluid findings in various stages of human immunodeficiency virus infection. *Arch Neurol* **45**: 954–8.

Masdeu JC, Yudd A, Van Heertum RL *et al.* (1991). Single photon emission computed tomography in human immunodeficiency virus encephalopathy: a preliminary report. *J Nucl Med* **32**: 1471–5.

Mastroianni CM, Liuzzi GM, Jirillo E *et al.* (1991). Cerebrospinal fluid markers for the monitoring of AIDS dementia complex severity; usefulness of anti-myelin basic protein antibody detection. *AIDS* **5**: 464–5.

McArthur JC, Cohen BA, Seines OA *et al.* (1989). Low prevalence of neurological and neuropsychological abnormalities in otherwise healthy HIV-1 infected individuals: results from the multicentre AIDS cohort study. *Ann Neurol* **26**: 601–11.

McArthur JC, Hoover R, Bacellar H *et al.* (1993). Dementia in AIDS patients: incidence and risk factors. *Neurology* **43**: 2245–52.

McArthur JC, McClernon DR, Cronin MF *et al.* (1997). Relationship between human immunodeficiency virus – associated dementia and viral load in cerebrospinal fluid and brain. *Ann Neurol* **42**: 689–98.

McArthur JC, Yiannoutsos C, Simpson D *et al.* (1998). Trial of recombinant human nerve growth factor for HIV-associated sensory neuropathy. *J Neurovirol* **4**: 359.

McConnell JR, Swindells S, Ong CS et al. (1994). Prospective utility of cerebral proton magnetic resonance spectroscopy in monitoring HIV infection and its associated neurological impairment. *AIDS Res Hum Retrovir* **8**: 977–82.

Merrill PT, Paige GD, Abrams RA et al. (1991). Ocular motor abnormalities in human immunodeficiency virus infection. *Ann Neurol* **30**: 130–8.

Michaels J, Price RW, Rosenblum MK, (1988). Microglia in the giant cell encephalitis of acquired immune deficiency syndrome: proliferation, infection and fusion. *Acta Neuropathol* **76**: 373–9.

Mileno M, Tashima K, Farrar D et al. (1997). Resolution of AIDS-related opportunistic infections with addition of protease inhibitor treatment. In: *program and abstracts of the Fourth Conference on Retroviruses and Opportunistic Infections*, Washington DC, USA, 129.

Mirsattari S, Power C, Nath A. (1998). Primary headaches in HIV infected patients in a neuro AIDS clinic. *J Neurovirol* **4**: 360.

Moulignier MD, Authier FJ, Baudrimont M et al. (1997). Peripheral neuropathy in human immunodeficiency virus-infected patients with the diffuse infiltrative lymphocytosis syndrome. *Ann Neurol* **41**: 438–45.

Mizusawa H, Hirano A, Llena JF et al. (1989). Cerebrovascular lesions in acquired immune deficiency syndrome (AIDS). *Acta Neuropathologica* **76**: 451–7.

Navia B, Jordan BD, Price RW. (1986a). The AIDS dementia complex: clinical features. *Ann Neurol* **19**: 517–24.

Navia B, Cho ES, Petito CK et al. (1986b). The AIDS dementia complex: II. Neuropathology. *Ann Neurol* **19**: 525–35.

Navia BA, Gonzalez RG. (1997). Functional imaging of the AIDS dementia complex and the metabolic pathology of the HIV-1 infected brain. *Neuroimaging Clin N Am* **7**: 431–45.

Norton GR, Sweeney J, Marriott D. (1996). An association between HIV distal symmetrical polyneuropathy and *Mycobacterium avium* complex infection. *J Neurol Neurosurg Psychiatr* **61**: 606–9.

Nuovo GJ, Gallery F, MacConnell P. (1994). *In situ* detection of polymerase chain reaction-amplified HIV-1 nucleic acids and tumor necrosis factor-RNA in the central nervous system. *Am J Pathol* **144**: 659–66.

Nuwer MR, Miller EN, Visscher BR et al. (1992). Asymptomatic HIV infection does not cause EEG abnormalities: results from the multi-centre AIDS cohort study (MACS). *Neurology* **42**: 1214–9.

Parisi A, Di Perri G, Strosselli M et al. (1989). Usefulness of computerized electroencephalography in diagnosing, staging and monitoring AIDS dementia complex. *AIDS* **3**: 209–13.

Pemberton LA, Kerr SJ, Smythe G. (1997). Quinolinic acid production by macrophages stimulated with interferon γ tumor necrosis factor α and interferon α. *J Interferon Cytokine Res* **17**: 589–95.

Perdices M, Cooper DA. (1989). Simple and choice reaction time in patients with human immunodeficiency virus infection. *Ann Neurol* **25**: 460–7.

Perry VH, Lawson LJ, Reid DM. (1994). Biology of the mononuclear phagocyte system of the central nervous system and HIV infection. *J Leukoc Biol* **56**: 399–406.

Petito CK, Navia BA, Cho ES et al. (1985). Vacuolar myelopathy pathologically resembling subacute combined degeneration in patients with acquired immunodeficiency syndrome (AIDS). *N Engl J Med* **312**: 874–9.

Petito CK, Cash KS. (1992). Blood brain barrier abnormalities in the acquired immune deficiency syndrome: immunohistochemical localization of serum proteins in postmortem brain. *Ann Neurol* **32**: 658–66.

Portegies P. (1995). HIV-1, the brain, and combination therapy. *Lancet* **346**: 1244–5.

Portegies P, Epstein LG, Hung ST, de Gans J, Goudsmit J. (1989). Human immunodeficiency virus type 1 antigen in cerebrospinal fluid. Correlation with clinical neurological status. *Arch Neurol* **46**: 261–4.

Portegies P, Enting RH, de Gans J et al. (1993). Presentation and course of AIDS dementia complex: 10 years of follow-up in Amsterdam, The Netherlands. *AIDS* **7**: 669–75.

Power C, Kong PA, Crawford TO et al. (1993). Cerebral white matter changes in acquired immunodeficiency syndrome dementia: alterations of the blood brain barrier. *Ann Neurol* **34**: 339–50.

Power C, McArthur JC, Johnson RT et al. (1994). Demented and non-demented patients with AIDS differ in brain-derived human immunodeficiency virus type 1 envelope sequences. *J Virol* **68**: 4643–9.

Price RW, Brew BJ. (1988). The AIDS dementia complex. *J Infect Dis* **158**: 1079–83.

Price RW, Sidtis JJ. (1990). Evaluation of the AIDS dementia complex in clinical trials. *J AIDS* **3**: S51.

Resnick L, Berger JR, Shapshak P et al. (1988). Early penetration of the blood-brain barrier by HIV. *Neurology* **38**: 9–14.

Rottenberg DA, Moeller JR, Strother SC et al. (1987). The metabolic pathology of the AIDS dementia complex. *Ann Neurol* **22**: 700–6.

Sacktor NC, Bacellar H, Hoorer DR et al. (1996). Psychomotor slowing in HIV infection: a predictor of dementia, AIDS and death. *J Neurovirol* **2**: 404–10.

Sacktor N, Lyles RH, Skolasky R et al. (2001). HIV-associated neurologic disease incidence changes: Multicenter AIDS Cohort Study. *Neurology* **56**: 257–60.

Said G, Lacroix C, Chemouilli P et al. 1991. Cytomegalovirus neuropathy in acquired immunodeficiency syndrome: a clinical and pathological study. *Ann Neurol* **29**: 139–46.

Santosh CG, Bell JE, Best JK. (1993). Abnormalities of the spinal tracts in AIDS: correlation of post-mortem MR findings with neuropathology. *Clin Neuropathol* **12**: S23.

Schielke E, Tatsch K, Pfister HW et al. (1990). Reduced cerebral blood flow in early stages of human immunodeficiency virus infection. *Arch Neurol* **47**: 1342–5.

Sharer LR, Prineas JW. (1988). Human imunodeficiency virus in glial cells continued. *J Infect Dis* **157**: 204.

Sharer LR, Dowling PC, Michaels J et al. (1990). Spinal cord disease in children with HIV-1 infection: a combined molecular biological and neuropathological study. *Neuropathol Appl Neurobiol* **16**: 317–31.

Simpson DM, Wolfe DE. (1991). Neuromuscular complications of HIV infection and its treatment. *AIDS* **5**: 917–26.

Simpson DM. Olney R, McArthur JC et al. (1998). A placebo controlled study of lamotrigene in the treatment of painful sensory polyneuropathy associated with HIV infection. *J Neurovirol* **4**: 366.

Sidtis JJ, Gatsonis C, Price RW et al. (1993). Zidovudine treatment of the AIDS dementia complex: results of a placebo controlled trial. *Ann Neurol* **33**: 343–9.

Singer EJ, Kim J, Fahy-Chandon B et al. (1996). Headache in ambulatory HIV-1 infected men enrolled in a longitudinal study. *Neurol* **47**: 487–94.

Smith TW, DeGrirolami U, Henin D et al. (1990). Human immunodeficiency virus (HIV) leukoencephalopathy and the microcirculation. *J Neuropathol Exp Neurol* **49**: 357–70.

Surtees R, Hyland K, Smith I. (1990). Central nervous system methyl-group metabolism in children with neurological complications of HIV infection. *Lancet* **335**: 619–21.

Stern Y, Marder K, Albert SM *et al.* (1998). The DANA cohort: predictors of HIV dementia. *J Neurovirol* **4**: 367.

Sweeney J, Brew BJ, Keilp J *et al.* (1991). Impairment of smooth pursuit in human immunodeficiency virus infection and its relationship to AIDS dementia complex. *J Psych Neurosci* **16**: 247–52.

Szeto E, Freund J, Pocock N *et al.* (1998). Cerebral perfusion scanning in AIDS dementia. *J Nucl Med* **39**: 298–302.

Takahashi K, Wesselingh SL, Griffin DE *et al.* (1996). Localization of HIV-1 in human brain using polymerase chain reaction/*in situ* hybridization and immunocytochemistry. *Ann Neurol* **39**: 705–11.

Tashima K, Caliendo AM, Ahmad M *et al.* (1998). Cerebrospinal fluid HIV-1 RNA levels and Efavirenz concentrations in patients enrolled in clinical trials. *J Neurovirol* **4**: 368.

Tozzi V, Narciso P, Galgani S *et al.* (1993). Effects of zidovudine in 30 patients with mild to end-stage AIDS dementia complex. *AIDS* **7**: 683–92.

Tracey I, Carr CA, Guimaraes AR *et al.* (1996). Brain choline-containing compounds are elevated in HIV-positive patients before the onset of AIDS dementia complex: a proton magnetic resonance spectroscopic study. *Neurology* **46**: 783–8.

Tross S, Price RW, Navia B *et al.* (1988). Neuropsychological characterization of the AIDS dementia complex: a preliminary report. *AIDS* **2**: 81–8.

Tyor W, Glass JD, Griffin JW *et al.* (1992). Cytokine expression in the brain during the acquired immune deficiency syndrome. *Ann Neurol* **31**: 349–60.

Van Gorp WG, Mandelkern MA, Gee M *et al.* (1992). Cerebral metabolic dysfunction in AIDS: findings in a sample with and without dementia. *J Neuropsychiatr Clin Neurosci* **4**: 280–7.

Vazeux R, Lacroix-Claudo C, Blanche S *et al.* (1992). Low levels of human immunodeficiency virus replication in the brain tissue of children with severe acquired immunodeficiency syndrome encephalopathy. *Am J Pathol* **140**: 137–44.

Wiley CA. (1996). Polymerase chain reaction in situ hybridization – opening Pandora's box. *Ann Neurol* **39**: 689–90.

Working Group of the American Academy of Neurology AIDS Task Force (1991). Nomenclature and research case definitions for neurologic manifestations of human immunodeficiency virus type 1 (HIV-1) infection. *Neurology* **41**: 778–85.

Yazdanian M, Ratigan S, Joseph D *et al.* (1997). Nevirapine, a nonnucleoside RT inhibitor, readily permeates the blood brain barrier. *Program and abstracts of the Fourth Conference on Retroviruses and Opportunistic Infections*, Washington DC, USA.

FIONA JUDD AND ANNE MIJCH

Psychiatric disorders are common among individuals with HIV infection. Some are the result of pre-existing psychiatric illness and may lead to behaviours predisposing to the transmission of HIV. Many patients develop psychiatric disorders secondary to HIV infection: as a result of the neuropathic effects of the virus, as a consequence of cerebral opportunistic infections or malignancy, as a psychological reaction to stresses associated with this disease, or as a side-effect of therapy. Drug-induced psychoses are common among injecting drug users (IDUs), particularly when associated with the use of amphetamines and hallucinogens. Psychiatric illness complicating HIV infection may lead to increased morbidity and mortality. Early detection and treatment of concurrent psychiatric disturbance will greatly enhance the patient's quality of life, and in some instances the patient's longevity.

Psychosocial factors and acquisition of HIV infection

Taking risks often reflects personality style. This may be the result of certain personality traits such as the belief in personal invulnerability or the perception that vulnerability is due to luck or fate, or it may be a feature of a particular personality disorder. For example, a central feature of borderline personality disorder is potentially self-damaging impulsiveness occurring in a variety of situations, such as sexual interactions and substance abuse. Antisocial personality disorder is characterized by a failure to conform to social norms, impulsivity, irresponsibility, and recklessness regarding the safety of oneself and others.

Perceived social norms regarding peer acceptability of safer sex practices, such as attitude toward the use of condoms and situational circumstances associated with episodic risk behaviour, have been identified as factors associated with risk-taking behaviour. The belief that safer sex is not an acceptable norm within one's peer group, younger age, and high levels of sexual activity with multiple partners (Kelly et al., 1990) all predict continued high-risk behaviour. Episodic, unprotected intercourse among those who generally practice safer sex may be associated with factors such as affectionate feelings towards one's partner, seeing condom use as a lack of trust, spontaneity of sex, or a strong desire to please one's partner (Kelly et al., 1991).

Intoxication or recreational drug use before or during sex has also been associated with high-risk sexual activity. Possible reasons for this association include impairment of judgement by drugs, the fact that both drug use and risk-taking behaviour may both result from personality style, or simply the pursuit of maximum sexual enjoyment. Alcohol consumption could be expected to influence safer sex practices in a similar fashion, and because alcohol use is widespread it is likely to have a marked effect on sexual practices.

Factors associated with safe practices among IDUs have been studied less than those with safer sex. Some risk factors, such as the disinhibiting effects of the drugs and impulsive and antisocial personality traits, are shared between the two. Injecting practices have been safest among IDUs who are older, use drugs infrequently, and those using opiates rather than cocaine (Kelly and Murphy, 1992). IDUs who use alcohol (Saxon and Calsyn, 1992) and benzodiazepines (Darke et al., 1992) share needles more than other IDUs. Interestingly, consistent use of condoms by IDUs and their sexual partners is uncommon, leading to a disparity between safe injection practice and sexual behaviour that increases the risk of sexual transmission of HIV (Des Jarlais et al., 1987).

The mentally ill have been identified as a group particularly at risk of acquiring HIV (Checkley et al., 1996). Those with chronic psychiatric disorders have been most studied. The reported seroprevalence of HIV among people with severe mental illness varies from 4 to 22.9%; findings across samples suggest that seroprevalence varies with geographical concentration of HIV and presence of comorbid psychiatric substance use disorders, but is consistently high (Cournos and McKinnon, 1997). Of note, in their analysis of the literature Cournos and McKinnon (1997) found that unsafe sex, and drug use (whether by injection or not) were associated with HIV infection, and that women were as likely to be infected as men.

Individuals with psychiatric disorders are vulnerable to HIV because they are frequently also substance abusers (Drake and Brunette, 1998; Weinhardt *et al.*, 1998) and because of the effects of their illness on social and interpersonal behaviour. Disinhibition, increased sexual activity, and sexual promiscuity occurring as a result of hypomania, lack of care for personal safety in patients with depression, and impaired problem solving and poor planning and judgement seen in patients with chronic schizophrenia place all these groups at risk. Patients with chronic mental illness show a remarkable lack of knowledge about AIDS and risk reduction measures (Kelly *et al.*, 1992). In addition, many patients report trading sex for drugs, money, or accommodation and coercion to engage in unwanted sex, or casual sex, following the use of drugs or intoxicants (Kelly *et al.*, 1992). Despite this, health-care workers in some psychiatric settings have demonstrated a lack of awareness of risk activities for HIV transmission among their patients with psychiatric illness (Thompson *et al.*, 1997).

Psychopathology in at-risk groups

The two groups identified as being most at risk for acquiring HIV infection in developed countries, IDUs and homosexual and bisexual men, have also been shown to have a greater prevalence of psychiatric disorders than the general population (Atkinson *et al.*, 1988; Williams *et al.*, 1991). Psychiatric comorbidity is common in patient groups seeking treatment for substance use. Among opiate addicts, the most common psychiatric diagnoses are depression, alcoholism, and antisocial personality disorder. Studies have consistently noted both a high rate of depression among opiate addicts presenting for treatment and also a high lifetime rate of depression (Rounsaville *et al.*, 1982). The observation that subgroups of drug users tend to prefer particular classes of drugs has led to the hypothesis, supported by clinical experience, that some of these individuals are medicating themselves: psychostimulant users treating depression, those who abuse depressants and sedatives treating anxiety, while those using hallucinogens and amphetamines may unmask previously latent psychotic disorders.

Two studies reported assessments of current and lifetime diagnoses of a variety of psychiatric disorders in homosexual and bisexual men with HIV infection (Table 11.1). In the first, Atkinson and colleagues (1988) found homosexual men, irrespective of HIV antibody status or stage of HIV infection, to have higher lifetime prevalence of anxiety, depression, and non-alcohol substance use disorders com-

Table 11.1 Lifetime prevalence of psychiatric disorders in homosexual and bisexual males

| Disorder | Prevalence (%) in indicated group | | | | |
| | Atkinson *et al.*[a] | | Williams *et al.*[b] | | |
	Homosexual men (*n* = 56)	Heterosexual men (*n* = 22)	HIV-infected men (*n* = 124)	HIV-uninfected men (*n* = 84)	Community sample males
Alcohol abuse or dependence	32.1	36.4	41	30	24
Non-opiate substance abuse (cannabis, psychostimulants)	32.1	4.5	56	38	7
Major depression	30.3	9.1	32	33	3
Generalized anxiety	39.3	0			
Panic disorder			4	2	1

[a]Adapted from Atkinson *et al.* (1988).
[b]Adapted from Williams *et al.* (1991).

pared with heterosexual controls matched for social and demographic factors. Furthermore, the psychiatric morbidity appeared to have preceded the AIDS epidemic. Similar findings were reported by Williams and associates (1991), who assessed 208 homosexual men whose HIV serology was known. Compared to the general population, high lifetime rates of depression and alcohol and other substance abuse or dependence disorders were reported (Table 11.1). The prevalence of psychiatric disorders in HIV-infected and uninfected groups did not differ significantly.

Coping with HIV infection

The way in which an individual copes with HIV infection and disease will be influenced by a variety of factors, which generally fall into three categories: intrapersonal, disease-related, and environmental (Lipowski, 1970).

Intrapersonal factors

Intrapersonal factors affecting how an individual copes with HIV infection include the person's age, sex, personality, body image, philosophical and religious beliefs, prior illness experiences, and previously employed coping mechanisms. The individual's ability to cope is also influenced by the timing of the illness in the life cycle. Most children cope well with illness, while illness during adolescence poses additional stresses on an individual dealing with important developmental tasks. In old age, cognitive impairment may reduce coping capacity. It has been suggested that women find disfiguring illness more difficult, while men have greater trouble coping with disabling illness (Peterson, 1974) Separation anxiety, fear of loss of love and approval, and fear of loss of control are additional stresses.

Personality structure may also be an important determinant of how an individual responds to illness. The meaning of illness varies from one individual to another according to their basic needs, the threat they are trying to cope with, and the kinds of defensive and adaptive behaviours that become intensified under such stress. For example, the compulsive personality may find illness a threat to their need for control, and as a result question every medical decision or nursing procedure. Providing specific and detailed information, setting a predictable routine (preferably written) for treatment, and involving the patient in discussions regarding any changes in management may prevent or minimize battles for control. The paranoid person tends to blame others for their illness

and its complications and may be fearful, controlling, and suspicious of others. Here, an empathic approach, taking care not to agree or disagree with complaints, and maintaining a uniform approach to management, are important. For the narcissistic person, illness is a threat to their self-image of perfection and invulnerability. Any (objectively) mild defect may be perceived as a catastrophe for the patient and lead to concerns that the treating physician may find difficult to understand. For example, a patient with Kaposi's sarcoma (KS) was devastated when he developed a small lesion on his forearm, because it would be visible when he wore a T-shirt, but was far less concerned by a larger lesion on his back, which his physician saw as a clear priority for treatment. Conflict between patient and therapist developed when the physician directed treatment to the objectively more serious lesion, rather than to the psychologically important lesion, which the patient wished to be treated first.

Disease-related factors

Disease-related factors impacting on how one copes with HIV infection include the type, location, rate of onset and progression of symptoms, degree of reversibility, and functional impairment (Lipowski, 1970). Certain body regions or organs have special significance for some patients. Impairment, disability, and handicap are important concepts in determining the effects of disease. Impairment occurs at the organ level and is defined as 'any loss or abnormality of psychological, physiological or anatomical structure or function' (WHO, 1980). Disability is 'any restriction or lack (resulting from an impairment) of ability to perform an activity in the manner or within the range considered normal for a human being'. Handicap occurs at the social level and has been defined as 'disadvantage for a given individual resulting from an impairment or a disability that limits or prevents the fulfilment of a role that is normal (depending on age, sex and social and culture factors) for that individual' (WHO, 1980). It should be noted that the same impairment may result in different degrees of disability and handicap, determined by the individual's situation. Early skin changes, in the presence of well-maintained general health, may cause significant handicap for an individual working in the entertainment or beauty industry. Muscle wasting may be particularly distressing for the individual who enjoys physical activities. Changes in body shape, such as the lipodystrophy related to protease inhibitor (PI) therapy are perceived by many to be identifying features of HIV infection and treatment and may pose such risks of disclosure as to limit an individual's ability to comply with life-prolonging treatment. For others, it is not physical change but the development of cognitive impairment that is most threatening.

Environmental factors

Environmental factors that may influence coping with illness include features of the hospital environment, relationships with staff, response of family and friends, and aspects of the patient's work environment (Lipowski, 1970; Moos and Schaefer, 1984). The societal approach to HIV disease and the populations most at risk of infection may substantially influence an individual's coping abilities (Cassens et al., 1983). General features of the hospital environment such as loss of privacy, separation from family, the prospect of painful procedures, and exposure to other ill and dying patients, as well as special stresses such as those of the intensive care unit (Moos and Schaefer, 1984) influence the patient's responses to this illness. The discrimination and stigma faced by many individuals with HIV infection is of particular importance here.

To cope successfully with illness requires the individual to address a series of general and illness-related tasks, the relative importance of which depend on the disease, the individual, and on general circumstances. Illness-related tasks include dealing with symptoms such as pain, dealing with the hospital environment and treatments, and interacting with hospital staff. General tasks include maintaining one's emotional state, maintaining one's self-image and sense of control, preserving relationships, and making provision for a changed future (Moos and Schaefer, 1984).

Coping with HIV infection also requires the individual to overcome a variety of crises during an illness that may last decades. Initially, the individual must cope with the news of the diagnosis of an ultimately fatal illness, together with the varied psychosocial implications of being HIV-infected. As the illness progresses, a variety of crises must be faced: falling CD4 counts, the initiation of antiretroviral treatment, the use of prophylaxis against opportunistic infections, dermatological and other 'minor' manifestations of HIV infection, the first AIDS-defining opportunistic infection or malignancy, cessation of work, weight loss, and progressive disfigurement and disability. The psychosocial and interpersonal accompaniments of these illness-related events will stress the individual further.

The 'second life' dilemma

The introduction of the PIs in 1995 and their use in combination with other antiviral medications has led to a new level of treatment efficacy, with physicians and patients speaking of the possibility of HIV/AIDS as a 'chronic controllable condition'. These treatment developments have created a new type of crisis for patients who experience major improvements, and extreme disappointment for those who do not.

Patients who do improve have frequently been on disability payments, having left work, used up savings and prepared themselves for premature death. Some may, after years of unemployment and poor health, be expected to return to work. 'Second life' dilemmas include whether to return to work, decisions about personal relationships and changes in family role and responsibilities (Rabkin and Ferrando, 1997). Further fears of new toxicities (diabetes, lipodystrophy and atherosclerotic vascular disease) make managing the good news, the second life stresses and the unknown future a substantial challenge.

Those whose hopes are raised, but who do not respond to new combination therapies must deal with feelings of disappointment, frustration and injustice. The distress of treatment failure may be exacerbated by seeing the improvement in friends. Thus, there may be not only the loss of hope for one's own health status, but also the loss of one's peer group and social circle as friends change their lifestyle commensurate with their improvement in health and well-being.

Adjustment disorder

Difficulty in coping may occur at any stage of HIV infection. The diagnosis of adjustment disorder is made when there is a persistent maladaptive response to an identified psychosocial stressor. The particular symptoms of the adjustment disorder may be quite varied; depressed or anxious mood are common, as are physical symptoms such as fatigue, headache, and abdominal and other pains. Determining how the individual has coped with previous crises and how the illness has impacted on the individual and their environment is useful in predicting the outcome of the disorder.

One patient, a 41-year-old man, first began to experience panic attacks following the initiation of zidovudine (ZDV) therapy. Although quite well, he interpreted the initiation of treatment as evidence of imminent poor health. Discussion with him revealed that his main support was his mother, and that he feared that illness would lead to abandonment by her.

A healthy 33-year-old man who had been HIV-infected for 9 years presented with depressed mood. Over the past decade many of his friends had died as a result of AIDS. He described increasing anxiety in anticipation of developing an AIDS-defining illness, because of the mistaken impression that all HIV-infected patients were dead within 10 years and guilt that he was well while most of his friends were very ill or had died. To date he had coped largely by using denial, but the experience of his friends becoming ill, together with constant confrontation by media reports of treatment successes and failures, had led to this previously adaptive and successful coping mechanism no longer being effective.

Treatment generally focuses on improving the individual's level of adaptation, using both environmental manipulation to remove or modify the stressors and psychotherapeutic techniques to explore attitudes and change the patient's perspective. Education will dispel the patient's misconceptions about the implications of particular symptoms or treatment strategies. Often family or partners will be included to ensure that there is a shared view of the disease and its effects. Strengthening social supports and strategies to change environmental stressors, such as housing or financial problems, are often helpful. Previously successful coping strategies, such as appropriate denial, should be encouraged.

Depressive disorders

Depression is common during medical illness, occurring in between one-quarter and one-third of patients with a variety of disorders. Mood disturbance may reflect a normal reaction to illness, it may be a manifestation of the underlying physical illness, occur as a side-effect of a variety of drugs, be part of a depressive syndrome, or be secondary to another psychiatric disorder.

In general, individuals may be predisposed to the development of depression as a result of both psychological and biological vulnerabilities. Strong evidence exists for a genetic predisposition to both bipolar affective disorder and to depression. There also appears to be an association between early loss of, or prolonged absence of, a parent during early life and the subsequent development of depression. An association between major life events and onset of affective illness has also been demonstrated.

In the context of HIV infection, depressive illness may be an independent and pre-existing problem, a psychological response to this disease, a direct result of central nervous system infection by HIV, or caused by drug therapy (Table 11.2). The diagnosis of a depressive illness is made when there is a sustained lowering of mood, with associated cognitive, affective and somatic symptoms. Many of the symptoms of depression may also be either symptoms of HIV infection or the result of treatment (e.g. fatigue, insomnia, and anorexia). Given that somatic symptoms may have multiple causes, the diagnosis of depression in a patient with more advanced HIV infection should rely primarily on cognitive or affective symptoms, using somatic symptoms only if severe, not readily explained by the effects of HIV infection or its treatment, and temporally related to the affective or cognitive symptoms.

The prevalence of depressive illness in patients with HIV infection has been studied in both inpatient and outpatient settings. Among outpatients, the prevalence of depressive illness has been reported to be between 15 and 25% (King, 1989; Catalan et al., 1992; Morriss et al., 1992; Judd et al., 1997b). Studies of inpatients have reported variable rates of affective illness. A retrospective chart review of 52 patients with AIDS found depression in nine (17%) patients and made a presumptive diagnosis of depression in

Table 11.2 Medications commonly associated with depression

Drug class	Examples
Antihypertensive drugs	Reserpine, methyldopa, guanethidine, bethanidine, propranolol, prazosin, clonidine, hydralazine, nifedipine
Glucocorticoids	
Anabolic steroids	
Oral contraceptives	
Nonsteroidal anti-inflammatory drugs	Phenylbutazone, indomethacin, ibuprofen
Neurological drugs	Levadopa, amantadine, baclofen, tetrabenazine, bromocriptine
Antiviral drugs	Interferon
Miscellaneous	Cimetidine, ranitidine, metoclopramide, salbutamol, methysergide, cyproheptadine, appetite suppressants, dapsone

another 34 (65%) (Perry and Tross, 1984). Subsequently, several prospective studies have documented the rate of affective disturbance among inpatients referred for psychiatric assessment (Dilley *et al.*, 1985; Seth *et al.*, 1991). Depression was diagnosed with varying frequency, and often a diagnosis of adjustment disorder with depressed mood was made. For example, of 22 patients with AIDS-related complex (ARC) or AIDS referred for psychiatric consultation over a 16-month period, four patients were found to have an adjustment disorder with depression and one to have a depressive illness (Buhrich and Cooper, 1987). Baer (1989) found that one-third of patients referred for psychiatric inpatient care were depressed (adjustment disorder with depressed moods, 13 with major depression) and Judd *et al.* (1997a) identified mood disorder as the most common psychiatric diagnosis among HIV/AIDS in patients referred for psychiatric assessment. By contrast, Wright and Perkins (1990) found no cases of major depression among 51 patients referred for psychiatric consultation over a 15-month period, but 14 patients with adjustment disorder and depressed mood were identified. Because these studies rely on patients being referred for assessment, they may seriously underestimate the true prevalence of depression among inpatients. For example, one study assessed all patients admitted with a diagnosis of AIDS by psychiatric interview and found 9.5% with a major depressive syndrome (Snyder *et al.*, 1992a). This is significantly less than the 'average' rate of depression in medically ill patients of 15–25%.

Longitudinal studies have differed in estimated rates of incident depressive illness and symptoms and the relationship of depression to HIV/AIDS symptomatic disease. Joseph *et al.* (1990) found stable rates of depressive illness over 3 years among subjects enrolled in the Chicago Multi-Center AIDS Cohort Study (MACS), despite progressive HIV illness. Perry *et al.* (1993) found a decrease in depressive symptoms in patients with AIDS over 12 months of follow-up, not different from HIV-uninfected controls. Lyketsos *et al.* (1996), Hoover *et al.* (1992) and Ickovics *et al.* (2001) demonstrated that the prevalence of depressive symptoms increases in the later stages of HIV infection, before the development of clinical AIDS. Neither these authors nor Rabkin *et al.* (1997) showed any increase in depressive symptoms in relation to physical illness developing over time. However, Griffin *et al.* (1998) found that while there was no difference in depression among men who were asymptomatic, symptomatic or diagnosed with AIDS, the degree of physical limitation predicted depression.

When it occurs, depression may amplify symptoms, increasing somatic complaints such as fatigue and nausea, and decreasing tolerance of disability. Depression is also associated with increased physical morbidity (poor compliance with treatment, poor self-care) and increased mortality (suicide).

For patients with HIV infection, depression may develop in response to a variety of illness-related factors. Multiple psychological stresses can be identified through the course of the illness. The initial diagnosis and its implications, together with stages of deteriorating physical health, are the most obvious. The rate of progression of the illness, together with the actual and perceived severity of symptoms, may profoundly influence the patient's mood. The lifestyle changes forced on the individual as a result of deteriorating health, together with increasing dependency on others and the reaction of family and friends, may all contribute to the development of depression.

A particularly striking example of depression developing late in the course of HIV infection concerned a 30-year-old man with severe cryptosporidial diarrhoea. The patient had previously coped well with a variety of HIV-related symptoms but became increasingly depressed as the diarrhoea failed to respond to multiple therapies. The depth of his depression appeared to result from his realization that he was unlikely to be able to survive outside the hospital and from his family's callous response, 'If he was a dog you'd shoot him.'

A variety or organic factors may also cause depression. Opportunistic infections affecting the central nervous system (CNS), cerebral tumours, and drugs used in the treatment of HIV and its complications have all been associated with the development of depression. Frontal lobe pathology (e.g. cerebral toxoplasmosis, lymphoma) should always be considered in an immunocompromised patient who develops depression, particularly where withdrawal and poor motivation are prominent symptoms. In addition, some non-HIV-related medical conditions and treatments are commonly associated with the onset of depression. Undue focus on HIV and its effects may lead to neglect of consideration of these factors.

A 51-year-old man with AIDS and severe impairment of immune function (CD4 lymphocyte count of less than 10 cells/μl) was extensively investigated for an organic cause of his depression. Computerized tomography (CT) and magnetic resonance imaging (MRI) scans were normal, neuropsychological assessment revealed no evidence of cognitive impairment, and treatment with adequate doses of antidepressants was ineffective. Reassessment after antidepressant therapy had failed included thyroid function tests (previously omitted from the organic investigations), which revealed that he was hypothyroid. Thyroid replacement therapy was commenced and his depression resolved.

Management of the patient with depressive symptoms

Assessment

Initially, the clinician must establish whether the patient has a depressive syndrome and whether there is an organic cause for the depression. Key steps in this assessment are shown in Table 11.3. All patients who develop depression should be reviewed by their treating physician, and consideration must be given to possible organic causes of the mood disorder. It is especially important to exclude reversible conditions that are directly related to HIV or to other illness. An organic cause of depression should be suspected when there is no family history or past history of depression, in the absence of obvious precipitants, when the presentation is atypical, when cognitive symptoms are unduly severe compared to the degree of affective disturbance, when the patient is severely immunocompromised, or when the patient has not responded to standard treatment for depression. Particularly important aspects of the medical assessment of a depressed patient with HIV infection are shown in Table 11.4. A thorough history and physical examination are essential for all patients present-

Table 11.3 Initial assessment of the patient with depressive symptoms

Are the symptoms described indicative of depression or any of the following? • Somatic symptoms due to HIV • Cognitive symptoms due to early dementia • Symptoms secondary to another medical condition • Part of another psychiatric syndrome **Is the patient describing transient or sustained depressive symptoms?** **Is there any organic cause for the depression, such as the following?** • Organic factors unrelated to HIV • Organic factors related to HIV • Medications (Table 11.2)

Table 11.4 Medical assessment of the depressed patient

History • Personal or family history of endocrine disease, particularly thyroid or pituitary • Any recent change in prescribed or non-prescribed medication • Alcohol consumption • Illicit drug use • Any new medical conditions or physical symptoms **Physical examination, particularly evidence of:** • Neurological disorder • Hypothyroidism • Unsuspected sepsis • Hypoxaemia • Liver or renal impairment **Screening investigations (most or all patients)** • Haemoglobin, liver and renal function, serum calcium, blood glucose, B_{12} and folate, erythrocyte sedimentation rate • Review past and recent serology for *Treponema pallidum*, *Toxoplasma gondii*, *Cryptococcus neoformans* • Thyroid function tests, including TSH • T-cell subsets • HIV viral load **Further assessment (as indicated)** • CT or MRI examination of the brain • Lumbar puncture to exclude meningeal disease

CT: computerized tomography; MRI: magnetic resonance imaging.

ing with depression; further investigations will depend on the patient's physical state, degree of immunocompetence, and the physician's index of suspicion of an organic cause.

Once a diagnosis of depression is established, the severity of depression must be determined (Table 11.5). In particular, the risk of self-harm by either self-neglect or suicide must be determined. Many depressed patients describe suicidal thoughts (e.g. 'I've thought I'd rather not wake up in the morning') or suicidal wishes. Patients with more severe depression may have developed a clear plan for suicide. Depressed patients who describe a plan for suicide, especially where they have access to the means (e.g. have a gun or stored medication) and particularly where there are few social supports, represent a psychiatric emergency and should be treated in an inpatient psychiatric unit.

Table 11.5 Clinical classification of severity of depressive illness[a]

	Mild	Moderate	Severe
Affective	Lowered mood	Inability to experience pleasure	Apathy and social withdrawal
	Crying	Pessimistic about future	See no future
	Anxious	Social withdrawal	Poor self-care
	Irritable	Self-reproach, feel worthless	Ideas of guilt
		Feel like a failure	Illness as punishment
		Hypochondriasis	Paranoid, hypochondriacal, or
		Paranoid ideas	nihilistic delusions
Cognitive	Impulsive	Work impairment	Marked work impairment
	Loss of confidence	Indecisiveness	Unable to make decisions
	Impaired concentration	Forgetful	Slowed mentation, impression of
	Loss of interest or poor motivation		cognitive impairment
Somatic	Low energy	No energy	Agitation or psychomotor retardation
	Restless	Eat with encouragement	Unable to eat
	Lowered libido	Loss of libido	Marked weight loss
	Loss of interest in food	Mild weight loss	Sleep only a few hours
	Mild initial insomnia	Initial insomnia	
	Wake once or twice a night	Wake several times a night	
Suicidal	Life not worth living	Thoughts of suicide	Plan or attempt suicide

[a]Not all clinical features are necessarily present in every patient.

Treatment

Treatment of the depressive disorder is determined by severity. Patients with mild depression are generally treated with one or more of the several varieties of short-term psychotherapy available. Supportive therapy, which provides advice, encouragement, and practical help to achieve environmental change, is used most often. Interpersonal therapy, which provides strategies to deal with current social and interpersonal problems associated with the onset of depression, may be particularly useful in some cases (Table 11.6) (Markowitz et al., 1992). Mild depression will generally be treated by the clinician managing other aspects of the patient's illness.

For patients with moderately severe depression, antidepressant medication is usually required, in addition to psychotherapy. As is the case more generally for medically ill patients, treatment of depression among patients with HIV infection has received little systematic study. Data are available from small, open studies and from placebo-controlled trials; overall response rates to active drug range from 45 to 80% (Elliott et al., 1998). High placebo response rates have been noted (Zisook et al., 1998) and generally interpreted as due to the benefits of concomitant psychological treatment. A variety of different classes of antidepressants

are available (Table 11.7). While of equal efficacy, antidepressants vary greatly in side-effect profile. Fluoxetine has been shown to be effective in a population of men with HIV infection (57% fluoxetine versus 41% placebo responded in the intention to treat analysis and 74% fluoxetine versus 47% placebo responded in the treatment analysis) (Rabkin et al., 1999). The additional effect of antidepres-

Table 11.6 Major areas of interpersonal difficulty causing depression amenable to interpersonal therapy

Area	Example
Grief	Mourning the loss of others' death
	Anticipatory mourning of one's own death
Role transition	Acceptance of HIV infection
	Starting antiretroviral therapy
	First physical symptoms
	Cessation of paid employment
	Developing AIDS
Interpersonal disputes	Conflict with friends, partner or family
Interpersonal deficits	Failure to tell others of HIV sero-positivity and subsequent isolation
	Negative responce of family and others, or shrinking of support system

Table 11.7 Side-effects of antidepressant medications

Organ system	Side-effects	Drug class						
		TCA	MAOI	RIMA	Mianserin	SSRI	SNRI	SARI
Automonic nervous system	Anticholinergic, e.g. dry mouth, blurred vision, urinary retention, constipation or tachycardia	+	+	+	Mild	–	–	–
	Excessive perspiration	+	–	–	Mild	–	+	–
	Sexual dysfunction	+	+	–	Mild	+	+	–
Cardiovascular	Postural hypotension	+	+	Variable	Mild	–	–	–
	Quinidine-like effect	+	–	–	–	–	–	–
Gastrointestinal	Anorexia	–	–	–	–	+	+	–
	Nausea and vomiting	–	–	+	–	+	+	–
Endocrine	Weight gain	+	–	–	Mild	–	+	+
CNS	Sedation	+	Variable	Variable	Mild	–	+	+
	Lower seizure threshold	+	–	–	–	–	–	–
	Anxiety and agitation	–	Occasionally	–	–	+	+	+
Notes		a	b	c	d	e	f	g

TCA: tricyclic antidepressants; MAOI: monoamine oxidase inhibitors; SNRI: serotonin and noradrenaline re-uptake inhibitors; RIMA: reversible inhibitor of monoamine oxidase A; SSRI: selective serotonin re-uptake inhibitors; SARI: serotonin antagonist and re-uptake inhibitors; +: commonly found.

Notes [a]Cardiotoxic with overdoses.
[b]Hypertensive response with tyramine containing foods, opiates, indirect-acting sympathomimetic amines, TCAs.
[c]No tyramine reactions, but agitation may occur following co-administration of opiates.
[d]Greater propensity to produce agranulocytosis than other antidepressants; frequency unclear; best detected by suggestive symptoms; routine blood counts of little value; full recovery on cessation of drug.
[e]Variable serum half lives: fluoxetine 1–4 days, norfluoxetine 7–9 days; SSRIs inhibit cytochrome p450 enzymes and may elevate plasma levels of co-administered drugs that are metabolized in the liver (e.g. rifampicin, ketoconazole). Special care is required when SSRIs and protease inhibitors are used together.
[f]May increase blood pressure at doses greater than 225 mg/day.
[g]Inhibition of cytochrome p450 3A4 isoenzymes; lower incidence of sexual dysfunction than withother antidepressants.

sants over psychotherapy has been shown to be particularly apparent in severe depression (Zisook *et al.*, 1998). Choice of drug is determined by past favourable response to a particular drug; by the particular physical manifestations of HIV, which may be worsened by drug side-effects, and by the possibility of potential interactions with other drugs.

Tricyclic antidepressants (TCAs) have been most widely used in patients with organic disease. Monoamine oxidase inhibitors (MAOIs) are very rarely used because of the necessity for a tyramine-free diet and potentially hazardous drug interactions. Reversible inhibitors of monoamine oxidase (RIMAs) do not interact with tyramine and have few drug interactions, although co-administration with opiates is not advised. Mianserin, which has fewer anticholinergic side-effects, less propensity to produce postural hypotension, and relative lack of cardiovascular effects compared to the TCAs and MAOIs, may be more suitable for use in the medically ill. However, these advantages must be weighed against two significant adverse effects: a reversible polyarthropathy, sometimes associated with fever and rash, and haematological toxicity. Mianserin appears to have a greater propensity to cause agranulocytosis than the other antidepressants, but the true frequency of this adverse reaction is unknown. Complete recovery occurs within 2–3 weeks of withdrawing the drug.

The selective serotonin re-uptake inhibitors (SSRI) have several advantages that make them suitable for use in medically ill patients, including lack of anticholinergic, sedative, and cardiovascular side-effects. The lack of anticholinergic and cardiovascular side-effects of the SSRIs is shared by the serotonin antagonist and re-uptake inhibitor (SARI) nefazadone. However, nefazadone can cause sedation, with complaints of fatigue and a 'drugged' feeling. Of note, nefazadone appears to cause less sexual dysfunction than other antidepressants. Venlafaxine, the first selective serotonin and noradrenalin re-uptake inhibitor (SNRI) has some side-effects in common with the SSRIs (nausea), and at higher doses other side-effects consistent with its effects on neuroadrenal function (increased blood pressure, sweating, tremors). The effect of venlafaxine on blood pressure is dose dependent and is rarely seen at a dose of less than 225 mg/day.

When using antidepressants in patients with medical illnesses, great care must be taken to consider possible pharmacokinetic interactions. TCAs are not known to affect the pharmacokinetics of other drugs to any appreciable extent, although many other drugs do affect the metabolism of TCAs (e.g. carbamazepine, phenytoin). Little is known of the effects of MAOIs on the pharmacokinetics of other drugs. The SSRIs are potent inhibitors of several different isoenzymes of the cytochrome P450 family of enzymes (Table 11.8) and so may cause potentially serious drug–drug interactions mediated through inhibition of specific cytochrome P450 enzyme pathways (Nemeroff *et al.*, 1996). The SARI nefazadone inhibits the cytochrome P450 3A4 subfamily of enzymes and is a weak inhibitor of P450 2D6. Venlafaxine is also a weak inhibitor of P450 2D6. Knowledge of the effects of the newer antidepressants on the cytochrome P450 system is of particular importance when prescribing these drugs together with PIs; all PIs are metabolized via the

Table 11.8 Classification of antidepressants based upon potency of inhibition of cytochrome p450 isoenzyme system

Antidepressant	Cytochrome p450 isoenzyme			
	2D6	3A3/4	IA2	SC19
Fluoxetine	+++	++	0/–	++
Paroxetine	+++	0/+	0/+	?
Fluvoxamine	0/+	+++	+++	+++
Sertraline	++	0/+	0/+	?
Citalopram	0/+	0/+	0/+	0/+
Nefazadone	0/+	+++	0/+	0/+
Venlafaxine	0/+	0/+	0/+	0/+

+++: potent inhibitor; ++: moderate–weak inhibitor; 0/+: low–minimal inhibitor; ?: unknown.

P450 isoenzymes, primarily the 3A subfamily and some to a lesser extent by P450 2D6. It should also be noted that the PIs inhibit some of the cytochrome P450 isoenzymes involved in drug metabolism (see Chapters 5 and 6). Ritonavir has the most potent effect on cytochrome P450 and is most likely to have significant drug interactions. Ritonavir has a high affinity for several cytochrome P450 (CYP) isoforms with the following rank order: CYP3A4 > CYP2D6 > CYP2C9,　CYP2C19 > CYP2A6, CYP1A2, CYP2E1. There are some indications that ritonavir may increase the activity of glucuronyltransferases; thus, loss of therapeutic effects from directly glucuronidated agents during ritonavir therapy may signify the need for dosage alteration of these agents also.

In general, a TCA or an SSRI will be first-line treatment for HIV-infected patients with moderate to severe depression. Severely depressed patients with strong suicidal ideation should not be given antidepressants as an outpatient, as the risk of overdose or suicide by other means is high. Antidepressants should be started at a low dose (Table 11.9), which is increased slowly (no more than every 3–4 days) with careful monitoring of side-effects, taking into account any change in the patient's medical condition and other drugs prescribed. There is a delay in onset of effect of 2–4 weeks with all classes of antidepressants. The dosage required in patients with concurrent organic disease is variable. While some patients are best treated with doses comparable to those used in patients without organic disease, others require a lower daily dose to achieve a therapeutic plasma level because of renal or hepatic impairment, drug interactions, or reduced serum albumin levels. Underdosing is a common cause of 'treatment-resistant

Table 11.9 Recommended dosage of antidepressants in patients with concurrent organic disease

Antidepressant (class and example)	Starting dose	Incremental doses	Usual final daily dose	Maximum daily dose[a]
TCA (e.g. imipramine)	25–50 mg at bedtime	25 mg every 3–4 days[b]	150–200 mg	300 mg
MAOI (e.g. phenelzine)	15 mg in the morning	15 mg every 3–4 days[b]	60–90 mg	120 mg
Mianserin	20–30 mg at bedtime	10 mg every 3–4 days[c]	60–90 mg	120 mg
Moclobemide	150 mg in the morning	150 mg every 3–4 days[d]	600 mg	900 mg
SSRI (e.g. fluoxetine)	20 mg every other day	To 20 mg daily after 1 week[e]	20 mg	80 mg
SNRI (venlafaxine)	37.5 mg twice daily	37.5 mg[f]	75 mg	375 mg
SARI (nefazadone)	50 mg twice daily	To 100 mg twice daily after 1 week, then to 200 mg twice daily after another week	200 mg twice daily	600 mg

TCA: tricyclic antidepressants; MAOI: monoamine oxidase inhibitors; SSRI: selective serotonin re-uptake inhibitors; SNRI: serotonin and noradrenaline re-uptake inhibitors; SARI: serotonin antagonist and re-uptake inhibitors.

[a]If this dose is not effective seek psychiatric review.
[b]Monitor closely for sedation; postural hypotension.
[c]Monitor closely for sedation; always check for any symptoms suggestive of haematological toxicity.
[d]Nausea may occur as dose increases.
[e]If initial anxiety/agitation occurs, increase dose more gradually; short-term co-administration of benzodiazepines may be of benefit.
[f]The usual therapeutic dose is 37.5 mg twice daily. Increases beyond this should be delayed for 2–4 weeks to enable drug to be of benefit, and blood pressure should be monitored at doses greater than 225 mg/day.

depression'. Antidepressant effects usually require a medication dosage that also causes side-effects, such as a dry mouth with TCAs.

Try to find a drug and dose that provides maximal antidepressant effect and minimum toxicity. Once the depressed mood improves, which usually takes at least 2 weeks but may take 6–8 weeks in some patients, the antidepressants should be continued for a further 4–6 months. Premature cessation of medication often results in relapse. When a decision to cease the medication is made, the dose should be gradually reduced, monitoring the patient for any signs of recurrent depression. The risk of relapse is greatest in the first 8 weeks after cessation of medication.

Table 11.10 Situation in which depressed patients should be referred for psychiatric assessment

- Diagnostic uncertainty
- Atypical presentation
- Past history of recurrent depression
- Past difficulty tolerating side-effects of antidepressants
- Patients express clear suicidal intent
- Particularly troublesome side-effects of drugs or problematic drug interactions
- Failure to respond to an adequate trial of a first-line antidepressant – 4 or more weeks of treatment at usual therapeutic doses (see Table 11.9)

While many patients with moderately severe depression are appropriately managed by their general physician, certain patients should be referred for psychiatric assessment and treatment (Table 11.10). Patients with severe depression or those with suicidal ideation usually require psychiatric inpatient treatment. For patients with severe or life-threatening depression (substantial suicide risk, severe anorexia, substantial weight loss or self-neglect, depressive stupor, delusions, or hallucinations) and where antidepressants are ineffective, electroconvulsive therapy (ECT) is the treatment of choice. Other therapeutic modalities utilized in patients with advanced disease include dextroamphetamine and occasionally testosterone in hypogonadal males.

Manic disorders

Mania is characterized by a persistently elevated, expansive, or irritable mood, described as unusually good, cheerful, euphoric, or high. Associated symptoms include grandiosity or inflated self-esteem, which in severe forms of the illness is delusional. Religious delusions (e.g. having a special relationship with God) or the conviction of possessing certain powers or skills are common. Increased energy and activity, increased talkativeness, and decreased need for sleep are commonly reported. Disinhibition and lack of good judgment may lead to poor financial planning, reckless spending, poor business decisions, reckless driving, and particularly relevant for HIV/AIDS, promiscuous sexual activity (Table 11.11). While the extreme forms of the illness are readily recognized, milder degrees of illness are easily overlooked. Close acquaintances of the patient are obviously in the best position to recognize mild symptoms. Patients with milder degrees of illness (hypomania) are cheerful, usually pleasant to interact with, and may appear to have normal behaviour in the confined interaction in the consulting room. However, their potential for self-destructive behaviour is high, especially if the disorder is not detected early.

Mania may occur as part of a bipolar affective disorder or secondary to a variety of medical or pharmacologic causes. A variety of drugs (e.g. glucocorticoids, amphetamine, cocaine, isoniazid, and levadopa) have been reported to cause mania, as have metabolic disturbances, infections (e.g. influenza, encephalitis, Q fever) and cerebral neoplasma (Krauthammer and Klerman, 1978).

Early case reports documented the occurrence of mania in patients with AIDS and noted that the patients generally had late-stage disease, objective evidence of cognitive impairment, and, in some, cerebral atrophy demonstrated on CT scan (Kermani et al., 1985; Gabel et al., 1986; Perry and Jacobsen, 1986; Dauncey, 1988; Schmidt and Miller, 1988). By contrast, mania may also occur during an HIV seroconversion illness (see Chapter 1).

Kieburtz et al. (1991) described the clinical, neuropsychological, laboratory, and brain imaging data in eight patients with AIDS (mean CD4 lymphocyte count 60/μl, with a range from 10 to 170) who developed a manic syndrome. Patients presented with typical manic symptoms, such as decreased sleep, pressured speech and disorganized thinking, and irritability was more common than elevated mood. Neuropsychological testing showed memory deficits, impaired cognitive flexibility and slowed perceptual speed. MRI scans were abnormal in all eight patients, with the most common abnormalities being found in the fornix and corpus callosum. More recently, Ellen et al. (1999) have provided similar data for 19 patients, with mania occurring in patients with advanced HIV disease. Clinical features and treatment responses were similar to those associated with bipolar affective disorder in the absence of HIV infec-

Table 11.11 Classification of severity of mania based on clinical features[a]

	Mild (hypomania)	Moderate	Severe (manic psychosis)
Mood	Cheerful or mild irritability	Unusually good or marked irritability	Euphoric or irritable and aggressive
Thought	Pressure of thought and speech	Racing thoughts, speech loud, rapid, difficult to interrupt Flight of ideas: changes topic based on understandable associations, distracting stimuli, plays on words	Jokes, puns, frequent irrelevancies Clanging: sounds rather than meaningful connections govern word choice Speech may be disorganized and incoherent
	Increased self-confidence and self-esteem	Grandiose ideas, unrealistic over-estimation of abilities	Grandiose delusions Paranoid delusions
Cognitive	Poor concentration	Distractable	Distractable, disorganised
Somatic	Mild insomnia Mild overactivity Increased libido	Reduced need for sleep Awake early and full of energy Increased sexuality	Minimal sleep without resulting fatigue Indiscriminate sexual activity Self-neglect Exhaustion
Social	Overly familiar Increased social confidence and interaction	Increased sociability – telephone calls, letter writing, visits to friends Fiscal irresponsibility Unwarranted optimism Increased sexual activity	Intrusive, domineering, demanding, social interactions Poor judgement – reckless spending, poor business decisions, reckless driving Activities are disorganized, flamboyant or bizarre

[a]Not all clinical features are necessarily present in every patient.

tion; while neuroradiological abnormalities were common, they were deemed not to be clinically relevant.

The association between mania and cognitive impairment in patients with HIV infection was further described in a group of 33 patients with AIDS or ARC referred for neuropsychological examination (Boccellari *et al.*, 1988). One-third of the sample met criteria for secondary mania, and these patients were significantly more impaired than those without affective disturbance by several neuropsychological measures (trail-making test part B, fine motor speed, and verbal fluency). Whether these areas of greater cognitive impairment were caused by the affective disorder, or whether those with greater cognitive deficits were more prone to the development of mania, is unknown.

At least in the era prior to combination antiretroviral therapy, development of mania in a patient with HIV appeared to be a poor prognostic sign. El-Mallakh (1991) reported that one-quarter of the 14 patients studied died within 6 months of the onset of psychiatric symptoms. Similarly, Seth *et al.* (1991) reported that all three patients with mania seen in their series died within 9 months of referral.

Mania secondary to ZDV is well-documented in patients with HIV infection, and may appear up to several months after beginning therapy (Maxwell *et al.*, 1988; O'Dowd and McKegney., 1988; Wright *et al.*, 1989). The doses of ZDV prescribed at the time of these reports (600–1200 mg/day) were generally higher than those currently used. Other causes of mania in patients with HIV should always be considered. Neurosyphilis can present with mania, and delayed development of, or even negative, syphilis serology has been reported (see Chapter 22 on bacterial infections). Other CNS pathology, especially mass lesions, may present with mania, and mania caused by cryptococcal meningitis has also been reported (Johannessen and Wilson, 1988). The association of mania with AIDS dementia complex (Lyketsos *et al.*, 1997) and the reported protective effect of ZDV therapy in a recent case–control study (Mijch *et al.*, 1999) raise the possibility that mania in these patients is a manifestation of HIV neuropathology.

Management of the patient with mania

Assessment

The initial steps in managing a patient with mania are to establish the diagnosis of a manic syndrome and to determine whether there is any organic basis for the mood disturbance (Table 11.12). All patients presenting with a manic illness require thorough assessment and

Table 11.12 Initial assessment of the patient with manic symptoms

Are the patient's symptoms indicative of mania, or of:
- disinhibition occurring as part of dementing process?
- affective and behavioural disturbance as part of schizophreniform disorder?

Does the patient have a sustained mood syndrome or transient elevation of mood?

Is there any organic cause for the mood disturbance that is:
- unrelated to HIV infection?
- drug-induced (e.g. glucocorticoid)?
- caused by HIV?

investigation to exclude any treatable organic cause. Key features of history, examination, and investigation are similar to those in the assessment of possible organic causes of depression (see Table 11.3). Following this evaluation, the clinician should assess the severity of the mood disorder (see Table 11.5) and the risk of harm to the patient and others; in particular, the risk of harm due to lack of self-care, exhaustion, and potentially self-destructive behaviours (e.g. disinhibition, sexual promiscuity, excessive spending).

Treatment

All patients presenting with mania should be assessed by a psychiatrist, and further management carried out jointly by the primary care provider and psychiatrist. Treatment of mania will be dictated by the cause and severity of the mood disturbance. When symptoms are mild (hypomania), support and stress reduction may be adequate for symptom relief. Careful observation is required to ensure that symptoms do not worsen. However, most patients with mania require medication. Several classes of drugs may be used: the neuroleptics (phenothiazines, butyrophenones and atypical antipsychotic drugs, e.g. risperidone), the high potency benzodiazepines (e.g. clonazepam), or lithium carbonate (Table 11.13).

The choice of drug for treatment of mania will be determined by past favourable response and the drug's toxicity profile (Table 11.13). Neuroleptics are widely used for the treatment of mania but should be used cautiously, particularly in patients with weight loss (risk of postural hypotension) and evidence of cognitive impairment (risk of confusion), which are frequently accompanying conditions in patients with HIV infection. A high incidence of extrapyramidal side-effects in patients with HIV treated with neuroleptics has been reported, and increased sus-

Table 11.13 Comparison of side-effect profile of neuroleptics used for treatment of mania and schizophrenia

Drug class (examples)	Relative severity of indicative toxicity					
	Sedation	Anticholinergic[a]	Postural hypotension	Acute extrapyramidal[b]	Initial dose for treatment of mania in medically ill patients[c]	Maximum dose for treatment of mania[d]
Phenothiazines Aliphatic (chlorpromazine)	+++	+++	+++	+	25–100 mg nocte up to four times daily	800 mg/day
Piperidine (thioridazine)	+	+++	+++	+	25–100 mg nocte up to four times daily	800 mg/day[e]
Piperazine (trifluoperazine)	+	±	±	+++	0.5–2 mg nocte up to four times daily	20 mg/day
Butyrophenones (haloperidol)	+	±	±	+++	0.5–2 mg nocte up to four times daily	20 mg/day
Diphenylbutylpiperidines (pimozide)	–	±	±	+++	2 mg nocte up to four times daily	20 mg/day[f]
Thioxanthenes (flupenthixol) (thiothixene)	+	±	±	+++	1 mg nocte up to four times daily 2 mg nocte up to four times daily	40 mg/day 30 mg/day
Risperidone	+	–	++	+	1 mg nocte up to 2 mg twice daily	8 mg/day
Olanzapine	++	+	++	+	5 mg nocte up to 5 mg twice daily	20 mg/day[g]

+: mild; ++: moderate; +++: severe; ±: variable; –: absent.

[a]Dry mouth, blurred vision, constipation, urinary retention.
[b]Dystonia, akathisia, parkinsonism.
[c]Dose determined by severity of mania, patient's physical condition and other currently used medications.
[d]Larger doses may be used with caution; always seek psychiatric assessment.
[e]Larger doses may cause retinal toxicity.
[f]Check ECG – may cause prolongation of Q–T interval.
[g]May cause hypersalivation.

ceptibility to neuroleptic malignant syndrome has been suggested. The neuroleptics vary in their potency and their propensity to produce anticholinergic, sedative, and hypotensive side-effects (Table 11.13). Generally, there is an inverse relationship between risk of sedation, anticholinergic effects, and extrapyramidal effects. The atypical antipsychotic agents (e.g. risperidone, olanzapine) are much less likely than conventional neuroleptics to cause extrapyramidal side-effects. Thus, these drugs, particularly risperidone, may be the treatment of choice for patients

with HIV-related mania (Singh et al., 1997). Benzodiazepines may be used alone or as an adjunct in the treatment of mania. Sedative effects are dose dependent and care should be taken to ensure that confusion does not develop, particularly when giving high doses, or in treated patients with cognitive impairment.

Although lithium is best known for its ability to prevent mania, it is also frequently used for acute management of elevated mood. As lithium has an entirely different side-effect profile to the neuroleptics, it may be particularly useful in patients unable to tolerate the extrapyramidal, sedative, or anticholinergic effects of these agents. Lithium is not suitable for patients with severe organic disease, as changes in fluid and electrolyte balance and drug interactions may result in lithium toxicity because of its low therapeutic ratio. Particular care must be taken when lithium is prescribed for patients with diarrhoea, as dehydration commonly precipitates lithium toxicity. When lithium is used, serum levels should be carefully monitored. The usual therapeutic range for control of mania is 1.2 mmol/l, while a lower level of 0.6–1 mmol/l is used for maintenance or prophylaxis.

Optimizing antiretroviral therapy should be a priority for patients with HIV-associated mania, although compliance is frequently a problem and directly observed therapy may need consideration.

Any therapy for mania should be continued for several months following recovery and then be slowly tapered, decreasing the dose by 5–10% every few weeks, while carefully observing the patient for evidence of relapse.

Schizophreniform and paranoid disorders

Schizophreniform disorder (schizophrenia-like psychosis) is characterized by disturbance of perception, thought, affect, volition, and psychomotor behaviour (Table 11.14). The relationship between HIV infection and the development of schizophreniform psychosis is poorly understood. Unlike hypomania and mania, schizophreniform disorders occur at all stages of HIV infection. Psychosis may occur as a reaction to the knowledge of having HIV infection and its implications, may by caused by drugs used by patients with HIV, or may be the result of neurotoxic effects of the virus or opportunistic intracerebral infections or tumours. However, many instances of schizophreniform disorder in HIV-infected patients may be coincidental. Schizophrenia is common (1% prevalence in the general population) and it usually begins between the ages of 15 and 25 years old, an age group at high risk for HIV infection. Differentiating the coincidental occurrence of schizophrenia from schizophreniform disorder linked to HIV disease is difficult, and is often only possible with longitudinal follow-up.

Data on the frequency of schizophreniform psychoses in HIV infection are sparse and conflicting. One retrospective review found five cases of new onset schizophreniform psychosis among 124 patients with Centre for Disease Control (CDC) group 2 or 3 disease followed since 1984 (Harris

Table 11.14 Clinical features of schizophreniform disorder

Perceptual disturbance	
Hallucinations	Most frequently auditory, but may be visual, tactile, olfactory or gustatory
Affective disturbance	Often labile, incongruous or inappropriate affect; may be perplexed, suspicious
Disturbance of thought	
Content	Delusions – paranoid, grandiose, religiose, somatic or of external control
Form	Loosening of associations (i.e. loss of logical links between concepts); when severe, incoherence of speech
Possession	Thought insertion or withdrawal or broadcasting
Volition	Lack of volition
Psychomotor behaviour	Psychomotor excitation Catatonic behaviour

et al., 1991). Halstead and associates (1988) reported five cases (four CDC group 2 or 3, one with CDC group 4) of 'florid and apparently functional psychosis' in a population of over 2200 HIV-infected patients, while Navia *et al.*, (1986), in a retrospective chart review, reported that seven of 46 patients with AIDS dementia experienced 'prominent' psychotic symptoms during the course of their illness.

There are numerous case reports of first-episode psychoses occurring in HIV-infected individuals. One group comprises patients with AIDS and cognitive impairment (Nurnberg *et al.*, 1984; Palan *et al.*, 1985: Perry and Jacobsen, 1986; Cummings *et al.*, 1987; Maccario and Scharre, 1987; Thomas and Szabadi, 1987; Halstead *et al.*, 1988). A second group includes HIV-infected patients with schizophreniform psychosis who are organically and cognitively normal (Thomas *et al.*, 1985; Halevie-Goldman *et al.*, 1987; Jones *et al.*, 1987; Buhrich *et al.*, 1988; Halstead *et al.*, 1988; Harris *et al.*, 1991). In this latter group particularly, a coincidental association cannot be excluded. Both those with and without evidence of cognitive impairment present with typical, schizophreniform symptoms (Halstead *et al.*, 1988). In the absence of cognitive impairment, its presentation is indistinguishable from schizophrenia. Delusions are the most common psychotic symptom, usually of paranoid, grandiose, or somatic type (see Table 11.14). Both auditory and visual hallucinations are also commonly described. Affective disturbance occurs in most patients, and labile, inappropriate, and flat effects have all been noted. Anxiety, agitation, formal thought disorder, and bizarre behaviour also occur frequently (Harris *et al.*, 1991). Two cases of catatonia, both occurring in association with organic cerebral impairment, have also been reported (Volkow *et al.*, 1987; Snyder *et al.*, 1992b).

Management of the patient with a schizophreniform disorder

Assessment

The clinician must first establish the diagnosis of schizophreniform disorder and determine whether the clinical findings are indicative of schizophreniform disorder, an acute organic brain syndrome (delirium), or paranoid ideation occurring secondary to dementia. The physician should also determine whether the symptoms are sustained or simply a brief disturbance brought on by drug use or another cause (Table 11.15). For those patients with a confirmed schizophreniform disorder, the clinician must also exclude organic causes for the disorder (Table 11.15).

The severity of disorder must also be assessed, particularly the risk to self resulting from disorganization, self-neglect, delusions (e.g. trying to escape from harm or persecution, or risky behaviour in response to grandiose delusions) or hallucinations (particularly command hallucinations where the voices instruct the patient to kill or harm themselves). Despite popular misconception, delusions and hallucinations rarely result in harm to others.

Treatment

All patients presenting with schizophreniform disorders should be referred for psychiatric assessment, and the psychiatrist and primary care giver should manage the patient jointly. Treatment will be determined by the degree to which behaviour is disorganized and patients are distressed by their psychotic symptoms. When patients are acting in response to their delusions or hallucinations inpatient psychiatric care is mandatory. Medication is generally required, and neuroleptics are the treatment of choice (see Table 11.13). Drugs should be chosen according to the severity of the patient's symptoms (more disturbed patients may benefit from a more sedating drug), organic comorbidity, and the propensity for particularly troubling side-effects (Table 11.13). Drug–drug interactions should be considered, especially if ritonavir is being utilized.

Suicide

Studies have shown that suicidal ideation and suicide are common among individuals with HIV infection (McKegney and O'Dowd, 1992; Kizer *et al.*, 1988; Perry *et al.*, 1990; Cote *et al.*, 1992). However, studies of suicidal behaviour generally tend to underestimate the magnitude of the problem. Many individuals who unsuccessfully attempt suicide do not come to medical attention. Many deaths from suicide are not identified as such because in many countries a finding of suicide requires irrefutable evidence that this was the cause of death. Some patients die as a result of 'passive suicide' by failing to seek or to comply with treatment.

Perry and colleagues (1990) found that one-third of patients seeking HIV testing described suicidal ideation, decreasing to about 10–15% for both sero-positive and sero-negative individuals 2 months after notification of their test result. The frequency of suicidal thoughts among patients with HIV infection varies according to the stage of infection. In patients with AIDS it was the same as that of uninfected patients with organic illness (9%), while for patients with CDC stage II–III disease it was twice as high (18%) (McKegney and O'Dowd, 1992).

The rate of suicide among patients with AIDS has consistently been shown to be much greater than that of the general population. In New York City in 1985 it was 66 times that for the city's general population (Marzuk *et al.*, 1988); in California in 1986 the rate was 21 times that of the state's general population (Kizer *et al.*, 1988). Between 1987 and 1989 in the USA, the national rate of suicide for men with AIDS was 7.4 times higher than for men in the general population (Cote *et al.*, 1992). Of note is the fact that the rate declined by nearly half over this

Table 11.15 Organic causes of schizophreniform disorder

Intracerebral pathology
- direct neuropathic effects of HIV infection
- cerebral tumour, psychosis associated with epilepsy, encephalitis, opportunistic infections and neoplasms

Drug induced[a]
- prescribed drugs (e.g. L-dopa, amantadine, bromocryptine, corticosteroids, aciclovir, interferon, dapsone, baclofen)
- illicit drugs (e.g. amphetamines, hallucinogens, marijuana, cocaine, phencyclidine)

[a]Drug-induced psychoses are generally self-limiting, usually resolving within days or weeks following cessation of the drugs. Amphetamine-induced psychosis may persist for several weeks.

time period – from 10.5 in 1987, to 7.4 in 1988 and to 6.0 in 1989 – perhaps because of the development of anti-retrovirals (ZDV was licensed in 1987), improved prophylaxis and treatment for opportunistic infections, and greater optimism regarding prognosis.

While demonstrating the increased rate of suicide, studies have not examined possible factors contributing to the high suicide rate in patients with AIDS. The incidence of suicide is increased in a variety of other debilitating and potentially fatal illnesses, such as end-stage renal disease, multiple sclerosis and cancer, and might also be expected to be so in individuals with HIV. Pre-existing personality plays a role, however, as HIV-infected individuals who are involved in acts of deliberate self-harm more often have a history of such behaviour or a past psychiatric history (Gala *et al.*, 1992) than those who have not so acted.

Assessment

The assessment and management of suicidal intent among HIV-infected patients (as well as those with other chronic diseases) involves clinical, ethical, and legal considerations. Generally, there are three situations in which patients express suicidal ideation: as part of a psychiatric illness, in response to a crisis, and as a rational choice.

Studies of patients who commit suicide suggest that up to 90% have a psychiatric disorder at the time of death. The most common of these is depression. 'Risk' factors for suicide in the context of depression include social isolation, male gender, advanced age, previous suicide attempts, and a painful illness. Patients with psychotic disorders may harm themselves in response to delusional beliefs or auditory hallucinations. Alcohol and drug use are also risk factors for suicide. Suicide may also occur in response to interpersonal crises, such as relationship conflicts or the death of a loved one, or in response to an illness-related crisis (e.g. a painful or debilitating new symptom, particularly one that proves resistant to treatment).

Many people contend that suicide can be a rational choice for individuals with a terminal illness such as AIDS. Determining whether such a decision is rational is never easy for the clinician (Table 11.16). When in doubt, seek psychiatric assessment.

Treatment

All patients who describe suicidal ideation should be carefully evaluated by their primary care provider and a psy-

Table 11.16 Evaluating the patient who is contemplating suicide as a rational choice

- Is the patient suffering from a psychiatric disorder (especially depression) that may be influencing their decision making?
- Does the patient have a correct and complete understanding of their illness and any available treatments?
- Are there any temporary conditions (psychosocial or illness related) influencing the patient's decision?
- Are there any 'external pressures' influencing the patient's decision (e.g. friends or relatives encouraging the patient to make this choice)?

chiatrist to determine whether they suffer from a psychiatric disorder, particularly depression. When severe depression is found, the patient should be treated as described above (see section on treatment of depressive disorders, p. 187), making provisions to ensure their safety. Likewise, where there is an acute crisis precipitating their suicidal intent, measures to ensure the patient's safety, together with interventions to assist in dealing with the crisis, are required. In general, suicidal patients should be managed by a psychiatrist, either alone or in concert with the patient's primary care giver.

Psychiatric disorder focused on HIV infection or AIDS in uninfected persons

Unfounded concern about HIV infection or AIDS may occur in a variety of psychiatric disorders. Depressed patients with hypochondriacal preoccupations may fear they have, or believe they have (delusion), a variety of illnesses such as cancer, syphilis, or AIDS. Patients with schizophrenia or monosymptomatic hypochondriacal delusional states may also believe that they have AIDS. Individuals with obsessional disorders may have obsessional fears about the possibility of developing HIV infection and constantly seek medical assessment and repeated serological testing to reassure them that this is not the case. A variety of terms have been used to describe these conditions, such as 'AIDS panic' (Schwartz, 1983), 'AIDophobia' (Freed, 1983), the 'worried well' (Miller *et al.*, 1986), and 'pseudo-AIDS' (Miller *et al.*, 1985). Because the underlying psychiatric condition causes these conditions, not HIV or AIDS, these terms are best avoided. Treatment should be directed to the underlying psychiatric disorder.

Factitious disorder (otherwise known as Munchausen's syndrome) presenting as AIDS has also been described (Baer, 1987). While uncommon, this is an important disorder to recognize. Physical symptoms are fabricated, self-inflicted, or exaggerated. In its severe and chronic form, multiple presentations with factitious symptoms and multiple hospitalizations occur. The many and varied physical manifestations of HIV infection explain how cases of factitious disorder could be misdiagnosed as cases of AIDS, resulting in inappropriate treatment, financial waste, and delay in psychiatric intervention. Where there is doubt about the diagnosis, usually resulting from inconsistent physical and laboratory findings, the patient's consent to check HIV serology should be sought. Such a request often precipitates the patient's abrupt recovery and departure from the hospital.

References

Atkinson HJ, Grant I, Kennedy CJ et al. (1988). Prevalence of psychiatric disorders among men infected with human immunodeficiency virus. Arch Gen Psychiatry 45: 895.

Baer JH. (1987). Munchausen's AIDS. Gen Hosp Psychiatry 9: 75–6.

Baer JH. (1989). Study of 60 patients with AIDS or AIDS-related complex requiring psychiatric hospitalisation. Am J Psychiatry 146: 1285–8.

Boccellari A, Dilley JW, Shore MD. (1988). Neuropsychiatric aspects of AIDS dementia complex: a report on a clinical series. Neurotoxicology 9: 381–90.

Buhrich N, Cooper DA. (1987). Requests for psychiatric consultation concerning 22 patients with AIDS or ARC. Aust NZ J Psychiatry 21: 346–53.

Buhrich N, Cooper DA, Freed E. (1988). HIV infection associated with symptoms indistinguishable from functional psychosis. Br J Psychiatry 152: 649–53.

Cassens BJ. (1983). Social consequences of the acquired immunodeficiency syndrome. Ann Intern Med 103: 765–7.

Catalan J, Klimes I, Day A et al. (1992). The psychological impact of HIV infection in gay men: a controlled investigation and factors associated with psychiatric morbidity. Br J Psychiatry 161: 774–8.

Checkley GE, Thompson SC, Crofts NC et al. (1996). HIV in the mentally ill. Aust NZ J 30: 184–94.

Cote T, Biggar RJ, Dannenberg AL. (1992). Risk of suicide among persons with AIDS: a national assessment. JAMA 268: 2066–8.

Cournos F, McKinnon K (1997). HIV seroprevalence among people with severe mental illness in the United States: a critical review. Clin Psychol Review 17: 259–69.

Cummings MA, Cummings KL, Rapaport MH et al. (1987). Acquired immunodeficiency syndrome presenting as schizophrenia. West J Med 146: 615–7.

Darke S, Hall W, Ross M et al. (1992). Benzodiazepine use and HIV risk taking behaviour among injecting drug users. Drug Alcohol Depend 31: 31–6.

Dauncey K. (1988). Mania in early stages of AIDS. Br J Psychiatry 152: 716–7.

Des Jarlais DC, Wish F, Friedman SR et al. (1987). Intravenous drug use and the heterosexual transmission of the human immunodeficiency virus: current trends in New York City. NY State J Med 87: 283–6.

Dilley JW, Ochititt HN, Perl M et al. (1985). Findings in psychiatric consultations with patients with acquired immune deficiency syndrome. Am J Psychiatry 142: 82–6.

Drake RE, Brunette MF. (1998). Complications of severe mental illness related to alcohol and drug use disorders. Recent Develop Alcohol 14: 285–99.

El-Mallakh RS (1991) Mania and paranoid psychosis in AIDS. Psychosomatics 32: 362.

Ellen S, Judd FK, Mijch AM et al. (1999). Secondary mania in patients with HIV infection. Aust NZ J Psychiatry 33: 353–60.

Elliott AJ, Vidoll KK, Bergam K et al. (1998). Randomized placebo-controlled trial of paroxetine versus imipramine in depressed HIV positive outpatients. Am J Pschiatry 155: 367–72.

Freed E. (1983). AIDophobic. Med J Aust 2: 479.

Gabel RH, Bernard N, Norko M et al. (1986). AIDS presenting as mania. Comp Psychiatry 27: 251–4.

Gala C, Pergami A, Catalan J et al. (1992). Risk of deliberate self harm and factors associated with suicidal behaviour among asymptomatic individuals with human immunodeficiency virus infection. Acta Psychiatr Scand 86: 70–5.

Griffin KW, Rabkin JG, Remien RH et al. (1998). Disease severity, physical limitations and depression in HIV-infected men. J Psychosom Res 44: 219–27.

Halevie-Goldman BD, Potkin SG, Poyourow P. (1987). AIDS-related complex presenting as psychosis. Am J Psychiatry 144: 964.

Halstead S, Riccio M, Harlow P et al. (1988). Psychosis associated with HIV infection. Br J Psychiatry 153: 618–23.

Harris MJ, Jeste DV, Gleghorn A et al. (1991). New onset psychosis in HIV-infected patients. J Clin Psychiatry 52: 369–76.

Hoover DR, Saah A, Bacellar H et al. (1992). The progression of untreated HIV-1 infection prior to AIDS. Am J Pub Health 82: 1538–41.

Ickovics JR, Hamburger ME, Vlahor D et al. (2001). Mortality, CD4 cell count decline, and depressive symptoms among HIV-seropositve women. JAMA 285: 1466–74.

Johannessen DJ, Wilson LG. (1988). Mania with cryptococcal meningitis in two AIDS patients. J Clin Psychiatry 49: 200–1.

Jones GH, Kelly CL, Davies JA (1987). HIV and onset of schizophrenia. Lancet i: 982.

Joseph JG, Caumartin S, Tal M et al. (1990) Psychological functioning in a cohort of gay men at risk for AIDS. J Nerv Ment Dis 178: 607–15.

Judd FK, Cockram A, Mijch A et al. (1997a). Liaison psychiatry in an HIV/AIDS unit. Aust NZ J Psychiatry 31: 391–7.

Judd FK, Mijch A, McCausland J, Cockram A. (1997b). Depressive symptoms in patients with HIV infection: a further exploration. Aust NZ J Psych 31: 862–8.

Kelly JA, Murphy DA. (1992). Psychological interventions with AIDS and HIV: prevention and treatment. J Consult Clin Psychology 60: 576–85.

Kelly JA, St Lawrence JS, Brashfield TL et al. (1990). Psychological factors that predict AIDS high-risk and AIDS precautionary behaviour. J Consult Clin Psychology 58: 117–20.

Kelly JA, Kalichman SC, Kauth MR et al. (1991). Situational factors associated with AIDS risk behaviour lapses and coping strategies used by gay men who successfully avoid lapses. Am J Pub Health 81: 1335–8.

Kelly JA, Murphy DA, Bahr R et al. (1992). AIDS/HIV risk behaviour among the chronically mentally ill. Am J Psychiatry 149: 886–9.

Kermani EJ, Borod JC, Brown PH et al. (1985). New pathologic findings in AIDS: case report. J Clin Psychiatry 46: 240–1.

Kieburtz K, Zettelmaier AE, Ketonen L et al. (1991). Manic syndrome in AIDS. Am J Psychiatry 148: 1608–70.

King MB. (1989). Psychosocial status of 192 outpatients with HIV infection and AIDS. Br J Psychiatry 154: 237–42.

Kizer KW, Green M, Perkins CI et al. (1988). AIDS and suicide in California. JAMA 260: 1881 [letter].

Krauthammer C, Kierman GI. (1978). Secondary mania: manic syndromes associated with antecedent illness or drugs. Arch Gen Psychiatry 35: 1333–9.

Lipowski ZJ. (1970). Physical illness: the individual and the coping process. Psychiatry in Med 1: 91–102.

Lyketsos CG, Hoover DR, Guccione M et al. (1996). Changes in depressive symptoms as AIDS develops. The Multicenter AIDS Cohort Study. Am J Psychiatry 153: 1430–7.

Lyketsos CG, Schwartz J, Fishman M et al. (1997). AIDS Mania. J Neuropsych Clin Neurosci 9: 277–9.

Maccario M, Scharre E. (1987). HIV and the acute onset of psychosis. Lancet ii: 342.

Markowitz JC, Klerman GL, Perry SW. (1992). Interpersonal psychotherapy of depressed HIV-positive outpatients. Hosp Comm Psychiatry 43: 885–90.

Marzuk PM, Tierney H, Tardiff K et al. (1988). Increased risk of suicide in persons with AIDS. JAMA 259: 1333–7.

Maxwell S, Scheftner WA, Kessler HA et al. (1988). Manic syndrome associated with Zidovudine treatment. JAMA 259: 3406–7.

McKegney FP, O'Dowd MA. (1992). Suicidality and HIV status. Am J Psychiatry 149: 396–8.

Miller D, Green J, Farmer R et al. (1985). A 'pseudo-AIDS' syndrome following fear of AIDS. Br J Psychiatry 146: 550–1.

Miller F, Welden P, Sacks M et al. (1986). Two cases of factitious acquired immune deficiency syndrome. Am J Psychiatry 143: 1843.

Mijch AM, Judd F, Lyketsos C et al. (1999). Secondary mania in patients with HIV infection: are antiretrovirals protective? J Neuropsychiatry Clin Neurosci 11: 475–80.

Moos RH, Schaefer JA. (1984). The crisis of physical illness: an overview and conceptual approach. In: R. Moos (ed.). Coping with physical illness 2: new perspectives. New York: Plenum Press, 3–25.

Morriss R, Schaerf F, Brandt J et al. (1992). AIDS and multiple sclerosis: neurological and mental features. Acta Psychiatr Scand 85: 331–6.

Navia BA, Jordan BD, Price RW. (1986). The AIDS dementia complex: 1. Clinical features. Ann Neurol 19: 517–24.

Nemeroff CB, de Vane CL, Pollock BG. (1996). Newer antidepressants and the cytochrome P450 system. Am J Psychiatry 153: 311–20.

Nurnberg HG, Prudic J, Flori M et al. (1984). Psychopathology complicating acquired immune deficiency syndrome. Am J Psychiatry 141: 95–6.

O'Dowd MA, McKegney FP. (1988). Manic syndrome associated with Zidovudine. JAMA 260: 3587–8.

Palan HJ, Hellerstein D, Amchin J. (1985). The impact of AIDS-related cases on inpatient therapeutic milieu. Hosp Comm Psychiatry 36: 173–6.

Perry S, Jacobsen P. (1986). Neuropsychiatric manifestation of AIDS spectrum disorders. Hosp Comm Psychiatry 37: 135–42.

Perry S, Tross S. (1984). Psychiatric problems of AIDS inpatients at the New York Hospital: preliminary report. Pub Health Rep 99: 200–5.

Perry S, Jacobsberg K, Fishman B. (1990). Suicidal ideation and HIV testing. JAMA 263: 679–82.

Perry S, Jacobsberg L, Card CAL et al. (1993). Severity of psychiatric symptoms after HIV testing. Am J Psychiatry 150: 775–9.

Peterson BH. (1974). Psychological reactions to acute physical illness in adults. Med J Aust 1: 311–6.

Rabkin JG, Ferrando S. (1997). A 'Second Life' Agenda. Arch Gen Psychiatry 54: 1049–53.

Rabkin JG, Goetz RR, Remien RH et al. (1997). Stability of mood despite HIV illness progression in a group of homosexual men. Am J Psychiatry 154: 231–8.

Rabkin JG, Wagner GJ, Rabkin K. (1999). Fluoxetine treatment for depression in patients with HIV and AIDS. A randomized placebo controlled trial. Am J Psychiatry 156: 101–7.

Rounsaville BJ, Weissman MM, Crits-Christoph K et al. (1982). Diagnosis and symptoms of depression in opiate addicts: course and relationship to treatment outcome. Arch Gen Psychiatry 39: 151–6.

Saxon AJ, Calsyn DA. (1992). Alcohol use and high risk behaviour by intravenous drug users in an AIDS education paradigm. J Stud Alcohol 53: 611–8.

Schmidt V, Miller D. (1988). Two cases of hypomania in AIDS. Br J Psychiatry 152: 839–42.

Schwartz R. (1983). AIDS panic. Psychiatry News, 17 August.

Seth R, Granville-Grossman J, Goldmeier D et al. (1991). Psychiatric illnesses in patients with HIV infection and AIDS referred to the liaison psychiatrist. Br J Psychiatry 159: 347–50.

Singh AN, Golledge H, Catalan J. (1997). Treatment of HIV-related psychotic disorders with risperidone: a series of 21 cases. J Psychsom Res 42: 489–93.

Snyder S, Reyner A, Schmeidler J et al. (1992a). Prevalence of mental disorders in newly admitted medical inpatients with AIDS. Psychosomatics 33: 166–70.

Snyder S, Prenzlaver S, Maruyama N et al. (1992b). Catatonia in a patient with AIDS related dementia. J Clin Psychiatry 53: 414 [letter].

Thomas C, Szabadi E. (1987). Paranoid psychosis as the first presentation of a fulminating lethal case of AIDS. Br J Psychiatry 151: 693–5.

Thomas C, Toone BK, El Komy A et al. (1985). HTLV-III and psychiatric disturbance. Lancet ii: 395–6.

Thompson S, Checkley G, Hocking J et al. (1997). HIV risk behaviour and HIV testing of psychiatric patients in Melbourne. Aust NZ J Psychiat 31: 566–76.

Volkow ND, Harper A, Munnisteri D et al. (1987). AIDS and catatonia. J Neurol Neurosurg Psychiatr 50: 104 [letter].

Weinhardt LS, Carey MP, Carey KB et al. (1998). HIV-risk behaviour and the public health context of HIV/AIDS among women living with a severe and persistent mental illness. J Nerv Ment Dis 186: 276–82.

Williams JBW, Rabkin JG, Remian RH et al. (1991). Multidisciplinary baseline assessment of homosexual men with and without human immunodeficiency virus infection: standardised clinical assessment of current and lifetime psychopathology. Arch Gen Psychiatry 48: 124–30.

World Health Organization (WHO). (1980). International classification of impairments, disabilities and handicaps. Geneva: WHO.

Wright JM, Perkins RJ. (1990). The role of liaison psychiatry in an AIDS unit. Aust NZ J Psychiat 24: 391–6.

Wright JM, Sachdev PS, Perkins RJ et al. (1989). Zidovudine related mania. Med J Aust 150: 339–41.

Zisook S, Peterkin J, Goggin KJ et al. (1998). Treatment of major depression in HIV-seropositive men. HIV Neurobehavioural Research Center Group. J Clin Psychiatry 59: 217–24.

12

DEBORAH GREENSPAN AND JOHN GREENSPAN

Oral manifestations of AIDS were described in the very first reports of the syndrome and continue to be an important cause of HIV-related morbidity (Gottlieb *et al.*, 1981; Greenspan, 1997). There is growing evidence that several relatively innocuous oral opportunistic infections are indicators of marked immunosuppression in HIV-infected patients and may predict the ultimate development of AIDS (Katz *et al.*, 1992, 1993). The mouth is the site of residence of extremely varied and complex microbial flora with marked potential to produce disease when host defenses are compromised. Examples include the frequent and troublesome episodes of fungal, bacterial, and viral infections in patients with primary immunodeficiency, immunosuppressed graft recipients, and patients receiving immunosuppressive chemotherapy for malignancy. The prevalence and incidence of oral lesions seen in association with the AIDS epidemic have again drawn attention to the importance of this group of diseases (Greenspan *et al.*, 1990b; Greenspan and Greenspan, 1996). Oral examination is a critical part of any physical examination, and nowhere is this more important than in the case of suspected HIV infection. All mucosal surfaces should be assessed using a mouth mirror, examination gloves, gauze squares for tongue extension, and an adequate light source. Any undiagnosed oral lesion should be subjected to further investigation using techniques such as smears, cultures, and biopsy.

Fungal and bacterial lesions

Candidiasis
The frequency of oral candidiasis increases as the CD4 lymphocyte count falls (Crowe *et al.*, 1991). A study of 10 patients with AIDS and oral candidiasis showed that all the patients had concomitant oesophageal candidiasis (Tavitian *et al.*, 1986). This extensive involvement has not been confirmed by others, and 30% of cases of oesophageal can-

didiasis have no associated oral candidiasis. In association with HIV infection, oral candidiasis, even the fairly innocuous-appearing erythematous form, is predictive of the subsequent development of AIDS.

Candida albicans is frequently part of the normal oral flora and is the species most often found in oral candidal infections. Other less common species produce similar oral lesions. Oral candidiasis associated with HIV infection may have several different clinical appearances. These include pseudomembranous candidiasis, erythematous candidiasis, and angular cheilitis. Pseudomembranous candidiasis, sometimes called thrush, is characterized by the presence of white or creamy plaques on the oral mucosa (Figure 12.1) (all the figures appear in the colour plate section). These white plaques can be removed, often revealing a bleeding surface. The erythematous form of candidiasis appears as a flat red lesion that may be found on the hard or soft palate, dorsal surface of the tongue, or other mucosal locations (Figure 12.2). When candidiasis affects the dorsal surface of the tongue, patchy depapillated areas appear. Angular cheilitis may appear as cracking, fissuring, ulceration, or erythema at the corner of the mouth and may be seen either alone or in conjunction with the intraoral lesions.

The prevalence of oral candidiasis in HIV infection is high, with up to 15% of the otherwise asymptomatic HIV population experiencing this infection. Increasing incidence of oral candidiasis occurs with advancing immunodeficiency (especially fewer than 200 CD4 lymphocytes/μl), so that the prevalence among those with severe HIV disease may be 80% or higher. Pseudomembranous candidiasis is slightly more common than the erythematous form, which can readily be missed, whereas angular cheilitis is even less common. The diagnosis of oral candidiasis is usually based on clinical appearance, although for confirmation smears examined by potassium hydroxide suspension or Gram stain show hyphae and blastospores. Culture of the organism is not necessary unless speciation and antifungal susceptibility testing is desired, as may be the case in recalcitrant cases that are unresponsive to therapy.

Little is known of the pathogenesis of HIV-associated oral candidiasis. Defective macrophage uptake and killing of the organism (Crowe et al., 1994), neutrophil defects, inadequate lymphocyte cytotoxicity, and antibody or complement defects may all play roles.

Treatment involves the use of systemic or topical antifungal drugs (Greenspan and Greenspan, 1991; Greenspan and Shirlaw, 1997). The currently available antifungal medications fall into two categories: the polyenes or the azoles. The polyene drugs commonly used include nystatin and amphotericin B. Oral topical medications include the topical troches or pastilles that are dissolved slowly in the mouth over a 20–30-min period. Water can be sipped during use to help dissolve the medication. Efficacy is dependent on the length of time the medication is held in the mouth. Topical solutions are often not helpful because of the short duration of contact time between the rinse and the affected mucosa. Nystatin is available as nystatin vaginal tablets, 100 000 units, one tablet dissolved slowly in the mouth three times a day, nystatin oral pastilles, 200 000 units, one or two tablets dissolved in the mouth five times a day, and an oral rinse. The nystatin pastille and the nystatin rinse contain sucrose, which may lead to an increased risk of dental caries if used frequently. If these medications are used frequently, topical fluoride rinses or gels should be used twice daily. Amphotericin B is available as a cream, lotion, oral suspension (100 mg/ml, 1 ml swished and swallowed three or four times a day) and solution for intravenous administration. In some countries, amphotericin B is available in oral troches. Amphotericin B oral suspension may be used for oral candidiasis that has failed to respond to other antifungal agents. The flavour and texture of the topical medications vary, and patient preference should be considered.

The azoles include the imidazoles, clotrimazole and ketoconazole, and the newer triazoles, fluconazole and itraconazole. Many drug interactions have been reported with the azoles. These drugs include antacids, H_2 receptor antagonists, phenytoin, rifampin, cyclosporin, terfenadine, astemizole, and warfarin, among others. The oral azole drugs are effective against C. albicans but may not be as effective against some Candida species, such as Candida krusei and Candida glabrata (Powderly, 1992; Como and Dismukes, 1994).

Clotrimazole is available as an oral 10 mg troche, one tablet dissolved slowly in the mouth five times a day. It has also proved useful when used as a prophylactic medication in patients with leukaemia (Cuttner et al., 1986). Ketoconazole is a systemic antifungal imidazole that is effective in a dose of one or two 200 mg tablets taken once daily with food. Ketaconazole may not be adequately absorbed in persons with reduced gastric acidity. Fluconazole is a systemic antifungal agent, effective when used as a 50–100 mg tablet taken once daily (Pons et al., 1993). However, cases have been reported of oral and oesophageal candidiasis that are resistant to fluconazole (Warnock et al., 1988; Akova et al., 1991; Heald et al., 1996; Maenza et al., 1996; Walmsley et al., 2001). Some of these cases are related to the emergence of strains known to be less sensitive to fluconazole, such as C. glabrata, and other cases are due to the emergence of resistant strains of C. albicans (Heinic et al., 1993b). Some of the cases of fluconazole-resistant candidiasis have been shown to be due to strains that are resistant to all azoles. Such cases may require treatment with intravenous amphotericin B (Ng and Denning, 1993). Oral candidiasis recurs frequently as the CD4 lymphocyte count falls. Fluconazole is effective for use as a prophylactic agent in doses ranging from 50 mg a day and 50 mg every other day to 100 mg a day (Hay, 1990; Stevens et al., 1991). Long-term prophylaxis with low-dose fluconazole may cause emergence of resistant strains of C. albicans (see Chapter 28). Itraconazole is a triazole antifungal agent that also requires normal gastric acidity for absorption but is effective in the treatment of oral candidiasis (Smith et al., 1991).

Topically applied creams or gels may be useful as adjunctive treatment for angular cheilitis. Clotrimazole, ketoconazole, and miconazole are examples of such agents.

Isolated case reports of a number of other opportunistic infections that cause oral lesions in HIV-infected persons have been described. These include Mycobacterium avium complex (MAC), tuberculosis, Cryptococcus neoformans, and Histoplasma capsulatum and Sporothrix schenkii (Volpe et al., 1985; Fowler et al., 1989; Heinic et al., 1992; Aarestrup et al., 2001).

Virus-associated lesions

Several viruses may reactivate, producing lesions in the mouth. These include the herpes group of viruses and papilloma viruses.

Herpes simplex virus

Herpes simplex virus (HSV) can produce recurrent painful episodes of ulceration intraorally and circumorally (see Chapter 32). Lesions most commonly occur on the vermilion border, and occasionally the adjoining facial skin may be involved. Intraoral lesions may appear on the palate or the gingival margin. The patient may report small vesicles, which erupt to form ulcers. Diagnosis can be made clinically, by virus culture, by cytological smears showing characteristic viral giant cells (Tzanck preparation), and by detection of viral antigens using monoclonal antibodies. Intraoral ulceration can be a difficult diagnostic problem in patients with HIV infection. Recurrent HSV produces vesicles and ulcers that occur on the keratinized mucosa, such as the hard palate or the attached gingiva. The ulcers usually heal within 10 days, but resolution of the lesions may take longer when associated with HIV infection and waning immunity. In cases of delayed healing, aciclovir capsules (200 mg taken five times a day) are useful, as are famciclovir and valaciclovir. Rarely, aciclovir-resistant HSV may cause serious progressive disease, but episodes usually respond to foscarnet (MacPhail *et al.*, 1989).

Zoster

Zoster, caused by varicella zoster virus (VZV, another member of the herpes group), presents with oral ulceration and pain. The prodromal symptoms may mimic dental pain. The vesicles and ulcers may occur intraorally before the appearance of skin lesions. All mucosal surfaces may be involved, including the vermilion border. The lesions, however, are always unilateral. Diagnosis is by clinical appearance. Treatment of herpes zoster requires high-dose aciclovir, 800 mg administered orally five times a day, or valaciclovir or famciclovir (see Chapter 32).

Cytomegalovirus

Cytomegalovirus (CMV) has been described in association with oral ulcers in several studies. The oral ulcers caused by CMV can appear on any mucosal surface and may mimic aphthous ulcers or can mimic periodontal disease when they occur on the periodontium (Dodd *et al.*, 1992b; Heinic *et al.*, 1993a). Ulcers can be co-infected with CMV and HSV. CMV ulcers in the oral cavity usually occur with disseminated CMV disease, and therefore diagnosis of CMV-infected oral ulcers should be followed by examination for systemic disease.

Hairy leukoplakia

Oral hairy leukoplakia is a white lesion of the oral mucosa, which is found predominantly on the lateral margins of the

tongue. The condition was first seen in San Francisco in 1981 in a group of homosexual men (Greenspan *et al.*, 1984). Oral hairy leukoplakia complicates HIV-infected persons worldwide. It is a group B (symptomatic HIV disease) condition according to the Center for Disease Control and Prevention (CDC) 1993 revised AIDS definition.

Oral hairy leukoplakia appears on the lateral margin of the tongue, either bilaterally or unilaterally, and sometimes on the buccal or labial mucosa and floor of the mouth, palate and oropharynx. It has been seen in these locations without co-existent tongue lesions in only a minority of patients. Oral hairy leukoplakia is white and does not rub off (Figure 12.3). The surface may be smooth, corrugated, or markedly prolific, with projections giving a 'hairy' appearance. The corrugations tend to run vertically along the lateral margin of the tongue. The leukoplakia may extend onto the ventral surface of the tongue where it may appear flat, and also onto the dorsal surface of the tongue, where it appears 'hairy'. Microscopically, there are characteristic appearances of folds or 'hairs', hyperparakeratosis, acanthosis, vacuolation of prickle cells, and little, if any, subepithelial inflammation.

Hairy leukoplakia has been aetiologically linked with Epstein-Barr virus infection (Raab-Traub *et al.*, 1997; Webster-Cyriaque *et al.*, 1997). Immunohistochemistry using monoclonal antibodies or polyvalent antisera to Epstein-Barr virus, Southern blot, or *in situ* hybridization with probes for Epstein-Barr virus all reveal the presence of the virus (Greenspan *et al.*, 1985; DeSouza *et al.*, 1990). Intraepithelial Langerhans cells are reduced or absent in the oral hairy leukoplakia lesion, and this decrease correlates with the presence of viral antigens (Daniels *et al.*, 1987). Virtually all patients with oral hairy leukoplakia are infected with HIV. Rare cases occur in HIV-negative persons, usually in association with other forms of immunodeficiency, notably organ and bone marrow graft recipients (Greenspan *et al.*, 1989; King *et al.*, 1994). Patients with oral hairy leukoplakia have a high risk of progression to AIDS (Greenspan *et al.*, 1987; Katz *et al.*, 1992). Originally, oral hairy leukoplakia was reported only in homosexual men and had not been reported prior to the AIDS epidemic. The lesion has now been described in all risk groups, including children (Greenspan *et al.*, 1988b). The lesion is usually asymptomatic, and treatment may not be indicated. However, patients with oral hairy leukoplakia are often concerned about the appearance of the lesion, and there may be soreness associated with co-existing *Candida* infection. Eliminating

Candida species with antifungal therapy may reduce the symptoms, but no drug is known to eliminate the lesion permanently. Oral hairy leukoplakia responds to high doses of aciclovir (Resnick *et al.*, 1988). A trial with the experimental drug desciclovir, an analogue given orally, which produces blood levels equivalent to intravenous aciclovir, showed temporary elimination or almost complete resolution in the clinical extent of the lesion. However, the lesions recurred within 1–4 months after desciclovir was stopped (Greenspan *et al.*, 1990a). Treatment for oral hairy leukoplakia is usually unnecessary, but if the lesion becomes extensive, uncomfortable, or unsightly, aciclovir capsules, 800 mg taken four times a day for 2 weeks, will usually result in the disappearance of the lesion and may be followed by a lower maintenance dose to prevent recurrence.

Oral warts

Human papilloma viruses (HPV) cause warts, including oral papillomas, condylomas, and focal epithelial hyperplasia. Focal epithelial hyperplasia is associated with HPV type 13, which is only found in the oral mucosa. Immunosuppressed persons show an increased tendency to develop skin warts, whereas anogenital warts occur as a sexually transmitted disease in male homosexuals and heterosexuals of both sexes. Many cases of oral warts of varying clinical appearance have been seen in HIV-infected persons (Figure 12.4). Some warts have a raised, cauliflower-like appearance, whereas others are well circumscribed, have a flat surface, and almost disappear when the mucosa is stretched. Some of the flat warts may be confused with small fibromas, and the diagnosis is made by biopsy and histopathological examination. The histological appearance may show multiple finger-like projections covered by hyperkeratotic epithelium, with a prominent granular layer, blunt projections covered by parakeratotic epithelium, or solitary areas of focal acanthosis (focal epithelial hyperplasia). Some koilocytosis may be seen. Identification of the virus type is performed by Southern blot, *in situ* hybridization, or newer molecular biology techniques. New and unusual types of papilloma viruses have been found in oral warts from HIV-infected persons, including HPV types 7, 13 and 32 (Greenspan *et al.*, 1988a; Syrjanen *et al.*, 1989). The oral warts can be quite troublesome, with multiple lesions occurring throughout the oral cavity. They frequently recur after surgical removal, whether by laser, cryosurgery, or knife. Warts showing atypical morphology are seen (Regezi *et al.*, 1994), but malignant change has not been described.

Periodontal disease

Even in health, the gingival crevice contains a diverse microflora. Many HIV-infected persons show a tendency to develop severe gingival inflammation and progressive destructive periodontal disease (Lamster *et al.*, 1996; Lamster *et al.*, 1997; Winkler *et al.*, 1988). Their gingivitis may resemble acute necrotizing ulcerative gingivitis, but is prolonged and severe. The gingiva appear bright red and swollen, with ulcers at the tips of the interdental papillae. Pain is often severe, and halitosis is common. The HIV-associated periodontitis presents as rapid and progressive destruction of the supporting tissues, periodontal ligament, and alveolar bone, with loosening of and even exfoliation of teeth (Figure 12.5). This is known as necrotizing ulcerative periodontitis. Plaque cultures show mixed flora, not unlike that seen in conventional chronic periodontal disease. The pathogenesis of these lesions is also poorly understood. The relative contributions to tissue damage made by the microbial products and by the host response to infection, notably polymorphs, macrophages, lymphocytes, and humoral factors, remain unclear. Treatment of periodontal disease involves removal of plaque, calculus, and necrotic tissue (Winkler *et al.*, 1989). Irrigation of affected sites with 10% povidone iodine mucosal solution and use of an appropriate antibiotic such as metronidazole, augmentin, or clindamycin is effective if careful oral hygiene is maintained.

Neoplasia

Both Kaposi's sarcoma (KS) and non-Hodgkin's lymphoma may manifest first as oral lesions. There are no data as yet that suggest that other oral neoplasias are also seen with increased frequency in persons with HIV infection.

Kaposi's sarcoma

The oral lesions of KS may be the first presentation of the disease and occur most commonly on the palate, with the second most common location being the gingiva (Figure 12.6). The tongue and other oral mucosal sites may also be involved. Similar to the lesions on the skin, the oral lesions are purple or dark red and may be flat or nodular (Ficarra *et al.*, 1988). A few are covered with a thick layer of uninvolved mucosa and therefore do not show abnormal colour. These lesions affect the gingiva and the tongue. Symptoms of oral KS are uncommon unless the nodular stage becomes ulcerated, when bleeding and pain from secondary infection may be present. The oral lesions of KS should be treated if they become nodular and involve gingival mucosa such that oral hygiene is compromised, there is interference with speech or other oral function, they are unsightly, or pain and bleeding become troublesome. In such cases, effective modes of therapy (Epstein, 1997) have included local excision, intralesional chemotherapy, use of sclerosing agents, and localized radiation therapy (Epstein and Scully, 1989; Lucatorto and Sapp, 1993).

Non-Hodgkin's lymphoma

Non-Hodgkin's lymphoma (Jordan et al., 1997) in association with HIV infection can present as oral ulcers or nodules, often of sudden onset with pain due to ulceration, that grow rapidly. Diagnosis may be difficult and delayed because of confusion with chronic major aphthous ulcers caused by opportunistic infection. In rare instances, the lesions may disappear and then reappear, and multifocal lesions have been described (Dodd et al., 1992a, 1993).

Other lesions

Recurrent aphthous ulcers are common oral lesions. The cause of these lesions is unknown, but hormonal factors, food allergy, stress, and viral factors have been implicated. A role for cellular immune dysfunction in the pathogenesis has been suggested. There may be recurrence of aphthous ulcers in association with HIV infection (MacPhail et al., 1991, 1992). These lesions may occur in people with a history of recurrent aphthous ulcers and also in those who have never had an episode of oral ulceration. The ulcers occur on the non-keratinized mucosa and are usually quite painful (Figure 12.7). The lesions usually have the typical appearance of recurrent aphthous ulcers: well-circumscribed ulcers with an erythematous margin. Sometimes, the ulcers persist and may become large with irregular margins and be locally quite destructive. They are usually of acute onset and heal in the course of 10 days to 2 weeks. Sometimes recurrent aphthous ulcers, particularly of the major type, may persist for a month or longer. In association with HIV infection, the ulcers may last for long periods of time, and outbreaks may occur frequently. Some patients complain that they are never without an ulcer. The local and systemic host defects in HIV infection may be the cause of recurrent aphthous ulcers in this group of patients. Diagnosis may be made from the clinical appearance, but persistent lesions should be biopsied to rule out other diagnoses. Differential diagnosis of recurrent aphthous ulcers includes squamous cell carcinoma, trauma, vesiculo-erosive disease, HSV infection and syphilis. Treatment with topical steroids, such as 0.05% flucinonide ointment mixed with 50% orabase, applied topically several times daily, will usually shorten the duration of the ulcers. Thalidomide has been reported as useful in shortening the duration and recurrence of these ulcers (Ryan et al., 1992; Jacobson et al., 1997).

Salivary gland enlargement has been reported in some HIV-infected adult and paediatric patients (Itescu et al., 1990; Schiødt et al., 1992). The cause is unknown, and both parotid and submandibular gland involvement have been seen. Histological examination of minor labial salivary glands reveals changes similar to those seen in Sjögren's syndrome, but with CD8 rather than CD4 lymphocytes predominating (Patel and Mandel, 2001). The ensuing changes of salivary function with reduced flow rates can be a significant problem, leading to increased dental caries. Symptomatic relief can sometimes be obtained with the use of salivary stimulants such as sugarless mints. Oral care should include the use of daily fluoride rinses or gels.

References

Aarestrup FM, Guerra RO, Vieira BJ et al. (2001). Oral manifestation of sporotrichosis in AIDS patients. Oral Dis **7**: 134–6.

Akova M, Akalin HE, Uzun O et al. (1991). Emergence of Candida krusei infections after therapy of oropharyngeal candidiasis with fluconazole [letter]. Eur J Clin Microbiol Infect Dis **10**: 598–9.

Como JA, Dismukes WE. (1994). Oral azole drugs as systemic antifungal therapy. N Engl J Med **330**: 263–72.

Crowe SM, Carlin JB, Stewart KI et al. (1991). Predictive value of CD4 lymphocyte numbers for the development of opportunistic infections and malignancies in HIV infected persons. J AIDS **4**: 770–6.

Crowe SM, Vardaxis N, Maerz A et al. (1994). HIV infection of monocyte-derived macrophages in vitro reduces phagocytosis of Candida albicans. J Leukoc Biol **56**: 318–27.

Cuttner J, Troy KM, Funaro L et al. (1986). Clotrimazole treatment for prevention of oral candidiasis in patients with acute leukemia undergoing chemotherapy. Results of a double-blind study. Am J Med **81**: 771–4.

Daniels TE, Greenspan D, Greenspan JS et al. (1987). Absence of Langerhans cells in oral hairy leukoplakia, an AIDS-associated lesion. J Invest Dermatol **89**: 178–82.

DeSouza YG, Freese UK, Greenspan D et al. (1990). Diagnosis of Epstein Barr virus infection in hairy leukoplakia by using nucleic acid hybridization and noninvasive techniques. J Clin Microbiol **28**: 2775–8.

Dodd CL, Greenspan D, Schiodt M et al. (1992a). Unusual oral presentation of non-Hodgkin's lymphoma in association with HIV infection. Oral Surg Oral Med Oral Pathol **73**: 603–8.

Dodd CL, Winkler JR, Heinic GS et al. (1992b). Cytomegalovirus infection presenting as acute periodontal infection in a patient infected with the human immunodeficiency virus. *J Rheumatol* **19**: 26–9.

Dodd CL, Greenspan D, Katz MH *et al.* (1993). Multifocal oral non-Hodgkin's lymphoma in an AIDS patient. *AIDS* **5**: 1339–43.

Epstein JB. (1997). Management of oral Kaposi's sarcoma and a proposal for clinical staging. *Oral Dis* **3**: S124–8.

Epstein JB, Scully C. (1989). Intralesional vinblastine for oral Kaposi's sarcoma in HIV infection. *Lancet* **2**: 1100–1.

Ficarra G, Person AM, Silverman S *et al.* (1988). Kaposi's sarcoma of the oral cavity: a study of 134 patients with a review of the pathogenesis, epidemiology, clinical aspects, and treatment. *Oral Surg Oral Med Oral Pathol* **66**: 543–50.

Fowler CB, Nelson JF, Henley DW *et al.* (1989). Acquired immune deficiency syndrome presenting as a palatal perforation. *Oral Surg Oral Med Oral Pathol* **67**: 313–8.

Gottlieb MS, Schroff R, Schantez HM *et al.* (1981). *Pneumocystis carinii* pneumonia and mucosal candidiasis in previously healthy homosexual men: evidence of a new acquired cellular immunodeficiency. *N Engl J Med* **305**: 1425–31.

Greenspan JS. (1997). Sentinels and signposts: the epidemiology and significance of the oral manifestations of HIV disease. *Oral Dis* **3**: S13–7.

Greenspan D, Greenspan JS. (1991). Management of the oral lesions of HIV infection. *J Am Dent Assoc* **122**: 26–32.

Greenspan D, Greenspan JS. (1996). HIV-related oral disease. *Lancet* **348**: 729.

Greenspan D, Shirlaw PJ. (1997). Management of the oral mucosal lesions seen in association with HIV infection. *Oral Dis* **3**: S229–34.

Greenspan D, Greenspan JS, Conant M *et al.* (1984). Oral 'hairy' leukoplakia in male homosexuals: evidence of association with both papillomavirus and a herpes-group virus. *Lancet* **2**: 831–4.

Greenspan JS, Greenspan D, Lennette ET *et al.* (1985). Replication of Epstein-Barr virus within the epithelial cells of 'hairy' leukoplakia, an AIDS associated lesion. *N Engl J Med* **313**: 1564–71.

Greenspan D, Greenspan JS, Hearst NG *et al.* (1987). Relation of oral hairy leukoplakia to infection with the human immunodeficiency virus and the risk of developing AIDS. *J Infect Dis* **155**: 475–81.

Greenspan D, de Villiers EM, Greenspan JS *et al.* (1988a). Unusual HPV types in the oral warts in association with HIV infection. *J Oral Pathol* **17**: 482–7.

Greenspan JS, Mastrucci T, Leggott P *et al.* (1988b). Hairy leukoplakia in a child. *AIDS* **2**: 143.

Greenspan D, Greenspan JS, DeSouza YG *et al.* (1989). Oral hairy leukoplakia in an HIV-negative renal transplant recipient. *J Oral Pathol Med* **18**: 32–4.

Greenspan D, DeSouza Y, Conant MA *et al.* (1990a). Efficacy of desciclovir in the treatment of Epstein-Barr virus infection in oral hairy leukoplakia. *J AIDS* **3**: 571–8.

Greenspan D, Greenspan JS, Pindborg JJ *et al.* (1990b). *AIDS and the mouth.* Copenhagen: Munksgaard.

Hay RJ. (1990). Overview of studies of fluconazole in oropharyngeal candidiasis. *Rev Infect Dis* **3**: S334–7.

Heald AE, Cox GM, Schell WA *et al.* (1996). Oropharyngeal yeast flora and fluconazole resistance in HIV-infected patients receiving long-term continuous versus intermittent fluconazole therapy. *AIDS* **10**: 263.

Heinic G, Greenspan D, MacPhail LA *et al.* (1992). Oral *Histoplasma capsulatum* in association with HIV infection: a case report. *J Oral Pathol Med* **21**: 85–9.

Heinic G, Greenspan D, Greenspan JS *et al.* (1993a). Oral CMV lesions and the HIV infected: early recognition can help prevent morbidity. *J Am Dent Assoc* **124**: 99–104.

Heinic GS, Stevens DA, Greenspan D *et al.* (1993b). Fluconazole-resistant Candida in AIDS patients. Report of two cases. *Oral Surg Oral Med Oral Pathol* **76**: 711–5.

Itescu SL, Brancato J, Buxbaum J *et al.* (1990). A diffuse infiltrative CD8 lymphocytosis syndrome in human immunodeficiency virus (HIV) infection: a host immune response associated with HLA-DR5. *Ann Intern Med* **112**: 3–10.

Jacobson JM, Greenspan JS, Spritzler J *et al.* (1997). Thalidomide for the treatment of oral aphthous ulcers in patients with human immunodeficiency virus infection. National Institute of Allergy and Infectious Diseases AIDS Clinical Trials Group. *N Engl J Med* **336**: 1487–93.

Jordan RCK, Chong L, DiPierdomenico S *et al.* (1997). Oral lymphoma in HIV infection. *Oral Dis* **3**: S135–7.

Katz MH, Greenspan D, Westenhouse J *et al.* (1992). Progression to AIDS in HIV-infected homosexual and bisexual men with hairy leukoplakia and oral candidiasis. *AIDS* **6**: 95–100.

Katz MH, Mastrucci MT, Leggott PJ *et al.* (1993). Prognostic significance of oral lesions in children with perinatally acquired HIV infection. *Am J Dis Child* **147**: 45–8.

King GN, Healy CM, Glover MT *et al.* (1994). Prevalence and risk factors associated with leukoplakia, hairy leukoplakia, erythematous candidiasis and gingival hyperplasia in renal transplant recipients. *Oral Surg Oral Med Oral Pathol* **78**: 18–26.

Lamster I, Grbic J, Fine J *et al.* (1996). A critical review of periodontal disease as a manifestation of HIV infection. In: JS Greenspan, D Greenspan (eds.) *Oral manifestations of HIV infection: proceedings of the second international workshop.* Chicago, IL: Quintessence Publishing.

Lamster IB, Grbic JT, Bucklan RS *et al.* (1997). Epidemiology and diagnosis of HIV-associated periodontal diseases. *Oral Dis* **3**: S141–8.

Lucatorto FM, Sapp JP. (1993). Treatment of oral Kaposi's sarcoma with a sclerosing agent in AIDS patients. *Oral Surg Oral Med Oral Pathol* **75**: 192–8.

MacPhail LA, Greenspan D, Schiødt M *et al.* (1989). Acyclovir-resistant, foscarnet-sensitive oral herpes simplex type 2 lesion in a patient with AIDS. *Oral Surg Oral Med Oral Pathol* **67**: 427–32.

MacPhail LA, Greenspan D, Feigal DW *et al.* (1991). Recurrent aphthous ulcers in association with HIV infection: description of ulcer types and analysis of T-cell subsets. *Oral Surg Oral Med Oral Pathol* **71**: 678–83.

MacPhail LA, Greenspan D, Greenspan JS *et al.* (1992). Recurrent aphthous ulcers in association with HIV infection: diagnosis and treatment. *Oral Surg Oral Med Oral Pathol* **73**: 283–8.

Maenza JR, Keruly JC, Moore RD *et al.* (1996). Risk factors for fluconazole-resistant candidiasis in human immunodeficiency virus-infected patients. *J Infect Dis* **173**: 219.

Ng TT, Denning DW (1993). Fluconazole resistance in Candida in patients with AIDS – a therapeutic approach. *J Infect* **26**: 117–25.

Patel S and Mandel L (2001). Parotid gland swelling in HIV diffuse infiltrative CD8 lymphocytosis syndrome. *NY State Dent J* **67**: 22–3.

Pons V, Greenspan D, Debruin M. (1993). Therapy for oropharyngeal candidiasis in HIV-infected patients; a randomized, prospective multicenter study of oral fluconazole versus clotrimazole troches. The Multicenter Study Group. *J AIDS* **6**: 1311–6.

Powderly WG. (1992). Mucosal candidiasis caused by non *albicans* species of *Candida* in HIV-positive patients. *AIDS* **6**: 604–5.

Raab-Traub N, Webster-Cyriaque J. (1997). Epstein-Barr virus infection and expression in oral lesions. *Oral Dis* **3**: S164–70.

Regezi JA, Greenspan D, Greenspan JS *et al.* (1994). HPV-associated epithelial atypia in oral warts in HIV+ patients. *J Cutan Pathol* **21**: 217–23.

Resnick L, Herbst JHS, Ablashi DV *et al.* (1988). Regression of oral hairy leukoplakia after orally administered acyclovir therapy. *JAMA* **259**: 384–8.

Ryan J, Colman J, Pedersen J *et al.* (1992). Thalidomide to treat oesophageal ulcer in AIDS [letter]. *N Engl J Med* **327**: 208–9.

Schiødt M, Dobb CL, Greenspan D *et al.* (1992). Natural history of HIV-associated salivary gland disease. *Oral Surg Oral Med Oral Pathol* **74**: 326–31.

Smith DE, Midgley J, Allan M *et al.* (1991). Itraconazole versus ketoconazole in the treatment of oral and oesophageal candidosis in patients infected with HIV. *AIDS* **5**: 1367–71.

Stevens DA, Greene I, Lang OS *et al.* (1991). Thrush can be prevented in patients with acquired immunodeficiency syndrome and the acquired immunodeficiency syndrome-related complex. *Arch Intern Med* **151**: 2458–64.

Syrjanen S, von Krogh G, Kellokoski J *et al.* (1989). Two different human papillomavirus (HPV) types associated with oral mucosal lesions in an HIV-seropositive man. *J Oral Pathol Med* **18**: 366–70.

Tavitian A, Raufman JP, Rosenthal LE *et al.* (1986). Oral candidiasis as a marker for oesophageal candidiasis in the acquired immunodeficiency syndrome. *Ann Intern Med* **104**: 54–5.

Volpe F, Schimmer A, Barr C *et al.* (1985). Oral manifestations of disseminated *Mycobacterium avium intracellulare* in a patient with AIDS. *Oral Surg Oral Med Oral Pathol* **5**: 567–70.

Walmsley S, King S, McGeer A *et al.* (2001). Oropharyngeal candidiasis in patients with human immunodeficiency virus: correlation of clinical outcome with in vitro resistance, serum azole levels and immunosuppression. *Clin Infect Dis* **32**: 1554–61.

Warnock DW, Burke J, Cope NJ *et al.* (1988). Fluconazole resistance in *Candida glabrata* [letter]. *Lancet* **2**: 1310.

Webster-Cyriaque J, Edwards RH, Quinlivan EB *et al.* (1997). Epstein-Barr virus and human herpesvirus 8 prevalence in human immunodeficiency virus-associated oral mucosal lesions. *J Infect Dis* **175**: 1324–32.

Winkler JR, Grassi M, Murray PA *et al.* (1988). Clinical description and etiology of HIV-associated periodontal diseases. In: *Perspectives on oral manifestations of AIDS: diagnosis and management of HIV-associated infections*. Littleton, MA: PSG, 49–70.

Winkler JR, Murray PA, Grassi M *et al.* (1989). Diagnosis and management of HIV-associated periodontal lesions. *J Am Dent Assoc* **119**: S25–34.

13

Evaluation and management of respiratory complications of HIV infection

ALISON MORRIS AND LAURENCE HUANG

Respiratory complications are frequent in HIV-infected persons and may be due to a wide spectrum of illnesses, both HIV-associated and non-HIV-associated (Table 13.1). The spectrum of HIV-associated illnesses encompasses opportunistic infections, neoplasms, and other respiratory disorders. The relative frequencies of each of these disorders depends on a number of factors, which will be discussed. Although each disorder has a characteristic presentation, these can vary and overlap. A careful evaluation of the individual patient will often suggest a specific diagnosis or a few diagnoses to consider. The first part of this chapter will review the evaluation of respiratory complications of HIV infection, while the second part will discuss intensive care of the HIV-infected patient.

Evaluation of respiratory complications

The initial evaluation of respiratory complications usually focuses on the diagnosis of HIV-associated opportunistic infections because of the need for prompt therapy of these

Table 13.1 Spectrum of respiratory complications of HIV infection and AIDS

Infections (most frequently identified organisms)	Neoplasms
Bacteria	KS
Streptococcus pneumoniae	NHL
Haemophilus influenzae	Lung carcinoma
Haemophilus species	
Gram-negative bacilli	*Other respiratory disorders*
Pseudomonas aeruginosa	Upper respiratory tract
Klebsiella pneumoniae	Colds
Staphylococcus aureus	Sinusitis
Fungi	Pharyngitis
Pneumocystis carinii	Lower respiratory tract
Cryptococcus neoformans	LIP
Histoplasma capsulatum	NIP
Coccidioides immitis	Acute bronchitis
Aspergillus species	Obstructive lung disease
Mycobacteria	Pulmonary vascular disease/pulmonary emboli
Mycobacterium tuberculosis	Primary pulmonary hypertension
Mycobacterium kansasii	BOOP
MAC	
Virus	
CMV	
Parasite	
Toxoplasma gondii	

MAC: *Mycobacterium avium* complex; CMV: cytomegalovirus; KS: Kaposi's sarcoma; NHL: non-Hodgkin's lymphoma; LIP: lymphocytic interstitial pneumonitis; NIP: non-specific interstitial pneumonitis; BOOP: bronchiolitis obliterans organizing pneumonia.

diseases. Remember that HIV-infected patients, especially those on highly active antiretroviral therapy (HAART), may have respiratory disorders (e.g. asthma, pulmonary embolism, lung carcinoma) that are unrelated to their HIV infection. In addition, risk factors for HIV infection, such as injecting drug use, may also contribute to respiratory disease (e.g. endocarditis with septic pulmonary emboli, pulmonary vascular disease). Therefore, clinicians should consider the possibility of non-HIV-associated respiratory disorders before embarking on an exhaustive search for an HIV-associated opportunistic infection or neoplasm.

The evaluation of respiratory complications begins with a thorough history and physical examination. Laboratory testing and chest radiography are performed in selected patients. Frequently, the clinical, laboratory, and chest radiographic presentation will suggest a specific diagnostic and management plan. Occasionally, additional tests such as chest computed tomography (CT) scan, chest high-resolution CT scan, pulmonary function tests, nuclear medicine studies or other tests may be needed. The most useful laboratory tests are those that provide a definitive microbiological or pathological diagnosis. Specimens from sites such as skin, lymph node, bone marrow, and cerebrospinal fluid (CSF) will at times provide the diagnosis of extrapulmonary or disseminated disease responsible for the pulmonary complaint. For certain opportunistic infections, blood or urine serologies (e.g. serum cryptococcal antigen, urine *Histoplasma* antigen) or molecular techniques such as polymerase chain reaction (PCR)-based analyses can provide or strongly suggest the diagnosis. The decision of which diagnostic test(s) to obtain and which treatment(s) to initiate relies on an accurate differential diagnosis derived from a thorough history and physical examination, selected laboratory data, and imaging studies.

History and physical examination
Clinical setting
The clinical setting in which the patient is evaluated impacts upon the relative frequency of respiratory disorders seen (Table 13.2). The Pulmonary Complications of HIV Infection Study (PCHIS) was a large, prospective, observational cohort study that followed over 1150 HIV-infected subjects for approximately 5 years at six sites across the USA (Pulmonary Complications of HIV Infection Study Group, 1993). The PCHIS found that ambulatory patients presenting to an outpatient clinic usually had illnesses such as colds, sinusitis, pharyngitis, and acute bronchitis, rather

Table 13.2 Evaluation of respiratory complications: diagnostic clues

Clinical setting
Outpatient clinic: colds, sinusitis, acute bronchitis
Hospital: bacterial, *Pneumocystis carinii*, mycobacterial, or fungal pneumonia
Intensive care unit: PCP

CD4 lymphocyte count (see Table 13.3)
　Current and/or lowest

History of present illness (see Table 13.3)
　Respiratory symptoms: duration
　Constitutional symptoms

Past medical history
HIV transmission category
　Injection drug use: bacterial pneumonia, tuberculosis
　Sex with men: KS
Habits
　Cigarettes: bacterial bronchitis or pneumonia, COPD, lung carcinoma
Travel and residence
　Endemic fungal diseases
　Tuberculosis
Non-adherence with prophylaxis
　PCP
　Systemic fungal diseases
　Tuberculosis

Physical examination
Vital signs
Lung examination
　Normal: PCP
　Focal: bacterial pneumonia
Cardiac examination
　S3 gallop, jugular venous distension: congestive heart failure
Neurological examination
　Altered mental status: *Cryptococcus neoformans*
　Focal neurological examination: *Toxoplasma gondii*
Skin examination
　KS
　Disseminated fungal disease
Abdominal examination
　Hepatosplenomegaly: disseminated fungal or mycobacterial disease, NHL

Laboratory tests
WBC count
　Elevated: bacterial pneumonia
　Left shift: bacterial pneumonia
　Neutropenia: bacterial pneumonia, *Aspergillus* species
LDH
　Elevated: PCP
ABG
Chest radiograph (see Table 13.5)

PCP: *Pneumocystis carinii* pneumonia; KS: Kaposi's sarcoma; COPD: chronic obstructive pulmonary disease; NHL: non-Hodgkin's lymphoma; WBC: white blood cell; LDH: serum lactate dehydrogenase; ABG: arterial blood gas.

than bacterial, tuberculous, fungal or *Pneumocytis carinii* pneumonia (PCP) (Wallace *et al.*, 1993, 1997). In contrast, patients requiring hospital admission more often had pneumonia, and those requiring critical care specifically had PCP (Wachter *et al.*, 1992; Rosen *et al.*, 1997). The geographical location of the clinic or hospital may also influence the common diagnoses in HIV-infected patients. In specific populations or geographical regions, mycobacterial and fungal pneumonias become important considerations.

CD4 lymphocyte count

The CD4 lymphocyte count is a critical piece of clinical information which should be obtained for every HIV-infected patient being evaluated for respiratory complications. The CD4 lymphocyte count is an excellent indicator of an HIV-infected patient's risk of developing a specific opportunistic infection or neoplasm. Each of the HIV-related respiratory complications is typically seen within a characteristic CD4 lymphocyte count range and uncommonly above that range (Table 13.3). Diseases such as colds, sinusitis, pharyngitis, acute bronchitis, bacterial pneumonia, tuberculosis, and non-Hodgkin's lymphoma (NHL), which are seen in non-immunocompromised persons, can be seen at any CD4 lymphocyte count in HIV-infected patients, although their incidence increases as the CD4 lymphocyte count declines. The Centers for Disease Control and Prevention's (CDC's) Adult and Adolescent Spectrum of HIV Disease Project provided statistics on which conditions occurred within certain CD4 lymphocyte count ranges, as well as which conditions were more common within a specific CD4 lymphocyte count range (Hanson *et al.*, 1995). For example, this study found that the vast majority (> 80%) of bacterial and tuberculous pneumonias occurred in subjects with a CD4 lymphocyte count of less than 500 cells/μl, suggesting that, although both these diseases should be considered in an HIV-infected patient regardless of the CD4 lymphocyte count, they are more common when the CD4 lymphocyte count is less than 500 cells/μl.

At CD4 lymphocyte counts of less than 200 cells/μl, bacterial pneumonia is often accompanied by bacteraemia, and *M. tuberculosis* infection is often associated with extrapulmonary, disseminated disease. In addition, at this CD4 lymphocyte count, PCP and *Cryptococcus neoformans* pneumonia become significant considerations, whereas neither would be common in a patient with a CD4 lymphocyte count greater than 200 cells/μl. At CD4 lymphocyte counts less than 100 cells/μl, pulmonary Kaposi's sarcoma (KS)

and pneumonia due to *Toxoplasma gondii* and bacterial pathogens such as *Pseudomonas aeruginosa* and *Staphylococcus aureus* are increasingly diagnosed. Finally, diseases caused by endemic (*H. capsulatum*, *C. immitis*) and non-endemic (*Aspergillus* species) fungi, certain viruses (cytomegalovirus; CMV), and non-tuberculous mycobacteria (*M. avium* complex; MAC) almost always occur at the lowest CD4 lymphocyte count ranges (less than 50 cells/μl). Often these diseases are disseminated and the extrapulmonary sites can dominate the clinical presentation.

Table 13.3 HIV-associated respiratory complications according to CD4 lymphocyte count

---

Any CD4 lymphocyte count
Upper respiratory tract illness
  Colds
  Sinusitis
  Pharyngitis
Acute bronchitis
Bacterial pneumonia (usually *Streptococcus pneumoniae*, *Haemophilus* species)
Mycobacterium tuberculosis pneumonia
NHL

CD4 lymphocyte count less than 500 cells/μl
  Bacterial pneumonia (recurrent)
  Nontuberculous mycobacterial pneumonia

CD4 lymphocyte count less than 200 cells/μl
PCP
Cryptococcus neoformans pneumonia
Bacterial pneumonia associated with bacteraemia/septicaemia
Mycobacterium tuberculosis associated with extrapulmonary/disseminated disease

CD4 lymphocyte count less than 100 cells/μl
  Pulmonary Kaposi's sarcoma
  Bacterial pneumonia (especially Gram-negative bacilli and *Staphylococcus aureus*)
Toxoplasma gondii pneumonitis

CD4 lymphocyte count less than 50 cells/μl
Histoplasma capsulatum associated with extrapulmonary/disseminated disease
Coccidioides immitis associated with extrapulmonary/disseminated disease
Aspergillus species pneumonia
CMV pneumonitis associated with extrapulmonary/disseminated disease
MAC associated with extrapulmonary/disseminated disease

NHL: non-Hodgkin's lymphoma; PCP: *Pneumocystis carinii* pneumonia; CMV: cytomegalovirus; MAC: *Mycobacterium avium* complex.

Lowest or current CD4 lymphocye count. Current antiretroviral combinations can produce dramatic and sustained rises in the CD4 lymphocyte counts of many patients. Some controversy exists over which CD4 cell count should be used to assess risk of disease, either the current count or the lowest. Several reports indicate that if, in response to HAART, patients sustain high CD4 cell counts ($>250/\mu l$) over the course of 3–6 months, the risk of many opportunistic infections is reduced (Furrer *et al.*, 1999; Weverling *et al.*, 1999; Kovacs and Masur, 2000). These findings may not hold true for all patients, and those with a history of particular opportunistic infections or of advanced AIDS before starting therapy may remain at increased risk of developing these disorders (Miller *et al.*, 1999). In general, however, the patient's most recent CD4 cell cound seems to be the most accurate predictor of disease risk (Kovacs and Masur, 2000).

Symptoms

The PCHIS demonstrated that respiratory symptoms are a frequent complaint of HIV-infected persons and increase in frequency as the CD4 lymphocyte count declines. In this study, HIV-infected subjects reported cough at 27%, shortness of breath at 23%, and fever at 9% of more than 12 000 routine visits (Huang, unpubl. data). These symptoms increased in frequency in the subset of subjects with a CD4 lymphocyte count of less than 200 cells/μl.

In many hospital settings, the two most frequent HIV-related respiratory complications are PCP and bacterial pneumonia (most commonly due to *Streptococcus pneumoniae* and *Hemophilus influenzae*). An autopsy series of HIV-infected patients found that bacterial pneumonia was almost twice as common as PCP (Afessa *et al.*, 1998). As bacterial pneumonia and PCP account for the majority of the respiratory complications seen in HIV-infected patients, the clinical evaluation often focuses on distinguishing between these two diseases (Table 13.4). PCP and bacterial pneumonia typically differ by the presence or absence of purulent sputum and the symptom duration (Huang and Stansell, 1996). PCP characteristically presents with fever, dyspnoea, and a dry, non-productive cough. When the cough is productive, it is usually clear, rather than purulent. Respiratory symptoms are usually subacute in onset and present for 2–4 weeks before diagnosis, or longer. The median duration of symptoms was 28 days in one early study (Kovacs *et al.*, 1984). In contrast, pneumonia due to *S. pneumoniae* or *H. influenzae* typically presents with fevers, shaking chills or rigors, pleuritic chest pain, and a productive cough with purulent sputum. Respiratory symptoms are usually acute in onset and present for 3–5 days. In an HIV-infected patient with a CD4 lymphocyte count of less than 200 cells/μl (at risk for both types of pneumonia), the absence of purulent sputum and symptom duration of a few weeks strongly favour the diagnosis of PCP, rather than bacterial pneumonia. In contrast, the presence of purulent spu-

Table 13.4 Comparison of clinical, laboratory, and chest radiographic findings in *Pneumocystis carinii* and bacterial pneumonias

	Pneumocystis carinii	Bacteria
CD4 lymphocyte count	Less than 200 cells/ul	Any
Symptoms	Non-productive cough	Productive cough
		Purulent sputum
Symptom duration	Subacute: 2–4 weeks or more	Acute: 3–5 days
Signs	Non-focal or normal lung examination	Focal lung examination
Laboratory data	WBC varies	WBC elevated
		Neutrophilia
	Serum LDH elevated	LDH varies
Chest radiograph		
Distribution	Diffuse > focal	Focal > diffuse
Location	Bilateral > unilateral	Unilateral > bilateral
	Perihilar	Segmental/lobar
Pattern	Reticular–granular	Consolidation
Cysts	15–20%	Rare
Pleural effusions	Very rare	25–30%

WBC: white blood cell; LDH: lactate dehydrogenase.

tum and symptom duration of a few days favour the diagnosis of bacterial pneumonia. Patients with mixed clinical findings may well have dual infections (PCP and bacterial pneumonia).

Past medical history

HIV transmission category and habits. A patient's HIV transmission category and habits impact upon the relative frequency of various HIV-related and non-HIV-related respiratory complications. Bacterial pneumonia and TB are more common in HIV-infected patients who are injecting drug users (IDU) than in HIV-infected patients without a history of injecting drug use (Hirschtick *et al.*, 1995). KS is seen almost exclusively in men who report sex with other men. Furthermore, injecting drug use or other illicit drugs can cause a variety of non-HIV-related pulmonary diseases such as aspiration pneumonia secondary to respiratory depression, endocarditis-related septic pulmonary emboli, pulmonary vasculitis, and drug-induced pulmonary oedema.

As in the general population, HIV-infected patients who are cigarette smokers are at an increased risk for a variety of respiratory illnesses. Both bacterial bronchitis and bronchopneumonia are more common in HIV-infected cigarette smokers than in HIV-infected non-smokers or former smokers (Hirschtick *et al.*, 1995). In addition, HIV-infected patients who report a long history of cigarette use may present with manifestations of chronic obstructive pulmonary disease (COPD) as the aetiology of their respiratory symptoms. Although HIV infection itself is probably not associated with an increased risk of lung carcinoma, HIV-infected smokers are more likely than HIV-infected non-smokers to develop this disease (Johnson *et al.*, 1997).

Travel and residence. Travel to or residence in a geographical region that is endemic for fungi such as *H. capsulatum* or *C. immitis* is a strong determinant of the risk of exposure, infection and, ultimately, disease. HIV-infected patients without such a history are unlikely to have been exposed and infected and, therefore, are unlikely to develop these diseases.

Tuberculosis (TB) is more common in certain geographical areas and in certain populations. HIV-infected patients who were born in or have travelled to a country with a high prevalence of TB and patients who are homeless, unstably housed, or previously incarcerated are at high risk of *M. tuberculosis* infection. IDUs, especially if anergic, are another population at increased risk for TB (Selwyn *et*

al., 1992). Patients who have a positive (defined as ≥ 5 mm induration in HIV-infected persons) tuberculin skin test are also at risk for developing TB (Markowitz *et al.*, 1997).

Prior pulmonary conditions and use of prophylaxis. Many HIV-related opportunistic infections are recurrent, and knowledge of a patient's prior pulmonary history may suggest the aetiology of the current illness. Recognition that bacterial pneumonias are common in HIV-infected patients and frequently recur led to the inclusion of recurrent pneumonia (two or more episodes within a 12-month period) as an AIDS-defining condition (CDC, 1993). Patients with a history of PCP are at high risk of recurrence and must be offered secondary *P. carinii* prophylaxis (Wallace *et al.*, 1997). Use of secondary prophylaxis after a sustained rise in the CD4 cell count from antiretroviral therapy is more controversial. Recent data suggest that stopping secondary prophylaxis for PCP is probably safe, but physicians and patients need to make this decision individually (Furrer *et al.*, 1999; Weverling *et al.*, 1999; Kovacs and Masur, 2000). HIV-infected patients with a history of cryptococcosis, coccidioidomycosis, or histoplasmosis are at high risk of relapse and should receive lifelong maintenance therapy with fluconazole (cryptococcosis and coccidioidomycosis) or itraconazole (histoplasmosis) after completing treatment of the acute infection (Wallace *et al.*, 1997). As with PCP, the recommendations for patients on HAART with improved CD4 cell counts are less clear; however, current data are not sufficient to warrant discontinuation of prophylaxis regardless of CD4 cell count. Similarly, HIV-infected patients with a history of cryptococcosis, coccidioidomycosis, or histoplasmosis are at high risk for relapse and should receive lifelong maintenance therapy with fluconazole (cryptococcosis and coccidioidomycosis) or itraconazole (histoplasmosis) after completing treatment of the acute infection (Wallace *et al.*, 1997). Patients with a positive tuberculin skin test who do not reliably take chemoprophylaxis (e.g. isoniazid) are at high risk of developing TB. Respiratory complications in an HIV-infected patient who does not adhere to the recommended therapy will frequently be due to recurrent or relapsed disease.

Signs

HIV-infected patients with pneumonia may be febrile, tachycardic, and tachypnoeic. Evidence of systemic hypotension suggests a fulminant disease process (e.g. bacterial septicaemia). Pulse oximetry often reveals a decrease in the oxygen saturation and provides an estimate of the severity of the disease. The presence of exercise-induced oxygen desaturation, hypoxia, and/or an increase in the alveolar–arterial oxygen gradient are all reported to be sensitive findings for PCP (Stover *et al.*, 1989).

Examination of the lungs may point to an aetiology for the respiratory symptoms. At least half of the patients with PCP have normal clinical respiratory examination findings (Table 13.4). In contrast, patients with bacterial pneumonia often have focal lung findings. Wheezing in an HIV-infected patient with a history of asthma indicates an exacerbation of that condition, whereas findings of decreased breath sounds in a patient who has a long history of cigarette use may indicate emphysema. In a patient with the sudden onset of pleuritic chest pain and/or shortness of breath, findings of absent breath sounds suggest a pneumothorax. Occasionally, abnormal findings on lung examination are the result of extrapulmonary disease. For example, rales in association with a cardiac gallop (specifically, a third heart sound noise) and elevated jugular venous pressure implies a cardiac aetiology for the respiratory symptoms.

The remainder of the physical examination may also indicate an aetiology for the respiratory symptoms since many of the opportunistic infections and neoplasms that affect the lung also cause extrapulmonary or disseminated disease. For example, headache or altered mental status in an HIV-infected patient with pulmonary disease whose CD4 lymphocyte count is less than 200 cells/μl suggests *C. neoformans* as the cause of both the neurological and pulmonary diseases. A patient with focal neurological findings and pulmonary disease may have *T. gondii* encephalitis and pneumonitis. Patients with new cutaneous lesions may have a disseminated fungal disease. Patients with cutaneous KS may have pulmonary disease; however, the absence of mucocutaneous disease does not exclude the possibility of pulmonary KS. In fact, we found that 15% of 168 consecutive HIV-infected patients diagnosed with pulmonary KS on bronchoscopy had no evidence of mucocutaneous disease at the time of bronchoscopy (Huang *et al.*, 1996). In these patients, pulmonary disease was the only manifestation of KS. Abdominal examination revealing hepatosplenomegaly can be found in either disseminated mycobacterial or fungal disease or NHL.

Laboratory tests

Laboratory tests may provide important clues to the diagnosis of respiratory complications; however, HIV-infect-ed patients often have a host of laboratory abnormalities that may be either non-specific or due to unrelated conditions. The clinician must be cautious before attributing a laboratory abnormality to a specific pulmonary disorder.

In general, laboratory tests that may be useful include complete blood count with white blood count and differential, serum lactate dehydrogenase (LDH) concentration, and arterial blood gas values. These tests serve as prognostic markers and as a baseline value for subsequent measurements. Serial measurements are useful in any patient who fails to exhibit a clinical response or who is worsening despite appropriate therapy.

White blood cell count (WBC). In persons with bacterial pneumonia, the WBC is frequently elevated relative to the patient's baseline value, and a left shift is commonly present as well (Table 13.4). HIV-infected patients with neutropenia are at higher risk for bacterial and certain fungal infections such as *Aspergillus*. Persons with PCP may have an elevated, normal, or even decreased WBC. In these patients, the WBC more frequently reflects the degree of the underlying immunosuppression, the use of bone marrow suppressive medications, and/or the presence of an infiltrative bone marrow process, rather than the presence of *P. carinii*.

Serum lactate dehydrogenase (LDH). The serum LDH is often elevated in patients with PCP (Table 13.4) (Kales *et al.*, 1987; Zaman and White, 1988; Garay and Greene, 1989). It may also be elevated in many other pulmonary (including bacterial pneumonia and TB) and non-pulmonary conditions, making this test more useful for prognosis than for diagnosis. As patients with PCP may also have a normal or a minimally elevated serum LDH level, a normal serum LDH does not rule out the possibility of PCP. Most of the published studies of serum LDH elevation in PCP consisted of hospitalized patients, some of whom had acute respiratory failure and were mechanically ventilated. The study that reported the lowest diagnostic sensitivity of an elevated serum LDH for PCP examined outpatients presenting to an urgent care clinic (Katz *et al.*, 1991). These results suggest that the severity of PCP and the patient population studied affect the diagnostic sensitivity of the test.

Despite its diagnostic limitations, the degree of elevation of the serum LDH has been shown to correlate with prognosis and response to therapy (Garay and Greene, 1989). Patients with PCP and an initial markedly elevated serum LDH or a rising serum LDH despite PCP treatment have a poor prognosis.

Table 13.5 Characteristic chest radiographic findings in selected HIV-associated respiratory complications listed in order of decreasing frequency (San Francisco General Hospital)

Normal
  Pneumocystis carinii
  Fungi (e.g. *C. neoformans* meningitis, disseminated *H. capsulatum*, *C. immitis*)
  Tuberculosis (extrapulmonary or disseminated)
  KS (only involving the trachea)
Focal infiltrate
  Bacteria
  Tuberculosis
  Fungi
  NHL
  Pneumocystis carinii
Multifocal or diffuse infiltrates
  Pneumocystis carinii
  Bacteria
  Tuberculosis
  Fungi
  KS
  NHL
  CMV
Reticular or granular pattern
  Pneumocystis carinii
  Cryptococcus neoformans
  Bacteria (*H. influenzae*)
  Tuberculosis
  Other fungi (*H. capsulatum*)
  CMV
  NHL
Consolidation pattern
  Bacteria
  Tuberculosis (low CD4 lymphocyte count)
  Cryptococcus neoformans
  NHL
  Pneumocystis carinii (uncommon unless severe, diffuse disease)
Miliary pattern
  Tuberculosis
  Fungi (*H. capsulatum*, *C. immitis*, *C. neoformans*)
  Pneumocystis carinii (uncommon)
Nodules or nodular pattern
  Tuberculosis
  Fungi (*C. neoformans*, *H. capsulatum*, *C. immitis*, *Aspergillus* species)
  KS
  NHL (nodules/masses)
  Bacteria
  Pneumocystis carinii (uncommon)
Cystic lesions
  Pneumocystis carinii
  Fungi (especially *C. neoformans* and *C. immitis*)
Cavitary lesions
  Tuberculosis (usually high CD4 lymphocyte count)
  Bacteria (especially *P. aeruginosa*, *S. aureus*, *R. equi*)
  Fungi (*Aspergillus* species, *C. neoformans*, *C. immitis*)

Table 13.5 Continued

  Mycobacterium kansasii
  Pneumocystis carinii (uncommon)
Pneumothorax
  Pneumocystis carinii
  Bacteria (uncommon)
  Tuberculosis (uncommon)
Intrathoracic lymphadenopathy
  Tuberculosis (usually low CD4 lymphocyte count)
  MAC
  Fungi (*C. neoformans*, *C. immitis*, *H. capsulatum*)
  KS
  NHL
Pleural effusions
  Bacteria
  Tuberculosis (all CD4 lymphocyte count ranges)
  Fungi (especially *C. neoformans*)
  KS
  NHL

KS: Kaposi's sarcoma; NHL: non-Hodgkin's lymphoma; CMV: cytomegalovirus; MAC: *Mycobacterium avium* complex.
The ranking in this table does not take CD4 lymphocyte counts or other clinical or demographic information into account.

Arterial blood gases. Arterial blood gases are frequently abnormal in patients with respiratory complications. Patients with acute lower respiratory disease typically have hypoxaemia, an increased alveolar–arterial oxygen difference, and hypocarbia with respiratory alkalosis. As these abnormalities are non-specific, they are more useful for prognosis than diagnosis.

Chest radiography The chest radiograph is the cornerstone of the evaluation of respiratory complications in HIV-infected patients. Because each of these complications has a characteristic radiographic presentation, the radiograph (combined with information from the history, physical examination, and selected laboratory tests) can narrow the diagnostic possibilities and suggest a diagnostic approach.

Characteristic chest radiographic findings for the most common HIV-associated respiratory complications are presented in Table 13.5. For each radiographic finding, the opportunistic infections and neoplasms are listed in order of decreasing frequency at our institution. The relative frequencies at other institutions may be different and altered by such factors as regional differences, a history of injecting drug use and other epidemiological factors, as discussed previously.

Patients often present with combinations of radiographic findings that can alter the differential diagnosis. For example, any severe opportunistic infection or neoplasm can cause diffuse pulmonary infiltrates. At our institution, PCP is the most common cause of diffuse radiographic disease. Pleural effusions are uncommon findings in PCP. As pleural effusions are usually caused by bacterial pneumonias, tuberculosis, fungal pathogens or pulmonary KS, patients with diffuse infiltrates and pleural effusions are more likely to have one of these diseases than PCP.

The patient's CD4 lymphocyte count should also be considered when evaluating the chest radiograph. For example, PCP is uncommon in HIV-infected patients with CD4 lymphocyte counts above 200 cells/μl, and virtually unheard of above 350 cell/μl. In patients with these near-normal CD4 lymphocyte counts, a chest radiograph with diffuse infiltrates may be more suggestive of a fulminant bacterial pneumonia than of PCP.

Presentations of common opportunistic infections

The characteristic chest radiographic presentations of the most common opportunistic infections – PCP and bacterial pneumonia – should be familiar to clinicians, because of their frequency. Given the implications of a missed or delayed diagnosis, clinicians should also be familiar with the two most characteristic radiographic presentations of TB. Finally, the presentation of the most common pulmonary neoplasm, pulmonary KS, should also be well known. The following is a brief summary of classic radiographic findings for these four pulmonary diseases.

Pneumocystis carinii pneumonia (PCP)

PCP classically presents with reticular or granular opacities (Figure 13.1) (DeLorenzo et al., 1987). In mild cases, the radiograph may be normal. Infiltrates due to PCP are characteristically bilateral and symmetrical. Occasionally, infiltrates are unilateral or asymmetric. In our experience, the pattern seen (reticular or granular) is more important than the distribution (bilateral/unilateral, symmetric/asymmetric, or diffuse/focal). All patients with reticular or granular opacities should undergo a diagnostic procedure for PCP.

In patients with milder disease, the radiographic findings may be limited to the perihilar region. As the disease progresses, the chest radiograph will progress from predominantly perihilar involvement to more diffuse involvement, and an alveolar or mixed reticular–alveolar pattern can result. Thin-walled, air-containing cysts or pneumatoceles are seen in approximately 15–20% of cases of PCP. The findings of either intrathoracic adenopathy or pleural effusions are rarely due to PCP. In a patient with documented PCP, these radiographic findings usually represent a concurrent process.

In patients with clinically suspected PCP who have a normal chest radiograph, high-resolution CT scanning of the chest is useful, and it will usually show patchy areas of ground glass opacities. These opacities are sensitive, but not specific for PCP, and thus further specific diagnostic tests for PCP should be performed. Gruden et al. (1997) reported that all six patients with PCP in a small series had typical opacities on high-resolution CT scanning,

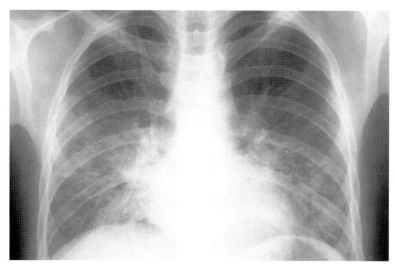

Figure 13.1 *Frontal chest radiograph of an HIV-infected patient with* Pneumocystis carinii *pneumonia (PCP). The bilateral, predominantly perihilar granular opacities are characteristic of PCP (with permission from L. Huang).*

and the specificity of the test was 89% (Gruden *et al.*, 1997). The negative predictive value was 100% in a series of 40 patients (Gruden *et al.*, 1997). Thus, high-resolution CT scanning of the chest can be a useful test to rule out or at least make unlikely the diagnosis of PCP, but it cannot be used to diagnose this disease. Other tests that have been used to evaluate patients with clinically suspected PCP who have a normal chest radiograph include exercise oximetry, measurement of the diffusing capacity for carbon monoxide, and a variety of nuclear medicine studies.

Bacterial pneumonia

Bacterial pneumonia due to *S. pneumoniae* typically presents with a patchy or focal, consolidation in a segmental or lobar distribution. Often, there is an associated pleural effusion. This presentation is similar to pneumococcal pneumonia in an HIV-negative person. Occasionally, the radiographic presentation is indistinguishable from other opportunistic infections (Magnenat *et al.*, 1991). In severe cases of pneumonia, the findings may be multifocal or diffuse.

Patients with a chest radiograph consistent with bacterial pneumonia should have sputum and blood cultures sent for microbiological analysis. Thoracentesis should also be considered for patients with pleural effusions, especially if the effusion is large or there is concern for possible empyema. Bacterial pneumonia due to *H. influenzae* may be indistinguishable from *S. pneumoniae*, but it has also been reported to present with diffuse infiltrates similar to PCP (Polsky *et al.*, 1986). In patients with advanced immunosuppression, pneumonias due to *P. aeruginosa* and *S. aureus* increase in frequency and may present with cavitary infiltrates (Burack *et al.*, 1994).

Tuberculosis

Tuberculosis has a number of different radiographic findings and presentations (Pitchenik and Rubinson, 1985; Sunderam *et al.*, 1986; Chaisson *et al.*, 1987; Jones *et al.*, 1993). The characteristic presentation depends to a large extent on the degree of immunosuppression. In early HIV disease, when the CD4 lymphocyte count is relatively high, tuberculosis presents with the well-known pattern of reactivation disease, namely upper lung zone infiltrates (apical and posterior segments of the upper lobes and superior segment of the lower lobes), often with cavities (Figure 13.2).

In contrast, cavities are a less common presentation of tuberculosis in advanced HIV disease. These patients are more likely to present with either diffuse radiographic

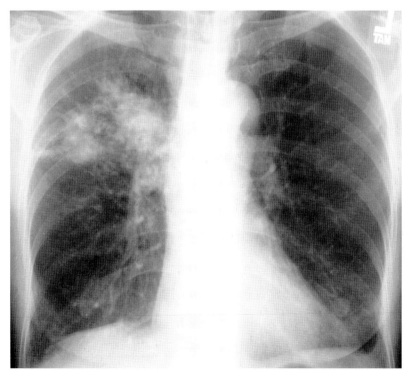

Figure 13.2 *Frontal chest radiograph of an HIV-infected patient with tuberculosis. The unilateral right upper lobe infiltrate is typical for tuberculosis in patients with high CD4 lymphocyte counts (with permission from L. Huang).*

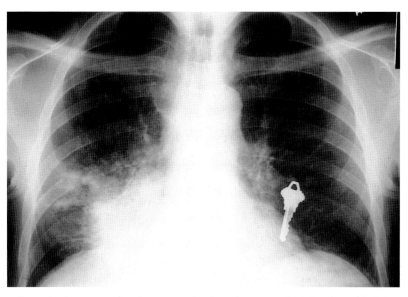

Figure 13.3 *Frontal chest radiograph of an HIV-infected patient with tuberculosis. A unilateral right middle lobe infiltrate is present, typical of tuberculosis in patients with CD4 lymphocyte count of less than 50 cells/μl. This patient was ultimately diagnosed with mono-rifampin resistant tuberculosis by sputum mycobacterial culture. The key shown was in the patient's shirt pocket when the radiograph was taken (with permission from L. Huang).*

disease or with predominantly middle and lower lung zone infiltrates that may be mistaken for a bacterial pneumonia (Figure 13.3). In the case illustrated in Figure 13.3, the key to the diagnosis of tuberculosis was knowledge of the patient's CD4 lymphocyte count and realization that this pattern was consistent with tuberculosis in a patient with a low CD4 lymphocyte count. Pleural effusions can be seen with TB at both high and low CD4 lymphocyte counts, but intrathoracic adenopathy is seen much more commonly in patients with low CD4 lymphocyte counts (see also Chapter 23).

Patients with clinically suspected tuberculosis and a consistent radiographic presentation should have three examinations and cultures of sputum for acid-fast organisms, as well as blood cultures for mycobacteria. Occasionally, more invasive diagnostic procedures such as bronchoscopy with bronchoalveolar lavage and transbronchial biopsies or mediastinoscopy with biopsy, are necessary. Thoracentesis with pleural biopsy should be considered for patients with pleural effusions. Tuberculosis may also present predominantly with extrapulmonary disease, especially in patients with low CD4 lymphocyte counts. Careful physical examination may reveal peripheral lymph nodes amenable to biopsy. Laboratory evidence of an infiltrative bone marrow disease should prompt bone marrow biopsy. In these patients, the absence of parenchymal disease on chest radiograph should not preclude obtaining

sputum specimens, as a number of these patients will have positive sputum cultures and even positive acid-fast smear examinations.

Pulmonary Kaposi's sarcoma (KS)

Pulmonary KS characteristically presents with bilateral opacities in a central or perihilar distribution (Figure 13.4). Gruden and colleagues reviewed the chest radiographic presentation of 76 consecutive patients with pulmonary KS diagnosed by bronchoscopy (Gruden *et al.*, 1995). All the patients had a bronchoalveolar lavage that was negative for infectious organisms. In this study, 95% of the chest radiographs had peribronchial cuffing and 'tram track' opacities with or without more extensive perihilar coalescent opacities. Small nodules or nodular opacities were seen in 78%, Kerley B lines in 71%, and pleural effusions in 53% of the radiographs. Of note, no patient presented with either Kerley B lines or pleural effusions without concurrent parenchymal findings. Sixteen per cent of these patients had hilar or mediastinal lymph node enlargement. Patients with these radiographic findings (especially if there is a history of male-to-male sexual encounters) should undergo bronchoscopy as part of the evaluation. Visualization of the characteristic tracheobronchial KS lesions will confirm the diagnosis, and bronchoalveolar lavage will serve to exclude a concurrent opportunistic infection.

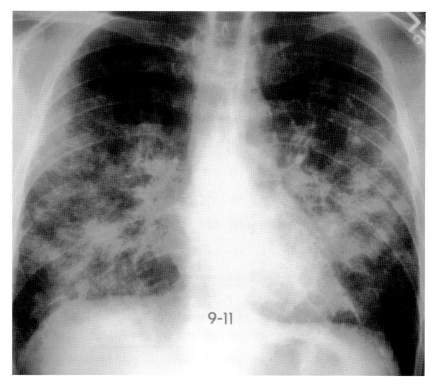

Figure 13.4 *Frontal chest radiograph of an HIV-infected man with pulmonary Kaposi's sarcoma (KS). Kerley B line and bilateral, predominantly middle and lower lung zone abnormalities with nodular opacities are typical of KS (with permission L. Huang).*

The risk of lung cancer appears to be increased in patients with HIV infection, and survival was short (Ricaurte *et al.*, 2001).

Critical care

HIV-infected patients may require critical care for a number of reasons. Acute respiratory failure accounts for 50–75% of intensive care unit (ICU) admissions in studies of the critical care of HIV-infected patients (Schein *et al.*, 1986; Wachter *et al.*, 1986; Smith *et al.*, 1989; Rogers *et al.*, 1989; Wachter *et al.*, 1992; De Palo *et al.*, 1995; Lazard *et al.*, 1996). PCP is present in 55–90% of these patients (Schein *et al.*, 1986; Wachter *et al.*, 1986; Rogers *et al.*, 1989; Smith *et al.*, 1989; Wachter *et al.*, 1992; De Palo *et al.*, 1995; Lazard *et al.*, 1996;). Patients with other HIV-associated infections or with HIV-associated neoplasms are also at risk of developing respiratory failure. Other frequent causes of ICU admissions include central nervous system (CNS) dysfunction (approximately 10–15%) and sepsis (approximately 10%). Finally, a number of HIV-infected patients, particulary those on HAART, are admitted to an ICU for reasons unrelated to their HIV infection (e.g. asthma or COPD, cardiac disease, GI bleed, drug overdose, trauma or following invasive procedures or surgery).

Respiratory complications of AIDS in the ICU

The management of patients with HIV-associated respiratory complications in the ICU is similar to the management of any patient requiring intensive care (Leifeld *et al.*, 2000). Special considerations in HIV-infected patients include evaluation for HIV-associated opportunistic infections (especially PCP) and careful attention to pharmacological interactions between the patient's HIV-related medications and those prescribed for critical care.

Non-invasive ventilatory support

HIV-infected patients with acute respiratory failure may occasionally be managed by non-invasive means. Continuous positive airway pressure (CPAP) delivered by a tight-fitting mask has been successful in improving arterial oxygenation in patients with PCP-associated acute respiratory failure (Gregg *et al.*, 1990). Unfortunately, patients with PCP have increased work in breathing and many (perhaps most) patients with moderate to severe PCP who begin CPAP therapy will eventually require intubation and mechanical ventilation. Nevertheless, CPAP therapy may be considered in carefully selected patients. First, all patients treated with CPAP should be awake, cooperative, and fully able to protect their airway. They should also be stable haemodynamically and must be closely observed in a monitored setting in case further respiratory deterioration should occur. Three groups of patients seem to benefit the most from CPAP therapy: patients with acute and presumably short-lived respiratory deterioration following bronchoscopy, recently extubated patients who require a temporary 'bridge' until further lung recovery occurs, and patients who request no intubation but otherwise wish full supportive care (Gregg et al., 1990). In these cases, a trial of CPAP may spare the patient intubation/re-intubation or may be life-saving.

Invasive ventilatory support – mechanical ventilation

Most HIV-infected patients with severe, acute respiratory failure require invasive ventilatory support (intubation and mechanical ventilation). For patients requiring mechanical ventilation, assist control or intermittent mandatory ventilation (IMV) modes are usually the initial modes of ventilation. Occasionally, a pressure control ventilation mode is needed. Positive end-expiratory pressure (PEEP) will often increase oxygenation (Wachter et al., 1992). Careful attention must be paid to the development of barotrauma and possible pneumothorax. Pneumothorax in patients with PCP-associated acute respiratory failure who are on mechanical ventilation is an extremely poor prognostic sign. In addition to the severe respiratory dysfunction caused by the PCP, these patients develop bronchopleural or bronchopleural-cutaneous fistulas that rarely heal while on positive pressure (and on the high-dose corticosteroids that are used as an adjunct to PCP therapy). In our experience, only a small proportion of these patients (less than 5%) will recover.

In terms of ventilator-associated complications, the rate of secondarily acquired nosocomial pneumonias in intubated HIV-infected patients with PCP appears to be less than that of intubated non-HIV-infected patients without PCP. One possible explanation is the incidental antibacterial activity of trimethoprim-sulfamethoxazole (TMP-SMX) (Peruzzi et al., 1990).

Pneumocystis carinii pneumonia (PCP)

PCP accounts for the majority of HIV-associated ICU admissions. Over the span of the AIDS epidemic, there has been a dramatic reduction in PCP-associated respiratory

failure and death. Survival rates may continue to fluctuate over the next decade as incidence, management, and demographics of the population at risk change. Current reported survival rates for PCP-associated acute respiratory failure are within the range of survival for acute respiratory failure in non-HIV-infected patients.

AIDS patients with PCP who are admitted to hospitals with low familiarity with HIV disease (as determined by total admissions for AIDS patients) may have a worse outcome than those patients who are admitted to hospitals experienced at managing HIV-infected patients (Bennett et al., 1989; Stone et al., 1992; Curtis et al., 1998). The PCP mortality in low familiarity hospitals was twice that in the experienced hospitals. Although average patient charges were the same for the two types of hospitals, the hospitals with high familiarity tended to spend more money, including more for bronchoscopy, on survivors. The hospitals with low familiarity tended to spend more money on non-survivors (Curtis et al., 1998; Bennett et al., 1989; Stone et al., 1992).

APACHE (Acute Physiology and Chronic Health Evaluation) II scores have been evaluated as predictors of outcome in PCP-associated acute respiratory failure. The APACHE II classification, based on observed mortalities in more than 5000 critically ill patients, was validated between 1979 and 1982, before the explosion of the AIDS epidemic (Knaus et al., 1985). In a 1989 study of HIV-infected patients with PCP-associated acute respiratory failure, APACHE II scores predicted a mortality of 44%; the actual mortality was 86% (Smith et al., 1989). In a study from the early 1990s of HIV-infected patients with acute respiratory failure, mean APACHE II scores for survivors were only slightly better than for non-survivors (Chu, 1993). Brown and Crede, in data accumulated from 1986 to 1991, found that the APACHE II scoring system significantly underestimated ICU mortality from all causes in severely immunosuppressed (CD4 lymphocyte count less than 200 cells/μl) HIV-infected patients (Brown and Crede, 1995). For less severely immunosuppressed HIV-infected patients, the APACHE II scores were predictive of estimated mortality (Brown and Crede, 1995). Recent data has found better correlation of the APACHE II score with actual mortality, particularly if the serum LDH level is included in the evaluation (Forrest et al., 1998).

Other causes of acute respiratory failure in HIV disease

Pneumonias secondary to bacteria, mycobacteria, fungi, CMV, and T. gondii have all been associated with acute respiratory failure in HIV-infected patients. The risk and predictors of acute respiratory failure for these pathogens are unknown (Stover et al., 1985; Schein et al., 1986; Rogers et al., 1989; Wachter et al., 1992; De Palo et al., 1995; Lazard et al., 1996). KS, NHL, and lymphocytic interstitial pneumonia (LIP) have also been reported as occasional causes of acute respiratory failure (Stover et al., 1985; Schein et al., 1986; Rogers et al., 1989; Wachter et al., 1992; De Palo et al., 1995; Lazard et al., 1996). Acute respiratory failure unrelated to HIV disease, such as accompanies an exacerbation of asthma or COPD, congestive heart failure, drug overdose, or trauma, accounts for a small proportion of patients in most case series (Wachter et al., 1986; Rogers et al., 1989; Smith et al., 1989; Wachter et al., 1992; De Palo et al., 1995; Lazard et al., 1996).

Women and the ICU

In a study of more than 3000 HIV-infected patients in New York City hospitals presenting with their first episode of PCP, women were less likely to undergo bronchoscopy (55.7% versus 61.2%, $p = 0.02$), but were more likely to be intubated for acute respiratory failure (13.6% versus 9.9%, $p = 0.01$) (Bastian et al., 1993). The mortality rate for women who required ICU care was 84%, compared to 57% for men (p-value = 0.05).

Infants and children and the ICU

Acute respiratory failure due to PCP is the primary reason for admission of infants to an ICU (Notterman, 1993). Infants with PCP who require mechanical ventilation have a very poor outcome. In one study, less than 20% of patients survived beyond 5 weeks, and only 8% survived beyond 1 year (Notterman, 1993). As noted in the adult population, data from the early 1990s have suggested some improvement in survival of infants with acute respiratory failure due to PCP (Notterman, 1993).

For children beyond infancy, PCP remains the primary reason for ICU admission, although the incidence of bacterial sepsis and systemic mycobacterial and fungal infections increases. The incidence of gastrointestinal (GI) bleeding and pancytopenia are also increased (Notterman, 1993). LIP is a common manifestation of HIV disease in children, which generally produces a slowly progressive pulmonary syndrome and rarely precipitates acute respiratory failure (Marolda et al., 1989). Adolescents seem to be similar to adults in admission patterns to ICUs (Marolda et al., 1989).

Advance directives and durable power of attorney

Decisions with regard to ICU care of HIV-infected patients, similar to all other ICU admissions, involve estimation of short-term prognosis and goals, risks and benefits, and patient wishes for life-sustaining treatment. In a study by Steinbrook and colleagues (1986), about 75% of HIV-infected patients wanted to discuss life-sustaining treatment with their physicians and thought that the most appropriate time to discuss these issues of future care was in the outpatient setting (Steinbrook et al., 1986). Only one-third of the surveyed persons in this outpatient AIDS clinic had ever had such a discussion with their physicians. Patients who had been hospitalized within the past year were more likely to have a living will than those never hospitalized and were more likely to have discussed life-sustaining treatments, at least with family members and partners.

A fundamental part of a patient's right to autonomy includes the right of a competent and informed patient to refuse care in terminal as well as non-terminal diseases. An advanced directive is the expression of a patient's preferences about future medical care, including life-sustaining measures. The advanced directive is made while the patient possesses decision-making capacity (Wachter and Lo, 1993). Generally, advance directives take the form of either a living will detailing the patient's preferences or a durable power of attorney (DPOA), designating some trusted person with decision-making authority for medical decisions. Because living wills, as a written instrument, may not address all of the medical scenarios encountered, a DPOA may provide more flexibility for the patient (Wachter and Lo, 1993). Additionally, a person holding the DPOA, by using his or her perception of the patient's wishes, can include new relevant medical advances in weighing decisions. Patients should be encouraged to discuss such issues with the person designated to hold their DPOA, as well as with their primary care physician before some medical situations common to AIDS, such as PCP-associated acute respiratory failure or AIDS dementia, limit their decision-making capacity.

Conclusion

Respiratory complications of HIV infection are quite common, especially as the CD4 count declines. Accurate diagnosis of respiratory disease requires integration of information from the history and physical, laboratory data, and the chest radiograph. Because of the diversity of findings in HIV-associated respiratory illnesses, no disease has a single pathognomonic presentation. Therefore, empirical therapy should be avoided and definitive diagnosis pursued whenever possible. The clinician should be aware of the typical presentations of the most common respiratory diseases and focus the diagnostic evaluation appropriately. Once respiratory disease has progressed to the point of respiratory failure, survival is now similar to that for non-HIV-associated conditions. Issues concerning end-of-life care should be addressed early by the physician and the patient, ideally in the outpatient setting.

References

Afessa B, Green W, Chiao J et al. (1998). Pulmonary complications of HIV infection: autopsy findings. Chest 113: 1225–9.

Bastian L, Bennett CL, Adams J et al. (1993). Differences between men and women with HIV-related Pneumocystis carinii pneumonia: Experience from 3070 cases in New York City in 1987. J Acquir Immune Defic Syndr Hum Retrovirol 6: 617–23.

Bennett CL, Garfinkle JB, Greenfield S et al. (1989). The relation between hospital experience and in-hospital mortality for patients with AIDS-related PCP. JAMA 261: 2975–9.

Brown MC, Crede WB. (1995). Predictive ability of acute physiology and chronic health evaluation II scoring applied to human immunodeficiency virus-positive patients. Crit Care Med 23: 848–53.

Burack JH, Hahn JA, Saint-Maurice D et al. (1994). Microbiology of community-acquired bacterial pneumonia in persons with and at risk for human immunodeficiency virus type 1 infection. Implications for rational empiric antibiotic therapy. Arch Intern Med 154: 2589–96.

Centers for Disease Control and Prevention (CDC). (1993). Revised classification system for HIV infection and expanded case definition for AIDS among adolescents and adults. JAMA 269: 729–39.

CDC. (1997). USPHS/IDSA guidelines for the prevention of opportunistic infections in persons infected with human immunodeficiency virus. MMWR 46: 1–48.

Chaisson RE, Schecter GF, Theuer CP et al. (1987). Tuberculosis in patients with the acquired immunodeficiency syndrome. Clinical features, response to therapy, and survival. Am Rev Respir Dis 136: 570–4.

Chu DY. (1993). Predicting survival in AIDS patients with respiratory failure. Application of the APACHE II scoring system. Crit Care Clin 9: 89–105.

Curtis JR, Bennett CL, Horner RD et al. (1998). Variations in intensive care unit utilization for patients with human immunodeficiency virus-related Pneumocystis carinii pneumonia: importance of hospital characteristics and geographical location. Crit Care Med 26: 668–75.

DeLorenzo LJ, Huang CT, Maguire GP et al. (1987). Roentgenographic patterns of Pneumocystis carinii pneumonia in 104 patients with AIDS. Chest 91: 323–7.

De Palo VA, Millstein BH, Mayo PH et al. (1995). Outcome of intensive care in patients with HIV infection. Chest 107: 506–10.

Forrest DM, Djurdev O, Zala C et al. (1998). Validation of the modified multisystem organ failure score as a predictor of mortality in patients with AIDS-related Pneumocystis carinii pneumonia and respiratory failure. Chest 114: 199–206.

Furrer H, Egger M, Opravil M et al. (1999). Discontinuation of primary prophylaxis against Pneumocystis carinii pneumonia in HIV-1-infected adults treated with combination antiretroviral therapy. Swiss HIV Cohort Study. N Engl J Med 340: 1301–6.

Garay SM, Greene J. (1989). Prognostic indicators in the initial presentation of Pneumocystis carinii pneumonia. Chest 95: 769–72.

Gregg RW, Friedman BC, Williams JF et al. (1990). Continuous positive airway pressure by face mask in Pneumocystis carinii pneumonia. Crit Care Med 18: 21–4.

Gruden JF, Huang L, Webb WR et al. (1995). AIDS-related Kaposi sarcoma of the lung: radiographic findings and staging system with bronchoscopic correlation. Radiology 195: 545–52.

Gruden JF, Huang L, Turner J et al. (1997). High-resolution CT in the evaluation of clinically suspected Pneumocystis carinii pneumonia in AIDS patients with normal, equivocal, or nonspecific radiographic findings. Am J Roentgenol 169: 967–75.

Hanson DL, Chu SY, Farizo KM et al. (1995). Distribution of CD4+ T lymphocytes at diagnosis of acquired immunodeficiency syndrome-defining and other human immunodeficiency virus-related illnesses. The Adult and Adolescent Spectrum of HIV Disease Project Group. Arch Intern Med 155: 1537–42.

Hirschtick RE, Glassroth J, Jordan MC et al. (1995). Bacterial pneumonia in persons infected with the human immunodeficiency virus. Pulmonary Complications of HIV Infection Study Group. N Engl J Med 333: 845–51.

Huang L, Stansell JD. (1996). AIDS and the lung. Med Clin N Am 80: 775–801.

Huang L, Schnapp LM, Gruden JF et al. (1996). Presentation of AIDS-related pulmonary Kaposi's sarcoma diagnosed by bronchoscopy. Am J Respir Crit Care Med 153: 1385–90.

Johnson CC, Wilcosky T, Kvale P et al. (1997). Cancer incidence among an HIV-infected cohort. Pulmonary Complications of HIV Infection Study Group. Am J Epidemiol 146: 470–5.

Jones BE, Young SM, Antoniskis D et al. (1993). Relationship of the manifestations of tuberculosis to CD4 cell counts in patients with human immunodeficiency virus infection. Am Rev Respir Dis 148: 1292–7.

Kales CP, Murren JR, Torres RA et al. (1987). Early predictors of in-hospital mortality for Pneumocystis carinii pneumonia in the acquired immunodeficiency syndrome. Arch Intern Med 147: 1413–17.

Katz MH, Baron RB, Grady D. (1991). Risk stratification of ambulatory patients suspected of Pneumocystis pneumonia. Arch Intern Med 151: 105–10.

Knaus WA, Draper EA, Wagner DP et al. (1985). APACHE II: a severity of disease classification system. Crit Care Med 13: 818–29.

Kovacs JA, Hiemenz JW, Macher AM et al. (1984). Pneumocystis carinii pneumonia: a comparison between patients with the acquired immunodeficiency syndrome and patients with other immunodeficiencies. Ann Intern Med 100: 663–71.

Kovacs JA, Masur H (2000). Prophylaxis against opportunistic infections in patients with human immunodeficiency virus infection. N Engl J Med 342: 1416–29.

Lazard T, Retel O, Guidet B et al. (1996). AIDS in a medical intensive care unit: immediate prognosis and long-term survival. JAMA 276: 1240–5.

Magnenat JL, Nicod LP, Auckenthaler R et al. (1991). Mode of presentation and diagnosis of bacterial pneumonia in human immunodeficiency virus-infected patients. Am Rev Respir Dis 144: 917–22.

Markowitz N, Hansen NI, Hopewell PC *et al.* (1997). Incidence of tuberculosis in the United States among HIV-infected persons. The Pulmonary Complications of HIV Infection Study Group. *Ann Intern Med* **126**: 123–32.

Marolda J, Pace B, Bonforte RJ *et al.* (1989). Outcome of mechanical ventilation in children with acquired immunodeficiency syndrome. *Pediatr Pulmonol* **7**: 230–4.

Miller V, Mocroft A, Reiss P *et al.* (1999). Relations among CD4 lymphocyte count nadir, antiretroviral therapy, and HIV-1 disease progression: results from the EuroSIDA study. *Ann Intern Med* **130**: 570–7.

Notterman DA. (1993). Pediatric AIDS and critical care. *Crit Care Med* **21**: S319–21.

Peruzzi WT, Shapiro BA, Noskin GA *et al.* (1990). Concurrent bacterial lung infection in patients with AIDS, PCP, and respiratory failure. *Chest* **18**: 21–4.

Pitchenik AE, Rubinson HA. (1985). The radiographic appearance of tuberculosis in patients with the acquired immune deficiency syndrome (AIDS) and pre-AIDS. *Am Rev Respir Dis* **131**: 393–6.

Polsky B, Gold JW, Whimbey E *et al.* (1986). Bacterial pneumonia in patients with the acquired immunodeficiency syndrome. *Ann Intern Med* **104**: 38–41.

Pulmonary Complications of HIV Infection Study Group. (1993). Design of a prospective study of the pulmonary complications of human immunodeficiency virus infection. *J Clin Epidemiol* **46**: 497–507.

Ricuarte JC, Hoerman MF, Nord JA, Tietjen PA. (2001). Lung cancer in HIV-infected patients: a one-year experience. *Int & STD AIDS* **12**: 100–2.

Rogers PL, Lane HC, Henderson DK *et al.* (1989). Admission of AIDS patients to a medical intensive care unit: Causes and outcome. *Crit Care Med* **17**: 113–17.

Rosen MJ, Clayton K, Schneider RF *et al.* (1997). Intensive care of patients with HIV infection: utilization, critical illnesses, and outcomes. Pulmonary Complications of HIV Infection Study Group. *Am J Respir Crit Care Med* **155**: 67–71.

Schein RM, Fischl MA, Pitchenik AE *et al.* (1986). ICU survival of patients with the acquired immunodeficiency syndrome. *Crit Care Med* **14**: 1026–7.

Selwyn PA, Sckell BM, Alcabes P *et al.* (1992). High risk of active tuberculosis in HIV-infected drug users with cutaneous anergy. *JAMA* **268**: 504–9.

Smith RL, Levine SM, Lewis ML. (1989). Prognosis of patients with AIDS requiring intensive care. *Chest* **96**: 857–861.

Steinbrook R, Lo B, Moulton J *et al.* (1986). Preferences of homosexual men with AIDS for life-sustaining treatment. *N Engl J Med* **314**: 457–60.

Stone VE, Seage GD, Hertz T *et al.* (1992). The relation between hospital experience and mortality for patients with AIDS. *JAMA* **268**: 2655–61.

Stover DE, White DA, Romano PA *et al.* (1985). Spectrum of pulmonary diseases associated with the acquired immune deficiency syndrome. *Am J Med* **78**: 429–37.

Stover DE, Greeno RA, Gagliardi AJ. (1989). The use of a simple exercise test for the diagnosis of *Pneumocystis carinii* pneumonia in patients with AIDS. *Am Rev Respir Dis* **139**: 1343–6.

Sunderam G, McDonald RJ, Maniatis T *et al.* (1986). Tuberculosis as a manifestation of the acquired immunodeficiency syndrome (AIDS). *JAMA* **256**: 362–6.

Wachter RM, Lo B. (1993). Advance directives for patients with human immunodeficiency virus infection. *Crit Care Clin* **9**: 125–36.

Wachter RM, Luce JM, Turner J *et al.* (1986). Intensive care of patients with the acquired immunodeficiency syndrome. Outcome and changing patterns of utilization. *Am Rev Respir Dis* **134**: 891–6.

Wachter RM, Luce JM, Hopewell PC. (1992). Critical care of patients with AIDS. *JAMA* **267**: 541–7.

Wallace JM, Rao AV, Glassroth J *et al.* (1993). Respiratory illness in persons with human immunodeficiency virus infection. The Pulmonary Complications of HIV Infection Study Group. *Am Rev Respir Dis* **148**: 1523–9.

Wallace JM, Hansen NI, Lavange L *et al.* (1997). Respiratory disease trends in the Pulmonary Complications of HIV infection study cohort. Pulmonary Complications of HIV Infection Study Group. *Am J Respir Crit Care Med* **155**: 72–80.

Weverling GJ, Mocroft, Ledergerber B *et al.* (1999). Discontinuation of *Pneumocystis carinii* pneumonia prophylaxis after start of highly active antiretroviral therapy in HIV-1 infection. EuroSIDA Study Group. *Lancet* **353**: 1293–8.

Zaman MK, White DA. (1988). Serum lactate dehydrogenase levels and *Pneumocystis carinii* pneumonia. Diagnostic and prognostic significance. *Am Rev Respir Dis* **137**: 796–800.

BRIAN KAYE

The clinical manifestations of HIV infection are myriad. Musculoskeletal problems plague up to 72% of HIV-infected persons (Berman *et al.*, 1988). Rheumatological complications can occur at any time during the course of HIV disease, and rheumatological conditions such as Reiter's syndrome, psoriatic arthritis, polymyositis, and necrotizing vasculitis may sometimes be the first clinical clue to the presence of HIV infection (Kaye, 1996; Casado, 2001). Non-specific arthralgias and myalgias are also common features of primary HIV infection. The rate of development of rheumatological manifestations of HIV infection is not affected by the use of antiretroviral therapy (Berman *et al.*, 1997). Rheumatological manifestations of HIV infection are much less common in children than in adults (Schuval *et al.*, 1993; Lopez-Longo *et al.*, 1994).

This chapter will focus on the rheumatological manifestations of HIV infection including arthritis, myopathies, vasculitis, sicca syndrome, and other auto-immune phenomena. Although some of these features, such as necrotizing vasculitis, can be life-threatening, others, such as severe arthritis or polymyositis, may greatly impair the quality of the patient's life. Furthermore, drugs such as methotrexate, azathioprine, and cyclophosphamide, which are commonly used to treat rheumatological conditions, may in fact hasten the development of opportunistic infections in HIV-infected persons. Consequently, one must be especially vigilant in managing these conditions.

Arthritis

Reiter's syndrome and reactive arthritis
Epidemiology
Reiter's syndrome and other spondyloarthropathies are probably the most common types of arthritis to affect HIV-infected individuals (Table 14.1). In careful studies of consecutive unselected HIV-infected patients performed in Tampa, Florida, New York City, Cleveland, Buenos Aires, and Toronto, the prevalence of Reiter's syndrome has been estimated at 2–10% (Espinoza *et al.*, 1992). However, large-scale epidemiological studies performed by questionnaire in San Francisco, Baltimore and Cincinnati have indicated a prevalence of Reiter's syndrome of 0.1–0.5%, figures similar to those found in the general population (Clark *et al.*, 1992; Solinger and Hess, 1993).

Clinical features
Reiter's syndrome in HIV-infected persons has similar clinical manifestations to idiopathic Reiter's syndrome (Kaye, 1996; Winchester *et al.*, 1987). Patients tend to have a severe persistent oligoarthritis, primarily affecting the large joints of the lower extremities. Enthesopathies of the Achilles' tendon, plantar fascia, and anterior and posterior tibial tendons are common and can be quite severe. These enthesopathies, combined with multidigit dactylitis of the toes, may prevent weight bearing or cause the patients to walk with a characteristic gait with the feet in inversion and extension in an attempt to distribute weight on the lateral margins of the feet. This gait has been termed the 'AIDS gait' (Brancato *et al.*, 1989). A few HIV-infected patients with Reiter's syndrome have been reported to have sacroiliitis, although the majority do not (Winchester *et al.*, 1987; Keat and Rowe, 1991). Urethritis has been found in 59% of HIV-infected persons with Reiter's syndrome, conjunctivitis in 47%, keratodermia blennorrhagicum in 25%, and circinate balanitis in 29% (Kaye, 1996). Oral ulcers have also been noted (Kaye, 1996).

The signs and symptoms of Reiter's syndrome have occurred before or simultaneous with the onset of clinical immunodeficiency in about two-thirds of patients with HIV infection (Kaye, 1996). Thus, the presence of Reiter's syndrome may be a clinical clue to the diagnosis of HIV infection in some persons. Consequently, patients presenting to

Table 14.1 Arthropathies associated with HIV infection

Disease	Relative prevalence	Helpful clinical features	Supportive diagnostic studies
Reiter's syndrome	2–10%	Oligoarthritis, mucocutaneous involvement, conjunctivitis, enthesitis, urethritis	HLA-B27; sacroiliitis on X-ray film
Psoriatic arthritis	2–6%	DIP arthritis, onycholysis, psoriasis	Pencil-in-cup deformities on DIP X-ray film
Undifferentiated spondyloarthropathy	Less common	Enthesitis, oligoarthritis	HLA-B27; sacroiliitis on X-ray film
HIV-associated arthritis	Rare	Extreme pain for 1–4 weeks; arthritis for 6 weeks–6 months	Non-inflammatory synovial fluid; HLA-B27, RF, ANA all negative
Septic arthritis	Common	Acute monarthritis	Synovial fluid culture and Gram stain
Fungal or myco-bacterial arthritis	Less common	Subacute or chronic monarthritis	Synovial biopsy and culture
Still's disease	Rare	Rash, spiking fevers, hepatosplenomegaly	None
Painful articular syndrome	Less common	Acute severe pain in one joint lasting < 24 h; normal joint examination	Normal X-ray films and laboratory tests
Rifabutin-induced arthralgias/arthritis	90% on doses > 1050 mg/day of rifabutin	Symmetric polyarthralgias and polyarthritis; uveitis; aphthous stomatitis	None
Arthralgias	30–40%	Non-specific arthralgias; may be part of primary HIV infection	None
Aseptic necrosis	Rare	Severe, sudden pain in knee or hip	MRI, bone scan
Hypertrophic osteoarthropathy	Rare	Associated PCP; digital clubbing	CXR, bone X-rays, bone scan
Dupuytren's contracture	6–30%	Contractures of flexor tendons of hand	None

DIP: distal interphalangeal joints; RF: rheumatoid factor; ANA: antinuclear antibodies; MRI: magnetic resonance imaging; CXR: chest X-ray; PCP: *Pneumocystis carinii* pneumonia.

a physician with Reiter's syndrome or reactive arthritis should be questioned about HIV risk factors.

Seventy-three per cent of HIV-infected persons with Reiter's syndrome from North America are HLA-B27 positive, a proportion similar to that found in patients with idiopathic Reiter's syndrome (Kaye, 1996). In contrast, HLA-B27 was not detected in any of 13 black African patients with Reiter's syndrome and HIV infection (Davis *et al.*, 1989), possibly reflecting either the low prevalence of HLA-B27 in blacks in general and in black patients with Reiter's syndrome in particular, or different causative agents or mechanisms in African patients (Kaye, 1996).

Some patients with a Reiter's-like arthritis lack urethritis and conjunctivitis and thus are more properly classified as having 'reactive arthritis'. The articular manifestations and triggering organisms found in patients with reactive arthritis are similar to those in Reiter's syndrome. Reiter's syndrome is in fact a part of the reactive arthritis spectrum (Khan and van der Linden, 1990). Clinical features that tend to differentiate reactive arthritis, including Reiter's syndrome, from other types of arthritis include oligoarticular involvement of the lower extremities, enthesopathies, antecedent diarrhoea or urethritis illnesses, and the presence of HLA-B27.

Aetiology

Although organisms known to trigger Reiter's syndrome or reactive arthritis, such as *Salmonella*, *Shigella*, *Campylobacter*, *Ureaplasma urealyticum*, and *Yersinia* species, have been found in less than one-third of HIV-infected patients with reactive arthritis, many HIV-infected persons with Reiter's syndrome and reactive arthritis have an antecedent culture-negative diarrhoeal illness (Winchester *et al.*, 1987; Brancato *et al.*, 1989; Keat and Rowe, 1991; Kaye, 1996).

The relationship between Reiter's syndrome, reactive arthritis, and HIV infection suggests a biological association, although the actual connection is unknown and subject to speculation. It is certainly possible that a coincident infection by sexually transmitted agents such as *Chlamydia trachomatis* or *U. urealyticum*, together with HIV, could cause both Reiter's syndrome and HIV infection (Winchester *et al.*, 1987; Kaye, 1996).

It is possible that either the HIV-induced immunodeficiency itself or the increase in CD8 lymphocytes associated with HIV infection can help to initiate aberrant immune responses that lead to Reiter's syndrome or reactive arthritis. Alternatively, immunodeficiency due to HIV infection may predispose to the acquisition of arthritogenic organisms. Furthermore, a novel enteric pathogen that can trigger the onset of Reiter's syndrome or reactive arthritis may be more prevalent in HIV-infected patients with diarrhoea than in other patients. Finally, activation of the immune responses in persons with Reiter's syndrome may accelerate progression of HIV infection (Winchester *et al.*, 1987; Kaye, 1996).

Management

Management of HIV-infected patients with Reiter's syndrome and reactive arthritis can be difficult. Because there have been no studies of the treatment of HIV-infected patients with this syndrome, treatment has usually paralleled treatment of Reiter's syndrome in HIV-uninfected persons.

Many patients with HIV infection and reactive arthritis do not respond well to non-steroidal anti-inflammatory drugs (NSAIDs), and maximum or near-maximum doses need to be employed for optimum clinical benefit. If traditional NSAIDs in maximal doses prove to be ineffective, some authorities have used phenylbutazone, starting with 100 mg three times a day and increasing to 400–600 mg daily if needed (Solomon *et al.*, 1991). The complete blood count needs to be monitored every 2 weeks for the first 2 months of therapy and then monthly thereafter in patients taking phenylbutazone, and the drug should be discontinued if the total granulocyte count falls below 3000 cells/μl. Despite having several patients taking either zidovudine (ZDV) or sulphasalazine concomitantly with phenylbutazone, Solomon and colleagues did not find any evidence of cytopaenia (Solomon *et al.*, 1991).

In general, low-dose corticosteroids have not been found to be beneficial in HIV-infected persons with Reiter's syndrome. Although Solomon and colleagues noted symptomatic relief with 40 mg or more of oral prednisone daily (Solomon *et al.*, 1991), the prompt and frequent development of candidiasis limits the use of this therapy. Intra-

articular corticosteroid injections usually provide effective symptomatic control, and can be a very practical treatment when one or two joints or entheses are involved. The benefits from corticosteroid injections can be augmented by immobilizing the injected joint with a splint for 5–7 days after injection (Solomon *et al.*, 1991). Although secondary septic arthritis from intra-articular steroid injections does not seem to be a significant problem in HIV-infected individuals, the patient should be instructed to watch carefully for signs of infection.

Disease-modifying antirheumatic drugs have been employed in the treatment of HIV-infected individuals with Reiter's syndrome. Although no controlled study has been performed, Solomon and colleagues report that about one-third of HIV-infected patients with Reiter's syndrome respond favourably to sulphasalazine in doses ranging from 1–3 g daily (Solomon *et al.*, 1991). Others have reported similar results (Youssef *et al.*, 1992; Disla *et al.*, 1994). Although sulphonamide allergies are common in HIV-infected persons, sulphasalazine-allergic patients can be desensitized to the drug (Solomon *et al.*, 1991).

Intramuscular administration of gold was reported to be effective in two patients with HIV-associated Reiter's syndrome (Solomon *et al.*, 1991; Shapiro and Masci, 1996). Anecdotal reports suggest that hydroxychloroquine fails to ameliorate symptoms in this condition (Solomon *et al.*, 1991). At least four patients with Reiter's syndrome and AIDS benefitted from treated with etretinate (Belz *et al.*, 1989; Williams and du Vivier, 1991; Louthrenoo, 1993).

Methotrexate should not be used to treat Reiter's syndrome or psoriatic arthritis in HIV-infected patients, because almost every patient treated has developed *Pneumocystis carinii* pneumonia (PCP) or Kaposi's sarcoma (KS) shortly after institution of methotrexate therapy (Lambert and Kaye, 1987; Winchester *et al.*, 1987; Arnett *et al.*, 1991; Keat and Rowe, 1991; Solomon *et al.*, 1991; Kaye, 1996). There are, however, three reports of successful treatment with methotrexate in patients with psoriatic arthritis and HIV infection who did not develop opportunistic infections (Mauer *et al.*, 1994; Masson *et al.*, 1995). One azathioprine-treated patient had development of profound fatigue and weight loss that resolved on discontinuation of this drug (Winchester *et al.*, 1987). Thus, methotrexate and azathioprine should not be used in HIV-infected patients with reactive arthritis. Prophylaxis with cotrimoxazole should be considered.

Solomon and associates employed cyclosporin A under an experimental protocol in five HIV-infected patients with Reiter's syndrome and persistent articular symptoms non-responsive to phenylbutazone and sulphasalazine. They used an initial dose of 1 mg/kg, with careful titration to 2–4 mg/kg, as needed. Two patients showed complete remission and three patients demonstrated partial remission. CD4 lymphocyte counts did not drop. None of the patients developed renal insufficiency, hypertension, cytopenia, or opportunistic infections while on cyclosporin A (Solomon et al., 1991).

Treatment with ZDV has generally not proven to be beneficial for Reiter's syndrome in HIV-infected persons (Solomon et al., 1991; Duvic et al., 1994). Physical therapy and adaptive devices such as canes and walkers can greatly enhance the quality of many of these patients, especially those with an 'AIDS gait'.

Psoriatic arthritis

Psoriatic arthritis occurs more often in HIV-infected persons than in the general population. Prevalences of 2–6% in unselected HIV-infected patients have been reported (Espinoza et al., 1992). Psoriasis without arthritis is also more common in HIV-infected persons than in the general population.

HIV-infected patients with psoriatic arthritis tend to have severe painful oligoarthritis predominantly affecting the lower extremities, a clinical picture similar to Reiter's syndrome and reactive arthritis (Njobvu et al., 2000). Sausage digits in the feet, as well as heel and foot enthesitis, are commonly present (Arnett et al., 1991). Psoriatic lesions of various types, including vulgaris, guttate, sebopsoriasis, pustular, and exfoliative erythroderma, may all be found in HIV-infected patients with psoriatic arthritis. Sometimes, more than one type of psoriatic skin lesion may be found in the same patient (Arnett et al., 1991). Interestingly, sacro-iliac involvement and uveitis, in association with psoriatic arthritis, may occur less commonly in the HIV-infected patient than in the HIV-uninfected patient (Arnett et al., 1991).

Management of psoriatic arthritis in the HIV-infected person is empirical, as no well-controlled studies have been published. Many patients will obtain symptomatic relief from the use of NSAIDs. Frequently, the maximum recommended dose of these medications is needed to provide effective symptomatic relief. On occasion, phenylbutazone in doses of 100 mg two or three times a day is effective when safer NSAIDs are ineffective. Patients receiving phenylbutazone should have complete blood counts performed at least every 2 weeks for the first 2 months of phenylbutazone therapy and monthly thereafter; the drug should be discontinued if the total granulocyte count falls below 3000 cells/μl (Arnett et al., 1991; Solomon et al., 1991).

Etretinate may be helpful in some HIV-infected patients with psoriatic arthritis (Solomon et al., 1991). The use of psoralen and pulsed ultraviolet actinotherapy benefited the skin and joints of one HIV-infected patient with psoriatic arthritis (Keat and Rowe, 1991). ZDV has produced skin clearing in some patients with psoriasis, but has been less consistently successful in treating psoriatic arthritis (Arnett et al., 1991). Cyclosporin A has been used successfully in one patient with both joint and skin manifestations of psoriasis (Durez et al., 1994; Tourne et al., 1997). As previously mentioned, methotrexate and azathioprine should be avoided in HIV-infected persons because of the high incidence of subsequent opportunistic infections and cancers (Lambert and Kaye, 1987; Winchester et al., 1987; Arnett et al., 1991; Solomon et al., 1991; Kaye, 1996); however, one group has successfully treated three HIV-infected patients with psoriatic arthritis without the development of opportunistic infections (Maurer et al., 1994). Etanercept may be of value (Aboulafia et al., 2000)

Other spondylarthropathies

There are some HIV-infected patients with spondyloarthropathic features such as enthesopathies, oligoarthritis, and onychodystrophy who lack the full clinical features of Reiter's syndrome or psoriatic arthritis. These patients are often referred to as having an undifferentiated spondyloarthropathy, and are probably part of a spectrum of spondyloarthropathic conditions, including Reiter's syndrome, reactive arthritis, and psoriatic arthritis. The management of undifferentiated spondyloarthropathies in the setting of HIV infection is identical to that of HIV-infected persons with Reiter's syndrome, reactive arthritis, and psoriatic arthritis. Ankylosing spondylitis and the arthritis of inflammatory bowel disease, two other forms of spondyloarthropathy, do not seem to be associated with HIV infection (Arnett et al., 1991).

HIV-associated arthritis
Clinical features
In 1988, Rynes and colleagues described the first four cases of a new, apparently HIV-associated arthritis (Rynes et al.,

1988). Their patients had subacute oligoarthritis, primarily involving the knees and ankles. The arthritis was characterized by relatively brief bouts of extreme disability and pain. The pain was maximal 1 to 4 weeks after onset, although the arthritis persisted for between 6 weeks and 6 months. Synovial fluid specimens were non-inflammatory, but synovial biopsies showed chronic mononuclear infiltrates, in contrast to the granulocytic infiltrates typically seen in inflammatory arthritis. None of these patients had antecedent infections, mucocutaneous lesions, or radiographic evidence of sacroiliitis. All patients tested negative for the HLA-B27 antigen, rheumatoid factor, and antinuclear antibodies (Rynes et al., 1988). Similar cases of HIV-associated arthritis have been described subsequently (Withrington et al., 1987; Berman et al., 1988; Forster et al., 1988; Davis et al., 1989; Ornstein and Sperber, 1996). Avascular necrosis in multiple sites may mimic HIV-associated arthritis (Gerster and Rossetti, 1998).

Pathophysiology

The pathophysiological mechanism of HIV-associated arthritis is unknown. Low synovial leucocyte counts and tubuloreticular inclusions, seen by electron microscopy in some patients with HIV-associated arthritis suggest direct viral infection of the synovium (Rynes et al., 1988). Furthermore, not only have researchers isolated HIV from synovial fluid of HIV-infected patients, but electron microscopy has also revealed retroviral-like particles in the synovial fluid (Withrington et al., 1987; Forster et al., 1988). Other viruses, including rubella virus, cytomegalovirus (CMV), and herpes simplex virus (HSV) type 1, are known to cause arthritis by direct invasion of synovial tissue (Kaye, 1996).

Immune-complex deposition in the joint, which occurs with hepatitis B and rubella virus-induced arthritis, may be another possible mechanism for the pathogenesis of HIV-related arthritis (Kaye, 1996). Rynes and associates have noted immunoglobulin depositions in the synovial biopsy specimens of patients with this form of arthritis (Rynes et al., 1988). Except for one patient with anticardiolipin antibodies, no serological tests indicative of auto-antibodies or immune complexes have been noted in these individuals (Rynes et al., 1988; Kaye, 1996).

A final proposed mechanism for the occurrence of HIV-associated arthritis is that it may in fact represent a form of reactive arthritis. However, as noted earlier, patients with HIV-associated arthritis have not had any of the usual laboratory and clinical concomitants of reactive arthritis such

as mucocutaneous lesions and sacroiliac erosion (Berman et al., 1988; Rynes et al., 1988; Kaye, 1996).

Treatment

The NSAIDs have promptly and successfully ameliorated pain and inflammation in some series of patients with HIV-associated arthritis (Rynes et al., 1988; Davis et al., 1989), but not in others (Forster et al., 1988). No other management strategies have been reported. Because of occasional past success with NSAIDs, we favour a 3–6 week trial of at least three different NSAIDs, discontinuing them if no benefit is observed. Intra-articular corticosteroid injections can be used for particularly symptomatic joints. Two patients with HIV-associated arthritis have benefited from treatment with hydroxychloroquine (Ornstein and Sperber, 1996). With our current understanding of HIV-associated arthritis, other disease-modifying antirheumatic drugs, such as parenteral gold, methotrexate and sulphasalazine, cannot be recommended.

Infectious arthritis

Not surprisingly, infectious arthritis may complicate HIV disease. Septic (bacterial) arthritis should be suspected in any HIV-infected person with acute mono- or oligoarthritis, particularly if there are associated signs of infection, such as fever and leukocytosis. Joints suspected of harbouring infectious agents should always be aspirated, and the synovial fluid sent for Gram stain and culture. In addition, synovial fluid from HIV-infected persons with subacute acute chronic arthritis should be aspirated and cultured before attributing such arthritides to a non-infectious cause. Sometimes synovial biopsies are necessary to isolate fungi and mycobacteria from joints.

Many types of bacteria, mycobacteria, and fungi have been isolated from joints in HIV-infected persons (Table 14.2). *Staphylococcus aureus* is the most common aetiological agent in HIV-infected patients with septic arthritis (Casado et al., 2000). Organisms such as fungi and mycobacteria, which usually cause chronic infectious arthritis in HIV-uninfected persons, may result in acute or subacute infectious arthritis in HIV-infected patients (Vassilopoulos et al., 1997). Bacterial arthritis is relatively rare in HIV-infected patients who do not use intravenous drugs. One study found only 14 cases of bacterial arthritis in 4023 HIV-infected patients admitted to a large Italian university hospital (Ventura et al., 1997). Another report from Spain found 10 cases of bacterial arthritis in 2718

Table 14.2 Organisms reported to cause infectious arthritis in HIV-infected patients

---

Bacteria
    Borrelia burgdorferi
    Haemophilus influenzae type B
    Klebsiella pneumoniae
    Neisseria gonorrhoeae
    Pseudomonas aeruginosa
    Rhodococcus erythropolis
    Salmonella choleraesuis
    Salmonella typhimurium
    Staphylococcus aureus
    Staphylococcus epidermidis
    Streptococcus agalactiae
    Streptococcus pneumoniae
    Treponema pallidum
Mycoplasmata
    Ureaplasma urealyticum
Mycobacteria
    Mycobacterium avium
    Mycobacterium haemophilum
    Mycobacterium kansasii
    Mycobacterium tuberculosis
Fungi
    Candida albicans
    Coccidioides immitis
    Cryptococcus species
    Cunninghamelia bertholletiae
    Histoplasma species
    Mucor species
    Nocardia asteroides
    Sporothrix schenckii

---

consecutive hospitalized HIV-infected patients (Polo *et al.*, 1996).

The same organisms that cause septic arthritis in HIV-infected patients have also been noted to cause septic bursitis and osteomyelitis. Septic arthritis and osteomyelitis sometimes coexist; therefore, imaging studies such as serial radiographs or radionuclide bone scans, or both, should be performed in patients with septic arthritis to eliminate the possibility of coexistent osteomyelitis.

Therapy for infectious arthritis in HIV-infected patients does not differ from the treatment of infectious arthritis in other immunocompromised hosts. The HIV-infected patient with septic arthritis should be treated parenterally with appropriate antibiotics for 4–8 weeks. Some physicians may choose to treat septic arthritis patients who are doing well clinically with oral antibiotics after 2–3 weeks of treatment with parenteral antibiotics. However, the efficacy of oral antibiotic therapy for septic arthritis has not been well established for all bacterial pathogens. Infections with fungi or mycobacteria invariably require longer periods of antimicrobial therapy.

Patients with septic arthritis should have arthrocentesis with complete drainage of the joint fluid performed once or twice a day as long as the synovial fluid continues to reaccumulate. The synovial fluid leucocyte count should be performed daily or every other day A decrease in the synovial fluid leucocyte count usually indicates satisfactory treatment of septic arthritis. If the synovial fluid leucocyte count does not continue to decrease or if closed-needle aspiration does not provide complete drainage of the synovial fluid, surgical drainage of the infected joint fluid, either by arthroscopy or by open arthrotomy, should be considered (Broy and Schmid, 1986). Open arthrotomy is usually required for infectious arthritis of the hip. Patients with septic bursitis can be managed frequently with closed-needle drainage and antibiotic therapy alone, with no need for surgery.

Rheumatoid arthritis

Rheumatoid arthritis has not been associated with HIV infection. Considering that the prevalence of rheumatoid arthritis is about 1% in the general population, it is surprising that there are only 16 case reports of rheumatoid arthritis in HIV-infected persons in the medical literature (Furie 1991; Jaffer 1991; Kerr and Spiera, 1991; Muller-Lander *et al.*, 1995; Ornstein *et al.*, 1995; Golden *et al.*, 1996; Stein and Davis, 1996). One possible reason for the lack of association is epidemiological. Rheumatoid arthritis occurs more frequently in women, whereas in Western countries, HIV infection mostly afflicts men (Kaye, 1996). However, there may be a direct relationship between HIV infection and the paucity of patients with rheumatoid arthritis. Rheumatoid joints have an increase in CD4 lymphocytes and a decrease in CD8 lymphocytes. This lymphocyte ratio may be of significance in the pathogenesis of rheumatoid arthritis. Infection with HIV is associated with a decrease in CD4 lymphocytes and a relative increase in CD8 lymphocytes, a phenomenon that may prevent development of rheumatoid synovitis (Kaye, 1996). In fact, many of the HIV-infected rheumatoid arthritis patients appear to go into remission as the result of the HIV infection (Furie, 1991). It is of interest that treatment of rheumatoid arthritis with anti-CD4 monoclonal antibodies has induced remission in patients with rheumatoid arthritis (Furie, 1991). Other patients with co-existent HIV infection and rheumatoid arthritis, have had continued joint destruction from rheumatoid arthritis, suggesting that rheumatoid arthritis activity does not require the presence of significant numbers of CD4 lymphocytes (Muller-Lander *et al.*, 1995; Ornstein, 1995).

Arthralgias

Diffuse arthralgias are a common manifestation of primary HIV infection, which causes an infectious mononucleosis-like syndrome (Kaye, 1996) (see Chapter 1). Arthralgias may occur at other times during the course of the HIV infection as well. Such arthralgias typically last from a few days to 2 weeks, and usually involve the small joints of the hands and feet, wrists, elbows, shoulders, hips, knees, and ankles.

Arthralgias in HIV-infected patients can usually be well controlled with simple analgesics such as acetaminophen or with NSAIDs. Physical measures such as the localized application of heat or ice can also add symptomatic relief.

Painful articular syndrome

Berman and colleagues described 10 HIV-infected patients in Florida with acute, severe, and intermittent articular pain (Berman *et al.*, 1988). These patients developed the sudden onset of debilitating arthralgias in three or fewer joints without exhibiting clinical evidence of synovitis. The articular pain lasted from 2 to 24 h. In many cases, NSAIDs did not adequately control the pain, and it was necessary to administer narcotics (Berman *et al.*, 1988). Others have confirmed this painful articular syndrome (Calabrese, 1989; Pouchot *et al.*, 1992), which appears to be unique in HIV-infected patients, but needs to be differentiated from avascular necrosis (Gerster *et al.*, 1991; Belmonte *et al.*, 1993; Chevalier *et al.*, 1993; Stovall and Young, 1995; Rademaker *et al.*, 1997).

Myopathies

Polymyositis

Clinical features

Several different types of myopathies have been reported in people infected with HIV (Table 14.3). Inflammatory myopathies resembling idiopathic polymyositis are most common (Kaye, 1996). Patients with HIV-associated inflammatory myopathy typically have a subacute onset of proximal muscle weakness (especially in the lower extremities), myalgias,

Table 14.3 Myopathies associated with HIV infection

Disease	Relative prevalence	Key clinical and laboratory features	Key pathological features
Polymyositis	More common	Proximal muscle weakness, creatine phosphokinase, abnormal electromyogram	Lymphocytic infiltrates of muscles; fibre degeneration and regeneration
Dermatomyositis	Rare	See polymyositis; skin rash; Gottron's papules	See polymyositis
Zidovudine-induced myopathy	More common	See polymyositis	Ragged-red fibres on electron microscopy
Necrotizing myopathy	Rare	See polymyositis	Focal muscle necrosis
Pyomyositis	Less common	Indurated, tender muscle mass; muscle aspirate culture; ultrasound; computerized tomography; magnetic resonance imaging	Bacteria on Gram stain of aspirate
Nemaline (rod) myopathy	Rare	Proximal muscle weakness, creatine phosphokinase	Nemaline (rod) bodies
Rhabdomyolysis	Less common	Acute muscle pain, creatine phosphokinase, myoglobinuria	Fragmented muscle fibres
Myositis ossificans	Rare	Uptake on gallium scan near joints; X-ray films with heterotopic ossification	Periarticular calcifications
Subclinical myopathy	73%[a]	Abnormal electromyogram	
Muscle-wasting degeneration	Common	Generalized cachexia	Axonal
Myalgias	Common	May be part of primary HIV infection	None

[a]Percentages based on the results of only one study.

and some limb muscle wasting (Espinoza *et al.*, 1991; Kaye, 1996). In contrast to idiopathic polymyositis, dysphagia and shortness of breath have not been reported (Espinoza *et al.*, 1991). Typical skin lesions of dermatomyositis on both the face and hands have also been seen (Gresh *et al.*, 1989; Espinoza *et al.*, 1991). In some individuals, the symptoms of polymyositis have been the first clinical feature of HIV infection (Dalakas *et al.*, 1986b). Almost all cases of polymyositis in HIV-infected patients have been associated with serum creatinine kinase levels more than five times higher than the normal range (Kaye, 1996). Electromyographic studies in these patients showed evidence of myopathy, and clinical testing usually showed muscle weakness (Kaye, 1996).

The pathological features seen in muscle biopsy specimens in patients with HIV-associated polymyositis strongly resemble those of idiopathic polymyositis, including inflammatory infiltrates with evidence of phagocytosis of muscle fibres and fibre necrosis (Kaye, 1996). Other pathological features that have been reported include cytoplasmic bodies, variation in fibre size, multinucleated giant cells, and central rod bodies (Kaye, 1996).

Pathogenesis

The exact pathogenic mechanism of polymyositis in HIV-infected persons is not known. Other viruses, such as influenza types A and B, coxsackievirus, echovirus, and rubella, have been associated with polymyositis (Kaye, 1996). One possible pathogenetic explanation is direct infection of muscle cells by HIV; *in vitro* studies appear to support this hypothesis (Espinoza *et al.*, 1991). In contrast, *in vivo* experiments using monkeys infected with simian immunodeficiency virus (SIV; a lentivirus closely related to HIV, which produces polymyositis in monkeys) have shown that SIV can be found in inflammatory cells surrounding or invading muscle fibres but not directly in the muscle fibres themselves (Dalakas *et al.*, 1986a). Furthermore, with the exception of one report of the presence of HIV p24 antigen in the cytoplasm of degenerating muscle fibres (Espinoza *et al.*, 1991), most investigators have not detected viral antigens or particles by immunocytochemical analysis or by electron microscopy in muscle fibres, nor have they successfully cultured HIV from affected muscle tissue in patients with HIV-associated polymyositis (Dalakas *et al.*, 1986b; Simpson and Bender, 1988; Espinoza *et al.*, 1991; Leon-Monzon *et al.*, 1993).

A second postulated aetiological mechanism for polymyositis in HIV-infected patients is an HIV-triggered immune mechanism leading to the invasion of muscle fibres by lymphoid cells. The presence of a mononuclear inflammatory cell infiltrate with both CD4 and CD8 lymphocytes in the involved muscle lends support to this hypothesis (Espinoza *et al.*, 1991). Dalakas reported that the predominant cells found in muscle in patients with HIV-associated polymyositis are CD8, non-viral-specific cytotoxic T lymphocytes. These cells, together with macrophages, invade or surround (MHC) class I antigen-expressing non-necrotic muscle fibres (Dalakas, 1995).

A third possible cause of polymyositis in HIV-infected persons is an inflammatory response to an antigen from an opportunistic organism, HIV, or both. This conjectured antigen, which would be present in the interstitial fibroblast as well as on the infecting organism, may serve as a cross-reacting antigen, which in turn would trigger an attack on the myocytes by cells of the immune system leading to necrosis and phagocytosis of myocytes (Dalakas *et al.*, 1986b; Dalakas *et al.*, 1987; Espinoza *et al.*, 1991). Finally, myositis may be a direct consequence of immunodeficiency itself (Dalakas *et al.*, 1987).

Treatment

Most patients with HIV-related polymyositis have responded to treatment with prednisone in doses ranging from 30 to 60 mg daily for 8–12 weeks, with improved strength and a decrease in serum creatinine kinase levels (Espinoza *et al.*, 1991; Kaye, 1996). Patients with HIV-associated polymyositis and dermatomyositis often take longer to show clinical and biochemical improvement in their disease than patients with the idiopathic form of the disease (Espinoza *et al.*, 1991). Although most patients have tolerated corticosteroids without the development of significant side-effects, two patients have developed opportunistic infections within a few weeks of taking steroids for polymyositis (Dalakas *et al.*, 1986b). As previously mentioned, methotrexate and azathioprine should not be used as steroid-sparing agents in HIV-infected patients because of the high incidence of subsequent opportunistic infections and cancers (Lambert and Kaye, 1987; Winchester *et al.*, 1987; Kaye, 1996; Arnett *et al.*, 1991; Solomon *et al.*, 1991).

Zidovudine-induced myositis

ZDV can induce a polymyositis-like clinical picture (Dalakas *et al.*, 1990). Proximal muscle weakness usually begins 3–21 months after starting therapy. Patients may complain of fatigue and myalgias and typically have a two-to sixfold elevation in serum creatinine kinase levels. Proximal muscle weakness is found on physical examination (Dalakas *et al.*, 1990; Chariot, 1994b; Cupler *et al.*, 1995).

Pathologically, ZDV-induced myositis is quite difficult to distinguish from idiopathic or HIV-associated polymyositis by light microscopy. It can be distinguished by the appearance of 'ragged-red fibres', indicative of a mitochondrial abnormality, on electron microscopy. This mitochondrial abnormality is probably induced by ZDV, perhaps through inhibition of mitochondria DNA polymerase gamma (Dalakas *et al.*, 1990). Diagnostically, histochemical reaction for cytochrome c oxidase has proved more sensitive than examination for 'ragged-red fibres' for the diagnosis of ZDV-induced muscular toxicity (Chariot *et al.*, 1993). Non-invasive detection is possible by evaluating the lactate–pyruvate ratio in blood (Chariot, 1994a).

The mechanism of mitrochondrial toxicity is not fully understood. ZDV is a thymidine analogue, which can act as a chain terminator when incorporated into a growing DNA strand. Phosphorylated ZDV also competitively and non-competitively inhibits mitochondrial DNA polymerase gamma, which could be a basis for toxicity of the drug (Chariot and Gherardi, 1995). A consistent depletion of mitochondrial DNA has been observed in patients with ZDV-induced myopathy (Arnaudo *et al.*, 1991). Other cofactors, such as selenium deficiency and interleukin-1, may be partially responsible for the development of ZDV myopathy (Chariot and Gherardi, 1995).

Seven of the 15 patients in Dalaka's study of ZDV-induced myositis showed muscle strength improvement and normalization of serum creatinine kinase levels 7–10 days after cessation of ZDV. Two patients showed clinical improvement with the use of NSAIDs, along with the discontinuation of ZDV. Four patients required the use of oral corticosteroids to achieve clinical improvement in their myopathies. These patients may have had HIV-associated polymyositis coexistent with ZDV-induced myositis. The remaining two patients in the study died of AIDS-related causes before their myopathy resolved (Dalakas *et al.*, 1990). Other investigators have shown a similarly good prognosis (Chalmers *et al.*, 1991; Mhiri *et al.*, 1991; Peters *et al.*, 1993; Simpson *et al.*, 1993).

Other myopathies

Pyomyositis, solitary or multiple muscle abscesses that are not formed by local extension from superficial subcutaneous tissues, have been reported in HIV-infected patients. These abscesses can be sterile, or may contain organisms including *Staphylococcus aureus*, *Salmonella*, *Escherichia coli*, *Morganella morganii* or microsporidia (Arranz-Caso *et al.*, 1996; Vassilopoulos *et al.*, 1997). Imaging techniques, such as ultrasound, computed tomography (CT), or magnetic resonance imaging (MRI) are helpful in identifying and localizing the abscess or abscesses, and may guide a needle aspiration for identification of the pathogenic organism. Treatment of pyomyositis should be promptly instituted using intravenous antibiotics, along with open surgical drainage and debridement when indicated (Goldenberg, 1991). In addition, muscle fibres can be directly infected by opportunistic organisms such as *Toxoplasma gondii*, *Cryptococcus neoformans*, *Mycobacterium avium* complex (MAC), microsporidia, *Escherichia coli*, *Trichinella spiralis*, group C streptococcus, *Citrobacter freundii*, and cytomegalovirus (CMV) (Chariot and Gherardi, 1995).

Comi and associates reported a subclinical myopathy in 11 of 15 consecutive unselected patients with AIDS (Comi *et al.*, 1986). These patients were characterized by abnormal electromyograms (EMG) in the presence of normal clinical examinations and no complaints of muscle pain or weakness. Biopsy samples from the biceps muscle showed non-specific signs of primary muscle involvement in four patients. Two of these patients also had findings that indicated associated muscle denervation (Comi *et al.*, 1986).

Several other types of myopathies have been reported in HIV-infected persons, including a necrotizing non-inflammatory myopathy, nemaline (rod) myopathy, rhabdomyolysis, and myositis ossifans (Table 14.3) (Kaye, 1996). Myalgia is a frequent symptom in patients with primary HIV infection (Kaye, 1996), and fibromyalgia-like symptoms have been reported in 11–29% of consecutive unselected HIV-infected patients (Buskila *et al.*, 1990; Sims *et al.*, 1992). Cocaine use is also a common cause of creatine kinase elevation in outpatients infected with HIV (Kazi *et al.*, 1994).

Vasculitis

Several different forms of vasculitis have been associated with HIV infection (Table 14.4) (Calabrese, 1991; Kaye, 1996; Cebrian *et al.*, 1997). Unlike vasculitic syndromes associated with infections such as hepatitis B, which represent well-defined clinical entities, the vasculitic conditions associated with HIV infection represent a microcosm of the entire vasculitic spectrum (Calabrese, 1991).

Table 14.4 Vasculitides associated with HIV infection

Disease	Relative prevalence	Key clinical or laboratory features	Pathology
Necrotizing vasculitis	More common	Necrotic skin lesions; foot and wrist drop; haematuria; proteinuria; urinary red blood cell casts	Medium and small muscular arteries affected
Leukocytoclastic vasculitis	More common	Palpable purpura; no visceral involvement; reported with zidovudine	Arterioles and venules affected
Henoch-Schönlein purpura	Less common	Palpable purpura; gastrointestinal symptoms; haematuria	Arterioles and venules affected
Eosinophilic vasculitis	Rare	Eosinophilia	Large arteries
Churg–Strauss vasculitis	Rare	Eosinophilia; asthma; allergic rhinitis; skin lesions, pulmonary infiltrates	Granulomas
Isolated angiitis of the central nervous system	Less common	Cognitive impairment, seizures; hemiparesis, headache; lack of systemic symptoms	Granulomas in central nervous system arteries
Behçet's disease	Rare	Oral and genital ulcers; uveitis, arthritis; skin lesions	Lymphocytic infiltrates
Relapsing poly-chondritis	Rare	Nasal, auricular and tracheal cartilage inflammation; eye inflammation	Chondrocyte degeneration, matrix discolouration; fibrosis
Cryoglobulinaemia	Rare	Distal digital infarcts, purpura; glomerulonephritis; cryoglobulinaemia	Arterioles and venules affected
Viral-induced vasculitis	Less common	Central nervous system infarcts and hemiplegia with varicella zoster, gastrointestinal tract involvement with cytomegalovirus	Viral inclusion bodies
Protozoan-induced vasculitis	Less common	Pulmonary cavities with *Pneumocystis carinii*, also reported with toxoplasma	Organisms seen in association with vasculitic changes
Angiocentric immunoprolifera-tive disorder	Less common	Brain involvement; occasionally affects internal organs	Continuum of benign lymphocytic angiitis to lymphomatold granulomatosis; angiocentric lymphoma

Syndromes resembling polyarteritis nodosa

Several HIV-infected patients have been described with a syndrome resembling polyarteritis nodosa (Calabrese, 1991; Gherardi *et al.*, 1993; Libman, 1995; Font *et al.*, 1996; Brannagan, 1997). These patients presented chiefly with peripheral neuropathies, including symmetrical sensori-motor neuropathies and mononeuritis multiplex. Digital ischemia with frank gangrene, other skin lesions, and evidence of gastrointestinal involvement on rectal biopsy have also been noted. Hepatitis B surface antigen was not detected in five HIV-infected patients with syndromes resembling polyarteritis nodosa who were tested for this antigen (Calabrese, 1991; Kaye, 1996).

Patients with HIV-associated polyarteritis nodosa syndromes have pathological changes that resemble typical polyarteritis nodosa, with necrotizing vasculitic lesions of medium-sized vessels. These histological findings have een most commonly demonstrated in small arteries within muscles, as well as in epineural arteries and arterioles. The infiltrates have generally been acute (Calabrese, 1991).

Treatment for the HIV-associated polyarteritis nodosa syndromes is usually with oral prednisone in doses of 40–60 mg daily. Such vasculitic syndromes usually respond well to oral corticosteroids. Cytotoxic drugs, such as cyclophosphamide and azathioprine, should be avoided whenever possible.

It is not known whether the necrotizing vasculitis in HIV-infected patients is a direct result of HIV or not. Other viruses, such as hepatitis B and CMV, have been implicated in the pathogenesis of necrotizing vasculitis; in some cases, these viruses may partially or wholly cause vasculitis in HIV-infected patients (Kaye, 1996). Several patients with AIDS who had CMV-induced necrotizing vasculitis have been described (Meiselman *et al.*, 1985; Burke *et al.*, 1987; Golden *et al.*, 1994). Alternatively, HIV antigens may form antigen–antibody complexes, causing vasculitis in a manner similar to that of hepatitis B surface antigen. Immunofluorescent studies performed in two cases of leucocytoclastic vasculitis occurring in HIV-infected persons suggested such immune complex mechanisms (Calabrese, 1991). HIV may also have a direct effect on the blood vessel wall, thus causing vasculitis in some way as yet unknown (Kaye, 1996). Calabrese and associates have cultured HIV from peripheral nerves of an HIV-infected patient with necrotizing vasculitis, but they could not demonstrate HIV in the vasculitic lesions (Calabrese *et al.*, 1988).

A single case of allergic granulomatosis or Churg-Strauss syndrome has been described in an HIV-infected patient. The patient was treated with high-dose prednisone alone and had a good clinical response at 1 month (Cooper and Patterson, 1989). A case of cryoglobulinaemia in a woman with chronic HIV and hepatitis C infection has been reported (Monsuez *et al.*, 1998).

Hypersensitivity vasculitis

Several reports of small-vessel vasculitis in HIV-infected patients, often referred to as the hypersensitivity vasculitides, have been reported (Calabrese, 1991). A variety of viral infections often associated with HIV infection, including CMV, Epstein–Barr virus, and hepatitis B virus, are known to cause leucocytoclastic vasculitis. CMV has been linked with hypersensitivity vasculitis in HIV-infected patients. Other well-studied cases of small-vessel vasculitis have not revealed any of the known causes of this type of vasculitis (Calabrese, 1991). ZDV has been demonstrated to induce leucocytoclastic vasculitis in at least one case (Torres *et al.*, 1992). Henoch-Schönlein purpura has been reported in adults and children infected with HIV (Veiji, 1986; Calabrese, 1991). No specific therapy is usually needed in these cases.

Primary angiitis of the central nervous system

Primary angiitis of the central nervous system (CNS) is an extremely rare disorder. Six of the 108 cases reported in the English literature up to January 1990 have been in HIV-infected persons (Calabrese, 1991). Fulminant CNS symptoms, including hemiparesis, cognitive impairment, dysphagia, seizures, and headaches, occur in primary angiitis of the central nervous system. Systemic necrotizing vasculitic symptoms, such as skin lesions, abdominal pain, foot and wrist drop, haematuria, and proteinuria, are absent. Histological examination reveals granulomatous involvement of cerebral arteries. A combination of cyclophosphamide and corticosteroids is usually necessary to treat primary angiitis of the central nervous system in HIV-uninfected patients. No treatment guidelines are available for the HIV-infected patient with this condition.

Lymphomatoid granulomatosis

Lymphomatoid granulomatosis is part of a spectrum of disorders known as angiocentric immunoproliferative lesions. It is a vasculitic disorder that often progresses to become angiocentric lymphoma. There have been at least six reports of this condition in HIV-infected persons. Lymphomatoid granulomatosis developing in the HIV-infected patient suggests that HIV-induced immune dysregulation may at times lead to uncontrolled lymphoproliferation of T-cell lineages with an angiocentric predisposition. This T-cell proliferation contrasts with the vast majority of lymphomatoid neoplasms in HIV infection, which originate from B cells (Calabrese, 1991).

In cases of lymphomatoid granulomatosis in HIV-infected patients, the CNS has been the primary site of involvement of the vasculitis. Muscle, peripheral nerve, heart, lung, and kidney have also been affected (Calabrese, 1991).

No controlled trials of treatment of vasculitis in HIV-infected patients have been undertaken. Each case of vasculitis needs to be treated individually. Certainly, high-dose corticosteroid therapy, such as 60–80 mg prednisone daily, should be employed in patients with potentially life-threatening disease. Cytotoxic drugs such as cyclophosphamide should be used with caution because of the high risk of developing opportunistic infection. Physicians at the Cleveland Clinic use combination chemotherapy for HIV-associated lymphoproliferative diseases in patients who have an absolute CD4 lymphocyte count of 400–500 cells/μl. They also advocate aggressive prophylaxis for opportunistic infections, including monthly intravenous immunoglobulin, monthly aerosolized pentamidine for *P. carinii* prophylaxis, and daily acyclovir for viral prophylaxis (Calabrese, 1991). Other investigators use cotrimoxazole for *P. carinii* and toxoplasma prophylaxis, as it is superior to aerosolized pentamidine.

Other rheumatological diseases

Sicca syndrome

Clinical features

Several authors have described HIV-infected persons with generalized lymphadenopathy and the sicca syndrome (xerophthalmia and xerostomia), termed diffuse infiltrative lymphadenopathy syndrome (DILS). At the time of development of sicca symptoms, none of these patients has met the criteria for AIDS (Itescu, 1991; Itescu and Winchester, 1992; Williams et al., 1998). These patients may resemble Sjögren's syndrome: clinically they had dry eyes, dry mouth, parotid gland enlargement, and lymphadenopathy (Itescu, 1991; Itescu and Winchester, 1992; Kaye, 1996). However, many important differences exist between HIV-associated generalized lymphadenopathy and sicca syndrome and idiopathic Sjögren's syndrome. In contrast to idiopathic Sjögren's syndrome, DILS is frequently associated with extraglandular manifestations, such as lymphocytic interstitial pneumonitis, and lymphocytic infiltration of the gastrointestinal, neurological and reticuloendothelial systems. Parotid gland and lymph node enlargement in patients with DILS is often massive, in contrast to those with idiopathic Sjögren's syndrome (Itescu, 1991; Itescu and Winchester, 1992). Peripheral neuropathy is quite common in these patients (Moulignier et al., 1997). In addition, the infiltrative T lymphocytes in DILS are CD8-positive, whereas in Sjögren's syndrome they are CD4-positive. Furthermore, auto-antibodies such as rheumatoid factor, antinuclear antibodies, anti-Ro/SS-A, and anti-La/SS-B, which are commonly seen in idiopathic Sjögren's syndrome, are absent in DILS. The HLA association with idiopathic Sjögren's syndrome is B8, DR2, DR3, and DR4 (when associated with rheumatoid arthritis). In contrast, black patients with DILS tend to be HLA-DR5 positive, whereas Caucasians are more commonly HLA-DR6- and DR7-positive. Finally, all DILS patients show evidence of HIV infection, whereas those with idiopathic Sjögren's syndrome do not have signs of HIV (Itescu, 1991; Itescu and Winchester, 1992). DILS is seen more commonly in African-american patients than in Caucasians (Williams et al., 1998).

The clinical course for HIV-infected patients with DILS appears to differ dramatically from that of HIV-infected patients as a whole. Itescu and colleagues followed 25 patients with DILS for a total of 822 patient months (range of follow-up, 12–144 months), and only one patient developed an opportunistic infection.

Two patients died, one as a result of pneumococcal pneumonia complicating severe lymphocytic interstitial pneumonitis and a second as a result of unrelated head trauma (Itescu, 1991).

Interestingly, 20–25% of HIV-infected patients do have decreased tear production, regardless of whether or not they have DILS (Geier et al., 1995).

Therapy

The most common symptoms in DILS relate to salivary gland infiltration, with ensuing facial pain and discomfort, sicca symptoms, and recurrent sinus, middle ear, and oral cavity infections. Therapy with antibiotics appropriate to the culture and infection site is usually effective for the latter problems. ZDV may diminish salivary gland enlargement in many patients. Dosages of 250 mg orally four times a day may lead to symptomatic responses as early as 1 week after starting ZDV, with maximal benefits usually occurring after 6 weeks. In general, discontinuation of ZDV has resulted in rapid re-enlargement of the parotid glands. There are no data regarding combination antiretroviral therapy. Artificial tears can be used for dry eyes. Chewing sugarless gum or sucking on sugarless candy may increase saliva production. Proper dental care is also essential in patients with DILS because the lack of saliva leads to more frequent dental caries (Itescu, 1991; Itescu and Winchester, 1992).

Progressive pulmonary, gastrointestinal, or renal lymphocytic infiltration needs to be evaluated further before instituting immununosuppressive therapy (Itescu, 1991). Tissue confirmation of pulmonary lymphocytic infiltration, either by transbronchial or open lung biopsy, as well as the use of gallium scans and pulmonary function tests, can aid in the evaluation of pulmonary status in DILS patients. Lymphocytic infiltration of the kidneys, which can manifest either by interstitial nephritis or renal tubular infiltration, may present with progressive renal insufficiency, hyperkalaemia, and type IV renal tubular acidosis (Itescu, 1991; Itescu and Winchester, 1992).

If the pulmonary or renal disease in DILS progresses and is symptomatic, Itescu and colleagues advocate treating with 40–60 mg of prednisone daily or with other immunosuppressive agents such as chlorambucil for 8–12 weeks. Patients are treated with antiretroviral agents in addition to prednisone. Although typical side-effects of high-dose corticosteroid therapy such as weight gain, hypertension, hyperglycaemia and oral candidiasis may be seen in patients with DILS, complicating opportunistic infections have not been noted (Itescu, 1991; Itescu and Winchester, 1992).

Auto-immune phenomena

Various auto-immune phenomena have been reported in HIV-infected patients (Table 14.5). The prevalence of these auto-antibodies varies greatly between clinical series (Solinger and Hess, 1991; Kaye, 1996). Two types of auto-antibodies – antiphospholipid antibodies and antinuclear antibodies – may have particular clinical and therapeutic significance. Several studies have noted a marked increase in prevalence of antiphospholipid antibodies (anti-cardiolipin antibodies and the lupus anticoagulant) in HIV-infected persons (Solinger and Hess, 1991; Kaye, 1996). In patients with rheumatological diseases such as systemic lupus erythematosus, antiphospholipid antibodies are associated with thrombotic events such as strokes and deep venous thromboses. There is no such association in HIV-infected patients, and thus there is no need for routine anti-coagulant therapy in these patients (Kaye, 1996).

About 45% of patients with AIDS are found to have the lupus anticoagulant (Kaye, 1996), and often have pro-longed partial thromboplastin times. The prolonged partial thromboplastin time cannot be corrected by mixing the patient's serum with normal serum, as can be done in haemophilia and other deficiencies of coagulation factors. Furthermore, the lupus anticoagulant is not associated with clinical bleeding problems. Thus, HIV-infected patients who are about to undergo an invasive procedure and have a prolonged partial thromboplastin time should be evaluated for the presence of the lupus anticoagulant, rather than be denied a necessary procedure because of a perceived risk of bleeding (Bloom et al., 1986).

HIV infection seems to be associated with an increased incidence of auto-antibodies. Although not related to the occurrence of rheumatological manifestations, the presence of auto-antibodies seems to be associated with lower CD4 lymphocyte counts and increased mortality, which implies prognostic significance to this phenomenon in the context of HIV infection (Massabki et al., 1997).

HIV infection and systemic lupus erythematosus share a number of clinical features in common (Table 14.6). Anti-nuclear antibodies have been reported in up to 13% of HIV-infected patients in one series (Kopelman and Zolla-Pazner, 1988), although many other investigators have not observed this association (Kaye, 1996). When a patient has the clinical symptoms outlined in Table 14.6 and a positive antinuclear antibody test, the diagnosis of systemic lupus erythematosus is often entertained, and treatment with cor-ticosteroid, antimalarial drugs, and even cytotoxic agents may be considered. Although up to 10% of patients with systemic lupus erythematosus may have antibodies to HIV detected by the enzyme-linked immunoabsorbant assay (Calabrese et al., 1986), false-positive tests in lupus patients are extremely rare when western blot is employed (McDougal et al., 1985; Esteva et al., 1992; Barthel and Wallace, 1993).

There are only 11 case reports of systemic lupus erythe-matosus occurring in HIV-infected persons reported in the medical literature (Furie, 1991; Molina et al., 1995; Kudva et

Table 14.5 Auto-immune phenomena associated with HIV infection

Auto-immune phenomena	Relative prevalence	Clinical significance
Antinuclear antibodies	Less common	None
Antiplatelet antibodies	Common	Disease (immune thrombocytopenic purpura)
Antilymphocyte antibodies	Common	Disease (immunodeficiency)
Antigranulocyte antibodies	Less common	Disease (immunodeficiency)
Direct antiglobulin (Coombs') test	Common	None
Lupus anticoagulant	Common	None (not associated with bleeding or thrombosis)
Anticardiolipin antibodies	Common	May parallel *Pneumocystis carinii* pneumonia activity; not associated with thrombosis
Antineutrophil cytoplasmic antibodies	Rare	None
Circulating immune complexes	Common	None
Rheumatoid factor	Less common	None
Cryoglobulins	Rare	Disease (cryoglobulinaemia)

Table 14.6 Similarities between systemic lupus erythematosus and HIV infection

---

Skin
    Malar rash (from seborrhoeic dermatitis)
Joint
    Arthritis and arthralgias
    Oral ulcers
Kidney
    Proteinuria
Blood
    Thrombocytopenia
    Leucopenia
    Lymphopenia
    Neutropenia
    Coombs' positive haemolytic anaemia
Nervous system
    Seizures
    Headaches
    Dementia
    Mononeuritis multiplex
    Peripheral and cranial neuropathies
    Myositis
Vasculitis
    Sicca syndrome
Constitutional
    Fever
    Lymphadenopathy
    Weight loss
Laboratory
    Antiphospholipid antibodies
    Antinuclear antibodies

---

al., 1996; Byrd and Sergent, 1996; Fox and Isenberg, 1997). The reasons for the lack of association between HIV infection and systemic lupus erythematosus are not fully known. One possibility is epidemiological; systemic lupus erythematosus occurs primarily in women, whereas in Western countries, HIV mostly afflicts men (Kaye, 1996). Second, the resulting immunological abnormalities from HIV infection may attenuate the clinical manifestations of systemic lupus erythematosus, thus making the disease less obvious. In two documented cases, patients with systemic lupus erythematous improved with concomitant lymphocyte depletion from the HIV infection. One patient was treated with ZDV, with a subsequent increase in the number of lymphocytes. At the same time, arthritis and pleuritis reappeared and anti-DNA antibody levels increased (Furie, 1991; Molina et al., 1995). Finally, the marked antibody production in patients with systemic lupus erythematous may somehow protect the patient from either developing HIV infection or expressing the immunodeficiency caused by HIV (Kaye, 1996). Because of the risk of further immunosuppression, cytotoxic drugs should not be used in the treatment of HIV-infected patients with systemic lupus erythematous. Azathioprine, methotrexate, and cyclophosphamide are therefore contraindicated in these patients.

References

Aboulafia DM, Bundow D, Wilske K et al. (2000). Etanercept for the treatment of HIV-associated psoriatic arthritis. *Mayo Clin Proc* **75**: 1098–8.

Arnaudo E, Dalakas, M, Shanske S et al. (1991). Depletion of muscle mitochondrial DNA in AIDS patients with zidovudine-induced myopathy. *Lancet* **337**: 508–10.

Arnett FC, Reveille JD, Duvic M. (1991). Psoriasis and psoriatic arthritis associated with human immunodeficiency virus infection. *Rheumatol Dis Clin N Am* **17**: 59–78.

Arranz-Caso JA, Cuadrado-Gomez LM, Romanik-Cabrera J et al. (1996) Pyomyositis caused by Morganella morganii in a patient with AIDS. *Clin Infect Dis* **22**: 372–3.

Barthel HR, Wallace DJ (1993). False-positive human immunodeficiency testing in patients with lupus erythematosus. *Semin Arthritis Rheum* **23**: 1–7.

Belmonte MA, Garcia-Partales R, Domenech I et al. (1993). Avascular necrosis of bone in human immunodeficiency virus infection and antiphosphospholipid antibodies. *J Rheumatol* **20**: 1425–8.

Belz J, Breneman DL, Nordlund JJ et al. (1989). Successful treatment of a patient with Reiter's syndrome and acquired immunodeficiency syndrome using etretinate. *J Am Acad Dermatol* **20**: 898–903.

Berman A, Espinoza LR, Diaz JD et al. (1988). Rheumatic manifestations of human immunodeficiency virus infection. *Am I Med* **85**: 59–64.

Berman A, Cahn P, Perez H et al. (1997). Prevalence and characteristics of rheumatic manifestations in patients infected with human immunodeficiency virus undergoing antiretroviral therapy. *J Rheumatol* **24**: 2492.

Bloom EJ, Abrams DI, Rodgers G. (1986). Lupus anticoagulant in the acquired immunodeficiency syndrome. *JAMA* **256**: 491–3.

Brancato LJ, Itescu S, Winchester R. (1989). Reiter's syndrome and related rheumatic conditions in HIV infection. *J Musculoskel Med* **6**: 14–32.

Brannagan TH. (1997). Retroviral-associated vasculitis of the nervous system. *Neurol Clin N Am* **15**: 927–44.

Broy SB, Schmid FR. (1986). A comparison of medical drainage (needle aspiration) and surgical drainage (arthrotomy or arthroscopy) in the initial treatment of infected joints. *Clin Rheum Dis* **12**: 501–22.

Burke G, Nichols L, Balogh K et al. (1987). Perforation of the terminal ileum with cytomegalovirus vasculitis and Kaposi's sarcoma in a patient with acquired immunodeficiency syndrome. *Surgery* **102**: 540–5.

Buskila D, Gladman DD, Langevitz P et al. (1990). Fibromyalgia in human immunodeficiency virus infection. *J Rheumatol* **17**: 1202–6.

Byrd VM, Sergent JS. (1996). Suppression of systemic lupus erythematosus by the human immunodeficiency virus. *J Rheumatol* **23**: 1295–6.

Calabrese LH. (1989). The rheumatic manifestations of infection with the human immunodeficiency virus. *Arthritis Rheum* **18**: 235–9.

Calabrese LH. (1991). Vasculitis and infection with the human immunodeficiency virus. *Rheum Dis Clin N Am* **17**: 131–47.

Calabrese LH, Proffitt MR, Segal AM *et al.* (1986). Clinical significance of serologic reactivity to human T cell lymphotropic virus type-III in patients with autoimmune disease [abstract]. *Arthritis Rheum* **29**: S21.

Calabrese LH, Yen-Lieberman B, Estes M *et al.* (1988). Systemic necrotizing vasculitis and the human immunodeficiency virus (HIV): an important etiologic relationship [abstract]. *Arthritis Rheum* **31**: S35.

Casado E, Olive A, Holgado S *et al.* (2001). Musculoskeletal manifestations in patients positive for human immunodeficiency virus: correlation with CD4 count. *J Rheumatol* **28**: 802–4.

Cebrian M, Miro O, Font C *et al.* (1997). HIV-related vasculitis. *AIDS Patient Care STDS* **11**: 245–58.

Chalmers AC, Greco CM, Miller RG. (1991). Prognosis in ZDV myopathy. *Neurology* **41**: 1181–4.

Chariot P, Gherardi R (1995). Myopathy and HIV infection. *Curr Opin Rheumatol* **7**: 497–502.

Chariot P, Monnet I, Gherardi R. (1993). Cytochrome c oxidase reaction improves histopathologic assessment of zidovudine myopathy. *Ann Neurol* **34**: 561–5.

Chariot P, Monnet I, Mouchet M *et al.* (1994a). Determination of the blood pyruvate:lactate ratio as a noninvasive test for zidovudine myopathy. *Arthritis Rheum* **37**: 583–96.

Chariot P, Ruet E, Gherardi R. (1994b). Zidovudine therapy and myopathies associated with human immunodeficiency virus infections. *Ann Neurol* **34**: 561–5.

Chevalier X, Larget-Piet B, Hernigou P, Gerardi R. (1993). A vascular necrosis of the femoral head in HIV-infected patients. *J Bone Joint Surg* **75**: 160.

Clark MR, Solinger AM, Hochberg MC. (1992). Human immunodeficiency virus infection is not associated with Reiter's syndrome. *Rheum Dis Clin N Am* **18**: 267–76.

Comi G, Medaglini S, Galardi G *et al.* (1986). Subclinical neuromuscular involvement in acquired immunodeficiency syndrome. *Muscle Nerve* **9**: 665.

Cooper LM, Patterson JAK. (1989). Allergic granulomatosis and angiitis of Churg-Strauss: cue report in a patient with antibodies to human immunodeficiency virus and hepatitis B virus. *Int J Dermatol* **28**: 597–9.

Cupler EJ, Danon MJ, Jay C *et al.* (1995). Early features of zidovudine-associated myopathy: histopathological findings and clinical correlations. *Acta Neuropathol* **90**: 1–6.

Dalakas MC. (1995). Immunopathogenesis of inflammatory myopathies. *Ann Neurol* **37**: S74–86.

Dalakas MC, London WT Gravell M *et al.* (1986a). Polymyositis in an immunodeficiency disease in monkeys induced by a type D retrovirus. *Neurology* **36**: 569–72.

Dalakas MC, Pezeshkpour GH, Gravell M *et al.* (1986b). Polymyositis associated with AIDS retrovirus. *JAMA* **256**: 2381–3.

Dalakas MC, Gravell M, London WT *et al.* (1987). Morphological changes of an inflammatory myopathy in rhesus monkeys with simian acquired immunodeficiency syndrome (42556). *Proc Soc Exp Biol Med* **185**: 368–76.

Dalakas MC, Illa I, Pezeshkpour GH *et al.* (1990). Mitochondrial myopathy caused by long-term zidovudine therapy. *N Engl J Med* **322**: 1098–105.

Davis P, Stein M, Latie A *et al.* (1989). Acute arthritis in Zimbabwean patients: possible relationship to human immunodeficiency virus infection. *J Rheumatol* **16**: 346–8.

Disla E, Rhim HR, Reddy A, Taranta A. (1994). Improvement in CD4 lymphocyte count in HIV-Reiter's syndrome in patients after treatment with sulphasalazine. *J Rheumatol* **21**: 662–4.

Durez P, Toume L, Van Vooren JR *et al.* (1994). Improvement in severe psoriatic arthritis associated with HIV infection by cyclosporine. *Arthritis Rheumatol* **37**: S235.

Duvic M, Crane MM, Conant *et al.* (1994). Zidovudine improves psoriasis in human immunodeficiency virus-positive males. *Arch Dermatol* **130**: 447–51.

Espinoza LR, Aguilar JL, Espinoza CG *et al.* (1991). Characteristics and pathogenesis of myositis in human immunodeficiency virus infection: distinction from azidothymidine-induced myopathy. *Rheumal Dis Clin N Am* **17**: 117–29.

Espinoza LR, Jara LJ, Espinoza CG *et al.* (1992). There is an association between human immunodeficiency virus infection and spondyloarthropathy. *Rheumatol Dis Clin N Am* **18**: 257–66.

Esteva MH, Blasini AM, Ogly D *et al.* (1992). False positive results for antibody to HIV in two men with lupus erythematosus. *Ann Rheumatol Dis* **51**: 1071–3.

Font C, Miro O, Pedrol E *et al.* (1996) Polyarteritis nodosa in human immunodeficiency virus infection: report of four cases and review of the literature. *Br J Rheumatol* **35**: 796–9.

Forster SM, Seifert MH, Keat AC *et al.* (1988). Inflammatory joint disease and human immunodeficiency virus infection. *Br Med J* **296**: 1625–7.

Fox RA, Isenberg DA. (1997). Human immunodeficiency virus infection in systemic lupus erythematosus. *Arthritis Rheum* **40**: 1168–72.

Furie RA. (1991). Effects of human immunodeficiency virus infection on the expression of rheumatic illness. *Rheum Dis Clin N Am* **17**: 177–88.

Geier SA, Libera S, Klauss V *et al.* (1995). Sicca syndrome in patients infected with the human immunodeficiency virus. *Ophthalmology* **102**: 1319–24.

Gerster JC, Rossetti G. (1998). Aseptic avascular osteonecrosis mimicking arthritis in HIV infection. *J Rheumatol* **25**: 604–5.

Gerster JC, Cammus JP, Chave JP *et al.* (1991). Multiple site avascular necrosis in HIV infected patients. *J Rheumatol* **18**: 300–2.

Gherardi R, Belec L, Mhiri C *et al.* (1993). The spectrum of vasculitis in human immunodeficiency virus-infected patients: a clinicopathologic evaluation. *Arthritis Rheum* **36**: 1164–72.

Golden MP, Hammer SM, Wanke CA *et al.* (1994). Cytomegalovirus vasculitis: case reports and review of the literature. *Medicine* **73**: 246–55.

Golden BD, Wong DC, Diconstanzo D *et al.* (1996). Rheumatoid papules in a patient with acquired immune deficiency syndrome and symmetric polyarthritis. *J Rheumatol* **23**: 760–2.

Goldenberg DL. (1991). Septic arthritis and other infections of rheumatologic significance. *Rheum Dis Clin N Am* **17**: 149–56.

Gresh J, Aguilar JL, Espinoza LR. (1989). Human immunodeficiency virus (HIV) infection-associated dermatomyositis. *J Rheumatol* **17**: 1397–8.

Itescu S. (1991). Diffuse infiltrative lymphocytosis syndrome in human immunodeficiency: a Sjögren's-like disease. *Rheumatol Dis Clin N Am* **17**: 99–115.

Itescu S, Winchester R. (1992). Diffuse infiltrative lymphocytosis syndrome: a disorder occurring in human immunodeficiency virus-1 infection that may present as a sicca syndrome. *Rheumatol Dis Clin N Am* **18**: 683–97.

Jaffer AM. (1991). Seronegative rheumatoid arthritis associated with AIDS [letter]. *Ann Rheum Dis* **50**: 134.

Kaye BR. (1996). Rheumatologic manifestations of HIV infections. *Clin Rev Allergy Immunol* **14**: 385–416.

Kazi S, Miller SM, Reveille JD (1994). Causes of creatinine kinase elevation in a large outpatient population infected with HIV-1. *Arthritis Rheum* **37**: S234.

Keat A, Rowe I. (1991). Reiter's syndrome and associated arthritides. *Rheum Dis Clin N Am* **17**: 25–42.

Kerr LD, Spiera H. (1991). The coexistence of acute classic rheumatoid arthritis and AIDS. *J Rheumatol* **18**: 1739–40.

Khan MA, van der Linden SM. (1990). A wider spectrum of spondyloarthropathies. *Semin Arthritis Rheumatol* **20**: 107–13.

Kopelman RG, Zolla-Pazner S. (1988). Association of human immunodeficiency virus infection and autoimmune phenomena. *Am J Med* **84**: 82–8.

Kudva YC, Peterson LS, Holley KE et al. (1996). SLE nephropathy in a patient with HIV infection: case report and review of the literature. *J Rheumatol* **23**: 1811–5.

Lambert RE, Kaye BR. (1987). Methotrexate and the acquired immunodeficiency. *Ann Intern Med* **106**: 773.

Leon-Monzon M, Lamperth L, Dalakas MC. (1993). Search for HIV proviral DNA and amplified sequences in the muscle biopsies of patients with HIV polymyositis. *Muscle Nerve* **16**: 408–13.

Libman BS, Quismorio FP, Stimmler MM. (1995). Polyarteritis-like vasculitis in human immunodeficiency virus infection. *J Rheumatol* **22**: 351–5.

Lopez-Longo FJ, Rodriguez-Mahou M, Monteagudo I et al. (1994). Manifestaciones reumática in niños infectados por el VIH. *Rev Esp Reumatol* **21**: 222–6.

Louthrenoo W. (1993). Successful treatment of severe Reiter's syndrome associated with human immunodeficiency virus infection with etretinate. Report of 2 cases. *J Rheumatol* **20**: 1243–6.

McDougal JS, Kennedy MS, Kalyanaraman VS et al. (1985). Failure to demonstrate (cross-reacting) antibodies to human T patients with rheumatic diseases. *Arthritis Rheumatol* **28**: 1170–4.

Massabki PS, Accetturi C, Nishie IA et al. (1997). Clinical implications of autoantibodies in HIV infection. *AIDS* **11**: 1845–50.

Masson C, Chennebault JM, Leclech C. (1995). Is HIV infection contraindication to the use of methotrexate in psoriatic arthritis? *J Rheumatol* **22**: 2191.

Maurer TA, Zackheim HS, Tuffanelli L et al. (1994). The use of methotrexate for treatment of psoriasis in patients with HIV infection. *J Am Acad Dermatol* **31**: 372–5.

Mauer TA, Zackheim HS, Tuffanelli L, Berger TG. (1994). The use of methotrexate for psoriasis in patients with HIV infection. *J Am Acad Dermatol* **31**: 372–5.

Meiselman MS, Cello JP, Margaretten W. (1985). Cytomegalovirus colitis: report of the clinical, endoscopic, and pathologic finding, in two patients with the acquired immunodeficiency syndrome. *Gastroenterology* **88**: 171–5.

Mhiri C, Baudrimont M, Bonne G. (1991). Zidovudine myopathy: a distinctive disorder associated with mitochondrial dysfunction. *Ann Neurol* **29**: 606–14.

Molina JF, Citera G, Rosler D et al. (1995). Coexistence of human immunodeficiency virus infection and systemic lupus erythematosus. *J Rheumatol* **22**: 347–50.

Monsuez J-J, Vittecoq D, Musset L et al. (1998). Arthralgias and cryoglobulinemia during protease inhibitor therapy in a patient infected with human immunodeficiency virus and hepatitis C virus. *Arthritis Rheumatol* **41**: 740–3.

Moulignier A, Authier FJ, Baudrimont M et al. (1997). Peripheral neuopathy in human immunodeficiency virus-infected patients with the diffuse infiltrative lymphocytosis syndrome. *Ann Neurol* **41**: 438–45.

Muller-Lander U, Kriegsmann J, Gay RE et al. (1995). Progressive joint destruction in a human immunodeficiency virus-infected patient with rheumatoid arthritis. *Arthritis Rheumatol* **38**: 1328–32.

Njobvu P, McGill P (2000). Psoriatic arthritis and human immunodeficiency virus infection in Zambia. *J Rheumatol* **27**: 1699–702.

Ornstein MH, Sperber K. (1996). The antiinflammatory and antiviral effects of hydroxychloroquine in two patients with acquired immunodeficiency syndrome and active inflammatory arthritis. *Arthritis Rheumatol* **39**: 157–61.

Ornstein MH, Kerr LD, Spiera H. (1995). A re-examination of the relationship between active rheumatoid arthritis and the acquired immunodeficiency syndrome. *Arthritis Rheumatol* **38**: 1701–6.

Peters BS, Winer J, Landon DN et al. (1993). Mitochondrial myopathy associated with chronic zidovudine treatment in AIDS. *Q J Med* **86**: 5–15.

Polo R, Verdejo J, Martinez M et al. (1996). Bacterial diseases in 2718 hospitalized HIV-patients. *Int Conf AIDS* **11**: 296.

Pouchot J, Simonpoli AM, Bortolotti V et al. (1992). Painful articular syndrome and human immunodeficiency virus infection. *Arch Intern Med* **152**: 646–7.

Rademaker J, Dobro JS, Solomon G. (1997). Osteonecrosis and human immunodeficiency virus infection. *J Rheumatol* **24**: 601–4.

Rynes RI, Goldenberg DL, DiGiacomo R et al. (1988). Acquired immunodeficiency syndrome-associated arthritis. *Am J Med* **84**: 810–6.

Schuval SJ, Bonagura VR, Ilowite NT. (1993). Rheumatologic manifestations of pediatric human immunodeficiency virus infection. *J Rheumatol* **20**: 1578–82.

Shapiro DL, Masci JR. (1996). Treatment of HIV associated psoriatic arthritis with oral gold. *J Rheumatol* **23**: 1818–20.

Simpson DM, Bender AN. (1988). Human immunodeficiency virus-associated myopathy analysis of 11 patients. *Ann Neurol* **24**: 79–84.

Simpson DM, Citak KA, Godfrey E et al. (1993). Myopathies associated with human immunodeficiency syndrome and zidovudine: can their effects be distinguished? *Neurology* **43**: 971–6.

Sims RW, Zerbini CAF, Perrante N et al. (1992). Fibromyalgia syndrome in patients with human immunodeficiency virus infection. *Am J Med* **92**: 368–74.

Solinger AM, Hess EV. (1991). Induction of autoantibodies by human immunodeficiency virus infection and their significance. *Rheumatol Dis Clin N Am* **17**: 157–76.

Solinger AM, Hess EV. (1993). Rheumatic diseases and AIDS – is the association real? *J Rheumatol* **20**: 678–83.

Solomon G, Brancato L, Winchester R (1991). An approach to the human virus-positive patient with a spondyloarthropathic disease. *Rheumatol Dis Clin N Am* **17**: 43–58.

Stein CM, Davis P. (1996). Arthritis associated with HIV infection in Zimbabwe. *J Rheumatol* **23**: 506–11.

Stovall D, Young TR. (1995). Avascular necrosis of the medial femoral condyle in HIV-infected patients. *Am J Orthop* **24**: 71–3.

Torres RA, Lin RY, Lee M *et al.* (1992). Zidovudine-induced leukocytoclastic vasculitis, *Arch Intern Med* **152**: 850–1.

Tourne L, Durez P, Van-Vooren J-P *et al.* (1997). Alleviation of HIV-associated psoriasis and psoriatic arthritis with cyclosporine. *J Am Acad Dermatol* **37**: 501–2.

Vassilopoulos D, Chalasani P, Jurado RL *et al.* (1997). Musculoskeletal infections with human immunodeficiency virus infection. *Medicine* **76**: 284–94.

Veiji AM. (1986). Leukocytoclastic vasculitis associated with positive HTLV-III serologic findings. JAMA **256**: 2196–7.

Ventura G, Gasparini G, Lucia MB *et al.* (1997). Osteoarticular bacterial infections are rare in HIV-infected patients. 14 cases found among 4,023 HIV-infected patients. *Acta Orthop Scand* **68**: 554–8.

Williams HC, du Vivier AWP. (1991). Etretinate and AIDS-related Reiter's disease. *Br J Dermatol* **124**: 389–92.

Williams FM, Cohen, PR, Jumshyd J *et al.* (1998). Prevalence of the diffuse infiltrative lymphocytosis syndrome among human immunodeficiency virus type 1-positive outpatients. *Arthritis Rheumatol* **41**: 863–8.

Winchester R, Bernstein DH, Fischer HD *et al.* (1987). The co-occurrence of Reiter's syndrome and acquired immunodeficiency. *Ann Intern Med* **106**: 19–26.

Withrington RH, Comes P, Harris JRW *et al.* (1987). Isolation of human from synovial fluid of a patient with reactive arthritis. *Br Med J* **294**: 484.

Youssef PP, Bertouch JV, Jones PD. (1992). Successful treatment of human virus-associated Reiter's syndrome with sulphasalazine. *Arthritis Rheumatol* **35**: 723–4.

Cardiovascular disease and HIV infection

15

ANURADHA AGGARWAL

Involvement of the cardiovascular system in human immunodeficiency virus infection is a clinically important problem. Autopsy and echocardiographic series have revealed a cardiac abnormality in over half of those examined (Anderson et al., 1988; Levy et al., 1989; Akhras et al., 1994; Patel and Frishman, 1996). After reviewing published US and European reports of HIV-related cardiac disease, Anderson and Virmani (1990) concluded that 6–7% of HIV-infected patients had symptomatic cardiac disease and that 95% of these had a prior diagnosis of acquired immunodeficiency syndrome. Furthermore, in autopsy series of patients who had died of AIDS between 1981 and 1985, 1.1% were found to have had cardiac cause of death. Similar series between 1986 and 1988 noted this to be 6.3% (Anderson and Virmani, 1990).

Since the first case of Kaposi's sarcoma affecting the heart was published in 1983 (Autran et al., 1983), there has been increasing recognition of cardiovascular complications. This apparent increase in incidence may reflect a heightened awareness by treating physicians, coupled with increased use of echocardiography, or it may reflect a change in HIV disease expression, which has been modified by antiretroviral and other adjunctive therapies, resulting in a dramatic increase in life expectancy. Palella et al. (1998) reported a decline in mortality in HIV infection from 29.4 per 100 person years in 1995 to 8.8 per 100 person years in 1997.

While there are several unresolved issues regarding the pathogenetic processes and the true incidence of cardiovascular abnormality, a number of generalizations (Herskowitz et al., 1994) can be made (Table 15.1). Although varying in incidence and severity, all cardiac structures and the pulmonary vasculature may be involved in HIV/AIDS (Table 15.2).

Table 15.1 Important generalizations regarding cardiovascular disease in HIV-infected patients

- The most common serious clinical manifestations of HIV-related cardiovascular involvement are congestive cardiac failure secondary to cardiomyopathy, and cardiac tamponade due to a pericardial effusion
- Asymptomatic left ventricular dysfunction and small pericardial effusions are common findings at autopsy or on echocardiography in HIV-infected patients and usually lead to no direct sequelae
- A cardiovascular cause of death in HIV infection remains uncommon
- Cardiac abnormalities occur in all risk groups of patients with HIV infection
- The incidence of cardiac pathology increases in the later stages of HIV infection
- A high index of suspicion needs to be present in order to diagnose cardiac pathology

Table 15.2 Overview of HIV-related cardiac disease

Myocardium
   Myocarditis
   Lymphocytic infiltrate without necrosis
   Myocyte necrosis without inflammation
   Dilated cardiomyopathy
Pericardium
   Pericarditis
   Effusion (cardiac tamponade)
Valves
   Non-bacterial thrombotic endocarditis (NBTE)
   Infectious endocarditis
Pulmonary vasculature
   Pulmonary hypertension
   Isolated right heart dilatation/failure
Accelerated atherosclerotic disease
Cardiac neoplasm
Arrhythmia

Myocardial disease

Myocarditis

The Dallas criteria are commonly used to define myocarditis and state that this condition is a 'process characterized by an inflammatory infiltrate of the myocardium with necrosis and degeneration of adjacent myocytes not typical of the ischemic damage associated with coronary artery disease' (Aretz *et al.*, 1987). Investigators examining the incidence of myocarditis in HIV infection have used somewhat modified definitions to that given above, including non-specific inflammatory infiltrates without myocyte damage or necrosis. The most commonly reported pattern of HIV-related myocarditis has been the latter definition (Anderson *et al.*, 1988). Another common pattern is isolated myocardial necrosis without inflammatory changes (Anderson and Virmani, 1990). The use of lymphocytic infiltration as a marker for myocarditis may be insensitive in this population because of accompanying lymphopenia. Herskowitz and colleagues (1994) have noted that in the absence of any histological criteria for myocarditis, a significant proportion of HIV-infected patients with cardiac disease had immunohistological evidence (e.g. increased expression of major histocompatibility class 1 antigen) of myocardial inflammation.

Hansen and colleagues (1992) found that myocarditis, according to the Dallas criteria, was present in 42% of 60 consecutive autopsies of patients with AIDS. Diffuse myocardial fibrosis was observed in 67% of the cases. The authors hypothesized that myocardium damaged by myocarditis resulting in diffuse fibrosis may undergo some degree of compensatory hypertrophy and dilatation, eventually resulting in dilated cardiomyopathy (Hansen, 1992). In a review of the HIV autopsy literature, the prevalence of 'myocarditis' was 33% of 656 autopsies conducted (Michaels *et al.*, 1997).

Cardiomyopathy

In 1986, Cohen and colleagues reported the first cases of fatal, dilated cardiomyopathy in three patients with AIDS (Cohen *et al.*, 1986). Since then, there have been numerous echocardiographic series examining the prevalence and incidence of this condition. Dilated cardiomyopathy is defined as a condition characterized by dilatation of both ventricular cavities and an increase in the weight of the heart, without any evidence of coronary artery disease, or of valvular heart disease, and with left ventricular hypo-

kinesia (ejection fraction less than 45%) (Roberts *et al.*, 1987). In a review of echocardiographic studies, the prevalence of left ventricular dysfunction in HIV disease was 103/484 (21%). Less than half of these patients went on to develop symptoms (Michaels *et al.*, 1997). Severe cardiac dysfunction occurs late in the course of HIV infection and therefore, with continuing improvement in prophylaxis and treatment of opportunistic infections and in antiretroviral therapies, more patients are likely to survive to develop such non-infectious complications (Levy *et al.*, 1989; Barbaro *et al.*, 1998a; Patel and Frishman, 1995).

In a prospective study, the prevalence of left ventricular (LV) hypokinesia was 14.5%, with an incidence of 18% per patient-year (Herskowitz *et al.*, 1993a). This contrasts with the annual incidence of cardiomyopathy in the USA of between 0.7 and 7.5 per 100 000 (Abelman, 1985). In the above-mentioned study, the incidence and prevalence of LV dysfunction was greater in the group with low CD4 lymphocyte counts. There was no significant difference between injecting drug users and those who did not use parenteral drugs. In a separate study of HIV-uninfected injecting drug users (Willoughby *et al.*, 1993), the prevalence of LV dysfunction was 1.2%, so that injecting drug usage *per se* would not seem to confer any increase in risk of development of dilated cardiomyopathy. Barbaro and colleagues (1998a) followed 952 asymptomatic HIV-infected patients over a period of 5 years and made an echocardiographic diagnosis of dilated cardiomyopathy in 8%. All of these patients developed symptoms of cardiac failure.

While severe, symptomatic cardiac dysfunction appears to occur late in the course of HIV infection, investigators have also demonstrated evidence of systolic dysfunction in asymptomatic subjects who are at an early stage of their HIV infection (Cardoso *et al.*, 1998a). In a large cohort study, echocardiograms were performed on 1236 asymptomatic HIV-infected patients who were functionally in category New York Heart Association Class 1, and findings were compared with those of 1230 matched healthy subjects. There was a significant reduction in the LV ejection fraction in the HIV-infected patients, compared with the control group. The prevalence of cardiac abnormalities was not correlated to the risk factor for HIV infection (Barbaro *et al.*, 1996a).

There is a broad spectrum in the severity of the dilated form of cardiomyopathy in HIV infection. It may be asymptomatic and present only echocardiographically; in these situations, it may resolve spontaneously and does not correlate with low CD4 lymphocyte counts (Currie *et al.*, 1994;

Herskowitz, 1996). There is a chronic presentation of LV dysfunction, which may be quite amenable to conventional heart failure therapy (Herskowitz, 1996). Most dramatically, severe global LV systolic dysfunction may be associated with fulminant cardiac failure, which is difficult to treat. The patients in this latter group tend to have a low CD4 lymphocyte count and more than 50% die from cardiac failure within 6–12 months of presentation (Currie et al., 1994; Patel and Frishman, 1995; Barbaro et al., 1998a). De Castro and colleagues (1994) found that 5.1% of patients developed clinical and echocardiographic findings of acute, severe global LV systolic dysfunction without LV dilatation. All of these patients had AIDS. The patients generally died of irreversible cardiac failure and autopsy showed acute myocarditis according to the Dallas criteria (De Castro et al., 1994). Others have also described the echocardiographic finding of LV diastolic dysfunction in the presence of normal systolic function. The clinical significance of this remains unclear (Cardoso et al., 1998a; Coudray et al., 1995).

Association between myocarditis and cardiomyopathy in HIV

In the Myocarditis Treatment Trial (Mason et al., 1995), 2233 non-HIV-infected patients with symptomatic LV global dysfunction underwent endomyocardial biopsy of the right ventricle. The prevalence of myocarditis, as defined by the Dallas criteria, was 10%. In contrast, autopsy and endomyocardial biopsy series of HIV-related cardiomyopathy have found a much higher prevalence of myocarditis. Herskowitz and colleagues (1994) reported that 51% of patients with symptomatic heart failure had evidence of myocarditis and another series concluded that myocarditis was present in all cases of LV dilatation and in all of those who died of congestive cardiac failure (Anderson et al., 1988; De Castro et al., 1994). In the study by Barbaro et al., (1998a), a histological diagnosis of myocarditis was made in 83% of cases of dilated cardiomyopathy. Reilly and colleagues (1988) evaluated 58 consecutive AIDS patients at autopsy and found that patients with myocarditis had a significantly higher incidence of symptomatic LV dysfunction than patients without myocarditis.

Pathogenesis of myocardial disease in HIV infection

The pathogenesis of myocarditis/dilated cardiomyopathy in HIV infection is uncertain. In a review by Kaul and

colleagues (1991), an opportunistic pathogen was identified in only 20% of patients with myocarditis. The following mechanisms for pathogenesis have been put forward.

HIV infection of the myocyte

It has not been established whether myocytes are the actual target cells for HIV and whether the virus is capable of replicating in the human cardiac myocyte. Myocardial cells lack the CD4 receptor, but Herskowitz and colleagues (1993b) have shown, in vitro, that a human fetal cardiac cell line can ingest HIV-1 using the Fc receptor. HIV transcripts in the cardiomyocyte have been demonstrated by various techniques, such as in situ hybridization, polymerase chain reaction (PCR), and southern blot. However, the significance of this is unclear, as HIV has been demonstrated in cardiac tissues from patients with and without cardiac disease. Rodriguez and colleagues (1991) used the technique of microdissection to show the presence of HIV sequences in myocytes of two of five patients with, and six of 10 without myocardial disease. Grody and colleagues (1990) demonstrated HIV nucleic acid sequences in myocytes of six of 22 patients using in situ hybridization on cardiac tissue obtained at autopsy. In these cases, there was no evidence of myocarditis or cardiomyopathy. However, another group failed to identify HIV genomic material by in situ hybridization in endomyocardial biopsy samples taken from patients with myocarditis and established cardiac failure (Beshorner et al., 1990).

In contrast, Herskowitz and colleagues (1994) showed that all patients who had positive in-situ hybridization for HIV-1 had histological and/or immunohistological evidence (induction of MHC class 1 antigen) of myocarditis. Specific myocyte hybridization was absent in those biopsy samples that had no evidence of myocarditis, but the majority of patients with myocarditis did not show positive hybridization findings. Furthermore, when specific hybridization was shown, it was found in rare, isolated myocytes. An autopsy series of 440 AIDS patients had more impressive findings. Of the 29 autopsy patients classified as demonstrating myocarditis, 25 had HIV nucleic acid sequences detectable in myocytes by in-situ hybridization (Barbaro et al., 1998b). However, as with the findings of Herskowitz and colleagues (1994) and others, the affected myocytes were sparse and not surrounded by inflammatory cells.

Thus, while the presence of HIV-1 within myocytes can be demonstrated in HIV-associated myocarditis, a direct pathogenic role of the virus has not yet been established (Barbaro *et al.*, 1998a).

Co-infection with other cardiotropic viruses

The common finding in AIDS of a monoclonal inflammatory myocardial infiltrate would suggest a viral or an auto-immune aetiology. Cytomegalovirus (CMV) is one of the most common opportunistic pathogens in AIDS, with its histological characteristic of intranuclear inclusion bodies. A lytic form of CMV infection of the heart with concurrent myocarditis has rarely been described in AIDS (Niedt and Schinella, 1985). The more common finding is the demonstration of the presence of CMV in the myocyte by *in-situ* hybridization, without the presence of inclusion bodies (Wu *et al.*, 1992). Herskowitz and colleagues (1994) found evidence for such latent infection, either alone or with HIV, in the hearts of patients who had histological and/or immunohistochemical evidence for myocarditis. However, infection was not demonstrated in the absence of myocarditis (Herskowitz *et al.*, 1994).

As mentioned earlier, a frequent finding at autopsy in AIDS cases is isolated myocardial necrosis in the absence of an inflammatory infiltrate. It is well-established that CMV infection can cause tissue necrosis without inflammation, providing a potential explanation of necrosis in the absence of an inflammatory infiltrate (Acierno, 1989). Necrosis may result from induction of CD8 lymphocytes in response to virus-infected myocytes expressing endogenous viral peptides in association with MHC Class 1 antigens.

Coxsackie B virus, the most common cause of non-AIDS myocarditis, has been linked to AIDS-related myocarditis in isolated case reports (Dittrich *et al.*, 1988).

Cytokine-mediated damage

Ho and colleagues (1987) proposed the model of 'innocent bystander destruction' in their explanation for the observed neuroglial cell damage in HIV-associated encephalopathy. As a corollary, authors have postulated that HIV-infected mononuclear cells release cytokines that are locally active and damaging to the myocyte (Wright *et al.*, 1988). TNF-α, interleukin-1 and interleukin-2 have been demonstrated to be elevated in HIV- and non-HIV-related cardiac failure (Lange and Schreiner, 1994; Herskowitz *et al.*, 1995). Animal studies have demonstrated that these cytokines have negative inotropic properties (Lange and Schreiner, 1994).

Auto-immunity

Various autoantibodies, for example to heavy-chain myosin and mitochondrial adenine nucleotide translocator (ANT), have been reported to occur in non-HIV and HIV-related cardiomyopathy (Kaul *et al.*, 1991; Lange and Schreiner, 1994). Patients who are HIV-infected but who do not have a cardiomyopathy do not have evidence of these autoantibodies (Kaul *et al.*, 1991; Lange and Schreiner, 1994). It is not clear whether these autoantibodies are pathogenic or an epiphenomenon. In support of an immunologically mediated mechanism is the observation that impaired myocardial growth and LV dysfunction in children with HIV can respond to the administration of intravenous immunoglobulin therapy (Lipshultz *et al.*, 1995).

Specific non-viral pathogens

It is unusual to find a specific opportunistic pathogen (Kaul *et al.*, 1991). When one is identified, it is usually in the setting of a disseminated process (Milei *et al.*, 1998). The most common non-viral organism to produce myocardial disease is *Toxoplasma gondii* (Michaels *et al.*, 1997). The heart is the most common extracerebral site of infection with this protozoan. It is important to note that the frequency of cardiac toxoplasmosis correlates closely with the prevalence of toxoplasmosis in the general population. It is markedly higher in southern Europe than in the USA. In a series of 182 autopsies of AIDS-related deaths performed in France between 1987 and 1991, evidence of cardiac toxoplasmosis was found in 21 patients (12%) (Hofman *et al.*, 1993). Myocardial lesions were generally asymptomatic and were not discovered until autopsy. Cardiac involvement was the cause of death in six of the 21 patients. The suggested lesions could arise when prophylaxis for toxoplasmosis was withdrawn, for example, because of drug toxicity. While the authors recommend the commencement of treatment for toxoplasmosis in patients who develop sudden heart failure from an area with a high prevalence of this parasite, only rare cases of successful treatment in AIDS have been documented (Grange *et al.*, 1990; Albrecht *et al.*, 1994).

Cryptococcal myocarditis has been described in the presence of a systemic infection. In a report of two cases, cardiac cryptococcosis was associated with cardiac failure with improvement in cardiac function after 1 week of anti-fungal treatment (Kinney *et al.*, 1989). Mycobacterial involvement of the myocardium appears to be extremely rare (Acierno, 1989).

Drugs

Alcohol and cocaine (Chokshi *et al.*, 1989) are well-established cardiomyopathic agents, and their abuse could contribute to a cardiomyopathy.

With the extensive range of supportive drug treatments used in the treatment of HIV infection, it is not surprising that hypersensitivity myocarditis with an eosinophilic infiltrate has been described. After withdrawal of the offending agent, cardiac function returns to normal (Herskowitz *et al.*, 1994).

Zidovudine (ZDV) has been implicated as a cause of myocardial damage. It is known to deplete the cell of mitochondrial DNA and has been shown to cause a cardiomyopathy in rats (Lewis *et al.*, 1991) and a skeletal myopathy in humans (Dalakas *et al.*, 1990). In a report of six patients who had cardiac dysfunction while on ZDV, didanosine (ddI) and zalcitabine, a significant improvement was seen in cardiac function after cessation of these agents (Herskowitz *et al.*, 1992). When antiretroviral treatment was re-introduced in some cases, recurrence of LV dysfunction was demonstrated. These authors recommend withdrawal of the nucleoside analogues in the setting of heart failure, and if the agents are re-introduced, that this be done under close supervision at a lower dose. In a retrospective study of 137 HIV-infected children, there was a strong association between the use of ZDV and the development of cardiomyopathy. The use of ddI was not associated with cardiomyopathy (Domanski *et al.*, 1995). However, the evidence against ZDV is by no means certain. In a smaller study, ZDV did not worsen or ameliorate cardiac dysfunction in a prospective comparison of two groups of children with and without this treatment (Lipshultz *et al.*, 1992).

A reversible congestive cardiomyopathy associated with the administration of interferon-α, used in the treatment of Kaposi's sarcoma, has also been described (Deyton *et al.*, 1989). Cardiomyopathy is a well-recognized dose-related effect of doxorubicin, used for treatment of AIDS-related lymphomas (Singal and Iliskovic, 1998).

Nutritional deficiency

HIV infection in its terminal stages is marked by anorexia and cachexia. Specific nutritional deficiencies, (of vitamin B and selenium, for example) can arise. Investigators have demonstrated low selenium levels in the cardiac tissue of patients with AIDS (Milei *et al.*, 1998). There is good evidence that such deficiencies can cause cardiomyopathy in the HIV-uninfected population (Patel and Frishman, 1995; 1996).

Pericardial disease

The pericardium is a common site of cardiac involvement in HIV infection. Indeed, the leading diagnosis associated with pericardiocentesis in urban American hospitals is AIDS (Eisenberg *et al.*, 1992; Flum *et al.*, 1995). The prevalence of pericardial effusions varies according to the population considered: pericardial effusions are much more common when a hospitalized, ill population is being examined than when an outpatient cohort is being studied. A review of available studies suggested a cumulative prevalence of 23% (Kaul *et al.*, 1991).

Pericardial effusions increase in frequency as the course of HIV infection approaches its terminal stages (Michaels *et al.*, 1997). The effusion itself is rarely a cause of death; rather, it appears to be an epiphenomenon of impending death. Most effusions are asymptomatic. When symptoms do occur, they are commonly dyspnoea and peripheral oedema (Herskowitz, 1996). An episode of clinical pericarditis is rare (Heidenreich *et al.*, 1995). Cardiac tamponade, the most dramatic presentation, occurs much less commonly than an asymptomatic effusion (Michaels *et al.*, 1997).

A prospective echocardiographic study of 231 ambulant subjects was performed over a 5-year period. Only those with AIDS at entry had the finding of an effusion on the initial echocardiogram, and the prevalence in this group overall was 5%. Thirteen subjects developed effusions during follow-up; 12 of these subjects had AIDS. The incidence of developing an effusion in AIDS patients was 11% per year. The survival for AIDS patients with effusions was significantly shorter (36% at 6 months) than survival for AIDS subjects without effusions (93% at 6 months). The effusion itself was not the cause of death. Eighty per cent of the effusions were small; only 6% were large. Eighty seven per cent were asymptomatic. The incidence of tamponade for AIDS subjects with effusion was 9% per year and for all AIDS subjects, 1% per year. Effusions were seen to resolve spontaneously in 13% of cases (Heidenreich *et al.*, 1995) (see Figure 15.1), but Blanchard and colleagues (1991) have reported a much higher rate of spontaneous resolution (Blanchard *et al.*, 1991).

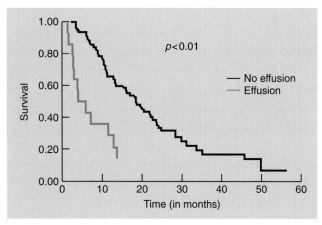

Figure 15.1 *Survival of AIDS patients by presence or absence of effusion.*

Table 15.3 Causes of pericardial effusion in AIDS

Bacteria
Staphylococcus aureus
Streptococcus pneumoniae
Listera monocytogenes
Nocardia asteroides
Chlamydia trachomatis
Rhodococcus equi
Mycobacteria
Mycobacterium tuberculosis
Mycobacterium avium complex (MAC)
Mycobacterium kansasii
Fungi
Histoplasma capsulatum
Cryptococcus neoformans
Protozoa
Toxoplasma gondii
Viral
Cytomegalovirus (CMV)
Herpes simplex
Malignancy
Kaposi's sarcoma
Non-Hodgkin's lymphoma
Adenocarcinoma
Metabolic
Uraemia
Hypoalbuminaemia
Capillary leak syndrome

While there are numerous case reports of pathogens causing a pericardial effusion, the majority are idiopathic and examination of the fluid and/or pericardial tissue is rarely enlightening (Table 15.3). There is no conclusive evidence to date to implicate HIV in a direct pathogenetic role. The fluid generally tends to be exudative. In an autopsy series of 115 patients with AIDS, Lewis (1989) found that no cause could be identified in all 35 patients with pericardial effusions. Zakowski and Ianuale-Shanerman (1993) examined effusions in 14 AIDS patients and biopsies in 10 of 14 of the patients. Two patients demonstrated a malignancy (lymphoma where a previous lymphoma diagnosis had been made); no cause was found in the remaining 87%.

A retrospective review of data on 29 patients with AIDS who had undergone the creation of a 'pericardial window' for management of pericardial effusions revealed that 24% of culture or biopsy specimens were diagnostic – adenocarcinoma (two), lymphoma (three), *S. aureus* (one), *M. tuberculosis* (one). However, there was no change in clinical management based on the operative findings in 94% of cases (Flum *et al.*, 1995). In Africa, *M. tuberculosis* accounts for the majority of the large and symptomatic effusions in AIDS patients (Cegielski *et al.*, 1990). Effusions caused by this organism tend to be larger, are more likely to be symptomatic, and more likely to require drainage.

The capillary leak syndrome has been proposed as a mechanism for the formation of an effusion, in the absence of an overt aetiology. Heidenreich and colleagues (1995) made the observation that there is frequent co-existence of serous pleural effusions, ascites and pericardial effusion. It has already been documented that cytokines such as TNF-

α and interleukin-2 are increased in HIV infection. These have been shown to induce a capillary leak syndrome in septic patients (Heidenreich *et al.*, 1995). Thus, this hypothesis may explain why, in the heightened cytokine activity seen in end-stage HIV infection, there is increased frequency of effusions that are associated with a poor prognosis, and in which a specific causative pathogen is not found.

Endocarditis

Infective endocarditis in HIV infection is usually related to the underlying risk factor. It is almost exclusively found in the injecting drug user (IDU) and is rare in the other risk groups (Currie *et al.*, 1995). In one of the earliest studies, the most common endocardial lesion seen with HIV infection was non-bacterial thrombotic endocarditis (NBTE), or marantic endocarditis (Cammarsono and Lewis, 1985). However, subsequent investigators have not noted such a high prevalence of this form of endocarditis, and it is possible that its prevalence may have been overestimated in the past. No evidence of NBTE was found in a series of 110 autopsies conducted on subjects from all major risk groups and at various stages of immune deficiency (Currie *et al.*, 1995). Endocarditis in HIV patients is usually bacterial (De Castro *et al.*, 1992). In North America, where homosexually acquired HIV predominates, endocarditis is uncommon. However, in southern Europe, where 75% of HIV-infected patients are IDU, endocarditis is more common. In a prospective echocardiographic study, infective endocarditis was diagnosed in five of 72 patients (6.9%) (De Castro *et al.*, 1992).

Staphylococcus aureus is the usual pathogen, as is the case in HIV-uninfected IDUs with endocarditis. In an autopsy series, cardiac involvement was examined in patients with a history of IDU with or without AIDS. The incidence of infective endocarditis (IE) was 5% in patients with AIDS and 87% in patients without AIDS. While such a study needs to be interpreted with caution, as it pre-selects patients with a fatal outcome, it would appear that HIV infection does not confer a special vulnerability for the development of infective endocarditis (Roberts *et al.*, 1989).

To address the question as to whether HIV infection alters the course of infective endocarditis, Vemuri and colleagues (1990) examined two groups of hospitalized patients with infective endocarditis, with and without co-existing HIV infection. In this study, the in-hospital mortality was not altered by the HIV status. However, evidence of LV dysfunction, in the presence of equivalent valvular involvement, was more frequent in the HIV-infected group, suggesting an HIV-related cardiomyopathy (Vemuri *et al.*, 1990). Similarly, Currie *et al.* (1995) concluded that asymptomatic HIV infection does not confer a particular susceptibility to the development of, or mortality from infective endocarditis (Currie *et al.*, 1995). However, IE was more rapidly progressive in the late stages of AIDS (Nahass *et al.*, 1990).

Pulmonary hypertension

Pulmonary hypertension is observed in HIV infection in the setting of lung pathology such as infection with *Pneumocystis carinii*, or in the absence of an apparent underlying cause. Kim and Factor (1987), were the first to describe the association between HIV infection and pulmonary hypertension and to date, there have been 88 reported cases. A review of these cases (Mesa *et al.*, 1998) showed a male predominance (61%). This is different from the female gender bias seen in non-HIV-related primary pulmonary hypertension, but one must remember that males constitute the vast majority of persons with HIV infection. Dyspnoea was the most common symptom (Mesa *et al.*, 1998). The mean systolic pressure was 68 mmHg. In 83% of the cases, no underlying cause, other than HIV infection, was found. This has led some investigators to include it in the syndrome of primary pulmonary hypertension (PPH) (Opravil *et al.*, 1997). The development of pulmonary hypertension (PH) is another example, along with pericardial effusions and cardiomyopathy, of the increased incidence of non-infectious complications due to longer survival and better prophylaxis against opportunistic infections in HIV infection.

The prevalence of pulmonary hypertension has been recorded as one in 200 (six of 1200 patients) by two investigators (Himelman *et al.*, 1989; Speich *et al.*, 1991). This observed rate for pulmonary hypertension is markedly higher than that which occurs in the general population (one in 200 000) (Petitpretz *et al.*, 1994). There appears to be no correlation between the degree of immunosuppression and the development of PH (Opravil *et al.*, 1997; Mesa *et al.*, 1998). It has been described in all major HIV risk groups (Mesa *et al.*, 1998). IDU *per se* appears unlikely to cause PH. Unless the individual is injecting crushed oral medications, the risk of developing foreign-body granulomas that could eventually lead to PH does not occur (Tomashefski and Hirsch, 1980). Another mechanism previously proposed has been that factor VIII infusions for haemophiliac patients may be linked to the subsequent development of PH. However, there is a scarcity of reports of PH in haemophiliacs not also infected with HIV (Mette *et al.*, 1992). Chronic liver disease with portal hypertension can also cause pulmonary hypertension. Of the total of 88 patients described, 13 (15%) have had concurrent hepatitis or cirrhosis (Mesa *et al.*, 1998).

The observed changes seen in HIV-related PH are generally indistinguishable from HIV-uninfected primary PH. The majority of patients demonstrate plexogenic pulmonary arteriopathy. The histopathological changes are confined to the precapillary muscular pulmonary arterioles with medial hypertrophy, fibroelastosis, and eccentric intimal fibrosis. Pulmonary veno-occlusive disease and PH secondary to recurrent emboli have been reported in a minority of cases (Mesa *et al.*, 1998).

It appears that, in most cases, HIV infection is the cause of PH. As with cardiomyopathy, this does not seem to be a result of direct pulmonary vascular infection. Rather, the 'innocent bystander' mechanism seems the most likely. Cytokines such as TNF-α, epidermal growth factor and platelet-derived growth factor have been implicated in the pathogenesis of this condition. Further, investigators have demonstrated that gp-120, an HIV envelope glycoprotein, stimulates the production of endothelin-1, a powerful pulmonary vasoconstrictor (Mesa et al., 1998). An autoimmune mechanism has also been postulated, with the finding that there is an increased incidence of certain HLA types in these patients (Morse et al., 1996).

In 63 of the 88 cases reviewed by Mesa et al. (1998), the 1-year survival rate was 51%. This compares with a 1-year survival rate of 68% for patients with non-HIV-related primary PH. Of the 38 fatal cases, death was directly due to the consequences of the PH (right heart failure, or respiratory failure) in 76% of cases (Mesa et al., 1998).

Opravil et al. (1997) prospectively followed 19 HIV-infected patients with PH. They utilized the non-invasive, echocardiographic approach to the assessment of pulmonary artery pressure. They found that antiretroviral treatment exerted a beneficial effect on the course of PH. Only those patients not treated with these agents showed continuous increases in the pressure gradient; ZDV or ddI seemed to halt the progress of PH (Opravil et al., 1997).

Thus, PH joins cardiomyopathy and pericardial effusions as a non-infectious cause of dyspnoea in the HIV-infected patient. Conversely, testing for HIV antibodies would appear advisable when a patient presents with these conditions and when there is no other aetiology apparent.

Premature atherosclerotic disease

The incidence of myocardial infarction in HIV-infected persons has increased since the introduction of HAART (Rickerts et al., 2001). Constans et al. (1997) reported that the lipid profile of HIV-infected patients, even early in the course of the disease, is atherogenic, with a reduction in high-density-lipoprotein cholesterol, and an increase in triglycerides and lipoprotein(a).

Until recently, the prognosis for people with HIV infection was so poor that concern about long-term sequelae was not a priority. With the advent of protease inhibitors (PIs), a dramatic improvement in prognosis has occurred, with declining morbidity and mortality in patients with advanced HIV infection (Carpenter et al., 1997). However, since the introduction of these PIs in 1996, an unexpected syndrome of vascular and lipid derangement has been described (see Chapter 18; also reviewed in Mooser and Carr, 2001). The syndrome consists of lipodystrophy, in which there is redistribution of fat from the limbs to the trunk, resulting in abnormal fat deposits in the abdomen and the formation of a 'buffalo hump'; insulin resistance; and, of most concern, the development of marked hypercholesterolaemia and hypertriglyceridaemia (SoRelle, 1998). It is with particular respect to this last abnormality that the onset of premature coronary artery disease may be attributed. While a strong association between this syndrome and the use of PIs is apparent, the mechanism is obscure: how does an agent that interferes with the final stages of the viral life cycle cause these metabolic derangements?

Susceptibility to the development of this syndrome depends on the duration of therapy with the PI (usually more than 1 year) and the type of PI. Ritonavir is most likely to be associated with this disturbance (SoRelle, 1998).

In a review of the 124 patients on PIs in their HIV clinic, Henry et al. (1998) found that 41 (31%) had hyperlipidaemia. Carr and colleagues (1998) noted that before the commencement of a PI, 59% of their patients had normal lipid values; after the treatment had begun, only 7% had normal values. In non-HIV-infected people, the levels of lipids found in this syndrome are associated with risk of angina and stroke. At this stage, it is difficult to quantify the extent of the problem in the HIV-infected population. However, an increasing number of case reports, describing acute ischemic coronary syndromes in HIV-infected patients treated with PIs, is being reported (Behrens et al., 1998; Gallet et al., 1998; Henry et al., 1998; Vittecoq et al., 1998; Depairon et al., 2001).

Aside from a metabolic basis for the development of premature atherosclerotic disease, there is also speculation on the role of an infective mechanism. There is evidence that chronic infections with such organisms as Chlamydia pneumoniae, CMV, and Helicobacter pylori, in the immunocompetent host, may be related to the development of coronary artery disease (Danesh et al., 1997; Siscovick et al., 2000). Using echoduplex, Constans (1997) found that HIV-infected patients more often had plaques in the carotid, iliac, or femoral arteries than HIV-uninfected matched controls. They, therefore, proposed that HIV-1 infection should be added to the list of infective agents that could be important in the development of atherosclerosis

(Constans, 1997). With HIV infection, as with CMV and *H. pylori*, von Willebrand factor is raised. There are other markers suggestive of endothelial dysfunction, such as elevation in thrombomodulin. In addition, the disease is also characterized by a systemic inflammatory state, as reflected by increased concentrations of cytokines such as TNF-α. These factors may play a role in the occurrence of ischemic events (Constans, 1997).

Cardiac neoplasm

Kaposi's sarcoma and non-Hodgkin's lymphoma are well known to involve the heart in patients with AIDS. This is usually in association with a systemic process, although isolated involvement of the heart is described. Kaposi's sarcoma involves the heart in 20% of patients at autopsy. However, this rarely produces significant clinical manifestations. Pericardial effusion with tamponade has been reported. Most often, the epicardium and pericardium are involved; infiltration of all layers of the myocardium is rarely described (Michaels *et al.*, 1997).

Non-Hodgkin's lymphoma in AIDS is usually of the B-cell-type, and the heart is generally involved in a systemic process. Chronic B-cell stimulation triggered by the Epstein-Barr virus and unchecked by T-helper lymphocytes has been suggested as a cause of cardiac lymphomas. Most of these lymphomas are high grade. In some cases, the Epstein-Barr virus genome may be demonstrated in the proliferating cells (Patel and Frishman, 1996). There may be diffuse infiltration of the myocardium, with the heart appearing large and pale. Resultant cardiac failure and conduction abnormalities are described. The other histological pattern of involvement is of the appearance of focal nodules in the epicardium, myocardium, and endocardium. Intra-cardiac masses, producing obstruction to flow, may also form. Pericardial involvement leading to tamponade is also rarely described. The involvement of the heart is probably silent in the majority of patients (Michaels *et al.*, 1997).

Arrhythmia

Involvement of the autonomic nervous system in HIV infection has been described from the beginning of the HIV epidemic, with reports of orthostatic hypotension, syncope, cardiac arrest, and urinary and bowel disturbance. Villa *et al.*, (1995) found that many of their HIV-infected patients had evidence of an autonomic neuropathy when tested non-invasively with techniques such as heart-rate variation during deep breathing. This finding correlated with a prolongation of the QT interval on the electrocardiograph (ECG). QT prolongation is a well-established risk factor for the development of ventricular tachyarrhythmias. If drugs that further prolong the QT interval are introduced in these individuals, there is an increased risk of sudden cardiac death.

Intravenous pentamidine therapy, has been associated with prolongation of the QT interval and the resultant occurrence of ventricular arrhythmias, especially Torsade de Pointes (TdP). In a prospective, open, non-randomized trial, the incidence of QT prolongation and TdP with the use of intravenous pentamidine was examined (Eisenhauer *et al.*, 1994). They studied 14 patients undergoing treatment for *Pneumocystis carinii*; all had normal baseline QT intervals. They were followed with daily ECGs for the duration of the pentamidine therapy. Five of this group developed significant QT prolongation; three of the five had TdP and one died of the arrhythmia. The development of the arrhythmia was independent of a co-existing cardiomyopathy; no serum electrolyte abnormality was recorded (Eisenhauer *et al.*, 1994). In a more recent study, Girgis *et al.*, (1997) found that QT prolongation with intravenous pentamidine was relatively uncommon. In 16 consecutive HIV-infected patients treated with pentamidine, there was no significant increase in QT interval and no significant increase in ventricular arrhythmias compared to premedication data or compared to therapy with trimethoprim-sulphamethoxazole (TMP-SMX). It is somewhat difficult to reconcile such diverse findings. The methods used in these two studies are different and both studies were relatively small, making it difficult to draw definitive conclusions. At present, it seems prudent to perform baseline ECGs and subsequent, daily ECGs on patients undergoing treatment with intravenous pentamidine. Concurrent factors that may prolong the QT interval, such as hypokalaemia and hypomagnesaemia, should be eliminated. If prolongation of the rate-corrected QT interval of greater than 480 ms is found, intravenous pentamidine should be discontinued or administered under continuous ECG monitoring. Ventricular arrhythmias with inhaled pentamidine have not been described.

Diagnosis of cardiovascular disease

While the reason for dyspnoea in an HIV-infected patient is likely to be an opportunistic infection of the lungs in the vast majority of cases, a cardiac pathology should also be borne in mind. Pericardial effusions, LV systolic dysfunction, and primary pulmonary hypertension may be explanations for the symptom and their presence should be actively sought when a more obvious cause is not apparent. An elevation in the jugular venous pressure, pulmonary oedema, a displaced apex beat and an S3 gallop are important clinical signs of a dilated cardiomyopathy. Pulmonary hypertension may lead to the findings of isolated right ventricular failure with peripheral oedema, in the absence of pulmonary congestion (Cardoso et al., 1998b). A chest X-ray can reveal an enlarged cardiac shadow consistent with an effusion or a dilated cardiomyopathy. Trans-thoracic echocardiography (TTE) has become an invaluable tool in examining cardiovascular involvement in the HIV infection (see Figure 15.2). It will provide information about ventricular function, the presence of pericardial effusions and whether the effusion is producing cardiac tamponade. It can also accurately determine the pulmonary artery pressure in most subjects. If the pulmonary artery pressure cannot be determined non-invasively, right heart catheterization may be undertaken. Lesions suggestive of endocarditis with any resultant derangement in valvular function will also be demonstrated by an echocardiogram. If, after a TTE study, there is still clinical suspicion of endocarditis, a trans-oesophageal study may be undertaken. This technique will detect vegetations as small as 2 mm in diameter. However, it is not possible to reliably distinguish infective from non-bacterial thrombotic endocarditis echocardiographically.

An ECG is rarely useful in diagnosing cardiovascular involvement in HIV infection. It is, however, important to perform an ECG prior to the commencement of, and for the duration of intravenous pentamidine therapy, with particular attention to the QT interval. An ECG should also be obtained, along with a baseline lipid profile, prior to the commencement of therapy with PIs, in order to detect any evidence of coronary ischaemia.

In a retrospective analysis of Holter electrocardiographic recordings, Barbaro et al. (1996b) found that the occurrence of ventricular ectopic activity could be correlated with the presence of HIV-related myocarditis (Barbaro

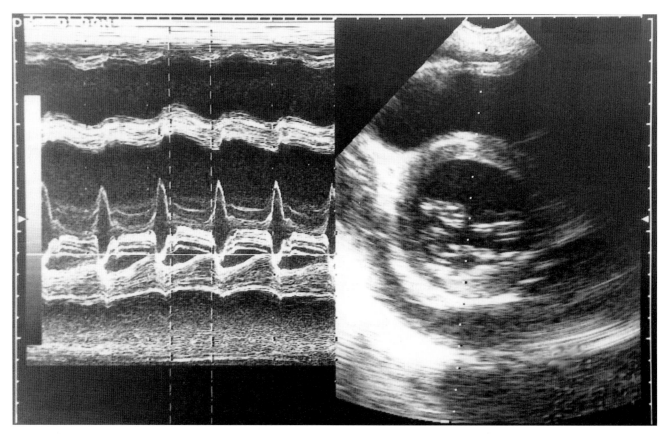

Figure 15.2 *Transthoracic 2D and M-mode usage showing a dilated hypokinetic left ventricle in a patient with AIDS who presented with left ventricular failure.*

et al., 1996b). The clinical utility of this observation remains uncertain. Right ventricular endomyocardial biopsies carry a significant mortality (0.4% in one meta-analysis) (Hrobon *et al.*, 1998) and are not justified in the investigation of LV systolic dysfunction in HIV. While there is a high prevalence of myocarditis in such cases, a specific pathogen responsible for this is rarely present, and it would be unusual to find information that leads to a change in management and outcome. Pericardiocentesis should be undertaken for relief of cardiac tamponade; however, drainage of asymptomatic effusions and pericardial biopsies are not justified, as the diagnostic yield and the likelihood of changing management on the basis of the findings is low.

The continued use of nucleoside analogues in patients with a cardiomyopathy should be diligently monitored with physical examination and echocardiographic studies. As there is no therapeutic benefit in identifying asymptomatic cardiac involvement in HIV infection, a case for routine screening with electrocardiograms and echocardiograms cannot be made.

Treatment of cardiovascular disease

Congestive cardiac failure should be managed with standard treatment consisting of fluid restriction, diuretics, digoxin and angiotensin-converting enzyme inhibitors. As in non-HIV-related cardiac failure, β-blockers may play an increasing part in the treatment (Packer *et al.*, 1996).

Some authors have noted that there is low systemic vascular resistance present in HIV-related cardiomyopathy. These patients may be more sensitive to treatment with afterload reduction (Herskowitz *et al.*, 1995). In the fulminant type of HIV-related cardiac failure, treatment can be difficult. A study examining the predictors of survival in HIV-infected patients admitted to the intensive care unit (ICU), (Casalino *et al.* (1998) found that the primary reason for admission to the ICU was heart failure in 4.5% of the patients. This admission diagnosis was associated with a particularly poor short- and long-term survival.

There appears to be a strong relationship between myocarditis and cardiomyopathy in HIV. The role of immunosuppression in non-HIV-related myocarditis is unclear (Mason *et al.*, 1995) and its place in a population that is already severely immunodepressed is even more dubious. However, as auto-immunity and cytokines may play a significant role in the pathogenesis of HIV-related myocarditis, immunosuppression may be of some benefit.

Levy *et al.* (1988) reported a patient with a dilated cardiomyopathy who had evidence of myocarditis on biopsy and who recovered after treatment with immunosuppressants. As cardiac failure secondary to a cardiomyopathy is likely to become an increasingly common problem in the HIV epidemic, a clinical trial examining the safety and efficacy of immunosuppression in proven myocarditis may be worthwhile.

If a pericardial effusion is large enough to produce symptoms, percutaneous drainage, with the placement of an *in situ* pigtail catheter for 24–48 h, can be performed. In a series of 29 patients who underwent surgical drainage and biopsy of the pericardium under a general anaesthetic, the mortality at 22 weeks was 100% (Flum *et al.*, 1995). Most of these procedures were done for diagnostic reasons. With a more conservative approach, other investigators have found a mortality of 62% at 6 months (Heidenreich *et al.*, 1995). Post-operative respiratory complications, and the lack of clinically significant findings in the former series, would appear to make the more aggressive approach inappropriate.

The treatment of infective endocarditis in the HIV-infected patient should be similar to the approach taken in the HIV-uninfected individual. The exception to this would be in the case of advanced immunosuppression, where the prognosis from AIDS would make the option of cardiac surgery inappropriate. Valve surgery, if indicated on the grounds of haemodynamic compromise or uncontrollable sepsis, should be offered if the prognosis from the HIV infection is reasonably good. The poor long-term prognosis in these patients seems to be related to ongoing injecting drug use, rather than HIV infection itself (Currie *et al.*, 1995). It would appear that cardiopulmonary bypass does not accelerate the progression from asymptomatic HIV infection to AIDS (Aris *et al.*, 1993).

Primary pulmonary hypertension generally has a high and early mortality, and this is even more marked in the setting of HIV infection. Long-term anticoagulation with warfarin has been found to improve survival without affecting symptoms; high-dose calcium-channel antagonists may improve symptoms and survival in a minority of patients. Recently, long-term intravenous treatment with prostacyclin (an agent with vasodilatory and anti-thrombotic properties) has been shown to improve symptoms and survival in an HIV-uninfected group (McLaughlin *et al.*, 1998). As the likelihood of response to short-term prostacyclin administration has been demonstrated to be independent of HIV-status in primary PH (Petitpretz et al., 1994), this therapy may also be useful in HIV-related PH.

Coronary artery disease in the HIV-infected individual has been treated with the same approaches as taken for the general population. Attention should be paid to the patient's lipid profile and the co-existence of any other risk factors for coronary artery disease.

Conclusions

The cardiovascular manifestations of HIV infection are likely to become more varied and prevalent as the management of the infective complications of the syndrome continue to improve. The first indication that a patient has been infected with HIV may be a presentation to a cardiologist with an unexplained dilated cardiomyopathy, pericardial effusion, or pulmonary hypertension. A cardiac cause of death is still rare in this epidemic, but appears to be increasing in incidence. Of the cardiovascular manifestations, HIV-related cardiomyopathy would be the most common cause of death.

The World Health Organization estimated that 38–110 million people worldwide would be infected with HIV by the year 2000. Therefore, even if 5% of these patients develop a symptomatic dilated cardiomyopathy, HIV will constitute an important cause of heart failure (Currie et al., 1994). The pathogenesis of HIV-related cardiomyopathy is not yet fully elucidated. It may be that as this becomes an increasingly common clinical problem worldwide, multicentre trials examining therapeutic options will be undertaken.

References

Abelman WH. (1985). Incidence of dilated cardiomyopathy. *Postgrad Med J* **61**: 1123–4.

Acierno JL. (1989). Cardiac complications in acquired immunodeficiency syndrome: a review. *J Am Coll Cardiol* **13**: 1144–54.

Akhras F, Dubrey S, Gazzard B et al. (1994). Emerging patterns of heart disease in HIV-infected homosexual subjects with and without opportunistic infections: a prospective color flow Doppler echocardiographic study. *Eur Heart J* **15**: 68–75.

Albrecht H, Stellbrink HJ, Fenske S et al. (1994). Successful treatment of *Toxoplasma gondii* myocarditis in an AIDS patient. *Eur J Clin Microbiol Infect Dis* **13**: 500–4.

Anderson WD, Virmani R. (1990). Emerging patterns of heart disease in human immunodeficiency virus infection. *Hum Pathol* **21**: 253–9.

Anderson DW, Virmani R, Reilly JM et al. (1988). Prevalent myocarditis at necropsy in the acquired immunodeficiency syndrome. *J Am Coll Cardiol* **11**: 792–9.

Aretz HT, Billingham ME, Edwards WD et al. (1987). Myocarditis – a histopathologic definition and classification. *Am J Cardiovasc Pathol* **1**: 3–14.

Aris A, Pomar JL, Saura E et al. (1993). Cardiopulmonary bypass in HIV-positive patients. *Ann Thorac Surg* **55**: 1104–8.

Autran BR, Gorin I, Leibowitch M et al. (1983). AIDS in a Haitian woman with cardiac Kaposi's sarcoma and Whipple's disease. *Lancet* **1**: 767–8.

Barbaro G, Barbarini G, Di Lorenzo G et al. (1996a). Early impairment of systolic and diastolic function in asymptomatic HIV-positive patients: a multicentre echocardiographic and echo-doppler study. *AIDS Res Hum Retrovir* **12**: 1559–63.

Barbaro G, Di Lorenzo G, Grisorio B et al. (1996b). Clinical meaning of ventricular ectopic beats in the diagnosis of HIV-related myocarditis: a retrospective analysis of Holter electrocardiographic recordings, echocardiographic parameters, histopathological and virologic findings. *Cardiologia* **41**: 1199–207.

Barbaro G, Di Lorenzo G, Grisorio B et al. (1998a). Incidence of dilated cardiomyopathy and detection of HIV in myocardial cells of HIV-positive patients. *N Engl J Med* **339**: 1093–9.

Barbaro G, Di Lorenzo G, Grisorio B et al. (1998b). Cardiac involvement in the acquired immunodeficiency syndrome: A multi-centre clinical-pathological study. *AIDS Res Hum Retrovir* **12**: 1071–7.

Behrens G, Schmidt H, Meyer D et al. (1998). Vascular complications associated with the use of HIV protease inhibitors. *Lancet* **351**: 1958.

Beshorner WE, Baughman KL, Turnicky RP et al. (1990). HIV associated myocarditis: pathology and immunopathology. *Am J Pathol* **137**: 1365–71.

Blanchard GD, Hagenhoff C, Chow LC et al. (1991). Reversibility of cardiac abnormalities in HIV-infected individuals: A serial echocardiographic study. *J Am Coll Cardiol* **6**: 1270–6.

Cammarsono C, Lewis W. (1985). Cardiac lesion in acquired immune deficiency syndrome (AIDS). *J Am Coll Cardiol* **5**: 703–6.

Cardoso SJ, Moura B, Martins L et al. (1998a). Left ventricular dysfunction in HIV-infected patients. *Int J Cardiol* **63**: 37–45.

Cardoso SJ, Moura B, Ferreira A et al. (1998b). Predictors of myocardial dysfunction in HIV-infected patients. *J Card Fail* **4**: 19–26.

Carpenter C, Fischl M, Hammer SM et al. (1997). Antiretroviral therapy for HIV infection in 1997. *JAMA* **277**: 1962–7.

Carr A, Samaras K, Burton S et al. (1998). A syndrome of peripheral hypodystrophy hyperlipidemia and insulin resistance in patients receiving HIV protease inhibitors. *AIDS* **12**: F51–8.

Casalino E, Mendoza-Sassi G, Wolff M et al. (1998). Predictors of short-and long-term survival in HIV-infected patients admitted to the ICU. *Chest* **113**: 412–29.

Cegielski PJ, Ramiya K, Lalinger GJ et al. (1990). Pericardial disease and HIV in Dar es Salaam, Tanzania. *Lancet* **335**: 209–12.

Chokshi SK, Moore R, Pandian NG et al. (1989). Reversible cardiomyopathy associated with cocaine intoxication. *Ann Intern Med* **111**: 1039–40.

Cohen IS, Anderson WD, Virmani R et al. (1986). Congestive cardiomyopathy in association with the acquired immunodeficiency syndrome. *N Engl J Med* **315**: 628–30.

Constans J, Seigneur M, Blann A et al. (1997). Chronic infections and coronary heart disease [letter]. *Lancet* **350**: 1030.

Coudray N, de Zultere D, Force G et al. (1995). Left ventricular diastolic function in asymptomatic and symptomatic human immunodeficiency virus carriers: an echocardiographic study. *Eur Heart J* **16**: 61–7.

Currie FF, Jacob JA, Foreman AR *et al.* (1994). Heart muscle disease related to HIV infection: prognostic implications. *Br Med J* **309**: 1605–7.

Currie PF, Sutherland GR, Jacob AJ *et al.* (1995). A review of endocarditis in acquired immunodeficiency syndrome and human immunodeficiency virus infection. *Eur Heart J* **16**: 15–8.

Dalakas MC, Illa I, Pezeshkpour GH *et al.* (1990). Mitochondrial myopathy caused by long-term zidovudine therapy. *N Engl J Med* **322**: 1098–105.

Danesh J, Collins R, Peto R *et al.* (1997). Chronic infections and coronary heart disease: is there a link? *Lancet* **350**: 430–6.

De Castro S, Migliau G, Silvestri A *et al.* (1992). Heart involvement in AIDS: a prospective study during various stages of the disease. *Eur Heart J* 1452–9.

De Castro S, Amati G, Gallo P *et al.* (1994). Frequency of development of acute global left ventricular dysfunction in HIV infection. *J Am Coll Cardiol* **24**: 1018–24.

Depairon M, Chessex S, Sudre P *et al.* (2001). Premature atherosclerosis in HIV-infected individuals – focus on protease inhibitor therapy. *AIDS* **15**: 329–34.

Deyton RL, Walker ER, Kovacs JA *et al.* (1989). Reversible cardiac dysfunction associated with Interferon-therapy in AIDS patients with Kaposi's sarcoma. *N Engl J Med* **321**: 1246–9.

Dittrich H, Chow L, Denaro F *et al.* (1988). Human immunodeficiency virus, coxsackievirus, and cardiomyopathy [letter]. *Ann Intern Med* **108**: 308–9.

Domanski MJ, Sloas MM, Follman DA *et al.* (1995). Effect of zidovudine and didanosine treatment on heart function in children infected with HIV. *Paediatrics* **127**: 137–46.

Eisenberg JM, Gordon A, Schiller NB. (1992). HIV-associated pericardial effusions. *Chest* **102**: 956–8.

Eisenhauer DM, Eliasson AH, Taylor AJ *et al.* (1994). Incidence of cardiac arrhythmias during intravenous pentamidine therapy in HIV-infected patients. *Chest* **105**: 389–94.

Flum RD, McGinn TJ, Tyras DH *et al.* (1995). The role of the 'pericardial window' in AIDS. *Chest* **107**: 1522–5.

Gallet B, Pulik M, Genet P *et al.* (1998). Vascular complications associated with use of HIV protease inhibitors. *Lancet* **351**: 1958–9.

Girgis I, Gualberti J, Langan L *et al.* (1997). A prospective study of the effect of intravenous pentamidine therapy on ventricular arrhythmias and QT prolongation in HIV-infected patients. *Chest* **112**: 646–53.

Grange F, Kinney EL, Monsuez JJ *et al.* (1990). Successful therapy for *Toxoplasma gondii* myocarditis in AIDS. *Am Heart J* **120**: 443–4.

Grody WW, Cheng L, Lewis W *et al.* (1990). Infection of the heart by the human immunodeficiency virus. *Am J Cardiol* **66**: 203–6.

Hansen BF. (1992). Pathology of the heart in AIDS: a study of 60 consecutive autopsies. *APMIS* **100**: 273–9.

Heidenreich AP, Eisenberg JM, Key LL *et al.* (1995). Pericardial effusions in AIDS. *Circulation* **92**: 3229–34.

Henry K, Melroe H, Huebsch J *et al.* (1998). Severe premature coronary artery disease with protease inhibitors. *Lancet* **351**: 1328.

Herskowitz A. (1996). Cardiomyopathy and other symptomatic heart diseases associated with HIV infection. *Curr Opin Cardiol* **11**: 325–31.

Herskowitz A, Willoughby SB, Baughman KL *et al.* (1992). Cardiomyopathy associated with antiretroviral therapy in patients with HIV infection: a report of six cases. *Ann Intern Med* **116**: 311–3.

Herskowitz A, Vlahov D, Willoughby S *et al.* (1993a). Prevalence and incidence of left ventricular dysfunction in patients with human immunodeficiency virus infection. *Am J Cardiol* **71**: 955–8.

Herskowitz A, Willoughby S, Wu TC *et al.* (1993b). Immunopathogenesis of HIV-1 associated cardiomyopathy. *Clin Immunol Immunopathol* **68**: 234–41.

Herskowitz A, Wu TC, Willoughby SB *et al.* (1994). Myocarditis and cardiotropic viral infection associated with severe left ventricular dysfunction in late-stage infection with HIV. *J Am Coll Cardiol* **24**: 1025–32.

Herskowitz A, Willoughby SB, Vlahov D *et al.* (1995). Dilated heart muscle disease associated with HIV infection. *Eur Heart J* **16**: 50–5.

Himelman RB, Dohrmann M, Goodman P *et al.* (1989). Severe pulmonary hypertension and cor pulmonale in AIDS. *Am J Cardiol* **64**: 1396–9.

Ho DD, Pomerantz RJ, Kaplan JC *et al.* (1987). Pathogenesis of infection with HIV. *N Engl J Med* **317**: 278–86.

Hofman P, Drici D, Gibelin P *et al.* (1993). Prevalence of toxoplasma myocarditis in patients with the acquired immunodeficiency syndrome. *Br Heart J* **70**: 376–81.

Hrobon P, Kuntz K, Hare JM. (1998). Should endomyocardial biopsy be performed for detection of myocarditis? *J Heart Lung Transplant* **17**: 479–86.

Kaul S, Fishbein M, Siegel RJ *et al.* (1991). Cardiac manifestations of acquired immune deficiency syndrome: a 1991 update. *Am Heart J* **122**: 535–44.

Kim KK, Factor SM. (1987). Membranoproliferative glomerulonephritis and plexogenic pulmonary arteriopathy in a homosexual man with acquired immunodeficiency syndrome. *Hum Pathol* **18**: 1293–6.

Kinney EL, Monsuez JJ, Kitzis M *et al.* (1989). Treatment of AIDS-associated heart disease. *Angiology* **40**: 970–6.

Lange GL, Schreiner FG. (1994). Immune mechanisms of cardiac disease. *N Engl J Med* **330**: 1129–35.

Levy WS, Varghese J, Anderson DW *et al.* (1988). Myocarditis diagnosed by endomyocardial biopsy in HIV infection with cardiac dysfunction. *Am J Cardiol* **62**: 658–9.

Levy WS, Simon GL, Rios JC *et al.* (1989). Prevalence of cardiac abnormalities in human immunodeficiency virus infection. *Am J Cardiol* **63**: 86–9.

Lewis W. (1989). AIDS: cardiac findings from 115 autopsies. *Prog Cardiovasc Dis* **32**: 207–15.

Lewis W, Papoian T, Gonzalez B *et al.* (1991). Mitochondrial ultrastructural and molecular changes induced by zidovudine in rat hearts. *Lab Invest* **65**: 228–36.

Lipshultz SE, Orav JE, Sanders SP *et al.* (1992). Cardiac structure and function in children with HIV infection treated with zidovudine. *N Engl J Med* **327**: 1260–5.

Lipshultz SE, Orav EJ, Sanders SP *et al.* (1995). Immunoglobulins and left ventricular structure and function in pediatric HIV infection. *Circulation* **92**: 2220–5.

Mason WJ, O'Connell JB, Herskowitz A *et al.* (1995). A clinical trial of immunosuppressive therapy for myocarditis. *N Engl J Med* **333**: 269–75.

McLaughlin VV, Genthner DE, Panella MM *et al.* (1998). Reduction in pulmonary vascular resistance with long-term Epoprostenol (Prostacyclin) therapy in primary pulmonary hypertension. *N Engl J Med* **338**: 273–7.

Mesa AR, Edell SE, Dunn WF *et al.* (1998). Human immunodeficiency virus infection and pulmonary hypertension : two new cases and a review of 86 reported cases. *Mayo Clin Proc* **73**: 37–45.

Mette AS, Palevsky IH, Pietra GG *et al.* (1992). Primary pulmonary hypertension in association with HIV infection. *Am Rev Respir Dis* **145**: 1196–1200.

Michaels DA, Lederman JR, MacGregor JS et al. (1997). Cardiovascular involvement in AIDS. Curr Prob Cardiol 22: 109–48.

Milei J, Grana D, Fernandez Alonso G et al. (1998). Cardiac involvement in AIDS – a review to push action. Clin Cardiol 21: 465–72.

Mooser V and Carr A (2001). Antiretroviral therapy-associated hyperlipidaemia in HIV disease. Curr Opin Lipidol 12: 313–9.

Morse JH, Barst RJ, Fotino M et al. (1996). Primary pulmonary hypertension in HIV infection: an outcome determined by particular HLA class 2 alleles. Am J Respir Crit Care Med 153: 1299–301.

Nahass RG, Weinstein MP, Bartels J et al. (1990). Infective endocarditis in intravenous drug users: a comparison of human immunodeficiency virus type 1-negative and – positive patients. J Infect Dis 162: 967–70.

Niedt GW, Schinella RA. (1985). Acquired immunodeficiency syndrome: clinicopathologic study of 56 autopsies. Arch Pathol Lab Med 109: 727–34.

Opravil M, Pechere M, Speich R et al. (1997). HIV-associated primary pulmonary hypertension. Am J Respir Crit Care Med 155: 990–5.

Packer M, Bristow MR, Cohn JN et al. (1996). The effect of carvedilol on morbidity and mortality in patients with chronic heart failure. N Engl J Med 334: 1349–55.

Palella FJ, Delaney K, Moorman AC et al. (1998). Declining morbidity and mortality among patients with advanced HIV infection. N Engl J Med 338: 853–60.

Patel RC, Frishman WH. (1995). AIDS and the heart: clinicopathologic assessment. Cardiovasc Pathol 3: 173–83.

Patel RC, Frishman WH. (1996). Cardiac involvement in HIV infection. Med Clin Nth Am 80: 1493–512.

Petitpretz P, Brenot F, Azarian R et al. (1994). Pulmonary hypertension in patients with HIV infection. Circulation 89: 2722–7.

Reilly JM, Cunnion RE, Anderson DW et al. (1988). Frequency of myocarditis and ventricular tachycardia in the acquired immune deficiency syndrome. Am J Cardiol 62: 789–93.

Rickerts V, Brodt H, Staszewski S et al. (2000). Incidence of myocardial infarctions in HIV-infected patients between 1983 and 1998: the Frankfurt HIV-cohort study. Eur J Med Res 5: 329–33.

Roberts WC, Siegel RJ, McManus BM et al. (1987). Idiopathic dilated cardiomyopathy: analysis of 152 necropsy patients. Am J Cardiol 60: 1340–55.

Roberts J, Navarro C, Johnson A et al. (1989). Cardiac involvement in intravenous drug abusers with and without acquired immunodeficiency syndrome [abstract]. Circulation 80: 1285.

Rodriguez R, Nasim S, Hsia J et al. (1991). Cardiac myocytes and dendritic cells harbor HIV in infected patients with and without cardiac dysfunction. Am J Cardiol 68: 1511–20.

Singal KP, Iliskovic N. (1998). Doxorubicin-induced cardiomyopathy. N Engl J Med 39: 900–5.

Siscovick PS, Schwartz SM, Corey L et al. (2000). Chlamydia pneumoniae, herpes simplex virus type 1 and cytomegalovirus and incident myocardial infarction and coronary heart disease death in older adults: the Cardiovascular Health Study. Circulation 102: 2335–40.

SoRelle R. (1998). Vascular and lipid syndromes in selected HIV-infected patients. Circulation 9: 829–30.

Speich R, Jenni R, Opravil M et al. (1991). Primary pulmonary hypertension in HIV infection. Chest 100: 1268–71.

Tomashefski JF, Hirsch CS. (1980). The pulmonary vascular lesions of intravenous drug abuse. Hum Pathol 11: 133–45.

Vemuri DN, Robbins JM, Boal HB. (1990). Does human immunodeficiency virus infection alter the course of infective endocarditis. J Am Coll Cardiol 15: 183A.

Villa A, Foresti V, Confalonieri F et al. (1995). Autonomic neuropathy and prolongation of QT interval in HIV infection. Clin Auton Res 5: 48–52.

Vittecoq D, Escaut L, Monsuez JJ et al. (1998). Vascular complications associated with use of HIV protease inhibitors [letter]. Lancet 351: 1959.

Willoughby SB, Vlahov D, Herskowitz A. (1993). Frequency of left ventricular dysfunction and other echocardiographic abnormalities in HIV-seronegative intravenous drug users. Am J Cardiol 71: 446–7.

Wright SC, Jewett A, Mitsuyasu R et al. (1988). Spontaneous cytotoxicity and tumor necrosis factor production by peripheral blood monocytes from AIDS patients. J Immunol 141: 99–104.

Wu TC, Pizzorno MC, Hayward GS et al. (1992). In-situ detection of human cytomegalovirus immediate-early gene transcripts within cardiac myocytes of patients with HIV-associated cardiomyopathy. AIDS 6: 777–85.

Zakowski MF, Ianuale-Shanerman A. (1993). Cytology of pericardial effusions in AIDS patients. Diagnostic Cytopathol 9: 266–9.

16

An approach to gastrointestinal and hepatobiliary disease in HIV infection

WILLIAM SIEVERT

Gastrointestinal disease

Gastrointestinal (GI) tract disorders are common in patients with HIV/AIDS. The lower GI tract may serve as a portal of entry for HIV infection in homosexual men. Alternatively, the intestine may be infected by recirculation of HIV-infected T cells. In addition to lymphocytes and monocytes, enterocytes also support HIV replication, although the absolute number of infected cells is usually small. Failure of both local and systemic immune responses plus constant exposure to environmental pathogens renders the intestine a common site for opportunistic infection and AIDS-related neoplasia. The commonly encountered gastroenterological signs and symptoms of dysphagia, abdominal pain, diarrhoea, weight loss and jaundice may reflect such HIV/AIDS-related complications.

Oesophageal disorders

Symptomatic oesophageal disease occurs in 20–30% of HIV-infected patients. Difficulty in swallowing (dysphagia) and pain on swallowing (odynophagia) are the cardinal signs of oesophageal involvement, and if sufficiently severe or prolonged they may have a detrimental effect on nutrition. Opportunistic infections include fungal oesophagitis, of which *Candida* sp. is the most common cause (see Chapter 28), and viral infections with either herpes simplex virus (HSV) (see Chapter 32) or cytomegalovirus (CMV), (see Chapter 21). These infections may co-exist in the same patient (Table 16.1).

Fungal oesophagitis

Candida oesophagitis may present with dysphagia or odynophagia, with or without concomitant oral involvement. The endoscopic appearance is quite characteristic, with plaques or columns of yellow-white pseudomembrane, which may be scattered focally throughout the oesophagus; in severe cases, the plaques become confluent and narrow the oesophageal lumen. Endoscopic biopsies provide a histological diagnosis.

Most clinicians treat patients empirically at first, based on characteristic symptoms. Fluconazole (100 mg/day) given for 2 weeks has acceptable levels of cure and appears to be less hepatotoxic than ketoconazole (200 mg/day) and more effective than alternative agents such as flucytosine (Barbaro *et al.*, 1995). In an Italian multi-centre study of over 2000 HIV-infected patients with *Candida* oesophagitis, short-term (2 weeks) endoscopic cure rates were higher with fluconazole than itraconazole. However, at 1 year follow-up, the combined clinical and endoscopic cure rates were greater than 95% in both groups, with a similar incidence of clinical relapse and treatment failure (Barbaro *et al.*, 1996).

Patients who do not respond to empirical therapy should undergo endoscopy with biopsy to confirm the diagnosis of

Table 16.1 Common causes of oesophageal disorders in patients with HIV infection

Fungal
Candida sp.
Histoplasmosis (in endemic areas)
Viral
Cytomegalovirus (CMV)
Herpes simplex virus (HSV)
Neoplastic
Lymphoma
Kaposi's sarcoma (KS)
Idiopathic ulcer (due to primary HIV infection?)
Unrelated to HIV infection
Pill-induced ulcers
Gastro-oesophageal reflux disease

fungal oesophagitis and exclude co-existing diseases. Wilcox *et al.*, (1996a) studied 74 patients with persistent symptoms despite empirical antifungal therapy, and found oesophageal ulceration (either idiopathic or due to CMV) to be the most common cause. If symptoms do not improve with empirical therapy and if no other diagnosis is identified endoscopically, the dose of fluconazole can be increased to 200 mg/day and treatment extended to 4 weeks. Alternatively, itraconazole (200 mg/day) can be tried (see also Chapter 28 for other treatment options). Relapse following cessation of any treatment regimen is not unusual.

Viral oesophagitis

CMV oesophageal infection causes dysphagia or odynophagia and occurs in patients with advanced immune deficiency (see Chapter 21). The endoscopic appearance can be variable but multiple small ulcers scattered throughout the distal oesophagus should prompt histological assessment for typical inclusion bodies. Giant (> 1 cm) ulcers due to CMV also occur. Ganciclovir (10 mg/kg per day) and foscarnet (90 mg/kg twice daily) are equally effective in promoting endoscopic and symptomatic improvement (Parente and Bianchi-Porro, 1998) (see Chapter 21 for full details of treatment). HSV oesophagitis occurs in HIV-infected patients with a median CD4 lymphocyte counts of 15/μl. The most common endoscopic appearance is that of diffuse ulcers, but occasionally pseudomembrane formation can occur. Aciclovir, administered either orally or intravenously, has a reported success rate of 70% (Genereau *et al.*, 1996) (see Chapter 32 for full details of treatment).

Idiopathic oesophageal ulcers

Large oesophageal ulcers can be a particularly difficult management problem if they cause severe odynophagia, resulting in malnutrition (see Chapters 12 and 18). The ulcers are usually in the distal oesophagus and require careful endoscopic technique for diagnosis, since the lack of contrast with surrounding mucosa may hide the ulcer from the inexperienced endoscopist. Multiple biopsies should be examined to exclude a viral aetiology (most commonly CMV) or lymphoma. Glucocorticoids, either injected intralesionally, or more commonly given orally, may lead to successful re-epithelialization of the ulcerated oesophagus and marked clinical improvement (Wilcox and Schwartz, 1994). A small, prospective placebo-controlled study has recently shown that thalidomide (200 mg/day for 4 weeks) is effective in healing idiopathic aphthous ulcers of the oesophagus in HIV-infected patients. Eight of 11 (73%) treated patients demonstrated complete healing endoscopically, with resolution of odynophagia. Adverse events were common and dose reduction or discontinuation was required in five (45%) patients (Jacobson *et al.*, 1999).

Diarrhoea

Diarrhoea is the most common gastrointestinal manifestation in patients with HIV infection. The clinical spectrum of diarrhoea in HIV-infected patients is broad and the definitions used are not uniform, so the true prevalence is uncertain. The degree of immune deficiency is an important determinant of illness, since patients with advanced immune deficiency are more likely to develop chronic diar-

Table 16.2 Etiological agents in HIV-related diarrhoea

	Commonly found or reported	Uncommon/rare	Unproven
Viruses	Cytomegalovirus (CMV)	Herpes simplex virus (HSV)	Adenovirus
Protozoa	Cryptosporidia	Cyclospora	*Blastocystis hominis*
	Microsporidia	*Giardia*[a]	
		Entamoeba histolytica[a]	
Bacteria	*Mycobacterium avium* complex (MAC)	*Helicobacter fetus*	*Helicobacter cinaedi*
	Salmonella spp.		*Histoplasma capsulatum*
	Campylobacter spp.		
	Shigella spp.		
	Yersinia spp.		
	C. difficile		
Other		Fungi	
		Intestinal spirochetes	
Non-infective		Lymphoma	
		Kaposi's sarcoma (KS)	

[a]Do not occur with increased frequency or virulence in HIV-infected patients.

rhoea. The most common pathogens are protozoa (see Chapter 30) and bacteria (see Chapter 17 and Table 16.2). Serious opportunistic infections with *Mycobacterium avium* complex (MAC) and CMV occur primarily in patients with CD4 lymphocyte counts of $< 100/\mu l$. Clinical management of HIV-infected patients with either an acute or chronic diarrhoeal illness should focus on identification of potentially treatable causes, relief of symptoms and correction of fluid and electrolyte imbalance. Prevention of malnutrition, an independent risk factor leading to increased mortality in HIV-infected patients, is also an important therapeutic goal.

The pathogenesis of diarrhoea in HIV infection is complex and reflects the multiple insults to the intestine. The CD4 lymphocyte depletion seen in peripheral blood also occurs as an early event in the lymphoid tissue within the intestinal mucosa (Lim *et al.*, 1993). Alterations in the mucosal immune system may predispose the gut to infection by opportunistic pathogens and could conceivably contribute to mucosal injury, although data to support either of these potential mechanisms are sparse. Overgrowth of bacteria in the stomach and proximal small intestine occurs more often in HIV-infected patients than in controls (Chave *et al.*, 1994) and may represent another mechanism for diarrhoeal illness. Finally, HIV can be detected in intestinal mononuclear cells (Kotler *et al.*, 1991) and thus primary HIV infection of the intestine may contribute to diarrhoea, especially in those patients in whom no other pathogen has been identified.

Bacteria

Salmonella, Shigella and *Campylobacter* spp. HIV-infected patients are susceptible to the common bacterial pathogens that also cause diarrhoea in the non HIV-infected population (Table 16.2; also, see Chapter 17). Transmission may occur via contaminated food or water or by oral–anal contact. Intestinal infection with *Salmonella, Shigella* and *Campylobacter* species is characterized by abdominal pain, fever and diarrhoea. Among HIV-infected patients, a diarrhoeal illness complicated by bacteraemia occurs most frequently in those who are immunosuppressed. The clinical course in bacteraemic HIV-infected patients can be severe and prolonged, and a high mortality in patients with *Campylobacter jejuni* bacteraemia has been reported (Tee and Mijch, 1998). Metastatic infection to lung and bone may occur.

Clostridium difficile. HIV-infected patients are at risk for *Clostridium difficile*-associated diarrhoea, primarily because of frequent antibiotic use, both prophylactic and therapeutic (Barbut *et al.*, 1997). Those patients who are hospitalized, particularly as immune deficiency advances, are also at risk of acquiring this nosocomial infection. *C. difficile* diarrhoea does not appear to be unusually severe in HIV-infected patients and commonly responds to conventional therapy.

Mycobacterium avium complex (MAC). MAC is the most serious opportunistic bacterial infection of the intestinal tract in patients with HIV infection (see Chapter 24). MAC infection of the gut is usually associated with systemic infection and occurs almost exclusively in patients with CD4 lymphocyte counts of $< 100/\mu l$. In addition to diarrhoea, other signs and symptoms of disseminated MAC infection include high swinging fevers, night sweats and weight loss (see Chapter 24). Abdominal pain is a prominent feature in patients with retroperitoneal adenopathy and extensive lymphatic obstruction may occur in some patients. Duodenal infection has a characteristic endoscopic appearance, with multiple raised, white plaques or nodules and large numbers of organisms demonstrated on histological examination. MAC infection may mimic Crohn's disease, with fistula formation and areas of stenosis. Examination of tissue biopsy specimens with appropriate histological techniques provides a more reliable diagnosis of infection than stool culture, since asymptomatic colonization of the gut may occur.

Viruses

Cytomegalovirus (CMV). CMV is the most serious viral opportunistic infection of the GI tract in HIV-infected patients (see Chapter 21). Virtually all patients were previously infected by the virus and active clinical infection represents reactivation in the setting of worsening immune deficiency. While CMV infection can affect the entire GI tract, causing mass lesions and ulceration in the oesophagus, stomach and small intestine, CMV colitis is the most commonly encountered clinical problem. Colonic infection ranges from a normal endoscopic appearance with CMV inclusions evident only on biopsy, through mild, patchy colitis, to severe pancolitis with perforation. Clinical presentation is equally variable, from a slight increase in stool frequency to severe diarrhoea requiring intravenous fluid and electrolyte replacement (Jacobson and Mills, 1988). Infection of vascular endothelial cells results in vasculitis, which may progress to localized ischemia, ulceration and in some patients to intestinal perforation. The HIV-infected patient presenting with severe abdominal pain, bloody diarrhoea and fever should be observed carefully for signs of intestinal perforation. CMV can occasionally present as a colonic mass lesion, which mimics colonic neoplasia at endoscopy, similar to the 'amoeboma' seen in amoebic colitis.

Diagnosis of intestinal CMV infection relies on demonstration of typical cytomegalic inclusion bodies in tissue biopsy specimens. The diagnostic yield is improved with examination of an adequate number of samples obtained from endoscopically identified lesions (rather than adjacent normal mucosa) by an experienced pathologist. Viral culture of biopsy specimens is not useful because of contamination with CMV, which may be present in blood. Serology is also useless, reflecting previous exposure rather than active infection. A randomized placebo-controlled trial has shown some evidence of clinical improvement with ganciclovir therapy (Dieterich et al., 1993) (see Chapter 21 for full treatment details).

Adenovirus. Adenovirus infection of the GI tract has been associated with diarrhoea in HIV-infected patients, as well as in other immunosuppressed patient groups, although the causal relationship is not firmly established. In a prospective survey conducted over 1 year, adenovirus was the detected in the faeces of 18 of 63 HIV-infected patients, but diarrhoea was reported in less than half of the adenovirus-infected group. Despite persistent faecal excretion of the virus, most patients remained asymptomatic (Khoo et al., 1995).

Protozoa

Microsporidiosis. Microsporidia are a group of obligate intracellular parasites, which have been implicated as a cause of chronic diarrhoea and malabsorption in 20–40% of HIV-infected patients (see Chapter 30). In severely immunosuppressed patients, the organisms can spread beyond the GI tract to involve the biliary, respiratory and urinary tracts. *Enterocytozoon bieneusi*, the most common infecting species, has been associated with transient diarrhoea in immunocompetent hosts, similar to *C. parvum*. Microsporidia can also be found in asymptomatic HIV-infected individuals, analogous to the asymptomatic intestinal infection seen with MAC. Controversy over the pathogenicity of microsporidia has arisen because of a high proportion of asymptomatic infection reported in some studies (Rabeneck et al., 1993), which has not been confirmed by other investigators (Coyle et al., 1996). While the mechanisms by which microsporidia cause diarrhoea and malabsorption remain unclear, most investigators accept these microorganisms as true pathogens.

The most common clinical presentation of intestinal microsporidiosis is chronic diarrhoea in a patient with a CD4 lymphocyte count of < 100 cells/μl, with signs of malabsorption and weight loss. Nausea, vomiting and abdominal pain are common, while a prolonged febrile illness is unusual. Diagnosis can be made in most laboratories from stool samples (Sobottka et al., 1998; see Chapter 30 for further information regarding diagnosis). The organisms may also be found in nasal secretions and urine, as well as histological samples from the biliary tract. Treatment of microsporidiosis remains unsatisfactory.

Cryptosporidiosis. Cryptosporidia are ubiquitous parasites, which cause a range of clinical manifestations in patients with HIV infection (see Chapter 30). GI infection can be asymptomatic or can resolve spontaneously in patients with preserved immunity. In patients with advanced immune deficiency, cryptosporidiosis can result in life-threatening diarrhoea with a daily faecal fluid loss exceeding 10–15 litres. Cryptosporidial infection of the gallbladder and biliary tree is a cause of AIDS-related cholangiopathy. Rarely, cryptosporidia have been reported to infect gastric mucosa and have been associated with gastroduodenal ulceration.

In patients presenting with diarrhoea, the diagnosis of cryptosporidiosis can be made from stool specimens using a modified, acid-fast stain. Faecal leukocytes are an unusual finding in diarrhoeal stool samples and there is only sparse inflammation seen in tissue specimens. Cryptosporidial diarrhoea is presumed to be due to increased epithelial chloride secretion or decreased sodium absorption, although the mechanisms have been difficult to demonstrate in human subjects (Kelly et al., 1996). Treatment of cryptosporidial diarrhoea remains largely symptomatic, with replacement of fluid and electrolyte losses and anti-diarrhoeal agents to decrease stool frequency.

Other protozoa. *Giardia lamblia* and *Entamoeba histolytica* infect the small and large bowel, respectively. Diarrhoea due to these protozoa is no more frequent in the HIV-infected population than in controls, although the prevalence in homosexual men may be higher, due to sexual practices. Typically, giardiasis causes a chronic diarrhoea associated with abdominal bloating. The infection is localized primarily to the small intestine and mucosal invasion does not occur. Thus faecal leukocytes and rectal bleeding are absent. Amoebiasis is a potentially more serious disease, which can present with colitis or focal ulceration associated with marked abdominal pain, fever and bloody diarrhoea. HIV-infected patients with giardiasis or amoebiasis are treated identically to HIV-uninfected patients.

Evaluation and management of HIV-infected patients with diarrhoea

Chronic diarrhoea has a significant impact on the quality of life of HIV-infected patients and, in some cases, results in mortality. Such patients should be evaluated carefully to search for a treatable pathogen and to exclude non-infectious causes of diarrhoea (Figure 16.1). The degree of immune suppression is an important clinical clue, because

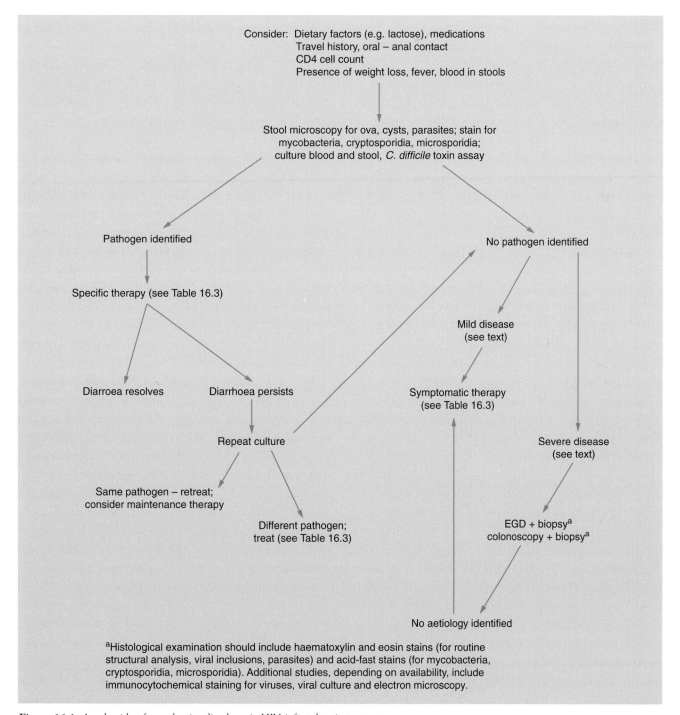

Figure 16.1 *An algorithm for evaluating diarrhoea in HIV-infected patients.*

pathogens such as MAC, CMV, cryptosporidia and microsporidia are found in patients predominantly with CD4 lymphocyte counts below 100 cells/μl. Fever and abdominal pain are more common with MAC and CMV, while high-volume diarrhoea is more suggestive of cryptosporidiosis. Weight loss and malabsorption are features of both MAC and microsporidiosis. Severe pain with bloody diarrhoea is more commonly associated with ischaemia resulting from CMV vasculitis, which can lead to intestinal perforation.

All HIV-infected patients with diarrhoea should have blood and stool specimens examined. Bacteraemia with common pathogens such as *Salmonella* sp. and *Shigella* sp. can be seen in HIV-infected patients and MAC may be isolated from blood in patients with advanced immunosuppression. Fresh stool specimens should be examined for cryptosporidia and microsporidia using special stains, which are readily available in most laboratories. The presence of red or white blood cells suggests mucosal inflammation due to invasion by bacteria or viruses such as CMV.

Stool cultures should be performed for *Salmonella*, *Shigella*, and *Campylobacter* species and the laboratory requested to perform acid-fast stains and cultures for MAC in patients with CD4 lymphocyte counts of < 100 cells/μl. The presence of *Clostridium difficile* toxin in stool establishes the diagnosis of *C. difficile*-associated diarrhoea or colitis, and permits appropriate therapy. In patients with an initially negative evaluation, it may be necessary to request cultures for relatively uncommon bacterial pathogens such as *Yersinia enterocolitica* or *Helicobacter fetus* and *cinaedi*. There are occasional reports of diarrhoea and colitis due to fungal infection with histoplasma or to protozoa such as pneumocystis and cyclospora. There is debate as to whether *Blastocystis hominis* is a true pathogen or a surrogate for exposure to other pathogens.

Endoscopy of the upper and lower GI tract is often used if initial diagnostic efforts are not rewarding. Gastroscopy with biopsy of the small intestine may demonstrate infection with cryptosporidia or MAC, or the presence of lymphoma. There has been controversy regarding the use of flexible sigmoidoscopy or colonoscopy as the initial diagnostic test. In a recent study of 317 HIV-infected patients with chronic diarrhoea and negative stool studies, a possible aetiology was identified in over one-third (112 subjects) at colonoscopy (Bini and Weinshel, 1998). A diagnosis was more commonly made in patients with advanced immune suppression (45% with CD4 lymphocyte counts of less than 100 cells/μl); CMV infection was identified in 24% and MAC in 6%. In one-third of the CMV-infected patients, the infection was seen only in the proximal colon, and three of four colonic lymphomas were located proximally. About 70% had a potential pathogen identified in the rectosigmoid colon, which is in keeping with a smaller study, which found rectosigmoid CMV disease in 10 of 11 patients with chronic diarrhoea and negative stool studies (Wilcox et al., 1996b).

Despite intensive efforts, a definitive diagnosis remains elusive in a large proportion of HIV-infected patients with chronic diarrhoea. This may occur because a pathogen was actually present but not detected or because another, non-infective, mechanism such as bile salt malabsorption or coeliac disease is present. There is also the possibility that primary HIV infection of enterocytes may be associated with mucosal damage and resulting diarrhoea; that is, a specific HIV enteropathy may exist (Greenson et al., 1991). The concept is neither new or widely accepted and 'AIDS enteropathy' remains a diagnosis of exclusion.

The extent and intensity of diagnostic evaluation of chronic diarrhoea in HIV-infected patients remains an area of debate (AGA Technical Review, 1996). With no prospective data to guide decision making, the clinician must prioritize several factors, such as the probability of identifying a treatable cause, especially in patients who may already be on empirical treatment, the degree of immune deficiency and the severity of co-existing illnesses and weight loss. A recent study failed to identify a potential cause for chronic diarrhoea in 27 of 48 HIV-infected patients, despite intensive evaluation (Wilcox et al., 1996b). These investigators and others (Blanshard and Gazzard, 1995) have observed that diarrhoea will eventually resolve in some patients in whom a pathogen is not identified. Idiopathic chronic diarrhoea also resolves frequently in patients who have a good response to combination antiretroviral therapy. It thus seems reasonable to target those patients with significant signs and symptoms, such as weight loss and a CD4 lymphocyte count of less than 100 cells/μl, for the most intensive evaluation (see Figure 16.1). Patients with mild disease may respond to empirical therapy or non-specific anti-diarrhoeal medications in the absence of an identifiable cause from stool culture and microscopy (see Table 16.3).

Table 16.3 Treatment of HIV-related diarrhoea

Specific therapy

CMV
    Ganciclovir 5 mg/kg/bd IV for 14 days, foscarnet 90 mg/kg/bd IV for 14 days; consider maintenance therapy (see Chapter 21).

MAC
    Multiple regimens (see Chapter 24)

***Salmonella* spp., *Shigella* spp.**
    Ciprofloxacin 500 mg orally twice daily for 14 days (see Chapter 17)
    (may be associated with bactaeremia)

***Campylobacter* spp.**
    Ciprofloxacin 500 mg orally twice daily for 7 days (see Chapter 17)
    (may be associated with bactaeremia)

C. difficile
    Vancomycin 125 mg orally four times daily for 7–14 days or
    metronidazole 400 mg three times daily for 7–14 days (see Chapter 17)

Cryptosporidiosis
    No proven effective therapy (see Chapter 30)

Microsporidiosis
    Albendazole 400 mg twice daily for 2–4 weeks
    No proven effective therapy (see Chapter 30)

Cyclospora
    Trimethoprim-sulfamethoxazole 160/180 mg orally four times daily for 10 days
    (consider maintenance therapy if relapse occurs) (see Chapter 30)

Non-specific or symptomatic therapy
    Loperamide (Imodium®)
    Diphenoxylate + atropine (Lomotil®)
    Codeine   Titrate dose by response
    Tincture of opium (DTO)

    Slow-release morphine

    Octreotide   50 µg subcutaneously every 8 h, titrate by response (over 24–48 h) to a maximum of
                500 µg subcutaneously every 8 h

Gastrointestinal bleeding

The true incidence of GI bleeding in association with HIV infection is unclear, but fortunately serious haemorrhage occurs in only a small percentage of patients (Parente *et al.*, 1991). When it does occur, significant haemorrhage is more likely in patients with advanced HIV disease, and thus the reported mortality in small series of patients approaches 40% (Cappell and Geller, 1992). In addition to the common causes of GI bleeding in the non-HIV-infected population, HIV-related causes must be considered. Upper GI haemorrhage may occur from gastroduodenal lymphoma or oesophageal infection with *Candida*, HSV or CMV (Parente *et al.*, 1991). Lower GI bleeding in HIV-infected patients may be due to CMV colitis, idiopathic colonic ulceration or Kaposi's sarcoma (Chalasani and Wilcox, 1998). Co-existing HIV-related thrombocytopenia may complicate effective management of active bleeding.

The clinical approach to either upper or lower GI haemorrhage in HIV-infected patients is the same as for non-infected patients. Haemodynamic stabilization, adequate resuscitation with blood products and correction of coagulation abnormalities should precede endoscopic or surgical intervention. If endoscopic therapy is not successful, patients should be considered for surgical intervention, bearing in mind that patients with more advanced HIV disease are at higher risk of surgical complications. A recent retrospective study of major abdominal surgery in 43 HIV-infected patients found that serious complications occurred in 49%, with a 37% overall mortality. Patients with a CD4 lymphocyte count of less than 200 cells/µl were at greater risk of complications than patients with relatively intact immunity (Albaran *et al.*, 1998).

Anal disease, including squamous carcinoma

Anal disease is common in homosexual men and the most frequent conditions are anal fistulae and peri-anal ulceration, which may be idiopathic or due to HSV, CMV or, rarely, spirochete infection. Neoplastic lesions include lymphoma, Kaposi's sarcoma (KS) and squamous carcinoma (see also Chapter 33).

Squamous carcinoma of the anus occurs in association with human papillomavirus (HPV) infection. HPV infection in homosexual men is sexually transmitted, as is HPV infection in women with cervical cancer. Risk factors for anal cancer include receptive anal intercourse and HIV infection (Palefsky et al., 1998a). Anal cytological abnormalities, including detection of HPV, can be identified in a greater proportion of HIV-infected men than in those without HIV infection. Detection of HPV increases with greater degrees of HIV-related immunosuppression (Palefsky et al., 1998b). Low-grade squamous intraepithelial lesions may progress to high-grade lesions, increasing the risk of developing anal carcinoma (Sayers et al., 1998). Some investigators have advocated cytological screening of high-risk individuals, although the accuracy of anal cytology and the natural history of intraepithelial lesions remain unclear.

Gastroinestinal and hepatobiliary neoplasia

Kaposi's sarcoma

KS is found predominantly in homosexual men but has been described in all risk groups for HIV infection (see Chapter 33). GI KS occurs in around half of the patients with cutaneous involvement and can be widespread throughout the upper and lower GI tract. The tumors are submucosal and therefore usually not a common cause of bleeding, unless there is superficial ulceration. While these tumors are most often asymptomatic, bulky tumors can occasionally lead to intussusception or obstruction. The diagnosis of GI KS is often made by the typical endoscopic appearance. The submucosal location makes standard endoscopic mucosal biopsy more difficult, but this remains the most common way to obtain histological specimens.

KS involves the liver in 8–15% of patients studied at postmortem, usually as part of disseminated disease, although rarely it may be the first manifestation of AIDS (Hasan et al., 1989). Imaging studies demonstrate multiple hepatic nodules. As with involvement of the luminal GI tract, most patients remain asymptomatic. The diagnosis is made incidentally on liver biopsy or more commonly at postmortem examination.

While treatment of hepatic KS is rarely indicated, GI KS may require treatment for obstruction or bleeding.

Lymphoma

The risk of developing non-Hodgkins lymphoma (NHL) is significantly higher in patients with HIV infection than in uninfected individuals (see Chapter 33). The most commonly involved extranodal sites are the central nervous system (CNS) and the GI tract. The tumors are usually high-grade, large-cell immunoblastic lymphomas of B-cell origin, which occur in patients with advanced HIV-related immunodeficiency. Patients with GI NHL are frequently symptomatic with abdominal pain and tenderness, weight loss and rectal bleeding. Tumor involvement occurs throughout the gut, including the oesophagus, stomach, small intestine, colon and rectum. Histological diagnosis is made from biopsy at the time of endoscopy or surgery or from computed-tomography (CT)-directed biopsy.

While the GI tract is commonly involved, hepatic disease occurs in only about 10–15% of patients with lymphoma. Most patients present with B symptoms – fever, night sweats and weight loss – and may have hepatomegaly or jaundice, the latter especially with bile duct involvement or lymphoma involving the head of the pancreas. Malignant ascites is rare. Hepatic involvement by NHL usually causes marked elevations of serum alkaline phosphatase (Schneiderman, 1987). The clinical presentation may mimic that of an opportunistic hepatic infection or AIDS-related cholangiopathy and therefore diagnosis requires tissue examination, either by directed biopsy of visceral lesions or biopsy of the papilla and bile cytology (in the case of bile duct lesions).

For patients with GI lymphoma, survival in small cohort studies has varied from 3 months (Cappell and Botros, 1994) to 2 years (Beck et al., 1996). Several chemotherapeutic regimens are available, which have resulted in high remission rates but short, disease-free intervals (see Chapter 33). The overall prognosis is poor.

Hepatobiliary disease

Hepatobiliary disease is common in HIV-infected patients and may present in a more subtle and insidious manner than opportunistic infections and neoplasia of the GI tract. Elevated serum alkaline phosphatase and aminotransferase levels are common, while jaundice, the cardinal sign of liver dysfunction, is an infrequent manifestation of HIV-related hepatic parenchymal disease. Hepatomegaly, in association with one or more abnormal liver function tests, is the most common clinical finding and autopsy studies have found an enlarged liver in over 80% of patients (Glasgow *et al.*, 1985). Traditionally, hepatobiliary disease has been grouped into those conditions primarily affecting liver cells (intrahepatic disease) and those affecting the biliary tract (extrahepatic disease). In HIV infection, the clinician must also consider the possibility of co-existing intra- and extrahepatic infection or neoplasia. Most hepatic parenchymal disease in HIV-infected patients is due to opportunistic infection, adverse reactions to therapeutic drugs, AIDS-related neoplasia and co-existing viral hepatitis. AIDS-related biliary tract disease can cause severe chronic pain.

Unlike the gut, the liver has not been considered a target organ for HIV infection, since hepatocytes do not express the CD4 molecule, the principal receptor for HIV. However, Kupffer cells (hepatic macrophages) and endothelial cells do express CD4 and support HIV replication. HIV RNA (but not p24 antigen) has been detected in hepatocytes by *in-situ* hybridization, suggesting that HIV may infect CD4 negative parenchymal liver cells (Housset *et al.*, 1993). Transplantation of livers from individuals with unrecognized HIV infection has resulted in transmission of HIV infection to the recipient, lending support to the concept of the liver as an HIV reservoir (Erice *et al.*, 1991). While not proven, HIV infection of hepatic cells may lead to altered function (such as impaired antigen processing and cytokine production by hepatic macrophages) and progressive hepatic disease.

Opportunistic infections of the liver
Mycobacteria

Mycobacterium avium complex. MAC is the most frequent hepatic opportunistic infection reported in clinical and autopsy series (Table 16.4; Cappell, 1991), with a postmortem prevalence ranging from 20–55% (Bonancini, 1992). MAC infection is typically found in patients with advanced HIV-induced immunosuppression (see Chapter 24). Clinical features of disseminated MAC infection include spiking fever, weight loss, diarrhoea, abdominal pain and enlargement of liver, spleen and mesenteric lymph nodes. Commonly, the serum alkaline phosphatase is strikingly elevated, with minimal abnormalities of serum bilirubin or aminotransferases. The diagnosis is made by liver biopsy, which shows poorly formed granulomata associated with

Table 16.4 HIV-related opportunistic infections of the liver

Bacteria
  Mycobacterium avium complex (MAC)
  M. tuberculosis
  Bartonella henselae
  B. quintana
Viruses
  Cytomegalovirus (CMV)
  Herpes simplex virus (HSV)
  (N.B. The hepatitis viruses are not classified as opportunists)
Fungi
  Histoplasma capsulatum
  Cryptococcus neoformans
  Coccidioides imitis
  Candida albicans
  Sporothrix schenckii
  Aspergillus fumigatus
  Pneumocystis carinii

mycobacteria. In some patients, there may be no granulomatous reaction at all in a liver biopsy swarming with mycobacteria. Cultures of liver tissue are usually positive, but the diagnosis is most often made from culture of blood or bone marrow (Hawkins *et al.*, 1986).

Mycobacterium tuberculosis. Extrapulmonary tuberculosis, an AIDS-defining illness, develops at an earlier stage of HIV infection than MAC, and is usually due to reactivation of prior M. *tuberculosis* infection (Selwyn *et al.*, 1989). The clinical presentation of tuberculous hepatitis is similar to that of disseminated MAC infection with fever, weight loss and hepatosplenomegaly. Diagnosis of tuberculous hepatitis is commonly made by culture of sputum, blood or tissue, including liver. AIDS patients with tuberculosis often have well-formed hepatic granulomata, reflecting an intact immune response in patients infected with a virulent organism at an earlier stage in their disease (Crowe *et al.*, 1991). An unusual manifestation of tuberculosis in AIDS patients is the development of visceral abscesses (Moreno *et al.*, 1988). Standard antituberculous therapy is usually effective (see Chapter 23).

Bacteria

Opportunistic pyogenic infection of the liver in patients with advanced HIV infection is rare, but *Salmonella* infections in such patients are often recurrent, with a high incidence of bacteraemia. Fever, abdominal pain and diarrhoea, accompanied by abnormal liver function tests, suggest seeding of the liver with salmonella. Diagnosis is readily made by blood and stool culture and patients should receive treatment with ampicillin, ciprofloxacin or trimethoprim-sulfamethoxazole (TMP-SMX).

Bacillary peliosis hepatis. Early reports of hepatic abnormalities in HIV-infected patients described blood-filled cystic spaces in both the liver and spleen. These histological abnormalities resembled peliosis hepatis, a rare disorder seen in patients with malignancy, tuberculosis or following treatment with anabolic steroids. Further studies demonstrated Gram-negative bacteria associated with the hepatic lesions (Perkocha *et al.*, 1990). *Bartonella* (formerly *Rochalimaea*) *henselae* and *B. quintana* are the aetiological agents of the peliotic lesions in liver and spleen and of bacillary angiomatosis, a vascular lesion of skin and bone first described in HIV-infected persons (Koehler *et al.*, 1997). Bacillary peliosis hepatis may occur without the co-existing skin lesions of bacillary angiomatosis (see Chapter 17).

Prolonged fever, weight loss and abdominal pain are the most common presenting symptoms of bacillary peliosis. In most patients, the liver is enlarged; abnormal liver function tests with raised alkaline phosphatase levels are common. Splenic infection and enlargement of mesenteric lymph nodes may also occur. Imaging studies may show hepatomegaly without focal abnormalities but multiple ring-enhancing lesions have been described (Slater 1992). Bacillary angiomatosis has been reported as a cause of fever, abdominal pain and GI haemorrhage from an intra-abdominal mass that communicated with the small intestine (Koehler and Cederberg, 1995).

Diagnosis of this uncommon opportunistic infection is currently made by histological examination of skin, liver or spleen. *B. henselae* may be recovered from blood cultures using special techniques. In the liver, typical blood-filled, dilated sinusoids are seen on routine H&E staining. However, the clumps of rod-shaped bacteria associated with the peliotic lesions are best demonstrated with the Warthin–Starry stain. The bacteria can also be identified by electron microscopy. Histological changes may be subtle, with only small areas of dilated capillaries in fibrous stroma (Perkocha *et al.*, 1990).

Systemic infection with *B. henselae* responds to prolonged antibiotic treatment. Erythromycin (2 g/day) given for 4–6 weeks is an effective regimen. Resolution of clinical symptoms with improvement of biochemical and histological changes has been reported in the small number of patients identified and treated (Perkocha *et al.*, 1990; Tappero *et al.*, 1993). Tetracycline (2 g/day) given orally for 4 months is also effective (Koehler and Cederberg, 1995) (see also Chapter 17).

Viruses

Cytomegalovirus. CMV causes a self-limited hepatitis in immunocompetent hosts usually associated with a glandular fever-like syndrome. Reactivation of CMV disease as the result of HIV-induced immunodeficiency occasionally results in hepatic infection, although clinical hepatitis is rare (see Chapter 21). Serious CMV hepatic infection is relatively rare compared with CMV ocular or GI disease and is uniformly associated with disseminated infection. CMV hepatitis is characterized by mild abnormalities in biochemical tests, and the diagnosis is made by identifying typical inclusion bodies in hepatocytes, Kupffer cells and biliary epithelium (Schneiderman *et al.*, 1987). Portal mononuclear cell infiltration is common and granulomas may occasionally be found. The virus can be identified in liver by *in-situ* hybridization or staining with monoclonal antibodies (Jacobson and Mills, 1988). There have been no prospective comparative trials of antiviral therapy for CMV hepatitis, but conventional antiviral therapy should be employed if treatment is warranted (see Chapter 21).

In a similar manner to CMV, disseminated HSV infection may rarely involve the liver; patients with HSV hepatitis should be treated with intravenous aciclovir (see Chapter 32).

Fungi

Disseminated fungal disease in AIDS patients may involve the liver. Histoplasmosis, cryptococcosis and coccidioidomycosis have all been described as occasionally causing hepatic infection, especially in patients living in endemic areas (see Chapters 27–29). The clinical presentation is usually that of a systemic infection, with hepatomegaly and variable abnormalities in biochemical tests of liver function. Large fungal abscesses may be visible on imaging studies. Liver biopsy will show the organisms in association with poorly formed granulomata or as free forms in sinusoids but the diagnosis is often made more readily from blood or bone marrow specimens. The liver infection will respond to appropriate antifungal therapy.

Disseminated candidiasis with hepatic microabcesses occurs in patients who are neutropenic secondary to cytotoxic therapy, but is rare in AIDS patients. Isolated cases of hepatic infection with disseminated *Sporothrix schenckii* and *Aspergillus fumigatus* have been reported in AIDS patients.

Pneumocystosis. Pneumocystis carinii pneumonia (PCP) is a common AIDS-defining disease in HIV infection and an important cause of AIDS-related morbidity and mortality (see Chapter 25). Many recent reports have described extrapulmonary pneumocystosis, which rarely may be an index AIDS diagnosis. GI involvement was initially described in the oesophagus and duodenum by Grimes *et al.* (1987). Infection of the liver and spleen was reported by Macher *et al.* (1987) and several patients with *P. carinii* hepatitis (including one with hepatic failure) have been subsequently described (Cohen and Stoeckle 1991; Sachs *et al.*, 1991).

The percentage of AIDS patients who develop disseminated *P. carinii* infection is small, but of those approximately 35% will have hepatic disease. GI infection with *P. carinii* may present as ascites or as abdominal pain and diarrhoea due to small intestinal or colonic involvement. Pulmonary disease at the time of diagnosis of extrapulmonary *P. carinii* infection is variable. Imaging studies may show diffuse small nodules in liver, spleen and kidneys, often with dystrophic calcification.

Diagnosis of *P. carinii* infection requires demonstration of the organism in tissue or body fluids. *P. carinii* may be seen in liver biopsies within foamy nodules containing numerous organisms, but no associated inflammatory cells (Poblete *et al.*, 1989) or within granulomatous lesions with multinucleated giant cells and calcification (Dieterich *et al.* 1992).

As hepatic and GI involvement by *P. carinii* is uncommon, no systematic studies of therapy for extrapulmonary disease have been performed. Although Dieterich *et al.* (1992) recommended treatment with intravenous pentamidine (200 mg/day for 3 weeks) followed by long-term intravenous prophylaxis (200 mg every 2 weeks), Northfelt *et al.* (1990) reported a good response to any systemic antipneumocystis therapy, with survival in 46% of patients. We recommend that patients with GI pneumocystosis are treated with conventional first-line therapeutic regimens (see Chapter 25). All patients should receive continuing secondary oral prophylaxis with systemic chemotherapeutics such as cotrimoxazole.

Interactions between HIV and hepatitis viruses

Interactions between viruses may occur as the result of co-infection of the same cell or through the diffusion of soluble factors including cytokines or viral proteins such as the hepatitis B virus X protein, which can stimulate HIV replication *in vitro*. In addition, HIV-induced immunodeficiency augments replication of many types of viruses. Peripheral blood mononuclear cells can be infected with both HIV and hepatitis B (Laure *et al.*, 1985), and hepatitis C replicative intermediates have also been found in those cells. Co-infection of hepatocytes with HIV and the hepatotrophic viruses has not been described, but Kupffer cells are infected with HIV, suggesting that interactions might occur through short-range diffusion of soluble factors. The clinical outcomes of such interactions are still being described. A recent prospective case–control study of 1894 HIV-infected patients studied prior to the institution of highly active antiretroviral therapy (HAART) identified 308 patient deaths while in hospital. Liver-related mortality, defined biochemically but not histologically, occurred in 35 patients (12%), and in 16 patients (5%) liver failure was the sole cause of death. Death from liver failure was independently associated with alcohol abuse and reactivity for HBsAg, although many patients were co-infected with HCV. Whether the introduction of HAART will decrease the incidence of liver-related deaths by inhibiting the replication of HBV or hepatitis C virus (HCV) remains unclear (Puoti *et al.*, 2000).

Hepatitis A virus (HAV)

HAV infection is common in homosexual men, due to faecal exposure. Epidemic HAV infection among homosexual men has been described in Australia and the USA (Centers for Disease Control and Prevention, 1992). HAV does not appear to be unusually virulent in this patient group and recovery from acute infection with long-term immunity is common, despite antecedent HIV infection. The hepatitis A vaccine is well tolerated and immunogenic in HIV-infected patients although seroconversion rates are lower than in uninfected persons. HIV-infected patients with low CD4 lymphocyte counts show lower seroconversion rates than those with intact immunity (Nielsen *et al.*, 1997).

Hepatitis B virus (HBV)

There is a high prevalence of HBV infection in homosexual men and injecting drug users, regardless of HIV status. However, HIV-infected patients are more likely to develop chronic infection with HBV than are HIV-uninfected persons. Because of the progressive immunodeficiency associated with HIV infection, HBV-infected patients subsequently infected with HIV may demonstrate a progressive reduction in hepatitis B surface antibody (HBsAb) titres (Biggar *et al.*, 1987) and hepatitis B surface antigen (HBsAg) may reappear. Individuals co-infected with HIV and HBV often have increased levels of hepatitis B viral DNA and hepatitis B e antigen (HBeAg). Thus, in HIV-infected chronic HBV carriers, HBV replication is generally poorly controlled by host immune mechanisms and body fluids are highly infectious (Hadler *et al.*, 1991). Does a greater degree of HBV replication affect liver fibrosis? Colin and colleagues studied a cohort of 132 homosexual men with untreated HBV infection; 65 were co-infected with HIV. No patient had chronic HCV infection. Co-infected patients were more likely than those infected only with HBV to be cirrhotic and to have greater HBV replication assessed by higher HBV DNA levels and a greater percentage of HBcAg-positive hepatocytes. No correlation was found between the degree of HIV-induced immunosuppression and the severity of liver disease, although only a small number of patients with advanced HIV infection were studied (Colin *et al.*, 1999). In contrast, other studies have found that HBV-induced liver cell injury, which is largely due to the host immune response to HBV-infected hepatocytes, may be ameliorated by HIV-induced immunosuppression (Bodsworth *et al.*, 1989). This divergence in outcomes raises questions regarding the mechanism of liver fibrosis in immunosuppressed patients and how immune restoration might influence the development of cirrhosis in co-infected patients.

HIV co-infection also frustrates attempts to prevent and treat HBV infection. The neutralizing antibody response to HBV vaccine is T-cell dependent and thus is generally impaired and of shorter duration in HIV-infected patients (Collier *et al.*, 1988), although there may be adequate protection if immunization occurs prior to significant HIV-induced immunosuppression. Zidovudine (ZDV) has not been shown to decrease HBV replication in HIV-infected patients (Gilson *et al.*, 1991). Patients co-infected with HIV and HBV are unlikely to respond to interferon (Wong *et al.*, 1995). A number of nucleoside analogues including lamivudine, and adefovir, initially developed to treat HIV infection, have shown activity against HBV and are now being further evaluated in HIV-uninfected individuals.

Lamivudine has been the most extensively studied nucleoside analogue. Lai *et al.* (1998) administered lamivudine or placebo for 12 months to 358 patients with chronic HBV infection without HIV co-infection. In the group of 140 patients treated with 100 mg daily there was a 98% reduction

in HBV DNA levels and a 16% HBeAg seroconversion rate at the end of treatment, which was accompanied by significant histological improvement. Ongoing studies may demonstrate higher HBeAg seroconversion rates following 2-year treatment regimens. In an open-label study of lamivudine in 40 HBV–HIV co-infected men, subgroup analysis of 27 patients with high baseline levels of HBV replication showed a 96% reduction in HBV DNA, with HBeAg loss in 19% (Benhamou *et al.*, 1996). A later study from the same group showed that development of the lamivudine-resistant YMDD mutant occurred with an annual incidence of 20%, despite the use of higher doses of lamivudine (300 mg/day) than are commonly used in patients with HBV alone. Development of resistance correlated with the duration of lamivudine therapy, as expected, but did not correlate with serum HBV DNA levels or CD4 lymphocyte counts (Benhamou *et al.*, 1999b). Thus, lamivudine is a promising agent for use in HBV–HIV co-infection. The use of lamivudine alone in HBV–HIV co-infected patients is not recommended; due to the development of HIV resistance, such patients should receive concurrent therapy for HIV infection.

While interactions between HIV and HBV have been demonstrated *in vitro*, there is no clinical evidence that concurrent HBV infection accelerates the progression of HIV immunosuppression (Soloman *et al.*, 1990). Scharschmidt *et al.* (1992) found a higher prevalence of serological markers of HBV in AIDS patients compared to patients with HIV infection who had not yet progressed to AIDS. Despite a higher rate of chronic infection (defined by the presence of HBsAg) in the AIDS patients there was no difference in survival between the two groups, suggesting that HBV does not accelerate the progression from asymptomatic HIV infection to AIDS. A cohort study of male homosexuals in the UK showed that HIV–HBV co-infected patients were more likely to have persistent and active HBV replication but not HIV progression compared to those infected only with HIV (Gilson *et al.*, 1997).

Hepatitis D (delta) virus (HDV)

HDV is a defective RNA virus, which depends upon HBV co-infection of liver cells in order to replicate. Delta hepatitis is more commonly seen in injecting drug users and haemophiliacs than in male homosexuals infected with HIV. HDV usually has an inhibitory effect on HBV replication, but it appears that in individuals who are also infected with HIV, there is increased replication of both HDV and HBV, compared to only HDV in HIV-uninfected individuals (Buti *et al.*, 1991). In an open study of high-dose, long-term interferon therapy (10 MU three times per week for 6 months followed by 6 MU three times per week for 6 months) no difference in sustained response was seen between HIV–HDV co-infected patients (one of 16) compared to patients infected with HDV alone (two of 21) (Puoti *et al.*, 1998).

Hepatitis C virus (HCV)

Infection with hepatitis C is more common after exposure to blood than by sexual transmission; thus, male homosexuals with HIV infection are less likely to be co-infected with HCV than injecting drug users or haemophiliacs. Heterosexual co-transmission of HCV and HIV has been described (Eyster *et al.*, 1991) and several studies have documented the increased likelihood of vertical transmission of HCV in HIV co-infected mothers compared to the low transmission of HCV to babies born to mothers with HCV infection alone (Novati *et al.*, 1992; Reinus *et al.*, 1992).

Do patients co-infected with hepatitis C and HIV develop liver fibrosis and liver failure more rapidly than patients infected with HCV alone? Early studies reported conflicting data. For example, Martin *et al.* (1989) reported progression to cirrhosis over 3 years in a small number of HCV–HIV co-infected patients with CD4 lymphocyte counts below 400 cells/μl. They had lower serum ALT levels and less histological inflammation than patients with HCV infection alone (Guido *et al.*, 1994), suggesting that HIV-induced immunosuppression lessened liver inflammation.

However, three recent studies have all shown that HCV-related liver disease can be more severe in HIV-infected patients. Soto and colleagues (1997) studied 547 HCV-infected patients (with HIV infection in 116) in whom progression to cirrhosis occurred more commonly and in significantly less time in HIV–HCV co-infected patients than in those with only HCV infection. A French study of 210 HCV-infected patients (of whom 60 were co-infected with HIV) found that histological inflammation was greater in co-infected patients. Cirrhosis was identified in 30% of HIV–HCV co-infected patients, compared to 15% of patients with HCV alone. Among HIV-infected patients, the percentage with cirrhosis was similar between heavy drinkers and those with lower alcohol intake (Pol *et al.*, 1998). Benhamou *et al.* (1999a) matched 122 HIV–HCV co-infected patients to 122 HCV-infected patients for age, duration of HCV infection and alcohol consumption. They found that hepatic fibrosis progressed at a greater rate

in the co-infected group and that alcohol consumption (> 50 g/day) and a CD4 cell count of less than 200 cells/μl were independently associated with more rapid progression to cirrhosis. Thus, it is very likely that HIV co-infection is a risk factor for developing advanced liver disease and that factors such as alcohol consumption and HCV genotype are as important in co-infected patients as they are in patients with chronic HCV infection alone.

Is the survival of patients with HIV–HCV co-infection worse than that seen in patients with chronic HCV infection alone? A study of HCV–HIV co-infected haemophiliacs found that 9% of co-infected patients developed liver failure compared to none of the patients infected with HCV alone (Eyster *et al.*, 1993). Most of the patients with liver failure had CD4 lymphocyte counts below 100 cells/μl. Whether the development of liver failure was related to HIV-induced immunosuppression, unrecognized opportunistic infection or to the adverse effects of antiretroviral therapy was not clear. Similarly, it is unclear whether the natural history of HCV–HIV co-infection in haemophiliacs can be generalized to other HIV-infected patients. For example, Wright and colleagues (1994) showed in a predominantly male homosexual population with HIV infection that HCV co-infection did not affect survival of patients with or without AIDS. Further prospective studies are needed to provide answers regarding the outcome of HIV–HCV co-infected patients (Ragni and Belle, 2001; Bica *et al.*, 2001).

Antiviral therapy for HCV has become a more relevant concept with the advent of highly effective antiviral therapy for HIV. However, there have been few large clinical trials of antiviral therapy for co-infected patients. One study of 119 HCV-infected patients (with HIV infection in 90) found no difference in sustained virological response between co-infected patients (22%) compared to patients with HCV alone (26%). A CD4 lymphocyte count of greater than 500 cells/μl was associated with a higher likelihood of response (Soriano *et al.*, 1996). Similar findings were recently reported by Causse *et al.* (2000). There have been no controlled studies of combination therapy with interferon and ribavirin in HCV–HIV co-infection.

The decision to treat HCV-related liver disease in patients co-infected with HIV is difficult due to the lack of controlled studies and the potential for serious drug interactions. Patients with mild histological changes (minimal inflammation, no fibrosis) may best be treated expectantly, as progression to cirrhosis in such patients is likely to be slow, if it occurs at all. Those patients with a greater degree of necro-inflammatory activity or fibrosis may be the group that will ultimately benefit from antiviral therapy for HCV. However, durability of response to interferon and the interactions among interferon, ribavirin, other nucleoside analogues and protease inhibitors (PIs) require further study.

Hepatitis G

The hepatitis G virus (HGV) is a recently described RNA virus with approximately 25% homology with HCV. Controversy surrounds the role of HGV as a cause of chronic hepatitis (Thomas et al., 1997). The virus appears to be transmitted by blood and by sexual contact and thus co-infection with HIV, HBV and HCV is relatively common. In 168 HIV-infected patients, the prevalence of HGV RNA was 18% (Ibanez et al., 1998). In a study of 235 HCV-infected patients, 30% were co-infected with HGV, although this did not seem to have an adverse effect on histological severity (Thiers et al., 1998).

Drug-induced hepatotoxicity

Patients with advanced HIV infection are often treated with a large number of medications and drugs must there-

Table 16.5 Potentially hepatotoxic drugs used in HIV infection

Drug/class
Antiretrovirals
Zidovudine
Didanosine
Zalcitabine
Stavudine
Indinavir
Nevirapine
Antifungals
Ketoconazole
Fluconazole
Antivirals
Ganciclovir
Antiprotozoal
Pentamidine
Dapsone
Antimycobacterial
Isoniazid
Rifampin
Azithromycin
Antibacterial
Trimethoprim-sulfamethoxazole (TMP-SMX)
Cytokines
G-CSF

fore be considered in the differential diagnosis of any hepatic injury (see Table 16.5 and Chapter 6). Cotrimoxazole (the combination of trimethoprim and sulfamethoxazole) was recognized early in the AIDS pandemic as a cause of elevated transaminases (Gordin et al., 1984) and hepatic granulomata (Lebovics et al., 1985), which may occur some months after therapy is initiated. Other sulfonamides and sulfones (e.g. dapsone) also may cause hepatitis.

Antiretroviral therapy may also result in hepatic dysfunction. Gradon et al. (1992) reported tender hepatomegaly, raised transaminases and mild jaundice in an AIDS patient treated with ZDV, which resolved with discontinuation of the drug (although the patient was not re-challenged). In a study of 1567 patients comparing two doses of ZDV to placebo, significant elevations of serum bilirubin, but not aminotransferases, were associated with ZDV therapy in 6% of patients (Koch et al., 1992). Lai et al. (1991) reported fulminant hepatic failure in a patient receiving didanosine (ddI). More recently, three patients were reported who developed acute severe hepatitis, with death in one cirrhotic patient, which was temporally related to indinavir therapy (Brau et al., 1997). A prospective cohort study of 298 HIV-infected patients on multiple antiretroviral regimens reported serious biochemical hepatotoxicity in 10% over 6 months – the greatest risk of developing raised serum aminotransferases was associated with ritonavir therapy. However, the majority of patients with chronic viral hepatitis did not experience significant toxicity (Sulkowski et al., 2000). Nonetheless, unexplained serum transaminase elevations and worsening hepatic synthetic function in patients treated with nucleoside analogues or PIs, especially in those with pre-existing chronic liver disease, should prompt serious consideration of stopping such antiretroviral therapy (see below).

The antifungal agents, ketoconazole and fluconazole, have both been linked to transient, usually asymptomatic, elevations of serum aminotransferases. Other commonly used and potentially hepatotoxic medication regimens include antituberculous agents and, less commonly, ganciclovir.

As in HIV-uninfected patients, the diagnosis of drug-induced hepatotoxicity should be considered when there is a likely temporal relationship between hepatic abnormalities and drug therapy. Drug withdrawal should only be followed by re-challenge with a potentially hepatotoxic drug if no suitable alternatives exist and the clinical circumstances mandate active therapy.

Hepatic steatosis

Macrovesicular steatosis (large droplet fat inclusions in liver cells) is a common nonspecific finding in AIDS patients (Lebovics, 1985; Schneiderman, 1987). The contribution of alcohol abuse to fatty change in the AIDS population is relatively small; in most patients, the steatosis remains unexplained but has been attributed to malnutrition from chronic disease. Grunfeld and Kotler (1992) have suggested that steatosis may be due to an interferon-mediated increase in hepatic lipogenesis in HIV infection, combined with a decrease in triglyceride clearance.

Hepatomegaly and extensive macrovesicular steatosis have been described in eight HIV-infected patients (seven female), none of whom used alcohol excessively or were malnourished. All patients had been treated for 6 months or longer with ZDV. Six patients with no history of liver disease developed an ultimately fatal syndrome characterized by raised serum aminotransferases and metabolic acidosis, with death attributed to hepatic failure. Postmortem examination showed extensive fatty deposition but no necro-inflammatory changes. Mitochondrial abnormalities were not reported (Freiman et al., 1993). A study of over 1800 HIV-infected patients identified two patients who had a rapidly fatal illness characterized by encephalopathy, metabolic acidosis and liver failure with large, fat-infiltrated livers found at autopsy (Fortang, 1995). The clinical presentation often includes signs of pancreatitis. A postulated cause is depletion of mitochondrial DNA by ZDV

through drug-induced inhibition of mitochondrial DNA polymerase. Long-term (over 4 months) treatment with other nucleoside analogues such as ddI and zalcitabine (ddC) have been linked anecdotally with this serious syndrome (Stein, 1994).

While a rare occurrence, 1.3 per 1000 person-years in the study by Fortang et al. (1995), the clinician should have a high index of suspicion in patients developing otherwise unexplained liver function abnormalities, especially in association with a raised serum lipase or low bicarbonate level. Cessation of nucleoside analogue therapy should be considered, with ongoing careful clinical assessment and monitoring.

AIDS-related cholangiopathy

A heterogeneous group of biliary tract disorders in patients with HIV infection has been labelled AIDS-related cholangiopathy. The earliest reports described acalculous cholecystitis secondary to cryptosporidial infection of the gallbladder, and subsequently a spectrum of bile duct abnormalities with variable clinical presentations has been described. Patients commonly present with upper abdominal pain, which may be severe, in association with low-grade fever and often striking elevations of alkaline phosphatase, while jaundice is less frequent. Weight loss and chronic diarrhoea are common. While generally seen in advanced HIV infection, bile duct disorders may also be the first sign of disease progression in patients with previously asymptomatic HIV infection (Bouche et al., 1993). Cello (1992) described four types of HIV-associated cholangiopathy seen during endoscopic retrograde cholangiography (ERCP) (Table 16.6).

Non-invasive imaging studies, including ultrasound and CT, are frequently abnormal, showing dilatation of the common bile duct and intra-hepatic biliary tree (Vakil et al., 1996). ERCP is useful in confirming ductal dilatation and thickening seen on CT or ultrasound scanning and in more precisely demonstrating discrete strictures or subtle changes in the bile duct wall. Biochemical abnormalities,

Table 16.6 Radiographical classification of AIDS cholangiopathy

Papillary stenosis
> The predominant abnormality is distal tapering of the bile duct at the papilla of Vater with proximal dilatation. This may be associated with delayed emptying of contrast from the bile duct.

Distal common bile duct structure
> This may be an extension of the pathological process in papillary stenosis in which the distal duct is narrowed over a 1–2 cm length with proximal dilation.

Sclerosing cholangitis
> The radiological picture is somewhat similar to primary sclerosing cholangitis with numerous focal strictures and proximal dilatation involving both the intra- and extrahepatic bile ducts.

Mixed
> The radiological appearance may combine features of both papillary stenosis and sclerosing cholangitis.

Table 16.7 Presumptive causes of AIDS cholangiopathy

Cytomegalovirus (CMV)
Cryptosporidia
Microsporidia
Mycobacterium avium complex (MAC)
Lymphoma

particularly a raised alkaline phosphatase, are common and if accompanied by pain or fever should lead to consideration of ERCP even if non-invasive imaging studies are normal.

AIDS-related cholangiopathy is commonly associated with opportunistic viral or protozoal infection of the intestine (Table 16.7). Cello (1992) reported the findings of histology and culture of ampullary biopsies (including postmortem studies) in 40 patients. He found evidence of CMV infection in seven, cryptosporidiosis in five, MAC in three and neoplasia in two; over half of the patients had acute or chronic inflammatory changes only, with no identifiable pathogen or neoplasm. Pol and colleagues (1993) documented microsporidia in biliary epithelium associated with inflammatory changes in HIV-infected patients presenting with cholangitis. A retrospective study of 82 HIV-infected patients following cryptosporidial contamination of a municipal water supply described diarrhoea in 58 and biliary symptoms in 24. CD4 lymphocyte counts were ≤ 50 cells/μl in 88% of the patients developing biliary symptoms (Vakil et al., 1996).

As with parenchymal liver disease, the clinician should try to identify treatable conditions and not expose patients to unnecessary intervention, although in this condition there is a paucity of controlled studies to guide clinical decisions. Endoscopic sphincterotomy may be useful in palliating severe upper abdominal pain. In the study reported by Vakil et al. (1996) endoscopic biliary sphincterotomy was performed in nine of 10 patients who underwent ERCP, resulting in partial relief in three patients and no relief in six. In contrast, a study reported in abstract form of 41 patients with AIDS-related cholangiopathy found that of 21 undergoing endoscopic sphincterotomy, 18 were pain free or 'moderately' pain free up to 3 months following the procedure (Wettstein et al., 1998).

No controlled trials of antibacterial or antiviral treatment of AIDS-related cholangiopathy have been reported. Anecdotal reports of therapy with metronidazole (Pol et al., 1993), ganciclovir or spiramycin (Bouche et al., 1993) have been disappointing, with no clear response noted. Dowsett et al., (1988) reported the onset of AIDS-related cholangiopathy in two patients on maintenance ganciclovir therapy for cytomegalovirus retinitis; no biliary pathogen was demonstrated in either patient. It seems likely that the incidence of opportunistic biliary infection will decrease following the introduction of highly active antiretroviral therapy (HAART).

Evaluation of HIV-infected patients with suspected hepatobiliary disease

In any patient with suspected liver or biliary tract disease, one must consider whether the current illness represents a new process, which in HIV-infected patients may be the first manifestation of AIDS, or whether there is reactivation or progression of pre-existing disease. Obtaining a history of viral hepatitis, alcohol abuse or the use of potentially hepatotoxic medications is a helpful first step. In patients with advanced HIV disease the systemic effects of sepsis, hypotension or malnutrition should be considered, in addition to disseminated opportunistic infections or HIV-related neoplasia. Initial diagnostic efforts should focus on whether the historical, biochemical and radiological evidence point to hepatic parenchymal disease or a biliary tract disorder.

Biochemical evaluation

A large proportion of patients with advanced HIV infection have non-specific elevations of serum aminotransferases (Lebovics et al., 1985). In patients without extrahepatic biliary tract obstruction, a marked elevation of serum alkaline phosphatase correlates with intra-hepatic MAC infection or lymphoma (Schneiderman et al., 1987). CMV hepatitis or intra-hepatic KS are not associated with a predictable pattern of biochemical abnormality. Drug-induced liver disease may present with a cholestatic, hepatocellular or mixed picture, which in some cases is accompanied by peripheral eosinophilia and eosinophilic infiltration of the liver. Appropriate viral serology may help distinguish among acute viral hepatitis, superinfection with a second viral agent or reactivation of a chronic infection (such as the change from a low to a high replication state for hepatitis B).

Imaging studies

CT and/or ultrasound scanning should be obtained early in the diagnostic process, looking specifically for focal hepatic lesions or dilated bile ducts. Imaging studies may be normal in patients with AIDS-related cholangiopathy (Cello, 1992) and may miss common bile duct stones, so if the clinical suspicion of biliary tract disease is high, ERCP should be the next step. Biopsy of the papilla and/or bile cytology may lead to a definitive diagnosis of infection with CMV, cryptosporidia or microsporidia. Endoscopic sphincterotomy may provide a degree of palliation in patients with abdominal pain and papillary stenosis, as discussed above.

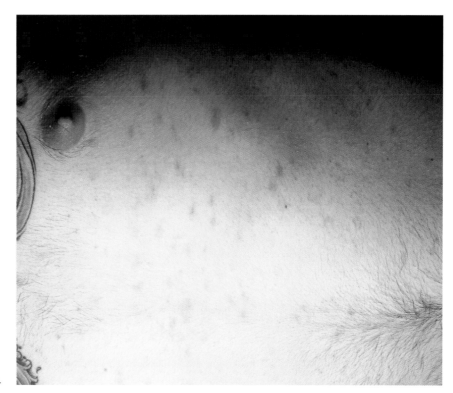

Figure 1.1 *Erythematous, maculopapular rash in a patient with primary HIV-1 infection.*

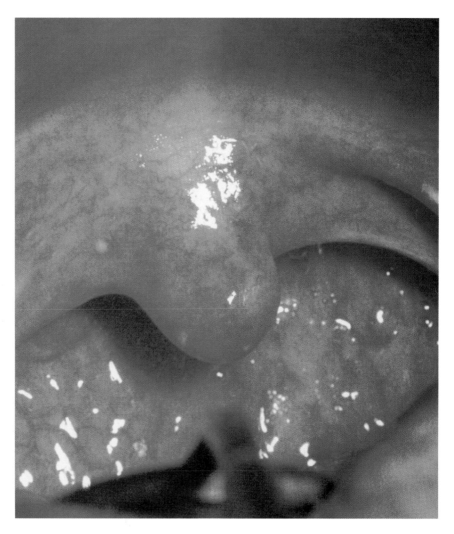

Figure 12.1 *Pseudomembraneous candidiasis. Creamy white patches on erythematous mucosa.*

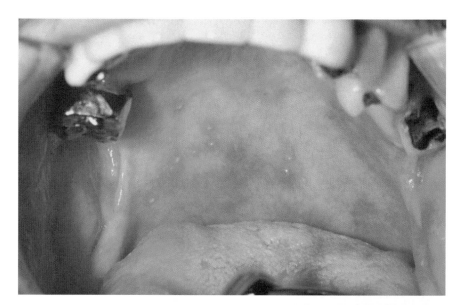

Figure 12.2 *Erythematous candidiasis appearing as palatal erythema.*

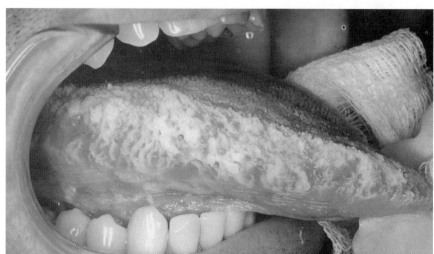

Figure 12.3 *Hairy leukoplakia appearing as corrugations on the lateral margin of the tongue.*

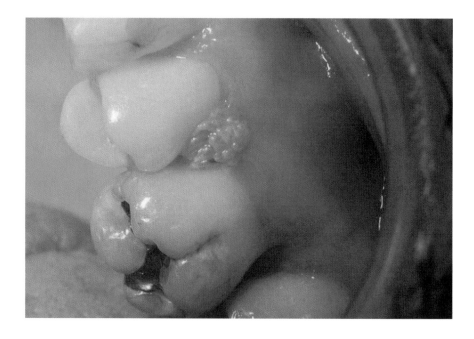

Figure 12.4 *Wart on gingiva.*

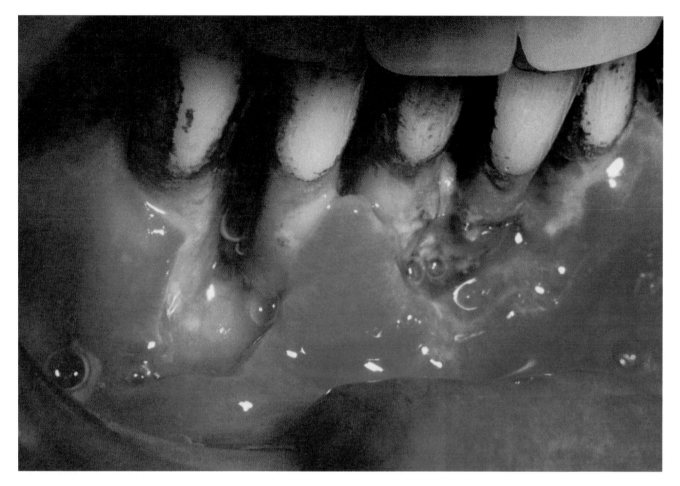

Figure 12.5 *HIV-associated peridontal disease showing extensive destruction of the gingival tissue.*

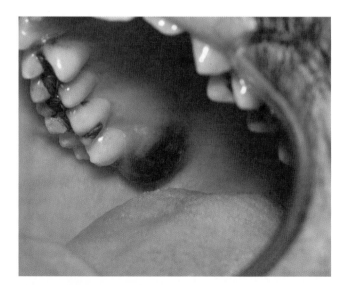

Figure 12.6 *Kaposi's sarcoma on the palate.*

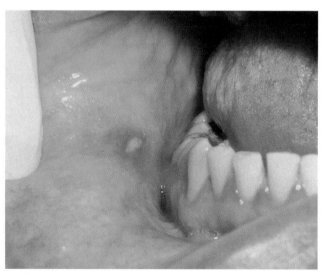

Figure 12.7 *Aphthous ulcer on the labial mucosa.*

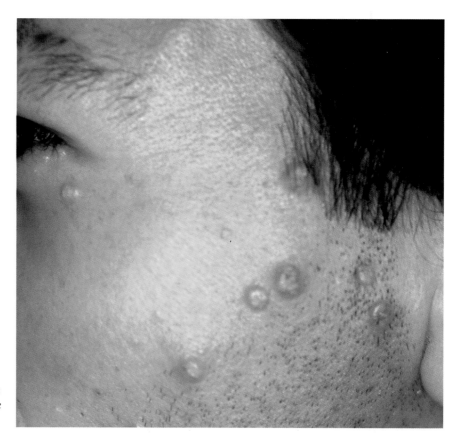

Figure 19.1 *Multiple facial molluscum contagiosum is virtually always seen in patients with fewer than 200 helper T cells/μl. Note the tendency for lesions to occur around the eyes.*

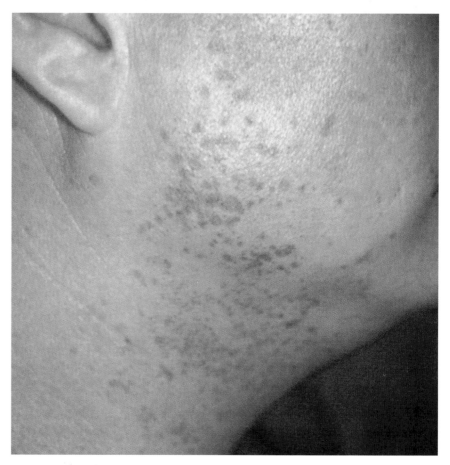

Figure 19.2 *Multiple facial warts are present.*

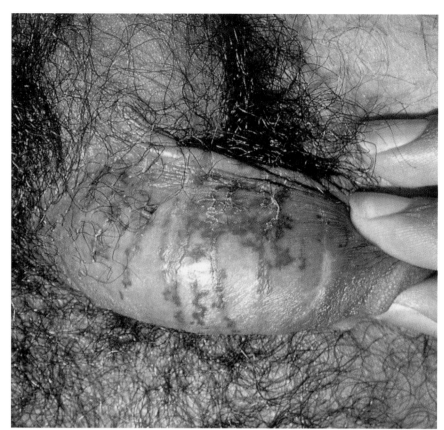

Figure 19.3 *Bowenoid papulosis due to human papillomavirus infection. Hyperpigmented plaques that histologically showed human papillomavirus infection and dysplasia. This lesion is potentially premalignant in the immunocompromised host.*

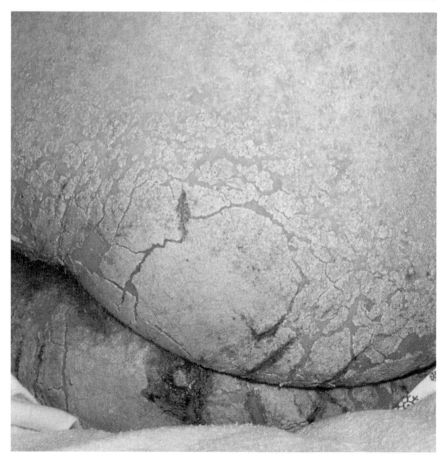

Figure 19.4 *This patient has Norwegian scabies and is highly contagious.*

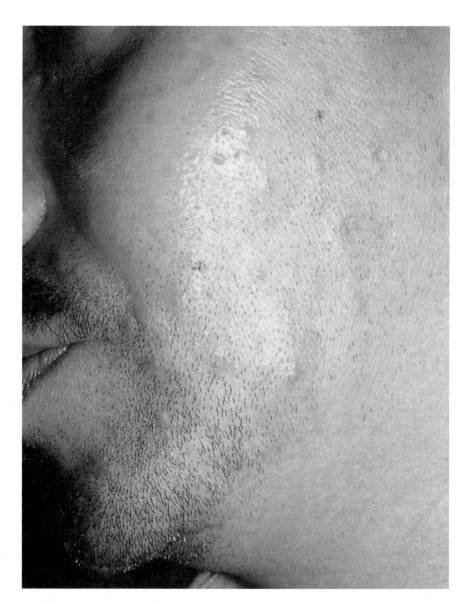

Figure 19.5 *Staphylococcal folliculitis of the face may include pruritic lesions mimicking eosinophilic folliculitis.*

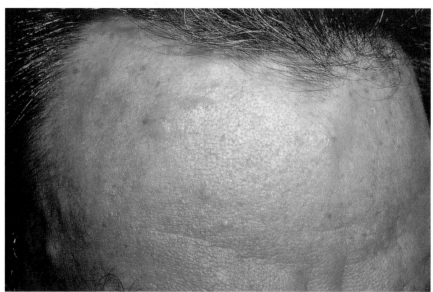

Figure 19.6 *Eosinophilic folliculitis with typical pruritic urticarial follicular papules. Pustules are rare.*

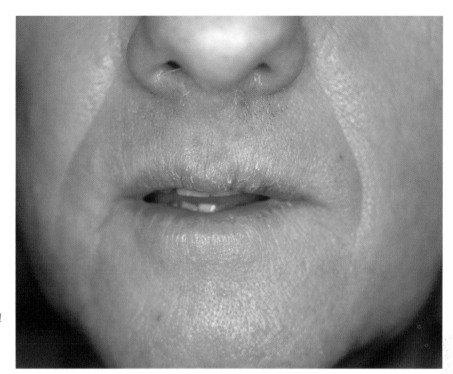

Figure 19.7 *Cheilitis and mild eczema associated with indinavir and itraconazole. Cheilitis, pruritis and asteototic eczema, as well as lipodystrophy, are being increasingly seen, particularly in association with the protease inhibitors.*

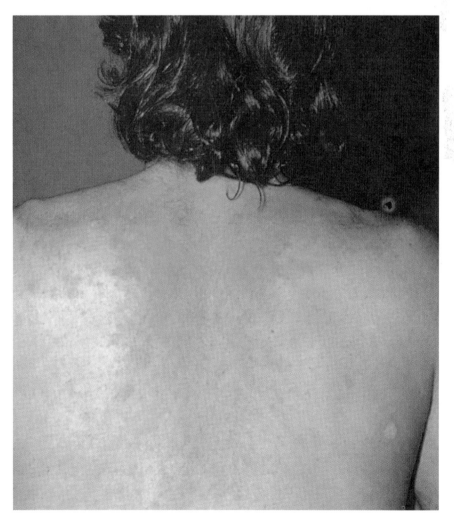

Figure 19.8 *This extensive form of seborrhoeic dermatitis may be very pruritic and spread down the back and upper arms, simulating an eczema.*

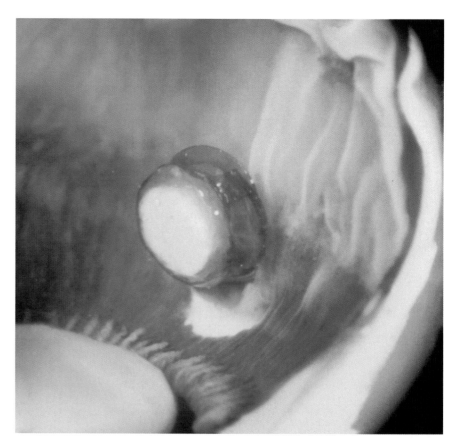

Figure 21.1 *Ganciclovir ocular implant.*

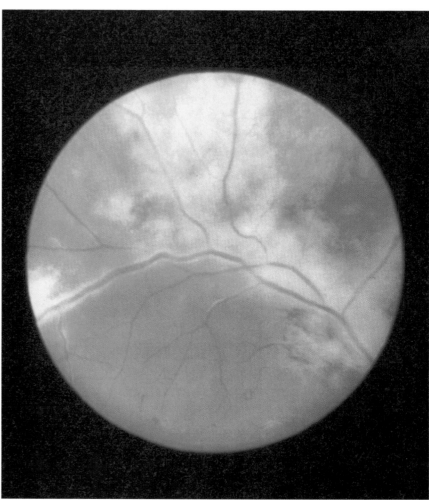

Figure 21.3 *Characteristic CMV retinitis with both yellow exudates sheathing the retinal vessels and haemorrhages.*

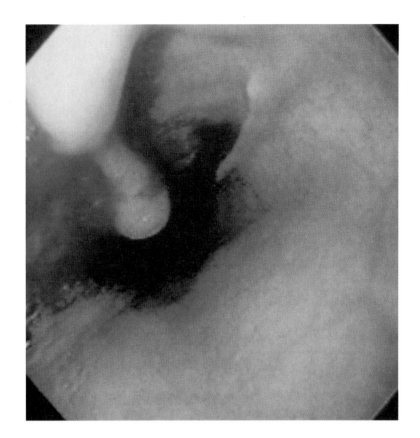

Figure 21.4 *CMV oesophageal ulcer.*

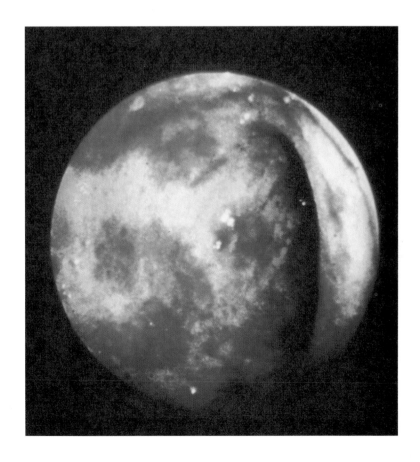

Figure 21.5 *CMV colitis.*

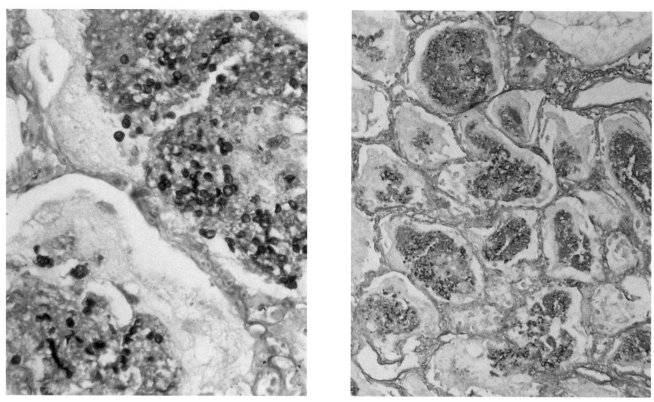

Figure 25.1 *Histopathology of Pneumocystis carinii pneumonia (PCP). The left panel shows lung tissue stained with haematoxylin and eosin from a patient with PCP. There are clumps of Pneumocystis organisms and proteinaceous material filling the alveolar lumen. In the right panel, a higher power view demonstrates clusters of cyst forms stained by methenamine silver (courtesy of R.D. Smith, MD).*

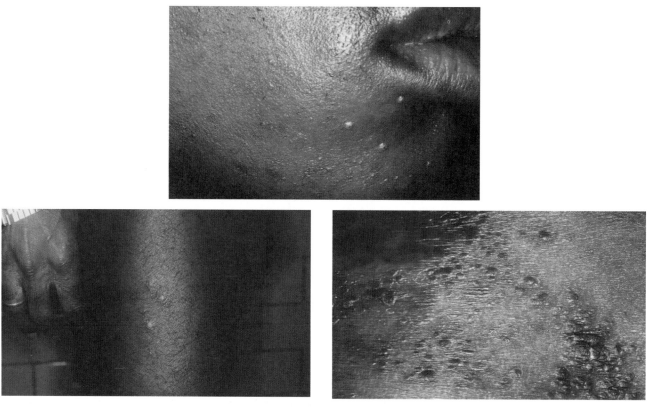

Figure 27.1 *Cryptococcal skin lesion in an African AIDS patient (reproduced with permission from M. Pancin, MD).*

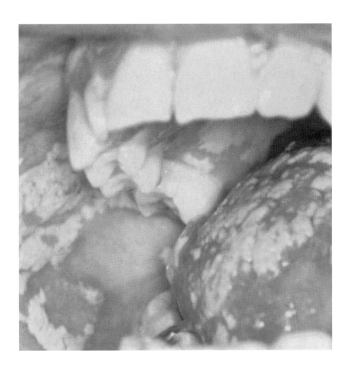

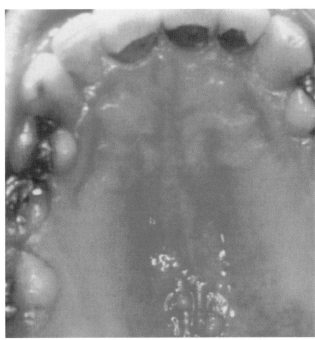

Figure 28.2 *Oral candidiasis; hypertrophic variety on the top and erythematous on the bottom (courtesy of J. Schaaf, Indiana University School of Dentistry).*

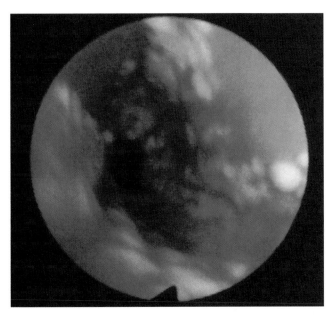

Figure 28.3 *Oesophageal candidiasis, showing white pseudomembrane as seen at endoscopy (courtesy of D. Dieterich, New York University Medical Center).*

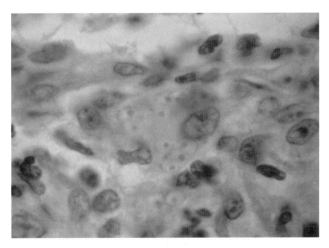

Figure 29.4 *Demonstration of H. capsulatum yeasts in tissues by haematoxylin and eosin stain.*

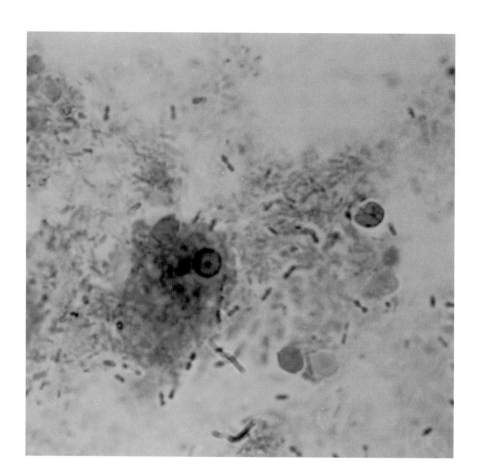

Figure 30.1 Cryptosporidium parvum *oocysts in stool specimen; modified Kinyoun iron haematoxylin stain.*

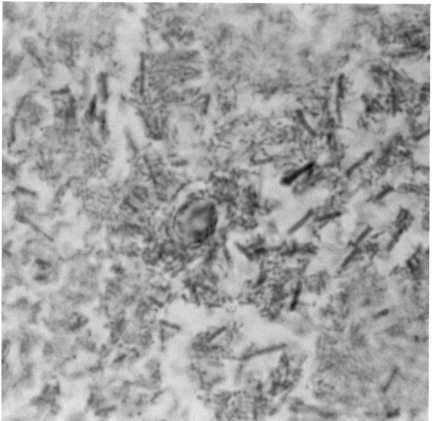

Figure 30.2 Cyclospora cayentanensis *oocysts in stool specimen; modified Kinyoun iron haematoxylin stain.*

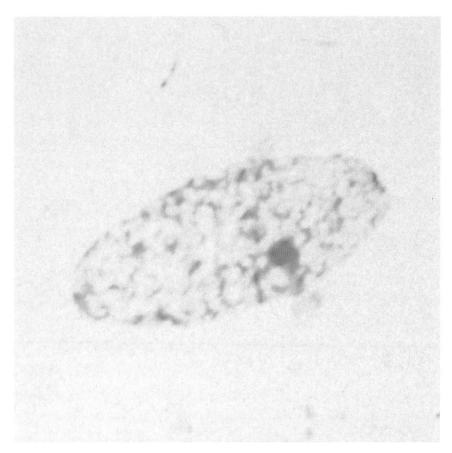

Figure 30.3 Isospora belli *oocyst in stool specimen; modified Kinyoun iron haematoxylin stain.*

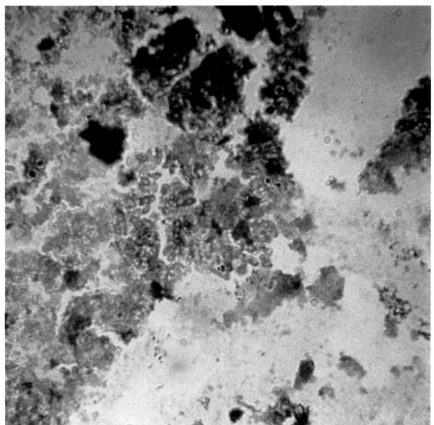

Figure 30.4 *Microsporidial spores in stool specimen; modified trichrome stain.*

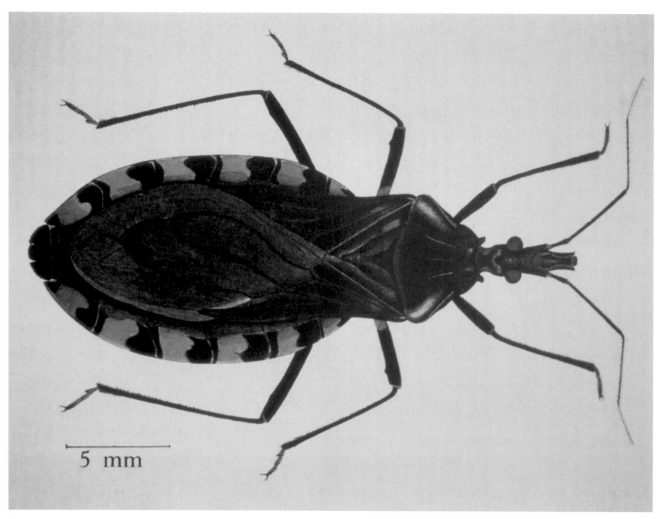

Figure 31.1 *Triatoma infestans (vinchuca)*.

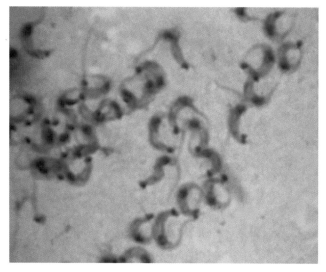

Figure 31.2 *T. cruzi in cerebrospinal fluid (courtesy of Dr David Lewi)*.

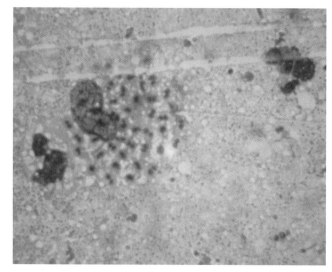

Figure 31.3 T. cruzi *amastigotes in brain biopsy*.

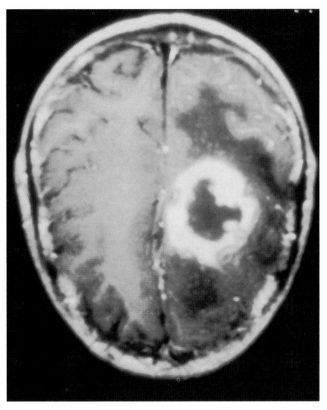

Figure 31.4 *Large cerebral granulomatous mass in NMR ('Chagoma'), enhancing with gadolinium.*

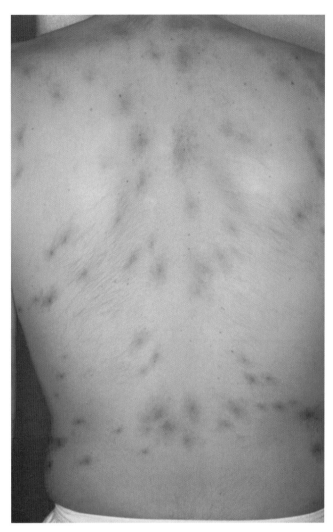

Figure 31.5 *A patient with visceral leishmaniasis and HIV infection. Exotic skin manifestations of leishmaniasis mimic Kaposi's sarcoma lesions (photograph courtesy of Dr Anatacio Queiroz de Souza).*

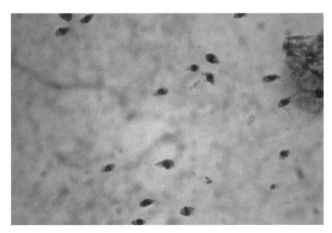

Figure 31.6 Leishmania *amastigotes in the peripheral blood of patients with visceral leishmaniasis and HIV infection (Giemsa skin, original magnification ×1000).*

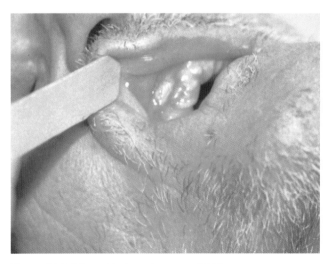

Figure 31.7 *Mucosal leishmaniasis in an AIDS patient.*

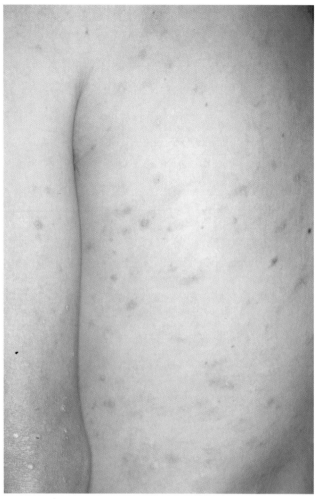

Figure 36.1 *Clinical appearance of pruritic papular eruptions in a Thai HIV-infected patient (photo courtesy of Dr Wiwut Kokit, Department of Dermatology, Chulalungkorn Hospital, Bangkok, Thailand).*

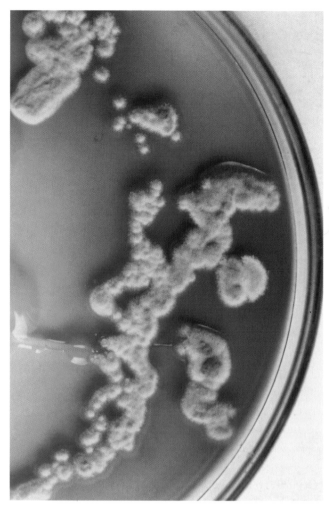

Figure 36.3 P. marneffei *culture appearance (photo courtesy of Dr Wiwut Kokit, Department of Dermatology, Chulalongkorn Hospital, Bangkok, Thailand).*

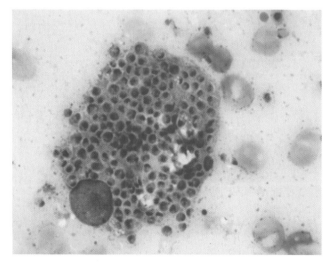

Figure 36.2 P. marneffei *seen on Wright's stain (photo courtesy of Dr Wiwut Kokit, Department of Dermatology, Chulalongkorn Hospital, Bangkok, Thailand).*

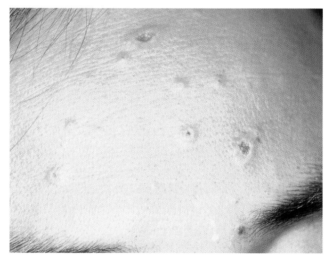

Figure 36.4 *Clinical appearance of penicilliosis in a Thai HIV-infected patient (photo courtesy of Dr Wiwut Kokit, Department of Dermatology, Chulalongkorn Hospital, Bangkok, Thailand).*

Table 18.3 Body composition changes in patients with AIDS during home parenteral nutrition

	Initial	Final
Body weight (kg)	51 ± 1.5	54 ± 3.0
Total body potassium (mM)	2620 ± 99	2644 ± 129
Body fat content (kg)	7.3 ± 1.4	11.2 ± 1.7[a]

(Adapted from Kotler et al., 1990.)
[a] $p = 0.0076$.
Note: Pre-treatment and final body compositions were compared while patients were receiving parenteral nutrition. As a primarily intracellular constituent, increases in total body potassium reflect increases in lean body mass. Data as mean ± SEM.

gained with refeeding. Kotler and colleagues, (1990) administered home total parenteral nutrition to 12 AIDS patients with prior weight loss (Table 18.3). Despite an increase in body weight, there was no change in LBM in the group; the increase in weight was accounted for entirely by changes in body fat stores. Retrospectively, the subjects could be divided into those who had gastrointestinal conditions (i.e. impaired intake of food) and those with opportunistic infections. The former group showed increased LBM, while the latter group did not, suggesting that nutrient-responsive starved and nutrient-unresponsive (abnormal metabolism) subgroups exist.

Results of studies using the appetite stimulant megestrol acetate in HIV-infected patients with significant weight loss have been similar (Hellerstein et al., 1990; Oster et al., 1994; Von Roenn et al., 1994). Megestrol acetate is a progesterone-agonist, oestrogen-antagonist, semi-synthetic steroid hormone that has been shown to increase food intake and body weight in women with breast cancer (Tcheckmedyian et al., 1987). The high-progesterone milieu of pregnancy is known to be associated with increased food intake and weight gain, and progesterone has long been recognized as having anabolic, as well as possible appetite stimulating, properties (Landau, 1953). In one study in men with AIDS-related weight loss, megestrol acetate (800 mg daily) caused a 22% increase in food intake and an average weight gain of 3.2 kg; however, at least 70% of the weight gained was fat (Hellerstein et al., 1990). Other investigators have reported that close to 100% of the weight gained was fat (4.2 kg body fat versus 4.1 kg weight gain) (Oster et al., 1994; Von Roenn et al., 1994). In addition, megestrol acetate at this dose had significant side-effects, particularly erectile impotence, which occurred in most subjects

(Hellerstein et al., 1990). Of interest, megestrol acetate causes marked hypogonadism with a large drop in serum total testosterone (Hellerstein, unpubl. observations, 1995). Reversal of megestrol acetate-induced hypogonadism may provide a strategy for improving the lean tissue response to this treatment. Preliminary results (Strawford et al., 1997) failed to show significant improvements in LBM by adding testosterone 200 mg by intramuscular injection every 2 weeks to megestrol acetate therapy, but this approach has not been fully explored. Studies to date with dronabinol (a cannabinoid with appetite-stimulating effects) have not evaluated changes in body composition. Nutritional studies in cancer have similarly revealed a preferential increase in body fat without gains in lean body mass (Shike et al., 1984; Streat et al., 1987).

The most likely explanation for failure of these patients to increase lean body mass with feeding is that infections, including HIV and the associated opportunistic infections, alter intracellular metabolism in a fashion that favours accrual of fat over lean tissue. There are a number of potential sites of metabolic dysregulation that could have this effect (Table 18.4). By using newly developed stable isotope-mass spectrometric techniques, it has been possible to study most of these metabolic pathways in HIV-infected humans (Hellerstein et al., 1993; Mulligan et al., 1993; Hoh et al., 1998). Some AIDS patients with weight loss have relatively normal metabolism, consistent with simple starvation (e.g. low energy expenditure, no synthesis of fat, low gluconeogenesis), but others have striking metabolic disturbances. The most consistent metabolic abnormality so far documented (Hellerstein, 1993; Hellerstein et al., 1993; Hellerstein et al., 1996; Hoh et al., 1998) is increased synthesis of fat, which may reflect the actions of

Table 18.4 Potential sites of metabolic dysregulation in HIV infection that could favour fat deposition over increases in lean body mass

Abnormal lipid metabolism
    Excess fat synthesis or storage
    Impaired fat mobilization or oxidation
Primary increase in gluconeogenesis
Primary abnormality of protein metabolism
    Decreased synthesis
    Increased breakdown
Energy-wasteful substrate cycles

cytokines in tissues and could contribute to abnormalities of body composition.

Differentiating between the nutrient-responsive (starved) and nutrient-unresponsive (abnormal metabolism) groups has been achieved by use of a research tool (mass spectrometric measurement of lipogenesis (Hoh *et al.*, 1998). Other routinely available clinical tests have not been able to discriminate between the two groups. The former group does well with nutritional therapy alone, while the latter group may require alternative anabolic therapies in addition to nutrient provision, perhaps because of the presence of an abnormal metabolic milieu. Failure to increase LBM after provision of nutrients may be taken as presumptive evidence that a patient falls into the nutrient-unresponsive category.

Because providing nutrients often fails to increase LBM in AIDS patients with wasting, a number of alternative anabolic therapies have been considered. The first of these to be tested was recombinant human growth hormone (rGH) therapy (Mulligan *et al.*, 1993; Schambelan *et al.*, 1996; Paton, 1997). Growth hormone has a direct effect on lipolysis, which could stimulate mobilization and oxidation of fat, thereby reducing oxidation of protein (Randle, 1986). This hormone also stimulates lean tissue metabolism indirectly through insulin-like growth factor-1 (IGF-1) (Guler *et al.*, 1987). Use of rGH had been previously shown to increase LBM in a variety of clinical settings, including hypocaloric postoperative patients (Jian *et al.*, 1989), and men over 60 years old (Rudman *et al.*, 1990). Treatment of HIV-infected patients maintained on a constant diet with rGH resulted in immediate weight gain and nitrogen retention. The positive nitrogen balance was sizeable (4–5 mg/day, representing 125–160 mg lean tissue/day) and was associated with the appropriate retention of potassium and phosphate for repletion of muscle tissue (Mulligan *et al.*, 1993). The HIV-infected patients gained weight and retained nitrogen at the same rate as the HIV-uninfected controls. In long-term studies of rGH treatment (Schambelan *et al.*, 1996), LBM increased by 3 kg over 12 weeks, while total weight increased by only 2 kg, due to loss of body fat. Some evidence for functional improvement (increased treadmill exercise performance in association with the increased LBM) was also presented (Schambelan *et al.*, 1996). LBM gains appear to persist only as long as recombinant growth hormone treatment is continued; withdrawal of therapy has generally resulted in reversal of lean tissue gains in most clinical settings, although formal dose reduction or withdrawal studies have not been reported. The need for continued growth hormone therapy is problematic, because long-term use of rGH is extremely expensive (currently US$1000 per week for the dose used), requires daily subcutaneous administration, and has adverse effects (diabetes, hypertriglyceridemia, carpal tunnel syndrome). A potentially more cost-effective use of rGH might be to administer it during acute opportunistic infections, such as pneumocystis pneumonia, to prevent the rapid weight loss often observed in this setting (MaCallan *et al.*, 1993). A recent report (Paton, 1997) suggests that this approach might be effective. The optimal dose and duration of rGH therapy is yet to be defined.

Other anabolic strategies have also been evaluated (Bhasin *et al.*, 1996; Coodley and Coodley, 1997; Bhasin *et al.*, 1998; Grinspoon *et al.*, 1998; Miller *et al.*, 1998a; Roubenoff *et al.*, 1999; Sattler *et al.*, 1999; Strawford *et al.*, 1999a, b). Recent studies using gonadal steroids (testosterone or its derivatives), either alone or in combination with exercise, have provided additional therapeutic options for repletion of LBM. Hypogonadism is the most common endocrine abnormality in men with AIDS and weight loss (Dobs *et al.*, 1988). Physiological testosterone replacement in frankly hypogonadal men has clearly been shown to be effective for restoring muscle mass, in HIV-wasting as well as in HIV-uninfected men (Bhasin *et al.*, 1997; Sih *et al.*, 1997; Bhasin *et al.*, 1998; Grinspoon *et al.*, 1998). Until recently the efficacy of administering androgens to these patients, especially to those with serum testosterone concentrations in the low–normal rather than the frankly hypogonadal range, had not been established. However, Strawford *et al.* (1999a) surveyed total serum testosterone levels in men with HIV-associated weight loss compared to HIV-uninfected healthy men in the San Francisco Bay Area (Figure 18.1). The most common levels in healthy men were in the range between 450 and 700 ng/dl, whereas in the HIV-weight loss group the most common levels were in the 200–450 ng/dl range (the lower limit of laboratory normal was 200 ng/dl). A placebo-controlled, randomized and blinded study of androgen therapy in these borderline hypogonadal men was then performed, comparing nandrolone decanoate (a testosterone derivative considered to be an 'anabolic' steroid) at 67–200 mg/week with placebo injections. While maintaining a constant diet and controlled activity under metabolic ward conditions, subjects who received either dose of nandrolone exhibited significant nitrogen retention (approximately 4 g nitro-

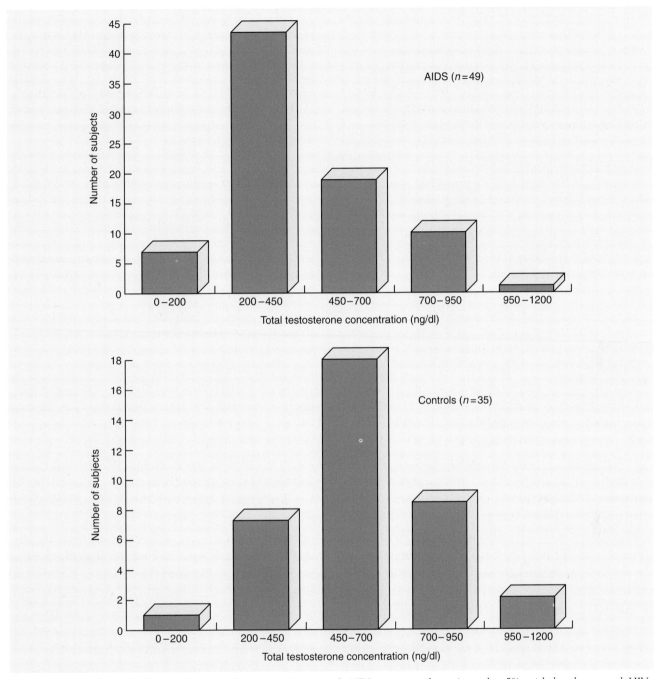

Figure 18.1. *Population distribution of serum total testosterone in men with AIDS-wasting syndrome (more than 5% weight loss documented, HIV-1 sero-positive, age less than 50 years of age, no acute opportunistic infections within past 60 days, no use of androgens or other nutritional/anabolic therapies within previous 3 months, n = 79) and normal HIV-1 seronegative men (n = 35, age less than 50 years of age) in the San Francisco Bay Area. Total testosterone was measured by Nichols Laboratories. Normal controls were recruited by advertisement; AIDS subjects were consecutive eligible individuals recruited by advertisement for studies of wasting that did not mention androgen treatment or gonadal status (courtesy of Strawford et al., 1999a).*

gen/day, representing about 130 g lean tissue gained per day) and weight gain over the 14-day study period, compared to the placebo group (Figures 18.2 and 18.3). In the subsequent 12-week open label phase, subjects gained about 3 kg lean body mass, similar to the effects of recom-

binant growth hormone. These subjects also gained 1.5 kg fat mass, unlike growth hormone treatment, which reduces fat mass (Schambelan et al., 1996). Nandrolone deconoate treatment was associated with improvement in some functional measures of exercise and strength

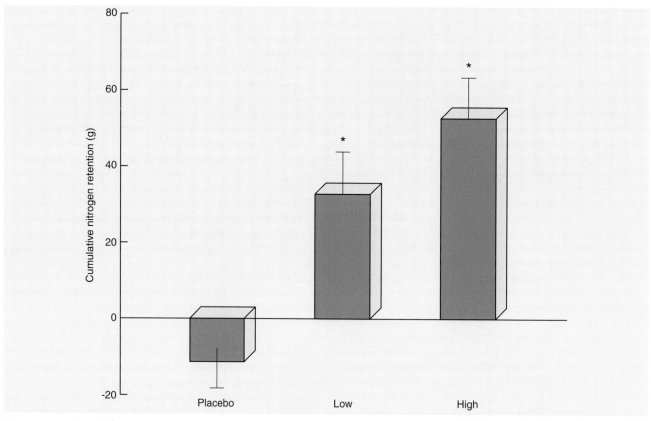

Figure 18.2. *Cumulative nitrogen retention (14-day total) during inpatient treatment phase for placebo group (n = 7), low-dose nandrolone group (n = 4) and high-dose nandrolone group (n = 7). *p < 0.05 versus placebo group (by ANOVA) (courtesy of Strawford et al., 1999a).*

(Strawford *et al.*, 1999a). In contrast to these results, and other studies using transferral of intramuscular testosterone therapy (Bhasin *et al.*, 1998; Grinspoon *et al.*, 1998), Coodley and Coodley (1997) reported no gains in weight or lean tissue with testosterone treatment in AIDS patients with prior weight loss. However, the latter study was performed in unselected AIDS patients rather than in those with reduced testosterone concentrations, and it suffered from a high drop-out rate. It appears likely, therefore, that treatment with androgenic agents is effective at restoring LBM but primarily in men with borderline–low or frankly low serum total testosterone levels (e.g. at or below the lowest quartile or tertile of normal range, typically less than about 500 ng/dl).

Administration of testosterone to eugonadal, healthy men in the absence of resistance exercise typically has modest effects on lean tissue mass or body composition. One reason for this is that, at physiological replacement doses (e.g. 100 mg testosterone/week by intramuscular injection), exogenous testosterone turns off endogenous testosterone production, resulting in no net change in androgen status (Wilson, 1990). At supraphysiological doses (e.g. testosterone 600 mg by intramuscular injection/week) in the absence of exercise, slight gains in lean tissue have been observed, without substantial effects on strength (Bhasin *et al.*, 1996). The combination of supraphysiological testosterone doses plus progressive resistance exercise, however, results in striking synergistic effects in normal men, with much greater gains in LBM, muscle size and muscle strength observed than with either exercise or testosterone alone (Bhasin *et al.*, 1996). The long-term safety and behavioural consequences of the very high doses of testosterone used by Bhasin *et al.* (1996) of 600 mg intramuscularly/week are not known and could pose serious risks (e.g. prostate cancer or hypertrophy, cardiovascular disease, baldness, acne, irritability, aggressive behaviour, etc). Strawford *et al.* (1999b) conducted a double-blind placebo-controlled study in 24 eugonadal men with HIV-associated weight loss to determine whether a moderately supraphysiological androgen regimen including an 'anabolic' steroid improves the lean tissue response to resistance exercise in HIV-1-infected men with prior weight

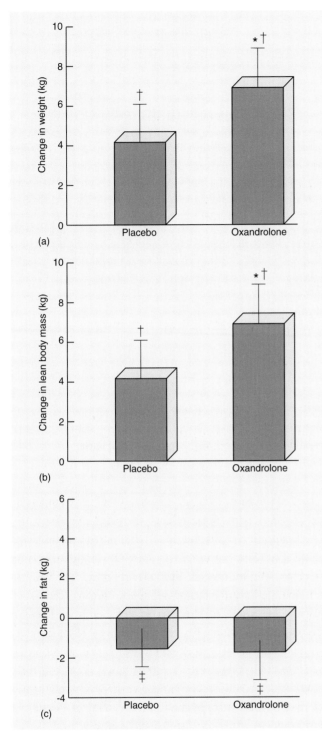

Figure 18.3. *Change in body weight and body composition (by DEXA) in patients with HIV-associated wasting receiving progressive resistance exercise plus placebo (placebo group) or 20 mg oxandrolone/day (oxandrolone group). Data are presented as mean ± SD. The asterisk indicates significantly different change from baseline between the groups, by repeated measures ANOVA (p < 0.05). The dagger indicates significant different change from baseline by the Tukey follow-up procedure (p < 0.05). The double dagger indicates significant change from baseline in both groups (p < 0.05), which is not significantly different between groups (courtesy of Strawford et al., 1999b).*

loss, and whether protease inhibitor (PI) antiretroviral therapy prevents lean tissue anabolism. All subjects received supervised progressive resistance exercise (PRE) with physiological testosterone replacement (100 mg by intramuscular injection/week) for 8 weeks, to suppress endogenous testosterone production. Men were randomized to anabolic steroid, oxandrolone (20 mg/day, OX/PRE) or placebo (P/PRE). Both intervention arms showed significant nitrogen retention and increases in LBM, weight, and strength (Figures 18.2 and 18.3). The gains were significantly greater in those randomized to OX/PRE than to P/PRE (5.6 ± 2.1 versus 3.8 ± 1.8 g nitrogen/day; 6.9 ± 1.7 versus 3.8 ± 2.9 kg LBM; greater upper and lower body muscle strength gains by maximum weight lifted and dynamometry; $p < 0.05$ for all parameters) (Table 18.4). High-density lipoprotein-cholesterol fell significantly in the OX/PRE group. The investigators concluded that a moderately supraphysiological androgen regimen that included an anabolic steroid, oxandrolone, substantially increases the lean tissue accrual and strength gains from PRE, compared to physiological testosterone replacement, in eugonadal men with HIV-associated weight loss. A *post-hoc* analysis for effect of HIV-PI therapy revealed that PIs do not prevent lean tissue anabolism. Recent studies with high-dose nandrolone deconoate combined with PRE (Sattler *et al.*, 1999) have shown similar additive results.

Anticytokine therapies have also been considered for prevention or reversal of body wasting. Although the hypothesis that TNF-α plays a role in HIV-associated wasting remains unproven, anti-TNF agents such as thalidomide have been considered (Sampaio *et al.*, 1991). Pentoxifylline inhibits cytokine effects *in vitro* but clinical results have not been impressive (DeZube *et al.*, 1993). Other anticytokine interventions, such as dietary supplementation with n-3 fatty acids, have also not proved efficacious in trials in advanced AIDS wasting (Hellerstein *et al.*, 1996).

Wasting in HIV-infected women is much less well-characterized than in men and exhibits distinct differences. A relatively greater loss of fat than lean body mass is lost in women with HIV-associated wasting, perhaps related to differences in gonadal steroid hormone (Grinspoon *et al.*, 1997). Low doses of testosterone (Miller *et al.*, 1998a) or perhaps anabolic steroids may improve function and increase lean body mass. More work needs to be done in women with HIV-associated weight loss.

In summary, at least some patients with HIV-associated wasting cannot increase their LBM by increasing food intake. To date, recombinant growth hormone (rGH), androgens (given to hypogonadal or borderline hypogonadal men), resistance exercise and moderately supraphysiological androgen treatment regimens combined with resistance exercise are proven to increase LBM in such patients. If there are indeed nutrient-responsive and -unresponsive subgroups of patients with HIV-associated wasting (Hoh et al., 1998; Kotler et al., 1990), routine diagnostic tests need to be developed that can differentiate the two groups. The use of adjunctive anabolic therapies should be considered in the nutrient-unresponsive group.

Prevention of weight loss

Prevention of weight loss involves different management strategies from those used for repletion of LBM already lost. Macallan and colleagues, (1995) measured food intake and total energy expenditure longitudinally during episodes of weight loss and found that acute weight loss was associated with reduced energy intake, rather than increased energy expenditure. Rapid weight loss is due in part to reduced calorific intake, because even in relatively severe chronic disease, energy expenditure is only increased by about 10–20%. A key question is whether reduction in LBM occurs as episodes of rapid weight loss or as a chronic, inexorable process. Macallan and colleagues (1993) showed that the most common pattern of weight loss in patients with AIDS involves episodes of acute weight loss, with only partial recovery in between. Because these episodes were associated with reduced intake, it might be possible to prevent them by provision of nutrients. Thus, dietary efforts to prevent loss of LBM should probably focus on avoiding periods of reduced food intake, whatever the causes (e.g. anorexia, oropharyngeal pathology), whereas once LBM has been lost, repletion may require adjunctive anabolic therapies in addition to supplemental nutrients. Alternatively, pharmacological interventions designed to reduce net lean tissue catabolism during episodes of weight loss (e.g. by administration of rGH; Paton, 1997) may prove effective for prevention.

Practical implications

The practical implications for clinicians are quite straightforward. First, clinicians must be aware of the importance of HIV-associated wasting. At a minimum, this means documenting body weights longitudinally. However, it is preferable to assess LBM in some manner, either by BIA (cost of a BIA device is about US$2500), anthropometrics or dual-energy X-ray absorptiometry. Second, LBM must be treated as the primary treatment endpoint. This means that if therapies such as megestrol acetate, enteral supplementation or home parenteral nutrition are used, increases in body weight should not be accepted as sufficient evidence of therapeutic effect. Third, the clinician must evaluate all possible causes of wasting. Food intake can be optimally quantified by a dietitian, with 3-day or 7-day weighed food records. Diarrhoea and malabsorption should be considered and treated appropriately if present. Antimotility agents, elemental or other enteral formula diets, or somatostatin analogues can be effective for AIDS-related enteropathy. If food intake is adequate and gastrointestinal problems are absent, metabolic abnormalities are likely.

Finally, all clinicians should be aware of the full range of therapeutic options available for patients with HIV-related wasting syndrome. Megestrol acetate (and possibly dronabinol) increase the intake of food. Megestrol acetate given in doses between 240 and 800 mg daily produces a therapeutic effect. Dronabinol 10 mg at bed-time, can reduce the psycho-active effects that occur during waking hours, while maintaining an appetite-stimulating effect. Prescribing supplemental liquid formulas can also increase intake of nutrients. Recombinant growth hormone clearly increases LBM, although it is expensive and has side-effects. Anticytokine therapies show promise but are not yet clinically proven. Testosterone or related anabolic steroid analogues may be useful in hypogonadal or borderline hypogonadal patients (i.e. serum testosterone in lowest quartile). Exercise is a potentially effective option for increasing LBM, if the patient can comply. Providing a facility and someone to supervise the exercise (i.e. a trainer) may be necessary to achieve compliance with exercise programmes in this population. Administering moderately supraphysiological doses of androgens (e.g. oxandrolone 20 mg/day orally or nandrolone 100 mg by intramuscular injection/week) in addition to testosterone at replacement doses (100 mg by intramuscular injection/week) in combination with supervised resistance exercise can result in remarkable gains in LBM and performance.

The clinician should also be aware of the episodic nature of wasting in AIDS patients. This suggests that increased emphasis should be placed on preventing rapid weight loss during acute opportunistic infections and other acute intercurrent illnesses, rather than attempting to replete the LBM lost. However, the optimal strategy for achieving this goal has not been determined.

Endocrine abnormalities

Hypogonadism

Low serum testosterone is the most common endocrine abnormality in men with HIV infection (Dobs et al., 1988). Associated complaints of impotence or loss of libido are highly prevalent (33 and 67%, respectively, in some studies). Serum testosterone progressively falls with advancing stages of HIV infection and correlates with weight loss and low CD4 counts (Coodley et al., 1994). Low testosterone levels are associated with shortened survival, with over half the hypogonadal men dying in 12-month follow-up, compared with 26% of eugonadal men. These observations suggest that hypogonadism in HIV-infected men is a non-specific response to stress, malnutrition, or chronic infection, as has been frequently reported in other acute or chronic illnesses (Woolf et al., 1985). Consistent with this hypothesis, hypogonadism was present in 18 of 24 patients studied and did not respond to gonadotropin-releasing hormone in seven of eight patients, thereby implicating a central aetiology consistent with 'stress' or malnutrition-related hypogonadism. There is a report of elevated luteinizing hormone (LH) and follicular-stimulating hormone (FSH) in hypogonadal men with AIDS and AIDS-related complex ARC (Villette et al., 1990), as well as a pathological study showing testicular atrophy (De Paepe and Waxman, 1989). Primary testicular failure may also be observed in some patients with advanced HIV infection.

It might be postulated that hypogonadism is adaptive; that is, a survival benefit results from the reduction in reproductive hormones that almost universally occurs during illness or malnutrition in both men and women. However, the hypothesis remains to be proven. Recent studies (Bhasin et al., 1998; Grinspoon et al., 1998; Strawford et al., 1999a) demonstrate that androgen replacement therapy can be useful for specific indications, such as repletion of LBM (reviewed above).

Endocrine aspects of osmoregulation and electrolyte abnormalities

Vitting and colleagues (1990) reported hyponatraemia in over 50% of hospitalized AIDS patients. Others have reported serum sodium concentrations of less than 130 mEq/l in 31–36% of AIDS patients (Aggarwal et al., 1989; Cusano et al., 1990), with the highest incidence in acutely ill patients with opportunistic infections, especially pulmonary infections. The syndrome of inappropriate antidiuretic hormone (SIADH) was diagnosed in 15 hyponatraemic AIDS patients on the basis of measurable serum antidiuretic hormone (ADH) levels (Vitting et al., 1990). The association with high mortality in hospitalized patients, concurrent opiate or barbiturate therapy, active pulmonary disease and iatrogenic administration of hypotonic fluids led to the conclusion that SIADH is usually secondary to stress or drugs and is often exacerbated by inappropriate fluid management. In contrast, Cusano and colleagues (1990) reported that hypovolaemia, generally caused by clinically unsuspected renal sodium losses, was the most common cause of hyponatraemia (88% of cases) and responded to intravenous saline infusion. The elevated ADH levels in these hypovolaemic individuals were therefore appropriate and occurred in the context of elevated plasma renin and aldosterone levels, low central venous pressures, and volume-related reductions in creatinine clearance. A combination of both aetiologies was also reported; one-third of patients studied had volume-depletion correctable by saline infusion and two-thirds had SIADH (Aggarwal et al., 1989).

Thus, isolated hyponatraemia is very common in AIDS patients. It is usually related to severe illness and is associated with poor prognosis. In many cases, it is caused by cryptic hypovolaemia and responds to saline administration. In other cases it is the result of stress-related SIADH, often exacerbated by iatrogenic factors (e.g. administration of hypotonic fluids, opiates or barbiturates) that can be corrected. The clinician can differentiate SIADH from salt-wasting by measuring plasma renin or aldosterone concentrations or by assessing the clinical response to saline administration or water restriction. The simplest clinical manoeuvre is to infuse 1–2 litres of 0.9% saline over 6–8 h and measure the serum sodium response while monitoring fluid status.

Unexplained hyperkalaemia is also an extremely common problem in hospitalized AIDS patients. Much attention has been paid to adrenal insufficiency, but most studies have shown that the prevalence of frank or relative adrenal insufficiency is low (see below). If adrenal insufficiency has been ruled out, hyperkalaemia may be caused by hyporeninemic hypoaldosteronism (Kalin et al., 1987; Guy et al., 1989; Lachaal and Venuto, 1989). Typical findings in this syndrome include hyperkalaemia (with or without hyponatraemia), mild acidosis, normal basal and adreno-corticotrophic hormone (ACTH)-stimulated cortisol levels, low basal aldosterone levels (despite elevated serum potassium, a potent secretory signal), low renin, and impaired aldosterone response to furosemide natriuresis (Kalin et al., 1987). In a clinically important study (Lachaal and Venuto, 1989), 19 of 20 AIDS patients treated with pentamidine for Pneumocystis carinii pneumonia (PCP) exhibited hyperkalaemia. Serum potassium concentrations were 5.1–8.7 mEq/litre and were often disproportionately elevated relative to the degree of azotaemia present. Serum bicarbonate concentrations were 14–21 mEq/litre and low renin and aldosterone concentrations were found in two of two patients tested. Thus, life-threatening hyperkalaemia may result from hyporeninemic hypoaldosteronism or renal tubular defects in the setting of pentamidine treatment for PCP. Hyperkalaemia generally responds to mineralocorticoid therapy in pentamidine-treated patients (fludrocortisone 0.1–0.2 mg/day).

Hyperkalaemia is also commonly found in AIDS patients treated with trimethoprim-sulpha or trimethoprim-dapsone, because of a renal tubular sodium channel-blocking ('amiloride-like') effect of trimethoprim when given at high doses (Velazquez et al., 1993). Hyperkalaemia (> 5.0 mEq/litre) was observed in 15 out of 30 patients treated with high-dose co-trimoxazole for PCP (Velazquez et al., 1993). The average increase in serum potassium was 0.6 mEq/litre, and this occurred despite an unchanged glomerular filtration rate. Greenberg and associates (1993) reported an average increase of 1.1 mEq/litre occurring after 9.8 ± 0.5 days of co-trimoxazole therapy, in the presence of only 30% increase in creatinine concentrations. The hyperkalaemia resolved after discontinuation of co-trimoxazole therapy. The response to fludrocortisone in trimethoprim-induced hyperkalaemia has not yet been evaluated.

Adrenal insufficiency

Adrenal pathology is prevalent in AIDS patients at autopsy (Guardo et al., 1984; Bricaire et al., 1987; Klatt and Shibata, 1988). Abnormal glands were observed in 64 of 83 AIDS patients by Bricaire and colleagues (1987), most frequently showing inflammation or necrosis and often the presence

of cytomegalovirus (CMV). The adrenal gland was the third most common site for CMV cytopathology, after the lungs and gastrointestinal tract (Guardo et al., 1984). The degree of adrenal necrosis observed (about 55%), is well below the amount believed necessary for clinical adrenal impairment (of more than 90% destruction) (Glasgow et al., 1985). Evidence of clinical or biochemical adrenal insufficiency is found in only about 5% of AIDS patients. Dobs and colleagues (1988) found a normal response to ACTH (serum cortisol of greater than 20 µg/dl) in 36 out of 39 ambulatory AIDS patients. Others have reported similar results of adrenal cortical testing, although subclinical abnormalities of 17-deoxy steroids or elevations in serum cortisol may be present.

The diagnosis of adrenal insufficiency is made on the basis of basal cortisol levels or the cortisol response to ACTH administration. Basal cortisol concentration of less than 5 µg/dl with an ACTH-stimulated increase of less than 7 µg/dl indicates frank adrenal insufficiency. A post-ACTH peak value greater than 22 µg/dl virtually excludes both relative and absolute adrenal insufficiency (Membreno et al., 1987).

Many medications can significantly alter corticosteroid metabolism. Ketoconazole inhibits adrenal corticosteroid synthesis and reduces the response to ACTH (Pont et al., 1982). This is an under-recognized cause of impaired adrenal reserve or frank adrenal insufficiency. Rifampin also increases corticosteroid clearance, and this may lead to relative adrenal insufficiency in the setting of impaired adrenal reserve (Kyriazopoulou et al., 1984). Co-administration of rifampin or other rifamycins with corticosteroids may require adjustment of the steroid dosage upward for equivalent efficacy.

Empiric glucocorticoid therapy is often reasonable while awaiting the results of adrenal function testing. Stress doses (180–200 mg hydrocortisone in divided doses) may be administered in the presence of acute illness. Most commonly, adrenal corticosteroid function will prove to be normal and the clinical abnormality that caused the suspicion of adrenal insufficiency – hyperkalaemia, hyponatraemia, hypotension – will remain. Mineralocorticoid therapy (fludrocortisone 0.1–0.2 mg/day) can be useful in these situations to avoid unnecessary glucocorticoid therapy. The causes of and the diagnostic approach to fluid and electrolyte abnormalities that prove not to be caused by adrenal insufficiency have been discussed earlier.

Endocrine pancreas

Pentamidine is a potent β-cell toxin (Bouchard *et al.*, 1982). Initially, therapy with pentamidine can result in unregulated release of insulin resulting in hypoglycaemia that may be life-threatening. Later, islet β-cell injury from prior pentamidine therapy may result in insulin deficiency and diabetes (Bryceson and Woodstock, 1969; Bouchard *et al.*, 1982). Pentamidine-induced hypoglycaemia has been reported in between 14 and 28% of AIDS patients treated for PCP (Stahl-Bayliss *et al.*, 1986; Waskin *et al.*, 1988). These estimates are recognized to be on the low side because mild hypoglycaemia may be unrecognized and can occur days or weeks after a therapeutic course, due to the long tissue half-life of pentamidine. Criteria have been developed for predicting patients who are at greatest risk for pentamidine hypoglycemia (Stahl-Bayliss *et al.*, 1986; Waskin *et al.*, 1988). The presence or development of azotaemia, increased total dose or duration of pentamidine treatment, and a history of prior pentamidine therapy predict a high risk for hypoglycaemia. Renal insufficiency was present in 40–100% of hypoglycaemic patients (Stahl-Bayliss *et al.*, 1986; Waskin *et al.*, 1988). These clinical groups need to be carefully monitored for hypoglycaemia during and after a therapeutic course of pentamidine, and clinicians need to maintain an awareness of the risk for late diabetes.

Recently, diabetes has been observed after initiation of HAART regimens (Nightingale, 1997; Visnegarwala *et al.*, 1997; Carr *et al.*, 1998; Patterson and Singh, 1998). This metabolic complication of antiretroviral therapy appears to be related to the development of insulin resistance rather than a direct effect on pancreatic function (see below).

Thyroid

The thyroid gland does not seem to be affected by HIV infection itself, and the gland is only rarely involved in opportunistic infections such as CMV (Frank *et al.*, 1987; Krauth and Katz, 1987), *P. carinii* or coccidioidomycosis, and Kaposi's sarcoma (KS) (Gallant *et al.*, 1988). The major controversy over thyroid function in AIDS is whether the typical 'euthyroid sick' syndrome associated with malnutrition or infection in other diseases is also observed in AIDS. LoPresti and colleagues (1989) reported that AIDS patients failed to exhibit the usual increase in reverse T_3 associated with severe illness; however, these observations have not been confirmed (Tang and Kaptein, 1989; Fried *et al.*, 1990). Hospitalized patients with PCP had low triodothyronine (T_3) levels, which correlated with hypoalbuminaemia and hyponatraemia and predicted poor survival (Tang and Kaptein, 1989; Fried *et al.*, 1990). Although the possibility that AIDS is associated with a unique pattern of thyroid hormone levels has not been rigorously excluded, the expected response to undernutrition or inflammatory illnesses (reduced serum T_3, a low-to-normal thyroid-stimulating hormone (TSH), and variable values of thyroxine (T_4)) is the pattern reported by most investigators. More recently, occurrence of thyroid abnormalities in HIV-infected children have been reported. These include anti-thyroid auto-antibodies (Fundaro *et al.*, 1998) and hypothyroidism (low thyroxine and elevated TSH levels) (Hirschfield *et al.*, 1996).

Pituitary function

Pituitary involvement in HIV infection is rare. No increase in the incidence of nodules or adenomas was observed at autopsy in men with AIDS (Sano *et al.*, 1989). Although CMV was sometimes present, there was no evidence of KS (none of 23 patients), lymphoma (none of 12), or *Mycobacterium avium* complex (MAC). Pituitary infiltration with *Toxoplasma gondii* was reported as a cause of hypopituitarism in one patient (Milligan *et al.*, 1984). One study (Croxson *et al.*, 1986) reported increased serum prolactin levels in association with progressive disease, but this was not confirmed in another report (Chernow *et al.*, 1990). It is useful to recall that the pituitary gland is anatomically not part of the brain, but is separated from the central nervous system (CNS) by the blood–brain barrier. Therefore, the various pathogens that commonly invade the CNS of AIDS patients rarely involve the pituitary. The exception to this rule relates to non-specific effects of illness or undernutrition on pituitary function (e.g. hypogonadism, discussed above). The frequent occurrence of abnormal growth and delayed puberty in HIV-infected haemophiliac boys (Ratner-Kaufan *et al.*, 1997), which is associated with reduced growth hormone secretion in addition to low serum testosterone levels, represents an important example of non-specific effects on pituitary function.

Calcium metabolism

Hypercalcaemia with increased urine calcium excretion was reported in four AIDS patients with lymphoma (Adams *et al.*, 1989). The aetiology was unclear. Evidence for extrarenal 1,25 dihydroxyvitamin D_3 synthesis was presented in one patient, and calcium as well as 1,25-D_3 levels fell after successful treatment of the non-cleaved B-cell lymphoma with chemotherapy. Others have reported hypercalcaemia caused by disseminated CMV infection, with suppressed serum parathyroid hormone and 1,25-D_3 levels (Zaloga et al., 1985). Hypercalcaemia of unknown cause has also been reported (Jacobs, 1986). Drugs employed to treat HIV infection may also cause abnormalities of serum calcium. The most important of these is foscarnet, which may cause acute reductions in ionized calcium during rapid intravenous infusion (Jacobson et al., 1991), resulting in cases of fatal hypocalcaemia. The mechanism may be foscarnet complexing with ionized calcium. Therefore, clinicians should measure serum ionized calcium during foscarnet therapy whenever neurological or cardiological abnormalities occur.

Metabolic complications of antiretroviral therapy

A number of metabolic complications of antiretroviral therapy have emerged since the introduction of HIV-protease inhibitors and potent combination therapeutic regimens. These complications include abnormalities of lipid and carbohydrate metabolism, as well as alterations in body composition. The most important and common complications have been alterations in serum lipid concentrations (hypertriglyceridaemia, low HDL cholesterol), body fat (content and distribution) and tissue insulin sensitivity (hyperinsulinaemia and type II diabetes mellitus). Although neither the underlying metabolic mechanisms nor the long-term clinical impact of these abnormalities are currently known, it is already clear that the future of antiretroviral therapy and the spectrum of disease associated with HIV-infection will be affected by these alterations and by our capacity to manage them.

Serum lipid abnormalities

As noted above, HIV-1 infection itself is characterized by hypertriglyceridaemia (Grunfeld et al., 1989; Mulligan et al., 1993; Hellerstein et al., 1996). The triglyceride (TG) concentrations in untreated HIV-1 infection are typically only modestly elevated, however, to the 150–300 mg/dl range. From the first clinical trials with HIV PIs, much greater elevations in serum TG concentrations have been observed, often into the range of 800–1000 mg/dl (Danner et al., 1995; Markowitz et al., 1995; DiPerri et al., 1998). It is still not known with certainty whether antiretroviral agents other than PIs cause increases in serum TG (i.e., whether

it is an antiretroviral effect (Saint-Marc and Touraine, 1999) or a class effect of PIs), or whether differences between PI agents exist. These questions will be important to answer in the near future. Some recent studies suggest that PIs may have a greater effect on serum TG than PI-sparing regimens, but not all reports have confirmed this (Carr et al., 1999; Martinez et al., 1999; Moyle et al., 1999; Ruiz et al., 1999).

Higher serum TG concentrations are often associated with abdominal obesity in HIV-1 patients on HAART regimens. As in any other clinical state characterized by high serum TG concentrations, serum high-density lipoprotein (HDL) cholesterol concentrations are reduced through direct interactions between very-low-density lipoprotein (VLDL)-TG and HDL particles in the serum compartment. The LDL cholesterol concentrations may or may not be elevated; although total serum cholesterol is high, it is mainly in the form of VLDL-cholesterol.

The combination of high TG and low HDL cholesterol concentrations suggests an increased risk for atherosclerosis, particularly coronary artery disease (see Chapter 15). Recent anecdotal reports of myocardial infarctions in relatively young HIV-1 infected patients with high serum TG/low HDL cholesterol concentrations on HAART regimens make this a critical issue for the long-term morbidity and mortality of the antiretroviral-treated population (Friedl et al., 2000; Rickerts et al., 2000).

Treatment of hypertriglyceridaemia in antiretroviral-treated patients begins with restriction of dietary saturated fat, then proceeds to drug therapy. There is currently no ideal medication for high TG/low HDL in this setting. Gemfibrozil (Lopid®, 600 mg twice a day) is a reasonable first-line treatment option but is typically not a very potent agent. Niacin (up to 1000 mg three times a day) is extremely effective but difficult to tolerate in many patients, due to flushing, itching and vasodilation and further complicates the already very complex medication regimens present in these antiretroviral-treated patients. Atorvastatin (Lipitor®) is an HMG-CoA reductase inhibitor that also lowers TG concentrations up to 40%. Atorvastatin and gemfibrozil should not be combined except in exceptional circumstances, due to the high incidence of severe myositis. A recent abstract (Saint-Marc et al., 1999b) reported 30–40% lowering of serum TG by therapy with metformin, an agent used in type 2 diabetes for lowering blood glucose and TG concentrations. The most useful agent of the group at present may be atorvastatin, but definitive studies are lacking.

Alterations in body fat content or distribution

Changes in body fat represent a serious and troublesome side-effect of antiretroviral therapy, which has emerged over the past few years. The changes have been in body fat content (increased adiposity) or distribution (locally increased or depleted adipose stores), and collectively are termed 'antiretroviral lipodystrophy'.

Changes in body fat content

As discussed above, patients with HIV infection tend to preserve body fat inappropriately during weight loss and preferentially add body fat during weight gain (Kotler *et al.*, 1985; Kotler *et al.*, 1990; Hellerstein *et al.*, 1990; Oster *et al.*, 1994; Von Roenn *et al.*, 1994). The introduction of HAART regimens has led to a recognizable syndrome of increased abdominal adiposity (Carr *et al.*, 1998; Miller *et al.*, 1998b; Silva *et al.*, 1998). Sometimes called 'protease paunch,' it is not known with certainty whether only PIs or other antiretroviral agents may also cause this syndrome of abdominal fat accumulation. It is likely but not certain that antiretroviral treatment, or immune reconstitution can lead to the syndrome, but that PIs have additional, class-specific action in this setting (Carr *et al.*, 1999; Martinez *et al.*, 1999). Patients are characterized by an increased waist:hip ratio (normal values being less than 1.0 in men and 0.9 in women) with or without total body weight gain. Symptoms are often quite severe, including abdominal discomfort, a feeling of fullness, inability to sleep comfortably, and even difficulty breathing. Distress concerning personal appearance is also often a prominent feature.

The central adiposity may occur in the context of whole-body weight gain or weight stability. Silva *et al.* (1999) confirmed the clinical impression that the vast majority of the weight gained (2–4 kg in their series) by patients after starting HAART regimens was due to an increase in body fat. The generally lower incidence of AIDS-wasting syndrome, as defined by body weight, in the era of PIs may therefore be misleading: body fat has increased in these patients, but LBM is not altered (see above). The optimal management strategy for controlling or reversing body fat gain has not been established. Attempts at calorific restriction have proved frustrating. Patients who have low or low–normal serum testosterone concentrations with central obesity in the setting of HAART can increase their LBM and feel better by administration of testosterone replacement therapy, but body fat does not typically fall unless exercise is also performed (Hoh and Hellerstein, unpubl. observations;

Strawford *et al.*, 1999b). Use of rGH has a rational basis, in that growth hormone mobilizes fatty acids from adipose tissue and reduces body fat. Several studies of the efficacy of rGH at reducing abdominal obesity in this setting are in progress but definitive results have not yet been reported. The disadvantages of rGH therapy (expense, worsening of hypertriglyceridaemia, see above) must also be considered. Use of the antihyperglycaemic agent metformin has recently been reported (Saint-Marc and Touraine, 1999) to reduce visceral fat content in PI-treated patients with paunch. Metformin has similar effects on body fat in type 2 diabetes and may act by improving insulin resistance at the level of the liver (Christiansen and Hellerstein 1998; unpubl. observation). We have observed anecdotally that the combination of aerobic exercise with low-fat diet can reduce abdominal obesity, or at least prevent its progression (Hoh and Hellerstein, unpubl. observations). Patients should be actively supported in their continued use of effective antiretroviral therapy, since some patients become discouraged by the weight gain and consider reducing or discontinuing their antiretroviral agents.

Changes in body fat distribution

Several syndromes of altered fat distribution have been described in HIV-1-infected patients receiving HAART regimens (Carr *et al.*, 1998; Hengel *et al.*, 1998; Lo *et al.*, 1998; Miller *et al.*, 1998b; Roth *et al.*, 1998; Silva *et al.*, 1998; Viraben and Aquilina, 1998): interscapular fat pad ('buffalo hump'), benign symmetric lipomas, subcutaneous lipodystrophy, and central adiposity, including breast enlargement. The occurrence of an interscapular fat pad has previously been considered almost pathognomonic of glucocorticoid excess (e.g. in Cushing's syndrome or supraphysiological glucocorticoid therapy). Occasional subjects on HAART regimens and some not on HAART regimens (Lo *et al.*, 1998; Saint-Marc and Touraine, 1999; Saint-Marc *et al.*, 1999) develop an interscapular fat pad. When these subjects have been investigated endocrinologically (Lo *et al.*, 1998; Yanovski *et al.*, 1999) there has been no evidence of glucocorticoid excess; the dexamethasone suppression test is normal, plasma and urinary steroids are within their normal ranges, and serum ACTH is not suppressed. The aetiology of the interscapular fat pad in these individuals is therefore unexplained. When biopsied, normal adipose tissue (i.e. no evidence of a lipoma) is observed; anecdotal experience suggests that attempts at excision are ineffective and result in regrowth of the fat pad. Benign lipomas occur as a rare condition, which tends to be symmetrical (Hengel *et al.*, 1998).

More common is the subcutaneous lipodystrophy syndrome. Lipodystrophy is defined as the alteration or loss of a normally present fat depot. Many HIV-1 infected patients, particularly those on HAART regimens, develop striking loss of subcutaneous adipose tissue in their extremities and face, often concurrent with central accumulation of body fat (Carr *et al.*, 1998; Viraben and Aquilina, 1998). The typical appearance is of thin but sinewy lower and upper extremities, loss of gluteofemoral fat in women, and well-maintained muscle mass and tone in the extremities. There are no known adverse medical consequences of lipodystrophy but its appearance can be very disturbing to patients. No treatments have been shown to reverse lipodystrophy. Use of rGH, for example, is likely to worsen the condition, in that lipolysis is stimulated by growth hormone; female gonadal steroids (e.g. oestrogens) might be expected to increase subcutaneous fat in the extremities, at least in women. Clinical trials of rGH or other therapies have not yet been reported.

Central adiposity and breast hypertrophy are often observed together in women on HAART regimens. Some women need to increase their brassiere size by two or three sizes. Abdominal fat deposition is discussed above.

Insulin resistance and diabetes

The syndrome of central obesity, hyperlipidaemia, insulin resistance and hypertension has been called 'syndrome X' or the 'deadly quartet' (Kaplan, 1989; Reaven and Hoffman, 1989) and is considered to be the most common set of risk factors for macrovasular disease in the Western world. These risk factors tend to cluster in individuals. In HIV-1-infected people receiving HAART regimens, a similar clustering of risk factors is often observed. Fasting hyperinsulinaemia (serum insulin concentrations above approximately $15\,\mu$ units/ml) is commonly observed in patients on HAART, frequently combined with high TG concentrations and fat gain in an abdominal distribution. Hyperinsulinaemia implies an impairment of tissue insulin action, such that a secondary elevation in insulin secretion is required to maintain euglycaemia.

Type 2 diabetes mellitus typically occurs in the non-HIV-infected general population in the setting of long-standing insulin resistance. The pathophysiological sequence for development of type 2 diabetes is believed to begin with insulin resistance and hyperinsulinaemia, which ultimately progresses to pancreatic failure ('pancreatic exhaustion') in susceptible individuals. The result is hyperglycaemia (i.e. clinical diabetes).

According to this model, gestational diabetes is a powerful predictor of later development of diabetes (of more than 80% predictive power) because it represents an insulin resistance 'stress test' for the pancreas. Insulin resistance is therefore the primary physiological factor leading to diabetes, and the occurrence of HAART-related insulin resistance would be expected over the long-term to lead to diabetes mellitus. Numerous reports of diabetes mellitus (Nightingale, 1997; Visnegarwala *et al.*, 1997; Carr *et al.*, 1998; Patterson and Singh, 1998) in subjects treated with HAART confirms this prediction, although the current prevalence of diabetes mellitus in HAART-patients appears to be only about 2%. The true incidence of diabetes mellitus may not become apparent for several years, however, since the natural history of pancreatic failure in response to long-term insulin resistance may require many years to become apparent.

A number of interventions can improve tissue insulin insensitivity, but none are proven effective in the HIV-1-infected patient on HAART regimens. Dietary energy restriction improves tissue insulin sensitivity, often within the first 3–5 pounds of weight loss (Wing, 1995; Christiansen *et al.*, 1996). The biguanide agent metformin also reduces fasting blood glucose concentrations by improving hepatic (and to a lesser extent peripheral) insulin sensitivity (Christiansen and Hellerstein, 1998). Troglitazone, a recently approved member of the thiazolidinedione class, is also a tissue insulin sensitizing agent. No drug treatment has yet been approved by the United States Food and Drug Administration (US FDA) for prevention of diabetes, although there is currently an ongoing large National Institute for Health (NIH) trial for diabetes prevention, comparing metformin, diet and exercise interventions. Metformin has the advantage of not causing hypoglycaemia, while reducing body weight and serum TG concentrations; troglitazone has the disadvantage of causing rare but serious liver toxicity (Gitlin *et al.*, 1998) and typically increases body fat and weight.

Summary

More questions remain unanswered than have been answered regarding metabolic complications of antiretroviral therapy. We do know that some of these alterations are very common, especially hypertriglyceridaemia, body fat accrual, central redistribution of body fat and tissue insulin resistance. We do not yet know the metabolic mechanisms underlying these alterations, whether they are peculiar to any particular class of antiretroviral agents or are a general effect of suppressing viral replication, what the long-term clinical impact will be, or how to manage them optimally.

References

Adams JS, Fernandez M, Gacad MA et al. (1989). Vitamin D metabolite-mediated hypercalcemia and hypercalciuria patients with AIDS- and non-AIDS-associated lymphoma. Blood 73: 235–9.

Aggarwal A, Soni A, Ciechanowsku M et al. (1989). Hyponatremia in patients with acquired immunodeficiency syndrome. Nephron 53: 317–21.

Bhasin S, Storer TW, Berman N et al. (1996). The effects of supraphysiologic doses of testosterone on muscle size and strength in normal men. N Engl J Med 335: 1–7.

Bhasin S, Storer TW, Berman N et al. (1997). A replacement dose of testosterone increases in fat-free mass and muscle size in hypogonodal men. J Clin Endocrinol Metal 82: 407–13.

Bhasin S, Storer TW, Asbel-Sethi N et al. (1998). Effects of testosterone replacement with a non-genital transdermal system. Androderm, in human immunodeficiency virus-infected men with low testosterone levels. J Clin Endocrinol Metal 83: 3155–62.

Blackham M, Cesar D, Park OJ et al. (1992). Effects of recombinant monokines on hepatic pyruvate dehydrogenase, pyruvate dehydrogenase kinase, lipogenesis de novo and plasma triacyiglycerols. Abolition by prior fasting. Biochem J 284: 129–35.

Bouchard P, Sai P, Reach G et al. (1982). Diabetes mellitus following pentamidine-induced hypoglycemia in humans. Diabetes 31: 40–5.

Bricaire F, Marche C, Zoubi D et al. (1987). Adrenal lesions in AIDS: anatomopathological study. Ann Med Interne (Paris) 138: 607–9.

Brozek J, Wells S, Keys A. (1946). Medical aspects of semi-starvation in Leningrad (Siege 1941–1942). Ann Rev Soviet Med 4: 70–86.

Bryceson A, Woodstock L. (1969). The accumulative effect of pentamidine dimethane sulfonate on the blood sugar. East Afr Med J 46: 170–3.

Cahill GF. (1976). Starvation in man. Clin Endocrinol Metab 5: 397–415.

Carr A, Miller J, Eisman JA, Cooper DA (2001). Osteopenia in HIV-infected men: association with asymptomatic lactic acidemia and lower weight pre-antiretroviral therapy. AIDS 15: 703–9.

Carr A, Samaras K, Burton S et al. (1998). A syndrome of peripheral lipodystrophy, hyperlipidemia, and insulin resistance in patients receiving HIV-protease inhibitors. AIDS 12: F51–8.

Carr A, Thorisdottir A, Samaras K et al. (1999). Reversibility of protease inhibitor (PI) lipodystrophy syndrome on stopping PI's or switching to nelfinavir. Sixth Conference on Retroviruses and Opportunistic Infections, Chicago, IL, USA.

Centers for Disease Control and Prevention. (1987). Revision of the CDC surveillance case definition for acquired immunodeficiency syndrome. MMWR 36: 3–14S.

Chernow B, Schooley RT, Dracup K et al. (1990). Serum prolactin concentrations in patients with the acquired immunodeficiency syndrome. Crit Care Med 18: 440–1.

Christiansen M, Hellerstein MK. (1998). Effects of metformin on the liver in diabetes mellitus type 2. Curr Op Diab Endocrinol 5: 252–5.

Christiansen M, Linfoot P, Neese R et al. (1996). Effect of dietary energy restriction on glucose production and substrate utilization in diabetes mellitus type 2. Diabetes (in press).

Cohn SH, Gartenhaus W, Sawitsky A et al. (1980). Compartmental body composition of cancer patients by measurement of total body nitrogen, potassium and water. Metabolism 30: 222.

Coodley GO, Coodley MK. (1997). A trial of testosterone therapy for HIV-associated weight loss. AIDS 11: 1347–52.

Coodley GO, Loveless MO, Nelson HD et al. (1994). Endocrine function in the HIV wasting syndrome. J AIDS 7: 46–51.

Croxson TS, Chapman WE, Miller LK et al. (1986). Prolactin levels in men with AIDS. II International Congress on Acquired Immunodeficiency Syndrome, Paris, France.

Cusano AJ, Thies HL, Siegal FP et al. (1990). Hyponatremia in patients with acquired immunodeficiency syndrome. J AIDS 3: 949–53.

Danner SA, Carr A, Leonard JM et al. (1995). A short-term study of the safety, pharmakinetics, and efficacy of ritonavir, an inhibitor of HIV-1 protease. European-Australian Collaborative Ritonavir Study Group. N Engl J Med 333: 1528–33.

De Paepe ME, Waxman M. (1989). Testicular atrophy in AIDS: a study of 57 autopsy cases. Hum Pathol 20: 210–4.

Dezube B, Pardee A, Chapman B et al. (1993). Pentoxifylline decreases tumor necrosis factor expression and serum triglycerides in people with AIDS (ACTG). J AIDS 6: 787–94.

DiPerri G, Del Bravo P, Concea E. (1998). HIV-protease inhibitors [letter]. N Engl J Med 339: 773–4.

Dobs AS, Dempsey MA, Ladensen PW et al. (1988). Endocrine disorders in men infected with human immunodeficiency virus. Am J Med 84: 611–6.

Feingold KR, Soued M, Serio MK et al. (1989). Multiple cytokine stimulate hepatic lipid synthesis in vivo. Endocrinology 125: 267–74.

Fields ALA, Cheema-Ohadli S, Wolman SL et al. (1982). Theoretical aspects of weight loss in patients with cancer. Possible importance of pyruvate dehydrogenase. Cancer 50: 2183–8.

Fliederbaum J. (1979). Clinical aspects of hunger disease in adults. In: Winick M (ed.) Hunger Disease. New York: Wiley, 11–43.

Frank TS, LiVolsi VA, Connor AM. (1987). Cytomegalovirus infection of the thyroid in immunocompromised adults. Yale J Biol Med 60: 1–8.

Freidl AC, Jost CH, Schalcher C et al. (2000). Acceleration of confirmed coronary artery disease among HIV-infected patients on potent antiretroviral therapy. AIDS 14: 2790–2.

Fried JC, LoPresti JS, Micon M et al. (1990). Serum triiodothyronine values. Prognostic indicators of acute mortality due to Pneumocystis carinii pneumonia associated with the acquired immunodeficiency syndrome. Arch Intern Med 150: 406–9.

Fundaro C, Olivieri A, Rendeli C et al. (1998). Occurrence of anti-thyroid antibodies in children vertically infected with HIV-1. J Pediatr Endocrinol Metab 11: 745–50.

Gallant JE, Enriquez RE, Cohen KL et al. (1988). Pneumocystis carinii thyroiditis. Am J Med 84: 303–6.

Gitlin N, Julie NL, Spurr CL *et al.* (1998). Two cases of severe clinical and histological hepatotoxicity associated with troglitazone. *Ann Intern Med* **129**: 36–8.

Glasgow BJ, Steinsapir KD, Anders K *et al.* (1985). Adrenal pathology in the acquired immune deficiency syndrome. *Am J Clin Pathol* **84**: 594–7.

Gorbach S. (1998). Oral Sessions. *Twelfth World AIDS Conference,* Geneva, Switzerland.

Greenberg S, Reiser IW, Chou SY *et al.* (1993). Trimethoprim-sul-famethoxazole induces reversible hyperkalemia. *Ann Intern Med* **119**: 291–5.

Grinspoon S, Corcoran C, Miller K *et al.* (1997). Body composition and endocrine function in women with acquired immunodeficiency syndrome wasting. *J Clin Endocrinol Metab* **82**: 1332–7.

Grinspoon S, Corcoran C, Askorri H *et al.* (1998). Effects of androgen administration in men with the AIDS-wasting syndrome: a randomized, double-blind placebo controlled trial. *Ann Intern Med* **129**: 18–26.

Grunfeld C, Kotler DP, Hamadeh R *et al.* (1989). Hypertriglyceridemia in the acquired immunodeficiency syndrome. *Am J Med* **86**: 27–31.

Grunfeld C, Kotler DP, Shigenaga JK *et al.* (1991). Circulating interfer-on-α levels and hypertriglyceridemia in the acquired immunodeficiency syndrome. *Am J Med* **90**: 154–62.

Grunfeld C, Pang L, Shimazu L *et al.* (1992). Resting energy expenditure, caloric intake and short-term weight change in human immunodeficiency virus infection and in acquired immunodeficiency syndrome. *Am J Clin Nutr* **55**: 455–60.

Guardo LA, Luna MA, Smith JL *et al.* (1984). Acquired immunodeficiency syndrome: postmortem findings. *Am J Clin Pathol* **81**: 549–57.

Guler HP, Zapf J, Froesch ER. (1987). Short-term metabolic effects of recombinant human insulin-like growth factor I in healthy adults. *N Engl J Med* **317**: 137–40.

Guy RJC, Turberg Y, Davidson RN *et al.* (1989). Mineralocorticoid deficiency in HIV infection. *Br Med J* **298**: 496–7.

Hellerstein MK. (1993). Pathophysiology of lean tissue wasting in HIV infection: therapeutic implications. *HIV: Adv Res Ther* **3**: 8–16.

Hellerstein MK, Kahn J, Mudie H *et al.* (1990). Current approach to the treatment of HIV-associated weight loss: pathophysiologic considerations and a preliminary report on a double-blind placebo-controlled trial of megestrol acetate. *Semin Oncol* **17**: 17–33.

Hellerstein MK, Grunfeld C, Wu K *et al.* (1993). Increased de novo hepatic lipogenesis in human immunodeficiency virus infection. *J Clin Endocrinol Metab* **76**: 559–65.

Hellerstein MK, Wu K, McGrath M *et al.* (1996). Effects of dietary n-3 fatty acid supplementation in men with weight loss associated with the acquired immune deficiency syndrome : relation to indices of cytokine production. *J Acquired Immun Defic Syndr Hum Retroviral* **11**: 258–70.

Hengel RL, Geary JAM, Vuchetich MA *et al.* (1998) Multiple symmetrical lipomatosis associated with protease inhibitor therapy. *Fifth Conference on Retroviruses and Opportunistic Infections,* Chicago, IL, USA **407**: 156.

Hirschfield S, Laue L, Cutter G *et al.* (1996). Thyroid abnormalities in children infected with human immunodeficiency virus. *J Pediatr* **128**: 70–4.

Hoh R, Pelfini A, Neese RA *et al.* (1998). De novo lipogenesis predicts short-term body composition response by bioelectrical impedance analysis to oral nutritional supplements in HIV-associated wasting. *Am J Clin Nutr* **68**: 154–63.

Hommes MJT, Romijn JA, Endert E *et al.* (1991). Resting energy expenditure and substrate oxidation in human immunodeficiency virus (HIV)-infected asymptomatic men: HIV affects host metabolism in the early asymptomatic stage. *Am J Clin Nutr* **54**: 311–5.

Jacobs MB. (1986). The acquired immunodeficiency syndrome and hypercalcemia. *West J Med* **144**: 469–71.

Jacobson MA, Gambertolio JG, Aweeka FT *et al.* (1991). Foscarnet induced hypocalemia and foscarnet effects on calcium metabolism. *J Clin Endocrinol Metab* **72**: 1130–5.

Jian ZM, He GZ, Zhang SY *et al.* (1989). Low dose growth hormone and hypocaloric nutrition attenuate the protein catabolic response after major operation. *Am Surg* **210**: 513–25.

Kalin MF, Poretsky L, Seres DS *et al.* (1987). Hyporeninemic hypoaldosteronism associated with acquired immune deficiency syndrome. *Am J Med* **82**: 1035–8.

Kaplan N. (1989). The deadly quartet. *Arch Intern Med* **149**: 1514.

Klatt EC, Shibata D. (1988). Cytomegalovirus infection in the acquired immunodeficiency syndrome. Clinical and autopsy findings. *Arch Pathol Lab Med* **112**: 540–4.

Kotler DP, Wang J, Pierson RN. (1985). Body composition studies in patients with the acquired immunodeficiency syndrome. *Am J Clin Nutr* **42**: 1255–65.

Kotler DP, Tierney AR, Wang J *et al.* (1989). Magnitude of body-cell mass depletion and the timing of death from wasting in AIDS. *Am J Clin Nutr* **50**: 444.

Kotler DP, Tierney AR, Culpeppermorgan JA *et al.* (1990). Effect of home total parenteral nutrition on body composition in patients with acquired immunodeficiency syndrome. *J Ent Parent Nutr* **14**: 454–8.

Krauth PH, Katz JF. (1987). Kaposi's sarcoma involving the thyroid in a patient with AIDS. *Clin Nucl Med* **12**: 848–9.

Kyriazopoulou V, Parparousi O, Vagenakis AG. (1984). Rifampicin-induced adrenal crisis in Addisonian patients receiving corticosteroid replacement therapy. *J Clin Endocrinol Metab* **59**: 1204–6.

Lachaal M, Venuto RC. (1989). Nephrotoxicity and hyperkalemia in patients with acquired immunodeficiency syndrome treated with pentamidine. *Am J Med* **87**: 260–3.

Landau RL. (1953). The appetite of pregnant women. *JAMA* **250**: 33323.

Lo JC, Mulligan K, Tai VW *et al.* (1998). 'Buffalo hump' in men with HIV-1 infection. *Lancet* **351**: 867–70.

LoPresti JS, Fried JC, Spencer CA *et al.* (1989).Unique alterations of thyroid hormone indices in the acquired immunodeficiency syndrome (AIDS). *Ann Intern Med* **110**: 970–5.

Macallan D, Noble C, Baldwin C *et al.* (1993). Prospective analysis of patterns of weight change in stage IV HIV infection. *Am J Clin Nutr* **58**: 417–24.

Macallan DC, Noble C, Baldwin C *et al.* (1995). Energy expenditure and wasting in human immunodeficiency virus infection. *N Engl J Med* **333**: 83–8.

Markowitz M, Saag M, Powderly W *et al.* (1995). A preliminary study of ritonavir, an inhibitor of HIV-1 protease, to treat HIV-1 infection. *N Engl J Med* **333**: 1534–9.

Martinez E, Lozano L, Conget I *et al.* (1999). Reversion of lipodystrophy after switching HIV-1 protease inhibitors to nevirapine. *Sixth Conference on Retroviruses and Opportunistic Infections,* Chicago, IL, USA.

Membreno L, Irony I, Dere W et al. (1987). Adrenocortical function in acquired immunodeficiency syndrome. *J Clin Endocrinol Metab* **65**: 482–7.

Miller K, Corcoran C, Armstrong C et al. (1998a). Transdermal testosterone administration in women with acquired immunodeficiency syndrome wasting: a pilot study. *J Clin Endcrinol Metab* **83**: 2717–25.

Miller KA, Jones E, Yanofsky JA et al. (1998b). Visceral abdominal-fat accumulation associated with use of indinavir. *Lancet* **351**: 871–5.

Milligan SA, Katz MS, Craven PC et al. (1984). Toxoplasmosis presenting as panhypopituitarism in a patient with the acquired immunodeficiency syndrome. *Am J Med* **77**: 760–4.

Mulligan K, Grunfeld C, Hellerstein MK et al. (1993). Anabolic effects of recombinant growth hormone in patients with weight loss associated with HIV infection. *J Clin Endocrinol Metab* **77**: 956–62.

Moyle G, Baldwin C, Dent N et al. (1999). Management of indinavir-associated metabolic changes by substitution with Efavirenz in virologically controlled HIV+ persons. *Sixth Conference on Retroviruses and Opportunistic Infections*, Chicago, IL, USA.

Nightingale SL. (1997). From the Food and Drug Administration. *JAMA* **278**: 379.

Oster M, Enders S, Samuels S et al. (1994). Randomized double-blind study comparing high dose megestrol acetate and placebo in cachectic patients with acquired immunodeficiency syndrome. *Ninth International Conference on AIDS* Berlin, Germany, B36–2360.

Patterson DL, Singh N. (1998). Exacerbated hyperglycemia associated with nelfinavir. *Ann Pharmacother* **32**: 609–10.

Paton N. (1997). *Second International Conference on Nutrition in HIV Infection*, Cannes, France.

Pont A, Williams PL, Loose DS et al. (1982). Ketoconazole blocks adrenal steroid synthesis. *Ann Intern Med* **97**: 370–2.

Randle PJ. (1986). Fuel selection in animals. *Biochem Soc Trans* **14**: 799–806.

Ratner-Kaufman F, Gerdner JM, Sleeper LA et al. (1997). Growth hormone secretion in HIV-positive vs HIV-negative hemophiliac males with abnormal growth and pubertal development. The Hemophilia Growth and Development Study. *J AIDS Hum Retrovirol* **15**: 137–44.

Reaven GM, Hoffman BB. (1989). Hypertension as a disease of carbohydrate and lipoprotein metabolism. *Am J Med* **87**: 2–6S.

Rickerts V, Brodt H, Staszewski S, Stille W (2000). Incidence of myocardial infarctions in HIV-infected patients between 1983 and 1998: the Frankfurt HIV-cohort study. *Eur J Med Res* **5**: 329–33.

Roth VR, Angel JB, Kravcik S et al. (1998). Development of cervical fat pad following treatment with HIV-1 protease. *Fifth Conference on Retroviruses and Opportunistic Infections*, Chicago, IL, USA **411**: 157.

Roubenoff R, McDermott A, Weiss L et al. (1999). Short-term progressive resistance training increases strength and lean body mass in adults infected with human immunodeficiency virus. *AIDS* **13**: 231–9.

Rudman D, Feller AG, Nagrai HS et al. (1990). Effects of human growth hormone in men over 60 years old. *N Engl J Med* **323**: 1–6.

Ruiz L, Bonjoch A, Paredes R et al. (1999). A multicenter, randomized, open-label comparative trial of the clinical benefit of switching the protease inhibitor (PI) by nevirapine (NVP) on HAART-experienced patients suffering from lipodystrophy (LD). *Sixth Conference on Retroviruses and Opportunistic Infections*, Chicago, IL, USA.

Saint-Marc T, Touraine JL. (1999). Effects of metformin in insulin resistance and central adiposity in patients receiving effective protease inhibitor (PI) therapy. *Sixth Conference on Retroviruses and Opportunistic Infections*, Chicago, IL, USA.

Saint-Marc T, Poizot-Martin I, Partisani M, (1999). A syndrome of lipodystrophy in patients receiving a stable nucleoside-analogue therapy. *Sixth Conference on Retroviruses and Opportunistic Infections*, Chicago, IL, USA.

Sampiao EP, Sarno EN, Galilly R et al. (1991). Thalidomide selectively inhibits tumor necrosis factor alpha production by stimulated human monocytes. *J Exp Med* **173**: 699–703.

Sano T, Kovacs K, Scheithauer BW et al. (1989). Pituitary pathology in acquired immunodeficiency syndrome. *Arch Pathol Lab Med* **113**: 1066–70.

Sattler PR, Jaque SU, Schroeder ET et al. (1999). Effect of pharmacologic doses of nandrolone decanoate and progressive resistance training in immunodeficient patients infected with the human immunodeficiency virus. *J Clin Endocrinol Metab* **84**: 1268–76.

Schambelan M, Mulligan K, Grunfeld C et al. (1996). Recombinant human growth hormone in patients with HIV-associated wasting. *Ann Intern Med* **125**: 873–82.

Shike M, Russell DM, Detsky AS et al. (1984). Changes in body composition in patients with small cell lung cancer. The effect of total parenteral nutrition as an adjunct to chemotherapy. *Ann Intern Med* **101**: 303–9.

Sih R, Marley JE, Kaiser FE et al. (1997). Testosterone replacement in older hypogonadal men: a 12-month randomized controlled trial. *J Clin Endocrinol Metal* **82**: 1661–7.

Silva M, Skolnick P, Gorbach S et al. (1999). Effects of protease inhibitors on weight and body composition in HIV-infected patients. *AIDS* **2**: 1645–51.

Stahl-Bayliss CM, Kalman CM, Laskin OL. (1986). Pentamidine-induced hypoglycemia in patients with the acquired immune deficiency syndrome. *Clin Pharmacol Ther* **39**: 271–5.

Strawford A, Hoh R, Neese RA et al. (1997). Effects of combined megestrol acetate and testosterone therapy in AIDS-Wasting Syndrome. *Presented at Second International Conference on Nutrition and HIV Infection*, Cannes, France.

Strawford A, Van Loan M, King J et al. (1999a). Effects of nandrolone decanoate on nitrogen balance, lean body mass, metabolic abnormalities and performance in borderline hypogonadal men with HIV-associated weight loss. *J AIDS Hum Retrovirol* **20**: 137–46.

Strawford A, Barbieri T, Van Loan M et al. (1999b). Effects of resistance exercise combined with supraphyscologic androgen therapy in eugonadal man with HIV-related weight loss. A randomized, controlled trial. *JAMA* **281**: 1282.

Streat SJ, Beddoe AH, Hill GL. (1987). Aggressive nutritional support does not prevent protein loss despite fat gain in septic intensive care patients. *J Trauma* **27**: 262–6.

Tang WW, Kaptein EM. (1989). Thyroid hormone levels in the acquired immunodeficiency syndrome (AIDS) or AIDS-related complex. *West J Med* **151**: 627–31.

Tcheckmedyian NS, Tait N, Moody M et al. (1987). High-dose megestrol acetate: a possible treatment for cachexia. *JAMA* **257**: 1195–8.

Velasquez H, Perazda MA, Wright FS et al. (1993). Renal mechanism of trimethoprim-induced hyperkalemia. *Ann Intern Med* **119**: 296–301.

Villette JM, Bourin, P, Doinel C et al. (1990). Circadian variations in plasma levels of hypophyseal, adrenocortical and testicular hormones in men infected with human immunodeficiency virus. *J Clin Endocrinol Metab* **70**: 572–7.

Viraben R, Aquilina C. (1998). Indinavir-associated lipodystrophy. *AIDS* **12**: F37–9.

Visnegarwala F, Krause KL, Musher DM. (1997). Severe diabetes associated with protease inhibitor therapy. *Ann Intern Med* **127**: 947.

Vitting KE, Gardenswartz MH, Zabetakis PM et al. (1990). Frequency of hyponatremia and nonosmolar vasopressin release in the acquired immunodeficiency syndrome. *J Am Med Assoc* **263**: 973–8.

Von Roenn JH, Armstrong D, Kotler DP et al. (1994). Megestrol acetate in patients with AIDS-related cachexia. *Ann Intern Med* **121**: 393–9.

Wanke CA, Silva M, Knox TA et al. (2000). Weight loss and wasting remain common complications in individuals infected with HIV in the era of highly active antiretroviral therapy. *Clin Infect Dis* **31**: 803–5.

Waskin H, Stehr-Green JK, Helmick CG et al. (1988). Risk factors for hypoglycemia associated with pentamidine therapy for pneumocystis pneumonia. *J Am Med Assoc* **260**: 345–7.

Wilson J. (1990). Androgens. In: TW Rall, AS Niew, P Taylor (eds.) *Goodman and Gilman's the pharmacological basis of therapeutics*. 8th edition. New York: Pergamon, 1413–30.

Wing RR. (1995). Use of very low calorie diets in the treatment of obese persons with non-insulin dependent diabetes mellitus. *J Am Diet Assoc* **95**: 569–72.

Woolf PD, Hamill RW, McDonald JV et al. (1985). Transient hypogonadotropic hypogonadism caused by critical illness. *J Clin Endocrinol Metab* **60**: 444–50.

Yanovski JA, Miller KD, Kino T et al. (1999). Endocrine and metabolic evolution of human immunodeficiency virus-infected patients with evidence of protease inhibitor-associated lipodystrophy. *J Clin Endocrinol Metab* **84**: 1925–31.

Zaloga GP, Chernow B, Eil C. (1985). Hypercalcemia and disseminated cytomegalovirus infection in the acquired immunodeficiency syndrome. *Ann Intern Med* **102**: 331–3.

MARGOT WHITFELD

Diseases of the skin affect more than 90% of people with HIV infection, and an even higher percentage of those with less than 200 CD4 lymphocytes/μl. The most common HIV-related problems are endogenous dermatoses, including seborrhoeic dermatitis and xerosis, unclassified pruritus and infections including herpes simplex and varicella, tinea and onychomycosis, molluscum contagiosum and viral warts, as well as bacterial and eosinophilic folliculitis (Goldstein et al., 1997; Uthayakumar et al., 1997). Less common but important problems include scabies, Kaposi's sarcoma (KS), atopic eczema, acne and psoriasis.

In many patients, the successful use of combination anti-retroviral therapies is reducing the incidence and severity of many of the traditional dermatological manifestations associated with HIV infection. In its place we are seeing an increase in the cutaneous adverse effects of the skin, including lipodystrophy, xerosis and dermatitis (Carr et al., 1998; MacKenzie-Wood et al., 1999). As patients with HIV infection live longer, recognition of other important skin conditions, including sun-related skin malignancies, is now even more important for these patients.

Molluscum contagiosum

Molluscum contagiosum virus (MCV) is a poxvirus distantly related to vaccinia and smallpox viruses. MCV occurs in 10–20% of persons with untreated AIDS, but is unusual in patients with asymptomatic HIV infection (Petersen and Gerstoft, 1992). Since the use of highly active antiretroviral therapy (HAART), its incidence has dropped dramatically, although some patients still have disease that is extensive or difficult to treat. Eighty per cent of those with MCV have a CD4 lymphocyte count below 200 cells/μl, but those with extensive MCV usually have less than 50 CD4 lymphocytes/μl (Schwartz and

Myskowski, 1992). Subclinical infection is probably common in patients with advanced HIV disease, as evidenced by the finding of microscopic changes of molluscum on biopsies for other conditions in the absence of visible lesions, and the finding by electron microscopy of MCV in apparently normal skin.

Clinical manifestations and diagnosis

The typical dome-shaped, umbilicated, pearly, 2–4 mm papules may occur on any part of the body, but preferentially affect the genital area and face, especially around the eyes (Fivenson et al., 1988) and beard area (Figure 19.1, all of the figures appear in the colour plate section). Lesions along the eyelid may induce a keratoconjunctivitis. In the beard area, lesions often begin at the follicular opening as barely visible skin-coloured papules, and may produce a viral folliculitis extending down into the dermis (Weinberg et al., 1997). Some patients may have more than 100 lesions and individual lesions may become greater than 1 cm in diameter. Large solitary lesions may simulate basal cell carcinomas, and multiple lesions may resemble disseminated fungal infections, especially cryptococcosis. In these latter cases, the onset is usually more rapid, and the lesions tend to be of a more uniform size (Picon et al., 1989). The diagnosis is usually made solely on clinical grounds, but it can be confirmed by biopsy.

Treatment

MCV lesions are usually treated with ablative cryotherapy. This method is usually successful, especially if repeated every few weeks until lesions are resolved, although residual hypopigmentation may occur. Alternative treatments include gentle electrosurgery (to avoid scarring), application of topical wart preparations, especially cantharidin (for 4–6 h, not in the genital area), and removal by curette. The latter method is most effective, virtually non-scarring (unless the lesions extend down the follicles to the dermis), and often preferred by the patient. MCV will almost always recur in patients with advanced HIV disease, and the patient's tolerance for aggressive therapy may be limited. Conversely, however, the improved immune function that is seen following combination antiretroviral therapy may clear even extensive lesions (Hicks et al., 1997). Cidofovir, a nucleotide analogue used primarily to treat cytomegalovirus (CMV) infection, is highly effective for treatment of MCV when used intravenously or topically as a 3% cream (Meadows et al., 1997). Cidofovir is very expensive compared with conventional therapies, but may be useful in patients with refractory disease.

Additional general measures for MCV include discontinuation of blade shaving if lesions are in the beard area, showering instead of bathing, avoiding the use of face cloths and the nightly application of topical retinoic acid at the highest strength tolerated. The latter appears to reduce the rate of appearance and size of new lesions, and is most useful in patients with moderate numbers of facial lesions who are not severely ill.

Human papilloma virus infection (warts)

Epidemiology

Immunosuppressed patients have greater numbers of warts than the general population and may be infected by multiple types. Numerous studies have linked certain human papilloma virus (HPV) types (types 16, 18, 33–35) with cervical, anal, penile and subungual squamous cell carcinoma (Macnab et al., 1986; Gal et al., 1987). Anal squamous cell carcinoma is more common in homosexual than in heterosexual men or women (Daling et al., 1982).

Anogenital warts occur in 20% of HIV-infected homosexual men and 27% of homosexual men with AIDS (Matis et al., 1987). When anal swabs are examined by the dot blot technique for HPV DNA, 48% of HIV-infected homosexual men and 54% of homosexual men with AIDS have evidence of HPV infection (Palefsky et al., 1990). If specimen DNA is amplified by PCR, HPV DNA will be found in anal swabs of 61% of HIV-uninfected homosexual men and 93% of those who are HIV-infected (Palefsky et al., 1998). The frequency of HPV types in anal lesions varies widely in different studies. In contrast to non-immunosuppressed patients, where HPV types 6 and 11 are the most common types isolated from condylomata, HPV 16 and 18

are most frequently detected in AIDS patients. Multitype infections are common (Rudlinger et al., 1988; Palefsky et al., 1990, 1998). Of major importance is the finding of anal intraepithelial neoplasia in 38% of anal swabs (Papanicolau smear equivalent) and in 15% of biopsies from AIDS patients. Multitype HPV infections are associated with a higher rate of abnormal cytological findings (Palefsky et al., 1990, 1998).

Cervical dysplasia or neoplasia related to HPV infection is common in symptomatic HIV-infected women, and increases in frequency and severity with advancing immune suppression (Shafer et al., 1991). Cervical carcinoma is an index AIDS diagnosis, and is discussed in more detail elsewhere in the book (see Chapters 8 and 33).

Clinical manifestations

Common warts of the hands and plantar warts are frequent in HIV-infected persons. Multiple, large and treatment-resistant warts are one of the hallmarks of advanced HIV infection. Flat warts may also be seen, particularly involving the beard area (Figure 19.2).

In the anogenital area, both typical condylomata as well as large vegetating masses occur, especially if there is a history of receptive anal intercourse. Lesions may extend into the anal canal, requiring anoscopy to evaluate the full extent of the infection. On the penile shaft and vulvar skin, typical condylomatous papules are most common. They may be few or quite numerous, and are usually slightly darker than the surrounding skin. Genital warts in this area must be distinguished from MCV, which are pearly, and usually lighter than the surrounding skin.

Bowenoid papulosis is a term used to describe HPV-related genital papules, which histologically show features of squamous cell carcinoma in situ (Patterson et al., 1986; Rudlinger and Buchmann, 1989). Lesions usually appear as flat to slightly elevated, hyperpigmented papules, patches or plaques (Figure 19.3). On the penis they tend to be 2–5 mm in size. While similar small lesions may be seen peri-anally, often lesions in this location are large, velvety patches with an irregular border. While usually behaving benignly in non-immunosuppressed persons, squamous cell carcinoma of the anus can develop from bowenoid papulosis in association with HIV infection (Goldstone et al., 2001; Sobhani et al., 2001). HPV type 16 is the most common type associated with bowenoid papulosis, although similar histological features have been seen with 'benign'

HPV types in both HIV-infected and uninfected persons (Rudlinger and Buchmann, 1989; Sanchez-Carazo et al., 1989). This is not surprising because HPV types 6 and 11 may be found in carcinoma in situ and frank neoplasia of the genital tract. Histology, not HPV typing, appears to be the best technique for predicting the potential behaviour of a given anogenital HPV-induced lesion. HPV typing is primarily a research tool, of little additional value to cervical or anal biopsy in patient management.

Treatment

As with other infectious conditions in the HIV-infected patient, treatment of warts is difficult and recurrence is to be anticipated. It appears that therapy failure is highest in those with the most advanced immune suppression, but the improvement in immunity associated with the new combination antiretrovirals has resulted in refractory lesions responding in some patients. Common and plantar warts in HIV-infected patients are managed by the usual methods: cryotherapy, keratolytics, cantharidin, bleomycin injections, electrodesiccation, or laser ablation. Treatment of warts with contact sensitization (dinitrochlorobenzene; DNCO) may be effective even when HIV disease is advanced. Flat warts of the beard area require less aggressive management, and may respond to topical 13-cis retinoic acid or 5-fluorouracil. Razor blade shaving should be discontinued until the beard area is free of lesions.

The most effective treatment of condylomata appears to be frequent (weekly) destructive therapy with liquid nitrogen, trichloroceticic acid, or cautery. Podophyllin is effective on moist areas, and podophyllotoxin, a derivative of podophyllin available as an 0.5% solution, is available for home treatment. Laser cautery carries a theoretical risk of dispersing HPV in the laser plume, but adequate precautions appear to minimize that risk (Sawchuk et al., 1989). 5-Fluorouracil can be used topically to treat bowenoid dysplasia of the genitalia and to reduce recurrence of treated lesions (Silman et al., 1985). Imiquimod, a topical immunomodulator, has been effective in HIV-uninfected patients, but in our experience is less effective in those with HIV infection (Edwards et al., 1998). Intralesional interferon injections are currently being studied. In one study, interferon was no more effective than placebo in HIV-infected persons (Douglas et al., 1986). In patients with AIDS, treatment of genital warts by any method is often followed by recurrence, and wart-free periods are rarely achieved.

Several aspects of the treatment of warts deserve emphasis. Patients should be evaluated for other sexually transmitted diseases. Sexual partners should be examined and, if necessary, treated. The technique of acetowhitening using 3–5% acetic acid will highlight clinically inapparent warts. The technique is non-specific, but multiple small, white papules adjacent to an apparent wart should be treated as HPV-infected lesions. Recalcitrant lesions should be biopsied, since bowenoid papulosis or squamous cell carcinoma may be clinically indistinguishable from benign papillomas. Histology is probably the best predictor of biological behaviour, and lesions with atypical histology should be considered for more aggressive management. At a minimum, patients with atypical biopsies require regular evaluation and a low threshold for biopsy of new or changing lesions.

Due to the high risk of cervical dysplasia in HIV infected women, annual Pap smears are recommended (see Chapters 8 and 33). Once cervical dysplasia is detected or the patient has had an AIDS-defining illness or a CD4 lymphocyte count below 200/μl, the frequency of Pap smears should increase to every 3 or 6 months, respectively (see Chapter 8).

Scabies

Epidemiology

Most cases of scabies are associated with close personal contact, including sexual exposure. In the setting of advanced HIV infection, however, our experience has been that a source of infection is frequently not found. Virtually all patients with a CD4 lymphocyte count over 200/μl will have typical scabies and a normal response to therapy. Unusual manifestations and treatment failures are usually seen only in patients with fewer than 200 CD4 lymphocytes/μl (Funkhouser et al., 1993).

Clinical features

Most patients with HIV infection have a clinical presentation similar to HIV-uninfected persons, except that staphylococcal pyoderma complicates at least 50% of all scabies cases in HIV-infected patients. Atypical variants of scabies seen in patients with a CD4 lymphocyte count of less than 200/μl include exaggerated scabies (Sadick et al., 1986), bullous scabies, papular scabies and crusted scabies (Funkhouser et al., 1993).

Exaggerated scabies is a widespread eruption, which may spare the typical scabies areas and involve the head and neck. Individual lesions are small papules, and scrapings for scabies are often positive from many of the lesions. Exaggerated scabies is frequently misdiagnosed as an inflammatory dermatosis or drug eruption. Bullous scabies presents in a typical scabies distribution, but large blisters are found on the palms and soles at the sites of mites. This hyperinflammatory blistering form is also seen in HIV-uninfected children but is rare in uninfected adults.

Papular scabies is an eruption consisting solely of papules on the trunk. Each papule is the site of a burrow and there is no associated hypersensitivity reaction. Pruritus may be minimal.

Crusted (Norwegian, or hyperkeratotic) scabies is usually non-pruritic and is characterized by sand-like, thick, tan crusts, which flake off, revealing underlying normal skin (Figure 19.4) (Moss, 1991; Hulbert and Larsen, 1992; Funkhouser et al., 1993). Lesions are usually generalized resembling dry skin, ichthyosis, or psoriasis. Fissures may form and be the source of fatal bacterial infection (Hulbert and Larsen, 1992). Localized lesions of the feet are rarely seen (Arico et al., 1992). Microscopic examination of any of the crusted material reveals numerous mites. Crusted scabies appears to be associated with HIV neuropathy or dementia (Funkhouser et al., 1993). Crusted scabies patients may be the source of epidemics of scabies in hospitals, hospices and nursing homes due to their high mite burden (Moss, 1991).

Treatment

Virtually all patients with a CD4 lymphocyte count of over 200 cells/μl will respond to standard therapy with topical permethrin (Walker and Johnstone, 2000). Permethrin failures are seen in patients with lower CD4 lymphocyte counts with and without atypical features. Lindane is now infrequently used due to its neurotoxicity (Meinking, 1996). There is no evidence that the mites themselves become resistant to scabicides, since healthy persons who contract scabies from patients failing therapy respond normally. Treatment failure appears to be related to immune suppression, high mite burden, and perhaps associated central nervous system (CNS) disease.

Initial therapy for scabies should be 5% permethrin cream, applying the cream to the whole body, including the head and neck. Individuals with exaggerated scabies and bullous scabies usually respond satisfactorily; however, patients with papular scabies may require multiple treatments. Ivermectin can be used for refractory disease. Crusted scabies is extremely difficult to eradicate and may require either repeated applications of scabicides for weeks to months or oral ivermectin (Alberici et al., 2000). Usually a single dose of 200 μg/kg is sufficient; however, a second dose 2 weeks later may be necessary (Meinking et al., 1995). Physical removal of the crusts, keratolytics and 5% permethrin cream can be used as adjunctive therapy. Because patients with crusted scabies shed mite-infested scale into their environments, extensive housekeeping measures are required, including treatment of bedding, carpets, drapes, clothing, and furniture. A patient with crusted scabies should never be transferred to a hospice or long-term care facility until they are cured, since the risk of precipitating a scabies epidemic among the residents and staff is high.

Superficial fungal infections (TINEA)

Clinical features

Tinea pedis is the most common dermatophytosis seen in patients with asymptomatic HIV disease. It is usually manifested by the typical interdigital maceration with scaling and diffuse hyperkeratosis of the sole. Bullous lesions, involvement of both feet and only one hand, or onychomycosis (fungal involvement of the nail) especially of the great toenails, are sometimes also present. The prevalence of dermatophytosis is not greater in HIV-infected patients than in control groups of uninfected, healthly athletes (Di Silverio et al., 1991).

Once patients develop AIDS, the pattern of dermatophytosis appears to change. Toenail dystrophy of a few or many nails frequently occurs. White subungual infection, often beginning at the proximal end of the nail, leads to thickened nails. This pattern of proximal subungual onychomycosis, which represents 90% of onychomycosis in AIDS, is otherwise unusual (Dompmartin et al., 1990). Patients with toenail onychomycosis may not have evidence of tinea elsewhere on the feet. Fingernail onychomycosis occurs ten times less frequently than toenail involvement, and is virtually always asymmetrical, being limited to, beginning or being more severe on one hand. Fingernail onychomycosis is often accompanied by diffuse dermatophytosis of both soles and the palm of the hand with the most affected nails. Candida albicans or other Candida sp. may also cause onychomycosis of the fingernails, and should be suspected if this 'two feet–one hand' pattern of involvement is not seen.

Tinea cruris follows tinea pedis and onychomycosis in frequency, presenting as an expanding scaling plaque of the upper thighs and groin with central clearing and a red, elevated border. Scrapings are mandatory in groin rashes, since seborrhoeic dermatitis of the groin is common and may simulate tinea. Tinea corporis in the setting of HIV disease virtually always represents tinea cruris, which has extended beyond the groin onto the trunk. This extensive form of tinea occurs in hot, humid climates (Wright et al., 1991), and may be seen at all levels of immunosuppression. In severely immunosuppressed AIDS patients lesions may have little inflammation, and often lack the elevated border and central clearing typical of tinea. They are recognized as sharply marginated areas of hyperkeratosis resembling dry skin. Tinea capitis in the adult and tinea facei are other less common patterns of dermatophytosis reported in HIV infection.

Treatment

For uncomplicated tinea pedis, a topical broad-spectrum imidazole (tinadazole, ketoconazole) or allylamine antifungal cream (see Table 19.1) will help to control the fungal infection and aid in preventing secondary Gram–positive bacterial infections.

Tinea corporis often also requires systemic therapy with oral griseofulvin, an imidazole (ketoconazole, fluconazole, or itraconazole) or an allylamine (Table 19.2). As in HIV-uninfected persons, fingernail infection can usually be cured with 3–6 months of an oral agent. Toenail infection is more difficult to resolve. Low gastric acidity in AIDS patients may reduce absorption of ketoconazole, markedly decreasing the efficacy of this drug (Lake-Bakaar et al., 1988), whereas fluconazole is well absorbed at any gastric pH. Care must be taken when the imidazoles are used in conjunction with the protease inhibitors (PIs), as each will inhibit the metabolism of the other and toxicity is more likely (MacKenzie-Wood, 1999) (see Chapters 5 and 6).

Inflammatory cutaneous complications of HIV infection

Since HIV infection causes immunosuppression, it could logically be assumed that inflammatory or 'immune-mediated' eruptions of the skin would be uncommon in HIV-infected patients. The opposite is the case. HIV-infected patients frequently experience pruritic eruptions which are often severe. The frequency of these eruptions increases as the CD4 lymphocyte count falls; most patients with severe pruritic eruptions have fewer than 200 CD4 lymphocytes/μl.

HIV infection appears to facilitate the expression of immunological conditions to which the person is genetically predisposed, rather than causing new diseases. Individuals with HLA-B27 or related antigens may develop psoriasis for the first time. In addition, cutaneous drug eruptions become more common and insect bite reactions become more pronounced. Paradoxically, at extremely low CD4 lymphocyte counts (less than 25 cells/μl) the probability of trimethoprim-sulphamethoxazole reactions again begins to fall (Smith et al., 1997), as does the prevalence of atopic dermatitis. We still know very little regarding the pathogenesis of theses HIV-related inflammatory skin diseases.

From a practical standpoint, most cutaneous conditions seen in HIV-infected persons are known cutaneous disorders, perhaps with an unusual or exaggerated presentation, e.g. seborrhoeic dermatitis and maculopapular drug eruptions. There seem to be very few inflammatory cutaneous disorders that are unique to HIV infection. Although the term 'papular pruritic eruption of AIDS' is commonly given as a diagnosis, we believe it is the dermatologists' analogue of 'chronic fatigue syndrome', a condition for which one or more causes obviously exists, although as yet are not identified. Insect bite hypersensitivities may account for a significant subgroup of these patients, particularly those with pruritic papules distributed principally in exposed areas. Our diagnostic algorithm is based on the morphology of the primary skin lesion (Table 19.3). In HIV-infected persons with an inflammatory, pruritic dermatosis the diagnoses listed should be correct in about 75% of cases. Should the diagnoses listed not seem appropriate, or the condition not respond to therapy, consultation with a dermatologist is warranted.

Follicular eruptions
Bacterial folliculitis

The lesions of S. aureus folliculitis consist of erythematous papules with a central pustule, and they may be extremely pruritic in the setting of HIV infection (Figure 19.3) (Duvic, 1987). As in atopic dermatitis, staphylococcal infection of the skin may complicate and exacerbate the eczematous or herpetic eruptions of HIV. The diagnosis of staphylococcal folliculitis is confirmed by bacterial culture. Folliculitis should be treated with a penicillinase-resistant semisynthetic penicillin (flucloxacillin or dicloxacillin, 0.5 g four times a day) or a first-generation cephalosporin (e.g. cephalexin, 0.5 g three times a day). Clindamycin (0.3 g three times per day) or erythromycin (250–400 mg four times per day) is a suitable alternative for the penicillin-allergic patient. Prolonged treatment courses are often necessary to eradicate the infection. About 50% of all HIV-infected persons without skin disease are nasal carriers of S. aureus. The rate of nasal carriage is much higher in those with active staphylococcal infection. For this reason, if the eruption is severe, continues to recur after treatment, or fails to respond to initial therapy, rifampin 600 mg daily for at least 5 days may be required. Once resolved, prophylaxis might include reducing blade shaving of the affected areas, the use of antibacterial skin cleansing agents (i.e. benzyl peroxide or hexachlorophane), intranasal mupirocin or bacitracin ointment, or low-dose sulpha-methoxazole-trimethoprim or clindamycin.

Eosinophilic folliculitis

Most patients with a chronic, pruritic, follicular eruption of the central trunk or face have eosinophilic folliculitis (Figure 19.6). The primary lesion is an edematous, almost urticarial, follicular papule, often without a central pustule (Rosenthal *et al.*, 1991). The most common areas of involvement are the forehead, neck, central back and chest. In more severe cases, the cheeks and proximal upper extremities may be involved. The eruption classically waxes and wanes independent of treatment. Uncomplicated eosinophilic folliculitis does not respond to antistaphylococcal antibiotics, but secondary staphylococcal infection may exacerbate it.

Table 19.1 Commonly used topical antifungals

Drug	Activity against		
	Candida	Tinea	Tinea versicolor
Nystatin	+		
Clotrimazole	+	+	+
Miconazole	+	+	+
Ketoconazole	+	+	+
Cicloproxolamine	+	+	+
Haloprogin		+	
Naftifine		+	
Terbinafine		+	
Tolnaftate		+	

Table 19.2 Oral antifungals and their dosages for the treatment of dermatophytosis resistant to topical therapy

Medication	Recommended dose for indicated form of tinea+		
	Corporis/cruris[a]	Pedis[b]	Unguium[c]
Griseofulvin (microsize)	500 mg daily	500 mg twice daily	500 mg to 1 g twice daily
Griseofulvin (ultramicrosize)	325 mg daily	250 mg twice daily	250 mg three times daily
Ketoconazole	200 mg daily	200 mg daily	200 mg daily or twice daily[d]
Fluconazole	100 mg daily	100 mg daily or twice daily	100 mg daily or twice daily[e]
Itraconazole			
Daily	200 mg daily	200 mg daily	200 mg daily[f]
Pulse	200 mg twice daily	200 mg twice daily	200 mg twice daily[f]
Terbinafine	250 mg daily	250 mg daily	250 mg daily

[a]Duration of therapy 4–6 weeks for griseofulvin and 2–4 weeks for other antifungals.
[b]Duration of therapy 6–12 weeks for griseofulvin, 1–8 weeks for other antfungals.
[c]Duration of therapy for fingernails 6 months, toenails 12 months; itraconazole fingernails 2 months. toenails 3 months; terbinafine finger and toenails 3 months.
[d]Due to hepatotoxicity with long-term use, ketoconazole is not recommended for the treatment of onychomycosis if the newer imidazoles or ally-lamines are available.
[e]The ideal treatment dose for fluconazole for the treatment of onychomycosis has not been determined.
[f]Treatment can be given as either daily therapy or as a pulse therapy, with medication given 1 week per month.

+ qd: daily; did: twice daily; tid: thrice daily.

The pathogenesis of eosinophilic folliculitis is unknown. Routine bacterial, viral and fungal cultures are negative. The diagnosis is established by skin biopsy, which shows perifollicular inflammation with eosinophils. Sometimes demodex hair mites are seen. Treatment is difficult. For mild cases, potent topical steroids and antihistamines may be tried. In more severe cases or if initial therapy is unsuccessful, ultraviolet light therapy often provides relief (Buchness *et al.*, 1988). UV-B phototherapy can be useful in pruritus of many aetiologies (Lim *et al.*, 1997). Itraconazole in a dose of 200–400 mg daily causes dramatic resolution within 10 days in about 70% of patients, but maintenance therapy is often required. PIs may increase the levels of itraconazole (MacKenzie-Wood *et al.*, 1999) and dideoxyinosine may reduce them (Moreno *et al.*, 1993). Other treatments that may benefit are topical steroids, oral antihistamines, isotretinoin and topical 5% permethrin cream applied regularly for 3–6 weeks.

Non-follicular papular eruptions

Insect bite reactions

Hypersensitivity to insect bites is extremely common in HIV disease (Diven *et al.*, 1988; Penneys *et al.*, 1989).

Patients note exaggerated and persistent lesions following bites of potentially sensitizing insects. In San Francisco, fleas are the most common cause of pruritic papules on the legs. Mosquitoes probably represent a common cause of pruritic papular eruptions, which are found on exposed sites, especially the arms, legs and face (Diven *et al.*, 1988). The diagnosis may be confirmed by skin biopsy. Should diagnostic confusion exist, simply wrap the involved extremity with an Unna boot. If biting insects are the cause, the occluded extremity will resolve over several weeks, while exposed sites continue to be affected (this is also an effective means of excluding self-induced skin diseases). Treatment consists of the extermination of biting insects from the patient's environment, insect repellents and clothing to deter the insects, topical corticosteroids to the individual lesions, and chronic potent antihistamines to reduce the hypersensitivity. Scabies has been discussed earlier in this chapter.

Photodermatitis

While most cases of photodermatitis are eczematous (see below), on the extremities HIV-related photosensitivity may present as firm pruritic papules, most commonly of the extensor forearms and dorsal hands. The diagnosis is a

Table 19.3 Differential diagnosis of pruritic eruptions commonly seen in HIV-infected patients

Principle rash morphology	Common diagnoses	Other diagnostic clues or tests
Papular: follicular	S. *aureus* folliculitis	Central papule; smear and culture shows staph
	Eosinophilic folliculitis	No central papule; typical distribution (forehead, face, chest and back), (biopsy shows eosinophils)
non-follicular	Insect bites (incl. scabies)	Grouped lesions, typical distribution, scrape for scabies (skin biopsy)
	Photodermatitis	Exposed locations; resolves with protection
	Granuloma annulare	Annular lesions on upper extremities and body (biopsy shows typical histopathology)
Morbilliform	Drug reactions	Responds (sometimes slowly) to discontinuing offending drug
Eczematous	Atopic dermatitis	Common in atopic patients, flexural lesions common; rare on scalp
	Nummular dermatitis	Coin-shaped lesions, often infected with staph; rare on scalp
	Asteatotic eczema	Dry skin on posterior arms and calves, rare on scalp; common in cold climates and winter; itching temporarily relieved by water
	Eczematous seborrheic dermatitis	Extension of pre-existing seborrhoeic dermatitis; scalp involvement common
Papulosquamous	Seborrhoeic dermatitis	Typical distribution. Greasy, red, scaling patches
	Psoriasis	Typical morphology (well-circumscribed plaques with silvery scale); typical distribution on elbows and knees
	Reiters syndrome	Arthritis, urethritis and conjunctivitis plus typical skin lesions; males predominate
	Secondary syphilis	Rarely pruritic, serological tests for syphilis virtually always positive

clinical one, based on distribution. Biopsy will usually show 'prurigo nodularis', a non-specific end-stage chronically excoriated papule. Prurigo nodularis in HIV is almost always a reaction to insect bites or photosensitivity, and the occlusion test (Unna boot) mentioned above is useful in confirming these diagnoses. Treatment is by sun avoidance, sunscreen and protective clothing, topical steroids, and oral antihistamines. Thalidomide can be helpful in resistant cases.

Granuloma annulare

Granuloma annulare is a mildly pruritic dermal inflammatory process of unknown cause. Histologically, a dermal infiltrate composed of macrophages surrounds areas of collagen, which are less cellular and contain excess tissue mucin. Granuloma annulare is relatively common, presenting in non-infected persons as annular lesions usually located on the dorsum of the hands or elbows.

Granuloma annulare may occur in all stages of HIV disease; typical lesions are 1–5 mm non-erythematous papules. These lesions may coalesce to form large circles up to several centimetres in diameter, so called-common pattern granuloma annulare. Rarely granuloma annulare may be localized to sun-exposed areas only (actinic granuloma). In HIV-infected patients, however, granuloma annulare lesions usually occur diffusely as single papules over the hands, elbows and knees, or over the whole body, so-called generalized granuloma annulare (Ghadially et al., 1989). Fewer than 10% of granuloma annulare cases seen in HIV-uninfected patients are extensive, and these patients usually have diabetes mellitus. In contrast, this generalized or locally diffuse pattern of granuloma annulare is the most common type seen in HIV disease, and it is not associated with diabetes mellitus.

Granuloma annulare is refractory to therapy. Localized disease may be treated with potent topical or intralesional steroids. Anecdotal reports have suggested that dapsone or niacinamide therapy is beneficial in HIV-uninfected patients, but in our experience they rarely work.

Morbilliform eruptions

Morbilliform, maculopapular, or exanthematous eruptions in HIV-infected patients are virtually always drug-induced. Occasional patients have widespread morbilliform rashes, which are apparently not drug related, but the causes of these eruptions are unknown. As a general rule, any patient who looks like they have a drug eruption probably has one. Medications can induce many other less common cutaneous eruptions, which are not addressed in this section. Guidelines regarding treatment of drug reactions and the risk of rechallenge apply only to patients with maculopapular eruptions.

Epidemiology

The frequency of drug reactions is increased in HIV-infected patients, especially to co-trimoxazole (37–45%), clindamycin 20–30%, antituberculosis chemotherapy 10–20%) and amoxicillin-clavulinic acid (Bayard et al., 1992). The risk of cutaneous drug reactions increases with decreasing CD4 lymphocyte numbers, becoming particularly high in patients with fewer than 200 lymphocytes/μl.

The rate of drug reactions appears to be partially dose-dependent, and is also related to ethnicity. For instance African, Haitian, and American black patients with HIV infection have much less frequent co-trimoxazole reactions than white patients (Murray and Mills, 1990). The increased rate of cutaneous reactions is probably directly due to HIV infection, because patients with Pneumocystis carinii pneumonia (PCP) treated with trimethoprim-trimoxazole have a lower rate of adverse reactions than those with HIV (Murray and Mills, 1990).

Clinical features and treatments

Morbilliform drug reactions usually begin during the second week of drug therapy. The eruption frequently begins in the groin and central chest and spreads to involve the whole body. Fever and eosinophilia may occur, but there is little correlation between severity of the eruption and the presence of these two findings. Moderate to severe pruritus is usually present and about 20% of patients will require a change in therapy due to pruritus. In those in whom the eruption is mild and controllable with topical and systemic therapy, the medication may be continued to the end of the course. Conversion of a maculopapular drug reaction to a more severe form during the same course of treatment has not been observed. Rechallenge with the drug at a later date may, however, result in a more severe reaction, such as Stevens-Johnson syndrome. If reinstitution of a medication to which the patient developed a maculopapular eruption is required, it should probably be done using a desensitization protocol (Finegold, 1986).

Once the offending medication is stopped, the eruption will usually fade in 3–5 days. With some medications, particularly those with long elimination half-lives, such as phenytoin and dapsone, resolution may take much longer. A small but important subset of AIDS patients have multiple, sequential, morbilliform reactions to unrelated medications (Ong and Mandal, 1989). Some of these patients will have increasingly severe reactions with each exposure, which may culminate in erythema multiforme major (Stevens–Johnson syndrome) or toxic epidermal necrolysis.

Medications administered by unusual routes may also cause cutaneous reactions. Aerosolized pentamidine may induce a widespread reaction. This complication is difficult to diagnose, since in most patients the eruption does not flare with each treatment. If aerosolized pentamidine is suspected, it must be discontinued for at least 8 weeks. The eruption will usually clear 6–7 weeks after the last treatment. Since these patients are usually also allergic to trimethoprim-sulphamethoxazole (TMP-SMX), pentamidine desensitization is probably warranted. We have had success rechallenging with 30 mg (one-tenth the treatment dose). A mild eruption with itching occurs at 3–5 days following the challenge, and clears in less than 1 week. In the three patients we have studied, we have not had a severe complication of low-dose rechallenge.

Sulphonamides and sulphones are among the most common medications causing drug eruptions in patients with HIV infection. For this reason, sulphonamide-containing eyedrops and creams (e.g. silvadene) should be avoided in these patients, and should definitely not be used if there is a prior history of TMP-SMX reactions. Long-acting sulphonamides (e.g. sulphadoxine found in combination with pyrimethamine in Fansidar®) are particularly troublesome and prone to life-threatening cutaneous reactions, which may take weeks to resolve when the offending medication has been discontinued. These drugs should therefore be avoided if possible.

Eczematous eruptions

The eczematous eruptions include those eruptions in which the primary skin lesion is a small pruritic papule. Multiple lesions commonly form confluent plaques. The classic morphology is seen in atopic dermatitis, and this section describes those conditions that look similar. Dermatologists use the word 'dermatitis' synonymously with eczema. Some pathologists may use the word 'dermatitis' for non-diag-nosable inflammation of the dermis, so a biopsy report stating the patient has 'dermatitis' does not necessarily mean that the patient has an eczematous eruption. All eczematous conditions are treated similarly and the treatment guidelines have been placed at the end of this section.

Pathogenesis

HIV-infected patients, especially those with CD4 lymphocyte counts of less than $200/\mu l$, have elevated levels of IgE (Wright et al., 1990). This may be related to a change in the cytokine environment of advanced HIV disease, with a decreased interleukin-2 (IL-2) and increased IL-4 and IL-10 production. These latter cytokines stimulate IgE production by B lymphocytes and downregulate IL-2-driven immune responses (Clerici and Shearer, 1993). It is unknown at present whether the elevated IgE and occasional eosinophilia seen in advanced HIV disease is related to atopy, the presence of skin disease, a reaction to infectious agents or medications, or is a direct result of HIV infection itself.

Xerosis and eczematous drug eruptions

Dry skin (xerosis, asteatosis) is extremely common in HIV disease, especially AIDS. The cause of xerosis is unknown. Dry skin can itch, and frequently accompanies or is the basis for eczematous eruptions.

Skin eruptions have occurred in a few patients related to PI therapy (Bonfanti et al., 1997; Calista and Boschini, 2000). Some of these eruptions are maculopapular and some eczematous. A syndrome involving asteotosis, eczema, and cheilitis (Figure 19.7), sometimes in association with paronychia and/or lipodystrophy has also been recognized at our hospital. The mechanism of these cutaneous changes, as well as the lipodystrophy, remain unclear. Possible mechanisms for the lipodystrophy include inhibition of the cytochrome p450 pathway, or binding to cytoplasmic retinoic acid-binding protein type 1, leading eventually to impaired differentiation of adipocytes (Carr et al., 1998a). In addition, in AIDS patients any pruritic eruption may induce scratching and secondary eczematous eruptions of the skin, so eczematous plaques may accompany scabies, staphylococcal folliculitis or eosinophilic folliculitis. Some of the non-eczematous drug eruptions may be due to an immune reconstitution phenomenon, and presentation or representation of a TMP-SMX or other drug sensitivity (Bonfanti et al., 1997).

Atopic dermatitis

Atopic eczema is common in children with HIV disease, and it preferentially affects certain sites (face and extensors in young children; antecubital, popliteal fossae and neck in older children). In HIV-infected adults, atopic dermatitis may appear in those with a prior history of atopy (allergic rhinitis, asthma) (Parkin et al., 1987) and the rash may not involve these diagnostic areas, instead presenting as widespread dermatitis or nummular eczema (see below).

Asteatotic eczema (dry skin eczema, winter itch)

The underlying xerosis of HIV disease is a major cause of pruritus in this population, analogous to the geriatric population. Xerosis is more common in winter, when there is less moisture in the interior air. Most patients with relatively normal skin who complain of itching have either dry skin or scabies incognito. Many HIV-infected patients bathe excessively, either to prevent folliculitis or to soothe their itching skin. Hot water and the use of antibacterial or deodorant soaps worsen xerosis. The diagnosis of dry skin pruritus is made by history. Ask the patient what happens to the itching when he/she is submerged in water or bathes. Invariably the pruritus stops for some period, only to recur once the patient is dry. The worse the dry skin, the shorter the pruritus-free period. Often the patient will say that bathing at one time prevented itching for several hours, but now he/she is forced to bathe more frequently to stop the itching. Initial submersion in water may be accompanied by stinging, as water contacts the microscopic fissures in the skin.

Dry skin itch usually begins on the driest areas of the body, the calves, outer thighs, and posterior arms. The face, and constantly moist areas (axillae, groin, and feet) almost never itch (in contrast to scabies). As the disease progresses, itching affects the lateral trunk, outer buttocks, then generalizes. On physical examination there is very little erythema. The skin is slightly scaly and may appear shiny. Small fissures filled with fine crusts may be seen on the most severely affected areas. These fissures characteristically form small circles (0.5–1.0 cm) and are frequently misdiagnosed as tinea corporis. (They improve with any moisturizing cream, so they appear to go away with topical antifungal therapy, apparently confirming the errant diagnosis!) Untreated xerotic eczema may progress to nummular dermatitis.

Nummular dermatitis

Nummular dermatitis is usually a consequence of atopic dermatitis or xerotic eczema (see above). Individual lesions are round (coin-shaped) and between 1 and 5 cm in diameter. Lesions may be dry, with attached scale and crust, or weepy. There is no central clearing, and scale cannot be removed easily (as in tinea). Secondary infection with S. aureus is almost always present. The first lesion(s) appears on the extremities, especially the forearm or calf, and if untreated new lesions are added, eventually covering large areas of the body. As disease activity increases, individual lesions also expand by developing a peripheral erythema followed by small papules, which coalesce into the main plaque. Itching is usually very intense. Treatment often requires several months, and there is a high likelihood of relapse if good skin hydration is not continued.

Eczematous seborrhoeic dermatitis

An unusual form of seborrhoeic dermatitis is seen occasionally in HIV-infected patients, which has a pattern resembling nummular eczema. The seborrhoea spills down the central back and chest, forming confluent plaques (Figure 19.8), and down the forearms as scattered annular lesions. Itching is much more severe than with typical seborrhoea. Seborrhoea dermatitis of the scalp is invariably present, and may be severe. This form of seborrhoea is unrelated to dry skin. The diagnosis is made by observing the distribution of lesions, since the other eczemas described in this section tend to spare the scalp, central chest and back. It is relatively easy to treat (see below).

Photodermatitis

Photosensitivity eruptions are extremely common in HIV-infected persons, but have largely gone unreported (Toback et al., 1986). In my opinion, many cases of 'prurigo' described in HIV-infected patients in the tropics represent photodermatitis. Since scientific documentation of photosensitivity requires sophisticated equipment, appropriate investigations are only now being performed. We encourage all HIV-infected persons to use broad-spectrum sunscreens daily, appropriate protective clothing, and to avoid recreational sun exposure.

Photosensitivity in the setting of HIV may either be induced by medication (photosensitive drug reaction or photodrug) or endogenous (possibly directly caused by

HIV). Morphologically, photodermatitis is usually eczematous, but can be lichenoid or have prurigo nodules as an early or late manifestation.

The diagnosis of photodermatitis is made by noting the initial distribution of the skin lesions, and the season of onset. Photoeruptions usually present following a period of increased sun exposure, during the spring or following a tropical holiday. Itching is usually moderate to severe. Lesions initially appear on the extensor arms and the dorsa of the hands. Finding a sharp demarcation between normal and abnormal skin at the base of the neck and the mid arm is virtually diagnostic of photodermatitis. The posterior, lateral, and anterior 'vee' of the neck may also be involved, along with the face (sparing the upper eyelids, below the nose, and sun-protected areas). The tip of the nose is characteristically involved in photoeruptions and is almost always spared in seborrhoeic dermatitis. Over time, the eruption may spread to sun protected areas, so the distribution at the time of examination may be misleading if the case is advanced. Endogenous pigmentation is not protective for photosensitivity eruptions, and in fact most of the severe photoeruptions we and others have seen have occurred in coloured patients. People with inherited endogenous photosensitivity (Native Americans and Hispanics with Native American heritage) are at special risk for photodermatitis.

Drug-induced photoeruptions may occur at any season. In HIV-infected patients, sulphonamides, sulphones, and non-steroidal anti-inflammatory agents are the most common photosensitizers used and consequently the most common causes of photodrug eruptions. Non-prescription medications, such as quinine may also induce photodrug reactions. Since photodrug eruptions require light plus the medication, the onset of the eruption may not correlate with when the medication was begun. Both drug-induced and endogenous photosensitivity are usually due to short-wave ultraviolet light, but as the eruption progresses the spectrum of reaction may increase, leading to long-wave ultraviolet sensitivity as well. Thus initially, in most patients, sunscreens and window glass are protective, but eventually patients may continue to react even if they remain indoors.

Treatment of eczematous eruptions

The most important factor in effective therapy of eczematous eruptions is establishing a correct diagnosis. Photodermatitis must, of course, be treated with sun protection and sunscreens, as well as general management. Xerotic, atopic, and nummular dermatitis are all complicated by dry skin, and adequate hydration with tub soaks and moisturizers are key in inducing and maintaining a remission. Eczematous seborrhoeic dermatitis is the easiest to manage, and mild topical steroids (hydrocortisone, 1–2.5%, triamcinolone, 0.25%, or the brand-name equivalent) are usually sufficient, especially when combined with aggresive treatment of the scalp seborrhoea (see below).

Topical corticosteroid preparations are the mainstay of management of eczematous eruptions. Treatment is begun using medium-potency typical steroids (e.g. triamcinolone acetonide, 0.1%) applied two to three times daily. For xerotic patients, ointments are preferred to creams. In addition, soaking with colloidal oatmeal or dilute (1:40) aluminum acetate in a tub of cool water twice daily is helpful. For refractory eczematous process (especially photoeruptions or nummular eczema), high potency topical corticosteroids are often required (e.g. clobetasol or betamethasone). A sedating dose of antihistamine (e.g. benadryl 50–100 mg) is given nightly and lower doses during the day as needed, for itch. Non-sedating antihistamines are of absolutely no benefit in suppressing eczema-associated pruritus. Co-existent staphylococcal infection should be treated in patients experiencing exacerbation of atopic and nummular dermatitis. Patients not responding to these general measures should be referred to a dermatologist for management.

Papulosquamous eruptions

Papulosquamous eruptions are very common in HIV-infected persons. Seborrhoeic dermatitis, the most common, is seen in up to 80% of AIDS patients. Whether the other papulosquamous diseases are increased in HIV is unknown, but roughly 1–2% of HIV-infected persons have psoriasis and 0.5–1.7% have Reiter's syndrome, usually incomplete (Calabrese *et al.*, 1991; Obuch *et al.*, 1992). These three disorders form a spectrum of disease, and patients may be found at any point along the spectrum. Sebopsoriasis, for example, describes extensive seborrhoea involving mostly the intertriginous areas, with features of psoriasis as well (scattered plaques on the elbows, for instance). HIV-infected patients with psoriasis not uncommonly have skin lesions, also seen in Reiter's syndrome, i.e. keratotic papules of the palms and soles, and patients with psoriasis may also have arthritis.

All papulosquamous eruptions are characterized by sharply marginated scaling lesions, usually with limited pruritus. Biopsies are usually not very helpful in diagnosing these disorders. Classic cases, which can be easily clinically diagnosed, have characteristic histology; but atypical cases, which present diagnostic problems may have non-diagnostic histology. These papulosquamous disorders do not appear to be different from the same conditions seen in non-infected patients, although they may be more severe than the same conditions in HIV-uninfected patients. In other words, there is no specific psoriasiform dermatitis of AIDS; it is merely psoriasis in a person with AIDS.

Seborrhoeic dermatitis

Seborrhoeic dermatitis usually affects hair-bearing areas, especially the scalp, eyebrows, moustache, beard and central chest, as well as the nasolabial fold and behind and in the ears. Involvement of the axillae and groin (including the penis and scrotum) is also common. Lesions may also extend from the scalp onto the central back. The scale is characteristically fine and may be greasy but red, non-scaling patches without central clearing also occur. Pruritus is usually absent or mild, but occasionally severe, especially on the scalp. Patients with erythematous papules and pustules over the nose and cheeks often have concurrent rosacea, and can be helped with topical metronidazole or oral tetracyclines.

We recommend applying a mild topical steroid (e.g. hydrocortisone, 1–2.5% cream) twice daily for facial seborrhoeic dermatitis, along with a topical imidazole cream. In severe cases, the addition of oral ketoconazole can be helpful. Although the mechanism is unknown, alterations in skin lipids and pityrosporum appear to play a contributing role (Aly and Berger 1996; Ostlere et al., 1996). Scalp involvement is treated with the frequent (daily) use of a shampoo containing selenium sulphide, tar or ketoconazole twice weekly. Topical steroid solutions, or creams containing tar, sulphur or salicylic acid may also be helpful. Recurrences are common, and maintenance therapy may be required.

Psoriasis

Psoriasis is seen in HIV-infected persons with at least as great a frequency as the general population (1–2%). About one-third of people with psoriasis and HIV have clinical evidence of psoriasis prior to HIV infection, and two-thirds note skin lesions only after they are HIV-infected (Obuch et al., 1992). This suggests that HIV somehow permits or enhances expression of psoriasis in an at-risk person. HIV-infected persons with psoriasis have either HLA-B27 or a B27-crossreactive HLA antigen (Reveille et al., 1990). The appearance of psoriasis in an individual at risk for HIV infection, especially if they are over 30 years, should therefore prompt HIV testing. All clinical patterns of psoriasis may be seen in HIV-infected persons, but axilla and groin involvement (inverse pattern) and palm and sole involvement seem to be especially common. These patterns are more common in Reiter's patients with and without HIV disease.

The classic lesions of psoriasis are well circumscribed plaques with silvery scales. Lesions favour the elbows and knees, lumbosacral area, and the gluteal fold. Nail involvement with pitting, onycholysis, and even marked thickening and crumbling is common and may mimic tinea. Factors that exacerbate common psoriasis may worsen HIV-associated psoriasis as well, for example streptococcal colonization or infection of the throat and certain medications primarily lithium and β-blockers. HIV-associated psoriasis may flare severely in association with staphylococcal sepsis, and in any HIV-infected person with sudden worsening of psoriasis this must be considered. Treatment of sepsis will often result in dramatic improvement of the psoriasis.

Psoriasis may appear at any stage of HIV disease and may worsen as HIV disease progresses. The reason is unknown, but most patients with HIV disease and severe psoriasis seem to have more advanced HIV disease. Articular symptoms are also more common in those with advanced disease. With worsening, lesions begin to generalize to the whole body, but usually spare the face. About 10% of HIV-infected patients with psoriasis have some joint involvement similar to the joint disease seen in psoriasis unassociated with HIV disease.

Psoriasis treatment is more art than science, and is best supervised by a dermatologist in moderate to severe cases. In mild cases, topical steroids, anthralin, calcipotriene, tar and salicylic acid are all used in various combinations. For any response, the topical steroids used must generally be equal to or stronger than triamcinolone 0.1% in non-intertriginous areas. Chronic steroid treatment may lead to relapse or rebound (tachyphylaxis). Of the antiretroviral therapies, zidovudine (ZDV) in particular has been helpful in improving psoriasis, and may be added or increased as a part of psoriasis treatment (Kaplan *et al.*, 1989). The mechanism of action is unknown. When topical measures fail, ultraviolet light therapy, in combination with tar (Goeckermann regimen) or acitretin, are useful (Buccheri *et al.*, 1997) and may be used simultaneously. Acitretin may be helpful in patients with extensive psoriasis, although hypertriglyceridaemia needs to be watched, particularly in those whose levels are already raised due to their PIs. The long -term risk of UV exposure in HIV-infected persons is unknown, but short-term data indicate no significant change in viral load or CD4 count (Gelfland *et al.*, 1998) *In vitro* activation of HIV by ultraviolet light has been documented. Immuno-suppressives, such as methotrexate and cyclosporin A are of potentially high risk. They are currently not recommended.

Reiter's syndrome

The characteristic skin lesions of Reiter's syndrome, keratoderma blenorrhagica and circinate balanitis, may be seen in HIV-infected persons in association with arthritis, urethritis and conjunctivitis (see Chapter 14). Most patients have only some of these features at one time (incomplete Reiter's). Between 30 and 75% of persons with Reiter's and HIV disease are HLA-B27 positive. HLA testing showing a B27 allele supports a diagnosis of Reiter's; a negative test for B27 has no significance. The skin lesions in Reiter's patients at sites other than the soles and penis are identical to psoriasis clinically and histologically and are treated identically. The arthritis of HIV-associated psoriasis and Reiter's may be quite difficult to manage. Etretinate and sulphasalazine have anecdotally been reported as useful. Non-steroid anti-inflammatory agents do not appear to exacerbate psoriasis or Reiter's and are frequently used in this setting. Antimalarials such as primaquine or chloroquine can cause severe flares of psoriasis and must be used with caution in treating the associated arthritis (see Chapter 14).

Cutaneous skin malignancies

Although an increased incidence of skin malignancies has not yet been demonstrated with HIV infection, the dramatic increase in squamous cell carcinomas seen with prolonged immunosupression in renal and cardiac transplant recipients reminds us that this potential problem should not be neglected. The risk factors for basal cell carcinoma and squamous cell carcinoma in those with HIV infection include excessive sun exposure and fair skin (Maurer *et al.*, 1997). As patients live longer and opportunistic infections are being seen less, cutaneous malignancies are being seen more, particularly in our Australian clinic.

References

Alberici F, Pagani L, Ratti G, Viale P (2000). Ivermectin alone or in combination with benzyl benzoate in the treatment of HIV-associated scabies. *Br J Dermatol* **142**: 969–72.

Aly R, Berger T. (1996). Common superficial fungal infections in patients with AIDS. *Clin Infect Dis* **22**: S128–32.

Arico M, Noto, G, La Rocca E *et al.* (1992). Localized crusted scabies in the acquired immunodeficiency syndrome. *Clin Exp Dermatol* **17**: 39–341.

Bayard P, Berger TG, Jacobson MA. (1992). Drug hypersensitivity reactions and human immunodeficiency virus disease. *J Acquir Immune Defic Syndr* **5**: 1237–57.

Buccheri L, Katchen BR, Karter AJ *et al.* (1997). Acitretin therapy is effective therapy for psoriasis associated with human immuno-deficiency virus infection. *Arch Dermatol* **133**: 711–5.

Buchness MR, Lim HW, Hatcher VA *et al.* (1988). Eosinophilic pustular folliculitis in the acquired immunodeficiency syndrome. *N Engl J Med* **318**: 1183–6.

Calabrese LH, Kelley DM, Myers A *et al.* (1991). Rheumatic symptoms and human immunodeficiency virus infection. *Arthritis Rheum* **34**: 257–63.

Calista D, Boschini A (2000). Cutaneous side effects induced by indinavir. *Eur J Dermatol* **10**: 292–6.

Carr A, Samaras, K Burton S *et al.* (1998a). A syndrome of peripheral lipodystrophy, hyperlipidaemia, and insulin resistance in patients receiving HIV protease inhibitors. *AIDS* **12**: F51–8.

Carr A, Samaras K, Chisolm DJ *et al.* (1998b). Pathogenesis of HIV-1 protease-associated peripheral lipodystrophy, hyperlipidaemia and insulin resistance. *Lancet* **31**: 1881–3.

Clerici M, Shearer GM. (1993). A TH1→ TH2 switch is a critical step in the etiology of HIV infection. *Immunol Today* **14**: 107–11.

Daling JR, Weiss NS, Klopfenstein LL *et al.* (1982). Correlates of homosexual behavior and the incidence of anal cancer. *J Am Medical Assoc* **247**: 1988–90.

Di Silverio A, Brazzelli V, Brandozzi G *et al.* (1991). Prevalence of dermatophytes and yeasts – (Candida spp., Malassezia furfur) in HIV patients. A study of former drug addicts. *Mycopathologia* **114**: 103–7.

Diven DG, Newton RC, Ramsey KM. (1988). Heightened cutaneous reactions to mosquito bites in patients with acquired immunodeficiency syndrome receiving zidovudine. *Arch Intern Med* **148**: 2296.

Dompmartin D, Dompmartin A, Deluol AM *et al.* (1990). Onychomycosis and AIDS – clinical and laboratory findings in 62 patients. *Int J Dermatol* **29**: 337–9.

Douglas JM, Rogers M, Judson FN. (1986). The effect of asymptomatic infection with HTLV-III on the response of anogenital warts to intralesional treatment with recombinant alfa2 interferon. *J Infect Dis* **154**: 331–4.

Duvic M. (1987). Staphylococcal infections and the pruritus of AIDS-related complex. *Arch Dermatol* **123**: 1599.

Edwards L, Ferenczy A, Eron L et al. (1998). Self administered 5% imiquimod cream for external anogenital warts. *Arch Dermatol* **134**: 25–30.

Finegold I. (1986). Oral desensitization to trimethoprim-sulfamethoxazole in a patient with acquired immunodeficiency syndrome. *J Allergy Clin Immunol* **78**: 905–8.

Fivenson DP, Weltman RE, Gibson SH. (1988). Giant molluscum contagiosum presenting as basal cell carcinoma in an acquired immunodeficiency syndrome patient. *J Am Acad Dermatol* **19**: 912–4.

Funkhouser ME, Omohundro C, Ross A et al. (1993). Management of scabies in patients with HIV disease. *Arch Dermatol* **129**: 911–3.

Gal AA, Meyer PR, Taylor CR. (1987). Papillomavirus antigens in anorectal condyloma and carcinoma in homosexual men. *J Am Med Assoc* **257**: 337–404.

Gelfland JM, Rudikoff D, Lebowhl M et al. (1998). Effect of UV-B phototherapy on plasma type 1 RNA viral level: a self-controlled prospective study. *Arch Dermatol* **134**: 940–5.

Ghadially R, Sibbald RG, Walter JB et al. (1989). Granuloma annulare in patients with human immunodeficiency virus infections. *J Am Acad Dermatol* **20**: 232–5.

Goldstein B, Berman B, Sukenik E et al. (1997). Correlation of skin disorders with CD4 lymphocyte counts in patients with HIV/AIDS. *J Am Acad Dermatol* **36**: 262–4.

Goldstone SE, Winkler B, Ufford LJ et al. (2001). High prevalence of anal squamous intraepithelial lesions and squamous cell carcinoma in men who have sex with men as seen in a surgical practice. *Dis Colon Rectum* **44**: 690–98.

Hicks CB, Myers SA, Giner J. (1997). Resolution of intractable molluscum contagiosum in a HIV-infected patient after institution of antiretroviral therapy with ritonavir. *Clin Infect Dis* **24**: 1023–5.

Hulbert TV, Larsen RA. (1992). Hyperkeratotic (Norwegian) scabies with gram-negative bacteremia as the initial presentation of AIDS. *Clin Infect Dis* **14**: 1164–5.

Kaplan MH, Sadick NS, Wieder J et al. (1989). Antipsoriatic effects of zidovudine in human immunodeficiency virus-associated psoriasis. *J Am Acad Dermatol* **20**: 76–82.

Kohn SR. (1987). Molluscum contagiosum in patients with acquired immunodeficiency syndrome. *Arch Ophthalmol* **105**: 458.

Lake-Bakaar G, Tom W, Lake-Bakaar D et al. (1988). Gastropathy and ketoconazole malabsorption in the acquired immunodeficiency syndrome (AIDS). *Ann Intern Med* **109**: 471–3.

Lim HW, Vullaurupalli S, Meola T et al. (1997). UVB Phototherapy is an effective treatment for pruritus in patients infected with HIV. *J Am Acad Dermatol* **37**: 414–7.

MacKenzie-Wood A, Ray JE, Whitfeld MJ. (1999). Itraconazole and HIV protease inhibitors – an important interaction. *Med J Aust* **170**: 46–7.

Macnab JCM, Walkinshaw SA, Cordiner JW et al. (1986). Human papillomavirus in clinically and histologically normal tissue of patients with genital cancer. *N Engl J Med* **315**: 1052–8.

Matis WL, Triana A, Shapiro R et al. (1987). Dermatologic findings associated with human immunodeficiency virus infection. *J Am Acad Dermatol* **17**: 746–51.

Meadows KP, Tyring SK, Pavia AT et al. (1997). Resolution of recalcitrant molluscum contagiosum virus lesions on human immunodeficiency virus-infected patients treated with cidofovir. *Arch Dermatol* **133**: 987–90.

Meinking TL. (1996). Safety of Permethrin vs Lindane for the treatment of scabies. *Arch Dermatol* **132**: 959–62.

Meinking TL, Taplin D, Hermida JL et al. (1995). The treatment of scabies with ivermectin. *N Engl J Med* **333**: 26–30.

Moreno F, Hardin TC, Rinaldi MG et al. (1993). Itraconazole–didanosine excipient interaction. *J Am Med Assoc* **269**: 1508.

Moss VA. (1991). Scabies in an AIDS hospice unit. *Br J Clin Pathol* **45**: 35–6.

Murray JF, Mills J. (1990). Pulmonary infectious complications of human immunodeficiency virus infection. Part II. *Am Rev Respir Dis* **141**: 1582–98.

Obuch ML, Maurer TA, Becker B et al. (1992). Psoriasis and human immunodeficiency virus infection. *J Am Acad Dermatol* **27**: 667–73.

Ong ELC, Mandal BK. (1989). Multiple drug reactions in a patient with AIDS. *Lancet* **2**: 976–7.

Ostlere LS, Taylor CR, Harris DW et al. (1996). Skin surface lipids in HIV-positive patients with and without seborrhoeic dermatitis. *Int J Dermatol* **35**: 276–9.

Palefsky JM, Gonzales J, Greenblatt RM et al. (1990). Anal intraepithelial neoplasia and anal papillomavirus infection among homosexual males with Group IV HIV disease. *J Am Med Assoc* **263**: 2911–6.

Palevsky JM, Holly EA, Ralston ML et al. (1998). Prevalence and risk factors for human papillomavirus infection of the anal canal in HIV positive and HIV negative homosexual men. *J Infect Dis* **177**: 361–7.

Parkin JM, Eales LJ, Galazka AR et al. (1987). Atopic manifestations in the acquired immune deficiency syndrome: response to recombinant interferon gamma. *Br Med J* **294**: 1185–6.

Patterson JW, Kao GFR, Graham JH et al. (1986). Bowenoid papulosis: a clinicopathologic study with ultrastructural observations. *Cancer* **57**: 823–36.

Penneys NS, Nayar JK, Bernstein H et al. (1989). Chronic pruritic eruption in patients with acquired immunodeficiency syndrome associated with increased antibody titers to mosquito salivary gland antigens. *J Am Acad Dermatol* **21**: 214–25.

Petersen CS, Gerstoft J. (1992). Molluscum contagiosum in HIV-infected patients. *Clin Lab Invest* **184**: 19–21.

Picon L, Vaillant l., Duong T et al. (1989). Cutaneous cryptococcosis resembling molluscum contagiosum: A first manifestation of AIDS. *Acta Derm Venereol* **69**: 365–7.

Reveille JD, Conant MA, Duvic M. (1990). Human immunodeficiency virus-associated psoriasis, psoriatic arthritis, and Reiter's syndrome: a disease continuum? *Arthritis Rheum* **33**: 1574–8.

Rosenthal D, LeBoit PE, Klumpp L. et al. (1991). Human immunodeficiency virus-associated eosinophilic folliculitis. A unique dermatosis associated with advanced human immunodeficiency virus infection. *Arch Dermatol* **127**: 206–9.

Rudlinger R, Buchmann P. (1989). HPV 16-positive Bowenoid papulosis and squamous-cell carcinoma of the anus in an HIV-positive man. *Dis Colon Rectum* **32**: 1042–5.

Rudlinger R, Grob R, Buchmann P et al. (1988). Anogenital warts of the condyloma acuminatum type in HIV-positive patients. *Dermatologica* **176**: 277–381.

Sadick N, Kaplan MH, Pahwa SG et al. (1986). Unusual features of scabies complicating human T-lymphotropic virus type III infection. *J Am Acad Dermatol* **15**: 482–6.

Sanchez-Carazo JL, Hernandez M, Vilata JJ et al. (1989). HPV types detected by *in situ* hybridization in Bowenoid papulosis. In: *ASD Twenty-Seventh Annual Meeting*, San Francisco, CA.

Sawchuk WS, Weber PJ, Lowy DR et al. (1989). Infectious papillomavirus in the vapor of warts treated with carbon dioxide laser or electrocoagulation: Detection and protection. *J Am Acad Dermatol* **21**: 41–9.

Schafer A, Friedmann W, Mielke M *et al.* (1991). The increased frequency of cervical dysplasia-neoplasia in women infected with the human immunodeficiency virus is related to the degree of immunosuppression. *Am J Obst Gynecol* **164**: 593–9.

Schwartz JJ, Myskowski PL. (1992). Molluscum contagiosum in patients with human immunodeficiency virus infection. *J Am Acad Dermatol* **27**: 583–8.

Silman FH, Sedlis A, Boyce JG. (1985). A review of lower genital intra-epithelial neoplasia and the use of topical 5-fluorouracil. *Obstet Gynecol* **40**: 190–220.

Smith KJ, Skelton HG, Yeager J *et al.* (1997). Increased drug reactions in HIV-1-positive patients: a possible explanation based on patterns of immune dysregulation seen in HIV disease. *Clin Exp Dermatol* **22**: 118–23.

Sobhani I, Vuagnat A, Walker F *et al.* (2001). Prevalence of high-grade dysplasia and cancer in the anal canali in human papillomavirus-infected individuals. *Gastroenterology* **120**: 857–66.

Toback AC, Longley J, Cardullo AC *et al.* (1986). Severe chronic photosensitivity in association with acquired immunodeficiency syndrome. *J Am Acad Dermatol* **15**: 1056–7.

Uthayakumar S, Nandawi R, Drinkwater T *et al.* (1997). The prevalence of skin disease in HIV infection and its relationship to the degree of immunosupression. *Br J Dermatol* **13**: 595–8.

Walker GJ, Johnstone PW (2000). Interventions for treating scabies. *Cochrane Database Syst Rev* 3:CD000320.

Weinberg JM, Mysliwiec A, Turiansky GW *et al.* (1997). Viral Folliculitis. Atypical presentations of herpes simplex, herpes zoster and molluscum contagiosum. *Arch Dermatol* **133**: 983–6.

Wright DN, Nelson RP, Ledford DK *et al.* (1990). Serum IgE and human immunodeficiency virus (HIV) infection. *J Allergy Clin Immunol* **85**: 445–52.

Wright DC, Lennox JL, James WD *et al.* (1991). Generalized chronic dermatophytosis in patients with human immunodeficiency virus Type 1 infection and CD4 depletion. *Arch Dermatol* **127**: 265–6.

BRIAN McDONALD

Until recently the almost invariable long-term consequence of HIV infection was death. With the introduction of highly active antiretroviral therapy (HAART) there has been a dramatic reduction in morbidity and mortality due to HIV/AIDS in countries where these therapies are available (Wood *et al.*, 1997; Palella *et al.*, 1998; Lee *et al.*, 2001). A study of 1255 patients with at least one CD4 lymphocyte count of less than 100 cells/μl reports a decline in mortality rates from 29.4 per 100 person-years in 1995 to 8.8 per 100 person-years in 1997, the reduction being attributed to more intensive antiretroviral therapy, including protease inhibitors (PIs) (Palella *et al.*, 1998). Even with the reduction in the number of AIDS cases and AIDS-related deaths, a significant level of morbidity and mortality remains and there is the possibility, as yet unsubstantiated, that morbidity may be more protracted than has previously been the case. A question remains as to the long-term outcome for those currently on optimal treatment with good virological control.

This chapter will explore some of the issues peculiar to palliative care for people with HIV/AIDS and will address some of the symptom management problems.

> *AIDS is a series of shocks. No sooner has the victim recovered from one disease when another takes its place. It is as though the various diseases are competing to see which can do the most damage in the shortest possible time. AIDS is about watching the pieces fall off. The body slowly disintegrates, things that worked yesterday don't work today ...*

Damon died from AIDS on the 1st April 1991. The narration by Bryce Courtenay of his son's progression through AIDS to death (Courtenay, 1993) emphasizes the importance of a holistic approach to the care of the person with HIV/AIDS. Damon's story reveals the extent to which the health-care system can be a confusing maze to patients, their carers and their families and highlights the importance of integrated and accessible care, particularly in the more advanced stages of the disease.

When death occurs it is often after a protracted period of declining health punctuated by various disease processes, which are manifestations of the impaired immune status of the person living with HIV/AIDS. If we are genuine in our desire to ensure that people living with advanced HIV/AIDS are able to maximize the quality of their lives, a partnership between the acute, sometimes intensive, services and the holistic multidisciplinary model of palliative care is essential to meet the needs of patients and their carers. This partnership addresses the symptom management, spiritual and psychosocial issues associated with a progressive life-threatening disease, which, for many, in response to modern treatments, may have become a much more slowly progressive chronic disease (Goldstone *et al.*, 1995). Where treatment of HIV/AIDS has not been fully successful, or the patient has chosen not to pursue treatment, the aim of palliative care is to improve quality of life by focusing on management of symptoms and the provision of physical, psychological, social and spiritual support (Kuhl, 1995).

Philosophical issues

The World Health Organization describes palliative care as:

> *The total care of patients whose disease is not responsive to curative treatment. Control of pain, of other symptoms, and of psychological, social and spiritual problems, is paramount. The goal of palliative care is achievement of the best quality of life for patients and their families.' (World Health Organization, 1989)*

There is increasing recognition of the legitimacy of providing palliative care interventions in an episodic manner, based more on the intermittent care needs of the patient, rather than on the traditional expectation of a prognosis of less than 6 months in the terminal phase of disease. This development is consistent with the perspective that palliation should be provided as a continuum with acute care. However, it may not be consistent with health-care funding conditions in some countries (Moss, 1990; Foley *et al.*, 1995; Grothe, 1995).

Palliative care advice can often be helpful in the earlier stages of HIV infection in conjunction with acute treatments and plays an increasingly important role in advanced disease. It is important that psychosocial support is considered in conjunction with specific treatment of HIV itself or of its medical complications (Barnes *et al.*, 1993; Higginson, 1993). In HIV/AIDS, palliative care, focusing on symptom control and quality of life issues, should be an integral part of acute care, just as acute care, with its focus on treatment of disease processes, should be an integral part of palliative care. The transition from predominantly acute care to predominantly palliative care is not well defined (Foley *et al.*, 1995). The majority of people with HIV/AIDS choose to continue with active treatments – many of which are truly palliative – until they are very close to death (George, 1991). Palliative care for people with HIV/AIDS requires a concept of continuing care encompassing symptom management, respite or shared care, rehabilitation and terminal care.

People in the advanced stages of HIV/AIDS and their carers often have concerns that there will inevitably be severe pain, loss of independence and loss of dignity. With good symptom control and psychosocial support most can maintain independence and enjoy life even with very advanced disease (Kimball and McCormick, 1996; Koffman *et al.*, 1996). The concept of palliative care may be confronting to a patient who is part of a population that has widely held the view that palliative care is only for those close to death and for those who have discontinued active treatments (Grothe, 1995).

Who should provide palliative care?

AIDS is a multisystem disease and its treatment requires a co-ordinated and holistic approach (Malcolm and Sutherland, 1992; Wood *et al.*, 1997). Physicians and general practitioners caring for people with HIV/AIDS are generally aware of the issues impacting on the patient, their carers and family, but their natural focus on their own area of expertise and interest may mean that they do not have the time, skills, knowledge or breadth of approach that pallia-

tive medicine and palliative care may bring to the care team (Breitbart, 1996).

Palliative medicine practitioners may not have the specialist knowledge and expertise required for the proper assessment, diagnosis and treatment of the full range of conditions from which patients might suffer (Wood *et al.*, 1997). It is essential to have access to expert advice when appropriate but some understanding of the particular issues presented by patients with HIV/AIDS is necessary in order to recognize when other specialist assessment and intervention might be necessary (Grothe, 1995). The range of carers can include infectious diseases physicians, oncologists, gastroenterologists, ophthalmologists, dietitians, occupational therapists, physiotherapists, social workers, counsellors from various backgrounds, lay volunteer care workers, various support organizations and others (Figure 20.1).

Where should palliative care be provided?

Palliative care for people with HIV/AIDS is provided in a range of settings, including the acute medical unit, HIV-specific continuing care or palliative care unit, general hospices and at home or in supported accommodation facilities. There is no single model whereby palliative care might be provided, as local history, resources and culture will determine how to best meet the needs of particular

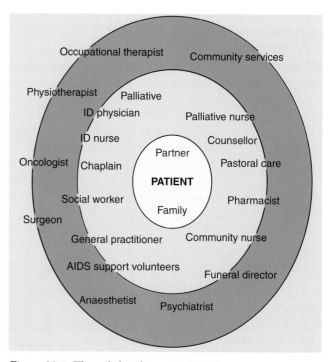

Figure 20.1 *The multidisciplinary HIV/AIDS care team.*

populations. A variety of models of care have developed including HIV/AIDS-specific services and services providing palliative care for HIV/AIDS integrated with other patient groups with cancer and other progressive life-threatening illnesses. Thus, the setting will depend on the care needs of the patient and availability of resources and care givers (Moss, 1990; Foley et al., 1995; Fraser, 1995; Johnson, 1995; Kimball and McCormick, 1996; Wood et al., 1997).

Issues impacting on provision of palliative care (Table 20.1)

Positive living philosophy

The concept of 'people living with AIDS' is part of many AIDS support organizations. People living with HIV/AIDS are often well informed about the various treatment options, which may have rescued their partners, their friends or themselves from acute or subacute life-threatening situations and provided extension of, and improvement in, the quality of life, sometimes for periods of months or years (Wood et al., 1997). Experienced advocates may be required to ensure that the patient is aware of treatment options in the advanced stages of illness.

Case profile

RG had severe wasting in the advanced stages of AIDS. At one stage, under the care of a hospice with limited experience with HIV/AIDS patients, he had been prescribed morphine and midazolam for relief of discomfort and anxiety. He required assistance in most activities, but spent periods of time at home. In response to concerns expressed by a community nurse, he was assessed by a general practitioner experienced in HIV/AIDS. The patient was admitted to an HIV/AIDS-specific palliative care unit which was part of a major HIV service. He was almost mute due to his cachexia and could barely stand unassisted. In response to the question as to whether he wished to attempt restorative care and rehabilitation or to be provided with support until he died, he expressed some surprise that there was the option of active treatment. He was not ready to die and responded positively to the suggested treatment interventions. Under the joint management of both infectious diseases and palliative care his rehabilitation included enteral feeding (eventually via gastrostomy), combination anti-retroviral therapies, physiotherapy, occupational therapy, nutritional and psychological support. After about 3 months he was discharged to community care with support from part-time attendant carers. His condition has remained stable and he has positively enjoyed life for over 3 years at the time of publication.

The outcomes of treatment in advanced cancer are relatively predictable compared with advanced AIDS (Fraser, 1995) and in the latter disease many patients and their physicians will pursue treatments with only a very small chance of success, rather than accept that treatment options have been exhausted.

Fears, phobias, stigmatization, confidentiality

Misunderstandings of the risks to close community or domestic contacts of people with HIV/AIDS persist, although anecdotally it is less common to observe overt discrimination from health-care workers than was the case earlier in the epidemic. Infection control issues may be a major concern to community health-care professionals and hospital staff unfamiliar with HIV/AIDS cases, particularly in isolated rural communities or hospitals, but expert advice will often allay any fears. Professional attitudes regarding involvement in the treatment of patients with HIV/AIDS appear to be relatively positive, although some physicians have concerns relating to their knowledge and the availability of expert support (Samuels et al., 1995).

Patients, carers and families may be reluctant to reveal their diagnosis of HIV/AIDS to friends or acquaintances or to bureaucrats because of concerns of stigmatization or discrimination. Patients may go to great lengths to conceal the diagnosis from close family members. It is necessary occasionally to collude with the patient to conceal the

Table 20.1 Issues impacting on palliative care

Positive living philosophy
Fears and phobias
Stigmatization and confidentiality
Homosexuality and gay issues
Age of patients and carers
Complex pharmacological treatments
Psychiatric issues
Autonomy and euthanasia

diagnosis from relatives, sometimes parents, and sensitivity to the particular customs of various cultural groups is essential (Perreault, 1995).

Patients may avoid local treatment centres and prefer to travel to or even live close to major metropolitan treatment centres for treatment and review (Foley et al., 1995). Maintaining confidentiality in small rural communities may be difficult. Some find that they receive additional support as a result of being known to have HIV/AIDS, while others report bigotry and prejudice from the unenlightened.

Homosexuality and gay issues

A substantial proportion of people with HIV/AIDS in the developed world are gay men or belong to other marginalized groups. Gay lifestyles may be alien to some health-care workers accustomed to a more conventional client group and awareness of and tolerance of 'alternative' lifestyles may take time to develop. For some members of the community, close relationships, partnerships and displays of affection between same-sex couples are natural. In order to provide optimum care it is necessary to gain the confidence of the gay community and to respect their rights and freedoms.

Gay male patients' care givers include lovers, family and friends, who provide both emotional and direct care. The 'families' of people with HIV/AIDS can be quite varied (Grothe, 1995). Lessons in acceptance and tolerance can be learned from observation of elderly parents who may have had to come to terms with the knowledge that their son is not only dying as a result of HIV/AIDS, but has a lifestyle and philosophy that challenges their own value systems.

Issues of 'ownership' of patient and property can be a source of conflict between the patient's family and his lover, particularly around the time of death. The health professional may have to negotiate very carefully with the various parties. Spiritual support from conventional sources may be compromised, as many of those affected by HIV/AIDS may feel that they cannot access organized religion because of the publicly dogmatic positions taken (Gray, 1995), but there are enlightened individuals from various religions who work well in the setting of HIV/AIDS.

Age of patients and carers – multiple loss

The average age of those dying from AIDS has been around 40 years (Butters et al., 1993; Goldstone et al., 1995; Kimball and McCormick, 1996), considerably less than the average age of 70 years of people traditionally admitted to

hospice (Briggs, 1992). Many patients from the gay community, drug users and haemophiliacs will have been exposed to multiple loss (Wood et al., 1997) having observed their lovers, friends and peers deteriorate with AIDS over 2–3 years. The carer may also be HIV-infected or have AIDS. Carers of people who have died from HIV/AIDS may be faced with social isolation, stigma and fear of contagion, complicating their grief (Perreault, 1995). Often elderly parents play a large part in the care and support of their adult children and demonstrate great courage in the face of imminent loss. They may require considerable support in dealing with untimely death.

Complex pharmacological treatments

People with advanced HIV/AIDS often require concurrent, often complex and continuous treatments for several AIDS-related conditions (Grothe, 1995), with a wide range of drugs with potential interactions and side-effects. Continuity of treatment into the palliative and terminal phase of the illness may be important to both staff and patient if the clinical and psychosocial needs are to be met. Palliative care service staff may not have the knowledge and training to provide support with pharmacological treatments (Wood et al., 1997), particularly in relation to intravenous drug infusions. Partnership with community or visiting nursing services who may be involved in the care of the patient for many weeks or months is essential.

Psychiatric and psychological issues

A significant number of people with HIV/AIDS have psychiatric disorders or cognitive impairment associated with HIV/AIDS (Foley et al., 1995; McKeogh, 1995; Baker, 1997). A number of people with primary psychiatric problems develop HIV/AIDS. In advanced disease people from both of these groups may require regular, sometimes 24-h supervision, which may not be available if they are single or their partner is working, and a system of shared care may be desirable in such situations. HIV/AIDS hospices or continuing care units may be in a position to provide care for such cases provided that behaviours are not unduly disruptive to other patients. The question as to where and how to best care for HIV/AIDS patients with psychiatric problems or for psychiatric patients with HIV/AIDS is unclear (Grothe, 1995).

Psychological distress to carers is a significant issue, with emotional support identified as the most difficult and demanding aspect of care (Clipp et al., 1995).

Recreational or illicit drug use

This particular group of patients, for whom HIV/AIDS may be but one of many challenges in a constant battle to survive, require special consideration as to the manner and place of care. Their problems may be compounded by homelessness, poverty, mistrust and the need for substitution drugs when hospitalized to prevent the effects of withdrawal or unmasked pain (Robb, 1995). A prospective study of 513 patients found that the 72% who had acquired HIV as a result of injecting drug use made relatively more use of the local AIDS hospice than those who had acquired HIV from other causes (Brettle *et al.*, 1997). Pain management of patients using illicit drugs presents a dilemma to many health-care providers and requires careful consideration. The fact that patients have been using or continue to use recreational drugs should not preclude the use of analgesics after careful evaluation (Foley *et al.*, 1995; Goldstone *et al.*, 1995). Patients with a history of illicit drug use and AIDS-related pain have been shown to achieve successful analgesia with morphine but may require higher doses than those without such a history (Kaplan *et al.*, 2000).

Autonomy and euthanasia

In common with many younger patients with progressive life-threatening illnesses such as cancer, AIDS patients are very involved in treatment decisions and value their rights to make informed choices, sometimes nominating a partner, friend or family member as their advocate in the event that they become cognitively impaired. The degree of the patient's knowledge of the treatment options and the effects and potential side-effects of drugs used for treating HIV/AIDS (Wood *et al.*, 1997) can facilitate discussions around treatment options. The autonomy promoted by palliative care in relation to withdrawing from active treatments must be respected where patients opt for active interventions. What may need promotion in the acute care environment and in the 'AIDS community' is a proper understanding of and opportunity to consider the option of discontinuing or not pursuing active treatment.

The concept of self-deliverance of drugs in the form of euthanasia or suicide is a concern for this group of patients. HIV/AIDS support groups and members of the gay community are generally advocates for legislation to permit euthanasia (Foley *et al.*, 1995). Euthanasia is practised in a proportion of HIV/AIDS cases (Meier *et al.*, 1998), although it is more frequently discussed than enacted. The provision of supportive palliative care and the assurance that all available measures will be taken to ensure the best possible symptom management including, if necessary, rendering the patient unconscious, will often allay fears of a painful distressing death (Goldstone, 1995; Grothe, 1995; Quill *et al.*, 1997). However, despite such assurances and vigorous attempts at symptom management, psychiatric, psychosocial and spiritual support, not all symptoms can be completely controlled or answers provided that allay the anguish felt by some patients. For some, euthanasia is seen as a legitimate answer to the relentless progress of the disease, loss of independence and concerns regarding the perceived burden they place on their carers, lovers and families. Doctors and health-care personnel working with people with advanced HIV/AIDS must determine their own individual response, but should at least be prepared to discuss the issues around requests for euthanasia (Voigt, 1995), whether or not they are prepared to assist. Euthanasia and physician-assisted suicide remain illegal but are condoned by particular legislatures, the most overt of which is Holland, where 22% of 131 deaths of people with HIV/AIDS were as a result of euthanasia or physician-assisted suicide (Bindels *et al.*, 1996).

Symptom management

Symptoms in patients with advanced HIV/AIDS have been documented and include debility and weight loss, pain, anorexia, nausea, depression, diarrhoea, constipation, dyspnea, cognitive impairment, dysphagia and neurological deficits (Table 20.2) (Moss, 1990; O'Neill and Sherrard, 1993; Kelleher *et al.*, 1997; Wood *et al.*, 1997). The following section does not provide detailed advice on the management of every symptom, but focuses on those areas that are considered to be of particular concern in HIV/AIDS. The management of symptoms should not be delayed while awaiting the outcome of assessment and active treatment (O'Neill and Sherrard, 1993). A number

Table 20.2 Symptoms in advanced HIV/AIDS

Wasting	Dyspnoea	Depression
Anorexia	Pain	Anxiety
Cognitive impairment	Diarrhoea	Dysphagia
Blindness	Constipation	Neurological deficits

Table 20.3 Opportunistic infections that may require continuing active treatment in advanced disease

Cytomegalovirus retinitis
Candidiasis
Herpes simplex infection
Mycobacterium avium complex
Pneumocystis carinii pneumonia
Cerebral toxoplasmosis

of opportunistic infections generally require continued medical treatment during palliative care (Table 20.3).

Caution must be exercised in the use of certain drugs that have utility in symptom management but may have significant interactions with antiretroviral drugs, particularly the PIs (see Chapter 6). Of particular concern are drugs that are frequently used for symptom management, including cisapride, non-sedating antihistamines, certain benzodiazepines and particularly midazolam and carbamazepine. This list is by no means exhaustive, and if there is any concern about particular combinations consultation with physicians or pharmacists experienced in HIV/AIDS treatments should be sought.

Pain management

Pain is common in the course of HIV/AIDS in both adults and children (Breitbart, 1996; Breitbart *et al.*, 1996; Hirschfeld *et al.*, 1996; Kimball and McCormick, 1996; Larue *et al.*, 1997). Estimates of the prevalence of pain as a feature of the illness in adults range from 25% in early HIV to 97% in later stages (O'Neill and Sherrard, 1993; Breitbart, 1996; Kimball and McCormick, 1996). In a survey of 61 children and their parents, more than 50% indicated pain as one component of the illness that impacted on their lives (Hirschfeld *et al.*, 1996).

Of greater concern is the alarming degree to which pain in HIV/AIDS is underestimated and undertreated (O'Neill and Sherrard, 1993; Breitbart *et al.*, 1996; Stephenson, 1996; Larue *et al.*, 1997). Breitbart reports inadequate analgesia in up to 85% of a series of 366 ambulatory AIDS patients with pain. Less than 8% of 110 patients reporting severe pain were treated with strong opioids. Women who were injecting drug users and poorly educated patients were more likely to be undertreated (Breitbart *et al.*, 1996; Breitbart *et al.*, 1997). In a study of 315 patients, 57% of whom reported moderate or severe pain, almost half received no analgesics and only 10 of 69

patients who reported severe pain were prescribed morphine (Larue *et al.*, 1997). Other studies indicate that satisfactory pain management is achievable for many HIV/AIDS patients (Kaplan *et al.*, 1994; Koffman *et al.*, 1996; Holzemer *et al.*, 1998). The principles of pain management in HIV/AIDS are similar to those applicable to cancer and other progressive life-threatening diseases. Pain in HIV/AIDS is multidimensional, the nature of and response to pain being the result of physical, sensory and nociceptive factors that are moderated to a variable degree by a range of psychosocial, spiritual, and cognitive factors (Breitbart, 1996). Drug therapy should thus only be one part of the management strategy. Non-drug treatments, which can contribute to symptom relief, include psychological support, relaxation, physiotherapy, massage, transcutaneous electric nerve stimulation (TENS) and acupuncture (Breitbart, 1996).

Analgesic drug use follows the WHO analgesic ladder guidelines (Figure 20.2), progressing in a stepwise manner from mild analgesics such as paracetamol (acetaminophen) to combinations with a weak opioid such as codeine, before using opioids. For specific types of pain the use of drugs such as non-steroidal anti-inflammatory drugs, antidepressants (principally tricyclics), anticonvulsants, antispasmodics, local anaesthetics and general anaesthetics may be more effective (Breitbart, 1996; Moss, 1990; O'Neill and Sherrard, 1993).

Opioids

Opioids used in pain management and palliative care include morphine, diamorphine, methadone, hydromorphone, oxycodone, and fentanyl (Gourlay *et al.*, 1986; Sawe, 1986; Fainsinger *et al.*, 1993; Maddocks *et al.*, 1996; Ravenscroft, 1996; Woodhouse *et al.*, 1996; Christrup,

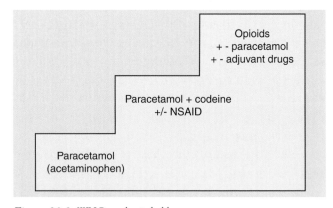

Figure 20.2 *WHO analgesic ladder.*

Table 20.4 Drugs used for management

Opioids used in palliative care	Drugs used for neuropathic pain
Morphine	Antidepressants – tricyclic
Diamorphine	Anticonvulsants – valproate, gabapentin
Methadone	
Hydromorphone	Anti-arrythmics – mexiletine
Oxycodone	Ketamine
Fentanyl	Clonidine

1997). Codeine has no analgesic effect until it is metabolized to morphine, and up to 10% of the Caucasian population are unable to convert it (Sindrup *et al.*, 1991; Ravenscroft, 1996). Availability varies in different countries, but the most commonly used opioid analgesic is morphine, against which the others are compared. Pethidine (meperidine) should not be used for chronic pain (Ravenscroft, 1996) as the metabolite norpethidine may cause central nervous system irritability with prolonged use or high doses (see Table 20.4).

Routes of administration for longer-term use include oral, subcutaneous, transdermal (fentanyl), and (rarely) intrathecal (Breitbart, 1996). When the oral route is not appropriate because of vomiting or reduced conscious state, the combination of opioids with certain other drugs (Chandler *et al.*, 1996) administered subcutaneously via a syringe driver has become established practice in palliative medicine. Medical and nursing staff in the acute care area may be unfamiliar with the drug combinations, dose ranges and methods of administration that are routine in palliative care and should be prepared to seek advice from specialists in the field.

Neuropathic pain

HIV-related symptomatic peripheral neuropathy is common, occurring in up to 30% of patients (Moss, 1990; O'Neill and Sherrard, 1993; Tyor *et al.*, 1995) and abolishing pain completely without unacceptable side-effects can be extremely difficult (see Chapter 10). The approach to pain management should follow the standard principles referred to earlier, with the exclusion of treatable reversible causes and trial of non-opioid analgesics.

Neuropathic pain was considered to be resistant to treatment with opioids, but it is now recognized that some patients can experience modification of their pain with morphine and other opioids, albeit in higher than normal

doses (Kaplan *et al.*, 1996; Warncke *et al.*, 1997). The total daily dose of morphine can range from 20 mg to as much as 3000 mg or more a day. There is no documented upper limit of dose for morphine, but further escalation of dosage is not warranted if no incremental improvement in pain management is demonstrated. Some patients may respond better to methadone rather than morphine, but the pharmacodynamics and risks of narcosis due to methadone are quite different from those of morphine (Gourlay *et al.*, 1986; Fainsinger *et al.*, 1993) and advice should be sought from specialists in pain management or palliative medicine. The use of adjuvant drugs such as antidepressants, anticonvulsants, local anaesthetic antiarrhythmics such as mexiletine (Galer *et al.*, 1996; Woolf and Mannion, 1999), in conjunction with analgesics, can significantly improve management but the response of individual patients is unpredictable. Some patients may require combinations of three or more drugs from different groups, which adds to the already high total daily drug burden common to people with advanced HIV/AIDS. The effect of ketamine, an N-methyl-D-aspartate (NMDA) receptor antagonist, has been shown to be superior to morphine for experimentally induced hyperalgesia (Warncke *et al.*, 1997) and may be considered for the treatment of neuropathic pain (Ravenscroft, 1996).

Intrathecal morphine has become a standard treatment option for intractable pain (Paice *et al.*, 1996, 1997) but there are no published studies of its use in HIV/AIDS. The use of intrathecal morphine in the management of HIV/AIDS-related pain is not established and its use for individual patients should only be considered after exhaustive titration of analgesics and adjuvant drugs, and assessment of the risks of infection in patients who are immunocompromised.

Case profile

SR, a 35-year-old man, had as his principal significant disability HIV myelitis, manifest as motor and sensory symptoms. His general health was stable and he was on combination antiretroviral therapy. He failed to respond to treatment with non-opioid analgesics, low-dose morphine and non-analgesic drugs and his mobility and comfort was severely compromised by hyperalgesia and occasional lancinating pain in his feet and legs. His quality of life improved significantly when his symptoms were considerably relieved with sustained-release morphine in doses of 2400 mg daily.

After much deliberation and joint assessment by his palliative medicine consultant, infectious diseases physician and a neurologist experienced in spinal disease and the use of intrathecal morphine, he had an intrathecal drug administration system implanted. His use of sustained-release morphine dropped to 200–400 mg daily as his intrathecal dose was gradually increased to 30 mg daily. After 12 months, the intrathecal administration device failed. Use of the intrathecal device was discontinued, as control of the dose was impossible and his oral morphine requirements gradually increased to the previous level of 2400 mg daily.

The failed device was replaced with a continuous infusion device, which has been delivering morphine 30 mg/24 h for over 2 years at the time of preparation of this manuscript.

Intractable diarrhoea

Diarrhoea is common in patients with advanced HIV/AIDS and has a variety of causes, which should be considered and treated appropriately (Moss, 1990; Wood et al., 1997). For many patients, diarrhoea will respond to conventional management, including treatment for susceptible pathogens, antidiarrheals and to dietetic measures. For some, the diarrhoea can be severe and intractable (Compean et al., 1994). Drugs that have been used conventionally for HIV/AIDS-related diarrhoea include loperamide, diphenoxylate, codeine phosphate, bulking agents, cholestyramine, morphine, and diamorphine. These remain the mainstay of symptom management, in addition to fluid replacement when dehydration is a problem. Total parenteral nutrition (TPN) is rarely used while 'resting' the gastrointestinal tract. The place of octreotide or alternative somatostatin analogues has been evaluated (Mosdell and Visconti, 1994; Beaugerie et al., 1996; Farthing, 1996) efficacy in HIV/AIDS has not been established. One small, randomized placebo-controlled trial of octreotide with only 10 patients in each arm claimed to demonstrate benefit (Compean et al., 1994), but this was not supported by another study involving 129 patients (Simon et al., 1995). With our current knowledge, it may be reasonable to consider the use of octreotide on an individual patient basis and to discontinue its administration in the absence of obvious benefit.

Wasting

Wasting is a common cause of debility in advanced HIV/AIDS and has a variety of causes, some of which may be reversible (Moss, 1990; Roubenoff et al., 2000; Sumpter 1997; Wanke et al., 2000; Wood et al., 1997; Young, 1997). Early dietetic intervention and support in combination with the treatment of specific disease processes may improve nutritional status. For those for whom medical and dietetic measures have failed, there may be benefits from the use of anabolic steroids or progestogens. Results of studies in HIV/AIDS patients have been equivocal with respect to the benefits or otherwise of these drugs (Berger et al., 1996; Gold et al., 1996; Grinspoon et al., 1996; Hengge et al., 1996; Strang, 1997). Many patients with wasting and other symptoms of advanced HIV/AIDS derive benefit from the use of cannabis and it may be that the therapeutic potential of this recreational drug could be further explored (Robson, 1998).

Terminal phase

Patients who die as a result of HIV/AIDS do so in various modes of care from aggressive, disease-orientated, life-preserving management to purely palliative symptomatic care. However, the cost is likely to be very high. Even where specific palliative care facilities are available, more than 50% of deaths occur in the acute care environment (Goldstone et al., 1995). It is incumbent on medical and nursing staff to have the skills and knowledge to manage patients in the terminal phase of their illness and/or to involve specialists in palliative care in the management of the dying patient.

Issues relating to nutrition and hydration and terminal sedation must be properly addressed. Some doctors and nurses may be unable to make the transition from active care to terminal palliative care and may be unable to come to terms with the withholding of hydration, even in an unconscious or heavily sedated patient (Quill et al., 1997). The patient may need strong advocacy and the staff and family may need intensive support through this period. Of paramount importance is the ability to relieve any sign of pain or other distressing symptoms, even if lucidity is compromised, unless the patient indicates to the contrary.

Restlessness or delirium may be a considerable cause of distress in the terminal stages of disease and it is essential to relieve such symptoms. Potentially correctable causes should be considered and treated (if appropriate and consistent with treatment objectives). Causes of restlessness include pain, which may be difficult to assess at this stage, retention of urine, constipation and faecal impaction, psychotic symptoms and anxiety (Table 20.5). Treatment

Table 20.5 Restlessness in the terminal stages of HIV disease

Terminal restlessness		
Possible signs	**Possible actions**	**Possible causes**
Physical agitation	History and examination	Pain
Mental confusion	X-ray, CT or MRI scans[a]	Drugs
Delirium	Metabolic Screen[a]	Metabolic abnormalities
Aggression	Psychiatric assessment[a]	Bladder distension
Withdrawal	Counsel partner/relatives	Encephalopathy
	Comfortable environment	Hypoxia
		Cerebral tumour/abscess
		Psychosis

[a]Do not investigate if there is no intention to treat!

of pain and other symptoms should be continued until death occurs. Restlessness in most patients can be well managed with benzodiazepines, including midazolam, clonazepam and diazepam, but it may require large doses if the period of sedation is prolonged (Table 20.6) (Burke, 1997; March, 1998).

Patients may choose to wait for a particular visitor or for a special event before accepting the symptom relief that must be available to them when necessary in their final few hours or days; they may indicate when they are ready for sedation. For those who are unable to participate in such decisions, guidance should be sought from the patient's advocate, if appointed, or their partner, family or friends. However, in many case, the decision will ultimately be entrusted to the treating doctors and nurses. Participation in the care of patients and their partners and families at this time is the ultimate compliment and privilege for those involved in palliative care.

Table 20.6 Pharmacological treatment of terminal restlessness – depending on cause and intent of treatment

Useful drugs	Single-dose range
Clonazepam	0.5–5 mg
Midazolam	2–15 mg
Diazepam	2–40 mg
Haloperidol	2–20 mg
Chlorpromazine	25–100 mg
Morphine	2.5–400 mg
Phenobarbitone	100–400 mg
Dexamethasone	2–16 mg

NB. Very high doses are necessary only in very exceptional circumstances. The correct dose is the lowest effective dose.

Palliative care in the setting of HIV in the developing world

Ensuring the provision of quality palliative care to people with HIV/AIDS in developed countries is complex and challenging at philosophical and resource levels. In areas of the world without access to sophisticated medical care, even the basics tools of palliative care, such as morphine to provide pain control, may not be accessible. In Uganda, with a population of about 17 million in 1993, for example, 411 000 AIDS deaths had occurred, with that number expected to double by 1998. Hospice Uganda, established in 1993, managed 450 patients over a 2-year period and was stated in 1996 to be one of only three hospice foundations in sub-Saharan Africa (Merriman, 1996).

References

Baker A. (1997). Dedicated palliative carers. *Nursing Times* **93**: 36–7.

Barnes R, LeBlanc E, Chan M et al. (1993). Hospital response to psychosocial needs of AIDS inpatients. *J Palliat Care* **9**: 22–8.

Beaugerie L, Baumer P, Chaussade S et al. (1996). Treatment of refractory diarrhea in AIDS with acetorphan and octreotide: a randomized crossover study. *Eur J Gastroenterol Hepatol* **8**: 485–9.

Berger JR, Pall L, Hall CD et al. (1996). Oxandrolone in AIDS-wasting myopathy. *AIDS* **10**: 1657–62.

Bindels PJ, Coutinho RA, van Griensven GP et al. (1996). Euthanasia and physician-assisted suicide in homosexual men with AIDS. *Lancet* **347**: 499–504.

Breitbart W. (1996). Pain management and psychosocial issues in HIV and AIDS. *Am J Hosp Palliat Care* **13**: 20–9.

Breitbart W, Rosenfeld BD, Passik SD et al. (1996). The under treatment of pain in ambulatory AIDS patients. *Pain* **65**: 243–9.

Breitbart W, Rosenfeld B, Passik S *et al.* (1997). A comparison of pain report and adequacy of analgesic therapy in ambulatory AIDS patients with and without a history of substance abuse. *Pain* **72**: 235–43.

Brettle RP, Atkinson FI, Wilcock J *et al.* (1997). Hospital and hospice resource use of HIV-positive patients in Edinburgh. *Int J STD AIDS* **8**: 234–42.

Briggs PG. (1992). Who needs a hospice? *Med J Aust* **156**: 417–20.

Burke AL. (1997). Palliative care: an update on 'terminal restlessness'. *Med J Aust* **166**: 39–42.

Butters E, Higginson I, George R *et al.* (1993). Palliative care for people with HIV/AIDS: views of patients, carers and providers. *AIDS Care* **5**: 105–16.

Chandler SW, Trissel LA, Weinstein SM. (1996). Combined administration of opioids with selected drugs to manage pain and other cancer symptoms: initial safety screening for compatibility. *J Pain Symptom Manage* **12**: 168–71.

Christrup LL. (1997). Morphine metabolites. *Acta Anaesthesiol Scand* **41**: 116–22.

Clipp EC, Adinolfi AJ, Forrest L *et al.* (1995). Informal care givers of persons with AIDS. *J Palliat Care* **11**: 10–8.

Compean DG, Jimenez JR, Guzman de la Garza F *et al.* (1994). Octreotide therapy of large-volume refractory AIDS-associated diarrhea: a randomized controlled trial. *AIDS* **8**: 1536–67.

Courtenay B. (1993). *April Fools Day: a modern tragedy.* W. Heinemann: Port Melbourne, Australia.

Fainsinger R, Schoeller T, Bruera E. (1993). Methadone in the management of cancer pain: a review. *Pain* **52**: 137–47.

Farthing MJ. (1996). The role of somatostatin analogues in the treatment of refractory diarrhea. *Digestion* **57**: 107–13.

Foley FJ, Cook D, Flintoft G *et al.* (1995). AIDS palliative care-challenging the palliative paradigm. *J Palliat Care* **11**: 19–22.

Fraser J. (1995). Sharing the challenge: the integration of cancer and AIDS. *J Palliat Care* **11**: 23–5.

Galer BS, Harle J, Rowbotham MC. (1996). Response to intravenous lidocaine infusion predicts subsequent response to oral mexiletine: a prospective study. *J Pain Symptom Manage* **12**: 161–7.

George RJD. (1991). Palliation in AIDS – where do we draw the line? *Genitourin Med* **67**: 85–6.

Gold J, High HA, Li Y *et al.* (1996). Safety and efficacy of nandrolone decanoate for treatment of wasting in patients with HIV infection. *AIDS* **10**: 745–52.

Goldstone I. (1995). Palliative care for HIV disease: the desirable vs the possible. *J Palliat Care* **11**: 54–7.

Goldstone I, Kuhl D, Johnson A *et al.* (1995). Patterns of care in advanced HIV disease in a tertiary treatment center. *AIDS Care* **7**: S47–56.

Gourlay GK, Willis RJ. (1986). A double blind comparison of the efficacy of methadone and morphine in post-operative pain control. *Anaesthesiology* **64**: 322–7.

Gourley GK, Cherry DA, Cousins MJ. (1986). A comparative study of the efficacy and pharmacokinetics of oral methadone and morphine in the treatment of severe pain in patients with cancer. *Pain* **25**: 297–312.

Gray N. (1995). 'Only Connect' – some thoughts towards the spiritual care of HIV disease. *J Palliat Care* **11**: 59–60.

Grinspoon S, Coscoran C, Lee K *et al.* (1996). Loss of lean body and muscle mass correlates with androgen levels in hypogonadal men with acquired immunodeficiency syndrome and wasting. *J Clin Endocrinol Metabolism* **81**: 4051–8.

Grothe TM. (1995). Palliative care for HIV disease. *J Palliat Care* **11**: 48–9.

Hengge UR, Baumann M, Maleba R *et al.* (1996). Oxymetholone promotes weight gain in patients with advanced human immunodeficiency virus (HIV-1) infection. *Br J Nutr* **75**: 129–38.

Higginson I. (1993). Palliative care: a review of past changes and future trends. *J Public Health Med* **15**: 3–8.

Hirschfeld S, Moss H, Dragisic K *et al.* (1996). Pain in pediatric human immunodeficiency virus infection: incidence and characteristics in a single-institution pilot study. *Pediatrics* **98**: 449–52.

Holzemer WL, Henry SB, Reilly CA. (1998). Assessing and managing pain in AIDS care: the patient perspective. *J Assoc Nurses AIDS Care* **9**: 22–30.

Johnson A. (1995). Palliative care in the home? *J Palliat Care* **11**: 42–4.

Kaplan BZ, Ksrishnamurthy U, Nori D. (1994). Opiate desensitization in a terminally ill cancer patient with pain: Physician assisted succour. *Am J Hosp Palliat Care* **Jan/Feb**: 34–9.

Kaplan R, Conant M, Cundiff D. (1996). Sustained-release morphine sulfate in the management of pain associated with acquired immune deficiency syndrome. *J Pain Symptom Manage* **12**: 150–60.

Kaplan R, Slywka, J, Slagl S *et al.* (2000). A titrated morphine analgesic regimen comparing substance users and non-users with AIDS-related pain. *J Pain Symptom Manage* **19**: 265–73.

Kelleher P, McKeogh M, Cox S (1997). HIV infection: the spectrum of symptoms and disease in male and female patients attending a London hospice. *Palliat Med* **11**: 152–8.

Kimball LR, McCormick WC. (1996). The pharmacologic management of pain and discomfort in persons with AIDS near the end of life: use of opioid analgesia in the hospice setting. *J Pain Symptom Manage* **11**: 88–94.

Koffman J, Naysmith A, Higginson I. (1996). Hospice at home – a new service for patients with advanced HIV/AIDS: a pilot evaluation of referrals and outcomes. *Br J Gen Pract* **46**: 539–40.

Kuhl D. (1995). Dancing across the lines: people in pain. *J Palliat Care* **11**: 26–9.

Larue F, Fontaine A, Colleau SM. (1997). Under estimation and under treatment of pain in HIV disease: multicentre study. *Br Med J* **314**: 23–8.

Lee LM, Karm JM, Selik R *et al.* (2001). Survival after AIDS diagnosis in adolescents and adults during the treatment era, United States, 1984–1997. *JAMA* **285**: 1308–15.

Maddocks I, Somogyi A, Abbott F *et al.* (1996). Attenuation of morphine-induced delirium in palliative care by substitution with infusion of oxycodone. *J Pain Symptom Manage* **12**: 182–9.

Malcolm JA, Sutherland DC. (1992). AIDS palliative care demands a new model [letter]. *Med J Aust* **157**: 572–3.

March PA. (1998). Terminal restlessness. *Am J Hosp Palliat Care* **15**: 51–3.

McKeogh M. (1995). Dementia in HIV disease – a challenge for palliative care? *J Palliat Care* **11**: 30–3.

Meier DE, Emmons CA, Wallenstein S *et al.* (1998). A national survey of physician assisted suicide and euthanasia in the United States. *N Engl J Med* **338**: 1193–201.

Merriman A. (1996). Uganda: status of cancer pain and palliative care. *J Pain Symptom Manage* **12**: 141–3.

Mosdell KW, Visconti JA. (1994). Emerging indications for octreotide therapy. *Am J Hosp Pharm* **51**: 1184–92.

Moss V. (1990). Palliative care in advanced HIV disease: presentation, problems and palliation. *AIDS* **4**: S235–42.

O'Neill WM, Sherrard JS. (1993). Pain in human immunodeficiency virus disease: a review. *Pain* **54**: 3–14.

Paice JA, Penn RD, Shott S. (1996). Intraspinal morphine for chronic pain: a retrospective, multicentre study. *J Pain Symptom Manage* **11**: 71–80.

Paice JA, Winkelmuller W, Burchiel K *et al.* (1997). Clinical realities and economic considerations of intrathecal pain therapy. *J Pain Symptom Manage* **14**: S14–26.

Palella FJ, Delaney MS, Moorman AC *et al.* (1998). Declining morbidity and mortality among patients with advanced human immuno-deficiency virus infection. *N Engl J Med* **338**: 853–60.

Perreault Y. (1995). AIDS grief: 'Out of the closet and into the boardrooms' – the bereaved caregivers. *J Palliat Care* **11**: 34–7.

Quill TE, Lo B, Brock DW. (1997). Palliative options of last resort: a comparison of voluntary stopping eating and drinking, terminal sedation, physician assisted suicide, and voluntary active euthanasia. *JAMA* **278**: 2099–104.

Ravenscroft PJ. (1996). Opioids – clinical applications in palliative care. *Aust Presc* **19**: 66–8.

Robb V. (1995). Working on the edge: palliative care for substance users with AIDS. *J Palliat Care* **11**: 50–3.

Robson P. (1998). Cannabis as medicine: time for the phoenix to rise? *Br Med J* **316**: 1034–5.

Roubenoff R. (2000). Acquired immune deficiency syndrome wasting, functional performance and quality of life. *Am J Man Care* **6**: 1003–16.

Samuels ME, Shi L, Stoskoph CH *et al.* (1995). Rural physicians: a survey analysis of HIV/AIDS patient management. *AIDS Pat Care* **Dec** 281–8.

Sawe J. (1986). High dose morphine and methadone in cancer patients. Clinical pharmacokinetic considerations of oral treatment. *Clin Phamacokinet* **11**: 87–106.

Simon DM, Cello JP, Valenzuela J *et al.* (1995). Multicentre trial of octreotide in patients with refractory acquired immunodeficiency syndrome-associated diarrhea. *Gastroenterol* **108**: 1753–60.

Sindrup SH, Brosen K, Bjerring P. (1991). Codeine increases pain thresholds to copper vapor laser stimuli in extensive but not poor metabolizers of sparteine. *Clin Pharmacol Ther* **49**: 686–92.

Stephenson J. (1996). Experts say AIDS pain 'dramatically under treated' [news]. *JAMA* **276**: 1369–70.

Strang P. (1997). The effect of megestrol acetate on anorexia, weight loss and cachexia in cancer and AIDS patients (review). *Anticancer Res* **17**: 657–62.

Sumpter J. (1997). Nutrition and HIV infection. *Nursing Times* **93**: 67–71.

Tyor WR, Griffin DE, McArthur JC *et al.* (1995). Unifying hypothesis for the pathogenesis of HIV-associated dementia complex, vacuolar myelopathy, and sensory neuropathy. *J Acquir Immune Defic Syndr Hum Retrovirol* **9**: 379–88.

Voigt RF, (1995). Euthanasia and HIV disease: how can physicians respond? *J Palliat Care* **11**: 38–41.

Wancke CA, Silva M, Knox TA *et al.* (2001). Weight loss and wasting remain common complications in individuals infected with HIV in the era of highly-active antiretroviral therapy. *Clin Infect Dis* **31**: 803–5.

Warncke T, Stubhaug A, Jorum E. (1997). Ketamine, an NMD receptor antagonist, suppresses spatial and temporal properties of burn-induced secondary hyperalgesia in man: a double-blind, cross-over comparison with morphine and placebo. *Pain* **72**: 99–106.

Wood CG, Whittet S, Bradbeer CS. (1997). ABC of palliative care. HIV infection and AIDS. *Br Med J* **315**: 1433–6.

Woodhouse A, Hobbes AF, Mather LE. (1996). A comparison of morphine, pethidine and fentanyl in the postsurgical patient controlled analgesia environment. *Pain* **64**:115–21.

Woolf CJ, Mannion RJ. (1999). Pain: neuropathic pain: aetiology, symptoms, mechanisms, and management. *Lancet* **353**: 1958–64.

World Health Organization (WHO), Regional Office for Europe (1989). *Palliative Care Policy Statement.* WHO, Geneva.

Young JS. (1997). HIV and medical nutrition therapy. *J Am Nutrition Therapy* **97**: S161–6.

CHARLES VAN DER HORST AND DAVID WOHL

First isolated by Margaret Smith in 1954, cytomegalovirus (CMV) is a herpes virus, which has become a major scourge of immunocompromised patients such as those infected with HIV. Prior to the availability of potent combination antiretroviral therapies, CMV-induced disease affected up to 44% of patients with AIDS, usually following a decline in CD4 lymphocyte count to below 50 cells/μl. However, the natural history of CMV disease has dramatically improved with new highly active antiretroviral therapies (HAART) capable of profoundly suppressing HIV replication and increasing CD4 lymphocyte numbers. While in the past, CMV disease usually necessitated lifelong treatment for suppression, there are now reports of patients with CMV retinitis who have experienced large increases in CD4 lymphocyte counts and have discontinued CMV therapy without reactivation of CMV disease.

Epidemiology and transmission

Transmission of CMV occurs perinatally, in childhood through close contact, and through sexual activity. In developed countries 10–15% of children are infected with CMV by adolescence. This varies by socio-economic status, with greater seroprevalence correlating with lower income. In developing nations, more than 90% of children are infected by 2 years of age (Drew, 1993).

During the reproductive years, the seroprevalence of CMV in the USA increases from 15 to 50% (Drew, 1993). CMV is frequently cultured from cervical washings and semen, thus accounting for this increased transmission. Heterosexual men shed CMV in semen at a lower rate (< 3%) than homosexual men, although this finding may reflect inadequate culturing methods (Collier et al., 1987; Hammitt et al., 1988; Bantel-Schaal et al., 1993). In addition to epidemiological evidence of sexual transmission of CMV, there have been numerous case reports of trans-

mission between sexual partners. There is little evidence of spread of CMV among adults other than by sexual means.

There is abundant evidence of sexual transmission of CMV among gay men. Over 95% of homosexual men are CMV sero-positive and close to 100% of gay men who are HIV-infected are also infected with the virus (Drew et al., 1981; Mintz et al., 1983; Lange et al., 1984; Quinnan et al., 1984). The frequency of CMV isolation from the semen of both asymptomatic HIV-infected gay males (47%) and from HIV-uninfected gay males (26%) is correlated with receptive anal sex and the number of partners (Collier et al., 1987; Rinaldo et al., 1992). CMV is also cultured from urine (12–22%) and throat washings (12–24%) of gay males, regardless of HIV serostatus (Rinaldo et al., 1992). Among HIV-infected men, the CD4 lymphocyte count decreases, the amount of CMV detected in semen increases (Quinnan et al., 1984; Howell et al., 1986; Leach et al., 1993).

In addition to sexual transmission, CMV can also be transmitted by blood transfusion (Prince et al., 1971). In situ cytohybridization studies suggest that CMV is maintained in a latent state in leucocytes, thus accounting for a transmission rate of 2.4 conversions per 100 units of transfused blood (Rice et al., 1984). CMV sero-negative, HIV-infected individuals should be transfused with blood from CMV sero-negative donors or leucocyte-depleted blood.

Natural history

The pre-HAART era

CMV retinitis usually develops when the CD4 lymphocyte count has dropped below 50 cells/μl (Crowe et al., 1991; Gallant et al., 1992; Pertel et al., 1992; Monforte et al., 1993). The risk increases with the duration of time the

CD4 lymphocyte count is less than 50 cells/μl, with a median time to retinitis diagnosis of 13 months (Pertel *et al.*, 1992). Prior to the availability of HAART, 21–44% of CMV sero-positive patients with AIDS could be expected to reactivate CMV and develop the disease (Gallant *et al.*, 1992; Hoover *et al.*, 1993).

In the era of HAART

Since protease inhibitors (PIs) became widely available in developed countries in early 1996, there has been a dramatic reduction in the incidence of CMV disease. In the USA, there has been an 83% decline in CMV retinitis (Palella *et al.*, 1998). A similar decline has been reported in Paris, where the incidence of CMV disease decreased by 73% from 1995 to late 1996 (Baril *et al.*, 1997).

The appearance of new CMV diagnoses at CD4 lymphocyte counts greater than 100 cells/μl in patients who have recently initiated PI therapy and whose CD4 lymphocyte count had been less than 80 cells/μl has been described (Gilquin *et al.*, 1997; Jacobson *et al.*, 1997). In all cases, CMV disease was diagnosed within 7 weeks of the initiation of HAART. It is possible that these patients had subclinical CMV disease at the time of HAART initiation. In addition, the partial immune restoration these patients experienced following suppression of HIV viral load may have led to an inflammatory reaction to previously undiagnosed CMV disease similar to that seen with mycobacteria (Dworkin *et al.*, 1998; Race *et al.*, 1998; Deayton *et al.*, 2000).

Before potent antiretroviral regimens became available, CMV retinitis was treated with lifelong therapy, aimed at prolonging the time between inevitable relapses and to prevent other systemic CMV disease. Potent combination antiretroviral therapy, has led to longer times to relapse and improved survival in patients with established CMV disease (Deayton *et al.*, 2000). In a retrospective analysis of 108 cases of CMV retinitis, there were fewer relapses in patients receiving combination antiretroviral therapy, including PIs compared with patients not taking these agents, and time to relapse was increased in the PI-treated group (1326 days versus 301 days) (Chiller *et al.*, 1998). Patients prescribed PIs or non-nucleoside reverse transcriptase inhibitors (NNRTIs) had a significantly longer survival compared with controls (1430 days versus 212 days).

Some patients with healed CMV retinitis who have responded to HAART have had anti-CMV therapy discontinued without reactivation of their retinitis during 1 year or more of follow-up (Mallolas *et al.*, 1997a; Macdonald *et al.*, 1998; Tural *et al.*, 1998). All the patients who have discontinued CMV maintenance therapy have been on HAART with a PI or NNRTI and have experienced an elevation in absolute CD4 lymphocyte number of at least 63 cells/μl. The achievement of HIV plasma viral load below the limits of assay detection may not be as important as the increased CD4 lymphocyte count in determining which patients can discontinue CMV maintenance therapy (Macdonald *et al.*, 1998). Preliminary reports indicate that reactivation of CMV retinitis following discontinuation of CMV maintenance therapy has occurred in patients experiencing a decline in CD4 lymphocyte count again below 50 cells/μl (Torriani *et al.*, 1998a).

Pathogenesis

CMV has the capacity to infect many cell types, transforming them into cytomegalic cells. After the initial infection the host mounts a vigorous humoral and cellular immune response, including neutralizing antibodies and complement-requiring cytolytic antibodies, and cellular immunity including HLA-restricted cytotoxic T cells and natural killer cells (Quinnan *et al.*, 1982). Lymphocytes and monocytes lyse CMV-infected cells in the presence of specific antibody by antibody-dependent cell-mediated cytotoxicity (ADCC) (Shore and Feorino, 1981). The importance of these cells in controlling CMV has been confirmed by attempts to reconstitute CMV-specific cellular immunity. In both bone marrow transplant recipients and patients with HIV infection, transfusions of clones of CD8 cytotoxic T cells specific for CMV structural proteins have successfully restored specific CMV immune responses (Walter *et al.*, 1995; Riddell *et al.*, 1996). In immunocompetent individuals, this multifaceted immune response results in suppression of the virus and restriction to certain cells.

CMV has been isolated from granulocytes, monocytes, both CD4 and CD8 lymphocytes, and circulating endothelial cells (Braun and Reiser, 1986; Boivin *et al.*, 1993; Grefte *et al.*, 1993). During HIV infection, immune suppression allows reactivation of CMV infection and eventually end-organ disease. Despite some *in vitro* evidence that CMV co-infection of cells transactivates the HIV long-terminal repeat and augments HIV replication, and that CMV infection itself can be immunosuppressive, there is little direct evidence that CMV co-infection accelerates progression of HIV infection in patients. Bidirectional interactions between HIV and CMV are suggested clinically. In a large clinical trial in patients with advanced AIDS, the presence of plasma CMV DNA was associated with a increase in risk of death of two-and-a half times during 12 months of follow-up (Spector et al., 1996; Spector et al., 1998). In another study, plasma HIV load was a strong predictor for the development of CMV end-organ disease, independent of CD4 lymphocyte count. Every $\log_{10}$ increase in HIV load was associated with a threefold increase in the risk of CMV disease (Swindells et al., 1997).

Unlike other immunosuppressed patients such as bone marrow or organ transplant recipients, who typically develop CMV pneumonitis (Gallant et al., 1992), 85% of CMV disease in persons with AIDS manifests as a retinitis. The affinity of CMV for the retina in HIV-infected individuals, compared to other immunosuppressed patients, may be a function of the profound nature and duration of the immunosuppression in HIV-infected individuals and perhaps of the differences in the immunological perturbations these different patient populations experience. HIV-mediated destruction of the CD4 lymphocyte pool is accompanied by disruption of the T-cell antigen receptor repertoire, narrowing the ability of T cells to respond to antigens, including pathogen proteins (Connors et al., 1997; Graziosi et al., 1998). With advanced HIV disease, the immune response to CMV and other pathogens wanes, favouring the development of opportunistic infections.

Potent antiretroviral therapy can lead to dramatic increases in CD4 lymphocyte counts, even among patients with nadir counts below 50 cells/μl (Gulick et al.,

1997). Initial reports suggested that the increase was solely in the quantity of pre-existing memory CD4 lymphocytes and not naive cells, which have not yet encountered antigen (Connors et al., 1997). This finding suggests that there would be limited significant reconstitution of the immune system if HAART merely expanded the remaining pool of memory CD4 cells. However, studies of patients treated for longer than 6 months with HAART suggest that naive cells also increase in number (Lederman et al., 1997; Feinberg et al., 1998; Li et al., 1998). These and other long-term studies have demonstrated normalization of the CD4 and CD8 repertoires in those subjects who have maintained very low HIV viral loads (Autran et al., 1997; Gorochov et al., 1998; Li et al., 1998). The presence of CMV-specific CD4 lymphocytes, as measured by flow cytometry, correlates with quiescence of CMV retinitis in patients treated with ganciclovir and HAART (Komanduri et al., 1998). Similarly, high levels of CMV-specific CD4 lymphocytes were observed in patients without CMV disease, despite overall low CD4 lymphocyte counts. In contrast, a paucity of CMV-specific CD4 lymphocytes were seen among patients with active CMV retinitis.

Therapeutic agents

Ganciclovir
Pharmacokinetics
Ganciclovir was first shown to be active against CMV in 1983 (Cheng et al., 1983). Like other nucleosides, ganciclovir is not active until it has been phosphorylated to the triphosphate. Initial monophosphorylation is catalyzed by the product of the CMV UL97 gene, a protein kinase

Table 21.1 Pharmacokinetics and CMV activity of selected antivirals

	Dose	Pharmacokinetics				CMV susceptibility	
		Serum peak (μM)	Serum trough (μM)	Serum $T^{1/2}$ (h)	Intracellular $T^{1/2}$ (h)	ID_{50} (μM)	ID_{90} (μM)
Ganciclovir	5 mg/kg twice daily i.v.	21–44	4	1.3–2.9	>18	0.4–5.9	2.8–7.9
	1000 mg three times daily p.o.	4.4	2.16	5.58	–		
Foscarnet	60 mg/kg three times daily	509	98	4.5	4.5	50–400	442–588
Cidofovir	5 mg/kg once per week for 2 weeks with probenecid	19.6		4	>65	0.5–2.8	

CMV: cytomegalovirus.
(From Cheng et al., 1983; Plotkin et al., 1985; Biron et al., 1986; Aweeka et al., 1989; Oberg, 1989; Chrisp and Clissold , 1991; Faulds et al., 1990; Leitman, 1992; Cundy et al., 1995; Spector et al., 1995.)

homologue (Sullivan *et al.*, 1993). Ganciclovir triphosphate is a semi-selective inhibitor of herpesvirus DNA polymerase. It is virustatic and thus replication resumes when drug is removed. For CMV, the ID_{50} for ganciclovir ranges from 0.54 to 5.9 μM (Table 21.1) (4 μM = 1 $\mu g/ml$) (Plotkin *et al.*, 1985; Erice *et al.*, 1989; Boivin *et al.*, 1993). Induction doses of intravenous ganciclovir (5 mg/kg twice per day) readily achieve peak values in excess of the ID_{50} required to inhibit CMV replication (Table 21.1).

The ID_{90} of CMV for ganciclovir is approximately double the ID_{50} (Table 21.1). Since the trough serum concentration of ganciclovir given intravenously, 5 mg/kg twice each day is only 4 μM, levels would not be adequate to prevent eventual reactivation, especially at the lower dose given during the maintenance phase. However, the intracellular half-life of ganciclovir triphosphate is far longer than the serum half-life (Biron *et al.*, 1985).

Following intravenous administration, cerebrospinal fluid (CSF) levels are 24–67% of serum levels, and aqueous fluid levels are 40% of serum levels (Faulds and Heel 1990; Price *et al.*, 1992). Ganciclovir concentrations in vitreous fluid averaged 0.96 $\mu g/ml$ in one study, below the ID_{50} for most strains.

The pharmacokinetics of ganciclovir explain the rationale for daily dosing during maintenance, and justify giving the drug five times each week at a slightly higher dose of 6–7 mg/kg instead of 7 days each week. Two small studies evaluated a maintenance dose of ganciclovir of 10 mg/kg three times a week, and no significant difference in time relapse was seen in comparison with historical controls (Hall *et al.*, 1991; Mallolas *et al.*, 1997b).

Alternate routes of ganciclovir administration

Oral ganciclovir has been approved for maintenance therapy but not induction therapy of CMV retinitis and for prophylaxis of CMV disease in persons with AIDS. The drug is poorly bioavailable, approximately 6%. Food minimally increases absorption (to 9%) as a result of lowering gastric pH. Despite the limited bioavailability of oral ganciclovir, peak plasma concentrations can be achieved that inhibit most CMV isolates *in vitro* (Plotkin *et al.*, 1985; Spector *et al.* 1995; Jacobson *et al.*, 1987) (Table 21.1). The drug is available in 250 mg and 500 mg capsules. The standard dose for treatment and prophylaxis is 1 g three times daily, requiring 6–12 pills a day. The adverse effects of oral ganciclovir are similar to those encountered when the drug is administered intravenously, but are less frequent (Spector *et al.*, 1996).

Ganciclovir can be administered intravitreally. Following intravitreal ganciclovir injection, vitreal drug levels exceeded the ID_{50} against CMV for 62 h (Henry *et al.*, 1987). The drug is usually given in the nasal or temporal superior quadrants, with slow injection of 0.1 ml (400 μg). Injections can lead to ocular pain, which usually disappears within 30 minutes, although this problem increases with increasing number of injections. Diastolic retinal intra-arterial flow is transiently interrupted in eyes with involvement of the posterior pole or with extensive retinal necrosis, but resumes within 2 min. The advent of the ganciclovir intraocular implant has largely obviated the need for intravitreal ganciclovir injections.

Ganciclovir can also be administered intravitreously via a sustained release intraocular implant. The ganciclovir implant is a surgically implantable device that is placed in the vitreous cavity and sutured to the eye wall (Figure 21.1, in the colour plate section). It contains approximately 4.5 mg of ganciclovir, released at an *in vitro* rate of approximately 1 $\mu g/h$ over 6–8 months (Sanborn *et al.*, 1992; Smith *et al.*, 1992; Anand *et al.*, 1993a, b).

After 6–8 months, the implant is depleted of drug (which cannot be determined by looking with an ophthalmoscope), and can be surgically removed and replaced with a new device. Both the initial placement and subsequent replacement is done in an outpatient surgical setting under local anesthesia and takes less than 1 h to perform. Repeated entry into the eye for exchange of implants has been associated with increased risk of transient vitreous haemorrhage (Martin *et al.*, 1997). With patients enjoying longer survival, many ophthalmologists are increasing the intervals between device re-implantation, especially when the patient experiences an increase in CD4 lymphocyte count.

Resistance

Isolates of CMV resistant to ganciclovir have been selected on laboratory passage and recovered from patients treated for long periods with ganciclovir (Erice *et al.*, 1989; Drew *et al.*, 1991; Sullivan *et al.*, 1993; Jabs *et al.*, 1998a, b; SOCA, 1997a). Most mutations have been in the UL97 gene. CMV isolates, which are ganciclovir resistant secondary to UL97 mutation, usually remain sensitive to foscarnet and cidofovir (Stanat *et al.*, 1991). Mutations of the viral DNA polymerase can also lead to ganciclovir resistance. Such polymerase mutations may confer cross-resistance to foscarnet and cidofovir (Baldanti *et al.*, 1996;

Cherrington *et al.*, 1996). After 3 months of intravenous maintenance therapy with ganciclovir, 8% of all patients and 38% of patients with chronic urinary CMV shedding will excrete isolates of ganciclovir-resistant CMV in the urine (Drew *et al.*, 1991). In a study of 76 patients with newly diagnosed CMV retinitis initially treated with intravenous ganciclovir, isolates resistant to ganciclovir were detected in either blood or urine in 5.4% at 3 months, 11.4% at 6 months and 27.5% at 9 and 12 months (Jabs *et al.*, 1998a, b). Resistance to ganciclovir was correlated with the development of contralateral retinitis among patients who presented with unilateral disease (OR = 9.06, $p = 0.003$).

Toxicity

The main toxicity of ganciclovir is haematological, with 16% of patients developing dose-limiting neutropenia (fewer than 500 cells/μl) and 9% developing thrombocytopenia (fewer than 20 000 cells/μl) (DeArmond, 1991). Other less frequent adverse events include nausea, vomiting, rise in liver enzymes, confusion, seizures, dizziness and headache. Some patients may be unable to tolerate both ganciclovir and zidovudine (ZDV) due to their shared bone marrow suppression, especially during the induction period. Judicious use of granulocyte-macrophage colony-stimulating factor (G-CSF) can alleviate neutropenia, but such therapy is very costly (Table 21.2).

Foscarnet

Pharmacokinetics

Foscarnet is a pyrophosphate analog, which is a broad-spectrum inhibitor of viral DNA polymerases. Unlike ganciclovir, foscarnet does not need to be phosphorylated before it is active; however, like ganciclovir it is merely virustatic. The median ID_{50} of foscarnet for most strains of CMV is approximately 200–250 μM (3.3 μM = 1 μg/ml), with the ID_{90} twice that (Drew, pers. com., 1994; Akesson-Johansson *et al.*, 1986). Trough levels of doses given during maintenance therapy are below those necessary for long-term suppression of CMV (see Table 21.1). Foscarnet also has activity against HIV, with 98% of HIV strains being inhibited by 33–150 μM (Oberg, 1989). This *in vitro* data has been confirmed clinically (Jacobson *et al.*, 1991b; SOCA, 1992).

Unlike ganciclovir, it does not have a prolonged intracellular half-life and thus must be given every day. Several small studies have compared induction therapy using foscarnet, at 90 mg/kg given twice each day or 60 mg/kg given three times each day, and have found no difference in clinical efficacy (Carosi *et al.*, 1993). Fletcher studied the effects of different foscarnet dosing regimens on CMV viraemia, as measured by quantitative cultures and measurement of CMV pp65 antigenaemia, and found a clear relationship between area under the curve exposure (AUC) to foscarnet and suppression of quantitative cultures and antigenaemia (Balfour *et al.*, 1996).

Resistance

Isolates resistant to foscarnet have been selected by *in vitro* passage and resistance to foscarnet has developed in patients (Sullivan and Coen, 1991; Wolf *et al.*, 1995; Baldanti *et al.*, 1996; Chou *et al.*, 1998). Mutations developing in the *pol* region of the DNA polymerase gene may lead to resistance to ganciclovir and cidofovir. In a prospective study of 44 patients with newly diagnosed CMV retinitis treated with foscarnet, resistance to foscarnet ($IC_{50} > 400 \mu$M) was detected in cultures of either blood or urine in 9% by 3 months, 26% by 6 months and 37% by 9 and 12 months (Jabs *et al.*, 1998b). Thus, there appears to be no significant difference in the the risk of development of foscarnet resistance compared with the risk of developing ganciclovir resistance during ganciclovir therapy.

Toxicity

Use of foscarnet requires careful management to avoid toxicity. Patients should receive at least 1 litre of saline prior to each dose to avoid renal toxicity, which can occur in 10–20% of patients (see Table 21.2) (Jacobson *et al.*, 1993). Doses must be adjusted weekly or more often, based on calculated creatinine clearance (see Table 21.3) (MacGregor *et al.*, 1991; S. Martin Munley; pers. com., 1994). In addition, during infusion foscarnet binds free ionized calcium, leading to abnormally low levels, while total serum calcium remains normal (Jacobson *et al.*, 1991a). The drop in ionized calcium is dose proportional with patients receiving 90 mg/kg, dropping a median of 0.15 mmol/l and those receiving 120 mg/kg dropping 0.30 mmol/l. The low ionized calcium can result in tetany, perioral numbness, finger paresthesias, weakness, seizures, hypercalcaemia, hyper- and hypo-phosphataemia, hypokalaemia. Foscarnet inhibits renal tubular reabsorption of phosphate, but during the first 2 weeks of induction therapy hyperphosphataemia is usually seen. In addition, hypomagnesaemia may occur, with

Table 21.2 Management guidelines for ganciclovir, foscarnet and cidofovir

	Induction therapy	Maintenance therapy	Management of relapses
Intravenous ganciclovir	5 mg/kg intravenously twice daily for 14 days Monitor haematological counts twice each week Transfuse if necessary and use G-CSF 300 μg daily subcutaneously for neutropenia (ANC of less than 750/μl) Titrate G-CSF to two to three times each week to keep ANC greater than 1000 μl If platelet counts drop below 25 000, switch to foscarnet	5 mg/kg daily (five times per week usually okay also), monitor haematology weekly	Look for clinical failure monthly Consider monthly urine cultures or CMV DNA PCR If positive after 3 months of therapy, the virus may be resistant to ganciclovir Patients should be re-induced with ganciclovir if reactivation diagnosed Alternatively, could switch to foscarnet or, cidofovir or, intraocular implant plus oral ganciclovir
Oral ganciclovir	Oral ganciclovir should not be used for induction therapy	1000 mg p.o. three times daily following induction therapy with intravenous regimen Monitor haematology every 1–2 weeks	As per intravenous ganciclovir, reinduce and maintain with ganciclovir or other intravenous agent or intraocular implant plus oral ganciclovir Assess adherence to oral ganciclovir
Intraocular ganciclovir implant	Induce with intravenous agent	Implant should be placed following induction course with intravenous agent Transient decreased visual acuity post-operatively for 4 weeks If bilateral disease present, insert implant in the most severely affected and salvageable eye first and then the other eye 1 week later Early retinal detachment may occur (12%) Concomitant oral ganciclovir (1000 mg three times daily) should be administered with monitoring as described above. Insert new implant in 6–8 months	Ganciclovir resistance is very likely if reactivation occurs before device is empty of drug Switch to foscarnet or cidofovir
Foscarnet	90 mg/kg intravenously twice daily for 14 days Monitor neutrophil count, electrolytes, creatinine, Ca^{2+} phosphates, Mg, twice weekly Hydrate patients well with at least 1l saline i.v. or 2l orally twice per day Also give calcium carbonate 500 mg three times daily and magnesium oxide 416 mg daily with initial therapy to prevent deficiency of these minerals	120 mg per kg daily. Monitor laboratory data weekly and adjust dose weekly	Consider re-inducing patient or switching to other agent

Table 21.2 (Continued)

	Foscarnet dose should be adjusted twice a week based on creatinine: men: 140 − age in years/creatinine 1 mg/dl × 72; women: men's calculated creatinine clearance × 0.85 (See Table 21.3 for dosing algorithm)		
Cidofovir	5 mg/kg i.v. once a week for 2 weeks	5 mg/kg i.v. once every 2 weeks, indefinitely	Consider re-inducing patient or switching to other agent
	Infuse 1 litre normal saline before cidofovir infusion and 1 litre normal saline post-infusion	Give with normal saline and probenicid as described above	
	2 g probenicid (4 × 500 mg tabs) 3 h prior to cidofovir infusion, 1 g probenicid 2 h post-cidofovir infusion and 1 g probenicid 8 h post-cidofovir infusion (for a total dose of 4 g probenicid)	Check creatinine and proteinuria before administering each dose.	
		If proteinuria >2+, serum creatinine increases >0.5 mg/dl, or serum creatinine is >2.0 mg/dl stop cidofovir	
	Half dose of probenicid for patients <50 kg	Some clinicians keep patients in the clinic for all the probenicid doses to ensure compliance and to prevent renal toxicity in those patients who skip the last dose	
	Hold zidovudine on days of cidofovir/ probenicid administration		
	Absolute contraindication to cidofovir are drugs that also cause renal toxicity	Conduct monthly opthalmologic exams	
	Agents such as aminoglycosides, intravenous pentamidine, amphotericin B, and diuretics must not be administered within 7 days of initiation of cidofovir or during cidofovir course		
	Cidofovir should only be used in patients with a serum creatinine < 1.5 mg/dl and a calculated creatinine clearance of ≤ 55 ml/min and < 2+ proteinuria (<100 mg/dl)		

CMV: cytomegalovirus; PCR: polymerase chain reaction.

symptoms similar to hypocalcaemia, namely, muscle tremors, agitation and confusion (Gearhart and Sorg, 1993).

Another complication of foscarnet is ulceration of the genitals, oropharynx and oesophagus (van der Pijl *et al.*, 1990; Saint-Marc *et al.*, 1992; Gross and Dretler, 1993). Because more than 90% of foscarnet is excreted unchanged in the urine, the genital ulceration is thought to be due to irritation of the mucosa by urine with foscarnet. The aetiology of the other ulcers is not known. In both cases, ulceration resolves within 2 weeks of cessation of drug. The genital ulcers may be prevented by patients cleaning themselves thoroughly after urination and applying an appropriate barrier agent such as petroleum jelly. Foscarnet is also associated with a mild anaemia.

Alternative routes for foscarnet administration
Intravitreal injections of foscarnet have been utilized for treatment of CMV retinitis, and appear to be efficacious in selected patients (Diaz-Llopis *et al.*, 1992, 1994). As the concentration of the intravenous solution of foscarnet is 24 mg/ml (2400 μg/0.1 ml), undiluted stock solution can be used for intravitreal administration. Induction treatment consists of two injections of foscarnet (1200 μg each week)

Table 21.3 Revised foscarnet dosing nomogram

Calculated CrCl (ml/min/kg)[a]	Dose
Induction dosing	
> 1.6	90 mg/kg Q12 h
1.4–1.6	85 mg/kg Q12 h
1.2–1.4	73 m/kg Q12 h
1.0–1.2	62 mg/kg Q12 h
0.8–1.0	50 mg/kg Q12 h
0.6–0.8	80 mg/kg Q24 h
0.4–0.6	56 mg/kg Q24 h
Maintenance	
> 1.6	120 mg/kg Q24 h
1.4–1.6	112 mg/kg Q24 h
1.2–1.4	98 m/kg Q24 h
1.0–1.2	82 mg/kg Q24 h
0.8–1.0	68 mg/kg Q24 h
0.6–0.8	105 mg/kg Q48 h
0.4–0.6	75 mg/kg Q48 h

[a] Creatinine clearance

(140 – age) / (creatinine × 72) (for men)

[(140 – age) / (creatinine × 72)] × 0.85 (for women)

for 3 weeks, followed by weekly injections of 1200 μg. High-dose (2400 μg/injection) intravitreal foscarnet for CMV retinitis (Diaz-Llopis et al., 1994) has been used as well. After a 3-week course of induction therapy, 62.5% of the subjects demonstrate complete resolution of the active retinitis, and the remainder of the patients display partial resolution. The rate of relapse on maintenance therapy (weekly injections) is 33% by 20 weeks. No local complications or drug toxicity were noted.

Cidofovir

Pharmacokinetics

Cidofovir is a nucleotide analog of deoxycytidine (dCMP) with broad activity against herpesviruses, including herpes simplex 1 and 2, varicella zoster, Epstein-Barr virus, human herpesvirus 6 and CMV. The drug suppresses CMV replication by exerting selective activity against the viral DNA polymerase. In vitro, the activity of cidofovir is 10–100 times greater than either ganciclovir or foscarnet (Snoeck et al., 1988). Unlike ganciclovir, cidofovir does not require viral-encoded enzymes in order to be phosphorylated to its active metabolite, cidofovir diphosphate; thus, the drug can be found in active form in uninfected cells. The ID_{50} of cidofovir against CMV strains is in the range of 0.69–2.8 μM

(Stanat et al., 1991). A long intracellular half-life of the active metabolite of 65 h permits infrequent dosing of cidofovir (once every 2 weeks) (Ho et al., 1992).

Cidofovir is administered intravenously. Intravitreous injection of cidofovir has been found to be efficacious for treatment of CMV retinitis but is associated with significant decreases in intraocular pressure (hypotony) and iritis (Banker et al., 1997; Chavez-da la Paz et al., 1997; Davis et al., 1997). Based on these toxicities, clinicians are strongly urged not to use intravitreal cidofovir.

Cidofovir is eliminated primarily by glomerular filtration, with some tubular secretion as well. The serum half-life increases with increasing dose, ranging from 3.36 h at 3 mg/kg to 8.11 h at 10 mg/kg.

Resistance

Detection of mutations at the pol region of the DNA polymerase conferring resistance to cidofovir from clinical CMV isolates has been reported (Erice et al., 1997; Jabs et al., 1998b). In 13 patients with newly diagnosed CMV retinitis treated with cidofovir, resistance to the drug (> 2.5 μM) was detected in 29% by 3 months (Jabs et al., 1998b). Cross-resistance of ganciclovir and cidofovir appears to be limited to isolates with high-level ganciclovir resistance (ID_{50} greater than 30 μM) (Smith et al., 1998). These isolates contain mutations in both UL97 and CMV DNA polymerase sequences. Cidofovir resistance can be associated with resistance to foscarnet, which also targets the viral DNA polymerase.

Toxicity

Cidofovir can cause neutropenia and renal insufficiency (usually preceded by glycosuria and proteinuria), and some patients have required dialysis or developed Fanconi's syndrome when this drug was given at doses higher than 10 mg/kg per week (Polis et al., 1995), without concomitant probenicid or with concommitant nephrotoxic drugs. Probenecid (4 g divided around the time of infusion) decreases total renal clearance of cidofovir by competing with the drug for uptake by the proximal convoluted tubule, reducing renal toxicity. Probenicid also decreases clearance of ZDV, leading to increased serum concentration of this antiretroviral drug.

Cidofovir should only be administered to patients with a serum creatinine less than 1.5 mg/dl, a calculated creatinine clearance of more than 55 ml/min and less than 2+ proteinuria (< 100 mg/dl). Urinalysis and serum creatinine should be checked prior to dosing of cidofovir and the drug discontinued if the creatinine increases by more than 0.5 mg/dl (44 μmol/l) above baseline and/or 2+ proteinuria develops. Care must be taken to ensure that concommitant nephrotoxic agents such as intravenous pentamidine, amphotericin B and aminoglycosides will not be administered. Additionally, there have been reports of neutropenia, anterior uveitis and decreased intraocular pressure associated with the use of intravenous cidofovir (Lalezari et al., 1997). Probenecid may also lead to treatment-limiting adverse events, including rash, vomiting and fever in 10–15% of patients (SOCA, 1997b; Lalezari et al., 1997).

Other drugs

Recently, Fomivirsen (ISIS 2922) was approved by the US Food and Drug Administration (FDA) for intravitreal treatment of CMV retinitis in patients who have a contraindication or are intolerant or unresponsive to other treatments for CMV retinitis. The drug is a phosphorothioate antisense oligonucleotide complementary to the human CMV immediate early region 2 messenger RNA, which inhibits viral replication in vitro (Azad et al., 1995). Antisense drugs are single-stranded oligonucleotide DNA anologs, which bind to target RNA gene copies, preventing synthesis of the protein encoded by the gene.

Adefovir dipivoxil or bis-(POM)-(PMEA) is an orally bioavailable prodrug of PMEA (9-[2-phosphonylmethoxyethyl] adenine) (Srinivas et al., 1993). PMEA is an acyclic nucleoside phosphonate of the same family as cidofovir, and also does not require viral kinases for activation. It has been shown to have potent in vitro activity against CMV and HIV, with an IC_{50} for ganciclovir-sensitive isolates of CMV of 1 μg/ml and 3.5 μg/ml for resistant isolates. Adefovir dipivoxil has an oral bioavailability in excess of 30% and an intracellular half-life of 16–18 h (Cundy et al., 1995; Barditch-Crovo et al., 1997); however, the serum level obtained after 14 days of 500 mg daily is only 0.64 μg/ml. Fanconi's syndrome (proximal renal tubular dysfunction) has been reported in 22% of recipients after 52 weeks of treatment (Fisher et al., 1999).

Pro-ganciclovir, or valganciclovir, is the valine ester of ganciclovir and is rapidly converted to ganciclovir in the intestinal wall, achieving drug levels equivalent to intravenous ganciclovir. Ongoing studies are evaluating the agent for treatment and prophylaxis of CMV retinitis.

Clinical manifestations and management of CMV retinitis

Clinical features
CMV retinitis

Common symptoms of retinitis include visual field defects (55%), floaters (11%) and, rarely, photophobia (Bachman et al., 1992). Macular or optic nerve involvement by CMV can cause rapid and precipitous decreases in visual acuity. Therefore, the appearance of CMV within the vascular arcade (Figure 21.2), 2 disc diameters (3000 μM) from the macula, or within 1 disc diameter of the optic disc (so-called Zone I lesions) warrants urgent treatment. Untreated CMV retinal lesions will display evidence of expansion within 2–3 weeks. Retinal expansion is defined as a new lesion of more than 750 μm (one-quarter of the disc diameter) or as an increase of an existing lesion by 750 μm (Palestine et al., 1991). The natural history of CMV retinal lesions is that they do not expand uniformly in all directions or in any given direction over time (Holland and Shuler, 1992). Even while being treated, many patients have slowly progressive retinal lesions by serial retinal photographs, which are not evident by routine indirect ophthalmoscopy (Gross et al., 1990).

Long-term complications of retinitis include no light perception in up to half of involved eyes after a mean of 15 months, retinal detachment in up to 33% of eyes, and papillitis/optic neuritis in 32% (Roarty et al., 1993; Kempen et al., 2001). Retinal detachment may occur when the lesions have extended anteriorly (away from the fovea).

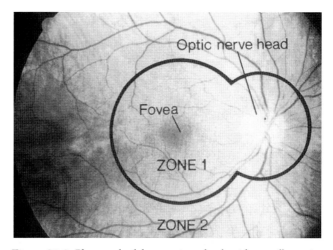

Figure 21.2 Photograph of the posterior pole of a right eye, illustrating zones used to identify the location of retinal lesions (reprinted with permission of the Archives of Ophthamology, Holland et al., 1989).

Immune recovery vitritis syndrome

While HAART has had a dramatic impact on the incidence and natural history of CMV disease in people with AIDS, an unforeseen development has been the emergence of a spectrum of sight-threatening intra-ocular inflammatory conditions in patients with healed CMV retinitis who have responded to HAART while on systemic CMV therapy or after stopping such therapy (Karavellas *et al.*, 1998; Torriani *et al.*, 1998a, 1998b; Zegans *et al.*, 1998; Deayton *et al.*, 2000). The inflammatory reactions reported include vitritis, papillitis, macular oedema and epiretinal membrane formation. Decreased visual acuity and progression to blindness has been reported. In all cases to date, intra-ocular inflammation developed in the eye with prior CMV retinitis 1–8 months after initiation of PI therapy. Most patients had had inactive CMV retinitis at the time the inflammatory reaction was diagnosed and all had responded to combination antiretroviral therapy, with an increase in CD4 lymphocyte count of 41–283 cells/μl.

The emergence of these inflammatory reactions following a partial restoration of CD4 lymphocyte counts suggests that the inflammation may be the result of a vigorous reaction to persistent intra-ocular CMV antigens (Nussenblatt and Lane, 1998; Torriani *et al.*, 1998a, b). At present there is no method to predict which patients with healed CMV retinitis will develop intra-ocular inflammation after initiating HAART. In all reported cases, the CD4 lymphocyte count has been above 60 cells/μl at the onset of inflammation. Treatment of these reactions with systemic or periocular corticosteroids provides only transient improvement (Holland, pers. com., December 1998).

Screening

Patients who are CMV sero-positive should undergo indirect ophthalomoscopy every 3 months when their CD4 lymphocyte count drops below 50 cells/μl. A retrospective review of 50 patients diagnosed with CMV retinitis at a university medical centre, where ophthalmologic screening of HIV-infected patients with CD4 lymphocyte counts below 50 cells/μl is standard of care, found that 42% of these patients were diagnosed during a routine scheduled eye clinic appointment (Wohl and Pedersen, 1998). Patients with CD4 lymphocyte counts between 50 and 100 cells/μl and those with a history of a nadir CD4 lymphocyte count below 50 cells/μl but now with counts exceeding this

Table 21.4 Schedule for ophthalmologic screening for CMV retinitis

CD4 count	Frequency of exam
No history of CMV retinitis	
Currently fewer than 50 cells/μl	Every 3 months
Currently 50–100 cell/μl	Every 6 months
Previously fewer than 50 cells/μl but now more than 50 cells/μl on HAART	Every 6 months
History of previous CMV retinitis	
Currently fewer than 50 cells/μl	Every month
Currently more than 50 cells/μl on HAART and CMV therapy	Every 2–3 months
Currently more than 50 cells/μl on HAART and CMV therapy Is discontinued	Every 2 weeks for 1 month, then monthly

HAART: highly active antiretroviral therapy;
CMV: cytomegalovirus.

level while receiving potent antiretroviral therapy appear to be at decreased risk of CMV disease and can be screened less frequently at 6-month intervals (see Table 21.4).

Diagnosis

Clinical examination

The diagnosis of CMV retinitis is made by examination of the optic fundus by an experienced clinician. The classic appearance, which is pathognomonic for CMV retinitis, is yellow exudates sheathing the retinal blood vessels and areas of focal haemorrhage (the so-called 'scrambled eggs and ketchup' appearance) (Figure 21.3, in the colour plate section). Not infrequently a patient will have cotton wool spots, which are yellow, small exudates. These are retinal infarcts, seen at all levels of CD4 lymphocyte counts in HIV-infected individuals, and can be difficult to distinguish from early CMV retinitis. Repeat examination in 2 weeks usually reveals progression of CMV retinitis compared with unaltered appearance of cotton wool spots. Although HIV can cause cotton wool spots on the retina, there is no evidence that these predispose to retinitis (Faber *et al.*, 1992). The patient who is sero-negative for CMV will not develop CMV retinitis, so serology should be obtained in doubtful cases.

Several cases of acute frosted retinal periphlebitis associated with CMV have been reported (Rabb *et al.*, 1992; Secchi *et al.*, 1992). In these cases there is a white exudate surrounding retinal veins. It responds to steroids plus ganciclovir or ganciclovir alone. This syndrome, which can be seen in non-immunocompromised or immunocompetent adults, is associated with possible immune complex disease of vessels in the eye.

CMV viraemia. As the diagnosis of CMV retinitis can be made only after damaged retinal tissue is obvious on clinical examination, the development of diagnostic tests with good predictive value for the development of CMV disease before end-organ destruction has been sought. Viral culture of the blood buffy coat, semen, or urine for CMV has not proved useful in predicting CMV disease in persons with AIDS. Many HIV-infected individuals shed the virus in their urine or have CMV cultured from blood without going on to develop CMV disease (Zurlo et al., 1993; MacGregor et al., 1995). Likewise, patients may not have culturable CMV from urine or blood at the time CMV end-organ disease is diagnosed (Shinkai et al., 1997).

Quantitation of CMV viraemia using molecular techniques, such as DNA polymerase chain reaction (PCR), has proved more predictive of CMV disease development and relapse than culture. There are several assays currently in use for quantifying CMV load: quantitative neutrophil associated CMV pp65 antigen assay, which requires a technician skilled in using fluorescent microscopy and preparation of the slides within 6 h of drawing the sample; qualitative and quantitative CMV DNA PCR, for either cell-free or cell-associated CMV; quantitative CMV branched DNA for cell-free CMV; and, quantitative hybrid capture assay on whole blood.

The ability of quantitative CMV DNA PCR to predict CMV disease development was studied using samples from 619 patients enrolled in a trial of oral ganciclovir for prophylaxis of CMV end-organ disease (Spector et al., 1996). Subjects had either CD4 lymphocyte counts of less than 50 cells/μl, or less than 100 cells/μl and a previous opportunistic infection. Of the total patient group, 55% had a negative CMV PCR test at baseline and 14% of this group went on to develop end-organ disease during the 12 months of follow-up. Forty-five per cent of the patient group had a positive baseline CMV PCR, and 43% of these patients developed end-organ disease. The quantitative results on patients with a positive baseline PCR revealed that the risk of CMV disease increased with higher PCR levels: 22% for patients with fewer than 2500 copies/ml, compared to 72% for those patients with greater than 50 000 copies/ml. For each $\log_{10}$ increase in CMV load at baseline, patients experienced a threefold increased risk of CMV disease and a twofold increase in risk of death (Spector et al., 1998).

Further studies are attempting to define the role of CMV viraemia assays in so-called, 'pre-emptive therapy' of CMV disease.

Treatment

Ganciclovir and foscarnet

Intravenous therapy. Ganciclovir and foscarnet are equally effective in the treatment of CMV retinitis. Used as secondary prophylaxis, these drugs delay the time to reactivation or progression after acute therapy from an average of 2–3 weeks with no therapy to more than 2 months (Jacobson et al., 1988; Palestine et al., 1991; SOCA, 1992; Jacobson et al., 1993; Spector et al., 1993).

The relative efficacy of ganciclovir and foscarnet was compared in one large trial of 234 patients, with CMV retinitis treated for a median of 9 months, the Study of Ocular Complications of AIDS (SOCA) trial (SOCA, 1992). Patients were randomly assigned to treatment with either foscarnet administered (60 mg/kg i.v. three times daily for 14 days followed by 90 mg/kg daily maintenance therapy) or ganciclovir (5 mg/kg i.v. twice daily for 14 days followed by 5 mg/kg/day maintenance). Both drugs had equivalent success in controlling the CMV disease and preventing relapses, with time to relapse being 56 to 59 days.

Intracellular ganciclovir implant

Two clinical trials have evaluated the safety and efficacy of the intraocular ganciclovir implant (Martin et al. 1999; Musch et al., 1997). Based on those results, the efficacy of the implant in controlling CMV retinal lesions is currently unrivalled by other treatment modalities. The median time to progression with the implant ranges from 182 to 226 days in these two studies and is essentially equal to the duration the drug is released from the device. Currently, the implant will release drug for up to 8 months after which the device can be replaced. The implant does have some adverse effects. Early retinal detachment occurs in 12–20% of patients treated, and there is also a transient (1-month) decrease in visual acuity postoperatively. Endophthalmitis has been reported and intravitreal haemorrhage is not uncommon, particularly following repeated replacements (Martin et al., 1997).

Because the implant only releases ganciclovir locally, disease can develop extraocularly or in the contralateral eye.

In a controlled trial comparing the implant to intravenous ganciclovir, contralateral CMV retinitis developed in 40% of patients with the implant, compared to 16% of patients receiving i.v. ganciclovir (Musch et al., 1997). Extraocular disease occurred in 11% of patients in this study and in 35% of subjects in a smaller trial (Martin et al., 1994).

The combination of local therapy (ganciclovir implant) plus systemic treatment (oral ganciclovir), was examined in a clinical trial of 375 patients with unilateral CMV retinitis, either newly diagnosed or stable on intravenous ganciclovir (Martin et al., 1997). Patients were randomly assigned to treatment with either the ganciclovir implant and oral ganciclovir (1500 mg three times daily), the ganciclovir implant plus oral placebo, or intravenous ganciclovir at standard induction and maintenance regimens. The combination of the ganciclovir implant plus oral ganciclovir was superior to the implant alone in preventing the occurrence of contralateral retinitis and extraocular CMV disease. The incidence of biopsy-proven extraocular CMV disease or contralateral CMV retinitis at 6 months was 37.8% in the implant plus placebo group, compared to 22.4% in the implant plus oral ganciclovir group ($p = 0.016$) and 17.9% in the intravenous ganciclovir group.

Thus, although the ganciclovir implant offers considerable advantage in terms of prolonged time until CMV progression and the avoidance of central venous catheters, it is associated with significant morbidity in terms of transient decreased visual acuity, risk of retinal detachment and risk of contralateral and/or systemic CMV disease. Concomitant oral ganciclovir reduces the risk of extension of CMV disease beyond the implanted eye. HAART reduces the risk of retinal detachment (Kempen et al., 2001)

Oral ganciclovir. Several studies have compared oral ganciclovir with intravenous ganciclovir for maintenance therapy of CMV retinitis responsive to an induction course of intravenous ganciclovir (Drew et al., 1995; The Oral Ganciclovir European/Australian Study Group, 1995; Squires, 1996). In these studies, 3000 mg of oral ganciclovir (500 mg six times a day or 1000 mg three times a day) was compared to 5 mg/kg once a day of intravenous ganciclovir. In each study, the mean time to progression of retinitis was several days to weeks shorter in the oral ganciclovir arms whether assessed by ophthalmological examination or fundus photographs. The toxicity associated with ganciclovir, particularly neutropenia, was much less frequent with oral than intravenous ganciclovir, and oral therapy avoided the placement of central venous catheters.

The benefits of oral ganciclovir (no central venous catheter, less frequent toxicity) must be weighed against the drug's poor bioavailability, large pill count and more rapid time to retinitis progression. Certainly, most authorities would not recommend oral ganciclovir for treatment or maintenance of zone 1 disease.

Cidofovir

Cidofovir has been studied in two randomized trials comparing immediate versus deferred therapy in patients with newly diagnosed non-sight-threatening retinitis (Lalezari et al., 1997; SOCA 1997b). The dose of cidofovir employed was 5 mg/kg, administered over 1 h i.v., once weekly for 2 weeks, then a dose of either 3 mg or 5 mg/kg infused every 2 weeks. Time to retinitis progression with immediate cidofovir treatment was 64–120 days, compared to 20–22 days without treatment. As with oral ganciclovir and the intraocular device, treatment with cidofovir precludes the use of a central venous catheter. However, the low toxic–therapeutic ratio of this agent may limit its use in some patients.

Management of relapses

The management of patients with CMV retinitis who have progressed on therapy is empirical, as the reasons for progression are usually obscure. Patients who have relapsed more than 3 months into therapy with ganciclovir and have positive urine cultures have a 40% chance of having ganciclovir-resistant CMV. However, results of susceptibility testing (if testing is accessible) will not be available for many weeks. Most relapses will not be caused by resistant virus but by inadequate antiviral doses used for maintenance therapy. One strategy is to re-induce the patient over 10–14 days, with the same agent being used for maintenance, and then to return to standard maintenance therapy. This strategy is effective in many patients. Alternatively, one may switch therapy from ganciclovir to foscarnet, especially in those patients with positive urine cultures who have been treated with ganciclovir for more than 3 months, while susceptibility testing is pending. However, in a large, randomized trial of patients with relapsed CMV retinitis, switching from ganciclovir to foscarnet, or vice versa, was no better than re-induction with the original agent (SOCA, 1996).

Combination ganciclovir and foscarnet has been studied both *in vitro* and *in vivo* using doses lower than standard dose. The two drugs are synergistic *in vitro* in suppressing CMV replication (Manischewitz *et al.*, 1990). A trial conducted by SOCA compared combination therapy with intravenous ganciclovir and intravenous foscarnet to the use of either drug alone (SOCA, 1996). Patients were assigned to treatment with either foscarnet (90 mg/kg twice a day induction, 120 mg/kg daily maintenance), ganciclovir (5 mg/kg twice daily induction, 10 mg/kg/day maintenance), or combination therapy (foscarnet dose 90 mg/kg per daily ganciclovir 5 mg/kg/day). Retinitis progression was most effectively prevented by combination therapy, with the median time to relapse 4.8 months with the use of combination therapy, compared to 1.6 months in the foscarnet arm and 2.1 months in the ganciclovir arm. There was no difference in the patients' visual acuity between the three arms; however, rate of visual field loss and change in retinal area involved by CMV was lowest in the combination arm. There was a significant negative impact on the quality of life for patients receiving the combination therapy. Few patients tolerate a daily 3–4 h pump infusion when provided with the option of a 1-hour infusion of ganciclovir prescribed as a single-agent treatment.

Salvage therapy with cidofovir has been studied in a trial involving 150 patients previously treated with ganciclovir, foscarnet or both (Lalezari *et al.*, 1998). The median time to progression in patients induced with 5 mg/kg of cidofovir weekly for 2 weeks and maintained with 5 mg/kg every other week was 115 days. For patients maintained with 3 mg/kg every other week, median time to progression was 49 days. The toxicity profile of cidofovir in this trial was not significantly different from that reported in other studies.

The intra-ocular ganciclovir implant has been used to treat relapsed CMV retinitis (Anand *et al.*, 1993b; Marx *et al.*, 1996). In these reports, progression of CMV retinitis was delayed; however, there was an 11–23% rate of retinal detachment in those patients with advanced CMV disease.

Fomivirsen has been evaluated in a series of studies involving 430 eyes in 330 patients. In one study of patients with new peripheral retinitis, 165 μg of intravitreal fomivirsen was administered weekly for 3 weeks, followed by injections every other week and compared with deferred therapy. The median time to progression for the 18 treated subjects was 71 days, compared to 13 days in the deferred arm (Muccioli *et al.*, 1998). In another study of 54 patients with recurrent central retinitis who had previously been treated with other agents, 34 subjects were administered 330 μg of fomivirsen weekly for 3 weeks and then every other week and the other 20 received 330 μg of drug on days 1 and 15 and then monthly thereafter. Median time to progression was reported to be 90 days in each group (Marwick, 1998). The less intensive regimen is the licensed recommendation. The agent's principal toxicity is intra-ocular inflammation and a limited number of patients have developed peripheral retinal pigment epithelial stippling. The frequency of intraocular inflammation following administration of fomivirsen remains unclear and warrants further study.

Stopping therapy

Some clinicians have recommended that discontinuation of maintenance CMV therapy is only considered in patients after 6 months of either treated and healed non-immediate sight-threatening CMV retinitis receiving potent antiretroviral treatment who have a CD4 lymphocyte count of more than 100 cells/μl, or who have a CD4 lymphocyte count between 50 and 100 cells/μl and a greater than 2 $\log_{10}$ decrease in plasma HIV viral load, or a plasma HIV viral load below the limit of detection (Holland, pers. com., 1998). The long-term safety of this approach and the risk of immune-mediated uveitis is currently being evaluated.

Prophylaxis

Development of a prophylactic strategy for CMV disease has been hampered by the absence of a potent and convenient oral anti-CMV agent. Several candidate drugs have been studied. Aciclovir was one of the first agents studied for CMV prophylaxis but was not found to be effective (Cooper *et al.*, 1993). A prophylactic trial of valaciclovir, the valine ester of aciclovir, using a dose of 8 gm/day, found that the drug did increase time to development of CMV disease compared to prophylaxis with aciclovir ($p = 0.03$); however, there was a trend towards earlier mortality in the valaciclovir arm, with a possible association with thrombotic microangiopathy ($p = 0.06$), leading to the premature halting of the study (Feinberg *et al.*, 1998).

Oral ganciclovir was studied as a prophylactic agent for CMV disease in patients with AIDS in two large clinical trials using a dose of 3 gm/day. The first study enrolled 725 CMV sero-positive patients without a history of CMV end-organ disease, and either a CD4 lymphocyte count of less than 50 cells/μl, or a CD4 lymphocyte count of less than 100 cells/μl and a prior AIDS-defining illness (Spector et al., 1996). Thirty-nine per cent of the patients receiving placebo versus 19% of patients receiving oral ganciclovir developed CMV disease ($p < 0.0001$) over 18 months of study follow-up. The relative risk for developing CMV end-organ disease while receiving oral ganciclovir was 0.49 compared to placebo dose. There was no difference in survival between the two study arms.

An analysis of CMV DNA PCR from 619 subjects enrolled in this study revealed the prophylactic benefit of oral ganciclovir to be greatest among PCR-negative patients and those with low PCR levels (of less than 2500 copies/ml) with up to an 84% reduction in risk (Spector et al., 1998). Patients with intermediate PCR levels (2500–50 000 copies/ml) displayed a moderate benefit (42% risk reduction), and for patients with high CMV DNA PCR levels (more than 50 000 copies/ml) there was no benefit from prophylaxis. Patients who cleared CMV DNA from their plasma had increased survival odds ratio of 2.4 after 12 months oral ganciclovir prophylaxis compared to non-responders. Patients on oral ganciclovir who were CMV PCR-positive at baseline and then became negative also had a lower risk of CMV disease compared to those who remained PCR-positive (Spector et al., 1998).

A second randomized study of oral ganciclovir was conducted by the Community Program for Clinical Research on AIDS (CPCRA) (Brosgart et al., 1998). The study was amended after the earlier ganciclovir prophylaxis results became available, at which time patients in both arms of the study were then allowed the option of oral ganciclovir, significantly altering study follow-up. In contrast to the first study, this trial found no difference between placebo and oral ganciclovir therapy in preventing the development of CMV disease. The relative risk for the development of retinitis on oral ganciclovir compared to placebo was 0.84 ($p = 0.37$).

The discrepancy between the results of the two studies can be ascribed to differences in study design: the lack of routine ophthalmological exams and photos in the CPCRA study, differences in the study patient populations, the longer blinded study follow-up on the first study and the effect of the amendment of the CPCRA study following the release of the results from the earlier study.

Although approved for the prophylaxis of CMV disease, oral ganciclovir has not been widely embraced. Many clinicians believe that oral ganciclovir reduces the incidence of CMV end-organ disease in patients at risk, but not all are in favour of using the agent indiscriminately in this group. While use of oral ganciclovir for prophylactic treatment in patients with a CD4 lymphocyte counts of less than 50 cells/μl would be expected to reduce the risk for CMV end-organ disease from 30 to 15%, some clinicians have adopted the converse argument that 70% of patients taking oral ganciclovir prophylactically would not benefit from the therapy, as they are not at high risk prior to therapy. An additional concern is the possibility of resistant viral strains in the subset of patients who do develop CMV end-organ disease despite receiving prophylactic oral ganciclovir. However, some preliminary studies report that the incidence of resistant CMV isolates from patients receiving oral ganciclovir is approximately 1% (Chou et al., 1997). These factors, plus the high pill count and the cost, continue to limit the popularity of prophylaxis with oral ganciclovir.

Upper gastrointestinal disease

Clinical disease

Approximately 7% of people with AIDS will develop CMV-induced gastrointestinal disease (Blanshard, 1992), most often when the CD4 lymphocyte count is less than 50 cells/μl (Nelson et al., 1991; Ramundo, 1993). CMV is most commonly associated with oesophageal or gastric disease, with oral lesions being relatively rare.

Oral lesions due to CMV can be found on the gingiva, lips, buccal mucosa, tongue and pharynx, and usually consist of single or multiple deep and very painful ulcers (Jones et al., 1993). In addition to CMV, similar lesions can be caused by herpes simplex, T. pallidum, and Histoplasma capsulatum, but most are idiopathic.

Approximately 4–13% of HIV-infected patients with odynaphagia, dysphagia or retrosternal pain will have CMV oesophagitis. Discrete gastric and colonic masses caused by CMV have been reported (Rich et al., 1992) as well as perforations (Ramundo, 1993), although these are usually associated with lymphoma or Kaposi's sarcoma (KS).

Diagnosis

The association of CMV with these upper gastrointestinal syndromes is complicated by the fact that occasional inclusion bodies due to CMV can be found in biopsies of apparently normal tissue in an HIV-infected patient. CMV should be cited as the aetiological agent only when there are numerous extensive CMV-specific cytological abnormalities with an inflammatory infiltrate on histology.

Half of the patients with characteristic CMV histology will have resolution of symptoms on antifungal therapy alone. When CMV is seen in association with candida oesophagitis, antifungal therapy should be used first, as 40% of patients with disease due to *Candida albicans* will have CMV identified by culture or histology (Laine *et al.*, 1992).

Endoscopy with biopsy is required for investigation of oesophagitis, as the differential diagnosis includes not only candida and CMV but also herpes simplex, KS and oesophageal reflux (Smith *et al.*, 1988; Kotler *et al.*, 1992). CMV oesophagitis is usually associated with either multiple small ulcers or a single large mucosal ulcer in the distal one-third of the oesophagus (Figure 21.4, in the colour plate section).

Treatment

Both foscarnet and ganciclovir have been used to treat oesophageal/gastric CMV disease, but the studies have been unrandomized and non-comparative (Dieterich *et al.*, 1988; Nelson *et al.*, 1991; Blanshard, 1992; Jones *et al.*, 1993; Ramundo, 1993; Smith *et al.*, 1993). Symptoms were found to abate within 2 weeks in over 75% of patients, but relapse occurred 1–7 months later in most. In a small study comparing foscarnet with ganciclovir in the treatment of both upper and lower gastrointestinal disease in 51 patients, there was no difference in efficacy between the two drugs and 90% of patients improved (Blanshard *et al.*, 1995). The length of induction therapy is determined by the clinical response but is usually 2–3 weeks. Antiviral doses are the same as those used for the treatment of CMV retinitis (Table 21.2). There are no large studies to help the clinician to decide whether or not to use maintenance therapy, and most clinicians do not, as relapses tend to occur many months after cessation of induction therapy. There are limited reports of successful treatment of CMV gastrointestinal disease with cidofovir (Blick *et al.*, 1997).

Colitis

Clinical features

Approximately half of all AIDS patients will have diarrhoea and of these, 15% or more will have CMV colitis (Smith *et al.*, 1988; Dieterich and Rahmin, 1991). The incidence of CMV colitis increases in patients with extracolonic CMV disease. CMV colitis is associated with watery, but not necessarily bloody diarrhoea, abdominal pain, fever, anorexia and weight loss (Dieterich and Rahmin, 1991; Nelson *et al.*, 1991; Ramundo, 1993). Two-thirds of patients will have persistent diarrhoea and one-third intermittent diarrhoea. On average, patients will pass seven liquid stools each day. Almost all patients with CMV colitis have fever and weight loss and two-thirds have crampy abdominal pain. CMV colitis also presents as discrete colonic masses (Rich *et al.*, 1992) or as colonic perforation. CMV-related mass lesions mimic lymphoma and KS lesions of the bowel, and may not be associated with fever and diarrhoea. CMV lesions can involve the small intestine as well as the colon.

Diagnosis

The diagnosis of CMV colitis must be made by colonoscopy with biopsy. The patient with diarrhoea is initially evaluated for both opportunistic and non-opportunistic enteric pathogens seen in patients with a CD4 lymphocyte count of less than 50 cells/μl, prior to doing colonoscopy to search for CMV colitis. If an abdominal computerized tomography (CT) scan is performed, diffuse bowel-wall thickening, luminal narrowing and inflammatory changes in the surrounding mesentery and pericolonic fat may be seen. Rarely, toxic megacolon may occur.

Sigmoidoscopy will miss 39% of cases, in whom disease is restricted to the right colon. Up to 25% of patients with diarrhoea will have normal-appearing colonic mucosa but will have CMV inclusions seen on biopsy. It is recommended that nine different randomly chosen areas of the entire colon be biopsied, even if normal in appearance (Dieterich and Rahmin, 1991). However, it remains unclear whether the aetiology of diarrhoea in those patients with a normal appearance of colon mucosa is CMV.

The usual endoscopic appearance of CMV colitis includes focal or diffuse mucosal erythema and extensive, deep, friable ulcerations with clearly defined borders and non-purulent bases (Figure 21.5, in the colour plate section). Biopsy usually reveals submucosal haemorrhage and ulceration. Intranuclear inclusions are more often associated with ulcerative CMV colitis than inflammatory CMV colitis (Mentec *et al.*, 1994). Patients with colon mucosa biopsies lacking CMV inclusions, but from which CMV is cultured, have increased risk of subsequent development of CMV colitis. CMV can lead to extensive mucosal ulceration with transmural necrosis and perforation, as well as fatal haemorrhagic colitis.

Treatment

Only one placebo-controlled study of ganciclovir for CMV colitis has been reported (Dieterich *et al.*, 1993). Although there was histological, virological and endoscopic improvement in the ganciclovir-treated patients as compared to placebo-treated controls, there were no statistically-significant changes in diarrhoea or other symptoms, despite trends towards improvement. The investigators felt that 14 days of therapy was probably insufficient to reverse the large amount of tissue destruction. However, the benefit of ganciclovir may have been obscured by including patients with a normal appearance on colonoscopy. A small comparative trial of foscarnet and ganciclovir for CMV colitis has shown no difference in efficacy between these two drugs (Blanshard *et al.*, 1995). Open-label studies of either ganciclovir or foscarnet have shown significant reduction of diarrhoea in 80% of patients and complete elimination of all symptoms in 40% (Dieterich *et al.*, 1988; Nelson *et al.*, 1991; Blanshard, 1992). Patients who do not have a complete response often have other organisms present.

Patients with histologically documented CMV colitis should be treated with either ganciclovir or foscarnet at the doses listed in Table 21.2; the duration of therapy should be determined by repeat colonoscopy after 2–3 weeks of treatment. As median time from termination of ganciclovir or foscarnet therapy to the onset of recurrent CMV disease is 3.4 months (Dieterich and Rahmin, 1991; Nelson *et al.*, 1991), most experts do not use routine maintenance therapy.

Sclerosing cholangitis

Clinical features

Patients with sclerosing cholangitis, usually experience right upper quadrant and epigastric pain and an elevated alkaline phosphatase. Serum concentrations of aspartate aminotransferase (AST) and alanine aminotransferase (ALT) can be normal. As in other manifestations of invasive CMV disease, the CD4 lymphocyte count is usually less than 50 cells/ml. Diarrhoea occurs in more than half of the patients (Forbes *et al.*, 1993) and one-quarter of patients will have hepatomegaly.

Diagnosis

Sonography of the right upper quadrant often reveals evidence of thickened bile ducts or dilatation of ducts associated with strictures, although this test may be normal in half of patients. The ultrasound findings should be confirmed by endoscopic retrograde cholangiopancreatography (ERCP), which reveals both intrahepatic and/or extrahepatic ductal involvement. Biopsy of the ampulla of Vater or brushings will yield CMV and/or cryptosporidia, or less often other gastrointestinal pathogens. Cryptosporidia is the most common cause of this syndrome, with only 10% having CMV isolated as the sole pathogen (Forbes *et al.*, 1993).

It is rare for a patient with right upper quadrant pain, an elevated alkaline phosphatase and a normal ERCP to progress to sclerosing cholangitis. However, it is well recognized that primary sclerosing cholangitis in patients without HIV infection may exist on histological criteria in the absence of cholangiographic abnormalities (Forbes *et al.*, 1993). Patients who have persistent right upper quandrant pain and elevation of alkaline phosphatase after 1 month with a negative ERCP and a negative work-up for other causes of right upper quandrant pain should probably have a liver biopsy.

Treatment

There is little evidence that antiviral chemotherapy for CMV-related sclerosing cholangitis is beneficial. Few studies have been done. The natural history is extremely variable, with some patients' symptoms resolving spontaneously within a median of 4 weeks and others requiring use of narcotics for pain control (Forbes *et al.*, 1993). The median survival is 7.5 months and a rising level of alkaline phosphatase portends a bad prognosis (van der Ende *et al.*, 1992; Forbes *et al.*, 1993).

CMV encephalitis

Clinical features

Autopsy series show that approximately 25% of patients who have AIDS will have evidence of CMV inclusions within the central nervous system (CNS) (Petito *et al.*, 1986). Nonetheless, few are symptomatic. Most patients have pre-existing CMV end-organ disease elsewhere at the time of presentation with CMV encephalitis (Kalayjian *et al.*, 1993; Holland *et al.*, 1994). Encephalitis has occurred in patients while they were receiving either therapy, ganciclovir or foscarnet.

Patients present with disorientation, delirium, apathy, withdrawal and occasionally cranial nerve defects and gaze-directed nystagmus. Symptoms progress over 4 weeks, in contrast to the indolent course of HIV dementia (Fiala *et al.*, 1993; Holland *et al.*, 1994). Many patients have associated hyponatraemia.

Diagnosis

Patients who present with an acute deterioration in mental status need both a CT or MRI brain scan and a lumbar puncture for evaluation. Severe cases have periventricular enhancement seen on MRI scans due to intense uptake of the gadolinium by ependymal cells. This is diagnostic of ventriculitis (see Figure 21.6) (Kalayjian *et al.*, 1993; Holland *et al.*, 1994). Periventricular rarefaction can be seen on CT brain scan. CSF protein is usually elevated but is only up to between two and four times normal and the glucose is almost always normal. Although a lymphocytic pleocytosis can occur, it is not common. If a pleocytosis is

present, CMV can sometimes be cultured from the CSF. The CSF findings of CMV encephalitis are in contrast with those seen in CMV polyradiculomyelitis, where there is a neutrophilic pleocytosis with hypoglycorachia and positive CMV cultures of the CSF in 60% of patients (de Gans *et al.*, 1990a; Kim and Hollander, 1993). CMV encephalitis and polyradiculomyelitis overlap in their presentation, and patients can present with encephalitis alone with a normal CSF, polyradiculomyelitis alone with CSF pleocytosis, or a combination of both.

Brain biopsy or autopsy examination reveals intranuclear inclusions associated with focal necrosis, microglial nodules and a necrotizing ventriculitis and/or encephalitis (Cinque *et al.*, 1992; Gozlan *et al.*, 1992; Fiala *et al.*, 1993; Kalayjian *et al.*, 1993; Holland *et al.*, 1994).

Because CMV is rarely isolated from CSF in encephalitis, detection of CMV DNA in CSF following PCR amplification has been evaluated as a diagnostic tool (Cinque *et al.*, 1992; Gozlan *et al.*, 1992). PCR amplification revealed CMV DNA in virtually 100% of patients, with documented CMV encephalitis if specimens were obtained within 3 months of diagnosis.

Treatment

Some patients with CMV encephalitis treated with ganciclovir have responded with either stabilization or improvement in their symptoms (Price *et al.*, 1992; Kalayjian *et al.*, 1993). However, since this is a necrotizing infection, improvement is rare. Patients who have had a long-term exposure to ganciclovir may progress despite therapy, suggesting the development of resistant virus. The average time to death is 9 weeks, compared to 45 weeks for patients with HIV dementia (Holland *et al.*, 1994).

Patients presenting with an acute deterioration in mental status, a benign CSF, evidence of periventricular inflammation on contrast MRI or CT or focal hypodensities in the absence of other causes of meningitis or encephalitis can be empirically treated with ganciclovir until PCR results return. If these symptoms develop in someone who has been on ganciclovir for more than 3 months foscarnet should be initiated, as ganciclovir resistance could have developed. Length of therapy is unknown, but if CSF or MRI scan is abnormal these can be followed for improvement, as neurological improvement will be limited.

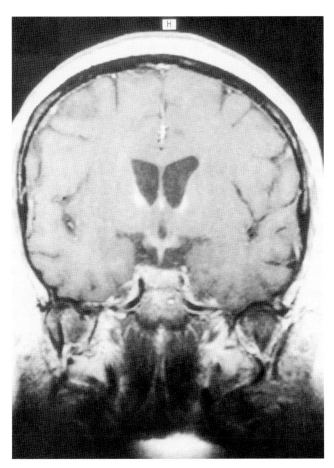

Figure 21.6 *MRI of the brain showing periventricular enhancement due to CMV ventriculitis.*

CMV polyradiculomyelopathy

Clinical findings

CMV involvement of the spinal cord and nerve roots is rare but devastating complication of AIDS. CMV polyradiculomyelopathy (PRAM) presents as a subacute ascending hypotonic lower extremity weakness preceded by pain and paresthesias in the legs and perineum in about one-half of patients. In addition, areflexia and urinary retention occur in two-thirds of patients, along with loss of sphincter control (Kim and Hollander, 1993). Progression occurs over days to weeks. Late in the disease the arms may be involved. Patients may have sensory levels and loss of tactile, vibratory and position senses. PRAM is often seen in association with CMV found elsewhere (de Gans *et al.*, 1990a; Kim and Hollander, 1993).

Diagnosis

Almost all patients with this syndrome will have CSF leucocytosis with neutrophilic predominance counts as high as 3400 cells reported (de Gans *et al.*, 1990a). All patients have high CSF protein concentrations and many will have a low

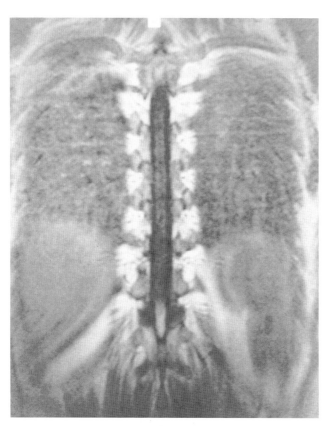

Figure 21.7 *MRI of the spine showing enhancement of cauda equina, which can occasionally occur in polyradiculomyelopathy.*

glucose concentration. CMV is often isolated from spinal fluid. Cytological examination of CSF reveals CMV inclusions, and immunohistochemistry confirms the presence of viral antigens in CSF leucocytes (de Gans *et al.*, 1990a).

Electromyographic studies show axonal neuropathy with denervation changes and compound muscle action potentials (Cohen *et al.*, 1993). Nerve conduction studies are usually normal but may show that F waves are delayed or absent, with conduction velocities normal or mildly slow. In some cases, MRI shows enhancement of the affected area (Figure 21.7).

On autopsy, patients have radicular necrosis or inflammation with polymorphonuclear and/or mononuclear infiltrates, necrotizing myelitis and/or anterior horn cell necrosis (Said *et al.*, 1991; Kim and Hollander, 1993).

PRAM should not be confused with inflammatory demyelinating polyneuropathy, which is seen early in the course of HIV disease in patients with high CD4 lymphocyte counts.

Treatment

Ganciclovir at the usual doses has been successfully used to treat CMV PRAM, with resolution of CSF abnormalities in 2 weeks and slow, steady improvement in neurological symptoms from inability to walk to walking within 3 months (Cohen *et al.*, 1993; de Gans *et al.*, 1990a; Kim and Hollander 1993). This slow improvement occurs as the axons regrow and form myelin. In a recent review of 17 treated patients, seven improved and three stabilized (Cohen *et al.*, 1993). All successfully treated patients started therapy within 2 weeks of onset of symptoms.

Failure to improve with ganciclovir therapy may be due either to resistant strains of CMV or necrotizing infection, which has destroyed neurons. To distinguish between these two possibilities a repeat spinal tap after 2 weeks of induction therapy is useful to assess changes in CSF parameters. In addition, if PRAM occurs in patients who are already being treated for CMV disease elsewhere, the physician can safely assume that the virus is resistant and they should therefore switch therapy to foscarnet. Conclusive evidence of foscarnet's efficacy in this disease is not available.

CMV adrenalitis

Clinical features

CMV adrenalitis is a little recognized disorder. Approximately 5–7% of patients who have progressed to AIDS will have evidence of adrenal dysfunction (M. Hellerstein, pers. com., April 1994). Although the classic presentation of hypotension, hyponatraemia, hyperkalaemia (due to mineralocorticoid deficit), eosinophilia and hyperpyrexia can be seen, patients may present only with severe fatigue or hypotension (Grutzmeier and Sandstrom, 1992). Other symptoms include nausea and abdominal pain, but less than half of the patients have darkening of skin.

Diagnosis

A single cortisol level will identify many patients. A single level greater than $20\,\mu$g/dl essentially rules out Addison's disease. Levels of less than $20\,\mu$g/dl may represent decreased adrenal reserve. A normal response to the rapid cosyntropin (synthetic ACTH) stimulation test rules out adrenal insufficiency.

Treatment

The principal treatment of CMV adrenalitis is corticosteroid replacement therapy, such as cortisone acetate 25 mg in the morning and 12.5 mg in the afternoon, supplemented with fludorcortisone acetate 0.1 mg daily for mineralocorticoid effect as needed (see Chapter 18). With maximal stimulation, as in the stress of an acute illness or surgery, the normal adrenal gland will produce 300 mg of cortisol each day. Thus stress doses of hydrocortisone (e.g. 100 mg three times by intravenous route daily) are required during these episodes. With mild stress such as a viral upper respiratory infection daily oral dose should be increased twofold. Response to therapy is dramatic, with improvement within hours. It is unknown whether anti-CMV chemotherapy has any role.

CMV pneumonia

Clinical presentation

CMV is often cultured or seen on cytology from bronchoalveolar lavage specimens associated with other causes of pneumonia in patients infected with HIV. Large studies have shown that in these clinical situations it does not impact on the course of disease and is merely a commensal, not a warranting therapy (Millar et al., 1990; Bozzette et al., 1992). In these studies, CMV-specific therapy or lack of such therapy does not alter the course of the pneumonia or patient survival. Bozzette and colleagues found that isolation of both CMV and *Pneumocystis carinii* pneumonia (PCP) was associated with a higher LDH and a lower CD4

lymphocyte count, fewer days in intensive care, higher short-term survival and fewer intubations than patients in whom PCP alone was identified. There was no difference in development of subsequent end-organ disease.

There have been several small case series reporting patients with pneumonia where CMV only is isolated. These patients usually have interstitial nodular densities seen on chest radiograph associated with hypoxaemia (Vasudevan et al., 1990; Aukrust et al., 1992; Squire et al., 1992). One prospective study described 85 patients with pneumonitis, of whom nine had CMV alone isolated (Squire et al., 1992). Seven had mild pneumonia, all had CD4 lymphocyte counts of less than 100 cells/μl and recovered without antiviral therapy. Two had severe pneumonia requiring ventilatory support and had CD4 lymphocyte counts of over 200 cells/μl. Viral inclusions were seen in three of the mild cases. Others have described cases of CMV pneumonitis in patients with low CD4 lymphocyte counts who respond to therapy (Aukrust et al., 1992).

References

Akesson-Johnsson A, Lernestedt JO, Ringden O et al. (1986). Sensitivity of cytomegalovirus to intravenous foscarnet treatment. *Bone Marrow Transplant* 1: 215–20.

Anand R, Nightingale SD, Fish RH et al. (1993a). Control of cytomegalovirus retinitis using sustained release of intraocular ganciclovir. *Arch Ophthalmol* 111: 223–7.

Anand R, Font RL, Fish RH et al. (1993b). Pathology of cytomegalovirus retinitis treated with sustained release intravitreal ganciclovir. *Ophthalmology* 100: 1032–9.

Aukrust P, Farstad OM. Frpland SS et al. (1992). Cytomegalovirus (CMV) pneumonitis in AIDS patients. The result of intensive CMV replication? *Eur Resp J* 5: 362–4.

Autran B, Carcelain G, Li TS et al. (1997). Positive effects of combined antiretroviral therapy on CD4+ T cell homeostasis and function in advanced HIV. *Science* 277: 112–6.

Aweeka F, Gambertoglio J, Mills J et al. (1989). Pharmacokinetics of intermittently administered intravenous foscarnet in the treatment of acquired immunodeficiency syndrome patients with serious cytomegalovirus retinitis. *Antimicrob Agents Chemother* 33: 742–5.

Azad RF, Brown-Driver V, Buckheit RW et al. (1995). Antiviral activity of a phosphorothioate oligonucleotide complementary to human cytomegalovirus RNA when used in combination with antiviral nucleoside analogs. *Antiviral Res* 28: 101–11.

Bachman DM, Bruni LM, Di Goia RA et al. (1992). Visual field testing in the management of cytomegalovirus retinitis. *Ophthalmology* 99: 1393–9.

Baldanti F, Underwood MR, Stanat SC et al. (1996). Single amino acid changes in the DNA polymerase confer foscarnet resistance and slow-growth phenotype, while mutations in the UL-97 encoded phophotransferase confer ganciclovir resistance in three double-resistant human cytomegalovirus strains recovered from patients with AIDS. *J Virol* 70: 1390–5.

Balfour HH, Fletcher CV, Erice A et al. (1996). Effect of foscarnet on quantities of cytomegalovirus and human immunodeficiency virus in blood of persons with AIDS. *Antimicrob Agents Chemother* **40**: 2721–6.

Banker AS, Arevalo JF, Munguia D et al. (1997). Intraocular pressure and aqueous humor dynamics in patients with AIDS treated with intra-vitreal cidofovir (HPMPC) for cytomegalovirus retinitis. *Am J Ophthalmol* **124**: 168–80.

Bantel-Schaal U, Newmann-Haefelin D, Schieferstein G. (1993). Cyto-megalovirus is absent from semen of a population of men seeking fertility evaluation. *J Infect Dis* **168**: 518–19.

Barditch-Crovo P, Toole J, Hendrix CW et al. (1997). Anti-human immunodeficiency virus activity, safety and pharmacokinetics of adefovir dipivoxil in HIV-infected patients. *J Infect Dis* **176**: 406–13.

Baril L, Jouran M, Caumes E et al. (1997). The impact of highly active antiretroviral therapy on the incidence of CMV disease in AIDS patients. *Thirty-seventh Conference on Antimicrobial Agents and Chemotherapy*, Toronto, Canada.

Biron KK, Stanat SC, Sorrell JB et al. (1985). Metabolic activation of the nucleoside analog 9-[2-hydroxy-1-(hydroxymethyl)ethoxy]methyl guanine in human diploid fibroblasts infected with human cytomegalovirus. *Proc Natl Acad Sci USA* **82**: 2473–7.

Biron KK, Fyfe JA, Stanat SC et al. (1986). A human cytomegalovirus mutant resistant to the nucleoside analog 9-[2-hydroxy-1-(hydroxy-methyl)ethoxy]methyl]guanine (BQ B759U) induces reduced levels of BW B759U triphosphate. *Proc Natl Acad Sci USA* **83**: 8769–73.

Blanshard C. (1992). Treatment of HIV-related cytomegalovirus disease of the gastrointestinal tract with foscarnet. *J AIDS* **5**: S25–8.

Blanshard C, Benhamou Y, Dohin E et al. (1995). Treatment of AIDS-associated gastrointestinal cytomegalovirus infection with foscarnet and ganciclovir; a randomized comparison. *J Infect Dis* **172**: 622–8.

Blick G, Garton T, Hopkins U et al. (1997). Successful use of cidofovir in treating AIDS-related cytomegalovirus retinitis, encephalitis, and esophagitis. *J Acquir Immune Defic Syndr Hum Retrovirol* **15**: 84–5.

Boivin G, Erice A, Crane DD et al. (1993). Ganciclovir susceptibilities of cytomegalovirus (CMV) isolates from solid organ transplant recip-ients with CMV viremia after antiviral prophylaxis. *J Infect Dis* **168**: 332–5.

Bozzette SA, Arcia J, Bartok AE et al. (1992). Impact of Pneumocystis carinii and cytomegalovirus on the course and outcome of atypical pneumonia in advanced human immunodeficiency virus disease. *J Infect Dis* **165**: 93–8.

Braun RW, Reiser HC. (1986). Replication of human cytomegalovirus in human peripheral blood T cells. *J Virol* **60**: 29–36.

Brosgart CL, Louis TA, Hillman DW et al. (1998). A randomized, placebo-controlled trial of the safety and efficacy of oral ganciclovir for prophylaxis of cytomegalovirus disease in HIV-infected individ-uals. Terry Beirn Community Programs for Clinical Research on AIDS. *AIDS* **12**: 269–77.

Carosi G, Castelli (Brescia) E, Italian Foscarnet/Retinitis Study Group. (1993). A randomized controlled trial of two dosage regimens of fos-carnet in AIDS patients with CMV retinitis. *Eleventh International Conference on AIDS in Affiliation with the Fourth STD World Congress*, Berlin, Germany.

Chavez-de la Paz E, Arevalo JF, Kirsch LS et al. (1997). Anterior non-granulomatous uveitis after intravitreal HPMPC (cidofovir) for the treatment of cytomegalovirus retinitis. Analysis and prevention. *Oph-thalmology* **104**: 539–44.

Cheng Y, Huang ES, Lin JC et al. (1983). Unique spectrum of activity of 9-[1,3-dihydroxy-2-propoxy)methyl]-guanine against herpesviruses *in vitro* and its mode of action against herpes simplex virus type 1. *Proc Natl Acad Sci USA* **80**: 2767–70.

Cherrington JM, Smith IL, Jiles RE et al. (1996). Ganciclovir resistant CMV: implications of UL97and polymerase mutations in cross resis-tance to cidofovir. *Antiviral Res* **30**: A44.

Chiller T, Park A, Chiller K et al. (1998). HIV protease inhibitor therapy is associated with increased time to relapse and death in AIDS pat-ients with cytomegalovirus retinitis. *Thirth-eight International Con-ference on Antimicrobial Agents and Chemotherapy*, San Diego, CA, USA.

Chou S, Marousek G, Guentzel S et al. (1997). Evolution of mutations conferring multidrug resistance during prophylaxis and therapy for cytomegalovirus disease. *J Infect Dis* **176**: 786–9.

Chou S, Marousek G, Parenti DM et al. (1998). Mutation in region III of the DNA polymerase gene conferring foscarnet resistance in cytomegalovirus isolates from three subjects receiving prolonged antiviral therapy. *J Infect Dis* **178**: 526–30.

Chrisp P, Clissold SP. (1991). Foscarnet: a review of its antiviral activ-ity, pharmacokinetic properties and therapeutic use in immuno-compromised patients with cytomegalovirus. *Drugs* **41**: 104–29.

Cinque P, Vago L, Brytting M et al. (1992). Cytomegalovirus infection of the central nervous system in patients with AIDS. Diagnosis by DNA amplification from cerebrospinal fluid. *J Infect Dis* **166**: 1408–11.

Cohen BA, McArthur JC, Grohman S et al. (1993). Neurologic progno-sis of cytomegalovirus polyradiculomyelopathy in AIDS. *Neurology* **43**: 493–9.

Collier AC, Meyers JD, Corey L et al. (1987). Cytomegalovirus infection in homosexual men. *Am J Med* **82**: 493–500.

Connors M, Kovacs JA, Krevat S et al. (1997). HIV infection induces changes in CD4+ T-cell phenotype and depletions within the CD4+ T-cell repertoire that are not immediately restored by antiviral or immune-based therapies. *Nat Med* **3**: 533–40.

Cooper DA, Pehrson PO, Pedersen C et al. (1993). The efficacy and safe-ty of zidovudine alone or as a cotherapy with aciclovir for the treat-ment of patients with AIDS and AIDS-related complex. A double-blind, randomized trial. *AIDS* **7**: 197–207.

Crowe SM, Carlin JB, Stewart KI et al. (1991). Predictive value of CD4 lymphocyte numbers for the development of opportunistic infections and malignancies in HIV-infected persons. *J AIDS* **4**: 770–6.

Cundy KC, Barditch-Crovo P, Walker RE et al. (1995). Clinical pharmacokinetics of adefovir in human immunodeficiency virus type 1-infected patients. *Antimicrob Agents Chemother* **39**: 2401–5.

Davis JL, Taskintuna I, Freeman WR et al. (1997). Iritis and hypotony after treatment with intravenous cidofovir for cytomegalovirus retinitis. *Arch Ophthalmol* **115**: 733–7.

De Armond B. (1991). Future directions in the management of cytomegalovirus infections. *J AIDS* **4**: S53–6.

Deayton JR, Wilson P, Sabin CA et al. (2000). Changes in the natural history of cytomegalovirus retinitis following the introduction of high-ly active antiretroviral therapy. *AIDS* **14**: 1163–70.

de Gans J, Portegies P, Tiessens G et al. (1990a). Therapy for cytomegalovirus polyradiculomyelitis in patients with AIDS: treat-ment with ganciclovir. *AIDS* **4**: 421–5.

de Gans J, Tiessens G, Portegies P et al. (1990b). Predominance of polymorphonuclear leukocytes in cerebrospinal fluid of AIDS patients with cytomegalovirus polyradiculomyelitis. J Acquir Immune Defic Syndr 3: 1155–8.

Diaz-Llopis M, Chipont E, Sanchez S et al. (1992). Intravitreal foscarnet for cytomegalovirus retinitis in a patient with acquired immune deficiency syndrome. Am J Ophthalmol 114: 742–7.

Diaz-Llopis M, Espana E, Munoz G et al. (1994). High dose intravitreal foscarnet in the treatment of cytomegalovirus retinitis in AIDS. Br J Ophthalmol 78: 120–4.

Dieterich DT, Rahmin M. (1991). Cytomegalovirus colitis in AIDS: presentation in 44 patients and a review of the literature. J Acquir Immune Defic Syndr Hum Retrovicol 4: S29–35.

Dieterich DT, Chachoua A, Lafleur F et al. (1988). Ganciclovir treatment of gastrointestinal infections caused by cytomegalovirus in patients with AIDS. Rev Infect Dis 10: S532–7.

Dieterich DT, Kotler DP, Busch DF et al. (1993). Ganciclovir treatment of cytomegalovirus colitis in AIDS: a randomized, double-blind, placebo-controlled multicenter study. J Infect Dis 167: 278–82.

Drew WL. (1993). Cytomegalovirus as a sexually transmitted disease. In: Y Becker, C Carai, (eds.) Molecular aspects of hyman cytomegalovirus disease. Heidelberg: Springer-Verlag, 92–100.

Drew WL, Mintz L, Miner RC et al. (1981). Prevalence of cytomegalovirus infections in homosexual men. J Infect Dis 143: 188–92.

Drew WL, Miner RC, Busch DF et al. (1991). Prevalence of resistance in patients receiving ganciclovir for serious cytomegalovirus infection. J Infect Dis 163: 716–9.

Drew WL, Ives D, Lalezari JP et al. (1995). Oral ganciclovir as maintenance treatment for cytomegalovirus retinitis in patients with AIDS. Syntex Cooperative Oral Ganciclovir Study Group. N Engl J Med 333: 615–20.

Dworkin MS, Fratkin MD. (1998). Mycobacterium avium complex lymph node abscess after use of highly active antiretroviral therapy in a patient with AIDS. Arch Intern Med 158: 1828.

Erice A, Chou S, Biron KK et al. (1989). Progressive disease due to ganciclovir resistant cytomegalovirus in immunocompromised patients. N Engl J Med 320: 289–93.

Erice A, Gil Roda C, Perez JL et al. (1997). Antiviral susceptibilities and analysis of UL97 and DNA polymerase sequences of clinical cytomegalovirus isolates from immunocompromised patients. J Infect Dis 175: 1087–92.

Faber DW, Lynn GB, Gross JG et al. (1992). Role of HIV and CMV in the pathogenesis of retinitis and retinal vasculopathy in AIDS patients. Investig Ophthalmol Visual Sci 33: 2345–53.

Faulds D, Heel RC. (1990). Ganciclovir. A review of its antiviral activity, pharmacokinetic properties and therapeutic efficacy in cytomegalovirus infections. Drugs 39: 597–638.

Feinberg J, Hurwitz S, Cooper D et al. (1998). A randomized, double-blind trial of valaciclovir (VACV) prophylaxis for Cytomegalovirus (CMV) end-organ disease in patients with AIDS. J Infect Dis 177: 48–56.

Fiala M, Singer EJ, Graves MC et al. (1993). AIDS dementia complex complicated by cytomegalovirus encephalopathy. J Neurol 240: 223–31.

Fisher E, Brosgart C, Cohn D et al. (1999). Placebo (PLC)-controlled, multicenter trial of adefovir dipivoxil (ADV) in patients (PE) with HIV disease. Sixth Conference on Retroviruses and Opportunistic Infection, Chicago, IL, USA.

Forbes A, Blanshard C, Gazzard B. (1993). Natural history of AIDS-related sclerosing cholangitis. A study of 20 cases. Gut 34: 116–21.

Gallant JE, Moore RD, Richman DD et al. (1992). Incidence and natural history of cytomegalovirus disease in patients with advanced human immunodeficiency virus disease treated with zidovudine. J Infect Dis 166: 1223–7.

Gearhart MO, Sorg TB. (1993). Foscarnet-induced severe hypomagnesemia and other electrolyte disorders. Ann Pharmacother 27: 285–9.

Gilquin J, Piketty C, Thomas V et al. (1997). Acute cytomegalovirus infection in AIDS patients with CD4 counts above $100 \times 10(6)$ cells/l following combination antiretroviral therapy including protease inhibitors. AIDS 11: 1659–60.

Gorochov G, Neumann AU, Kereveur A et al. (1998). Perturbation of CD4+ and CD8+ T-cell repertoires during progression to AIDS and regulation of the CD4+ repertoire during antiviral. Nat Med 4: 215–21.

Gozlan J, Salord JM, Roullet E et al. (1992). Rapid detection of cytomegalovirus DNA in cerebrospinal fluid of AIDS patients with neurologic disorders. J Infect Dis 166: 1416–21.

Graziosi C, Soudeyns H, Rizzardi GP et al. (1998). Immunopathogenesis of HIV infection. AIDS Res Hum Retrovir 14: S135–42.

Grefte A, Blom N, Van Giessen M et al. (1993). Ultrastructural analysis of circulating cytomegalic cells in patients with active cytomegalovirus infection. Evidence for virus production and endothelial origin. J Infect Dis 168: 1110–8.

Gross JC, Bozzette SA, Matthews WC et al. (1990). Longitudinal study of cytomegalovirus retinitis in acquired immune deficiency syndrome. Ophthalmology 97: 681–6.

Gross AS, Dretler RH. (1993). Foscarnet-induced penile ulcer in an uncircumcised patient with AIDS. Clin Infect Dis 17: 1076–7.

Grutzmeier S, Sandstrom E. (1992). Adrenal insufficiency is a common cause of fatigue and wasting in advanced CMV-infection in AIDS patients. Eighth International Conference on AIDS/III STD World Congress, Amsterdam, Holland.

Gulick RM, Mellors JW, Havlir D et al. (1997). Treatment with indinavir, zidovudine, and lamivudine in adults with human immunodeficiency virus infection and prior antiretroviral therapy. N Engl J Med 337: 734–9.

Hall AFH, Jennens ID, Lucas CR et al. (1991). Low frequency maintenance ganciclovir for cytomegalovirus retinitis. Scandinavian J Infect Dis 23: 43–6.

Hammitt DG, Aschenbrenner DW, Williamson RA. (1988). Culture of cytomegalovirus from frozen-thawed semen. Fertil Steril 49: 554–7.

Henry K, Contrill H, Fletcher C et al. (1987). Use of intravitreal ganciclovir for cytomegalovirus retinitis in a patient with AIDS. Am J Ophthamol 103: 17–23.

Ho HT, Woods KI, Bronson JJ et al. (1992). Intracellular metabolism of the antiherpes agent (S)-1-(3-hydroxy-2-phosphonylmethoxypropl) cytosine. Mol Pharmacol 41: 197–202.

Holland GN, Shuler JD. (1992). Progression rates of cytomegalovirus retinopathy in ganciclovir-treated and untreated patients. Arch Ophthalmol 110: 1435–42.

Holland GN, Buhles WC, Mastre B et al. (1989). Controlled retrospective study of ganciclovir treatment for cytomegalovirus retinopathy. Arch Ophthamol 107: 1759–66.

Holland NR, Power C, Matthews VP et al. (1994). Cytomegalovirus encephalitis in acquired immunodeficiency syndrome (AIDS). Clinical features and course. Neurology 44: 507–14.

Hoover DR, Saah AJ, Bacellar H et al. (1993). Clinical manifestations of AIDS in the era of Pneumocystis prophylaxis. N Engl J Med 329: 1922–6.

Howell CL, Miller MJ, Bruckner DA. (1986). Elimination of toxicity and enhanced cytomegalovirus detection in cell cultures inoculated with semen from patients with acquired immunodeficiency syndrome. J Clin Microbiol 24: 657–60.

Jabs DA, Enger C, Dunn JP et al. (1998a). Cytomegalovirus retinitis and viral resistance: ganciclovir resistance. CMV Retinitis and Viral Resistance Study Group. J Infect Dis 177: 770–3.

Jabs DA, Enger C, Forman M et al. (1998b). Incidence of foscarnet resistance and cidofovir resistance in patients treated for cytomegalovirus retinitis. The Cytomegalovirus Retinitis and Viral Resistance Study Group. Antimicrob Agents Chemother 42: 2240–4.

Jacobson MA, de Miranda P, Cederberg DM et al. (1987). Human pharmacokinetics and tolerance of oral ganciclovir. Antimicrob Agents Chemother 31: 1251–4.

Jacobson MA, O'Donnell JJ, Brodie HR et al. (1988). Randomized prospective trial of ganciclovir maintenance therapy for cytomegalovirus retinitis. J Med Virol 25: 339–49.

Jacobson MA, Gambertoglio JG, Aweeka FT et al. (1991a). Foscarnet induced hypocalcemia and effects of foscarnet on calcium metabolism. J Clin Endocrinol Metab 72: 1130–5.

Jacobson MA, van der Horst CA, Causey DM et al. (1991b). In vivo additive antiretroviral effect of combined zidovudine and foscarnet therapy for human immunodeficiency virus infection (ACTG Protocol 053). J Infect Dis 163: 1219–22.

Jacobson MA, Causey D, Polsky B et al. (1993). A dose ranging study of daily maintenance intravenous foscarnet therapy for cytomegalovirus retinitis in AIDS. J Infect Dis 168: 444–8.

Jacobson MA, Zegans M, Pavan PR et al. (1997). Cytomegalovirus retinitis after initiation of highly active antiretroviral therapy. Lancet 349: 1143–5.

Jones AC, Freedman PD, Phelan JA et al. (1993). Cytomegalovirus infections of the oral cavity. Oral Surg Oral Med Oral Pathol 76: 76–85.

Kalayjian RC, Cohen ML, Bonomo RA et al. (1993). Cytomegalovirus ventriculoencephalitis in AIDS. A syndrome with distinct clinical and pathologic features. Medicine 72: 67–77.

Karavellas MP, Lowder CY, Macdonald C et al. (1998). Immune recovery vitritis associated with inactive cytomegalovirus retinitis: a new syndrome. Arch Ophthalmol 116: 169–75.

Kempen JH, Jabs DA, Dunn JP et al. (2001). Retinal detachment risk in cytomegalovirus retinitis related to the acquired immunodeficiency syndrome. Arch Ophthalmol 119: 33–40.

Kim YS, Hollander H. (1993). Polyradiculopathy due to cytomegalovirus: report of two cases in which improvement occurred after prolonged therapy and review of the literature. Clin Infect Dis 17: 32–7.

Komanduri KV, Viswanathan M, Wieder E et al. (1998). Restoration of cytomegalovirus-specific CD4+ T-lymphocyte responses after ganciclovir and highly active antiretroviral therapy in individuals infected with HIV-1. Nat Med 4: 953–6.

Kotler DP, Reka S, Orenstein JM et al. (1992). Chronic idiopathic esophageal ulceration in the acquired immunodeficiency syndrome. J Clin Gastroenterol 15: 284–90.

Laine L, Boracini M, Sattler F et al. (1992). Cytomegalovirus and Candida esophagitis in patients with AIDS. J AIDS 5: 605–9.

Lalezari JP. Kuppermann BD. (1997). Clinical experience with cidofovir in the treatment of cytomegalovirus retinitis. J Acquir Immune Defic Syndr Hum Retrovirol 1: S27–31.

Lalezari JP, Stagg RJ, Kupperman BD et al. (1997). A randomized controlled trial of intravenous cidofovir for peripheral CMV retinitis in patients with AIDS. Ann Intern Med 126: 257–63.

Lalezari JP, Holland GN, Kramer F et al. (1998). Randomized, controlled study of the safety and efficacy of intravenous cidofovir for the treatment of relapsing cytomegalovirus retinitis in patients with AIDS. J Acquir Immune Defic Syndr Hum Retrovirol 17: 339–44.

Lange M, Klein EB, Kornfield H et al. (1984). Cytomegalovirus isolation from healthy homosexual men. JAMA 252: 1908–10.

Leach CT, Cherry JD, English PA et al. (1993). The relationship between T-cell levels and CMV infection in asymptomatic HIV-1 antibody-positive homosexual men. J AIDS 6: 407–13.

Lederman M, Connick E, Landay A et al. (1997). Partial immune reconstitution after 12 weeks of HAART (ZDV, 3TC, ritonavir). Preliminary results of ACTG 314. Fourth Conference on Retroviruses and Opportunistic Infections, Washington, DC, USA.

Li TS, Tubiana R, Katlama C et al. (1998). Long lasting recovery in CD4 T-cell function and viral-load reduction after highly active antiretroviral therapy in advanced HIV-1 disease. Lancet 351: 1682–6.

Macdonald JC, Torriani FJ, Morse LS et al. (1998). Lack of reactivation of cytomegalovirus (CMV) retinitis after stopping CMV maintenance therapy in AIDS patients with sustained elevations in CD4 T cells in response to highly active antiretroviral therapy. J Infect Dis 177: 1182–7.

MacGregor RR, Graziani AL, Weiss R et al. (1991). Successful foscarnet therapy for cytomegalovirus retinitis in an AIDS patient undergoing hemodialysis. Rationale for empiric dosing and plasma level dosing. J Infect Dis 164: 785–7.

MacGregor RR, Pakola SJ, Graziani AL et al. (1995). Evidence of active cytomegalovirus infection in clinically stable HIV infected individuals with CD4+ lymphocyte counts below 100/ml of blood: features and relation to risk of subsequent CMV retinitis. J Aquir Immune Defic Syndr Hum Retrovirol 10: 324–30.

Mallolas JJ, Arrizabalaga L, Montserrat M et al. (1997a). Cytomegalovirus disease in HIV-1 infected patients treated with protease inhibitors. Thirty-fifth Annual Meeting of the Infectious Diseases Society of America, San Francisco, CA, USA.

Mallolas JJ, Gatell JM, Gomez-Sirvent JL et al. (1997b). Prophylaxis secondary to retinitis by CMV in patients with AIDS. The efficacy of an intermittent schedule of three days/week. Enfermedades Infecciosas Y Microbiologia Clinica 15: 61–4.

Manischewitz JF, Quinnan GV, Lane HC et al. (1990). Synergistic effect of ganciclovir and foscarnet on cytomegalovirus replication in vitro. Antimicrob Agents Chemother 34: 373–5.

Martin DF, Parks DJ, Mellow SD et al. (1994). Treatment of cytomegalovirus retinitis with an intraocular sustained release ganciclovir implant. A randomized controlled trial. Arch Ophthamol 112: 1531–9.

Martin DF, Ferris FL, Parks DJ et al. (1997a). Ganciclovir implant exchange. Timing, surgical procedure, and complications. Arch Ophthalmol 115: 1389–94.

Martin DF, Kuppermann BD, Wolitz RA et al. (1999). Oral ganciclovir for patients with cytomegalovirus retinitis treated with a ganciclovir implant. Roche Ganciclovir Study Group. N Engl J Med 340: 1063–70.

Marwick C. (1998). First 'antisense' drug will treat CMV retinitis. *JAMA* **280**: 871.

Marx JL, Kapusta MA, Patel SS *et al.* (1996). Use of the ganciclovir implant in the treatment of recurrent cytomegalovirus retinitis. *Arch Ophthalmol* **114**: 815–20.

Mentec H, Leport C, Leport J *et al.* (1994). Cytomegalovirus colitis in HIV-1 infected patients. A prospective research in 55 patients. *AIDS* **8**: 461–7.

Millar AB, Patou G, Miller RF *et al.* (1990). Cytomegalovirus in the lungs of patients with AIDS. *Am Rev Respir Dis* **141**: 1474–7.

Mintz L, Drew WL, Miner RC *et al.* (1983). Cytomegalovirus infections in homosexual men. *Ann Intern Med* **99**: 326–9.

Monforte Ad'A, Mainini F, Vago L *et al.* (1993). Factors associated with increased risk of acquiring cytomegalovirus disease in AIDS patients. *J Infect Dis* **168**: 1071–2.

Muccioli C, Goldstein DA, Johnson DW *et al.* (1998). Fomivirsen safety and efficacy in the treatment of CMV retinitis: a phase three, controlled, multicenter study comparing immediate versus delayed treatment. *Fifth Conference Retroviruses and Opportunistic Infection*, Chicago, IL, USA.

Musch DC, Martin DF, Gordon JF *et al.* (1997). Treatment of AIDS related CMV retinitis with Ganciclovir implant: a multicenter randomized controlled trial. *N Engl J Med* **337**: 83–90.

Nelson MR, Connolly GM, Hawkins DA *et al.* (1991). Foscarnet in the treatment of cytomegalovirus infection of the esophagus and colon in patients with the acquired immune deficiency syndrome. *Am J Gastroenterol* **86**: 876–81.

Nussenblatt RB, Lane HC. (1998). Human immunodeficiency virus disease: changing patterns of intraocular inflammation. *Am J Ophthalmol* **125**: 134–382.

Oberg B. (1989). Antiviral effects of phosphonoformate (PFA, foscarnet sodium). *Pharmacol Ther* **40**: 213–85.

Palella FJ, Delaney KM, Moorman AC *et al.* (1998). Declining morbidity and mortality among patients with advanced human immunodeficiency virus infection. HIV Outpatient Study Investigators. *N Engl J Med* **338**: 853–60.

Palestine AG, Polis MA, De Smet MD *et al.* (1991). A randomized, controlled trial of foscarnet in the treatment of cytomegalovirus retinitis in patients with AIDS. *Ann Intern Med* **115**: 665–73.

Pertel P, Hirschtick R, Phair J *et al.* (1992). Risk of developing cytomegalovirus retinitis in persons infected with human immunodeficiency virus. *J AIDS* **5**: 1069–1074.

Petito CK, Cho ES, Lemann W *et al.* (1986). Neuropathology of acquired immunodeficiency syndrome (AIDS). An autopsy review. *J Neuropathol Exper Neurol* **45**: 635–46.

Plotkin SA, Drew WL, Felsenstein D *et al.* (1985). Sensitivity of clinical isolates of human cytomegalovirus to 9-(1,3-dihydroxy-2-propoxymethyl) guanine. *J Infect Dis* **152**: 833–4.

Polis MA, Spooner KM, Baird BF *et al.* (1995). Anticytomegaloviral activity and safety of cidofovir in patients with human immunodeficiency virus infection and cytomegalovirus viruria. *Antimicrobial Agents Chemother* **39**: 882–6.

Price TA, Digioia RA, Simon GL. (1992). Ganciclovir treatment of cytomegalovirus ventriculitis in a patient infected with human immunodeficiency virus. *Clin Infect Dis* **15**: 606–8.

Prince AM, Szmuness W, Millian SJ *et al.* (1971). A serologic study of cytomegalovirus infections associated with blood transfusion. *N Engl J Med* **284**: 1125–31.

Quinnan GV, Kirmani N, Rook AH *et al.* (1982). Cytotoxic T cells in cytomegalovirus infection. *N Engl J Med* **307**: 7–12.

Quinnan GV, Masur H, Rook AH *et al.* (1984). Herpesvirus infections in the acquired immune deficiency syndrome. *JAMA* **252**: 72–77.

Rabb MF, Jampol LM, Fish RH *et al.* (1992). Retinal periphlebitis in patients with acquired immunodeficiency syndrome with cytomegalovirus retinitis mimics acute frosted retinal periphlebitis. *Arch Ophthalmol* **100**: 1257–60.

Race EM, Adelson-Mitty J, Kriegel GR *et al.* (1998). Focal mycobacterial lymphadenitis following initiation of protease-inhibitor therapy in patients with advanced HIV-1. *Lancet* **351**: 252–5.

Ramundo MB. (1993). Cytomegalovirus gastrointestinal disease in patients with HIV infection. *Thirty-third Interscience Conference on Antimicrobial Agents and Chemotherapy*, New Orleans, LA, USA.

Rice GP, Schrier RD, Oldstone MB. (1984). Cytomegalovirus infects human lymphocytes and monocytes: virus expression is restricted to immediate-early gene products. *Proc Natl Acad Sci USA* **81**: 6134–8

Rich JD, Crawford JM, Kazanjian SN *et al.* (1992). Discrete gastrointestinal mass lesions caused by cytomegalovirus in patients with AIDS. Report of three cases and review. *Clin Infect Dis* **15**: 609–14.

Riddell SR, Elliott M, Lewinsohn DA *et al.* (1996). T-cell mediated rejection of gene-modified HIV-specific cytotoxic T lymphocytes in HIV-infected patients. *Nat Med* **2**: 216–23.

Rinaldo CR, Kingsley LA, Ho M *et al.* (1992). Enhanced shedding of cytomegalovirus in semen of human immunodeficiency virus seropositive homosexual men. *J Clin Microbiol* **30**: 1148–55.

Roarty JD, Fisher EJ, Nussbaum JJ. (1993). Long term visual morbidity of cytomegalovirus retinitis in patients with acquired immune deficiency syndrome. *Ophthalmology* **100**: 1685–8.

Said G, Lacroix C, Chemouilli P *et al.* (1991). Cytomegalovirus neuropathy in acquired immunodeficiency syndrome. A clinical pathological study. *Ann Neurol* **29**: 139–46.

Saint-Marc T, Fournier F, Touraine JL *et al.* (1992). Uvula and oesophageal ulcerations with foscarnet. *Lancet* **350**: 970–1.

Sanborn GE, Anand R, Torti RE *et al.* (1992). Sustained-release ganciclovir therapy for treatment of cytomegalovirus retinitis: use of an intravitreal device. *Arch Ophthalmol* **110**: 188–95.

Secchi AG, Tognon S, Turrini B *et al.* (1992). Acute frosted retinal periphlebitis associated with cytomegalovirus retinitis. *Retina* **12**: 245–7.

Shinkai M, Bozzette S, Powderly W *et al.* (1997). Utility of urine and leukocyte cultures and plasma DNA polymerase chain reaction for identification of AIDS patients at risk for developing human cytomegalovirus disease. *J Infect Dis* **175**: 302–8.

Shore SL, Feorino PM. (1981). Immunology of primary herpesvirus infections in humans. In: AJ Nahmias, WR Dowdle, RF Shinazi (eds.) *The human herpes viruses*. New York: Elsevier, 267–8.

Smith PD, Lane HC, Gill VJ *et al.* (1988). Intestinal infections in patients with the acquired immunodeficiency syndrome. *Ann Intern Med* **108**: 328–33.

Smith TJ, Pearson A, Blandford DL *et al.* (1992). Intravitreal sustained-release ganciclovir. *Arch Ophthalmol* **110**: 255–8.

Smith PD, Eisner MS, Manischewitz JF *et al.* (1993). Esophageal disease in AIDS is associated with pathologic processes rather than mucosal human immunodeficiency virus type 1. *J Infect Dis* **167**: 547–52.

Smith IL, Cherrington JM, Jiles RE *et al.* (1998). High-level resistance of cytomegalovirus to ganciclovir is associated with alterations in both the UL97 and DNA polymerase genes. *J Infect Dis* **177**: 1140–1.

Snoeck R, Sakuma T, De Clercq E et al. (1988). (S)-1-(3-hydroxy-2-phosphonylmethoxypropyl)cytosine, a potent and selective inhibitor of human cytomegalovirus replication. Antimicrob Agents Chemother 32: 1839–44.

Studies of Ocular Complications of AIDS Research Group (SOCA). (1992). Mortality in patients with the acquired immunodeficiency syndrome treated with either foscarnet or ganciclovir for cytomegalovirus retinitis. Studies of Ocular Complications of AIDS Research Group in collaboration with the AIDS Clinical Trials Group. N Engl J Med 326: 213–20.

SOCA. (1996). Combination foscarnet and ganciclovir therapy vs monotherapy for the treatment of relapsed cytomegalovirus retinitis in patients with AIDS. The Cytomegalovirus Retreatment Trial. The Studies of Ocular Complications of AIDS Research Group in Collaboration with the AIDS Clinical Trials Group. Arch Ophthalmol 114: 23–33.

SOCA. (1997a). Cytomegalovirus (CMV) culture results, drug resistance, and clinical outcome in patients with AIDS and CMV retinitis treated with foscarnet or ganciclovir. Studies of Ocular Complications of AIDS (SOCA) in collaboration with the AIDS Clinical Trial Group. J Infect Dis 176: 50–8.

SOCA. (1997b). Parenteral cidofovir for cytomegalovirus retinitis in patients with AIDS: the HPMPC peripheral cytomegalovirus retinitis trial. A randomized, controlled trial. Studies of Ocular complications of AIDS Research Group in Collaboration with the AIDS Clinical Trials Group. Ann Intern Med 126: 264–74.

Spector SA, Weingeist T, Pollard RB. (1993). A randomized, controlled study of intravenous ganciclovir therapy for cytomegalovirus peripheral retinitis in patients with AIDS. J Infect Dis 168: 557–63.

Spector S, Busch DF, Follansbee S et al. (1995). Pharmacokinetic, safety, and antiviral profiles of oral ganciclovir in persons infected with human immunodeficiency virus: a phase I/II study. J Infect Dis 171: 1431–7.

Spector SA, McKinley G, Lalezari JP et al. (1996). For the Roche Co-operative Ganciclovir Study Group. Oral ganciclovir for the prevention of cytomegalovirus disease in persons with AIDS. N Engl J Med 334: 1491–7.

Spector SA, Wong R, Hsia K et al. (1998). Plasma cytomegalovirus DNA load predicts CMV disease and survival in AIDS patients. J Clin Invest 101: 497–502.

Srinivas RV, Robbins BL, Connelly MC et al. (1993). Metabolism and in vitro antiretroviral activities of bis(pivaloyloxymethyl) prodrugs of acyclic nucleoside phosphonates. Antimicrob Agents Chemother 37: 2247–50.

Squire SB, Lipman MCI, Bagdades EK et al. (1992). Severe cytomegalovirus pneumonitis in HIV-infected patients with higher than average CD4 counts. Thorax 47: 301–4.

Squires KE. (1996). Oral ganciclovir for cytomegalovirus retinitis in patients with AIDS: results of two randomized studies. AIDS 10: S13–8.

Stanat SC, Reardon JE, Erice A et al. (1991). Ganciclovir resistant cytomegalovirus clinical isolates. Mode of resistance to ganciclovir. Antimicrob Agents Chemother 35: 2191–7.

Sullivan V, Coen DM. (1991). Isolation of foscarnet-resistant human cytomegalovirus patterns of resistance and sensitivity to other antiviral drugs. J Infect Dis 164: 781–4.

Sullivan V, Biron KK, Talarico C et al. (1993). A point mutation in the human cytomegalovirus DNA polymerase gene confers resistance to ganciclovir and phosphonylmethoxyalkyl derivatives. Antimicrob Agents Chemother 37: 19–25.

Swindells S, Currier JS, Williams P. (1997). DACS 071: correlation of viral load and risk for opportunistic infection. Fourth Conference on Retroviruses and Opportunistic Infections, Washington, DC, USA.

The Oral Ganciclovir European and Australian Co-Operative Study Group. (1995). Intravenous versus oral ganciclovir: European/Australian comparative study of efficacy and safety in the prevention of cytomegalovirus retinitis recurrence in patients with AIDS. AIDS 9: 471–7.

Torriani F, Havlir D, Freeman W et al. (1998a). Proliferative responses against CMV in AIDS patients on HAART and with healed CMV retinitis who stopped maintenance therapy. Fifth Conference on Retroviruses and Opportunistic Infections, Chicago, IL, USA.

Torriani F, Freeman WR, Durand D et al. (1998b). Evidence that HAART-induced immune recovery vitritis in CMV retinitis patients is immune-mediated. Twelfth World AIDS Conference, Geneva, Switzerland.

Tural C, Romeu J, Sirera G et al. (1998). Long-lasting remission of cytomegalovirus retinitis without maintenance therapy in human immunodeficiency virus-infected patients. J Infect Dis 177: 1080–3.

Van der Ende ME, van Buuren HR, Kroes ACM et al. (1992). Failure of antiviral therapy in AIDS-associated cytomegalovirus cholangitis. Infection 20: 371–2.

Van der Pijl JW, Frissen PHJ, Reiss P et al. (1990). Foscarnet and penile ulceration. Lancet 335: 286.

Vasudevan VP, Mascarenhas DAN, Klapper P et al. (1990). Cytomegalovirus necrotizing bronchiolitis with HIV infection. Chest 97: 483–4.

Walter EA, Greenberg PD, Gilbert MJ et al. (1995). Reconstitution of cellular immunity against cytomegalovirus in recipients of allogeneic bone marrow by transfer of T-cell clones from the donor. N Engl J Med 333: 1038–44.

Wohl D, Pedersen S. (1998). Routine ophthalmologic screening for detection of asymptomatic CMV retinitis. Int Conf AIDS, Geneva, Switzerland. 12: 312.

Wolf DG, Smith IL, Lee DJ et al. (1995). Mutations in human cytomegalovirus UL97 gene confer clinical resistance to ganciclovir and can be detected in patient plasma. J Clin Invest 95: 257–63.

Zhang ZQ, Schuler T, Cavert W et al. (1999). Reversibility of the pathological changes in the follicular dendritic cell network with treatment of HIV-1 infection. Proc Natl Acad Sci USA 96: 5169–72.

Zegans ME, Walton RC, Holland GN et al. (1998). Transient vitreous inflammatory reactions associated with combination antiretroviral therapy in patients with AIDS and cytomegalovirus retinitis. Am J Ophthalmol 125: 292–300.

Zurlo JJ, O'Neill D, Polis M et al. (1993). Lack of utility of cytomegalovirus blood and urine cultures in patients with HIV infection. Ann Intern Med 118: 12–17.

Bacterial infection and HIV infection

ALAN STREET

Patients with HIV infection can develop a wide range of bacterial infections in addition to the familiar opportunistic viral, parasitic and fungal pathogens typically associated with disorders of cellular immunity. The relative importance of bacterial infections has increased as effective prophylaxis has reduced the frequency of fungal and parasitic opportunistic infections and the pool of vulnerable patients with advanced AIDS has enlarged. Countering these trends, the advent of highly active antiretroviral therapy (HAART; see Chapter 7) has led to a substantial reduction in the incidence of a number of HIV-related infections, including bacterial infections.

Bacterial infections often occur at lesser degrees of immunosuppression than other opportunistic infections, and so account for a significant proportion of pre-AIDS morbidity. Infants and children with HIV infection are particularly vulnerable to these infections. Bacterial infections are also very common in patients with HIV infection in the developing world. As these infections can be serious but are usually easily treatable, they should be recognized promptly. Some bacterial infections can be transmitted to household, social or hospital contacts. In common with other infections seen in HIV-infected patients, bacterial infections frequently recur, and some require long-term prophylactic therapy.

Virulent organisms such as *Streptococcus pneumoniae*, *Haemophilus influenzae*, *Mycobacterium tuberculosis* (see Chapter 23) and *Treponema pallidum* typically affect immunocompetent individuals but are also important pathogens in patients with HIV infection. Somewhat unexpectedly, opportunistic bacteria such as *Nocardia* and *Listeria*, which are common in patients with iatrogenic immunosuppression, rarely cause infection in HIV-infected patients. Newly identified bacteria, such as *Bartonella henselae*, were first discovered in HIV-infected patients and have subsequently also been described in immunocompetent and other immunosuppressed patients.

The predisposition to bacterial infection is a consequence of a constellation of HIV-mediated immune defects and other factors. Dysfunction of B cells, characterized by impaired antibody production in response to acute infection despite higher total serum immunoglobulin levels, may account for the increased incidence of pneumococcal and *H. influenzae* pneumonia observed in these patients. Mycobacterial and *Salmonella* infections occur because of defects in cellular immunity due to destruction of CD4 lymphocytes and macrophage dysfunction resulting from HIV infection. Quantitative and qualitative neutrophil defects undoubtedly predispose HIV patients to many types of bacterial infection (Moore *et al.*, 1995). Long-term indwelling intravenous access devices, frequent hospitalization, use of antibiotics and cytotoxic agents and poor nutrition are general factors that increase the risk of infection in patients with serious underlying medical conditions, including those with HIV infection.

Bacterial pneumonia

Epidemiology and aetiology

Bacterial pneumonia (see Chapter 13) is many times more common in HIV-infected patients than in those without HIV infection. It often occurs in those who have not yet developed AIDS, although the risk of bacterial pneumonia increases as the CD4 count falls. HIV-infected children and injecting drug users are particularly at risk, and cigarette smoking confers an added risk of pneumonia to those with less than 200 CD4 lymphocytes/μl (Hirschtick *et al.*, 1995; Dworkin *et al.*, 2001).

Table 22.1 Bacteria usually causing pneumonia in HIV-infected patients

Organism	Stage of HIV infection	Pneumonia syndrome	Usual locale of infection	Important features
Streptococcus pneumoniae	Early and late	Acute	C	Common in children, injecting drug users
Haemophilus influenzae				Bacteraemia and recurrence common
Staphylococcus aureus Enteric Gram-negative rods	Late	Acute	N	Neutropenia may be present Course can be fulminant High mortality
Pseudomonas aeruginosa	Late	Acute or chronic recurrent	N or C	Nosocomial-acute necrotizing pneumonia Community -acquired – less severe, Cavitation on CXR, recurrence frequent
Mycobacterium tuberculosis (see Chapter 23)	Early or late	Sub-acute or chronic	C (N)	Atypical clinical and X-ray presentation Extra-pulmonary disease common
Rhodococcus equi	Late	Chronic cavitary	C	Organism can be isolated in sputum May disseminate (skin, CNS)
Nocardia asteroides	Late	Chronic ± cavitation	C (N)	Uncommon (in contrast to transplant patients) Extrapulmonary involvement (skin, CNS)
Legionella	Late	Acute	C or N	Uncommon, may co-exist with other pathogens, may cavitate (*L. micdadei*)
Chlamydia pneumoniae	Early or late	Acute or sub-acute	C	May present as mild pneumonia, or a fulminant process such as PCP

C: community acquired; N: nosocomial CXR: chest X-ray; CNS: central nervous system; PCP: *Pneumocystis carinii* pneumonia.

As in the general community, *S. pneumoniae* and *H. influenzae* are the leading causes of community-acquired bacterial pneumonia (Polsky *et al.*, 1986; Witt *et al.*, 1987; Burack *et al.*, 1994; Hirschtick *et al.*, 1995) (Table 22.1). Most *H. influenzae* infections are caused by non-type-b strains. *Pseudomonas aeruginosa*, a rare cause of pneumonia in most patients without HIV infection, is an important cause of both community-acquired and nosocomial pneumonia in patients with late-stage HIV infection (Baron and Hollander, 1993; Sorvillo *et al.*, 2001). *Staphylococcus aureus* pneumonia is seen in association with injecting drug use or as a nosocomial infection (Tumbarello *et al.*, 1998). Enteric Gram-negative bacillary pneumonia is usually nosocomially acquired and a complication of very advanced HIV infection.

Less common causes of pneumonia in HIV-infected patients are also listed in Table 22.1. Despite their frequency in other immunocompromised patients, *Nocardia* and *Legionella* are rarely isolated from HIV patients. The overall importance of 'atypical' organisms, notably *Chlamydia pneumoniae*, is uncertain but cases have been reported (Visco Comandini *et al.*, 1997).

Pneumococcal pneumonia is at least 20 times more common in patients with HIV infection than in age-matched uninfected individuals (Witt *et al.*, 1987). There is a similar relative risk of developing invasive *H. influenzae* among HIV-infected patients (Farley *et al.*, 1992). Pneumococci are among the most common blood culture isolates from HIV-infected patients (Table 22.2). The rate of pneumococcal bacteraemia is 40 times higher in HIV-infected patients (Plouffe *et al.*, 1996) and up to 300 times higher in AIDS patients (Redd *et al.*, 1990; Schuchat *et al.*, 1991) than in uninfected subjects. HIV infection may be an independent risk factor for infection with penicillin-resistant *S. pneumoniae* (Bedos *et al.*, 1996).

Table 22.2 Causes of bacteraemia in HIV-infected patients

Study[a]	A	B	C	D	E	F	G	
No. of episodes[b]	38	33	44	NS[c]	NS	51	71	
No. of patients	29	33	38	135	47	51	58	
No. of bacterial isolates (total = 461) in indicated study								% of all isolates
Staphylococcus aureus	12	4	10	66	5	17	19	29
Coagulase negative staph	5	10	2	–	4	4	10	8
Pneumococcus	2	1	9	20	10	6	12	13
Other Gram-positives[d]	6	3	7	10	7	1	7	9
Salmonella spp.	7	14	5	14	3	3	11	12
Haemophilus influenzae	1	–	–	8	–	3	–	3
Pseudomonas aeruginosa	3	1	4	42	13	8	6	17
Other Gram-negatives[e]	2	2	11	–	5	9	15	10
Any organism								100%

[a]Key to studies. A: Whimbey *et al.*, 1986; B: Eng *et al.*, 1986; C: Krumholz *et al.*, 1989; D: Simberkoff and Leaf, 1992; E: Shanson, 1990; F: Fairfield Hospital, Melbourne, unpublished; G: Meyer *et al.*, 1994.
[b]Some patients had more than one episode, and some episodes were polymicrobial.
[c]NS = not stated.
[d]Including β haemolytic streptococci, viridans streptococci, *Enterococcus faecalis*, *Listeria monocytogenes*, *Clostridium perfringens*, and *Corynebacterium jeikeium*.
[e]Including enteric Gram-negative rods, *Stenotrophomonas maltophilia*, and *Neisseria meningitidis*.

Clinical features

HIV infection does not usually modify the clinical presentation of pneumococcal or *H. influenzae* pneumonia. Patients generally present with the abrupt onset of fever, sometimes with a shaking chill, accompanied by headache and other constitutional symptoms. Productive cough and pleuritic chest pain, if present, develop early in the course of the illness. On examination, patients with staphylococcal or Gram-negative bacillary pneumonia generally appear more unwell than those with pneumococcal pneumonia. Chest findings vary from those of classic consolidation to localized coarse crackles, or in rare instances, a normal examination. A pleural effusion may be evident at presentation, or may develop later (Schlamm and Yancovitz, 1989; Janoff *et al.*, 1993). Some patients present with a longer history, prominent dyspnoea and a non-productive cough (Moreno *et al.*, 1991), but concurrent opportunistic infections such as tuberculosis or *Pneumocystis carinii* pneumonia (PCP) may account for some of these atypical presentations.

As in HIV-uninfected individuals, local complications of pneumococcal pneumonia include empyema, recurrent pleural effusions and chest wall abscesses (Rodriguez-Barradas, 1992a). Pneumococcal meningitis, endocarditis, pericarditis and brain abscesses have all been described, but are probably no more common in HIV-infected patients. *Haemophilus influenzae* rarely causes infections outside the lung in adults.

A notable feature of HIV-associated bacterial pneumonia is the tendency for repeated episodes of infection to occur. Up to 24% of HIV patients with pneumococcal pneumonia develop a recurrence within 6 months of the original episode, a much higher rate than for those without HIV infection. The risk of recurrence is highest in those with low CD4 lymphocyte numbers (Janoff *et al.*, 1992; Gilks *et al.*, 1996).

Diagnosis

Bacterial pneumonia can often be diagnosed with a reasonable degree of confidence on the basis of the clinical presentation and a chest X-ray showing a localized lobar, segmental or subsegmental alveolar infiltrate. The white cell count may be increased, but is often normal or low if patients have advanced HIV disease or are being treated with myelosuppressive drugs such as zidovudine (ZDV). Differentiation of the two most common causes of bacterial pneumonia, pneumococcus and *H. influenzae*, is not possible on clinical or radiological grounds. The sputum Gram stain may indicate the most likely pathogen, but a reliable diagnosis depends upon isolation of the organism

Table 22.3 Features useful for differentiating bacterial from *Pneumocystis carinii* pneumonia

	Bacterial pneumonia	PCP
Onset	Acute: hours–days	Sub-acute: days–weeks
Cough	Productive	Non-productive
Pleuritic chest pain	Common	Uncommon
Shortness of breath	With chest pain	Prominent, especially on exertion
Pleural effusion	Common	Rare
Focal CXR infiltrate	Usual	Rare
White cell count	May be increased	Normal or low
CD4 count	Not helpful	Usually less than 200/μl
PCP prophylaxis	Any (including TMP-SMX)	None, or not TMP-SMX

CXR: chest X-ray; PCP: *Pneumocystis carinii* pneumonia; TMP-SMX: trimethoprim-sulphamethoxazole.

from blood cultures. Up to 60% of HIV-infected patients with pneumococcal pneumonia are bacteraemic, compared to only 15%–20% of HIV-uninfected patients, while bacteraemia occurs in 10–15% of HIV-infected patients with *Haemophilus influenzae* pneumonia (Schlamm and Yancovitz, 1989; Gordon *et al.*, 2001).

Enteric Gram-negative or staphylococcal infection should be suspected if bacterial pneumonia is nosocomially acquired, pursues a fulminant course, develops in a neutropenic patient, or occurs in an already moribund patient. *Pseudomonas* pneumonia may present in a similar fashion, but also occurs in patients from the community with a sub-acute or chronic course (discussed subsequently). Haematogenous staphylococcal pneumonia is seen in injecting drug users with right-sided endocarditis.

Rhodococcus equi pneumonia almost always occurs in patients with a CD4 lymphocyte count of less than 200 cells/μl. Features suggesting this diagnosis include cavitation on chest X-ray (present in 70% of cases), and pleural effusion (Capdevila *et al.*, 1997). The organism can be readily isolated from sputum if the laboratory is alerted, and blood cultures are positive in up to one-half of cases.

Nocardiosis also occurs in those with advanced immunosuppression, and usually presents as a chronic pneumonia or occasionally as a brain abscess (Javaly *et al.*, 1992). The chest X-ray shows localized or multifocal air space disease, but cavitation is present in less than one-quarter of cases. Extra-pulmonary spread to sites such as brain is common. Diagnosis can be suspected on Gram-staining appropriate clinical specimens (beaded, branching filamentous Gram-positive rods) and is confirmed by culture

– again, the laboratory must be alerted to the possibility of this infection.

The clinical features of bacterial pneumonia and PCP are usually distinctive enough for the two conditions to be readily distinguished from one another. A short history (less than 1 week) with productive cough and pleuritic chest pain, signs of consolidation, a localized infiltrate on chest X-ray, the presence of pleural fluid and a rapid response to non-trimethoprim-sulphamethoxazole (TMP-SMX) antibacterial therapy are all suggestive of bacterial pneumonia (Table 22.3). However, as with any infection, the spectrum of clinical and radiological manifestations of both bacterial pneumonia and PCP is wide, and occasionally features of the two infections may overlap. For example, patients presenting with what appears to be bacterial pneumonia who do not respond to treatment may have 'atypical' PCP. The possibility of dual infection also needs to be kept in mind. In a patient with presumed or confirmed PCP, failure to respond to specific therapy or excessive systemic toxicity suggests the possibility of a concurrent bacterial pneumonia and should prompt the use of empirical antibacterial therapy.

Tuberculosis (see Chapter 23) must always be considered in patients with pneumonia because of its protean manifestations, particularly in areas where co-infection with HIV and *Mycobacterium tuberculosis* is common. A prolonged cough and fever, weight loss and a cavitary infiltrate all increase the likelihood of tuberculosis (Selwyn *et al.*, 1998). Less common pneumonic processes occurring in HIV patients that may also warrant consideration include cryptococcal or aspergillus pneumonia, pulmonary Kaposi's sarcoma (KS) and pulmonary lymphoma (Table 22.4).

Table 22.4 Causes of localized pulmonary infiltrates in HIV-infected patients

Infections	Bacterial pneumonia
	Mycobacterium tuberculosis
	Cryptococcus neoformans
	Rhodococcus equi
	Aspergillus spp.
	Nocardia asteroides
Non-infectious conditions	Pulmonary KS
	Pulmonary lymphoma

KS: Kaposi's sarcoma.

Treatment

Many factors influence the choice of an empirical anti-microbial regimen for treatment of bacterial pneumonia (Table 22.5).

Despite a growing tendency to use broad-spectrum agents such as third-generation cephalosporins or extended spectrum fluoroquinolones for both HIV and non-HIV-associated bacterial pneumonia, intravenous penicillin remains a very reasonable initial choice for the HIV-infected patient with community-acquired pneumonia of mild to moderate severity, especially if Gram-positive cocci are seen in sputum (Table 22.6). The presence of *in vitro* penicillin resistance does not appear to lessen the effectiveness of penicillin when treating pneumococcal pneumonia. If a diagnosis of *H. influenzae* is suggested by the sputum Gram stain, intravenous penicillin or ampicillin/amoxicillin is appropriate if β-lactamase-positive isolates are uncommon in the community, but otherwise a third-generation cephalosporin such as cefotaxime or ceftriaxone is recommended. Injecting drug users with severe community-

Table 22.5 Factors affecting choice of antimicrobials for pneumonia

- Whether the infection is community or nosocomially acquired
- The degree of immunosuppression, as reflected by the CD4 lymphocyte count
- The local prevalence of resistance of respiratory pathogens to antibiotics such as penicillin
- The presence of neutropenia
- The severity of pneumonia
- Epidemiological factors, such as injecting drug use

Table 22.6 Initial antibiotic treatment of bacterial pneumonia in HIV-infected patients

Clinical setting	Antibiotic
Community-acquired AND mild-to-moderate severity[a]	Penicillin G 1.2 g i.v. every 6 h or ceftriaxone 1 g i.v. daily[b]
Severe community-acquired[c] or penicillin allergy	Ceftriaxone 1–2 g i.v. daily[d] ± erythromycin 1 g i.v. every 6 h[e]
Nosocomial pneumonia or pneumonia with neutropenia	Ceftazidime 1–2 g i.v. every 8 h *and* antistaphylococcal penicillin[f] 2 g i.v. every 6 h

[a]Severity assessed by features including, but not limited to, blood pressure, extent of chest X-ray changes, arterial blood gases or oxygen saturation, presence of renal impairment (see Bartlett *et al.*, 1998).
[b]Choice will depend upon sputum Gram-stain result and local prevalence of penicillin resistance in *Haemophilus influenzae*.
[c]Coverage against *Pneumocystis carinii* pneumonia may be needed.
[d]Cefotaxime 1–2 g i.v. every 8–12 h is an alternative.
[e]Especially if clinical or epidemiological evidence of Legionnaire's disease (see text).
[f]If MRSA are prevalent, use vancomycin 1 g i.v. every 12 h instead.
MRSA: methicillin-resistant *Staphylococcus aureus*.

acquired pneumonia should receive antimicrobials active against staphylococci.

For neutropenic patients and those with nosocomial pneumonia, treatment should include an anti-staphylococcal agent (a β-lactamase-resistant penicillin, or vancomycin if methicillin-resistant *Staphylococcus aureus* [MRSA] is prevalent) and an anti-pseudomonal agent (usually ceftazidime with or without an aminoglycoside – see below). If features of both bacterial pneumonia and PCP are present, especially if the pneumonia is severe, a third-generation cephalosporin should be added to TMP-SMX. Once a specific organism is identified, treatment can be modified accordingly. As in HIV-uninfected patients, addition of erythromycin should be considered for those with severe community-acquired pneumonia, particularly if Legionnaire's disease is suggested by clinical features or local epidemiology.

Prevention

A reduction in bacterial infections, including bacterial pneumonia, occurs in patients being treated with potent combination antiretroviral treatment regimens (see Chapter 7) (Costagliola, 1998; Moore *et al.*, 1998), just as the incidence of other opportunistic infections has fallen with this therapy. Authorities such as the US Centers for

Disease Control and Prevention (1997) have recommended immunization of all HIV-infected patients with the 23-valent polysccharide pneumococcal vaccine. The results of a case–control study supported this recommendation (Beall et al., 1998). However, a recent randomized, placebo-controlled trial in Ugandan adults failed to demonstrate a protective effect of the vaccine against pneumococcal disease (French et al., 2000).

A satisfactory antibody response to the pneumococcal vaccine is more likely to occur in patients with a CD4 lymphocyte count of 500/μl or more (Rodriguez-Barradas et al., 1992b; Dworkin et al., 2001), although ZDV may augment responses at lower CD4 counts (Glaser et al., 1991). A new 5-valent pneumococcal polysaccharide protein conjugate vaccine does not appear to improve antibody responses in patients with lower CD4 counts (Ahmed et al., 1996). In patients being treated with one or two antiretroviral drugs, immunization with the pneumococcal polysaccharide vaccine can lead to transient, and usually minor increases in HIV viral load (Brichacek et al., 1996) but these increases are blunted or abolished if highly active combination antiretroviral drug regimens are used (Cutillar-Garcia et al., 1998).

The conjugate H. influenzae type b vaccine is immunogenic in HIV-infected patients (Steinhoff et al., 1991), but its routine use is not recommended at present because it can only confer protection against type-b infections, its efficacy is unknown in HIV-infected patients and the overall importance of H. influenzae infections in these patients is still unclear.

Life-long prophylaxis with penicillin V, 250 mg twice a day, should be considered for HIV-infected patients after a single bacteraemic or two or more non-bacteraemic pneumococcal infections. Similar indications (using amoxicillin or amoxicillin/clavulanic acid) apply for H. influenzae infections. The use of TMP-SMX prophylaxis for PCP also confers some protection against bacterial pneumonia (Hirschtick et al., 1995), but the prevalence of pneumococci resistant to folate antagonists is increasing.

Intravenous gamma globulin is expensive and inconvenient to administer but may have a role if vaccination and antibiotic prophylaxis fail. The recommended dose is 400 mg/kg, administered monthly. In patients with advanced HIV infection and neutropenia, administration of granulocyte-colony stimulating factor (G-CSF) has reduced the rate of bacterial infections (although not specifically bacterial pneumonia), and infection-related hospitalizations (Kuritzkes et al., 1998).

Sinusitis

Sinusitis is a frequent and troublesome complication of HIV infection. In common with bacterial pneumonia, sinusitis may occur in patients with relatively well-preserved immune function, but it becomes more common with advanced immunosuppression, and the disease frequently recurs.

Epidemiology and aetiology

Most patients with sinusitis have a CD4 lymphocyte count of less than 200 cells/μl. There are numerous causes of sinusitis (Table 22.7) and determination of the aetiological agent is confounded by the presence of colonizing organisms. The most commonly isolated bacteria are S. pneumoniae, Pseudomonas aeruginosa, Staphylococcus aureus and anaerobic organisms (Table 22.7). Occasional cases of sinusitis due to opportunistic bacteria such as mycobacteria and Legionella have been described. Aspergillus is the most important cause of fungal sinusitis, and sinusitis due to parasites such as Microsporidia has been reported (Dunand et al., 1997).

Clinical features

Most patients with sinusitis have a sub-acute or chronic illness and complain of fever, headache and nasal discharge, but only a small proportion have more specific findings such as facial pain or sinus tenderness (Godofsky et al., 1992). Notably, when the presenting syndrome is fever and headache alone, the diagnosis of sinusitis is often delayed. Some patients are discovered to have incidental sinusitis on

Table 22.7 Causes of sinusitis in HIV-infected patients

Bacterial	Streptococcus pneumoniae
	Pseudomonas aeruginosa
	Staphylococcus aureus
	Legionella pneumophila
Mycobacterial	MAC
	Mycobacterium kansasii
Fungal	Aspergillus spp.
Protozoal	Encephalitozoon intestinalis
	Encephalitozoon hellem
	Cryptosporidium parvum
	Acanthamoeba species
	Pneumocystis carinii
Viral	CMV

MAC: Mycobacterium avium complex; CMV: cytomegalovirus.

computed tomographic (CT) scanning. *Aspergillus* sinusitis can be complicated by local invasion of surrounding structures, leading to signs of orbital, cavernous sinus or brain involvement.

Diagnosis

CT scanning of sinuses is substantially more sensitive than plain sinus radiography in indicating the extent of sinus disease (Godofsky *et al.*, 1992). Specific signs of sinusitis are mucosal thickening, sinus opacification and the presence of an air–fluid level. Bony erosion suggests fungal or *Pseudomonas* sinusitis. More than 80% of patients have bilateral disease. The maxillary sinus is most commonly involved, but many patients will also have infection of ethmoid and sphenoid sinuses.

A microbiological diagnosis is not obtained at the outset in most cases. Examination of nasal discharge is generally not helpful, except for diagnosis of microsporidial sinusitis, where organisms can be visualized using a modified trichrome stain of a nasopharyngeal aspirate. When surgery is performed for diagnostic or therapeutic reasons, specimens from the involved sinus should be sent for routine, mycobacterial, fungal and microsporidial studies.

Treatment

Most patients with sinusitis can be treated medically. Amoxicillin (alone, or with clavulanic acid), a second- or third generation oral cephalosporin or a macrolide are reasonable empirical oral antibiotics, while a third-generation cephalosporin such as cefotaxime or ceftriaxone should be used if intravenous treatment is required. Antipseudomonal treatment (discussed subsequently) should be considered in patients with a low CD4 lymphocyte count not responding to first-line antibiotics. Patients should also be treated with adjunctive analgesics and decongestants.

Indications for early surgery include sinusitis with systemic toxicity not responding rapidly to medical therapy and the presence of complications such as extension of infection into the orbit. Surgery should also be considered for those with recurrent disease, in whom sinus drainage may not only be useful therapeutically but will also provide specimens for diagnosis of more unusual causes of sinusitis.

Patients with non-bacterial sinusitis should receive treatment directed against the specific cause. *Aspergillus* sinusitis requires a combined medical (amphotericin B or itraconazole) and surgical approach (Mylonakis *et al.*,

1997). Microsporidial sinusitis due to *Encephalitozoon intestinalis* responds well to albendazole (see Chapter 30).

Prognosis

Most patients with bacterial sinusitis will improve with an initial course of antibiotics, although complete clinical and radiological responses are unusual. Unfortunately, most patients will relapse, often within 3 months of the initial episode (Godofsky *et al.*, 1992). The optimal management of recurrent disease is unknown. Surgery should be considered, as discussed above. Prophylactic (or more accurately, suppressive) antibiotics are often used, but their effectiveness is unclear and development of antibiotic resistance or superinfection with a resistant organism is always a concern. Hopefully, HAART will provide some benefit for patients with this difficult-to-treat infection.

Aspergillus sinusitis is a very serious condition, and survival 6 months beyond diagnosis is uncommon, even with optimum medical therapy and aggressive surgery.

Bacterial gastroenteritis – *Salmonella*, *Campylobacter* and *Shigella* infections

Epidemiology

Salmonella, *Campylobacter* and *Shigella* are important pathogens in HIV-infected patients, as well as being common causes of bacterial gastroenteritis in the general community. *Salmonella* and *Campylobacter* infections are 20–40 times more common in HIV-infected patients than in those without HIV infection (Celum *et al.*, 1987; Sorvillo *et al.*, 1991). Both of these infections were part of the spectrum of the so-called 'gay bowel syndrome' in the pre-AIDS era, but they can occur in HIV-infected members of any risk group. In addition to specific immune abnormalities, factors such as antibiotic use, achlorhydria and chronic haemolysis (with elevated plasma iron concentrations) may also contribute to the increased risk of developing these infections.

The most common *Salmonella* isolates are *Salmonella enteritidis* and *Salmonella typhimurium* (Table 22.8). *Campylobacter jejuni* is the usual *Campylobacter* isolate, but infections with other species such as *C. lari* (previously *C. laridis*), *C. coli* and *C. upsaliensis*, and with organisms of the related *Helicobacter* genus also occur. *Shigella* infections are less common than *Salmonella* or *Campylobacter*. In the setting of HIV infection, infections caused by these bacteria are more likely to be complicated by a prolonged course, bacteraemia and recurrent disease.

Table 22.8 Causes of bacterial gastroenteritis in HIV-infected patients

Common	Salmonella enteritidis
	Salmonella typhimurium
	Campylobacter jejuni
	Shigella spp.
	Clostridium difficile
Other organisms	Other Salmonella spp., e.g. cholerae suis
	Campylobacter coli
	Campylobacter upsaliensis
	Campylobacter lari
	Campylobacter fetus
	Helicobacter cinaedi
	Helicobacter fennelliae

Clinical features

Patients with bacterial gastroenteritis usually present with the abrupt onset of fever, cramping abdominal pain and diarrhoea. The diarrhoea is often watery and voluminous at the onset of the illness, but symptoms of colitis such as blood or mucus in the stool and tenesmus may predominate later, particularly with Campylobacter and Shigella infections. Most infections are acute and self-limiting.

The syndrome of bacteraemia without prominent gastrointestinal symptoms occurs in up to 30% of Salmonella infections and may also occur with Campylobacter infections, particularly those due to less common species such as C. fetus, Helicobacter cinaedi and Helicobacter fennelliae (Costel et al., 1984; Ng et al., 1987). Metastatic foci of infection including endocarditis, osteomyelitis, pneumonia and central nervous system (CNS) infections can complicate these primary bacteraemic infections (Fernandez Guerrero et al., 1997).

Recurrent salmonellosis, manifest as either gastroenteritis or bacteraemia, occurs in up to 25% of patients, more commonly in patients with AIDS than in those without and in those who were bacteraemic initially (Nelson et al., 1992). Recurrent disease develops in a similar proportion of patients with Campylobacter jejuni infections (Nelson et al., 1992). Persistent (as opposed to recurrent) disease can complicate Campylobacter and Shigella infections (Perlman et al., 1988; Blaser et al., 1989).

Diagnosis

The diagnosis of bacterial gastroenteritis should be suspected in any patient presenting with an acute onset of fever and diarrhoea. The various bacterial causes of gastroenteritis cannot usually be differentiated on purely clinical grounds, although features of colitis are more common with Campylobacter and Shigella infections. A faecal smear will often contain leucocytes, although less commonly with Salmonella infections.

A specific diagnosis depends upon isolation of the causative organism from faecal cultures. Some non-jejuni Campylobacter and Helicobacter organisms require special techniques such as membrane filtration, prolonged incubation at temperatures above 37°C and molecular biological methods for their isolation and identification (Snidjers et al., 1997). Blood cultures should be obtained from all patients. They are positive in up to 50% of Salmonella infections and in 10–15% of Campylobacter infections (Nelson et al., 1992).

The differential diagnosis includes Clostridium difficile diarrhoea ('antibiotic-associated colitis'), particularly if antibiotics have been taken recently. Cytomegalovirus (CMV) colitis (see Chapter 21) may also mimic bacterial gastroenteritis, but occurs almost exclusively in patients with less than 50 CD4 lymphocytes/μl. Amoebic dysentery is an uncommon infection in HIV-infected patients. Cryptosporidial diarrhoea is usually chronic, profuse and not associated with fever (see Chapter 30). Because the clinical spectrum of bacterial gastroenteritis includes syndromes such as chronic or watery diarrhoea, and because bacterial infection can coexist with other causes of diarrhoea, cultures for bacterial pathogens should always be obtained in the initial evaluation of any HIV-infected patient with diarrhoea, and at the time of exacerbations of chronic diarrhoea, due to a known, non-bacterial cause.

Treatment

Empirical antimicrobial therapy is warranted in HIV-infected patients with a clinical diagnosis of acute bacterial gastroenteritis because early treatment shortens the duration of the disease, interrupts shedding and transmission, and because many patients are bacteraemic. Antimicrobial therapy is essential if the patient is immunodeficient (less than 200 CD4 lymphocytes/μl). The rare patients who require parenteral therapy can be treated with either intravenous ciprofloxacin or a third-generation cephalosporin (cefotaxime or ceftriaxone) and an aminoglycoside (gentamicin) (Table 22.9). Otherwise, oral ciprofloxacin or norfloxacin is begun, pending faecal culture results. If there is reason to suspect a quinolone-resistant Campylobacter

Table 22.9 Treatment of bacterial gastroenteritis in HIV-infected patients

Clinical setting	Recommended treatment
Empirical therapy	
Oral	Ciprofloxacin 500 mg orally every 12 h[a]
Parenteral	Ciprofloxacin 200 mg i.v. every 12 h
	OR cefotaxime 1 g i.v. every 8 h
	+ gentamicin 1 mg/kg i.v. every 8 h
Specific oral therapy	
Salmonella spp.	Ciprofloxacin 500 mg every 12 h for 3–5 days[b]
Campylobacter jejuni	Erythromycin 250 mg every 6 h for 10–14 days
Shigella spp.	Ciprofloxacin 500 mg every 12 h 3–5 days
Non-jejuni Campylobacter or Helicobacter spp.	Erythromycin 250 mg every 6 h for 10–14 days[c]

[a]Erythromycin indicated if suspicion for Campylobacter infection is strong – see text for details.
[b]If bacteraemic, treat for 14 days.
[c]Parenteral treatment with an aminoglycoside is recommended if these organisms are isolated from blood. Subsequent treatment will depend upon the clinical response, and the results of susceptibility testing – most infections can be treated with either erythromycin or ciprofloxacin.

infection (see below) (for example, if there is a high rate of quinolone resistance in the community or a past Campylobacter infection did not respond to or relapsed after quinolone treatment), erythromycin should be started instead.

For patients with proven salmonellosis, treatment with a quinolone agent should be continued, even if the isolate is sensitive to amoxicillin or TMP-SMX. Quinolones shorten the duration of the illness more effectively than other agents, and they may also reduce relapse rates (Jacobson et al., 1989). Quinolone resistance remains uncommon among non-typhi Salmonella isolates. The recommended duration of therapy is 3–5 days for uncomplicated infections, and 14 days if blood cultures are positive. Quinolones are also the treatment of choice for Shigella infections.

The preferred antimicrobial for treatment of Campylobacter jejuni infections is uncertain. Rates of quinolone resistance among Campylobacter jejuni are increasing in many areas of the world (Kuschner et al., 1995). In addition, there are reports of resistance to quinolones and macrolide agents developing during therapy of these infections in HIV-infected patients (Tee et al., 1995). The frequency with which such resistance develops is unknown. Erythromycin or another macrolide such as clarithromycin is preferred as the initial treatment for C. jejuni infections and should be continued for 10–14 days. Combination macrolide and quinolone treatment may lessen the rate of emergence of resistance and reduce the risk of relapse but has not been assessed in a systematic fashion.

Treatment of Helicobacter and drug-resistant Campylobacter infections is difficult, as third-generation cephalosporins are not uniformly active against these organisms. Initial treatment with an aminoglycoside such as gentamicin is recommended until the results of susceptibility tests become available. A 14-day treatment course can usually be completed with either erythromycin or a quinolone unless the organism is resistant to these drugs, in which case the aminoglycoside should be continued, or other drugs such as doxycycline or chloramphenicol considered.

Long-term ciprofloxacin is advised for patients with a single prior episode of Salmonella bacteraemia and for patients with two or more episodes of gastroenteritis. The role of prolonged therapy for Campylobacter infections is less clear because of concerns about the development of resistance.

Prevention

All HIV-infected patients should be counselled about food handling and preparation practices that will lessen the risk of infection and cross-contamination by enteric pathogens (Griffin and Tauxe, 1988). Patients with Salmonella or Campylobacter infection who are either food handlers or health-care providers must be given specific advice about the risk of transmission. HIV-infected patients should also follow simple measures that will lessen the risk of acquisition of enteric pathogens from animals (Centers for Disease Control and Prevention [CDC], 1997). HIV-infected travellers to developing countries will need specific advice about precautions to minimize the risk of travellers' diarrhoea (see Chapter 37).

In addition to its antiretroviral activity, ZDV has activity against coliforms, including *Salmonella* species, and ZDV may prevent relapses of *Salmonella* bacteraemia (Salmon *et al.*, 1991). A similar effect has not been observed with *Campylobacter* infections. Prophylactic antibiotics are not generally advised for HIV-infected travellers (see Chapter 37).

Staphylococcal infections

Epidemiology

Staphylococci are common pathogens in HIV-infected patients (Jacobson *et al.*, 1988). *Staphylococcus aureus* and coagulase-negative staphylococci are the most common blood culture isolates in this population (Table 22.2). Factors that predispose to staphylococcal infections in these patients include indwelling intravenous devices, neutropenia, abnormalities of neutrophil function (Ellis *et al.*, 1988), injecting drug use, prior hospitalization, increased rates of *Staphylococcus aureus* nasal carriage (Raviglione *et al.*, 1990) and pre-existing skin conditions, such as psoriasis.

Clinical presentation

Vascular catheter infections

Coagulase-positive and -negative staphylococci are the most common causes of vascular catheter-related infections in HIV-infected patients, as they are in other patient populations. Gram-negative organisms and fungi account for a smaller number of cases (Raviglione *et al.*, 1989; Skoutelis *et al.*, 1990). Infection rates of long-term venous catheters such as the Hickman catheter or Port-A-Cath® are generally higher in HIV-infected patients than other patients, probably because the catheters are manipulated more frequently and average neutrophil counts are lower in HIV-infected patients. Fever without any other obvious infected focus is the most common presentation. Patients may have signs of local inflammation (at the exit site, along the subcutaneous tunnel or around the implanted device) with or without bacteraemia, or bacteraemia may occur in the absence of local signs. Metastatic foci of infection such as endocarditis or pulmonary abscesses are uncommon.

Skin infections

Staphylococcus aureus causes troublesome skin infections that frequently recur or persist and may be difficult to treat. Examples include folliculitis, furunculosis, bullous impetigo and superinfection of other skin conditions such as psoriasis. These infections are more common with advanced HIV infection. They are not usually associated with fever, leucocytosis or lymphadenopathy and complications such as bacteraemia are rare. The lesions of staphylococcal folliculitis are pustular and pruritic. They are distributed on the face, upper trunk and upper arms and are difficult to differentiate from another common HIV-related skin complication, eosinophilic pustular folliculitis (see Chapter 19). Staphylococcal furuncles occur in warm, moist, hair-bearing areas such as the nape of the neck, axillae, groins and natal cleft.

Pyomyositis

This infection, an abscess of skeletal muscle, is common in tropical countries (hence the alternative name tropical pyomyositis), but until recently was rare in the Western world. There have now been numerous reports of pyomyositis in association with HIV infection (Gaut *et al.*, 1988; Schwartzman *et al.*, 1991). Involved muscles include those of the lower limbs, psoas, anterior chest wall, and paraspinal muscles. Patients present with fever and pain in the affected area. Some patients are critically ill, but most exhibit only mild-to-moderate systemic upset. Swelling may or may not be a prominent feature, and erythema is usually absent. Diagnosis is often delayed because of the non-specific early clinical features. The pathogenesis of these infections is unknown, but bacteraemic seeding seems more likely than direct inoculation. Most patients have low CD4 lymphocyte numbers, but they are usually not neutropenic. The majority of these infections are due to *Staphylococcus aureus*, but other organisms such as haemolytic streptococci have also been isolated (Schwartzman *et al.*, 1991).

Endocarditis

Endocarditis associated with HIV infection is usually seen in injecting drug users and the clinical presentation, response to treatment and prognosis resemble the course seen in HIV-uninfected patients (Nahass *et al.*, 1990). Tricuspid endocarditis is more common than mitral or aortic disease. *Staphylococcus aureus* is the most common aetiological agent, but fungi and many other bacteria are occasionally isolated. For practical purposes, all patients will have positive blood cultures.

Other infections

Other manifestations of staphylococcal infection occur late in the course of HIV infection. Staphylococcal bacteraemia in the absence of an indwelling vascular line or other obvious focus (primary bacteraemia) is usually a terminal event often associated with neutropenia. Staphylococcal pneumonia is usually nosocomially acquired and has a high mortality, but community-acquired staphylococcal pneumonia also occurs, chiefly in injecting drug users, and has a relatively good prognosis (Tumbarello et al., 1996). Focal staphylococcal infections can occasionally be complicated by the toxic shock syndrome.

Diagnosis

Staphylococci should be considered as potential pathogens in patients presenting with the illnesses and syndromes listed above. Many patients, particularly those with advanced HIV infection, do not have leucocytosis. Depending on the site of infection, cultures of pus, blood, tissue or catheter tips should be obtained. Blood cultures positive for *Staphylococcus aureus* almost always indicate true bacteraemia. For practical purposes, significant coagulase negative staphylococcal bacteraemia only occurs in patients with an indwelling vascular catheter or a prosthetic heart valve and in patients who are profoundly neutropenic. Ultrasound or CT scanning is needed to demonstrate intramuscular abscesses.

Treatment

The management of an infected intravenous catheter will depend on the clinical condition of the patient, the particular type of intravenous access device, the extent of local infection and the species of staphylococcus isolated. Catheter removal is usually necessary, especially under the circumstances outlined in Table 22.10.

In the absence of these features, a trial of antibiotics can be attempted, with the catheter left *in situ*, if the infection is due to a coagulase-negative staphylococcus.

Most localized collections need to be drained, and for pyomyositis, this can often be accomplished percutaneously under CT or ultrasound guidance. Rarely, open drainage may be required.

Anti-staphylococcal antibiotics are the mainstay of treatment (Table 22.11). Until identification and sensitivity

Table 22.10 Mandatory indications for removal of an indwelling intravenous catheter in a patient with staphylococcal bacteraemia

- If the patient is critically ill
- If a subcutaneous tunnel infection is present
- If infection is present around an implanted subcutaneous port
- If *Staphylococcus aureus* is isolated from blood cultures
- If the patient remains febrile 48–72 h after appropriate antibiotics are started
- If metastatic foci of infection are present, especially pulmonary emboli

results are available, vancomycin should be used for nosocomial infections where MRSA is likely, and for intravenous catheter infections (because of the high prevalence of methicillin resistance among coagulase-negative staphylococci). Methicillin-sensitive infections are treated with an anti-staphylococcal penicillin such as flucloxacillin or a first-generation cephalosporin such as cephalothin or cephalexin. Clindamycin or a macrolide agent are other options for therapy of these infections, especially in those allergic to β-lactams.

Prevention

Careful catheter insertion under prophylactic antibiotic cover and meticulous catheter care should help prevent catheter-related infections (Battan et al., 1990). Eradication of nasal carriage of *Staphylococcus aureus* is often difficult to achieve but is indicated for those with recurrent skin infections. Intranasal mupirocin ointment (applied twice a day for 5 days) is the treatment of choice (Martin et al., 1999) and may be combined with other measures such as regular washing with chlorhexidine and treatment of household contacts.

Pseudomonas infections

Epidemiology

Infections with *Pseudomonas aeruginosa* and related organisms such as *Stenotrophomonas* (previously *Xanthomonas*) *maltophilia* have become common in immunosuppressed HIV patients. They usually occur late in the course of HIV infection in patients with a preceding AIDS-defining illness (Roilides et al., 1992; Fichtenbaum et al., 1994). Additional risk factors include presence of urinary or long-term

Table 22.11 Recommended antimicrobials for staphylococcal infections

Drug	Dose
Parenteral agents	
Anti-staphylococcal penicillins	
flucloxacillin, oxacillin, nafcillin	1–2 g i.v. every 4–6 h[a]
Parenteral cephalosporins	
First generation, e.g. cephalothin	1–2 g i.v. every 6 h[a]
Second generation, e.g. cefuroxime[b]	0.75–1.5 g i.v. every 8 h
Third generation, e.g. cefotaxime[b]	1–2 g i.v. every 8 h
Vancomycin	1 g i.v. every 12 h[c]
Oral agents	
Anti-staphylococcal penicillins	
flucloxacillin, cloxacillin, dicloxacillin	250–500 mg orally every 6 h
Amoxicillin/clavulanic acid	250/125–500/125 mg orally every 8 h
Oral cephalosporins	
cephalexin	250–500 mg orally every 6 h
cefaclor	250–500 mg orally every 8 h
Clindamycin	300 mg orally every 8 h
Erythromycin	250–500 mg orally every 6 h

[a]The higher doses are recommended for treatment of endocarditis.
[b]These agents are not considered first-line anti-staphylococcal agents.
[c]The dose should be reduced in patients with renal impairment, guided by serum levels.
[d]Other macrolide agents (roxithromycin, azithromycin, clarithromycin) have similar anti-staphylococcal activity.

vascular catheters, steroid therapy and neutropenia (Dropulic et al., 1995). In contrast to other immuno-suppressed patient groups, many pseudomonal infections in HIV-infected patients are community-acquired, although most of these patients have been hospitalized previously (Fichtenbaum et al., 1994; Sorvillo et al., 2001).

Clinical features
Bacteraemia
Of this group of bacteria, Pseudomonas aeruginosa and Stenotrophomonas maltophilia are the most common causes of bacteraemia in HIV-infected patients (Table 22.2). Bacteraemias caused by these organisms commonly arise from infected venous catheters (Nelson et al., 1991; Mendelson et al., 1994; Dropulic et al., 1995), and such infections are more likely to be associated with severe signs of sepsis than are intravascular device infections caused by other organisms. Both removal of the catheter and antibiotics are essential for eradication of these infections. Pseudomonas aeruginosa bacteraemia may also complicate primary infections of lung, soft tissue or urinary tract and occurs occasionally in the absence of any readily identifiable focus, especially in the setting of pre-terminal HIV infection or neutropenia.

Bronchopulmonary infections
Two patterns of Pseudomonas aeruginosa respiratory tract infection occur. Nosocomial Pseudomonas aeruginosa pneumonia manifests as severe pneumonia with sepsis. The chest radiograph usually shows a non-cavitary infiltrate, blood cultures are often positive and the mortality rate is high. In contrast, patients with community-acquired infection present with a subacute or chronic illness with few systemic findings. An excavated pulmonary infiltrate is seen in up to one-half of patients. The condition is rarely fatal, but the organism is difficult to eradicate, and recurrent or persistent infection is common (Baron and Hollander, 1993; Schuster and Norris, 1994; Dropulic et al., 1995). This syndrome resembles that seen in cystic fibrosis patients with persistent Pseudomonas aeruginosa airways colonization. Some HIV-infected patients with Pseudomonas aeruginosa in sputum have a normal chest X-ray but improve with specific antipseudomonal therapy, suggesting that Pseudomonas tracheobronchitis is part of the spectrum of this syndrome.

Other sites of infection
Pseudomonas aeruginosa is an important cause of sinusitis in HIV-infected patients (discussed previously). Catheter-related urinary tract infections, malignant otitis externa, eye

infections and skin and soft-tissue infections due to *Pseudomonas aeruginosa* also occur, usually as late complications of HIV infection.

Diagnosis

Diagnosis ultimately rests on demonstration of the organism in blood, sputum, pus or other tissue. Pending laboratory confirmation, pseudomonal infections should be suspected in very ill patients with a vascular catheter-related infection, in patients with one of the two pneumonia syndromes described above and in febrile neutropenic patients or those with septic shock. *Pseudomonas aeruginosa* should not necessarily be dismissed as a contaminant or colonizer in sputum from patients with otherwise unexplained chronic respiratory symptoms, with or without a chest X-ray infiltrate.

Treatment

Vascular catheters suspected or documented as the source of sepsis must always be removed. Neutropenic patients should be treated with two antipseudomonal antibiotics; for example, an aminoglycoside in combination with either an extended-spectrum penicillin such as piperacillin, a third-generation antipseudomonal cephalosporin such as ceftazidime, or imipenem (Table 22.12). Monotherapy with either of the latter two agents is acceptable in non-neutropenic patients, although the risk of development of antibacterial resistance is probably higher than when two agents are used.

Providing the patient is afebrile, clinically stable and not neutropenic, treatment with oral ciprofloxacin can follow an initial course of intravenous therapy. This allows discharge from hospital, a highly desirable goal in this group of patients with late-stage HIV disease. Total treatment duration will vary, but needs to be prolonged (3–4 weeks) in cases of *Pseudomonas aeruginosa* pneumonia.

The place of chronic suppressive therapy is unknown, but emergence of resistance is an obvious concern. Some patients with chronic *Pseudomonas aeruginosa* pneumonia have been treated successfully with long-term administration of inhaled aerosolized antibiotics such as aminoglycosides or colistin (Zylberberg *et al.*, 1996). In common with some other infections, use of HAART with improvement in immune function has been reported to control this difficult-to-treat infection (Domingo *et al.*, 1998).

Stenotrophomonas maltophilia is resistant to most antibiotics except TMP-SMX. Antibiotic selection is difficult

Table 22.12 Recommended antimicrobials for pseudomonas infections

Drug	Dose
Anti-pseudomonal penicillins[a]	
Ticarcillin	3 g i.v. every 4 h
Mezlocillin	3 g i.v. every 4 h
Piperacillin	3 g i.v. every 6 h
Anti-pseudomonal cephalosporins[b]	
Ceftazidime	1–2 g i.v. every 8 h
Cefaperazone	1–2 g i.v. every 8 h
Cefipime	1–2 g i.v. every 12 h
Carbapenems[b]	
Imipenem	0.5–1 g i.v. every 6–8 h
Meropenem	0.5–1 g i.v. every 8 h
Ciprofloxacin	300 mg i.v. every 12 h
	500–750 mg orally every 12 h
Aminoglycosides[c]	
Gentamicin or tobramycin	1.0–1.5 mg/kg i.v. every 8 h
	or 4–6 mg/kg i.v. daily
Amikacin	5.0–7.5 mg/kg i.v. every 12 h
	or 15 mg/kg i.v. daily

[a]These agents should always be combined with an aminoglycoside, unless the infection is confined to the urinary tract.
[b]Generally combine with an aminoglycoside, especially if the patient is neutropenic (neutrophils less than 500 cells/μl), or has a life-threatening infection such as endocarditis or pneumonia.
[c]Dosage adjustment required with renal impairment.

if the patient is allergic to TMP-SMX, and must be guided by the results of antibiotic susceptibility testing.

Bacillary angiomatosis peliosis

History and bacteriology

Bacillary angiomatosis, also known as epithelioid angiomatosis, was first reported in an HIV-infected man with skin lesions resembling KS (Stoler *et al.*, 1983). On histological examination, organisms were noted with morphological and staining characteristics similar to those seen in cat-scratch disease, hence the early designation of this condition as disseminated cat-scratch disease. The DNA extracted from these skin lesions was found to contain ribosomal RNA gene sequences very similar to those of rickettsia-like organisms belonging to the genus *Rochalimaea* (Relman *et al.*, 1990).

The clinical spectrum of this disease has subsequently expanded. The varied clinical manifestations are due to one of two organisms, which have now been reclassified into the genus *Bartonella*. The organisms can be cultured from involved tissues (Slater *et al.*, 1992). Some infections are due to a newly recognized *Bartonella* species, *Bartonella henselae*, while *Bartonella quintana*, the agent of trench fever, is isolated from other patients (Koehler *et al.*, 1992). The disease is now referred to as bacillary angiomatosis-peliosis.

Epidemiology

Members of the cat family are the likely reservoir of *Bartonella henselae*. Many patients with bacillary angiomatosis-peliosis have pet cats and the organism can be cultured from the blood of these cats, as well as from fleas combed from the cats (Koehler *et al.*, 1994). It is not known whether the organism is transmitted by the bite or scratch of an infected cat, or by the bite of an infected flea. Many, if not all, cases of cat-scratch disease are due to *Bartonella henselae* (Dolan *et al.*, 1993).

From studies of trench fever in World War I, *Bartonella quintana* was known to be transmitted by the human body louse. Among HIV-infected patients, infection with *Bartonella quintana* is associated with exposure to lice, as well as with homelessness and low income (Koehler *et al.*, 1997).

Clinical presentation

Bacillary angiomatosis-peliosis is a rare complication of late-stage HIV infection. Most patients have a CD4 lymphocyte count of less than 50 cells/μl, and have had a prior AIDS-defining opportunistic infection or malignancy.

The cutaneous lesions (bacillary angiomatosis) are pinkish or red papules that can enlarge, become nodular and sometimes ulcerate. The number of lesions and their size is variable. They can resemble KS, but they can be usually differentiated on histological grounds. Both *Bartonella henselae* and *Bartonella quintana* cause these lesions (Koehler *et al.*, 1997). Subcutaneous nodules or masses with normal or erythematous overlying skin can also occur, especially with *Bartonella quintana* infections.

Some patients present with liver involvement, manifest histologically as numerous blood-filled spaces (peliosis hepatis) with organisms demonstrable on a silver stain. The spleen may also be involved. These patients may or may not have cutaneous lesions. Clinical features include fever, abdominal pain and hepatomegaly (Slater *et al.*, 1992). Peliosis hepatis is almost always due to *Bartonella henselae* infection (Koehler *et al.*, 1997).

Bacteraemia, producing persistent fevers and weight loss, may occur with or without cutaneous or visceral involvement. The clinical picture closely resembles that of other conditions causing fever and wasting such as disseminated *Mycobacterium avium* complex (MAC) infection.

Bacillary angiomatosis-peliosis has been described in many other organs and tissues, often without cutaneous disease. Involvement of long bones (almost always due to *Bartonella quintana*) manifests as bone pain and lytic lesions on X-ray. Polypoid and nodular lesions have been noted in the gastrointestinal and respiratory tract. Intracerebral space-occupying lesions similar to cerebral toxoplasmosis can occur and aseptic meningitis has been reported. Lymph node or tonsillar enlargement can accompany other forms of the disease or occur in isolation and is associated with *Bartonella henselae* infection. *Bartonella quintana* endocarditis has been described in a single HIV-infected patient.

Diagnosis

The possibility of bacillary angiomatosis-peliosis should be considered in patients with compatible clinical findings (Table 22.13). A biopsy of the involved tissue will often

Table 22.13 Manifestations of bacillary angiomatosis-peliosis

Feature	More usual causes
Cutaneous papules or nodules	KS, angiomas
Fevers, weight loss (wasting syndrome)	MAC
	Tuberculosis
	Lymphoma
Lytic (and usually painful) bony lesions	KS
	Lymphoma
Lymphadenopathy	HIV
	KS
	Mycobacteria
Hepatomegaly	MAC
	CMV
	KS
Peliosis hepatitis	KS
Endobronchial lesions	KS
Intracerebral space-occupying lesions	Cerebral toxoplasmosis
	Intracerebral lymphoma
Aseptic meningitis	Cryptococcal meningitis
	HIV
	Tuberculosis

KS: Kaposi's sarcoma; MAC: *Mycobacterium avium* complex; CMV: cytomegalovirus.

reveal characteristic histological changes – proliferation of small, capillary-sized blood vessels lined by cuboidal endothelial cells in involved skin, lymph nodes or bone, and dilated, thin-walled peliotic spaces in involved liver. Clumps of dark-staining, tangled bacilli are visible on silver stain. However, biopsies are not always diagnostic and the lesions can be confused with other conditions such as KS, pyogenic granuloma and angiosarcoma.

Definitive diagnosis rests on culture of the organism, which requires prolonged incubation in 5% CO_2 on chocolate or heart infusion agar (Slater et al., 1992). Up to one-half of patients with bacillary angiomatosis-peliosis will have positive blood cultures (Koehler et al., 1997), but the organism is difficult to grow from involved tissue. Molecular methods are used to identify organisms grown in culture or from paraffin-embedded tissue sections, by characterizing 16S ribosomal RNA gene sequences.

Serological assays (indirect immunofluorescence and enzyme immunoassay) can detect antibodies to Bartonella in patients with cat-scratch disease, but there is limited experience with these tests in HIV-associated bacillary angiomatosis-peliosis.

Treatment

Bartonella henselae and Bartonella quintana are sensitive to many antibacterial agents in vitro, but a macrolide agent (such as erythromycin 500 mg 6 hourly) or tetracycline 100 mg 12 hourly, either alone or in combination with rifampicin 300 mg 12 hourly, appear to be the agents of choice (Koehler et al., 1988). Treatment for 8–12 weeks is recommended for those who only have skin lesions or isolated bacteraemia. Response is usually satisfactory, but relapses can occur, in which case a longer course of therapy should be given. Patients with other forms of the disease should be treated for at least 3 months, and perhaps indefinitely, especially if clinical response is slow or relapse occurs (Koehler and Tappero, 1993).

Syphilis

Interactions between HIV and syphilis

Syphilis and HIV interact at multiple levels. Both are sexually transmitted diseases, and clinical or serological evidence of syphilis is reasonably common in individuals with sexually acquired HIV infection. In addition, early syphilis causes genital ulcer disease, which can facilitate HIV transmission or acquisition.

Most interest and controversy centres around whether HIV co-infection modifies the clinical course of syphilis, its serological expression or its treatment requirements (Musher et al., 1990). Early reports described unusual manifestations and treatment failures in HIV-infected patients with syphilis (Johns et al., 1987), and led some clinicians to advocate a different diagnostic and treatment approach when syphilis and HIV infection coexist. More recent prospective studies suggest that most cases of syphilis in HIV patients have clinical features virtually identical to those seen in HIV-uninfected patients (Gourevitch et al., 1993; Rolfs et al., 1997). Although unusual clinical and serological manifestations do occur, as do treatment failures, they are the exception rather than the rule.

Clinical presentation
Early syphilis

In most respects, HIV infection (regardless of the level of immusuppression) does not modify the clinical presentation of early (primary, secondary or early latent) syphilis. However, HIV-infected patients with early syphilis are more likely than non-HIV-infected patients to present with secondary disease, to have multiple chancres and to have coexistent secondary syphilis and a chancre (Hutchinson et al., 1994; Rolfs et al., 1997). Unusual manifestations of secondary syphilis, such as malignant syphilis (ulceronodular skin lesions and necrotizing vasculitis), are reported but rare (Rubinstein and Christie, 1995).

Neurosyphilis

Although comparative longitudinal studies have not been performed, reports of neurosyphilis in the USA indicate an increased proportion of cases of early neurosyphilis in the HIV era (Dowell et al., 1992; see Chapter 10). Early neurosyphilis manifests as aseptic meningitis, retinitis, cranial neuropathy (most commonly of cranial nerves II, VII and VIII), uveitis, polyradiculopathy or meningovascular syphilis. Some cases have occurred after treatment of early syphilis with the recommended dose of benzathine penicillin (see discussion below).

Asymptomatic cerebrospinal fluid (CSF) invasion by Treponema pallidum during primary or secondary syphilis occurs in up to 40% of patients with or without HIV infection (Rolfs et al., 1997). It is not known whether HIV-infected patients are more likely to develop asymptomatic neurosyphilis subsequently. Diagnosis of neurosyphilis has always been problematic, and in HIV-infected patients this issue is further complicated by the frequent occurrence of CSF abnormalities (abnormal cell count and raised protein level) unrelated to syphilis. Reported rates of asymptomatic neurosyphilis (variously defined) in latent syphilis have ranged from 9% (Holtom et al., 1992) to 17% (Tomberlin et al., 1994), to as high as 50% (Dowell et al., 1992).

Late neurosyphilis is much less common than early disease. Among 75 HIV-infected patients with neurosyphilis studied in San Francisco, only one had tabes dorsalis or general paresis, whereas 34 had early neurosyphilis (Flood et al., 1998).

Late syphilis

Non-neurological manifestations of late syphilis – cardio-vascular syphilis and gummatous disease – occur in HIV-infected patients but with an unknown frequency.

Diagnosis

Both non-treponemal (Venereal Disease Research Laboratory [VDRL] and rapid plasma reagin [RPR]) and treponemal (fluorescent treponemal antibody-absorbed [FTA-Abs] and microhaemagglutination-treponema palladium [MHA-TP]) tests can be affected by concurrent HIV infection. Biological false-positive non-treponemal tests are more common in patients with HIV infection than in those without (Rompalo et al., 1992), presumably because of polyclonal B-cell activation, and serum VDRL or RPR titres tend to be higher at each stage of syphilis in HIV-infected patients (Gourevitch et al., 1993). There have been a few reports of patients with secondary syphilis and negative VDRLs, but this phenomenon is very uncommon. Among those with a past history of syphilis, HIV infection has been associated with more frequent reversion of specific tests to negative in some (Johnson et al., 1991), but not all studies (Gourevitch et al., 1993). However, it is not known whether a negative-specific test can occur in patients with active disease.

As indicated above, diagnosis of neurosyphilis can be difficult in both HIV-infected and uninfected patients because of the varied clinical expression of this disease, the lack of a gold standard laboratory test and the relative insensitivity of the CSF VDRL test. Culture of the organism, by injection into rabbit testes, is limited to a few research laboratories. Viable Treponema pallidum organisms have been demonstrated in CSF with a negative VDRL test, and a normal cell count, protein and glucose (Lukehart et al., 1988). Recently, Treponema pallidum DNA has been detected in CSF following PCR amplification, but experience with the test is limited.

Treatment: regimens and results

Early syphilis

In the pre-AIDS penicillin era, early syphilis treatment failures (as indicated by the subsequent development of neurosyphilis) were exceedingly rare. However, a number of HIV-infected patients have developed early neurosyphilis after treatment of primary or secondary syphilis with the recommended doses of benzathine penicillin (Johns et al., 1987). It was hypothesized that standard treatment was relatively ineffective in HIV-infected patients because an impaired immune system was not able to act in concert with antibiotic therapy to control Treponema pallidum infection.

Fortunately, prospective studies have shown that HIV-infected patients with early syphilis respond as well to the recommended regimen of benzathine penicillin (2.4 million units i.m.) as do uninfected individuals (Gourevitch et al., 1993; Rolfs et al., 1997). Although an occasional treatment failure is possible, they are rare. Enhancement of the standard treatment regimen with a 10-day course of oral amoxicillin does not improve success rates (Rolfs et al., 1997). The non-treponemal (VDRL or RPR) titre falls more slowly in HIV-infected than in uninfected patients, leading to a higher proportion of serologically defined failures among HIV-infected patients (Rolfs et al., 1997), but the long-term clinical significance of this phenomenon is unknown.

Late syphilis

Just as with early syphilis, treatment failures have been reported in patients with late syphilis, predominantly neurosyphilis, despite adequate antibiotic therapy (Dowell et al., 1992; Gordon et al., 1994; Malone et al., 1995). However, other patients seem to respond well to such treatment (Flood et al., 1998).

Influential guidelines from the US CDC (1998) recommend similar syphilis treatment regimens for HIV-infected and uninfected patients (Table 22.14). For HIV-infected patients, more frequent serological monitoring of treatment response is advised, as is CSF examination in all those with latent syphilis present for more than 1 year or of unknown duration, and in those who do not exhibit a satisfactory serological response to treatment (Table 22.14). Treatment failure may not be a problem in countries such as the UK and Australia that have traditionally treated syphilis with daily intramuscular injections of procaine penicillin, rather than with benzathine penicillin as in the USA, but it seems prudent to follow the CDC recommendations concerning follow-up and CSF examination.

Table 22.14 Treatment of syphilis in HIV-infected individuals

Stage of syphilis	Treatment regimens	
	CDC guidelines[a]	Alternatives[b]
Primary Secondary	Benzathine penicillin 2.4×10^6 units i.m.	Procaine penicillin 1 g i.m. daily, 10 days
Early latent[c]	Single dose[d]	
Late latent[e]	Benzathine penicillin 2.4×10^6 units i.m. 3 weekly doses[d]	Procaine penicillin 1 g i.m. daily, 15 days
Neurosyphilis	Benzyl penicillin $10–20 \times 10^6$ units i.v. daily 10–14 days[d]	Procaine penicillin 2.4 g i.m. daily, 10–14 days, and Probenecid 500 mg every 6 h

[a]Centers for Disease Control and Prevention, 1998.
[b]For pregnant penicillin-allergic patients, or those with neurosyphilis, penicillin desensitization should be performed. For other penicillin-allergic patients, every effort should be made to verify the allergy, using skin testing if available. If penicillin cannot be given, alternatives are: (i) doxycycline 100 mg orally twice a day (or tetracycline 500 mg every 6 h), for 15 days for early syphilis and for 30 days for late syphilis, and (ii) ceftriaxone 1 g i.m. daily, for 7–10 days for early syphilis. Erythromycin is a less effective alternative.
[c]Within 1 year of secondary syphilis.
[d]Follow-up: early syphilis – clinical and serological at 3, 6, 9, 12 and 24 months; late latent – clinical and serological at 6, 12, 18 and 24 months; neurosyphilis – clinical, serological and cerebrospinal fluid at 6, 12, 18 and 24 months.
[e]Cerebrospinal fluid examination is recommended for latent syphilis of more than 1 year or of unknown duration, for clinical or serological treatment failures and for penicillin-allergic patients.

References

Ahmed F, Nelson KE, Musher DM *et al.* (1996). Effect of human immunodeficiency virus type 1 infection on the antibody response to a glycoprotein conjugate pneumococcal vaccine: results from a randomized trial. *J Infect Dis* **173**: 83–90.

Baron AD, Hollander H. (1993). Pseudomonas aeruginosa bronchopulmonary infections in late human immunodeficiency virus disease. *Am Rev Respir Dis* **148**: 992–6.

Bartlett JG, Breiman RF, Mandell LA *et al.* (1998). Guidelines from the Infectious Diseases Society of America. Community-acquired pneumonia in adults: guidelines for management. *Clin Infect Dis* **26**: 811–38.

Battan R, Raviglione MC, D'Amore T *et al.* (1990). Vancomycin prophylaxis for long term central venous catheter infections in AIDS patients. In: *Proceedings of the Sixth International Conference on AIDS*, San Francisco CA, USA, 254.

Beall G, Guerrero M, Kruger S *et al.* (1998). HIV-associated pneumonias: the efficacy of pneumococcal vaccine (PV). *Proceedings of the Twelfth International Conference on AIDS*, Geneva, Switzerland, abstract **22108**, p. 283.

Bedos J-P, Chevret S, Chastang C *et al.* (1996). Epidemiological features of and risk factors for infection by *Streptococcus pneumoniae* strains with diminished susceptibility to penicillin: findings of a French survey. *Clin Infect Dis* **22**: 63–72.

Blaser MJ, Hale TL, Formal SB. (1989). Recurrent shigellosis complicating human immunodeficiency virus infection: failure of pre-existing antibodies to confer protection. *Am J Med* **86**: 105–7.

Brichacek B, Stevenson M, Pirruccello S *et al.* (1996). Increased plasma human immunodeficiency virus type 1 burden following antigenic challenge with pneumococcal vaccine. *J Infect Dis* **174**: 1191–9.

Burack JH, Hahn JA, Saint-Maurice D *et al.* (1994). Microbiology of community-acquired pneumonia in persons with and at risk for human immunodeficiency virus type 1 infection. *Arch Intern Med* **154**: 2589–96.

Capdevila JA, Bujan S, Gavalda J *et al.* (1997). *Rhodococcus equi* pneumonia in patients infected with the human immunodeficiency virus. Report of two cases and review of the literature. *Scand J Infect Dis* **29**: 535–41.

Celum CL, Chaisson RE, Rutherford GW *et al.* (1987). Incidence of salmonellosis in patients with AIDS. *J Infect Dis* **156**: 998–1001.

Centers for Disease Control and Prevention. (1997). USPHS/IDSA guidelines for the prevention of opportunistic infections in persons infected with human immunodeficiency virus. *MMWR* **46**: 13–18.

Centers for Disease Control and Prevention (1998). Guidelines for treatment of sexually transmitted diseases. *MMWR* **47**: 38–40.

Costagliola D. (1998). Trends in incidence of clinical manifestations of HIV infection and antiretroviral prescriptions in French university hospitals. In: *Proceedings of The Fifth Conference on Retroviruses and Opportunistic Infections*, Chicago IL, USA, abstract **182**.

Costel EE, Wheeler AP, Gregg CR. (1984). *Campylobacter fetus* ssp. fetus cholecystitis and relapsing bacteremia in a patient with acquired immunodeficiency syndrome. *South Med J* **77**: 927–8.

Cutillar-Garcia M, Keller MA, Zangwill K *et al.* (1998). Pneumococcal and influenza immunization and HIV viral load in children. In: *Proceedings of the Fifth Conference on Retroviruses and Opportunistic Infections*, Chicago IL, USA, abstract **255**.

Dolan MJ, Wong MT, Regnery RL *et al.* (1993). Syndrome of Rochalimaea henselae adenitis suggesting cat scratch disease. *Ann Intern Med* **118**: 331–6.

Domingo P, Ferre A, Baraldes MA *et al.* (1998). Remission of relapsing Pseudomonas aeruginosa bronchopulmonary infection following antiretroviral therapy. *Arch Intern Med* **158**: 929–30.

Dowell ME, Ross PG, Musher DM *et al.* (1992). Response of latent syphilis or neurosyphilis to ceftriaxone therapy in persons infected with human immunodeficiency virus. *Am J Med* **93**: 481–8.

Dropulic LK, Leslie JM, Eldred LJ *et al.* (1995). Clinical manifestations and risk factors of Pseudomonas aeruginosa infection in patients with AIDS. *J Infect Dis* **171**: 930–7.

Dunand VA, Wanke CA, Piessens E *et al.* (1997). Parasitic sinusitis and otitis in patients infected with human immunodeficiency virus: report of five cases and review. *Clin Infect Dis* **25**: 267–72.

Dworkin MS, Ward JW, Hanson DL *et al.* (2001). Pneumococcal disease among HIV-infected persons. *Clin Infect Dis* **32**: 794–800.

Ellis M, Gupta S, Galant S *et al.* (1988). Impaired neutrophil function in patients with AIDS or AIDS-related complex. *J Infect Dis* **158**: 1268–76.

Eng RHK, Bishburg E, Smith SM *et al.* (1986). Bacteremia and fungemia in patients with acquired immune deficiency syndrome. *Am J Clin Path* **86**: 105–7.

Farley MM, Stephens DS, Brachman PS *et al.* (1992). Meningitis Surveillance Group. Invasive Haemophilus influenzae disease in adults: a prospective, population-based surveillance. *Ann Intern Med* **116**: 806–12.

Fernandez Guerrero ML, Ramos JM, Nunez A *et al.* (1997). Focal infections due to non-typhi Salmonella in patients with AIDS: report of 10 cases and review. *Clin Infect Dis* **25**: 690–7.

Fichtenbaum CJ, Woeltje KF, Powderly WG. (1994). Serious *Pseudomonas aeruginosa* infections in patients infected with human immunodeficiency virus: a case–control study. *Clin Infect Dis* **19**: 417–22.

Flood JM, Weinstock HS, Guroy ME *et al.* (1998). Neurosyphilis during the AIDS epidemic, San Francisco, 1985–92. *J Infect Dis* **177**: 931–40.

French N. Nakiyingi J, Carpenter LM *et al.* (2000). 23-Valent pneumococcal polysaccharide vaccine in HIV-1-infected Ugandan adults: double-blind, randomised and placebo-controlled trial. *Lancet* **355**: 2106–11.

Gaut P, Wong PK, Meyer RD. (1988). Pyomyositis in a patient with the acquired immunodeficiency syndrome. *Arch Intern Med* **148**: 1608–10.

Gilks CF, Ojoo SA, Ojoo JC *et al.* (1996). Invasive pneumococcal disease in a cohort of predominantly HIV-1 infected female sex-workers in Nairobi, Kenya. *Lancet* **347**: 718–23.

Glaser JB, Volpe S, Aguirre A *et al.* (1991). Zidovudine improves response to pneumococcal vaccine among persons with AIDS and AIDS-related complex. *J Infect Dis* **164**: 761–4.

Godofsky EW, Zinreich J, Armstrong M *et al.* (1992). Sinusitis in HIV-infected patients: A clinical and radiographic review. *Am J Med* **93**: 163–70.

Gordon MA, Walsh AL, Chapon da M *et al.* (2001). Bacteraemia and mortality among medical admissions in Malawi. *J Infect Dis* **42**: 44–9.

Gordon SM, Eaton ME, George R *et al.* (1994). The response of symptomatic neurosyphilis to high-dose intravenous penicillin G in patients with human immunodeficiency virus infection. *N Engl J Med* **331**: 1469–73.

Gourevitch MN, Selwyn PA, Davenny K *et al.* (1993). Effects of HIV infection on the serologic manifestations and response to treatment of syphilis in intravenous drug users. *Ann Intern Med* **118**: 350–5.

Griffin PM, Tauxe RV. (1988). Food counseling for patients with AIDS. *J Infect Dis* **158**: 668.

Hirschtick RE, Glassroth J, Jordan MC *et al.* (1995). Bacterial pneumonia in persons infected with the human immunodeficiency virus. *N Engl J Med* **333**: 845–51.

Holtom PD, Larsen RA, Leal ME *et al.* (1992). Prevalence of neurosyphilis in human immunodeficiency virus-infected patients with latent syphilis. *Am J Med* **93**: 9–12.

Hutchinson CM, Hook EW, Shepherd M *et al.* (1994). Altered clinical presentation of early syphilis in patients with human immunodeficiency virus infection. *Ann Intern Med* **121**: 94–9.

Jacobson MA, Gellermann H, Chambers H. (1988). *Staphylococcus aureus* bacteremia and recurrent staphylococcal infection in patients with acquired immunodeficiency syndrome and AIDS-related complex. *Am J Med* **85**: 172–6.

Jacobson MA, Hahn SM, Gerberding JL *et al.* (1989). Ciprofloxacin for *Salmonella* bacteremia in the acquired immunodeficiency syndrome (AIDS). *Ann Intern Med* **110**: 1027–9.

Janoff EN, Breiman RF, Daley CL *et al.* (1992). Pneumococcal disease during HIV infection: epidemiologic, clinical and immunologic perspectives. *Ann Intern Med* **117**: 314–24.

Janoff EN, Brecman RF, Daley CL *et al.* (1993). Streptococcus pneumoniae colonization, bacteremia and immune response among persons with human immunodeficiency virus infection. *J Infect Dis* **167**: 49–56.

Javaly K, Horowitz HW, Wormser GP. (1992). Nocardiosis in patients with human immunodeficiency virus infection: report of two cases and review of the literature. *Medicine* **71**: 128–38.

Johns DR, Tierney M, Felsenstein D. (1987). Alteration in the natural history of neurosyphilis by concurrent infection with the human immunodeficiency virus. *N Engl J Med* **316**: 1569–72.

Johnson PD, Graves SR, Stewart L *et al.* (1991). Specific syphilis serological tests may become negative in HIV infection. *AIDS* **5**: 419–23.

Koehler JE, LeBoit PE, Egbert BM *et al.* (1988). Cutaneous vascular lesions and disseminated cat scratch disease in patients with the acquired immunodeficiency syndrome (AIDS) and AIDS-related complex. *Ann Intern Med* **109**: 449–55.

Koehler JE, Quinn FD, Berger TG *et al.* (1992). Isolation of *Rochalimaea* species from cutaneous and osseous lesion of bacillary angiomatosis. *N Engl J Med* **327**: 1625–31.

Koehler JE, Tappero JW. (1993). Bacillary angiomatosis and bacillary peliosis in patients infected with human immunodeficiency virus. *Clin Infect Dis* **17**: 612–24.

Koehler JE, Glaser CA, Tappero JW. (1994). *Rochalimaea henselae* infection: a new zoonosis with the domestic cat as reservoir. *JAMA* **271**: 531–5.

Koehler JE, Sanchez MA, Garrido CA *et al.* (1997). Molecular epidemiology of *Bartonella* infections in patients with bacillary angiomatosis-peliosis. *New Engl J Med* **337**: 1876–83.

Krumholz HM, Sande MA, Lo B. (1989). Community-acquired bacteremia in patients with acquired immunodeficiency syndrome: clinical presentation, bacteriology and outcome. *Am J Med* **86**: 776–9.

Kuritzkes DR, Parenti D, Ward DJ *et al.* (1998). Filgrastim prevents severe neutropenia and reduces infective morbidity in patients with advanced HIV infection: results of a randomized, multicenter controlled trial. *AIDS* **12**: 65–74.

Kuschner RA, Trofa AF, Thomas RJ *et al.* (1995). Use of azithromycin for the treatment of *Campylobacter* enteritis in travellers to Thailand, an area where ciprofloxacin resistance is prevalent. *Clin Infect Dis* **21**: 536–41.

Lukehart SA, Hook EW, Baker-Zander SA *et al.* (1988). Invasion of the central nervous system by Treponema pallidum: implications for diagnosis and treatment. *Ann Intern Med* **109**: 855–62.

Martin JN, Perdreau-Remington F, Karbalija M *et al.* (1999). A randomised clinical trial of mupirocin in the eradication of *Staphylococcus aureus* nasal carriage in human immunodeficiency virus disease. *J Infect Dis* **180**: 896–9.

Malone JL, Wallace MR, Hendrick BB *et al.* (1995). Syphilis and neurosyphilis in a human immunodeficiency virus type-1 seropositive population: evidence for frequent serologic relapse after therapy. *Am J Med* **99**: 55–63.

Mendelson MH, Gurtman A, Szabo S *et al.* (1994). *Pseudomonas aeruginosa* bacteremia in patients with AIDS. *Clin Infect Dis* **18**: 886–95.

Meyer CN, Skinhoj P, Prag J. (1994). Bacteremia in HIV-positive and AIDS patients: incidence, species distribution, risk factors, outcome, and influence of long-term prophylactic antibiotic treatment. *Scand J Infect Dis* **26**: 635–42.

Moore RD, Keruly JC, Chaisson RE. (1995). Neutropenia and bacterial infection in acquired immunodeficiency syndrome. *Arch Intern Med* **155**: 1965–70

Moore RD, Chaisson RE, Keruly JC. (1998). Decline in CMV and other opportunistic disease with combination antiretroviral therapy. In: *Proceedings of The Fifth Conference on Retroviruses and Opportunistic Infections*, Chicago IL, USA, abstract no. 41S, p. 157.

Moreno S, Martinez R, Barros C *et al.* (1991). Latent Haemophilus influenzae pneumonia in patients infected with HIV. *AIDS* **5**: 967–70.

Musher DM, Hamill RJ, Baughn RE. (1990). Effect of human immunodeficiency virus (HIV) infection on the course of syphilis and response to treatment. *Ann Intern Med* **113**: 872–81.

Mylonakis E, Rich J, Skolnik PR *et al.* (1997). Invasive Aspergillus sinusitis in patients with human immunodeficiency virus infection. *Medicine* **76**: 249–55.

Nahass RG, Weinstein MP, Bartels J *et al.* (1990). Infective endocarditis in intravenous drug users: a comparison of human immunodeficiency virus type-1-negative and -positive patients. *J Infect Dis* **162**: 967–70.

Nelson MR, Shanson DC, Barter GJ *et al.* (1991). Pseudomonas septicaemia associated with HIV. *AIDS* **5**: 761–3.

Nelson MR, Shanson DC, Hawkins DA *et al.* (1992). *Salmonella, shigella* and *campylobacter* in HIV-seropositive patients. *AIDS* **6**: 1495–8.

Ng VL, Hadley WK, Fennell CL *et al.* (1987). Successive bacteremias with 'Campylobacter cinaedi' and 'Campylobacter fennelliae' in a bisexual male. *J Clin Microbiol* **25**: 2008–9.

Perlman DL, Ampel NM, Schifman RB *et al.* (1988). Persistent *Campylobacter jejuni* infection in patients infected with the human immunodeficiency virus (HIV). *Ann Intern Med* **108**: 540–6.

Plouffe JF, Breiman RF, Facklam RR. (1996). Bacteremia with Streptococcus pneumoniae: implications for therapy and prevention. *JAMA* **275**: 194–8.

Polsky B, Gold JW, Whimbey E *et al.* (1986). Bacterial pneumonia in patients with the acquired immunodeficiency syndrome. *Ann Intern Med* **104**: 38–41.

Raviglione MC, Battan R, Pablos Mendez A *et al.* (1989). Infections associated with Hickman catheters in patients with acquired immunodeficiency syndrome. *Am J Med* **86**: 780–6.

Raviglione MC, Taranta A, Ottuso P *et al.* (1990). High *Staphylococcus aureus* nasal carriage rate in patients with acquired immunodeficiency syndrome or AIDS-related complex. *Am J Infect Cont* **18**: 64–9.

Redd SC, Rutherford GW, Sande MA *et al.* (1990). The role of human immunodeficiency virus infection in pneumococcal bacteremia in San Francisco residents. *J Infect Dis* **162**: 1012–17.

Relman DA, Loutit JS, Schmidt TM *et al.* (1990). The agent of bacillary angiomatosis: an approach to the identification of uncultured pathogens. *N Engl J Med* **323**: 1573–80.

Rodriguez-Barradas MC, Musher DM, Hamill RJ *et al.* (1992a). Unusual manifestations of pneumococcal infection in human immunodeficiency virus-infected individuals: the past revisited. *Clin Infect Dis* **14**: 192–9.

Rodriguez-Barradas MC, Musher DM, Lahart C *et al.* (1992b). Antibody to capsular polysaccharides of *Streptococcus pneumoniae* after vaccination of human immunodeficiency virus-infected subjects with 23-valent pneumococcal vaccine. *J Infect Dis* **165**: 553–6.

Roilides E, Butler KM, Husson RN *et al.* (1992). Pseudomonas infections in children with human immunodeficiency virus infection. *Pediat Infect Dis J* **11**: 547–53.

Rolfs RT, Joesoeff MR, Hendershot EF *et al.* (1997). A randomized trial of enhanced therapy for early syphilis in patients with and without human immunodeficiency virus infection. *N Engl J Med* **337**: 307–14.

Rompalo AM, Cannon RO, Quinn TC *et al.* (1992). Association of biologic false positive reactions for syphilis with human immunodeficiency virus infection. *J Infect Dis* **165**: 1124–6.

Rubinstein R, Christie S. (1995). Malignant syphilis (lues maligna) and concurrent infection with HIV. *Int J Dermatol* **34**: 403–7.

Salmon D, Detruchis P, Leport C *et al.* (1991). Efficacy of zidovudine in preventing relapses of *Salmonella* bacteremia in AIDS. *J Infect Dis* **163**: 415–16.

Schlamm HT, Yancovitz SR. (1989). *Haemophilus influenzae* pneumonia in young adults with AIDS, ARC or at risk of AIDS. *Am J Med* **86**: 11–14.

Schuchat A, Broome CV, Hightower A *et al.* (1991). Use of surveillance for invasive pneumococcal disease to estimate the size of the immunosuppressed HIV-infected population. *JAMA* **265**: 3275–9.

Schuster MG, Norris AH. (1994). Community-acquired *Pseudomonas aeruginosa* pneumonia in patients with HIV infection. *AIDS* **8**: 1437–41.

Schwartzman WA, Lamberus MW, Kennedy CA *et al.* (1991). Staphylococcal pyomyositis in patients infected by the human immunodeficiency virus. *Am J Med* **90**: 595–600.

Selwyn PA, Pumerantz AS, Durante A *et al.* (1998). Clinical predictors of *Pneumocystis carinii* pneumonia, bacterial pneumonia and tuberculosis in HIV-infected patients. *AIDS* **12**: 885–93.

Shanson DC. (1990). Septicaemia in patients with AIDS. *Trans R Soc Trop Med Hyg* **84** (Suppl. 1): 14–16.

Simberkoff MS, Leaf HL (1992). Bacterial infections in patients with HIV infection. In: GP Wormser (ed.) *AIDS and other manifestations of HIV infection*. 2nd edition. New York: Raven Press, 269–75.

Skoutelis AT, Murphy RL, MacDonell KB *et al.* (1990). Indwelling central venous catheter infections in patients with acquired immunodeficiency syndrome. *J AIDS* **3**: 335–42.

Slater LN, Welch DF, Min K-W. (1992). *Rochalimaea henselae* causes bacillary angiomatosis and peliosis hepatis. *Arch Intern Med* **152**: 602–6.

Snidjers F, Kuijper EJ, de Wever B *et al.* (1997). Prevalence of *Campylobacter*-associated diarrhea among patients infected with human immunodeficiency virus. *Clin Infect Dis* **24**: 1107–13.

Sorvillo FJ, Lieb LE, Waterman SH. (1991). Incidence of campylobacteriosis among patients with AIDS in Los Angeles County. *J AIDS* **4**: 598–602.

Sorvillo F, Beall G, Turner PA *et al.* (2001). Incidence and determinants of pseudomonas aeruginosa infection among persons with HIV. *Am Infect Control* **29**: 79–84.

Steinhoff MC, Auerbach BS, Nelson KE *et al.* (1991). Antibody responses to *Haemophilus influenzae* type b vaccines in men with human immunodeficiency virus infection. *N Engl J Med* **325**: 1837–42.

Stoler MH, Bonfiglio TA, Steigbigel RT *et al.* (1983). An atypical subcutaneous infection associated with acquired immunodeficiency syndrome. *Am J Clin Path* **80**: 714–18.

Tee W, Mijch A, Wright E *et al.* (1995). Emergence of multidrug resistance in *Campylobacter jejuni* isolates from three patients infected with human immunodeficiency virus. *Clin Infect Dis* **21**: 634–8.

Tomberlin MG, Holtom PD, Owens JL *et al.* (1994). Evaluation of neurosyphilis in human immunodeficiency virus-infected individuals. *Clin Infect Dis* **18**: 288–94.

Tumbarello M, Tacconelli E, Lucia MB *et al.* (1996). Predictors of *Staphylococcus aureus* pneumonia associated with human immunodeficiency virus infection. *Respir Med* **90**: 531–7.

Tumbarello M, Tacconelli E, de Gaetano *et al.* (1998). Bacterial pneumonia in HIV-infected patients. *J AIDS* **18**: 39–45.

Visco Comandini U, Maggi P, Santopadre P *et al.* (1997). Chalamydia pneumoniae respiratory infections among patients infected with the human immunodeficiency virus. *Eur J Clin Microbiol Infect Dis* **16**: 720–6.

Whimbey E, Gold JW, Polsky B *et al.* (1986). Bacteremia and fungemia in patients with the acquired immunodeficiency syndrome. *Ann Intern Med* **164**: 511–14.

Witt DJ, Craven DE, McCabe WR. (1987). Bacterial infections in adult patients with the acquired immunodeficiency syndrome (AIDS) and AIDS-related complex. *Am J Med* **82**: 900–6.

Zylberberg H, Viard JP, Rotschild C *et al.* (1996). Prolonged efficiency of secondary prophylaxis with colistin aerosols for respiratory infection due to Pseudomonas aeruginosa in patients infected with human immunodeficiency virus. *Clin Infect Dis* **23**: 641–3.

CHRISTOPHER CARPENTER, CONSTANCE BENSON AND RICHARD CHAISSON

Tuberculosis is one of the most common opportunistic diseases in those with human immunodeficiency virus (HIV) infection worldwide. Although the impact of tuberculosis in HIV-infected populations is greatest in developing countries, it is also a major public health concern in urban areas in the USA and Europe. The rise in multidrug-resistant tuberculosis observed in populations with or at risk of HIV infection is in part related to insufficient public health infrastructure in some urban areas. There is a compelling need for new drug development, improved and more rapid diagnostic techniques, and innovative methods of creating a more effective public health response to tuberculosis in all areas of the world.

Persons with HIV infection will continue to be uniquely and adversely affected by tuberculosis co-infection. A number of measures are key to achieving a favourable outcome in this population. These include:

(1) maintenance of a high index of suspicion for the diagnosis;
(2) early institution of adequate infection control procedures for prevention of transmission;
(3) early and rapid diagnosis and initiation of effective antituberculous therapy, with appropriate modification based on susceptibility test results;
(4) assuring sustained compliance through the completion of treatment by directly observing or supervising administration of antituberculous chemotherapy; and
(5) providing effective screening and preventive measures.

The ongoing education of health-care workers and patients is necessary to assure that these goals are met while we await new drug development and improvements in the health-care infrastructure.

Epidemiology and geographical variability

Mycobacterium tuberculosis is one of the most prevalent infections of human beings and contributes considerably to illness and death around the world. Globally, it is estimated that approximately one-third of the world population is latently infected with M. tuberculosis and that eight million new cases of active tuberculosis occur each year (Dye, 1999). The World Health Organization (WHO) estimates that globally 1.9 million people die of tuberculosis each year, making it the second most common infectious cause of death in the world after HIV infection (WHO, 1999). HIV-related tuberculosis is growing in frequency as the HIV pandemic worsens, and the WHO estimates that 22% of all TB deaths occur in HIV-infected people. In Africa, where AIDS is the leading cause of death from any disease, tuberculosis is the leading AIDS-related opportunistic infection (Raviglione, 1997). In most developing countries, tuberculosis is the most common HIV-related opportunistic infection, and a leading cause of death in patients with AIDS (De Cock, 1992).

The impact of the HIV epidemic on tuberculosis control has been enormous. Although the interaction of HIV and tuberculosis was first noted in developed countries (Chaisson, 1987), the importance of tuberculosis as an opportunistic infection has escalated as the pandemic has blossomed. In countries where latent tuberculosis infection is highly prevalent, the spread of HIV infection has resulted in substantial increases in tuberculosis incidence. In northern Thailand, for example, the rapid increase in HIV prevalence that occurred in the early 1990s was accompanied by a doubling of the incidence of tuberculosis over a 4-year period (Yanai, 1996). In sub-Saharan Africa, the HIV epidemic has had a devastating impact on tuberculosis control, and case rates have increased in virtually all countries, overwhelming treatment capacity (Cantwell and Binkin, 1996, 1997; Harries, 1996). Even in those countries with well-organized and clinically effective tuberculosis control programmes, the marked rise in tuberculosis incidence in HIV-infected people results in escalating case rates that cannot be contained with current control strategies (De Cock and Chaisson, 1999).

The risk of developing tuberculosis is a function of the risk of becoming infected with M. tuberculosis and the likelihood that infection will progress to active disease. HIV infection alters tuberculosis dynamics in two important ways. In both industrialized and developing countries, people at risk for HIV infection are also at risk for latent tuberculosis infection. In developed countries, injection drug users, inner-city residents and immigrants from endemic areas have a higher prevalence of latent tuberculosis than other members of the population. In addition, people with HIV infection who attend clinics or are hospitalized are at risk for infection with M. tuberculosis spread within health-care institutions. As discussed below, HIV infection impairs the cellular immunity that is responsible for containing latent tuberculosis, leading to high rates of disease in individuals with both infections. It is estimated that more than 1% of the entire population of sub-Saharan Africa is co-infected with both HIV and M tuberculosis, and in many areas this figure is in fact greater than 10% (UNAIDS, 2000).

There are many reasons for the global increase in tuberculosis incidence. Infection with HIV, coupled with factors such as poverty, homelessness, drug abuse, deteriorating or absent public health infrastructure, lack of access to medical care, geographical relocation of persons born in areas where tuberculosis is endemic, and overcrowded housing or incarceration of persons at high risk for acquisition and spread of tuberculosis, all have had a major impact on the epidemiology of tuberculosis.

Parallel to the rise in the number of reported cases of tuberculosis has been an increase in the number of reported cases due to antimycobacterial drug-resistant strains of M. tuberculosis. These cases have been identified chiefly in urban areas of developed countries where co-infection with tuberculosis and HIV is common. In addition to the social and demographic factors responsible for the resurgence of tuberculosis, delays in treatment, poor compliance with treatment regimens, ineffective treatment regimens, delays in recognition of drug resistance and appropriate modification of drug regimens, lack of timely drug susceptibility testing, and ineffective infection control procedures in institutional facilities, have all served to create a milieu for the development and propagation of drug resistance (Iseman, 1993).

Transmission

Tuberculosis is spread from person to person through inhalation of infectious respiratory droplet nuclei aerosolized by coughing, sneezing, or talking. Rarely, infected secretions from draining wounds or other body fluids or tissues may be aerosolized and inhaled, or directly inoculated. The efficiency of transmission is determined by the inoculum size, the infectiousness of the contact case, and the duration and intimacy of contact. Those with cavitary pulmonary disease who expectorate sputum containing large numbers of mycobacteria are the most infectious. Prolonged close contact and large repetitive inocula are usually required for transmission to non-immunocompromised persons. It has been estimated that 2–4% of immunologically normal household contacts of acid-fast bacilli smear-positive cases develop tuberculosis within 12 months of exposure, although higher infection rates may be seen in crowded environments housing susceptible individuals (Bailey et al., 1983).

People co-infected with HIV and M. tuberculosis have a greater risk of developing active tuberculosis than those without HIV infection, although these rates vary widely according to the population studied (Selwyn et al., 1989, 1992; Daley et al., 1992; Hopewell, 1992). The majority of non-HIV-infected persons with intact cellular immunity never develop active tuberculosis; a small proportion (3–5%) will develop active disease within the first 1–3 years following infection, and an additional 5% develop active tuberculosis later in life, often decades after acquiring infection (Styblo, 1980; Bailey et al., 1983; Daley et al., 1992). However, for HIV-infected drug users with latent tuberculous infection, the observed rate of development of active tuberculosis was 14% over 2 years (Selwyn et al., 1989). Daley and colleagues reported that over a 12-week period following exposure to a source contact, 37% of susceptible residents of a housing facility for HIV-infected drug users developed active pulmonary tuberculosis with genetically identical M. tuberculosis strains, as determined by restriction fragment length polymorphism analysis (Daley et al., 1992). Finally, although rare among immunologically normal people, exogenous re-infection may occur in patients with advanced HIV disease. In a study of patients with AIDS being treated for known drug-susceptible tuberculosis, restriction fragment length polymorphism analysis documented subsequent development of active tuberculosis due to re-infection with a new strain of multidrug-resistant M. tuberculosis (Small et al., 1993).

The effect of HIV infection on the rate of transmission of tuberculosis to other non-immunosuppressed contacts is uncertain. In a study reported by Klausner and associates (1993) from Kinshasa, Zaire, tuberculin skin test reactivity was compared for 521 household contacts of 74 HIV-infected patients and 692 household contacts of 95 HIV-uninfected patients with sputum smear-positive pulmonary tuberculosis. The prevalence of M. tuberculosis infection increased with age for both household groups, such that by 16 years of age, 75% of household contacts were tuberculin skin test positive. No difference was seen in the prevalence of culture-positive pulmonary tuberculosis between contacts of HIV-infected or HIV-uninfected patients in any age group. In contrast, in a cross-sectional survey conducted in Zambia, 52% of contacts of HIV-seropositive pulmonary tuberculosis patients had a positive tuberculin response, compared with 71% of contacts of HIV-uninfected patients ($p < 0.001$) (Elliott et al., 1993). Tuberculin response in contacts was associated with age of the contact, intimacy of the contact with the index case, level of crowding in the household, and the number of acid-fast bacilli seen in the sputum smear of the index case. Active tuberculosis was diagnosed in 4% of contacts of HIV-infected cases.

Pathogenesis

Because of its virulence, M. tuberculosis may cause disease in individuals in all stages of HIV infection (Theuer et al., 1990; Barnes et al., 1991; Small et al., 1991; Hopewell, 1992). Theuer and colleagues reported that the median CD4 lymphocyte count for HIV-infected patients with tuberculosis was 326 cells/μl versus 928 cells/μl for HIV-

uninfected individuals with tuberculosis (Theuer et al., 1990). The timing and rate of development of active disease, however, are determined by the immunological status of the host. It is likely that the T-cell response to M. tuberculosis varies with the stage of both tuberculosis and HIV infection and depends on the interactions among multiple mycobacterial antigens, cytokines and effector cells.

Cell-mediated immune response

The acquired cellular immune response to tuberculosis in the immunologically intact person involves primarily CD4 lymphocytes and macrophages (Orme et al., 1993). Gamma delta T cells also appear to play a role (Orme et al., 1993). In vitro studies have demonstrated that gamma delta T cells recognize mycobacterial antigens and expand preferentially in response to live mycobacteria, a response mediated by antigen-presenting mononuclear phagocytes (Havlir et al., 1991; Boom et al., 1992). More recent studies suggest that the primary role of gamma delta T cells is in influencing local cellular traffic, by promoting the influx of lymphocytes and monocytes and limiting the influx of destructive inflammatory cells that do not contribute to host protection (D'Souza et al., 1997). The specific functions of various mononuclear cell subsets, how they inhibit mycobacterial growth, and how failure of cell-mediated immune responses in HIV-infected persons promotes progression of primary infection or reactivation of latent infection remain to be established (Orme et al., 1993).

On recognition of mycobacterial antigens, CD4 lymphocytes become activated to proliferate and produce cytokines, which in turn activate macrophages to inhibit the growth and survival of intracellular mycobacteria (Orme et al., 1993). Macrophages infected with or exposed to mycobacteria, when activated, also produce a number of cytokines, including tumour necrosis factor, interleukin-1, -6, -10, and tissue growth factor-β, each of which appear to have immunomodulatory functions (Orme et al., 1993). The CD4 lymphocyte populations produced by stimulation with M. tuberculosis antigens also release large amounts of interferon-γ (but little or no interleukin-4 or -5), consistent with a Th1-like cell phenotype (Boom et al., 1991; Haanen et al., 1991). However, interferon-γ may play only a minor role in containment of mycobacterial infection (Douvas et al., 1985). In addition to their ability to induce cytokine production, CD4 lymphocyte populations from persons infected with M. tuberculosis have been found to be directly cytotoxic for monocytes infected with mycobacteria or exposed to mycobacterial antigens (Ottenhof et al., 1987; Kumararatne et al., 1990; Orme et al., 1993). Recently, it has been shown that actively replicating mycobacteria are sequestered in monocytes, thus evading antigen presentation and subsequent immune surveillance by CD4 lymphocytes (Pancholi et al., 1993).

Based on these data, the intact immune response to M. tuberculosis may be summarized as follows. After acute primary infection with M. tuberculosis, blood-derived and tissue macrophages serve primarily as antigen-presenting cells; presentation of mycobacterial antigens to CD4 lymphocyte cells results in CD4 lymphocyte activation and clonal expansion. Ongoing mycobacterial replication within acutely infected macrophages results in formation of large numbers of sensitized CD4 lymphocytes. CD4 lymphocyte-induced cytotoxicity may subsequently result in lysis and destruction of acutely infected mononuclear cells. Cytokines released following cell lysis inhibit further mycobacterial replication and ultimately granuloma formation begins. The clonal expansion of sensitized CD4 lymphocytes may form both a circulating population of T cells that can mediate a delayed-type hypersensitivity response to mycobacterial antigens and a population of memory T cells that may protect against subsequent exogenous re-infection (Orme et al., 1993). In contrast to acutely infected macrophages, however, chronically infected macrophages appear to stimulate T cells poorly, chiefly because they do not present viable replicating organisms to circulating CD4 lymphocytes (Pancholi et al., 1993). Pancholi and colleagues (1993) suggest that this may be due to selective blockade of antigen presentation, possibly resulting from impaired or altered phagosome–lysosome fusion and acidification. Such 'sequestration' of viable mycobacteria from immune CD4 lymphocytes may contribute to the virulence of mycobacteria, allowing their persistence and providing a focus for reactivation during impaired immune surveillance.

One can hypothesize that HIV-associated defects in CD4 lymphocyte function or depletion result in failure of the CD4 lymphocyte responses necessary to contain M. tuberculosis infection and enhance risk of progressive primary infection or reactivation of latent infection. The CD4 cytolytic lymphocyte activity directed against mycobacterial antigens appears to be impaired in persons with HIV infection; the degree of impairment increases as the CD4 lymphocyte count declines (Forte et al., 1992). Productive HIV infection may also impair intracellular killing (Fauci, 1991).

Pathophysiology

Inhaled mycobacteria migrate initially to middle and lower lung fields, corresponding to the pattern of air flow in these areas, where they are ingested by alveolar macrophages. Before specific cell-mediated immune responses to mycobacteria develop, organisms multiply within macrophages and spread to regional lymph nodes. During this time, the organism can spread by bloodstream and lymphatics to lymph nodes, kidneys, epiphyseal areas of long bones, vertebral bodies, the central nervous system, and most frequently, the apical-posterior regions of the lung, where higher oxygen content may promote growth of aerobic mycobacteria (Des Prez and Goodwin, 1990).

Unrestricted mycobacterial replication within infected mononuclear phagocytes eventually destroys them; cytokine release is followed by recruitment of other phagocytes, which are in turn destroyed, ultimately forming an area of pneumonia. Quiescence or progression of disease is dependent on the antigen load and host immune factors as previously discussed. Development of cell-mediated immunity and tissue hypersensitivity between 6 and 12 weeks after infection in the normal host enables organization of activated mononuclear cells, epithelioid cells, Langhans' giant cells, fibroblasts, and capillaries into granulomas that can effectively contain infection. Lytic enzymes released from degenerating cells cause tissue necrosis and the formation of the classic 'caseous' exudate, which is unfavourable for mycobacterial growth. Mycobacterial replication is then arrested, and in most patients bacterial destruction occurs. However, in a small proportion, potentially viable bacteria persist in a quiescent state for many years. Reactivation of latent infection is thought to be the most common route by which tuberculosis develops in HIV-infected persons, though as discussed previously, primary progression occurs at higher rates than in persons without HIV infection. Those infected with HIV with advanced immunosuppression appear to be at greater risk for primary progression and for exogenous re-infection than those with early HIV disease.

Clinical presentation

The clinical manifestations of tuberculosis in persons co-infected with HIV are in large part dependent on the degree of underlying immunosuppression and on whether disease is due to reactivation or to primary progression.

As in HIV-uninfected subjects, the lung is the most frequently involved organ in patients with tuberculosis and HIV infection. Persons with high CD4 lymphocyte counts are likely to have clinical signs and symptoms of pulmonary tuberculosis similar to those described in patients without HIV disease (Theuer et al., 1990; Barnes et al., 1991; Small et al., 1991). Typical symptoms include fever, night sweats, malaise, fatigue, anorexia, weight loss, and persistent and usually productive cough. Chest pain may be present if there is pleural or pericardial disease. Haemoptysis may accompany endobronchial erosion, caused by inflammation or granuloma formation. Dyspnoea is generally seen later in the course of tuberculosis in patients with extensive pulmonary parenchymal destruction or anaemia interfering with oxygen exchange or delivery (see Chapter 22).

The chest radiographic abnormalities of pulmonary tuberculosis generally also correlate with the degree of HIV-related immunosuppression. Radiographic abnormalities in those who are minimally immunosuppressed are similar to the changes seen in the immunologically normal host with tuberculosis; upper lobe or apical posterior cavitary infiltration, hilar adenopathy, pleural effusion, and fibrosis with volume contraction are the most prevalent findings.

In patients with advanced HIV-associated immunodeficiency, pulmonary disease remains common but extrapulmonary manifestations increase in frequency (Lee et al., 2000). Seventy per cent of patients with an AIDS diagnosis prior to or soon after developing tuberculosis will have extrapulmonary involvement. About one-third of persons with extrapulmonary disease will have concomitant pulmonary disease (Pitchenik et al., 1984; Sunderam et al., 1986; Barnes et al., 1991; Small et al., 1991; Hopewell, 1992; Lee et al., 2000). The usual sites of extrapulmonary disease are the lymphoreticular system (lymph nodes, liver, spleen, bone marrow), the bloodstream and the central nervous system (CNS). Several studies have estimated that with the use of lysis centrifugation and radiometric culture techniques, 26–42% of HIV-infected patients with tuberculosis will have mycobacteria recovered from the blood (Modilevsky, et al., 1989; Shafer et al., 1989; Barnes et al., 1991; Antonucci et al., 1992). The incidence of tuberculous meningitis in HIV-infected patients may be as high as 10%, compared with 2% in persons with tuberculosis and no HIV infection. The reported incidence may be influenced by geographical variability (Berenguer et al., 1992).

Radiographic manifestations of pulmonary tuberculosis in those with advanced HIV-associated immunosuppression are more likely to be atypical (Pitchenik and Rubinson, 1985; Modilevsky et al., 1989; Theuer et al., 1990; Barnes et al., 1991). Diffuse bilateral infiltration without cavitation, alveolar or lobar consolidation, miliary patterns that mimic the interstitial infiltrates of Pneumocystis carinii pneumonia (PCP) or other opportunistic pathogens, and other abnormalities may make the differentiation of tuberculosis from other opportunistic infections more difficult.

Primary progressive pulmonary tuberculosis is more likely to occur in HIV-infected persons who acquire infection when they are profoundly immunosuppressed. These individuals appear to develop signs and symptoms of active disease rapidly, within weeks of contact with an infected source (Daley et al., 1992; Edlin et al., 1992; Fischl et al., 1992a; Hopewell, 1992). In such individuals, the disease appears to follow a more aggressive clinical course, with rapid development of fever, sweats, cough, dyspnoea, and weight loss accompanied by progressive, often bilateral, lower lobar consolidation or diffuse bilateral interstitial or miliary radiographic patterns. Cavitation is unusual. Spread to other organs may intervene if diagnosis and treatment are delayed.

Multidrug-resistant tuberculosis has had a unique impact among persons with HIV infection. In general, multidrug-resistant tuberculosis has occurred in the context of nosocomial or institutional outbreaks, in which those with HIV infection were housed or treated in contiguity with other persons with infectious multidrug-resistant tuberculosis (CDC, 1990a, 1991a, 1992; Edlin et al., 1992; Fischl et al., 1992b; Barnes and Barrows, 1993). The mortality rate among HIV-infected persons with multidrug-resistant tuberculosis reported in many of these outbreaks has ranged from 72 to 89%, with a median time to death of 4–16 weeks; approximately 50% of the deaths were thought to have been related to complications of tuberculosis.

In one case–control analysis of HIV-infected patients, some clinical features of multidrug-resistant tuberculosis differed from those of drug-susceptible tuberculosis (Fischl et al., 1992a). Case patients infected by drug-resistant strains of M. tuberculosis were twice as likely to have concomitant pulmonary and extrapulmonary disease than were HIV-infected controls infected with drug-susceptible strains. Chest radiographs in case patients were more likely to show alveolar infiltrates, cavitation or interstitial infiltrates with a reticular pattern at the outset than controls. The clinical course for patients with multidrug-resistant tuberculosis was more likely to follow an overwhelming miliary pattern with involvement of lungs, pleura, stool, meninges, bone marrow, bloodstream, lymph nodes and skin. The median survival was 1.5 months for patients with an AIDS diagnosis and multidrug-resistant tuberculosis, 14.8 months for HIV-infected patients with multidrug-resistant tuberculosis who did not have AIDS, 14.3 months for patients with AIDS and drug-susceptible tuberculosis, and 17.9 months for HIV-infected patients with drug-susceptible tuberculosis who did not have AIDS (Fischl et al., 1992a).

Diagnosis

The diagnosis of tuberculosis requires consideration of epidemiological, demographic, and exposure history, assessment of previous treatment or preventive therapy and of current clinical signs and symptoms, tuberculin skin testing, radiographic or other diagnostic imaging procedures, and microbiological demonstration of M. tuberculosis by smear and culture of appropriate clinical specimens.

Tuberculin skin testing

Tuberculin skin testing detects the presence of infection with M. tuberculosis but does not indicate active disease. Skin testing is not sensitive or specific; a number of host-related factors may cause decreased ability to respond to tuberculin, even in patients with active tuberculosis, and cross-reactivity with other non-tuberculous mycobacteria may occur (American Thoracic Society, 2000). In HIV-infected persons, the presence of skin-test reactivity depends on the degree of underlying immunosuppression. Cutaneous anergy is present in approximately 10% of asymptomatic HIV-infected persons with CD4 lymphocyte counts of greater than 500 cells/μl (CDC, 1991b). Anergy has been reported for approximately 66% of HIV-infected persons with CD4 lymphocyte counts of less than 200 cells/μl and 80% of persons with CD4 lymphocyte counts of less than 50 cells/μl (CDC, 1991b).

The rate of positive tuberculin skin tests among HIV-infected patients is lower than that for HIV-uninfected persons exposed to tuberculosis in comparable settings. In a study in Uganda among postpartum women, 82% of 27 women who were HIV-infected had a positive tuberculin skin test, compared with 48% of HIV-infected women (CDC, 1990b). Asymptomatic HIV-infected injection drug users in Switzerland and prisoners in Italy had significantly lower rates of tuberculin reactivity than similar HIV-uninfected groups (CDC, 1991b). In a study in Baltimore, 34% of 90 HIV-uninfected injection drug users were tuberculin skin test reactive, compared with only 9% of 22 HIV-infected injecting drug users (CDC, 1991b). Even among those with active tuberculosis, HIV infected persons have a lower rate of reactivity than those without HIV-infection. In a study conducted in Los Angeles, only 55% of 47 HIV infected persons with active tuberculosis had a positive skin test; the mean CD4 lymphocyte count for those who were positive was 220 cells/μl versus 66 cells/μl for those who were negative (CDC, 1991b).

It is recommended that tuberculin skin tests are administered by the standard Mantoux method using 0.1 ml of a 5-TU strength of purified protein derivative tuberculin antigen; the response should be interpreted after 48–72 h (American Thoracic Society, 2000; USPHS/IDSA Prevention of Opportunistic Infections Working Group, 1997). A reaction of 5 mm or more of induration to purified protein derivative indicates tuberculous infection in HIV-infected individuals, regardless of reactions to other antigens. The risk of tuberculosis increases markedly at 5 mm induration, as demonstrated in an HIV-infected cohort study (Markowitz et al., 1997). The rate of tuberculosis in those with a 0 mm reaction (negative reaction) was 0.5 cases/100 patient-years, and those with a 1–4 mm reaction had a rate of 0.0 cases/100 patient-years, whereas those with 5–9, 10–19, and $\geq$ 20 mm induration had substantially higher rates at 2.4, 2.5 and 5.4 cases/100 patient-years, respectively. To assist in diagnosis and preventive intervention, Mantoux skin testing should be done as early as possible in HIV-infected individuals to detect those with latent infection before HIV-related immunosuppression results in cutaneous anergy. Patients with low CD4 lymphocyte counts who respond to antiretroviral therapy should be retested if their initial test was negative.

In HIV-positive individuals who have negative (< 5 mm induration) tuberculin reactions, anergy testing is no longer recommended to identify false-negative results (CDC, 1997). The reliability of anergy testing was evaluated using serial skin testing with Candida, mumps, and tuberculin (Chin et al., 1996). Of subjects who initially had no reactions to any of the three antigens, 30% reacted to Candida or mumps when tested a year later, a result that is the opposite of what we would expect as the HIV infection progresses. Furthermore, of 50 subjects with false-negative purified protein derivative reactions after a previously positive result, mumps antigen test was reactive in 39% of subjects. These data show that cutaneous anergy testing has no clinical value when used in the evaluation of HIV-positive individuals with negative tuberculin tests.

Microbiologic diagnosis: staining, culture and identification of M. tuberculosis

Stained smears

The detection of acid-fast bacilli in a stained smear of pulmonary or other body-fluid secretions is presumptive evidence of mycobacterial infection. Smears of acid-fast bacilli are not specific for M. tuberculosis and may be positive in persons infected with other species of mycobacteria. From 50 to 80% of non-immunosuppressed patients with pulmonary tuberculosis have positive sputum smear for acid-fast bacilli. It had been suggested that HIV-infected persons with pulmonary tuberculosis are less likely to be smear-positive, but estimates in this population range from 30 to 70%, and most studies document an acid-fast bacilli smear rate that is not substantially different from that reported for HIV-uninfected persons with pulmonary tuberculosis (Chaisson et al., 1987; American Thoracic Society, 1990; Theuer et al., 1990; Small et al., 1991; Cauthen et al., 1996). The presence of acid-fast bacilli in sputum smears is contingent on the clinical syndrome present; positive smears are more likely in samples recovered from persons with extensive or diffuse pulmonary infiltrates or those with cavities containing heavy inocula of organism. The lower frequency of cavitary disease in HIV-infected patients with tuberculosis may be the reason for the decreased proportion of positive expectorated sputum examinations in some studies; because acid-fast bacilli smears are less likely to be positive in patients with non-tuberculous mycobacterial disease, a positive smear should be presumed to indicate tuberculosis.

Cultures

Isolation of M. tuberculosis from clinical specimens is the 'gold standard' for diagnosis. The organism can be recovered from sputum, gastric aspirate, urine, cerebrospinal fluid (CSF), pleural fluid, bronchial washings, bone marrow, blood, and other tissue. Culture is more sensitive than acid-fast bacilli smears (American Thoracic Society, 1990). Conventional culture systems require inoculation of concentrated, digested clinical specimens onto solid media such as Lowenstein-Jensen or Middlebrook 7H10 or 7H11 agar-based media (American Thoracic Society, 1990). It is recommended that specimens are inoculated on both types of solid media for improved yield. Specimens should be incubated in 5–10% CO_2 to further enhance the yield. The usual recovery time is 3–6 weeks, although drug-resistant strains may not grow as well on conventional media. M. tuberculosis can be readily identified by colonial appearance on agar, a positive niacin test, weak catalase activity, and a positive nitrate reduction test. As discussed later, DNA probes for M. tuberculosis and other mycobacteria are now commercially available and offer a rapid, inexpensive, and specific alternative for species identification.

At least three sputum samples for culture should be collected on different days, preferably the first morning specimen. When aerosol-induction of sputum is required, appropriate respiratory infection control procedures must be initiated to minimize the risk of transmission. Gastric aspirates may be useful for those who cannot produce sputum, particularly children. Fiberoptic bronchoscopy with bronchial washings, bronchoalveolar lavage, or transbronchial biopsy may be necessary when sputum cannot be induced and a diagnosis cannot be made through other modalities (American Thoracic Society, 1990).

It has been estimated that blood cultures are positive for M. tuberculosis in 26–42% of HIV-infected persons with tuberculosis. These estimates may be more applicable to those with advanced immunosuppression and other evidence of extrapulmonary disease (Modilevsky et al., 1989; Shafer et al., 1989; Theuer et al., 1990; Barnes et al., 1991; Antonucci et al., 1992). Bone-marrow aspirate and culture may provide a similar yield for those with disseminated disease. Other invasive procedures for obtaining clinical specimens should be directed by the clinical condition of the patient and the organ(s) or site(s) of involvement.

Radiometric systems detect early growth of mycobacteria in liquid media; a ^{14}C-labelled substrate incorporated into the medium is utilized by replicating bacteria, releasing $^{14}CO_2$, which can be quantitated. The most widely used system is the BACTEC system. Utilization of this system for culture and susceptibility testing can reduce the time to detection of a positive culture to 1–3 weeks (Ellner et al., 1988; Crawford, et al., 1989; Barnes and Barrows, 1993).

New diagnostic tests

New diagnostic techniques that are becoming available in commercial as well as reference and research laboratories include the polymerase chain reaction (PCR) and other nucleic acid amplification methods, although a clinical role for such tests is still being defined. Enzyme-linked immunoabsorbent assays or radioimmunoassays may be used for rapid detection of M. tuberculosis antigens in cerebrospinal fluid. Sensitivity of these assays ranges from 39 to 79% and the specificity from 98 to 100%, an improvement over those associated with acid-fast bacilli smear or culture of CSF in persons with tuberculous meningitis (Watt et al., 1988; Radhakrishnan and Mathai, 1991). Diagnosis of tuberculosis infection with immune-based assays is also under investigation. For example, measurement of interferon-γ responses to stimulation of peripheral blood mononuclear cells with M. tuberculosis antigens may be a potentially useful diagnostic technique (Converse et al., 1997).

Antituberculous drug susceptibility testing

The CDC recommends that all initial M. tuberculosis isolates and isolates obtained from patients who fail or relapse following therapy should be submitted for drug-susceptibility testing. The results should be used to guide choices of effective antituberculous agents for treatment (CDC, 1993a).

For radiometric susceptibility testing, a sample of a subculture from the primary isolation is inoculated into radiometric liquid media containing various concentrations of drug; the growth index measured in the drug-containing samples is compared with that obtained in the control sample. This technique, when combined with radiometric culture systems, substantially reduces the time to a susceptibility result to a total of 3–4 weeks from the time a sample is submitted for culture.

Treatment

The advent of highly active antiretroviral therapy (HAART) has been of great benefit in the management of the HIV-infected patient, but concomitantly it has further complicated therapy for patients who are also infected with M. tuberculosis. The CDC has addressed the issues of treatment and prevention for patients co-infected with HIV and M. tuberculosis in recently published guidelines, stressing the interactions of antiretroviral therapy and antituberculous therapy, as well as short-course preventative regimens (CDC, 1998). They provide an algorithm for assessing treatment options in the HIV-infected tuberculosis patient (Figure 23.1), with emphasis on the substitution of rifabutin for rifampin in patients on certain protease inhibitors (PIs) or non-nucleoside reverse transcriptase inhibitors (NNRTIs) because of the substantial drug interactions between the rifamycin class of antituberculous drugs and these agents (Table 23.1). Further details are provided below.

Because exposure of a growing mycobacterial population to a single antituberculous drug results in the selection and outgrowth of variants that are resistant to the drug, effective therapy for tuberculosis requires the combination of multiple drugs to which the organisms are susceptible. The simultaneous administration of two or more active drugs prevents emergence of resistance.

The current epidemiology of drug resistance in the community determines the choice of initial therapy, which must usually start prior to the availability of culture and susceptibility test results. Based on surveys of all tuberculosis cases

Table 23.1 Dosing of antiretroviral drugs and rifabutin

HIV drug and dose	Rifabutin daily	Rifabutin twice weekly
Indinavir 1200 mg q 8 h	150 mg	300 mg
Nelfinavir 1000 mg three times a day	150 mg	300 mg
Saquinavir soft-gel formulation (fortovase) 1200 mg three times a day	150 mg	300 mg
Amprenavir 1200 mg twice a day	150 mg	300 mg
Efavirenz 600 mg at bedtime	450–600 mg	600 mg

reported in the USA to the CDC through the first quarter of 1991, 3% of new cases were resistant to either isoniazid or rifampin and 6.9% of recurrent cases were resistant to both drugs (CDC, 1993a). This is in contrast to the preceding 5-year period, in which these proportions were 0.5% and 3%, respectively. From 1990 to 1992, the CDC has investigated a total of 22 institutional outbreaks of multi-drug-resistant tuberculosis in the USA, localized largely to urban areas of New York and Florida. Recently, a multi-national study of drug-resistant tuberculosis was conducted in 35 countries on five continents (Pablos-Mendez et al., 1998). This survey found that a median of 9.9% of all previously untreated tuberculosis patients had isolates resistant to at least one first-line drug (range 2–41%), with multidrug resistance found in 1.4% (range 0–14.4%). The prevalence of resistance to at least one first-line drug in previously treated patients was 36% (range 5.3–100%), with corresponding multidrug prevalence of 13% (range 0–54%).

Initial treatment regimen

In HIV-infected patients in whom HAART is not available or is not recommended because of clinical or adherence cri-

teria, treatment with a standard four-drug regimen of isoniazid, rifampin, pyrazinamide and either streptomycin or ethambutol is the preferred initial treatment for tuberculosis (Table 23.2) (Centers for Disease Control and Prevention, 1998). This regimen can be administered daily, intermittently three times a week from the beginning, or twice weekly following a 2-week induction phase of daily therapy. Given the influence of poor compliance on the development of drug resistance, directly observed or supervised therapy is recommended for all patients with tuberculosis (CDC, 1993a; Iseman, 1993). Based on the prevalence and characteristics of drug-resistant organisms in the USA, this regimen will provide at least 95% of patients with at least two drugs to which their organisms are susceptible (CDC, 1993a). This is likely to be an effective regimen for initial treatment in other areas of the world as well, although less expensive drugs such as amithiozone and streptomycin are more frequently substituted for rifampin, ethambutol or pyrazinamide in developing countries (Iseman, 1993).

The clinical and microbiological response, cure and relapse rates with effective therapy of drug-susceptible

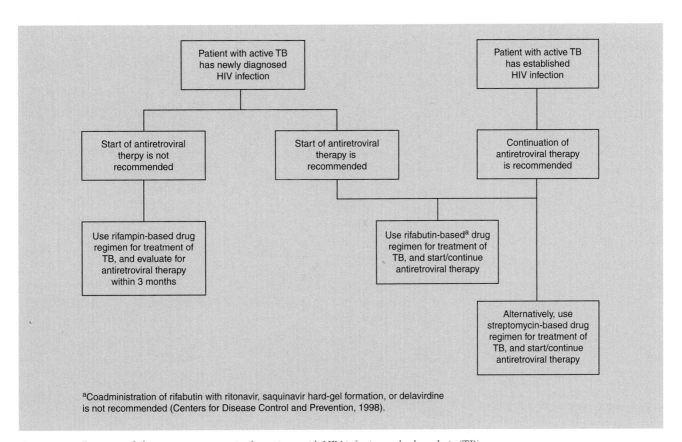

Figure 23.1 *Recommended management strategies for patients with HIV infection and tuberculosis (TB).*

tuberculosis in HIV-positive persons is similar to that in HIV-uninfected persons. Small and colleagues reported that a 6-month treatment course cured tuberculosis in patients with advanced HIV disease, with a relapse rate of 3%, similar to that seen in non-HIV-infected persons (Small *et al.*, 1991). In a recent study of tuberculosis therapy conducted in Haiti, intermittent therapy with isoniazid, rifampin, pyrazinamide and ethambutol, administered three times weekly for a total of 6 months, was as effective in HIV-infected patients (clinical response 82%) as in HIV-uninfected patients (clinical response 87%) (Chaus-

son *et al.*, 1996). A retrospective study of patients with HIV-related tuberculosis in Baltimore in the USA, showed that directly observed therapy was associated with better survival than self-administered therapy (Alwood *et al.*, 1994).

Four antituberculous drugs should be continued for the first 2 months of treatment; isoniazid and rifampin should then be continued for the duration. When drug-susceptibility results are available, the regimen should be amended as appropriate. Data specific to a given area can be used to guide initial therapy; in areas where isoniazid

Table 23.2 Doses and potential adverse effects of first-line antituberculous drugs

Drug	Usual adult dose	Paediatric dose[a]	Adverse effects
Isoniazid			
Daily	300 mg	10–20 mg/kg	Hepatitis
Twice weekly	900 mg	20–40 mg/kg	Peripheral neuropathy
Three times a week	900 mg	20–40 mg/kg	Rash or drug fever
			Lupus-like syndrome
Rifampin			
Daily	600 mg	10–20 mg/kg	Rash or drug fever
Twice weekly	Same	Same	Hepatitis
Three times a week	Same	Same	Neutropenia
			Thrombocytopenia
Rifabutin			Myalgia
Daily	150–300 mg	5 mg/kg	Red-orange body fluid discoloration
Twice weekly	300 mg	Same	Drug interactions
Three times a week	300 mg	Same	
Pyrazinamide			
Daily	2 g	15–30 mg/kg	Anorexia, nausea
Twice weekly	4 g	50–70 mg/kg	Hyperuricaemia
Three times a week	3 g	50–70 mg/kg	Arthralgia
			Hepatitis
			Rash
Ethambutol[b]			
Daily	15–25 mg/kg	15–25 mg/kg	Anorexia
Twice weekly	50 mg/kg	50 mg/kg	Headache
Three times a week	25–30 mg/kg	25–30 mg/kg	Retrobulbar neuritis
			Peripheral neuropathy
			Rash or drug fever
			Hyperuricaemia
Streptomycin			
Daily	1 g	20–30 mg/kg	Nephrotoxicity
Twice weekly	1.5 g	25–30 mg/kg	Ototoxicity
Three times a week	1 g	25–30 mg/kg	Rash
			Headache
			Nausea, vomiting

[a]Children < 12 years; maximum doses should not exceed the doses listed for adults.
[b]Maximum dose not to exceed 2.5g; not recommended for children when visual acuity cannot be adequately evaluated, but should be included in a four-drug regimen in children with HIV and tuberculosis, and should be considered when *M. tuberculosis* isolate is potentially resistant to other drugs (adapted from Centers for Disease Control, 1993a; Iseman, 1993)

resistance rates are known to be low, the use of fewer drugs is acceptable. If drug-susceptibility results are not available, the initial four-drug regimen should be modified by discontinuation of pyrazinamide after 8 weeks, but isonizid, rifampin and ethambutol or streptomycin should be continued for the duration of therapy (CDC, 1993a). Although the recommended duration of therapy for HIV-related tuberculosis is 6 months, a recent study in Haiti showed that the rate of relapse was reduced from 8% per year to 1% per year by giving secondary prophylaxis with INH (Fitzgerald et al., 2000).

HIV-infected patients already receiving HAART or who are candidates to start HAART should be initiated on a four-drug regimen as well, with rifabutin substituted for rifampin (exceptions noted below). This modification is necessary because of the effects that rifamycins and certain HAART agents have on the P-450 cytochrome oxidases. Of the available rifamycins, rifampin is the most potent inducer of cytochrome P-450, followed by rifapentine (not recommended in HIV-infected patients) with intermediate activity, and rifabutin, which has substantially less activity as an inducer. The nucleoside reverse transcriptase inhibitors (NRTIs) are not metabolized by the cytochrome P-450 pathway and do not have clinically significant interactions with rifabutin or rifampin. However, NNRTIs and PIs are metabolized by cytochrome P-450 oxidases. The PIs act as cytochrome P-450 inhibitors (ritonavir > amprenavir ≅ indinavir ≅ nelfinavir > saquinavir), whereas among the NNRTIs, nevirapine is an inducer, delavirdine is an inhibitor and efavirenz is both an inducer and an inhibitor of cytochrome P-450. In general, the interactions between rifamycin and HAART agents are bidirectional, with rifamycins lowering the serum concentrations of PIs and NNRTIs and rifamycin levels increased by PIs and lowered by efavirenz.

Because rifampin markedly lowers the serum concentration of NNRTIs (efavirenz may be an exception) and PIs, it is contraindicated in patients on these medications. Rifabutin should be substituted for rifampin except in patients taking ritonavir, the hard-gel formulation of saquinavir (invirase), and delavirdine, these agents are contraindicated with all rifamycins because of difficult-to-manage drug interactions. In patients on these contraindicated agents, possible management options may include either substituting streptomycin for the rifamycin or altering the HAART regimen. Notably, rifabutin levels are also increased by PIs and lowered by efavirenz. In patients who are on HAART agents not contraindicated for use with rifabutin, Table 23.1 lists recommended doses of antiretroviral agents and rifabutin, based on whether rifabutin, is given daily or twice weekly (CDC, 1998).

Rifapentine, a long-acting rifamycin, was recently approved in the USA for treatment of tuberculosis in HIV-uninfected patients. However, use of rifapentine in HIV-infected patients is not recommended at present, as emergence of rifamycin resistance during therapy was seen in one trial (Vernon et al., 1998).

Treatment of drug-resistant tuberculosis

For HIV-infected persons treated in settings where outbreaks or transmission of multidrug-resistant tuberculosis have occurred, or when retreating an HIV-infected patient with a prior history of antituberculous therapy, more aggressive treatment with five- or six-drug regimens may be initially required to circumvent the high mortality reported for those with HIV infection and multidrug-resistant tuberculosis. If the susceptibilities for outbreak or exposure strains are known, these can be used to guide initial choices. In the absence of these, the regimen should include a minimum of isoniazid, rifampin, pyrazinamide, and ethambutol or streptomycin; additional second-line drugs should be added such that at least two and possibly three drugs to which the strain may be susceptible or which the patient has not previously received are administered (Iseman, 1993). Data reported in a study evaluating treatment of multidrug-resistant tuberculosis in persons without HIV infection, in which most patients were retreated following relapse or failure of prior therapy, suggested that outcome was better when patients received at least three drugs to which their isolate was susceptible (Goble et al., 1993). Similar data were reported from an outbreak of multidrugresistant tuberculosis among HIV-infected persons in Florida (Fischl et al., 1992a). Response rates in general are poorer for persons with multidrug-resistant tuberculosis than in those patients infected with fully susceptible strains. This is probably related to the loss of the most active sterilizing drugs, isoniazid and rifampin (Goble et al., 1993; Iseman, 1993). Table 23.3 shows second-line agents and the usual doses for treatment of multidrug-resistant tuberculosis.

Three fluoroquinolones, ciprofloxacin, ofloxacin, and levofloxacin are active in vitro at standard doses against M. tuberculosis (Leysen et al., 1989). Their contribution to the efficacy of antituberculous therapy remains to be determined. Ofloxacin has been shown in a small, uncontrolled clinical trial to be active and well tolerated in doses up to 800 mg/day when used in multidrug regimens for treatment of drug-resistant tuberculosis (Yew *et al.*, 1990).

It is currently recommended that HIV-infected patients with fully susceptible organisms are treated with a 6-month antimycobacterial regimen consisting of isoniazid, rifampin, and pyrazinamide administered for 2 months, followed by isoniazid and rifampin for 4 months. Ethambutol or streptomycin should be included in the initial regimen until the results of drug susceptibility tests are available. If the response to initial therapy is judged to be slow or substandard, the duration of treatment should be prolonged. Using the prior recommendation of continuing therapy for 6 months after sputum culture conversion to negative may be a reasonable approach (CDC, 1993a). Regimens effective for treatment of pulmonary tuberculosis should be equally effective for treatment of extrapulmonary disease. Treatment for multidrug-resistant tuberculosis should be continued for 18–24 months and for at least 12 months after conversion to sputum culture negative (CDC, 1991a).

Studies completed to date do not support the need for indefinite continuation of isoniazid following completion of antimycobacterial treatment.

Adverse reactions to antituberculous chemotherapy

Adverse reactions to antimycobacterial therapy are reported with greater frequency among patients with HIV infection than among the general population (Small *et al.*, 1991; Hopewell, 1992). The incidence of such reactions may be higher in those with advanced immunosuppression, possibly reflecting poorer hepatic and bone marrow reserve. Rifampin appears to be the agent associated with the greatest frequency of hypersensitivity reactions; rash, drug fever, hepatitis, and thrombocytopenia are reported in up to 10% of patients (Small *et al.*, 1991). Adverse reactions to isoniazid, pyrazinamide, and ethambutol occur at rates near the age-associated rates of persons without HIV infection.

The potential interactions of antituberculous agents with other drugs further complicates the care of the HIV-infected patients with both active and latent tuberculosis (see

Table 23.3 Usual adult doses and potential adverse effects of second-line antituberculous drugs[a]

Drug	Usual adult dose	Adverse effects
Ethionamide	250 mg two or three times a day	Nausea, vomiting, anorexia Metallic taste Thrombocytopenia Peripheral neuropathy Optic neuritis Depression Hepatitis
Cycloserine	250 mg two or three times a day	Neurotoxicity (somnolence, tremor, dysarthria, confusion, seizures)
Capreomycin	1 g daily (i.m.)	Nephrotoxicity)
Kanamycin	1 g/day (i.m.)	Ototoxicity Nephrotoxicity
Para-aminosalicylic acid (PAS)	4–12 g/day	Nausea, vomiting, diarrhoea Anorexia, abdominal pain Anaemia, neutropenia Thrombocytopenia Hepatitis
Levofloxacin	500 mg/day	Nausea, vomiting, abdominal pain, anorexia
Ofloxacin	400 mg/day	Headache
Ciprofloxacin	750 mg/day	Anxiety, tremulousness

(Adapted from Iseman, 1993.)

Chapters 5 and 6). As elaborated above, the interaction between rifamycins and PIs and NNRTIs is bidirectional and requires either substitution of rifabutin for rifampin, use of a non-rifamycin-based antituberculosis regimen, or adjustment in the HAART regimen (CDC, 1998). The adverse effects of rifabutin are similar to those of rifampin (Table 23.2). Furthermore, there are important interactions between isoniazid and rifampin with the azole class of antifungal agents frequently used in patients who are HIV-infected. Both isoniazid and rifampin decrease ketoconazole and fluconazole levels, and ketaconazole interferes with the absorption of rifampin.

HAART has been associated with paradoxical worsening of signs and symptoms of tuberculosis; such 'reversal reactions' are felt to represent reconstitution of the immune response to mycobacteria (Behrens et al., 2000). One study found over one-third of patients developing such reactions (Narita et al., 1998). Treatment for 'reversal reactions' is generally supportive, with the caveat that treatment failure, non-adherence, and drug resistance must be ruled out.

Finally, the new guidelines from the CDC include two important differences in the treatment of HIV-infected individuals with tuberculosis relating to potential adverse drug reactions. First, pregnant women with HIV and tuberculosis should be treated with a four-drug regimen, including pyrazinamide. This drug was not endorsed in the USA (although its use was recommended throughout the world) because of perceived inadequate safety data. This potential risk is now felt to be outweighed by the likely benefit. Second, children with HIV and tuberculosis should be treated with a four-drug regimen, including ethambutol. Previously, this drug was discouraged in children too young to be evaluated for ocular toxicity, but again the benefit in this setting was felt to outweigh the potential risks (CDC, 1998).

Prophylaxis

Chemoprophylaxis

All patients with HIV infection should undergo Mantoux tuberculin skin testing to identify those with latent tuberculosis infection. Skin testing should be performed as early as possible after HIV serodiagnosis to avoid the problems of interpretation encountered in the anergic patient. Persons with HIV infection should receive preventative therapy for tuberculosis if they have a positive tuberculin test, as previously defined. It is imperative to rule out active tuberculosis before initiating chemo-prophylaxis, to assure that persons with active disease are not exposed to single-drug treatment, which may lead to resistance.

Prophylaxis should also be given to HIV-infected persons who are contacts of known infectious tuberculosis patients, regardless of skin testing results. Pape and co-workers (1993) showed that isoniazid prophylaxis reduced the risk of tuberculosis significantly in HIV-infected, tuberculin skin test-positive Haitian adults. The study also suggested that isoniazid prophylaxis may reduce the risk of HIV disease progression and death, though other studies have not confirmed this. In HIV-infected persons with repeated exposure to tuberculosis, prophylaxis should be prescribed with the same guidelines as the initial exposure.

Isoniazid remains the most frequently recommended preventative therapy, with dosing 300 mg/day and 10 mg/kg/day for children (not to exceed 300 mg/day) (CATS/CDC, 2000). The recommended duration of therapy has decreased to 9 months, with some experts believing that 6 months is adequate (the same as for tuberculosis patients not co-infected with HIV) (CDC, 1998). Isoniazid can also be administered intermittently in doses of 900 mg twice weekly to facilitate directly observed therapy.

Rifampin and pyrazinamide given for 2 months appears to be as effective as 12 months of isoniazid (Gordin et al., 2000; Halsey et al., 1998). Toxicity with this regimen is similar to isoniazid, though there is slightly less hepatotoxicity with the rifampin-based regimen, and adherence to this regimen is superior to that for 12 months of isoniazid. Drug interactions, as noted above, are a potential limitation for the use of rifampin for preventive therapy, and of note, rifampin can induce narcotic withdrawal in patients receiving opiates such as methadone. Methadone doses should be increased by 5–10 mg/day up to a 50% increase in total dose when rifampin is added. Furthermore, although no studies have been undertaken evaluating the use of rifabutin in tuberculosis prevention in HIV-infected patients, there is no reason to believe that the drug would not be effective for this indication. Thus, for patients on HAART, rifabutin may be substituted for rifampin, with the exceptions noted previously.

The 2-month combination of rifampin and pirazinamide mentioned above (Gordin et al., 2000; Halsey et al., 1998) is currently the only adequately tested option for preventive therapy for those exposed to an isoniazid-resistant isolate of *M. tuberculosis* or unable to tolerate isoniazid; other potential options include 4 months of rifampin or rifabutin alone, or rifampin combined with ethambutol (CDC, 1990a). There are no uniform recommendations for preventive therapy for those exposed to a multidrug-resistant strain of *M. tuberculosis*. Some experts have suggested that individuals infected with multidrug-resistant strains who have a high risk of developing active tuberculosis should receive at least two antimycobacterial drugs; pyrazinamide 25–30 mg/kg/day and ethambutol 15–25 mg/kg/day is one alternative regimen (CDC, 1992). Another potential regimen is the combination of pyrazinamide and a fluoroquinolone such as ciprofloxacin 750 mg twice daily or levofloxacin 500 mg daily (CDC, 1992).

Bacille Calmette Guérin (BCG) vaccination

BCG vaccine is derived from a strain of *Mycobacterium bovis* attenuated through serial passage in culture. Many BCG vaccines are available worldwide, and preparations vary because of genetic differences in bacterial strains and in techniques of production. They also vary widely in efficacy, with estimates ranging from 56 to 80% (CDC, 1988). Data collected from studies conducted in areas where tuberculosis is endemic and vaccination is performed at birth indicate that the incidence of tuberculous meningitis and miliary tuberculosis is reduced by 52–100% and that of pulmonary tuberculosis by 2–80% in vaccinated children, compared with unvaccinated control subjects (CDC, 1988). Randomized, controlled clinical trials assessing the efficacy of BCG vaccination in adults have not been performed.

In the USA, the general population in most areas remains at low risk of acquiring tuberculous infection, and tuberculosis control is maintained through case detection and preventive chemotherapy; BCG vaccination is not routinely recommended. However, BCG vaccination may contribute to tuberculosis control in some population groups. BCG may be recommended for:

(1) tuberculin skin test-negative infants and children who have the potential for close and prolonged exposure to untreated or ineffectively treated patients with infectious pulmonary tuberculosis and who cannot be removed from the source of exposure or be placed on long-term preventive therapy;

(2) tuberculin skin test-negative infants or children who are continuously exposed to persons with isoniazid- and rifampin-resistant tuberculosis; and

(3) groups with an excessive rate of new infection, such as those without regular access to or utilization of health care (CDC, 1988).

Adults infected with HIV are not considered candidates for BCG vaccination for several reasons, including the lack of proven benefit, the potential for later reactivation and development of active infection with BCG strains, and the potential risk of augmenting HIV replication by vaccine-induced CD4 lymphocyte activation (Weltman and Rose, 1993). Some experts have raised the possibility that health-care workers who are repeatedly exposed to multidrug-resistant tuberculosis strains may be candidates for BCG vaccination. Uniform recommendations must await further controlled trials in such settings. BCG vaccination continues to be a standard cornerstone of preventative care in countries where tuberculosis is prevalent.

References

Alwood K, Keruly J, Moore-Rice K *et al.* (1994). Effectiveness of supervised, intermittent therapy for tuberculosis in HIV-infected patients. *AIDS* **8**: 1103–8.

American Thoracic Society. (2000). Diagnostic standards and classification of tuberculosis in adults and children. *Am J Resp Crit Care Med* 2000; **161**: 1376–95.

American Thoracic Society/Centers for Disease Control and Prevention. (2000). Target tuberculin testing and treatment of latent tuberculosis infection. *Am J Resp Crit Care Med* **161**: S221–47.

Antonucci G, Girardi E, Armignacco O *et al.* (1992). Tuberculosis in HIV-infected subjects in Italy: a multicentre study. *AIDS* **6**: 1007–13.

Arachi A. (1991). The global tuberculosis situation and the new control strategy of the World Health Organisation. *Tubercule* **72**: 1–6.

Bailey WC, Albert RK, Davidson PT *et al.* (1983). Treatment of tuberculosis and other mycobacterial diseases: an official statement of the American Thoracic Society. *Am Rev Respir Dis* **127**: 790–6.

Barnes PF, Barrows SA. (1993). Tuberculosis in the 1990s. *Ann Intern Med* **119**: 400–10.

Barnes PF, Bloch AB, Davidson PT et al (1991). Tuberculosis in patients with human immunodeficiency virus infection. *N Engl J Med* **324**: 1644–50.

Behrens GM, Meyer D, Stoll M *et al.* (2000). Immune reconstitution syndromes in HIV infection following effective antiretroviral therapy. *Immunobiology* **202**: 186–93.

Berenguer J, Moreno M, Laguna F *et al.* (1992). Tuberculous meningitis in patients infected with the human immunodeficiency virus. *N Engl J Med* **326**: 668–72.

Boom WH, Chervenak KA, Wallis RS. (1991). Human Mycobacterium tuberculosis reactive CD4+ T cell clones: heterogeneity in antigen recognition, cytokine production and cytotoxicity for mononuclear phagocytes. *Infect Immun* **59**: 2737–43.

Boom WH, Chervenal KA, Mincek MA et al. (1992). Role of the mononuclear phagocyte as an antigen-presenting cell for human gamma delta T cells activated by live Mycobacterium tuberculosis. Infect Immun 60: 3480–8.

Cantwell MF, Binkin NJ. (1996). Tuberculosis in sub-Saharan Africa: a regional assessment of the impact of the human immunodeficiency virus epidemic by National Tuberculosis Control Program quality. Int J Tuberc Lung Dis 77: 220–5.

Cantwell MF, Binkin NJ. (1997). Impact of HIV on tuberculosis in sub-Saharan Africa: a regional perspective Int J Tuberc Lung Dis 1: 205–14.

Cauthen GM, Dooley SW, Onorato IM et al. (1996). Transmission of Mycobacterium tuberculosis from tuberculosis patients with HIV or AIDS. Am J Epidemiol 144: 69–77.

Centers for Disease Control and Prevention (CDC). (1988). Use of BCG vaccines in the control of tuberculosis: a joint statement by the ACIP and the Advisory Committee for Elimination of Tuberculosis. MMWR 37: 663–75.

CDC. (1990a). Nosocomial transmission of multidrug-resistant TB to health-care workers and HIV-infected patients in an urban hospital – Florida. MMWR 39: 718–22.

CDC. (1990b). Tuberculin reactions in apparently healthy HIV-seropositive and HIV-seronegative women – Uganda. MMWR 39: 638–46.

CDC. (1991a). Nosocomial transmission of multidrug-resistant tuberculosis among HIV-infected persons – Florida and New York, 1988–1991. MMWR 40: 585–91.

CDC. (1991b). Purified protein derivative (PPD)-tuberculin anergy and HIV infection: guidelines for anergy testing and management of anergic persons at risk of tuberculosis. MMWR 40: 27–33.

CDC. (1992). National action plan to combat multidrug-resistant tuberculosis: meeting the challenge of multidrug-resistant tuberculosis; Management of persons exposed to multidrug-resistant tuberculosis. MMWR 41: 1–71.

CDC. (1993a). Initial therapy for tuberculosis in the era of multidrug resistance. Recommendations of the Advisory Council for the Elimination of Tuberculosis. MMWR 42: 1–8.

CDC. (1997). Anergy skin testing and tuberculosis preventive therapy for HIV-infected persons: revised recommendations. MMWR 46: 1–10.

CDC. (1998). Prevention and treatment of tuberculosis among patients with human immunodeficiency virus: principles of therapy and revised recommendations. MMWR 47: 1–51.

Chaisson RE, Schecter GF, Theuer CP et al. (1987). Tuberculosis in patients with the acquired immunodeficiency syndrome: clinical features, reponse to therapy and outcome. Am Rev Respir Dis 136: 570–4.

Chaisson RE, Clermont HC, Holt EA et al. (1996). Six-month supervised intermittent tuberculosis therapy in Haitian patients with and without HIV infection. Am J Resp Crit Care Med 154: 1034–8.

Chin DP, Osmond D, Page-Shafer K et al. (1996). Reliability of anergy skin testing in persons with HIV infection. Am J Respir Crit Care Med 153: 1982–4.

Converse PJ, Jones SL, Astemborski J et al. (1997). Comparison of a tuberculin interferon-gamma assay with the tuberculin skin test in high-risk adults: effect of human immunodeficiency virus infection. J Infect Dis 176: 144–50.

Daley CL, Small PM, Schecter GF et al. (1992). An outbreak of tuberculosis with accelerated progression among persons infected with the human immunodeficiency virus. An analysis using restriction-fragment-length polymorphisms. N Engl J Med 326: 231–5.

De Cock KM, Chaisson RE. (1999). Can DOTS do it? A reappraisal of tuberculosis control in countries with high rates of HIV infection. Int J Tuberc Lung Dis 3: 457–65.

De Cock KM, Soro B, Coulibaly IM et al. (1992). Tuberculosis and HIV infection in sub-Saharan Africa. JAMA 268: 1581–7.

Des Prez RM, Goodwin RA. (1990). Mycobacterium tuberculosis. In: GL Mandell, RG Douglas Jr, JE Bennett (eds.) Principles and practice of infectious diseases. Third edition. New York: Churchill Livingstone, 1383–406.

Douvas GS, Looker DL, Vatter AE et al. (1985). Gamma interferon activates human macrophages to become tumoricidal and leishmanicidal but enhances replication of macrophage-associated mycobacteria. Infect Immun 50: 1–8.

D'Souza CD, Cooper AM, Frank AA et al. (1997). An anti-inflammatory role for gamma delta T lymphocytes in acquired immunity to Mycobacterium tuberculosis. J Immunol 158: 1217–21.

Dye C, Scheele S, Dolin P et al. (1997). Global burden of tuberculosis: estimated incidence, prevalence, and mortality by country. JAMA 282: 677–86.

Edlin BR, Tokars JI, Grieco MH et al. (1992). An outbreak of multi-drug resistant tuberculosis among hospitalized patients with the acquired immunodeficiency syndrome. N Engl J Med 326: 1514–21.

Elliott AM, Hayes RJ, Halwiindi B et al. (1993). The impact of HIV on infectiousness of pulmonary tuberculosis: a community study in Zambia. AIDS 7: 981–7.

Ellner PD, Kiehn TE, Cammarata R et al. (1988). Rapid detection and identification of pathogenic mycobacteria by combining radiometric and nucleic acid probe methods. J Clin Microb 26: 1349–52.

Fauci AS. (1991). NIH conference: immunopathogenic mechanisms in human immunodeficiency virus (HIV) infection. Ann Intern Med 114: 678–83.

Fischl MA, Daikos GL, Uttamchandani RB et al. (1992a). Clinical presentation and outcome of patients with HIV infection and tuberculosis caused by multiple-drug-resistant bacilli. Ann Intern Med 117: 184–90.

Fischl MA, Uttamchandani RB, Daikos GL et al. (1992b). An outbreak of tuberculosis caused by multiple-drug-resistant tubercle bacilli among patients with HIV infection. Ann Intern Med 117: 177–3.

Fitzgerald DW, Desvarieux M, Severe P et al. (2000). Effect of post-treatment isoniazid on prevention of recurrent tuberculosis in HIV-1-infected individuals: a randomized trial. Lancet 356: 1470–4.

Forte M, Maartens G, Rahelu M et al. (1992). Cytolytic T-cell activity against mycobacterial antigens in HIV. AIDS 6: 407–11.

Goble M, Iseman MD, Madsen LA et al. (1993). Treatment of 171 patients with pulmonary tuberculosis resistant to isoniazid and rifampin. N Engl J Med 328: 527–32.

Gordin F, Chaisson RE, Matts JP et al. (2000). Rifampin and pyrazinamide vs isoniazid for prevention of tuberculosis in HIV-infected persons: an international randomized trial. Terry Beirn Community Programs for Clinical Research on AIDS, the Adult AIDS Clinical Trials Group, the Pan American Health Organization, and the Centers for Disease Control and Prevention Study Group. JAMA 283: 1445–50.

Haanen JBAG, de Waal MR, Res PCM et al. (1991). Selection of human T helper type 1-like T cell subsets by mycobactria. J Exp Med 174: 583–92.

Halsey NA, Coberly JS, Desormeaux J et al. (1998). Randomized trial of isoniazid verses rifampin and pyrazinamide for prevention of tuberculosis in HIV-1 infection. Lancet 351: 786–92.

Harries AD, Nyong'Onya Mbewe L, Salaniponi FM et al. (1996). Tuberculosis programme changes and treatment outcomes in patients with smear-positive pulmonary tuberculosis in Blantyre, Malawi. Lancet 347: 807–9.

Havlir DV, Ellner JJ, Chervenak KA et al. (1991). Selective expansion of human gamma delta T cells by monocytes infected by live Mycobacterium tuberculosis. J Clin Invest 87: 729–33.

Hopewell PC. (1992). Impact of human immunodeficiency virus infection on the epidemiology, clinical features, management, and control of tuberculosis. Clin Infect Dis 15: 540–7.

Iseman MD. (1993). Treatment of multidrug-resistant tuberculosis. N Engl J Med 329: 784–91.

Klausner JD, Ryder RW, Baende E et al. (1993). Mycobacterium tuberculosis in household contacts of human immunodeficiency virus type 1-seropositive patients with active pulmonary tuberculosis in Kinshasa, Zaire. J Infect Dis 168: 106–11.

Kumararatne DS, Pithie AS, Drysdale P et al. (1990). Specific lysis of mycobacterial antigen-bearing macrophages by class II MHC-restricted polyclonal T cell lines in healthy donors or patients with tuberculosis. Clin Exp Immunol 80: 314–23.

Lee MP, Chan JW, Ng KK et al. (2000). Clinical manifestations of tuberculosis in HIV-infected patients. Respirology 5: 423–6.

Leysen DC, Haemers A, Pattyn SR. (1989). Mycobacteria and the new quinolones. Antimicrob Agents Chemother 33: 1–5.

Markowitz N, Hansen NI, Hopewell PC et al. (1997). Incidence of tuberculosis in the United States among HIV-infected patients. Ann Intern Med 126: 123–32.

Modilevsky T, Sattler FR, Barnes PF. (1989). Mycobacterial disease in patients with human immunodeficiency virus infection. Arch Intern Med 149: 2201–5.

Narita M, Ashkin D, Hollender ES et al. (1998). Paradoxical worsening of tuberculosis following antiretroviral therapy in patients with AIDS. Am J Respir Crit Care Med 158: 157–61.

Orme IM, Andersen P, Boom WH. (1993). T cell response to Mycobacterium tuberculosis. J Infect Dis 167: 1481–97.

Ottenhof THM, Kale V, van Embden JDA et al. (1987). The recombinant 65-kD heat shock protein of Mycobacterium bovis BCG/M tuberculosis is a target molecule of CD4+ cytotoxic T lymphocytes that lyse human monocytes. J Exp Med 168: 1947–52.

Pablos-Mendez A, Raviglione MC, Laszlo A et al. (1998). Global surveillance for antituberculosis-drug resistance, 1994–1997. World Health Organization International Union against Tuberculosis and Lung Disease Working Group on Anti-Tuberculosis Drug Resistance Surveillance. N Engl J Med 338: 1641–9.

Pancholi P, Mirza A, Bhardwaj N et al. (1993). Sequestration from immune CD4+ T cells of mycobacteria grown in human macrophages. Science 260: 984–6.

Pape JW, Jean SS, Ho JL et al. (1993). Effect of isoniazid prophylaxis on incidence of active tuberculosis and progression of HIV infection. Lancet 342: 628–33.

Pitchenik AE, Rubinson HA. (1985). The radiographic appearance of tuberculosis in patients with the acquired immune deficiency syndrome (AIDS) and pre-AIDS. Am Rev Respir Dis 131: 393–6.

Pitchenik AE, Cole C, Russell BW et al. (1984). Tuberculosis, atypical mycobacteriosis, and the acquired immunodeficiency syndrome among Haitian and non-Haitian patients in south Florida. Ann Intern Med 101: 641–5.

Radhakrishnan VV, Mathai A. (1991). Detection of Mycobacterium tuberculosis antigen 5 in cerebrospinal fluid by inhibition ELISA and its diagnostic potential in tuberculous meningitis. J Infect Dis 163: 650–2.

Raviglione MC, Harries AD, Msiska R et al. (1997). Tuberculosis and HIV: current status in Africa. AIDS 11 (Suppl. B): S115–23.

Selwyn PA, Hartel D, Lewis VA et al. (1989). A prospective study of the risk of tuberculosis among intravenous drug users with human immunodeficiency virus infection. N Engl J Med 320: 545–50.

Selwyn PA, Sckell BM, Alcabes P et al. (1992). High risk of active tuberculosis in HIV-infected drug users with cutaneous anergy. JAMA 268: 504–9.

Shafer RW, Goldberg R, Sierra M et al. (1989). Frequency of Mycobacterium tuberculosis bacteremia in patients with tuberculosis in an area endemic for AIDS. Am Rev Respir Dis 140: 611–13.

Small PM, Schecter GF, Goodman PC et al. (1991). Treatment of tuberculosis is patients with advanced human immunodeficiency virus infection. N Engl J Med 324: 289–94.

Small PM, Shafer RW, Hopewell PC et al. (1993). Exogenous reinfection with multidrug-resistant Mycobacterium tuberculosis in patients with advanced HIV infection. N Engl J Med 328: 1137–44.

Styblo K. (1980). Recent advances in epidemiological research in tuberculosis. Advan Tuberc Res 20: 1.

Sunderam G, McDonald RJ, Maniatis T et al. (1986). Tuberculosis as a manifestation of the acquired immunodeficiency syndrome (AIDS). JAMA 256: 362–6.

Theuer CP, Hopewell PC, Elias D et al. (1990). Human immunodeficiency virus infection in tuberculosis patients. J Infect Dis 162: 8–12.

Tuberculosis Control Division, City and County of San Francisco. (1997). Tuberculosis in San Francisco, 1996. San Francisco: Tuberculosis Control Division.

USPHS/IDSA Prevention of Opportunistic Infections Working Group. (1997). 1997 USPHS/IDSA guidelines for the prevention of opportunistic infections in persons infected with human immunodeficiency virus. MMWR 46: 1–46.

Vernon A, Burman W, Benator D et al. (1999). acquired rifamycin monoresistance in patients with HIV-related tuberculosis treated with once-weekly rifapentine and isoniazid. Tuberculosis Trials Consortium. Lancet 353: 1843–7.

Watt G, Zaraspe G, Bautista S et al. (1988). Rapid diagnosis of tuberculous meningitis by using an enzyme-linked immunosorbent assay to detect mycobacterial antigen and antibody in cerebrospinal fluid. J Infect Dis 158: 681–6.

Weltman AC, Rose DN. (1993). The safety of Bacille Calmette-Guerin vaccination in HIV infection and AIDS. AIDS 7: 149–57.

World Health Organization (WHO). (1999). World Health Report 1999: Making a difference. Geneva: WHO.

Yanai H, Uthaivoravit W, Panich V et al. (1996). Rapid increase in HIV-related tuberculosis, Ching Rai, Thailand, 1990–1994. AIDS 10: 527–31.

Yew WW, Kwan SY, Ma WK et al. (1990). In-vitro activity of loxacin against Mycobacterium tuberculosis and its clinical efficacy in multiply resistant pulmonary tuberculosis. J Antimicrob Chemother 26: 227–36.

Management and prevention of disseminated *Mycobacterium avium* complex infections

JENNIFER HOY

Mycobacterium avium complex (MAC) infection caused significant morbidity and contributed to mortality in HIV-infected patients, until the availability of effective prophylaxis and the advent of highly active antiretroviral therapy (HAART). It was the most common bacterial infection complicating AIDS in the developed world, and was one of the most common opportunistic infections overall. Since the availability of potent antiretroviral therapy (mid-1996), several observations have been made. First, there has been a marked reduction in the incidence of disseminated MAC infections. In addition, reports of unusual manifestations of MAC infection and an altered natural history of this AIDS-related opportunistic infection have been reported. Disseminated MAC infection occurs at an advanced stage of HIV-induced immunodeficiency. Anti-mycobacterial chemotherapy has been shown to improve the quality of life and prolong survival of AIDS patients with disseminated MAC infection. Several drug regimens have produced clinical benefit in 60–75% of patients and eradication of mycobacteria from blood in 40–88% of patients.

Microbiology

The *Mycobacterium avium* complex, which includes *M. avium* and *M. intracellulare*, is a group of slow-growing acid fast bacilli. Like *Mycobacterium tuberculosis*, MAC is a facultative intracellular pathogen able to survive and replicate within macrophages.

The majority of isolates that cause disease in AIDS patients are *M. avium* (97%) and of the 28 serovars, three are most commonly encountered in AIDS patients in the USA (serovars 4 [40%], 8 [17%] and 1 [9%] (Yakrus and Good, 1990). There is some geographical variation in the prevalence of serovars 4 and 8. For example, serovar 8 and serovar 4 occur in similar frequencies of 25–28% in California, while in New York serovar 4 accounts for 42% of isolates and serovar 8 for 17%. In Australia, the majority of typeable isolates belong to serovars 1, 4 and 8, and a similar geographical variability has also been noted. The dominant serovar in Victoria is serovar 4, while serovar 8 predominates in New South Wales (Dawson, 1990). The Australian study reported that of 45 patients with MAC isolates from different sites, 17 (38%) were infected with multiple serovars (Dawson, 1990).

M. intracellulare serotypes account for only 3% of isolates in HIV-infected patients and are recovered mainly from sputum (none identified from stool specimens). *M. intracellulare* is identified in only 1.4% of blood isolates (Yakrus and Good, 1990). This is in contrast to MAC infection in individuals with chronic obstructive airways disease, where the predominant serotype is *M. intracellulare*. This suggests that the respiratory tract is the route of infection for *M. intracellulare* and associated disseminated disease is uncommon.

MAC organisms are ubiquitous and commonly isolated from environmental sources such as water, soil, dust and aerosols. Contaminated water and aerosols of water are presumed to be the most likely source of organisms in HIV-infected patients who develop disseminated MAC (Inderlied and Young, 1990), although one environmental study performed on water, food and soil samples collected from the environs of HIV-1-infected individuals in San Francisco revealed less than 1% recovery of MAC organisms from food and water, but 55% recovery from soil samples from potted plants (Yajko *et al.*, 1995). No epidemiological relationship has been demonstrated for environmental exposure and MAC disease.

Over half the clinical isolates of MAC from AIDS patients contain plasmids. It is suspected but unproven, that these plasmids bear genes for virulence or drug resistance. Colony morphology reflects pathogenicity, as translucent colony variants appear to be more pathogenic in animal models and more resistant to antibiotics *in vitro* (Ellner *et al.*, 1991).

Epidemiology

Prior to 1980, *Mycobacterium avium intracellulare*, now usually called MAC, was most often recognized as the cause of slowly progressive fibrocavitary disease in individuals with chronic lung disorders. Disseminated infection was extremely rare, even in individuals with severe immuno-suppression (Horsburgh *et al.*, 1991), but the number of cases increased dramatically with the beginning of the HIV/AIDS epidemic.

The cumulative incidence of symptomatic disseminated MAC infection in HIV-infected patients reported from clinic-based studies varied from 15 to 30%, until the introduction of HAART. Up to half of autopsies performed in AIDS patients revealed evidence of MAC infection, although this could have been an overestimate due to referral of cases with undiagnosed clinical syndromes. Nightingale *et al.* (1992) prospectively determined the actuarial incidence of MAC bacteraemia in 1006 patients who had monthly blood cultures for mycobacteria after their first AIDS-defining event. They reported an incidence of MAC bacteraemia in 21% ± 2% at 12 months after an AIDS diagnosis and 41% ± 3% at 24 months (Nightingale *et al.*, 1992). In Melbourne, 42% of all AIDS patients seen from 1983 to 1993 had disseminated MAC infection diagnosed. MAC infection was the index diagnosis in 6% of AIDS patients, and 13% of all MAC infections were AIDS-defining. These percentages were slightly higher that those reported from the USA (Horsburgh, 1991; Havlik *et al.*, 1992), possibly due to more intensive surveillance for MAC infection.

The first reductions in incidence of disseminated MAC were noted from 1993 to 1994, following the widespread utilization of specific MAC prophylaxis. The Centers for Disease Control and Prevention (CDC) in the USA reported a 40% reduction in both confirmed and presumed diagnoses of atypical mycobacterial infection (Jacobson and French, 1998). In contrast, the Swiss HIV Cohort Study demonstrated an increased incidence of microbiologically confirmed disseminated MAC infection with a cumulative probability of MAC disease at 2 years in those with fewer than 50 CD4 lymphocytes/µl, increasing from 9.8% in 1987–1989 to 29.8% in 1993–1995 (Low *et al.*, 1997). A similar increase in risk of MAC infection was also noted over similar time periods in Australia, with a 2-year cumulative risk of 50% for 1991–1994 (Dore *et al.*, 1997). Reasons for an apparent increase in the incidence of MAC infection in Europe while the incidence decreased in the USA are unclear. There has been some speculation that disseminated MAC infection is more common in the USA than in Europe. Evidence supporting this observation can be found in the placebo-controlled trial of clarithromycin prophylaxis for prevention of MAC infection. MAC bacteraemia was identified in 11% of European patients randomized to the placebo arm, compared with 21% in participants from the USA (Pierce *et al.*, 1996).

Recent analysis of untreated men in the Multicenter AIDS Cohort Study has identified HIV RNA viral load as the significant predictor of subsequent MAC infection, with the relative hazard increasing from 1.29 for those with a viral load of 30 000–60 000 copies/ml to 14.97 for those with a viral load greater than 90 000 copies/ml (Lyles *et al.*, 1999). A similar observation was made in patients treated in several ACTG studies, where the risk of MAC infection was between three and six times greater in patients with high viral loads compared with those with the same CD4 lymphocyte counts and lower viral loads. Reductions in viral load were associated with reductions in risk of MAC infection (Williams *et al*, 1999).

Further significant reductions in MAC diagnoses occurred from 1994 to 1996, with the most dramatic reductions in incidence noted following the introduction of protease inhibitor (PI) therapy. Data from the HIV Outpatient Study show that the incidence of MAC fell from 20 infections per 100 person years to less than 5 per 100 person years in 1997 (Pallela *et al.*, 1998). In the setting of highly active antiretroviral therapy, the development of disseminated MAC infection occurs in the first 2 months of therapy with HAART in over 85% of patients (Baril *et al.*, 2000). Disseminated MAC remains one of the most common infective complications in AIDS.

All studies of the natural history of MAC infection in AIDS have confirmed a significantly reduced survival for MAC-infected AIDS patients (Chaisson and Hopewell, 1989; Jacobson *et al.*, 1991; Nightingale *et al.*, 1992; Chaisson *et al.*, 1992; Chaisson *et al.*, 1998). Horsburgh and Selik,

(1989) reported a median survival of 7.4 months in AIDS patients with non-tuberculous mycobacterial infection, compared with 13.3 months in AIDS patients without MAC infection, although confounding variables such as CD4 lymphocyte counts were not considered (Horsburgh and Selik, 1989). More recent studies, which did control for factors that influence survival, such as year of AIDS diagnosis, CD4 lymphocyte count, zidovudine (ZDV) therapy and *Pneumocystis carinii* and MAC prophylaxis, continue to report conflicting results on the influence of MAC infection on survival. One retrospective study revealed no difference in survival for patients with treated disseminated MAC compared with patients with other AIDS diagnoses (median survival for untreated disseminated MAC of only 4 months compared with 8 months for treated disseminated infection) (Horsburgh et al., 1991), whereas the Johns Hopkins HIV Clinic cohort study revealed a statistically significant increased risk of death associated with MAC infection (relative hazard 3.0), independent of CD4 lymphocyte count (Chaisson et al., 1998). The median survival following diagnosis of MAC infection was 7.9 months in the Swiss HIV cohort, and survival did not improve over the 10 years of observation (Low et al., 1997).

The risk of MAC infection is unrelated to gender, HIV transmission risk group and race (Chaisson et al., 1992). Hispanics have been reported to have a slightly lower prevalence (Horsburgh and Selik, 1989) and in the developing world, disseminated MAC infection is uncommon in AIDS patients compared to tuberculosis. The International MAC Study Group examined the prevalence of MAC infection in the USA, Finland, Trinidad and Kenya between 1991 and 1994. In those with advanced immunodeficiency (fewer than 25 CD4 lymphocytes/μl), the prevalence of MAC infection was 20–34% in the USA and Finland. This was in contrast to rates of 6.7–7.5% in the developing countries. Tuberculosis rates of 3.3% in Trinidad and 25% in Kenya were noted in the same profoundly immunocompromised patients (Okello et al., 1990; von Reyn et al., 1996).

Transmission

Acquisition of MAC is presumed to occur via exposure to contaminated water or aerosols. Unlike tuberculosis, there is no evidence for transmission of MAC from person to person and this route of infection is considered to be unimportant epidemiologically. Infection is usually initiated by ingestion of contaminated water, although respiratory colonization also occurs frequently.

The comparative significance of respiratory or gastrointestinal colonization prior to dissemination requires further study. Retrospective studies have suggested that anywhere between 17 and 77% of patients are colonized at respiratory or gastrointestinal sites before dissemination, but the number of individuals with appropriate cultures for evaluation in these studies is unknown (Ellner et al., 1991). However, a prospective study in which stool specimens were cultured 6 monthly, and blood and sputum cultures were performed at the time of development of symptoms, revealed that of those that developed disseminated MAC, 16% had MAC isolated from stool specimens prior to dissemination. These investigators also documented isolation of MAC from respiratory secretions at the time of pulmonary symptomatology, and of these 63% went on to develop disseminated MAC a mean of 170 days later (Bessesen et al., 1990). Jacobson and colleagues (1991) reported a 65% risk of subsequent MAC dissemination in AIDS patients who had respiratory colonization. This retrospective study emphasized the importance of CD4 lymphocyte counts on the subsequent development of disseminated MAC in colonized individuals. The median CD4 lymphocyte count was 10/μl in patients who developed subsequent dissemination compared with 84/μl in patients who did not (Jacobson et al., 1991). Finally, a recent prospective study determined that patients with a CD4 lymphocyte count of less than 50 cells/μl and MAC cultured from either the respiratory or gastrointestinal tract had a 60% risk of MAC bacteraemia within 12 months. However, the sensitivity of respiratory or stool cultures to identify which patients would go on to develop disseminated MAC was low at 21–22%, indicating that cultures at these sites were not useful as a screening test (Chin et al., 1994). From these studies and others, it is apparent that MAC colonization of respiratory and gastrointestinal tracts may progress to dissemination, and that the duration of antecedent colonization is variable and often prolonged. However, not all patients who are colonized will develop disseminated disease (Benson et al., 1990). In practice, the majority of patients with disseminated MAC infection do not have antecedent colonization documented, and routine surveillance cultures are not recommended.

The major risk factor for the development of disseminated MAC is the level of immunodeficiency, i.e. CD4 lymphocyte counts of less than 100 lymphocytes/μl (Crowe *et al.*, 1991; Ellner *et al.*, 1991; Jacobson *et al.*, 1991). Data from the placebo-controlled trials of rifabutin for the prevention of disseminated MAC, revealed that the risk of MAC infection correlated with the degree of immune deficiency. The 1-year probability of developing MAC bacteraemia was 34% for individuals with CD4 lymphocyte counts of less than 25 cells/μl, 23% for those with CD4 lymphocyte counts between 25 and 50 cells/μl, and 10% for those with CD4 lymphocyte counts of more than 100 cells/μl (Gordin *et al.*, 1997).

Pathogenesis

Whether disseminated MAC infection occurs as a consequence of reactivation similar to other opportunistic infections in AIDS (e.g. toxoplasmosis, CMV disease) or is secondary to recent acquisition of the organism is unknown (Ellner *et al.*, 1991). Epidemiological features such as similar prevalence of infection in different age groups, races and transmission categories suggest that recent acquisition of organisms is the most likely source of MAC. One study showed that almost half of AIDS patients studied with MAC colonization or infection were infected with multiple serotypes, suggesting frequent exposure to an environmental reservoir (Dawson 1990). Using an ELISA for detection of type-specific antibodies to M. *avium* glycopeptolipid antigens, Lee and collaborators (1991) found M. *avium* antibody in only 2–4% of a control population compared with 33% of HIV-uninfected homosexual men and 46% of HIV-infected patients without evidence of MAC infection (Lee *et al.*, 1991). The prevalence of antibodies to M. *avium* was independent of CD4 lymphocyte numbers (Lee *et al.*, 1991), suggesting that colonization with MAC increases with worsening immunodeficiency. These studies suggest that MAC colonization and/or infection are widespread in certain groups at risk for HIV infection, supporting reactivation of quiescent infection as a mechanism of disease. Despite this observation, the current majority view is that disseminated MAC occurs secondary to recent acquisition of the organism in a highly immunosuppressed individual.

The host defence mechanisms against MAC have not been fully elucidated. AIDS-related strains of MAC appear to attach to intestinal cells via mycobacterial adhesions and then invade the mucosa and submucosa (Malpother and Sanger, 1984). Intestinal macrophages ingest massive numbers of MAC organisms by phagocytosis, and act as an *in vivo* reservoir of mycobacteria. HIV-infected macrophages have impaired phagocytosis, activation and intracellular killing of MAC. The cytokines tumor necrosis factor (TNF-α), interleukin-2 (IL-2), and granulocyte macrophage-colony stimulating factor (GM-CSF) activate macrophages, which then kill or inhibit the replication of intracellular MAC (Bermudez and Young, 1988; Bermudez and Young, 1990a). Neutrophils from AIDS patients show increased antimycobacterial activity in the presence of exogenous G-CSF, and neutrophils harvested from AIDS patients without MAC infection, prior to treatment with G-CSF and after 5 days of treatment, showed a significant enhancement of MAC killing (George *et al.*, 1998). Intracellular killing of MAC is only variably stimulated by interferon-γ (Bermudez and Young, 1988, 1991; Rose *et al.*, 1991).

In HIV infection, macrophage activation is impaired by the reduction in number and function of T cells, with a secondary reduction in synthesis and release of cytokines (e.g. TNF-α, interferon-γ). *In vitro* studies of concurrent MAC and HIV-1 infection of macrophages reveal increased multiplication of MAC within the chronically infected macrophages, as well as uncontrolled cytokine overproduction with increased interleukin-6, interleukin-1B, and TNF-α levels (Newman *et al.*, 1993). Some evidence indicates that there is an inverse relationship between the load of intracellular mycobacteria and the ability of the macrophage to respond to stimulation with TNF-α (Bermudez *et al.*, 1990). Muller and colleagues (1998) hypothesized that the increased susceptibility to MAC infection in patients with advanced HIV disease was related to increased interleukin-10 production by monocyte/macrophages, with resultant reductions in TNF-α levels (Muller *et al.*, 1998).

Cytokine responses to MAC bacteraemia have been investigated *in vivo*, in a case–control study of placebo recipients of a MAC prophylaxis trial. Serum interleukin-6 levels rose significantly in those with early MAC bacteraemia, while TNF-α levels increased in both MAC bacteraemia patients and controls with advanced HIV disease. In this study, there was no associated increase in plasma HIV RNA levels associated with the onset of MAC bacteraemia (Haas *et al.*, 1998). In contrast, Havlir and colleagues (1998) observed a statistically significant, but modest median increase in plasma HIV RNA of 0.4 $\log_{10}$ copies/ml associated with MAC bacteraemia in a similar matched case–control study, but included individuals who had failed MAC prophylaxis. Prior to development of MAC bacteraemia there was no significant difference in HIV RNA changes between cases and controls (Havlir *et al.*, 1998).

Histological studies of the gastrointestinal tract show intestinal macrophages loaded with MAC organisms, with involvement of both Peyer's patches and the mesenteric lymph nodes, and intestinal mucosal erosion (Bermudez and Young, 1989). Dissemination occurs primarily to the reticuloendothelial system (liver, spleen, lymph nodes, and bone marrow).

Clinical presentation

Asymptomatic colonization of the gastrointestinal or respiratory tracts is usually identified when an HIV-infected patient presents with pulmonary or gastrointestinal symptoms for investigation. For example, after complete resolution of symptoms in patients following therapy for *Pneumocystis carinii* pneumonia (PCP), or campylobacter enteritis, isolation of MAC from the original sputum or stool sample may be reported by the laboratory. These patients are likely to have had MAC co-infection and/or colonization. If there is a recurrence of pulmonary or gastrointestinal symptoms or the development of symptomatic disseminated MAC, appropriate cultures, including blood, should be collected for confirmation.

Reports of detection of MAC in stool, duodenal biopsies or respiratory secretions including sputum, need to be considered in the context of the clinical findings as colonization at these sites is not always predictive of invasive disease or subsequent dissemination. As MAC colonization of the respiratory tract infrequently produces positive acid-fast bacillus (AFB) smears of sputum, AFB in sputum should never be assumed to be MAC and the author's experience has shown that they are commonly *M. tuberculosis*. Patients with AFB in sputum should be placed in respiratory isolation and antituberculous chemotherapy begun immediately until pulmonary tuberculosis has been excluded.

MAC disease usually presents as disseminated infection in HIV-infected patients at an advanced stage of immunodeficiency (CD4 lymphocyte count of less than 50 cells/μl). Symptoms of disseminated MAC are frequently non-specific, and the onset may be little more than an exacerbation of chronic constitutional symptoms. The patient complains of persistent, high swinging fevers to 39°C and above, drenching night sweats, fatigue and progressive weight loss. Rigors, anorexia, lethargy and weakness are generally present, while myalgias and headaches are variably present. Dissemination, primarily to the reticuloendothelial system, may be manifest by lymphadenopathy (fewer than 10% cases) and hepatosplenomegaly, although enlargement of these organs is often present prior to the onset of disseminated MAC symptoms (Table 24.1).

In a prospective evaluation of symptoms associated with MAC infection in two placebo-controlled trials of MAC prophylaxis, only 50% of patients had significant fever at the onset of MAC bactaeremia, and 24% had night sweats. These individuals were undergoing monthly blood cultures as part of the trial and therefore were identified with early disease. Significant numbers of individuals in all the MAC prophylaxis trials have been excluded because of asymptomatic MAC bacteraemia at screening for entry into the trials (Gordin *et al.*, 1997). It is likely that many individuals have asymptomatic MAC bacteraemia for weeks to months prior to the onset of symptoms and subsequent diagnosis. Gordin and colleagues also identified a clinical prodrome, which occurred up to 3 months prior to the first isolation of MAC from blood, and consisted of significant weight loss, fever, and low haemoglobin and elevated lactate dehydrogenase levels. They considered that this represented manifestations of localized MAC disease in the gastrointestinal or respiratory tracts (Gordin *et al.*, 1997).

Gastrointestinal symptoms may be present at the onset of fevers, sweats and weight loss. Chronic diarrhoea and malabsorption are due to infiltration of the lamina propria and intestinal lymphatics with macrophages resulting in blocked diffusion and exudative enteropathy (Roth *et al.*, 1985; Grunfeld and Kotler, 1992). Progressive weight loss resulting in cachexia may occur. Acute or chronic abdominal pain produced by mesenteric lymph node enlargement is reasonably common. MAC is not often identified as a cause of colitis (tenesmus, small-volume diarrhoea associated with mucus, fever and weight loss).

Although MAC is the most common infection to involve the liver parenchyma and produces striking elevations of cholestatic enzymes, hepatobiliary involvement by MAC is generally asymptomatic (see Chapter 16). Markedly elevated serum alkaline phosphatase levels are a sensitive indicator of disseminated disease. Anaemia and increasing blood transfusion requirements are also frequently associated with disseminated disease due to bone marrow involvement.

Table 24.1 Clinical manifestations of *Mycobacterium avium* complex infection

Condition	Clinical findings	Laboratory tests
Asymptomatic colonization	None	Stool culture positive Sputum culture positive (Rule out tuberculosis if AFB smear positive)
Focal pneumonia	Cough, fever	Repeated positive sputum culture Chest X-ray/CT scan – hilar/mediastinal lymph nodes
Enteropathy	Chronic/subacute diarrhoea Fever ± abdominal pain (may be predominant symptoms of disseminated disease)	Small bowel biopsy AFB stain/culture positive, stool culture positive, blood cultures frequently positive
Lymphadenitis	Lymphadenopathy, fever	Biopsy/aspirate of lymph node Blood cultures (rare)
Disseminated disease	Fever (85–90%) Night sweats (80%) Diarrhoea (50%) Abdominal pain (30%) Nausea (25%) Weight loss (50%) Lymphadenopathy (Peripheral and/or intra-abdominal 10–30%) Hepatosplenomegaly (20%)	Elevated alkaline phosphatase (70%) Anaemia (85 to 90%) Blood cultures positive (90%) Bone marrow AFB smear ± culture Sputum/stool culture positive (60%) CSF culture positive (rare)

AFB: acid-fast bacillus; CSF: cerebrospinal fluid.

Localized symptomatic infection may occur in the respiratory (rarely) and gastrointestinal (more commonly) tracts, without evidence of dissemination. Focal pneumonia (patchy or nodular infiltrates) with or without hilar or mediastinal lymphadenopathy is uncommon, but can occur in 5% of patients with disseminated MAC (Ruf *et al.*, 1990). MAC can be isolated from sputum in up to one-third of individuals with disseminated infection and represents respiratory colonization in the majority (Hocqueloux *et al.*, 1998). Patients with pulmonary MAC infection without dissemination also experience symptoms of fever, night sweats, and weight loss, in addition to respiratory symptoms of cough, chest pain and dyspnoea. Chest radiography generally reveals infiltrates involving one lobe only, with or without hilar or mediastinal lymphadenopathy (Hocqueloux *et al.*, 1998). Pulmonary MAC disease should always be differentiated from pulmonary tuberculosis.

Involvement of the small bowel results in a syndrome consisting of mid-epigastric cramping, abdominal pain, watery diarrhoea that is often voluminous and severe weight loss. Fever is generally absent. This may be the initial manifestation of MAC infection, with dissemination occurring shortly thereafter. The radiological appearance is similar to Whipple's disease. Endoscopic examination reveals a characteristic patchy yellow-white pseudomembrane on the duodenal mucosa. This appearance is due to massive numbers of mycobacteria within mucosal macrophages. The histological appearance varies from minimal inflammatory reaction to poorly formed granulomata. The classic granulomatous reaction occurs rarely.

Localized MAC lymphadenitis was noted to occur as an AIDS-defining illness in about 5% of HIV-infected individuals initiating zidovudine (ZDV) monotherapy when the CD4 lymphocyte count fell below 200 cells/μl (Hoy, unpubl. data). The illness generally occurred within 8 weeks of commencing ZDV, and was accompanied by fever and lethargy. Associated drenching sweats and weight loss was unusual. The diagnosis was made by needle aspirate of the clinically involved lymph nodes, and by detection of AFB in smear and culture of MAC from the aspirated material. This localized tissue infection was reported by French *et al.* (1992), who noted the onset of symptoms within 2 weeks of commencing zidovudine therapy. This manifestation of infection was not associated with MAC isolation from blood. These individuals may have had low grade mycobacteraemia resulting in localized infection when cellular immunity improved following ZDV therapy (French *et al.*, 1992).

Since the routine initiation of antiretroviral therapy at CD4 lymphocyte counts of less than 500 cells/μl, lymphadenitis has been infrequently observed, until the advent of potent antiretroviral therapy. Individuals with profound immunodeficiency, who experience suppression of HIV replication and some restoration of cellular immunity, appear to unmask previously subclinical MAC infection. In the setting of no MAC prophylaxis, these individuals show an inflammatory response to MAC with fever, leukocytosis and focal granulomatous lymphadenitis, without MAC bacteraemia (Race *et al.*, 1998). Some individuals with localization of MAC to abdominal lymph nodes have experienced severe abdominal pain, requiring narcotic analgesia for relief, and required laparotomy for differentiation of MAC lymphadenitis from lymphoma. A similar phenomenon of 'immune restoration disease' has also been reported for *Mycobacterium tuberculosis* and other opportunistic infections (John and French, 1998).

Other rare manifestations of MAC infection (Table 24.2) include terminal ileitis, pericarditis, endophthalmitis, cutaneous abscesses, septic arthritis and osteomyelitis (Horsburgh 1991). MAC organisms have been identified in a number of organs (including the thyroid, pancreas, adrenal glands, kidney, muscle and brain) following dissemination. Symptoms relating to involvement of these organs are extremely rare, probably due to the minimal inflammatory response elicited by the mycobacteria.

In children, the incidence of disseminated MAC has been reported to be 18% of AIDS cases with 10% presenting with gastrointestinal MAC without dissemination.

Table 24.2 Rare clinical presentations of *Mycobacterium avium* complex

Pulmonary
nodules
cavity
endobronchial lesions
diffuse infiltrates
Pericarditis
Skin and soft tissue abscesses
Skin lesions
Osteomyelitis, septic arthritis
Parenchymal brain abscess
Endophthalmitis

Chronic diarrhoea, abdominal distension and pain, and failure to thrive occurred in the majority of infected children. Just over half the children with disseminated MAC have prolonged fevers, anorexia, weight loss, abdominal pain and diarrhoea. Lymphadenitis and chronic subcutaneous nodules are uncommon. Anaemia and increasing blood transfusion requirements are also seen. The median survival is similar to that of adults with disseminated MAC (Rutstein *et al.*, 1993).

Recognition and diagnosis

Any HIV-infected severely immunocompromised patient (CD4 lymphocyte counts of less than 50 cells/μl) with persisting fever, recurrent night sweats, more than 10% body weight loss and symptoms persisting for 1 month, with no other cause identified, has a greater than 75% chance of having disseminated MAC infection (Young, 1988). Attempts to isolate the organism should begin and a presumptive diagnosis of disseminated MAC can be made. Empirical therapy may be instituted while waiting for culture confirmation.

MAC bacteraemia may be found serendipitously in asymptomatic HIV-infected individuals. Follow-up blood cultures are generally negative, although there is the occasional persistently mycobacteraemic patient who remains entirely asymptomatic. In this situation, the physician is left with the dilemma of whether or not to treat with multiple antimycobacterial agents. Our approach has been to withhold therapy unless the patient becomes symptomatic.

Laboratory diagnosis

The diagnosis of disseminated MAC is most easily made by recovery of mycobacteria from blood. The Bactec® radiometric culturing systems using Bactec 13A media has allowed early detection of mycobacteraemia. The majority of positive cultures will be evident from within 3–14 days. The sensitivity of this culture method is reported to be 86–96% (Ellner *et al.*, 1991). Lysis of peripheral blood mononuclear cells to release viable intracellular mycobacteria, which are then concentrated by centrifugation, is achieved by lysis centrifugation prior to inoculation into Bactec media; although this technique is labour intensive, it improves diagnostic yield (Gill *et al.*, 1985). Quantification of MAC colony counts by the lysis centrifugation culture system has been shown to be reproducible within and between laboratories and is ideal for clinical trial evaluation of therapeutic regimens for MAC bacteraemia (Havlir et al., 1993). The conventional culture methods for mycobacteria (plating specimen of blood onto Middlebrook 7H11 agar or Lowenstein-Jensen media) are used in combination with radiometric methods to improve yield. Commercially available DNA probes for the identification of M. tuberculosis and MAC result in earlier presumptive species identification but still require confirmation after subculture on solid media.

As mycobacteraemia is usually continuous once it develops, two blood cultures will detect 95% of cases of disseminated MAC infections (Barnes and Arevalo 1988; Yagupsky and Menegus 1990). Continuous bacteraemia has been observed in over 90% of patients, once a single positive culture is obtained (Agins et al., 1989; Ellner et al., 1991). The use of polymerase chain reaction (PCR) directly on blood specimens in an attempt to expedite the diagnosis has had variable results. In one study, peripheral blood polymorphonuclear and mononuclear cells isolated by Ficoll/Hypaque centrifugation were analysed using a commercial PCR assay, which targeted the first variable region of the 16s rRNA gene. The probe was specific for both M. avium and M. intracellulare. The sensitivity of the PCR assay was 43% and the specificity was 100% when tested on 200 blood samples, making this approach insensitive as a diagnostic tool for disseminated MAC infection (Ninet et al., 1997).

Buffy coat smears of blood for microscopic detection of mycobacteria are insensitive, result in a low diagnostic yield and are not recommended for diagnostic purposes. Mycobacteria can be detected by microscopy (after suitable staining) and culture of bone marrow, lymph nodes and liver. Several authors have questioned the utility of bone marrow examination for the investigation of patients with fever and cytopenias, possibly due to mycobacterial infection. In one study, over 80% of patients with MAC infection had concordant bone marrow and blood culture results, and only 7% had mycobacteria isolated from bone marrow without concomitant isolation from blood cultures. Time to diagnosis of mycobacterial infection was similar for bone marrow examination and blood culture. Therefore, bone marrow examination offers little additional information over the less invasive and cheaper blood culture investigation (Kilby et al., 1998).

Susceptibility testing

In vitro susceptibility testing of MAC is unstandardized and the results are of uncertain clinical significance. Both broth dilution and agar dilution techniques are used for MAC susceptibility testing, but the former consistently yields lower minimum inhibitory concentrations (MIC). Both agar and broth dilution methods test MAC grown in the absence of host cells, yet in patients this pathogen exists almost completely intracellularly. As tissue penetration and intracellular concentration of antimycobacterial drugs are important considerations, determination of MICs by these methods may not predict in vivo efficacy of the agent. There have been no studies attempting to correlate clinical efficacy and in vitro susceptibility testing. Currently, routine in vitro susceptibility of MAC is not recommended and should be reserved for clinical trial settings.

MAC strains are consistently resistant to isoniazid and pyrazinamide, unlike M. tuberculosis. Marked variability in the number of isolates susceptible to antimycobacterial drugs has been observed. There has been no correlation between susceptibility and MAC serotype. By agar dilution, Yajko et al. (1987) found that 88% of MAC isolates from AIDS patients were susceptible to clofazimine (1.0 μg/ml), 32% susceptible to ethambutol (15 μg/ml), and 27% susceptible to rifampicin (10 μg/ml) (Yajko et al., 1987). Rifabutin susceptibility was increased from 28% at 0.5 μg/ml to 92% at 2.0 μg/ml.

Khardori et al. (1989) determined that 95% MAC isolates were susceptible to ciprofloxacin, (2.0 μg/ml), 81% to clarithromycin (4.0 μg/ml) and 100% to amikacin (16.0 μg/ml) (Khardori et al., 1989). Heifets et al. (1988) reported 67% susceptible to ethambutol, 20–38% to rifabutin, 46% to clofazimine and 28% to ciprofloxacin (Heifets et al., 1988). In contrast to the in vitro results, clofazimine monotherapy did not reduce blood mycobacterial load over 2 weeks, while ethambutol monotherapy produced a 0.5 log reduction over the same time period (Kemper et al., 1994).

Combinations of antimycobacterial agents have been evaluated for evidence of in vitro synergy. The following combinations have demonstrated synergy in vitro: rifabutin plus ethambutol, clarithromycin plus ethambutol or rifabutin, ciprofloxacin plus ethambutol or amikacin. Synergy was observed in 28–71% of pairs of antibiotics that included ethambutol (Kent et al., 1992), suggesting that ethambutol should be considered in therapeutic combinations. Bactericidal activity was also assessed and comparative activity noted for rifabutin, ethambutol and clarithromycin. Combinations of these drugs produced an additive rather than synergistic effect (Kent *et al.*, 1992).

Macrophage models have been used to assess both the uptake of antimicrobial agents and intracellular bactericidal activity. Comparative studies reveal clarithromycin and rifabutin are bactericidal *in vitro* against MAC, and the combination of rifabutin and clarithromycin or the addition of ethambutol (Perronne *et al.*, 1990) potentiates this activity. There is evidence for facilitated uptake of rifabutin, rifampin, clofazimine, ethambutol, clarithromycin and ciprofloxacin into macrophages (Ellner *et al.*, 1991). In the human macrophage model, a post-antibiotic effect has been demonstrated for amikacin (15.2 h), clarithromycin (77.4 h), clofazimine (72.9 h) and rifampin (39.1 h), suggesting prolonged intracellular inhibition of mycobacterial replication after a single exposure to drug (Horgen *et al.*, 1998).

Currently, *in vitro* susceptibility testing of MAC isolates has limited value in the routine management of individual AIDS patient with disseminated MAC, as no correlation between *in vitro* testing and clinical efficacy has been established.

Treatment

Despite early impressions that MAC did not cause significant morbidity, or that therapy resulted in poor clinical responses and persistent mycobacteraemia, it is now recognized that effective therapy can relieve the debilitating constitutional symptoms associated with infection and control mycobacteraemia. Symptomatic localized disease and disseminated MAC are clear indications for treatment. There have been no placebo-controlled trials to establish the efficacy of the four and five drug regimens currently used for treatment of disseminated MAC, although there are now some conflicting data from prospective, randomized comparative trials of different regimens. There is no evidence to support the treatment of individuals colonized with MAC in an attempt to prevent disseminated disease, although the MAC prophylaxis studies, which reported significant reductions in the incidence of disseminated MAC, may in fact support such a strategy.

Treatment studies

Cohort studies

Early reports of treatment for disseminated MAC infection comprised mainly retrospective case series and cohort studies. Disappointing results were reported from retrospective studies using low-dose rifabutin (150–300 mg/day), in combination with other antimycobacterial agents for variable duration. One study showed persistent mycobacteraemia in the majority of patients, or a poor mycobacterial response rate of 46% (Hawkins *et al.*, 1986; Masur *et al.*, 1987). The quadruple regimen of isoniazid, clofazimine, ethambutol and rifabutin was evaluated for efficacy in three studies of disseminated MAC. Clearance of mycobacteria occurred in 64–88% of treated patients, but the number of patients evaluated was small, and relapse rates were high. There appeared to be a dose response relationship for rifabutin, with higher response rates observed when higher doses of rifabutin were employed in the combination (Agins *et al.*, 1989; Hoy *et al.*, 1990; Dautzenberg *et al.*, 1991b). In one of these studies (Hoy *et al.*, 1990), complete resolution of symptoms occurred in 18 (72%) of the 25 patients. Fever resolved first, generally within 2 weeks of treatment, followed by resolution of sweats and lethargy in 4 weeks. Peripheral lymphadenopathy resolved in 2–3 months, while intra-abdominal lymphadenopathy responded after 5–6 months of therapy (Hoy *et al.*, 1990).

Other four-drug regimens evaluated in small numbers of patients in uncontrolled studies include rifampin 10 mg/kg/day, ethambutol 15 mg/kg/day, ciprofloxacin 750 mg twice daily for 12 weeks, and amikacin 7.5 mg/kg/day for the first 4 weeks, (30% mycobacterial response and clinical benefit in 60%), and rifampin, clofazimine, ciprofloxacin and ethambutol for 12 weeks (41% mycobacterial response and clinical benefit in 70%) (Chiu *et al.*, 1990; Kemper *et al.*, 1992).

Macrolide monotherapy

Monotherapy with either clarithromycin or azithromycin has been evaluated in short duration studies, because of the potent intracellular activity of these drugs against MAC. Azithromycin administered in a dose of 500 mg/day for 10, 20 and 30 days in an uncontrolled phase I study resulted in reduction of MAC colony counts from blood culture in all patients, and three-quarters of them experienced resolution of clinical symptoms (Young *et al.*, 1991). Similar results were obtained with clarithromycin monotherapy using doses of either 500 mg, 1000 mg or 2000 mg twice daily, in a study performed by the AIDS Clinical Trials Group (Chaisson et al., 1994). The majority of patients who continued therapy were able to eradicate mycobacteria from blood; however, 20% of patients developed in vitro resistance to clarithromycin after 12 weeks of monotherapy. Dautzenberg et al., (1991a) performed a small controlled clinical trial of clarithromycin monotherapy for 6 weeks, in which eight patients had significant reduction in colony counts after 2 weeks of therapy and seven patients achieved eradication from blood.

Combination therapy

Combination therapy with clarithromycin appears necessary to prevent relapse with the emergence of clarithromycin-resistant isolates. Several prospective, randomized trials of combination regimens for disseminated MAC have now been published. The Canadian HIV Trials Network showed that the combination of rifabutin (600 mg daily), ethambutol (15 mg/kg daily to a maximum dose of 1000 mg) and clarithromycin (1000 mg twice daily) was significantly superior to the four-drug regimen of rifampin, ethambutol, ciprofloxacin and clofazimine in clearance of mycobacteria from blood (69% versus 29%) and improved survival (8.6 months versus 5.2 months). There were significantly greater numbers of patients withdrawn from the study in the four-drug arm by 4 weeks of treatment, which appeared to be the minimum duration of treatment required for sterilization of blood cultures. There were no mycobacterial relapses during the 16-week study. This study also confirmed the rifabutin dose response observed in previous retrospective cohort studies: eradication of mycobacteria reported in 79% on 600 mg rifabutin, and 58% on 300 mg rifabutin (Shafran et al., 1996). The four-drug arm in this study is clearly inferior to clarithromycin- and rifabutin-containing regimens.

The most appropriate dose of clarithromycin for inclusion in combination therapy studies has been influenced by the unexplained increased mortality in patients who received high doses. In the original clarithromycin monotherapy study, mortality was lower in the 500 mg twice daily arm, and the significantly lower mortality was observed in an interim analysis of a combination therapy study using 500 mg versus 1000 mg clarithromycin twice daily, resulting in modification of the clarithromycin dose (Chaisson et al., 1994; Cohn et al., 1996). However, when used in combination with rifabutin, the plasma concentration of clarithromycin is approximately halved.

Clarithromycin (500 mg twice daily) plus ethambutol was significantly more effective than azithromycin (600 mg daily) plus ethambutol in eradication of mycobacteraemia (86% versus 38%) and median time to clearance of mycobacteria from blood (4.4 weeks versus more than 16 weeks) in a small, randomized study (Ward et al., 1998).

Role of clofazimine

In a randomized, open-label trial of the two-drug combination of clarithromycin (500 mg twice daily) and ethambutol, compared with the same two drugs plus clofazimine, inclusion of clofazimine did not improve either the clinical or mycobacterial response rates of the clarithromycin–ethambutol combination (54% for the clarithromycin, ethambutol, clofazimine arm versus 65% for the clarithromycin, ethambutol arm). The clofazimine-containing arm was also associated with higher mortality. The study results were potentially biased by the significant imbalance of baseline mycobacterial load, with higher mycobacterial colony counts in the three-drug arm. Only one patient (in the two-drug arm) developed clarithromycin resistance on therapy, underscoring the effectiveness of combining ethambutol with clarithromycin in prevention of resistance (Chaisson et al., 1997). A similar study utilizing clarithromycin (1000 mg twice daily) plus clofazimine (100 mg daily) with or without ethambutol (400 mg twice daily) also showed no difference in mycobacterial response rates (69%) in each arm, but there was a significant reduction in relapse rate and time to relapse with a clarithromycin-resistant strain in the ethambutol-containing arm. There was no difference in median survival (Dube et al., 1997). It appears that clofazimine does not add appreciable activity to clarithromycin and is not recommended in the initial regimen for MAC therapy.

Role of rifabutin

The role of rifabutin in the combination regimen including clarithromycin and ethambutol is not clearly defined. Conflicting trial results have been reported in 1999/2000. Gordin and colleagues (1999) performed a randomized, placebo-controlled trial of clarithromycin (500 mg twice daily) plus ethambutol (1200 mg daily) with rifabutin (300 mg daily) or placebo. There was no difference in baseline mycobacterial load (18 cfu/ml and 24 cfu/ml), or rates of bacteriological response (63% versus 61%). However, there was a trend to faster eradication of mycobacteria from blood in the rifabutin-containing arm, and greater rates of development of clarithromycin resistance noted in the non-rifabutin arm (2% versus 14%). There was no difference in survival between the two arms (Gordin *et al.*, 1999). The second study (ACTG 223) compared clarithromycin (500 mg twice daily) plus ethambutol, clarithromycin (500 mg twice daily) plus rifabutin (initially 450 mg daily, with dose reduction to 300 mg daily), and clarithromycin, and rifabutin plus ethambutol. Enrolment into the study was adversely influenced by the effects of widespread adoption of MAC prophylaxis and HAART, extending the accrual period to 3.5 years. The week 12 complete microbiological response rates (two consecutive negative blood cultures) were 40%, 42% and 51%, respectively. There was also no statistically significant difference in rates of complete clinical and microbiological responses across the three arms. The clarithromycin, rifabutin and ethambutol arm had a significantly higher proportion of patients achieving a complete microbiological response in a shorter time than the other arms, and was associated with a significantly improved survival. Relapses were more common in the clarithromycin, rifabutin group (Benson *et al.*, 1999). Hence, unlike the former study, rifabutin conferred a survival advantage for those receiving treatment for MAC. The fail-ure rates in these studies are relatively high (40–60%), and although the current US Public Health Service Task Force recommendations for treatment of MAC suggest clarithromycin plus ethambutol plus/minus rifabutin, the optimal therapy remains to be definitively determined. It is possible that the doses of clarithromycin and rifabutin in these two studies were insufficient, due to the pharmacokinetic interactions between the two drugs (described below), or poor adherence to therapy. A pharmacokinetic substudy of ACTG 223 is yet to be analyzed and these results may explain the poor results achieved.

From these studies (Tables 24.3 and 24.4), it is evident that suppression of constitutional symptoms, improved quality of life, and reduction or eradication of mycobacteraemia are attainable in about 50–75% of patients with disseminated MAC infection. Combinations of drugs will be required to prevent the development of resistance and relapse of mycobacteraemia.

Treatment of patients who fail or relapse

What are the options for the significant proportion of individuals who either fail initial therapy or relapse? There are no clinical trial assessments of salvage strategies for disseminated MAC. Agents commonly added to combination regimens include clofazimine, amikacin, and

Table 24.3 Clinical and microbiological results of combination therapy for *Mycobacterium avium* complex bacteraemia in cohort studies

Author (year)	Type of study	Treatment regimen	No. of patients	Clinical improvement	Microbiological results. Blood culture negative
Hawkins (1986)	Retrospective	Rifabutin (150 mg/day) or rifampin or ethambutol or ethionamide or clofazimine ± isoniazid amikacin pyrazinamide cycloserine	26	Not evaluated	2 (8%)
Masur (1987)	Retrospective	Rifabutin (150–300 mg) clofazimine ± amikacin ciprofloxacin isoniazid cycloserine	13	Not evaluated	6 (46%) 2 relapse
Hoy (1990)	Retrospective	Rifabutin (300–600 mg/d) ethambutol clofazimine isoniazid	25	21 (84%) 18 complete resolution	22 (88%) 6 relapse
Agins (1989)	Retrospective	Rifabutin (150 mg/d) ethambutol clofazimine isoniazid	7	6 (86%)	6 (86%) 1 relapse
Dautzenberg (1991)	Prospective	Rifabutin (300–600 mg/d) ethambutol clofazimine isoniazid	14	–	9 (64%) 4 relapse
Chiu (1990)	Prospective	Rifampin ethambutol ciprofloxacin amikacin	17	7/15 (46%)	3/15 (20%)
Kemper (1992)	Prospective	Rifampin clofazimine ciprofloxacin ethambutol ± amikacin	31 22 (no amikacin)	27 (87%) 15 (68%)	13 (42%) 9 (41%)

Table 24.4 Randomized treatment studies in patients with disseminated *Mycobacterium avium* complex infection

Study	Comparators	Microbiological response	Relapse rate	Median survival
Chaisson (1997)	Clarithromycin + ethambutol (C + E)	65%	16%	38% (C + E) versus 61% (C+E + CI) mortality
	or			Baseline MAC colony counts
	Clarithromycin + ethambutol + clofazimine (C + E + CI)	54%	23%	> 1000 cfu/ml 199 days 100–1000 cfu/ml 303 days < 100 cfu/ml more than 465 days
Shafran (1996)	Clarithromycin + ethambutol + rifabutin	69%	0%	37 weeks
	or			
	Rifampin + ciprofloxacin + ethambutol + clofazimine	29%	1.1%	23 weeks
Dube (1997)	Clarithromycin + clofazimine	69%	22%	31 weeks
	or			
	Clarithromycin + clofazimine + ethambutol	69%	5%	39 weeks
May (1997)	Clarithromycin + clofazimine	21%	51%	32 weeks
	or			
	Clarithromycin + ethambutol + rifabutin	33%	14%	52 weeks
Gordin (1999)	Clarithromycin + ethambutol + rifabutin	63%	0%	57 weeks
	or			
	Clarithromycin + ethambutol	61%	1.5%	63 weeks
Benson (1999)	Clarithromycin + ethambutol	40%	7%	two fold greater hazard of death in two-drug arm
	or			
	Clarithromycin + rifabutin	42%	24%	compared with three-drug arm
	or			
	Clarithromycin + ethambutol + rifabutin	51%	6%	

ciprofloxacin. Amikacin has activity against MAC, which has been demonstrated *in vitro*, in animal models and in man. But an open, randomized, comparative study of the addition of amikacin 10 mg/kg administered either intravenously or intramuscularly for 5 days per week for the first 4 weeks of initial MAC therapy with a four-drug oral regimen of rifampin, ciprofloxacin, clofazimine and ethambutol, did not improve the clinical or microbiological response at 4 weeks (16% culture negative) or 12 weeks (38% culture negative). Median survival was 30 weeks in both groups (Parenti *et al.*, 1998). The contribution of fluoroquinolones, such as ciprofloxacin, to efficacy in the combination regimens is difficult to ascertain. Not all MAC isolates are susceptible to ciprofloxacin and monotherapy studies have shown a very modest effect on mycobacterial load, in a subset of patients only. Only one placebo-controlled study of ciprofloxacin (750 mg/day) in combination with rifampin and ethambutol has been performed. Mycobacterial load was decreased by greater than 1 log in 45% of patients receiving ciprofloxacin, and

no reduction occurred in the placebo recipients. No clinical benefit was noted in either group (Alangaden and Lerner, 1997).

Adjunctive immunomodulatory therapy

Immunomodulatory treatment may improve outcome in patients treated for disseminated MAC. Administration of granulocyte-colony stimulating factor (G-CSF) with combination therapy for MAC in neutropenic AIDS patients was associated with improved survival (355 days versus 211 days) in a retrospective cohort study (Keiser *et al.*, 1998). Recombinant granulocyte-macrophage colony-stimulating factor (GM-CSF) has also been evaluated in a small pilot study of eight patients with disseminated MAC. The addition of GM-CSF to azithromycin monotherapy did not have an effect on mycobacteraemia, but did induce activation of peripheral blood monocytes and enhanced mycobactericidal killing (Kemper *et al.*, 1998; Kedzierska et al., 2000). Interferon-γ may be useful for combination therapy with antimycobacterial drugs, following a report of resolution of refractory, disseminated MAC infection in non HIV-infected patients (Holland *et al.*, 1994). Clinical trials evaluating the role of interferon-γ as adjunctive therapy for MAC infection were terminated due to poor tolerance of the interferon-γ therapy.

Some clinicians advocate adjunctive corticosteroids for those patients with persistent or progressive symptoms despite antimycobacterial therapy. A retrospective study of 12 patients with persistent fatigue, fever, night sweats and weight loss, added dexamethasone (2–4 mg daily) to the combination antimycobacterial regimen for up to 5 months. Rapid improvement and resolution in clinical symptoms was observed in 11 of the 12 patients; however, seven patients developed a new opportunistic manifestation of AIDS (Dorman *et al.*, 1998). Initiation of HAART would be more appropriate than adjunctive steroids; however, there will be some patients who have failed most potent antiretroviral regimens for whom this therapy may be an option for symptomatic control. Pentoxifylline may also be useful for control of inflammatory cytokine-related symptoms induced by TNF-α as described in one patient with MAC and late-stage HIV disease (Reeves *et al.*, 1996).

Adverse drug reactions and interactions

The four- and five-drug regimens described above were found in clinical trials to be remarkably well tolerated by the patients, the majority of whom had advanced HIV infection. Anorexia, nausea and other gastrointestinal symptoms are the most common side-effects of therapy and may accelerate pre-existing weight loss. The adverse effects observed with antimycobacterial drugs at the doses utilized in treatment regimens are found in Table 24.5. Intolerance of rifampin is reported in 12% of AIDS patients and an increased incidence of rash and granulocytopenia has been observed with rifabutin in the placebo-controlled prophylaxis studies (Gordin *et al.*, 1992). Ototoxicity secondary to amikacin has been reported in 15% of patients (Kemper *et al.*, 1992).

Pseudo-jaundice (yellow pigmentation of skin associated with normal serum bilirubin concentration) was reported in 13 of 59 patients receiving high-dose rifabutin (600 mg) in combination with ethambutol and clarithromycin. In the same Canadian study, uveitis was diagnosed in 23 patients receiving the combination of clarithromycin, ethambutol and rifabutin (Shafran *et al.*, 1994). The risk of uveitis was significantly greater in those receiving 600 mg versus 300 mg rifabutin, and those with lower baseline body weight. It was not increased by concomitant fluconazole. Uveitis has also been reported in two patients who received 1800 mg of rifabutin daily, in a dose-limiting toxicity study of rifabutin. Management of uveitis includes prompt discontinuation of rifabutin, and topical administration of corticosteroids and mydriatic agents (Shafran *et al.*, 1998). A reversible syndrome of arthralgia and arthritis was noted in 90% of HIV-infected volunteers at doses greater than 1 g/day (Siegal *et al.*, 1990).

Two-way pharmacokinetic drug interactions occur with the combination of rifabutin and clarithromycin. Rifabutin reduces the serum clarithromycin concentrations by 50%, and increases the area under the plasma concentration time curve (AUC) of the 14-hydroxy-clarithromycin, the major metabolite by approximately 50%. This metabolite has no activity against MAC (Hafner *et al.*, 1998). Clarithromycin increases the AUC of rifabutin by 77–99% and the active metabolite of rifabutin by 236–375% (DATRI 001 Study Group, 1994, Wallace *et al.*, 1995; Hafner *et al.*, 1998). Concomitant administration of fluconazole and rifabutin also results in significantly increased serum concentrations of rifabutin and its major metabolite (Trapnell *et al.*, 1993). Cautious use of these combinations is recommended.

Rifabutin is an inducer of the hepatic cytochrome metabolizing enzymes P450 3A4, although it is a less potent inducer than rifampicin. Complex drug interactions therefore occur when rifabutin is administered with the protease inhibitors (PIs) and the non-nucleoside reverse transcriptase inhibitors (NNRTIs), which also induce or inhibit the cytochrome P450 3A4 enzymes (see Chapter 6). These enzymes are responsible for the metabolism of both the antiretroviral agents and rifabutin. The PIs inhibit the P450 3A4 enzyme to variable degrees, with ritonavir being the most potent inhibitor and saquinavir the weakest. Co-administration of rifabutin and ritonavir results in a four-fold increase in the AUC of rifabutin and a thirty-five-fold increase in the AUC of its metabolite, while co-administration of clarithromycin and ritonavir results in a 77% increase in the AUC of clarithromycin and a three-fold increase in its half-life (Cato *et al.*, 1996; Ouellet *et al.*, 1996). Rifabutin should be prescribed at half dose when co-administered with indinavir and

Table 24.5 Adverse effects observed with antimycobacterial agents at doses utilized in the treatment of disseminated *Mycobacterium avium* complex

Drug	Usual daily dose	Common adverse effects	Drug interactions	Dose adjustment for renal/hepatic insufficiency
Amikacin	7.5–10 mg/kg	Nephrotoxicity, ototoxicity	Foscarnet Amphotericin B	Yes/No
Azithromycin	600 mg	Nausea, vomiting, diarrhoea, abdominal pain, elevated liver enzymes, ototoxicity	Antacids	
Ciprofloxacin	1500 mg	Rash, anorexia, nausea, diarrhoea, headache, elevated liver enzymes	Antacids	No/No
Clarithromycin	1000–2000 mg	Nausea, vomiting, diarrhoea	Zidovudine rifabutin, carbamazepine, warfarin	Yes/Yes (severe)
Clofazimine	100 mg	Skin discoloration, anorexia, nausea		No/No
Ethambutol	15 mg/kg (maximum 1000 mg)	Anorexia, nausea, diarrhoea, rash, optic neuritis (rare at < 1000 mg/day), confusion, hepatitis (rare)		No/No
Rifampin	10 mg/kg (maximum 600 mg)	Anorexia, nausea, vomiting, diarrhoea, rash, hypersensitivity reaction (fever), hepatitis (rare)	Fluconazole Dapsone Ketoconazole Methadone Phenytoin Itraconazole Oral contraceptives Protease inhibitors Non-nucleoside reverse transcriptase inhibitors	No/Yes
Rifabutin	300–600 mg	Rash, leukopenia thrombocytopenia anorexia nausea, diarrhoea, fever, headache, hepatitis, abdominal pain, elevated liver enzymes, flu-like syndrome, (hypersensitivity), red discolouration of urine/faeces/tears/sweat, uveitis, pseudojaundice, arthralgia and arthritis	Warfarin Clarithromycin Zidovudine Ketoconnazole Oral contraceptives Protease inhibitors Non-nucleoside reverse transcriptase inhibitors	No/Yes

nelfinavir, and should be dosed at 150 mg second daily when administered with ritonavir. The combination of saquinavir and rifabutin should be avoided due to insufficient plasma levels of saquinavir resulting from the interaction.

Management recommendations

Some clinicians advocate the initiation of monthly blood cultures for isolation of mycobacteria in patients whose CD4 lymphocyte count falls below 100 cells/μl whether symptomatic or not. Our approach has been to culture blood only when patients develop symptoms suggestive of disseminated MAC. Routine monitoring of stool and respiratory tract secretions for MAC, in the absence of symptoms, is of little value. If MAC is persistently isolated from stool or sputum in symptomatic individuals and an alternative cause for symptoms referable to the gastro-intestinal or respiratory tracts has not been found, this probably represents localized disease, which may warrant treatment (Horsburgh et al., 1992). The risk of disseminated disease in patients with colonization or localized disease has not been established.

Disseminated disease should be treated with at least two antimycobacterial drugs, and a failing regimen should have two new drugs added. In the absence of consistent results from comparative or placebo-controlled trials of specific therapeutic regimens, several multidrug regimens could be recommended (Table 24.6). The optimal therapeutic regimen is yet to be determined. The US Public Service Health Task Force on Prophylaxis and Therapy for *Mycobacterium avium* complex has recommended that either azithromycin or clarithromycin is included in the chosen therapeutic regimen, and that ethambutol is included as the second drug. One or more of clofazimine, rifabutin, rifampicin, and ciprofloxacin can be added as third or fourth agents (USPHS/IDSA Prevention of Opportunistic Infections Working Group, 1997). A clinical response should occur within 2–4 weeks of beginning therapy. If there is no response, the clinician should evaluate the patient for the presence of a coexistent opportunistic infection. In our experience, patients with significant diarrhoea have a poor response to treatment. This could be due to

malabsorption of antimycobacterial agents or to the large load of organisms in the small bowel wall. Patients failing therapy should have two additional agents added to the regimen.

The duration of therapy required is uncertain, but is certainly longer than 2–3 months. Further, the concept of an 'induction treatment' regimen followed by 'suppressive maintenance' treatment (as is used for cytomegalovirus (CMV) disease and many other opportunistic infections) is poorly delineated for disseminated MAC. Relapse of mycobacteraemia following cessation of treatment is well documented. An initial regimen of three or four agents for 12 weeks, followed by maintenance treatment with two agents indefinitely is an option that requires evaluation in clinical trials. As with other opportunistic infections (e.g. CMV retinitis), clinicians have suggested that indefinite antimycobacterial therapy may not be necessary in patients who have a persistent improvement in their immunological status following initiation of HAART. There are anecdotal reports of eradication of MAC bacteraemia in four patients treated with 12 months or more of combination antimycobacterial therapy (containing a macrolide) and HAART. All patients had increases in CD4 lymphocyte counts of more than 135 cells/μl and three of the four patients had fewer less than 500 copies/ml of HIV RNA in plasma at the time of discontinuation of MAC therapy. No relapse of MAC bacteraemia occurred in the 8–13 months follow-up after discontinuation of MAC treatment. However, all patients have maintained CD4 lymphocyte counts well above the range that would put them at risk of disseminated MAC (Aberg et al., 1998).

Prophylaxis

After recognition of the impact of disseminated MAC on morbidity, quality of life and mortality, and that MAC infection affected up to 40% of HIV-infected individuals, a number of studies were initiated to evaluate the efficacy of different agents for prophylaxis. The first were two large placebo-controlled studies of rifabutin 300 mg daily in patients with counts of fewer than 200 CD4 cells/μl. These demonstrated a reduction in the incidence of MAC bacteraemia from 18% and 17% in the placebo-treated groups to 9% and 8% in the rifabutin groups (Nightingale et al., 1993). The prophylactic benefit appeared to be limited to individuals with fewer than 75 CD4 lymphocytes/μl. No

Table 24.6 Recommended therapeutic and prophylactic regimens for adults with disseminated *Mycobacterium avium* complex

---

Treatment of established infection
Initial regimen[a]
   Clarithromycin 500 mg twice daily[b]
   Ethambutol 15 mg/kg daily
     Plus/minus rifabutin 300–450 mg daily
Salvage regimen
   Clarithromycin 500 mg twice daily[b]
   Ethambutol 15 mg/kg daily
   Rifabutin 300–450 mg daily
   Amikacin 10 mg/kg daily
     Plus/minus ciprofloxacin 750 mg twice daily
Prophylaxis for MAC[c]
First-line regimen
   Azithromycin 1200 mg once weekly
   or
   Clarithromycin 500 mg twice daily
Second-line regimen
   Rifabutin 300 mg daily[d]

---

[a]Isoniazid 300 mg daily should be included for all patients in whom *Mycobacterium tuberculosis* has not been excluded; if the suspicion of *M. tuberculosis* is high, especially if multidrug resistant *M. tuberculosis* is considered, use isoniazid and pyrazinamide pending tests results.
[b]Azithromycin 500–600 mg daily can be alternated with clarithromycin if the latter is poorly tolerated.
[c]Indicated for individuals with CD4 lymphocyte counts of less than 50/μl, who do not have clinical or microbiological evidence of disseminated MAC.
[d]Active tuberculosis should be excluded prior to initiation of rifabutin prophylaxis.

overall survival benefit with rifabutin prophylaxis could be demonstrated in these studies; however, they were not designed to assess survival. Resistance to rifabutin did not appear to cause the prophylactic failures as the proportion of MAC isolates susceptible to rifabutin was the same in the placebo and rifabutin-treated groups (Wynne *et al.*, 1992). When MAC isolates obtained at baseline and MAC isolates obtained during the study were compared for susceptibility, no difference in susceptibility to rifabutin was found. The placebo-controlled trial of clarithromycin 500 mg twice daily in patients with fewer than 100 CD4 lymphocytes/μl was terminated early because of the significant reduction in the incidence of MAC in the clarithromycin arm (6% versus 16%), and improved survival. Of note, however, is that 58% of MAC isolates in the small number of patients that did develop MAC bacteraemia were resistant to clarithromycin (Pierce *et al.*, 1996). Azithromycin 1200 mg once weekly has also been shown to significantly reduce the incidence of MAC bacteraemia in a placebo-controlled trial in the same at-risk population (11% versus 25%), and to improve survival (Oldfield *et al.*, 1998).

Both azithromycin and clarithromycin have been compared with rifabutin and the combination of the macrolide and rifabutin in two large randomized, comparative studies. Azithromycin 1200 mg weekly was significantly superior to rifabutin in prophylactic efficacy (7.6% versus 15.3% incidence of MAC) and the combination had superior efficacy again (2.8% incidence of MAC), although was less well tolerated. There was no difference in survival between the three arms. Azithromycin resistance was detected in 11% of breakthrough isolates, which were also cross-resistant to clarithromycin (Havlir *et al.*, 1996). The comparison of clarithromycin 500 mg twice daily with rifabutin 300–450 mg daily and the combination of clarithromycin and rifabutin produced similar results. Clarithromycin was significantly more effective in preventing MAC infection than rifabutin (9% versus 15%) but the combination did not contribute much greater effect (7%). There was also no difference in survival between the three arms. Clarithromycin resistance was found in 29% of clarithromycin monotherapy and 27% of the combination therapy breakthrough isolates (Benson *et al.*, 2000; Cohn, 1997).

The most recent recommendations of the US Public Health Service Task Force for prophylaxis of MAC complex in HIV-infected adults and adolescents with lymphocyte counts of fewer than 50 CD4 ells/μl are azithromycin 1200 mg once weekly or clarithromycin 500 mg twice daily. The alternative recommended regimen is rifabutin 300 mg daily. Prior to initiation of MAC prophylaxis, the presence of disseminated MAC should be excluded by both clinical assessment and a baseline mycobacterial blood culture. In addition, active tuberculosis needs to be excluded in those patients who will receive rifabutin, as exposure to rifabutin has been implicated in the development of rifampin resistance in *M. tuberculosis* (USPHS/IDSA prevention of Opportunistic Infections Working Group, 1997).

It has also been shown in two randomized controlled trials that it is safe to discontinue primary MAC prophylaxis in individuals who have responded to combination antiretroviral therapy. In the first trial, patients with initial CD4 lymphocyte counts less than 50/ml that had subsequently been maintained above 100 cells/ml were randomized to azithromycin 1200 mg weekly or placebo. There were no episodes of confirmed MAC in either group over a median duration of follow-up of 12 months, although CD4 lymphocyte counts remained above 200 cells/ml during the observation period (El-Sadr *et al.*, 2000). The second trial from the AIDS Clinical Trials Group was of similar study design, and reported two cases of MAC infection in the placebo group, compared with no cases in the azithromycin group during a median follow-up of 16 months (Currier *et al.*, 2000). Both cases of MAC infection occurred in patients with CD4 lymphocyte counts greater than 200 cells/ml and MAC was isolated from vertebral bone and a paraspinal mass. In both studies, approximately one-third of patients had received no prior MAC prophylaxis, despite having a nadir CD4 lymphocyte count of below 50 cells/ml. In 1999, the US Public Health Service and Infectious Diseases Society of America (USPHS/IDSA Prevention of Opportunistic Infections Working Group) updated their recommendations to include criteria for discontinuation of primary MAC prophylaxis. It is appropriate to consider discontinuation in those patients who have responded to potent antiretroviral therapy with an increase in CD4 lymphocyte counts to greater than 100 cells/ml and suppression of HIV RNA for a sustained period of at least 3–6 months. It is also prudent to reinstitute MAC prophylaxis if the CD4 lymphocyte count declines to below 50 cells/ml again (USPHS/IDSA Prevention of Opportunistic Infections Working Group, 1999).

References

Aberg JA, Yajko DM, Jacobson MA. (1998). Eradication of AIDS-related disseminated *Mycobacterium avium* complex infection after 12 months of antimycobacterial therapy combined with highly active antiretroviral therapy. *J Infect Dis* **178**: 1446–9.

Agins BD, Berman DS, Spicehandler D *et al.* (1989). Effect of combined therapy with ansamycin, clofazimine, ethambutol, and isoniazid for *Mycobacterium avium* infection in patients with AIDS. *J Infect Dis* **159**: 784–7.

Alangaden GJ, Lerner SA. (1997). The clinical use of fluoroquinolones for the treatment of mycobacterial diseases. *Clin Infect Dis* **25**: 1213–21.

Baril L, Jouan M, Agher R *et al.* (2000). Impact of highly active antiretroviral therapy on onset of *Mycobacterium avium* complex infection and cytomegalovirus disease in patients with AIDS. *AIDS* **14**: 2593–6.

Barnes PF, Arevalo C. (1988). Blood culture positivity patterns in bacteraemia due to *Mycobacterium avium* intracellulare. *Southern Med J* **81**: 1059–60.

Benson C, Kerns E, Sha B *et al.* (1990). Relationship of respiratory and GI tract colonization with *Mycobacterium avium* complex (MAC) to disseminated MAC disease in HIV infected patients. In *Program and abstracts of the Sixth International Conference on AIDS*, San Francisco, CA, USA.

Benson C, Williams P, Currier J *et al.* (1999). ACTG 223: An open, prospective, randomized study comparing efficacy and safety of clarithromycin (C) plus ethambutol (E), rifabutin (R) or both for treatment (Rx) of MAC disease in Pts with AIDS. *Sixth Conference on Retroviruses and Opportunistic Infections*, Chicago, IL, USA.

Benson CA, Williams PL, Cohn DL *et al.* (2000). Clarithromycin of rifabutin alone or in combination for primary prophylaxis or *Mycobacterium avium* complex in patients with AIDS: randomized, double-blind, placebo-controlled trial, *J Infect Dis* **181**: 1289–97.

Bermudez LE, Young LS. (1988). Tumor necrosis factor, alone or in combination with IL-2, but not IFN-? is associated with macrophage killing of *Mycobacterium avium* complex. *J Immunol* **140**: 3006–13.

Bermudez LE, Young LS. (1989). Oxidative and non-oxidative intracellular killing of Mycobacterium avium complex. *Microbiol Pathogen* **7**: 289–97.

Bermudez LE, Young LS. (1990). Recombinant granulocytemacrophage colony stimulating factor activates human macrophages to inhibit or kill Mycobacterium avium complex. *J Leuk Biol* **48**: 67–74.

Bermudez LE, Kolonoski PT, Young LS. (1990). Natural killer cell activity and macrophage dependent inhibition of growth or killing of *Mycobacterium avium* complex in a mouse model. *J Leuk Biol* **47**: 135–40.

Bermudez LE, Young LS. (1991). Natural killer cell dependent mycobacteriostatic and mycobacterial activity in human macrophages. *J Immunol* **146**: 265–9.

Bessesen MT, Berry CD, Johnson MA *et al.* (1990). Site of origin of disseminated MAC infection in AIDS. In *Program and sbstracts of the Thirtieth Interscience Conference on Antimicrobial Agents and Chemotherapy (Atlanta)*, Washington, DC, American Society for Microbiology.

Cato A, Cavannaugh JH, Shi H *et al.* (1996). Assessment of multiple doses of ritonavir on the pharmacokinetics of rifabutin. *Eleventh International Conference on AIDS*, Vancouver, BC, USA.

Chaisson RE, Hopewell PC. (1989). Mycobacteria and AIDS mortality. *Am Review Respir Dis* **139**: 1–3.

Chaisson RE, Moore RD, Richman DD *et al.* (1992). Incidence and natural history of *Mycobacterium avium* complex infections in patients with advanced human immunodeficiency virus disease treated with zidovudine. *Am Rev Respir Dis* **146**: 285–9.

Chaisson RE, Benson CA, Dube M *et al.* (1994). Clarithromycin therapy for bacteremic *Mycobacterium avium* complex disease. A randomized double-blind, dose-ranging study in patients with AIDS. *Ann Intern Med* **121**: 905–11.

Chaisson RE, Keiser P, Pierce M *et al.* (1997). Clarithromycin and ethambutol with or without clofazimine for the treatment of bacteremic *Mycobacterium avium* complex disease in patients with HIV infection. *AIDS* **11**: 311–17.

Chaisson RE, Gallant JE, Keruly JC *et al.* (1998). Impact of opportunistic disease on survival in patients with HIV infection. *AIDS* **12**: 29–33.

Chin DP, Hopewell PC, Yajko DM *et al.* (1994). *Mycobacterium avium* complex in the respiratory or gastrointestinal tract and the risk of M. avium complex bacteraemia in patients with human immunodeficiency virus infection. *J Infect Dis* **169**: 289–95.

Chiu J, Nussbaum J, Bozzette S *et al.* (1990). Treatment of disseminated *Mycobacterium avium* complex infection in AIDS with amikacin, ethambutol, rifampin, and ciprofloxacin. *Ann Intern Med* **113**: 358–61.

Cohn DL. (1997). Prevention strategies for *Mycobacterium avium*-intracellulare complex (MAC) infection. *Drugs* **54**: 8–15.

Cohn DL, Fisher E, Franchino B *et al.* (1996). Comparison of two doses of clarithromycin in a randomized trial of four 3-drug regimens for treatment of disseminated *Mycobacterium avium* complex disease in AIDS: excess mortality associated with high-dose clarithromycin. In: *Program and abstracts of the Eleventh International Conference on AIDS*, Vancouver, BC, USA.

Crowe SM, Carlin JB, Stewart KL *et al.* (1991). Predictive value of CD4 lymphocyte numbers for the development of opportunistic infections and malignancies in HIV-infected persons. *J Acquir Immune Defic Syndr* **4**: 770–6.

Currier JS, Williams PL, Koletar SL *et al.* (2000). Discontinuation of *Mycobacterium avium* complex prophylaxis in patients with antiretroviral therapy-induced increases in CD4$^+$ cell count. A randomized, double-blind, placebo-controlled trial. *Ann Intern Med* **133**: 493–503.

DATRI 001 Study Group. (1994). Co-administration of clarithromycin (CL) alters the concentration-time profile of rifabutin (RFB). In: *Program and abstracts of the Thirty-fourth Interscience Conference on Antimicrobial Agents and Chemotherapy*, Orlando, FL, American Society for Microbiology.

Dautzenberg B, Truffot C, Legris S *et al.* (1991a). Activity of clarithromycin against *Mycobacterium avium* infection in patients with the acquired immune deficiency syndrome. *Am Review Respir Dis* **144**: 564–9.

Dautzenberg B, Truffot C, Mignon A *et al.* (1991b). Rifabutin in combination with clofazimine, isoniazid and ethambutol in the treatment of AIDS patients with infections due to opportunist mycobacteria. *Tubercle* **72**: 168–75.

Dawson DJ. (1990). Infection with *Mycobacterium avium* complex in Australian patients with AIDS. *Med J Aust* **153**: 466–8.

Dore GJ, Hoy JF, Mallal SA *et al.* (1997). Trends in incidence of AIDS illnesses in Australia from 1983 to 1994: The Australian AIDS cohort. *J Acquir Immune Defic Syndr Hum Retrovirol* **16**: 39–43.

Dorman SE, Heller HM, Basgoz NO et al. (1998). Adjunctive corticosteroid therapy for patients whose treatment disseminated Mycobacterium avium complex infection has failed. Clin Infect Dis 26: 682–6.

Dube MP, Sattler FR, Torriani FJ et al. (1997). A randomized evaluation of ethambutol for prevention of relapse and drug resistance during treatment of Mycobacterium avium complex bacteraemia with clarithromycin-based combination therapy. J Infect Dis 176: 1225–32.

Ellner JJ, Goldberger MJ, Parenti DM. (1991). Mycobacterium avium infection and AIDS: a therapeutic dilemma in rapid evolution. J Infect Dis 163: 1326–35.

El-Sadr WM, Burman WJ, Bjorling Grant L et al. (2000). Discontinuation of prophylaxis against Mycobacterium avium complex disease in HIV-infected patients who have a response to antiretroviral therapy. N Engl J Med 342: 1085–92.

French MAH, Mallal SA, Dawkins RL. (1992). Zidovudine induced restoration of cell mediated immunity to mycobacteria in immunodeficient HIV-infected patients. AIDS 6: 1293–7.

George S, Coffey M, Cinti S et al. (1998). Neutrophils from AIDS patients treated with granulocyte colony-stimulating factor demonstrate enhanced killing of Mycobacterium avium. J Infect Dis 178: 1530–3.

Gill VJ, Park CH, Stock F et al. (1985). Use of lysis-centrifugation (Isolator) and radiometric (BACTEC) blood culture systems for the detection of mycobacteraemia. J Clin Microbiol 22: 543–6.

Gordin FM, Cohn DL, Sullam PM et al. (1997). Early manifestations of disseminated Mycobacterium avium complex disease: a prospective evaluation. J Infect Dis 176: 126–32.

Gordin FM, Sullam PM, Shafran SD et al. (1999). A randomized, placebo-controlled study of rifabutin added to a regimen of clarithromycin and ethambutol for treatment of disseminated Mycobacterium avium complex. Clin Infect Dis 28: 1080–5.

Grunfeld C, Kotler D. (1992). Wasting in the acquired immunodeficiency syndrome. Sem Liver Dis 12: 175–87.

Haas DW, Lederman MM, Clough LA et al. (1998). Pro-inflammatory cytokine and human immunodeficiency virus RNA levels during early Mycobacterium avium complex bacteraemia in advanced AIDS. J Infect Dis 177: 1746–9.

Hafner R, Bethel J, Power M et al. (1998). Tolerance and pharmacokinetic interactions of rifabutin and clarithromycin in HIV-positive volunteers. Antimicrob Agents Chemother 42: 631–9.

Havlik JA, Horsburgh CR, Metchock B et al. (1992). Disseminated Mycobacterium avium complex infection: Clinical identification and epidemiologic trends. J Infect Dis 165: 577–80.

Havlir D, Kemper CA, Deresinski SC. (1993). Reproducibility of lysis-centrifugation cultures for quantification of Mycobacterium avium complex bacteraemia. J Clin Microbiol 31: 1794–8.

Havlir DV, Dube MP, Sattler FR et al. (1996). Prophylaxis against disseminated Mycobacterium avium complex with weekly azithromycin, daily rifabutin, or both. N Engl J Med 335: 392–8.

Havlir DV, Haubrich R, Hwang J et al. (1998). Human immunodeficiency virus replication in AIDS patients with Mycobacterium avium complex bacteraemia: a case control study. J Infect Dis 177: 595–9.

Hawkins CC, Gold JWM, Whimbey E et al. (1986). Mycobacterium avium complex infections in patients with the acquired immunodeficiency syndrome. Ann Intern Med 105: 184–8.

Heifets LB, Iseman MD, Lindholm-Levy PJ. (1988). Combinations of rifampin or rifabutine plus ethambutol against Mycobacterium avium complex. Am Rev Respir Dis 137: 711–5.

Hocqueloux L, Lesprit P, Herrmann J et al. (1998). Pulmonary Mycobacterium avium complex disease without dissemination in HIV-infected patients. Chest 113: 542–8.

Holland SM, Eisenstein EM, Kuhris DB et al. (1994). Treatment of refractory disseminated non-tuberculous mycobacterial infection with interferon gamma. N Engl J Med 330: 1348–55.

Horgen L, Jerome A, Rastogi N. (1998). Pulsed-exposure and postantibiotic leukocyte enhancement effects of amikacin, clarithromycin, clofazimine, and rifampin against intracellular Mycobacterium avium. Antimicrob Agents Chemother 42: 3006–8.

Horsburgh CR. (1991). Mycobacterium avium complex infection in the acquired immunodeficiency syndrome. New Engl J Med 324: 1332–8.

Horsburgh CR, Selik RM. (1989). The epidemiology of disseminated non-tuberculous mycobacterial infection in the acquired immunodeficiency syndrome (AIDS). Am Rev Respir Dis 139: 4–7.

Horsburgh CR, Havlik JA, Ellis DA et al. (1991). Survival of patients with acquired immune deficiency syndrome and disseminated Mycobacterium avium complex infection with and without antimycobacterial chemotherapy. Am Review Respir Dis 144: 557–9.

Horsburgh, CR, Metchock BG, McGowan JE et al. (1992). Clinical implications of recovery of Mycobacterium avium complex from the stool or respiratory tract of HIV-infected individuals. AIDS 6: 512–14.

Hoy J, Mijch A, Sandland M et al. (1990). Quadruple-drug therapy for Mycobacterium avium intracellulare bacteraemia in AIDS patients. J Infect Dis 161: 801–5.

Inderlied CB, Young LS. (1990). Disseminated Mycobacterium avium complex infection. In: PA Volberding, MA Jacobson (eds.) AIDS Clinical Review. New York: Marcel Dekker, 165–91.

Jacobson MA, French M. (1998). Altered natural history of AIDS-related opportunistic infections in the era of potent combination antiretroviral therapy. AIDS 12: S157–63.

Jacobson MA, Hopewell PC, Yajko DM et al. (1991). Natural history of disseminated Mycobacterium avium complex infection in AIDS. J Infect Dis 164: 994–8.

John M, French MAH. (1998). Exacerbation of the inflammatory response to Mycobacterium tuberculosis after antiretroviral therapy. Med J Aust 169: 473–4.

Kedzierska K, Mak J, Mijch A et al. (2000). GM-CSF augments phagocytosis of MAC by HIV-1-infected moncyte/macrophages in vitro and in vivo. J Infect Dis 181: 390–4.

Keiser P, Rademacher S, Smith J et al. (1998). G-CSF association with prolonged survival in HIV-infected patients with disseminated Mycobacterium avium complex infection. Int J STD AIDS 9: 394–9.

Kemper CA, Meng TC, Nussbaum J et al. (1992). Treatment of Mycobacterium avium complex bacteraemia in AIDS with a four-drug oral regimen. Annals Intern Med 116: 466–72.

Kemper CA, Havlir D, Haghighat D et al. (1994). The individual microbiologic effect of three antimycobacterial agents, clofazimine, ethambutol, and rifampin, on Mycobacterium avium complex bacteraemia in patients with AIDS. J Infect Dis 170: 157–64.

Kemper CA, Bermudez LE, Deresinski SC. (1998). Immunomodulatory treatment of Mycobacterium avium complex bacteraemia in patients with AIDS by use of recombinant granulocyte-macrophage colony-stimulating factor. J Infect Dis 177: 914–20.

Kent RJ, Bakhtlar M, Shanson DC. (1992). The in vitro bactercidal activities of combinations of antimicrobial agents against clinical isolates of Mycobacterium avium-intracellulare. J Antimicrob Chemother 30: 643–50.

Khardori N, Rolston K, Rosenbaum B et al. (1989). Comparative in-vitro activity of twenty antimicrobial agents against clinical isolates of Mycobacterium avium complex. J Antimicrob Chemother 24: 667–73.

Kilby JM, Marques MB, Jaye DL *et al.* (1998). The yield of bone marrow biopsy and culture compared with blood culture in the evaluation of HIV-infected patients for mycobacterial and fungal infections. *Am J Med* **104**: 123–8.

Lee BY, Chatterjee D, Bozic CM. (1991). Prevalence of serum antibody to the type specific glycopeptidolipid antigens of *Mycobacterium avium* in human immunodeficiency virus-positive and -negative individuals. *J Clin Microbiol* **29**: 1026–9.

Low N, Pfluger D, Egger M *et al.* (1997). Disseminated *Mycobacterium avium* complex disease in the Swiss HIV Cohort Study: increasing incidence, unchanged prognosis. *AIDS* **11**: 1165–71.

Lyles RH, Chu C, Mellors JW *et al.* (1999). Prognostic value of plasma HIV RNA in the natural history of *Pneumocystis carinii* pneumonia, cytomegalovirus and *Mycobacterium avium* complex. *AIDS* **13**: 341–9.

Malpother ME, Sanger JE. (1984). *In vitro* interaction of *Mycobacterium avium* with intestinal epithelial cells. *Infect Immun* **45**: 67–73.

Masur H, Tuazon C, Gill V *et al.* (1987). Effect of combined clofazimine and ansamycin therapy on *Mycobacterium avium-Mycobacterium intracellulare* bacteraemia in patients with AIDS. *J Infect Dis* **155**: 127–9.

May T, Brel F, Beuscart C *et al.* (1997). Comparison of combination therapy regimens for treatment of human immunodeficiency virus-infected patients with disseminated bacteraemia due to *Mycobacterium avium*. *Clin Infect Dis* **25**: 621–9.

Muller F, Aukrust P, Lien E *et al.* (1998). Enhanced Interleukin-10 production in response to *Mycobacterium avium* products in mononuclear cells from patients with human immunodeficiency virus infection. *J Infect Dis* **177**: 586–94.

Newman GW, Kelley TG, Gan H *et al.* (1993). Concurrent infection of human macrophages with HIV-1 and *Mycobacterium avium* results in decreased cell viability increased M. *avium* multiplication and altered cytokine production. *J Immunol* **151**: 2261–72.

Nightingale SD, Byrd LT, Southern PM *et al.* (1992). Incidence of *Mycobacterium avium* intracellulare complex bacteraemia in human immunodeficiency virus-positive patients. *J Infect Dis* **165**: 1082–5.

Nightingale SD, Cameron DW, Gordin FM *et al.* (1993). Two controlled trials of rifabutin prophylaxis against *Mycobacterium avium* complex infection in AIDS. *New Engl J Med* **329**: 828–33.

Ninet B, Auckenthaler R, Rohner P *et al.* (1997). Detection of *Mycobacterium avium-intracellulare* in the blood of HIV-infected patients by a commercial polymerase chain reaction kit. *Europ J Clin Microbiol Infect Dis* **16**: 549–51.

Okello DO, Sewankambo N, Goodgame R *et al.* (1990). Absence of bacteraemia with *Mycobacterium avium*-intracellulare in Ugandan patients with AIDS. *J Infect Dis* **162**: 208–10.

Oldfield EC, Fessel WJ, Dunne MW *et al.* (1998). Once weekly azithromycin therapy for prevention of *Mycobacterium avium* complex infection in patients with AIDS: a randomized, double-blind, placebo-controlled multicenter trial. *Clin Infect Dis* **26**: 611–19.

Ouellet D, Hau A, Granneman GR *et al.* (1996). Assessment of the pharmacokinetic interaction between ritonavir and clarithromycin. *Clin Pharmacol Therapeut* **59**: 143.

Pallela FJ, Delaney KM, Moorman AC *et al.* (1998). Declining morbidity and mortality among patients with advanced human immunodeficiency virus infection. *New Engl J Med* **338**: 853–60.

Parenti DM, Williams PL, Hafner R *et al.* (1998). A phase II/III trial of antimicrobial therapy with or without amikacin in the treatment of disseminated *Mycobacterium avium* infection in HIV-individuals. *AIDS* **12**: 2439–46.

Perronne C, Gikas A, Truffot-Pernot C *et al.* (1990). Activities of clarithromycin, sulfisoxazole, and rifabutin against *Mycobacterium avium* complex multiplication within human macrophages. *Antimicrob Agents Chemother* **34**: 1508–11.

Pierce M, Crampton S, Henry D *et al.* (1996). A randomized trial of clarithromycin as prophylaxis against disseminated *Mycobacterium avium* complex infection in patients with advanced acquired immunodeficiency syndrome. *New Engl J Med* **335**: 384–91.

Race EM, Adelson-Mitty J, Kriegel GR *et al.* (1998) Focal mycobacterial lymphadenitis following initiation of protease-inhibitor therapy in patients with advanced HIV-1 disease. *Lancet* **351**: 252–5.

Reeves GEM, Ferguson JK, Dobson P *et al.* (1996). Pentoxifylline to treat *Mycobacterium avium* complex exacerbation in late-stage HIV infection. *Med J Aust* **166**: 446.

Rose RM, Fuglestad JM, Remington L. (1991). Growth inhibition of *Mycobacterium avium* complex in human alveolar macrophages by the combination of recombinant macrophage colony-stimulating factor and interferon gamma. *Am J Respir Cell Molec Biol* **4**: 248–54.

Roth RI, Owen RL, Keren DF. *et al.* (1985). Intestinal infection with *Mycobacterium avium* in acquired immunodeficiency syndrome (AIDS): histological and clinical comparison with Whipple's disease. *Digestive Dis Sci* **30**: 497–504.

Ruf B, Schuermann D, Brehmer W *et al.* (1990). Pulmonary manifestations due to *Mycobacterium avium-Mycobacterium* intracellulare in AIDS patients. *Am Rev Respir Dis* **141**: 611.

Rutstein RM, Cobb P, McGowan KL *et al.* (1993). *Mycobacterium avium* intracellulare complex infection in HIV-infected children. *AIDS* **7**: 507–12.

Shafran SD, Deschenes J, Miller M *et al.* (1994). Uveitis and pseudojaundice during a regimen of clarithromycin, rifabutin and ethambutol. *New Engl J Med* **330**: 438–9.

Shafran SD, Singer J, Zarowny DP *et al.* (1996). A comparison of two regimens for the treatment of *Mycobacterium avium* complex bacteraemia in AIDS: rifabutin, ethambutol, and clarithromycin versus rifampin, ethambutol, clofazimine, and ciprofloxacin. *New Engl J Med* **335**: 377–83.

Shafran SD, Singer J, Zarowny DP *et al.* (1998). Determinants of rifabutin-associated uveitis in patients treated with rifabutin, clarithromycin, and ethambutol for *Mycobacterium avium* complex bacteraemia: a multivariate analysis. *J Infect Dis* **177**: 252–5.

Siegal FP, Eilbott D, Burger H *et al.* (1990). Dose limiting toxicity of rifabutin in AIDS-related complex, syndrome of arthralgia/arthritis. *AIDS* **4**: 433–41.

Trapnell CB, Narang PK, Li R *et al.* (1993). Fluconazole (FLU) increases rifabutin (RIF) absorption in HIV patients on stable zidovudine (ZDV) therapy [abstract]. *Ninth International Conference on AIDS*, Berlin, Germany.

USPHS/IDSA Prevention of Opportunistic Infections Working Group. (1997). USPHS/IDSA guidelines for the prevention of opportunistic infections in persons infected with human immunodeficiency virus: a summary. *Clin Infect Dis* **25**: S313–35.

USPHS/IDSA Prevention of Opportunistic Infections Working Group (1999). USPHS/IDSA guidelines for the prevention of opportunistic infections in persons infected with human immunodeficiency virus: US Public Health Service (USPHS) and Infectious Diseases Society of America (IDSA). *Morb Mortal Wkly Rep* **48**: 1–66.

Von Reyn CF, Arbeit RD, Tosteson ANA *et al.* (1996). The international epidemiology of disseminated *Mycobacterium avium* complex. *AIDS* **10**: 1025–32.

Wallace RJ, Brown BA, Griffith DE *et al.* (1995). Reduced serum levels of clarithromycin in patients treated with multidrug regimens including rifampin or rifabutin for *Mycobacterium avium*–*Mycobacterium intracellulare* infection. *J Infect Dis* **171**: 747–50.

Ward TT, Rimland DD, Kauffman C *et al.* (1998). Randomized, open-label trial of azithromycin plus ethambutol vs. clarithromycin plus ethambutol as therapy for *Mycobacterium avium* complex bacteraemia in patients with human immunodeficiency virus infection. *Clin Infect Dis* **27**: 1278–85.

Williams PL, Currier JS, Swindells S. (1999). Joint effects of HIV-1 RNA levels and CD4 lymphocyte cells on the risk of specific opportunistic infections. *AIDS* **13**: 1035–44.

Wynne B, Nightingale S, Cameron W *et al.* (1992). The development of *Mycobacterium avium* complex (MAC) bacteraemia in AIDS patients in the placebo (PLAC)-controlled MAC prophylaxis studies (087023 and 087027): drug, host or other factors? In: *Program and abstracts of the Thirty-second Interscience Conference on Antimicrobial Agents and Chemotherapy.*

Yagupsky P, Menegus MA. (1990). Cumulative positivity rates of multiple blood cultures for *Mycobacterium avium* intracellulare and Cryptococcus neoformans in patients with the acquired immunodeficiency syndrome. *Arch Pathol Lab Med* **114**: 923–5.

Yajko DM, Nassos PS, Hadley WK. (1987). Broth microdilution testing of susceptibilities to 30 antimicrobial agents of *Mycobacterium avium* strains from patients with acquired immunodeficiency syndrome. *Antimicrob Agents Chemother* **31**: 1579–84.

Yajko DM, Chin DP, Gonzalez PC *et al.* (1995). *Mycobacterium avium* complex in water, food, and soil samples collected from the environment of HIV-infected individuals. *J Acquir Immune Defic Syndr Hum Retrovirol* **9**: 176–82.

Yakrus MA, Good RC. (1990). Geographic distribution, frequency, and specimen source of *Mycobacterium avium* complex serotypes isolated from patients with acquired immunodeficiency syndrome. *J Clin Microbiol* **28**: 926–9.

Young LS. (1988). *Mycobacterium avium* complex infection. *J Infect Dis* **157**: 863–7.

Young LS, Wiviott L, Wu M. (1991). Azithromycin for treatment of *Mycobacterium avium* intracellulare complex infection in patients with AIDS. *Lancet* **338**: 1107–9.

PETER FRAME AND AIMEE WILKIN

Clusters of cases of *Pneumocystis carinii* pneumonia (PCP) without the usual risk factors for this opportunistic infection were the first indicators of the AIDS epidemic in 1981. Although many other opportunistic infections and neoplasms, as well as conditions caused directly by HIV, have been described subsequently, PCP remains the most common severe complication of AIDS in developed countries. In the early years of the AIDS epidemic, 60% of AIDS patients had PCP as their presenting illness, and 80% of AIDS patients eventually had PCP during their lifetime. In the 1990s, PCP became much less common as an opportunistic pathogen in patients with known HIV infection because of the widespread use of combination antiretroviral therapy and effective prophylactic regimens (Yarchoan *et al.*, 1991; Palella *et al.*, 1998), but it continues to be a common presenting illness in patients not receiving treatment. In our experience at the University of Cincinnati, the incidence of PCP has fallen from 23.5 cases/1000 patient-years in 1994 to 5.1 cases/1000 patient-years in 1997 (Martinez E, pers. comm.). Despite these treatment advances, PCP remains a common opportunistic infection, with a mortality rate of 10–20% (Dohn *et al.*, 1992; Hardy *et al.*, 1992).

Biology of *Pneumocystis carinii*

Pneumocystis carinii is a eukaryotic single-celled organism that was variously classified as a protozoan, a fungus, or an undifferentiated protist. Because it has not been cultured *in vitro*, our knowledge of the biology of *P. carinii* remains fragmented. However, during the 1990s, molecular tools rapidly expanded our understanding of *Pneumocystis* cell physiology, even without the ability to grow it in culture. Although its exact taxonomy is still unclear, *P. carinii* appears to be most closely related to ascomycetous fungi.

This relationship is supported by its ultrastructure and the close similarity between the ribosomal RNA thymidylate synthetase, dihydrofolate reductase and mitochondrial DNA sequences of *P. carinii* and fungi. Analysis of ribosomal RNA of *Pneumocystis* from different mammalian species has shown that *Pneumocystis carinii* is a heterogenous group of organisms with a specific strain causing disease only in its particular host. Rat and human *P. carinii*, which are morphologically identical, may be different species by this analysis. *Pneumocystis* differs from fungi in having cholesterol instead of ergosterol as the main structural lipid, and in being resistant to conventional antifungal agents.

P. carinii appears in several different forms in host tissues. There is a cyst form and a trophozoite form; the latter may be small (1.5–2 μM) or large (3–5 μM). The large trophozoites in turn may have either small or large nuclei. The most widely accepted model of the *Pneumocystis* life cycle in the animal host, based primarily on ultrastructural analysis, begins with a cyst containing eight haploid trophozoites. After excystment, the trophozoites multiply by binary fission, creating large haploid trophozoites with small nuclei in the alveolar lumen. These are the major pathogenic forms. Under stimuli that are as yet unknown, some of these haploid trophozoites can fuse to form diploid trophozoites. In this presumed sexual cycle, the large diploid cells then divide to form eight haploid daughter trophozoites within the original cell membrane; at the same time, a cyst wall forms, resulting in a cyst containing eight haploid trophozoites. It is unknown whether this is the complete life cycle of *Pneumocystis*, which would represent the cycle of an obligate animal parasite spreading directly from host to host. Alternatively, there could be a free-living form such as exists for some dimorphic fungi such as *Histoplasma*, *Blastomyces*, and *Coccidioides*.

The cell surface characteristics of *P. carinii* are important for the attachment of the organism to type I alveolar cells, a step required for disease pathogenesis. The thin cell wall of the trophozoite consists of a classic bilamellar membrane under a thin layer of material, which contains glucan and chitin and is rich in polysaccharides. Several lines of investigation have suggested that *P. carinii* may attach to multiple cell-surface molecules including fibronectin, and that carbohydrate-lectin and Fc-immunoglobulin interactions may mediate attachment to alveolar macrophages. The major surface glycoproteins of *Pneumocystis* are a heterogeneous family of fibronectin-binding proteins, which have some similarities to integrins, the mammalian proteins that normally bind to fibronectin. Although *P. carinii* can also bind to fibronectin on the surface of alveolar macrophages, such binding does not stimulate phagocytosis or killing.

The major surface glycoprotein of *Pneumocystis* also binds to mannose-fucose receptors (lectins) on alveolar macrophages. The abundant mannose and N-acetylglucosamine carbohydrate residues on the surface of *Pneumocystis* also bind to the lectins on alveolar macrophages. Lectin-mediated binding of *Pneumocystis* to macrophages activates them to ingest and kill the organism. Similarly, antibody-coated *Pneumocystis* binding to macrophage Fc receptors are ingested and killed. Unlike some other pathogens, *P. carinii* cannot survive within activated macrophages.

Pneumocystis carinii is an aerobic organism with mitochondria containing tricarboxylic acid cycle enzymes and an electron-transport chain containing cytochromes. An endoplasmic reticulum and free ribosomes are present, as are cytoplasmic vacuoles, as well as 'round bodies' of unknown significance. No cytoskeletal, microtubule, or microfilament structures have been consistently recognized, which suggests the absence of motility. No toxins or other extracellular pathogenic products have been described.

Pathogenesis of *P. carinii* infection

Pneumocystis carinii is an intra-alveolar extracellular parasite, and it is only very rarely tissue invasive. The tight binding of *Pneumocystis* trophozoites to type I alveolar epithelial cells (the cell primarily involved in gas exchange) probably allows the organism to extract nutrients from pulmonary capillary blood. The normal alveolar environment must be hostile to this organism because it is rarely identified in histological sections of normal lung. However, continuous human exposure to *P. carinii* is probably the rule, either because of residence of a small number of these organisms in the normal lung (i.e. human-to-human transmission) or repeated environmental exposure. *Pneumocystis* is ubiquitous in the human environment, as indicated by the appearance of antibody in more than 80% of humans during infancy or early childhood (Smulian *et al.*, 1993).

In hosts with defective cellular immunity, *P. carinii* can replicate in the alveolar environment. In animal models, CD4 lymphocyte depletion is the immunological abnormality most conducive to development of pneumocystosis. However, the mechanism by which CD4 lymphocytes protect the host from *P. carinii* pneumonia is unclear. Although not the case in adults, infants with isolated immunoglobulin deficiency are also predisposed to *Pneumocystis* infection, suggesting that although antibodies may also protect against PCP, they may not be required in the presence of an intact cellular immune system.

The earliest pathophysiological change noted in animal models of PCP is increased permeability of the alveolar-capillary membrane, with leakage of fluid into the alveolar space. Thereafter, the type I cell begins to degenerate, with denudation of the basement membrane. Restriction of lung compliance occurs as a result of loss of normal surfactant function. In both animal models and humans, PCP is associated with progressive impairment of oxygen exchange due to the destruction of type I alveolar cells followed by obliteration of alveolar space (Figure 25.1, in the colour plate section). Exuberant multiplication of *P. carinii* forms an eosinophilic foamy exudate, which fills the alveolar space. The exudate consists of *Pneumocystis* cysts and trophozoites in a heterogeneous matrix of surfactant, transudated serum proteins, cyst walls, and non-cellular cyst contents. A mild interstitial pneumonitis with a mononuclear-cell infiltrate is also seen. Occasional patients have a polymorphonuclear leucocyte alveolar and airway exudate, which has been reported to have a poor prognosis (Mason *et al.*, 1989). More advanced cases of PCP may have destruction of lung tissue with interstitial fibrosis and thin-walled parenchymal cavities. Most of these emphysematous cysts occur from progressive destruction of lung stroma, but some may represent excavation of nodular *Pneumocystis* infiltrates. These bullous cavities are predominant in the apices of the lung and are frequently subpleural (Feuerstein *et al.*, 1990; Kuhlman *et al.*, 1990). Cyst rupture leads to pneumothorax, a fairly common complication of PCP. During resolution of PCP, there may be extensive interstitial fibrosis and occasional intra-alveolar obliterative fibrosis, giving a pathological appearance similar to bronchiolitis obliterans with organizing pneumonia (Travis *et al.*, 1990).

P. carinii occasionally invades the pulmonary vasculature, and this is probably the mechanism for disseminated infection. Disseminated *P. carinii* infection is rare, but it may be seen in almost any tissue (see section on extrapulmonary pneuymocystosis). The disseminated lesions are also characterized by invasion of blood or lymphatic vessels with associated vessel necrosis and perivascular lymphocytic infiltration (Raviglione, 1990; Travis *et al.*, 1990).

Clinical features of *P. carinii* infection

Pneumocystis pneumonia

Clinical presentation

PCP develops predominantly in HIV-infected patients with severe immunosuppression. In a large cohort of asymptomatic HIV-infected homosexual men who were not receiving preventive therapy, 8.4% of those with CD4 lymphocyte counts of less than 200 cells/μl developed PCP within 6 months and 18.4% did so within 1 year. Conversely, of those with CD4 lymphocyte counts between 200 and 350 cells/μl, only 0.5% developed PCP in 6 months and only 4% did so within 1 year. Those with CD4 lymphocyte counts of more than 350 cells/μl had no PCP in 6 months and only 0.5% had PCP within the next year (Phair *et al.*,

1990) (Table 25.1). Previous episodes of fever, persistent fatigue, unintentional weight loss, or oral candidiasis are also risk factors for PCP (Phair *et al.*, 1990). Recent studies from the same cohort have shown that the predictive value of CD4 lymphocyte enumeration can be enhanced by measurement of HIV RNA in plasma (viral load) (Lyles *et al.*, 1999).

In contrast to PCP in other immunosuppressed patients, PCP associated with HIV infection most commonly has a subacute presentation, with respiratory symptoms or fever preceding the diagnosis by 3–6 weeks or more. In patients with undiagnosed HIV infection, the duration of illness is frequently longer and the patients are often severely ill when they come to medical attention. Even in those patients already under care for HIV infection, symptoms usually last more than 2 weeks before the diagnosis. However, occasional patients have an acute onset of respiratory distress lasting only a few days, similar to that seen in other immunosuppressed patients.

The usual symptoms of PCP are cough, chest tightness, and exertional dyspnoea. The cough is uniformly non-productive and is commonly triggered by deep breathing and exercise. Patients who have pre-existing conditions associated with chronic sputum production generally do not have a change in the quality or quantity of sputum. A sensation of 'tightness' in the chest frequently accompanies the cough and when described as substernal pain can occasionally be mistaken for a sign of oesophageal or cardiac disease. Night sweats are a frequent symptom of PCP but true rigors are rare, except when induced by intermittent

Table 25.1 Cumulative incidence of *Pneumocystis carinii* pneumonia (PCP) in patients with HIV infection according to CD4 lymphocyte count at entry into the MACS cohort[a]

CD4 lymphocytes at baseline (per μl)	Number of patients	Cumulative incidence (%) of PCP at[b]	
		6 months	12 months
< 100	16	22.2	44.4
101–150	26	8.9	18.6
151–200	35	2.9	9.5
201–350	217	0.5	4.0
351–500	389	0.0	1.4
501–700	483	0.0	0.4
> 700	499	0.0	0.0

[a]MACS: Multicenter AIDS Cohort Study. Participants who took prophylactic medicines were excluded from analysis (modified from Phair *et al.*, 1990).
[b]Kaplan Meier estimates.

antipyretic use. As the infection progresses, exertional dyspnoea worsens and shortness of breath at rest may develop. In a review of 93 consecutive patients with PCP, only 53% had the triad of cough, fever, and dyspnoea, confirming that symptoms can be quite subtle (Opravail *et al.*, 1994). Patients who have had a previous episode of PCP can often accurately identify a recurrent episode, whereas patients who have not had PCP often describe it as a 'bad cold that won't go away'. Occasional patients present with combined bacterial and *Pneumocystis* pneumonia, in which case the clinical features of bacterial pneumonia usually predominate (see Chapter 22). The fact that a patient has been prescribed *Pneumocystis* prophylaxis does not exclude the possibility of PCP. Although none of the prophylactic regimens are 100% effective, patients who are compliant with trimethoprim-sulfamethoxazole (TMP-SMX) prophylaxis very rarely develop PCP (Ioannidis *et al.*, 1996). Prophylaxis with aerosolized pantamidine is somewhat less effective than with TMP-SMX.

The physical examination is often abnormal but almost invariably non-specific. Fever is usually present and most commonly ranges between 38.5 and 40°C with an appropriate tachycardia. Shallow tachypnoea is common in more advanced cases. Severe pneumonia is associated with air hunger and cyanosis. A non-productive shallow cough is common, and is often exacerbated by deep breathing during the physical examination. Auscultation of the lungs rarely reveals abnormalities. Accompanying extrapulmonary physical findings suggesting significant immune deficiency include oral candidiasis, hairy leucoplakia of the tongue, moderate-to-severe periodontal disease, or oropharyngeal Kaposi's sarcoma (KS).

Radiological features

The most frequent pattern seen on the chest radiograph in patients with PCP is a bilateral diffuse infiltrate that appears interstitial in its early stages and becomes alveolar as the disease progresses (Figures 13.1 and 25.2). The infiltrates are usually perihilar but sometimes show an upper lobe distribution. Less commonly, infiltrates can be focal and mimic a segmental bronchopneumonia. (This may also occur in patients with combined *Pneumocystis* and bacterial pneumonia.) True lobar consolidation is extremely rare. Cavitation is uncommon but has been described, usually in patients with pre-existing chronic lung disease or in those with recurrent PCP. Pleural effusions are rare. Over one-third of patients with proven PCP may have a normal chest radiograph (Opravail *et al.*, 1994), or the only finding may be pneumothorax (Sepkowitz *et al.*, 1991). In situations where the patient or physician has a high index of suspicion

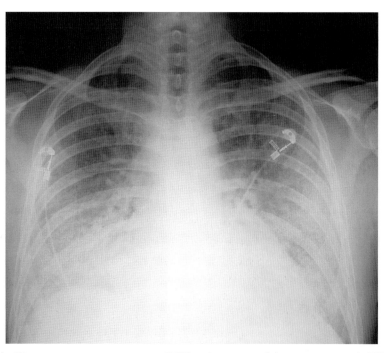

Figure 25.2 *Chest radiograph of* Pneumocystis carinii *pneumonia (PCP) with respiratory failure in a patient with AIDS. It illustrates the typical perihilar interstitial infiltrates seen in PCP. In addition, subcutaneous emphysema is visible. The patient later developed bilateral tension pneumothoraces.*

for *Pneumocystis*, a normal chest film is relatively common (Dohn *et al.*, 1992).

Although computed chest tomography is not recommended routinely for patients suspected of having PCP, it is useful in some cases. High-resolution computed chest tomography in patients suspected of having PCP with normal chest films can demonstrate patchy or nodular ground-glass attenuation. A review of computed tomographic (CT) findings in 39 patients with PCP revealed several patterns of disease: a 'ground-glass' appearance (26%), patchy bilateral infiltrates separated by normal-appearing lung tissue (56%), and interstitial disease (18%). Bullae and thin-walled cysts were present in more than one-third of the patients (Kuhlman *et al.*, 1990). Most of these cysts are apical and subpleural and are the cause of spontaneous pneumothorax (Feuerstein *et al.*, 1990; Kuhlman *et al.*, 1990). In one series, patients with clinical findings consistent with PCP but with normal chest tomograms either had no *P. carinii* on bronchoscopy or recovered without empirical treatment for PCP (Gruden *et al.*, 1997).

In the past, ^{67}Ga radionuclide lung scanning was used to identify some patients with PCP and normal chest radiographs. As this test is slow (72 h), expensive and non-specific, it is no longer employed for detection of PCP.

Laboratory findings

Hypoxaemia is almost always present in patients with PCP (Chouaid *et al.*, 1993). Although the resting arterial oxygen saturation and partial pressure can be within normal limits, hypoxaemia can virtually always be demonstrated after exercise. In a few centres, exercise-induced oxygen desaturation or widening of the alveolar–arterial oxygen pressure gradient is still used as a sensitive but non-specific diagnostic test (Stover *et al.*, 1989). Hypocarbia due to alveolar hyperventilation is very common. Occasionally, patients with PCP present with respiratory failure, although it is more common for this to develop during treatment.

All patients suspected of having PCP should have the adequacy of their oxygenation evaluated. Even if hypoxia is demonstrated by a transcutaneous oxygen electrode, arterial blood gases should be measured while the patient is breathing room air to assess the full extent of oxygenation and alveolar ventilation. The alveolar–arterial oxygen pressure gradient (PA-aO$_2$, or A-a gradient) is then determined from the blood gas values by the equation:

$$PA\text{-}aO_2 = 150 - [(PaCO_2/0.8) + PaO_2]$$

The PA-aO$_2$ has important prognostic significance, with PCP mortality being low in those with mild disease (PA-aO$_2$ < 35 mmHg), higher in those with moderate disease (35–45 mmHg), and highest in patients with severe disease (>45 mmHg) (Brenner *et al.*, 1987; Bozzette *et al.*, 1990; National Institutes of Health University of California Expert Panel, 1990). These categories are routinely used in the decision to administer adjunctive steroid therapy. Altitude, weather, and body temperature adjustments are of minor clinical significance in calculating the A–a gradient.

Depressed CD4 lymphocyte counts are universal in HIV-infected patients with pneumocystosis. Most patients with PCP have CD4 lymphocyte counts of less than 100 cells/μl, although 5% of cases will have counts of more than 200 cells/μl (Stansell *et al.*, 1997). Routine hematological studies are invariably non-specific. Anaemia, neutropenia, thrombocytopenia, and lymphopenia are common sequelae of HIV infection, and may be present but are not specific for *Pneumocystis*. Leucocytosis is unusual and if present warrants consideration of co-existent bacterial infection.

Most serum chemistry findings are non-specific. An elevated serum lactate dehydrogenase is common in patients with PCP and has some prognostic significance (Zaman and White, 1988; Forrest *et al.*, 1998). Although the mean serum lactate dehydrogenase concentration in patients with PCP is higher than in those with other respiratory conditions, there is too much overlap to make it useful in establishing the specific diagnosis of PCP, although it has prognostic significance (Forrest *et al.*, 1998). Some have used a normal enzyme level as a screening test to exclude the possibility of PCP, although mild cases may have low or normal values.

In summary, a patient with known HIV infection or with HIV risk should be suspected of having PCP when the CD4 lymphocyte count is low (usually less than 200 cells/μl), and fever and non-productive cough are present (Table 25.1). Dyspnoea on exertion, resting or exercise-induced hypoxia, and an abnormal roentgenogram with bilateral diffuse interstitial infiltrates (Figures 13.1 and 25.2) complete the classic presentation. One or more of these features may be absent in specific cases. Co-infections (e.g. with bacteria) are common, so the presence of another pathogen does not exclude PCP (see Chapter 13).

Extrapulmonary pneumocystosis

The true incidence of extrapulmonary pneumocystosis is hard to establish because only histopathological examination establishes the diagnosis with certainty, and if disseminated disease is present in patients with PCP, the extrapulmonary disease may respond to treatment and continue to be unrecognized (for review, see Ng *et al.*, 1997). Likewise, the incidence will be underestimated if the patient with extrapulmonary disease dies without an autopsy. Two reviews from New York suggest that extrapulmonary *Pneumocystis* occurs at a rate approximately 0.5–3% of the PCP rate. At one centre, five cases (0.5%) of extrapulmonary infection occurred during the time that 940 cases of PCP were diagnosed (Raviglione, 1990). At the other centre, seven (2.8%) of 253 autopsies of AIDS patients had extrapulmonary *Pneumocystis* infection (Telzak *et al.*, 1990).

Extrapulmonary pneumocystosis usually develops in patients who have had prior PCP and in those with profound HIV-related immunodeficiency (i.e. very low CD4 lymphocyte counts). It is extremely rare in patients receiving TMP-SMX prophylaxis, perhaps more common in those receiving alternative systemic prophylaxis, and most common (albeit still rare overall) in those not receiving prophylaxis or in those on aerosol pentamidine. Combination antiretroviral therapy reduces the risk of extrapulmonary *Pneumocystosis* dramatically.

Extrapulmonary *P. carinii* most frequently involves the reticuloendothelial system: lymph nodes, spleen, liver, and bone marrow. Isolated cases of involvement of nearly every other tissue have been reported, most often the gastrointestinal tract, genitourinary tract, eyes, and thyroid and adrenal glands. Osteomyelitis and subcutaneous soft-tissue masses have also been reported. Most cases of isolated disease have presented with nodules or masses involving the affected organ, such as chorioretinal fluffy nodules, polyps of the auditory canals, thyroid nodules, and space-occupying masses in soft tissues. Haematoxylin-eosin-stained biopsies of suspicious lesions demonstrate the same foamy eosinophilic exudate seen in the lung, and methenamine silver stain demonstrates the characteristic cysts.

Extrapulmonary *P. carinii* infection may develop concomitant with PCP or independently. The usual symptoms (e.g. fever and malaise) are highly non-specific, although localizing symptoms due to the organ involvement may occur. The cutaneous lesions of extrapulmonary *Pneumocystis* are usually described as nodules or polyps and are frequently seen on the cranium. Involvement of lymph nodes is common. Retinal involvement may cause visual symptoms. Fluffy white retinal exudates, which do not involve the retinal vessels and are not associated with haemorrhage, distinguish *Pneumocystis* from cytomegalovirus (CMV) retinitis (Raviglione, 1990).

Diagnostic procedures for *Pneumocystis* pneumonia

Obtaining material for diagnosis

Diagnosis of PCP depends almost entirely upon demonstration of the organism in pulmonary secretions or lung tissue by microscopy following special staining (Ng *et al.*, 1993). Patients with PCP generally do not have a productive cough, so respiratory specimens that reflect alveolar contents must be elicited. Airway fluid specimens may be obtained by induced expectorated sputum or tracheobronchial suction (30–90% sensitivity); by bronchoalveolar lavage (90–99% sensitivity); or lung biopsy via bronchoscopy or open-lung surgery (95–100% sensitivity) (Baughman *et al.*, 1994).

Sputum and tracheobronchial secretions

In patients who are not producing sputum, bronchoalveolar fluid can be induced by inhalation of a hypertonic saline mist. The patient is first asked to gargle with water to remove saliva, oral debris, and contaminating organisms. In a room or booth that meets the Public Health Service guidelines for tuberculosis control (Centers for Disease Control and Prevention, 1990), the patient breathes a mist of hypertonic (3%) saline generated by an ultrasonic nebulizer for 5–15 min. All material produced by coughing (usually 2–3 ml) is collected and diluted with an equal volume of sterile water. In the laboratory, the specimen is liquefied with dithiothreitol, centrifuged, and slides are prepared for staining and microscopic examination. This procedure has a diagnostic sensitivity of 30–90%, with lower yields obtained from patients receiving aerosolized pentamidine prophylaxis (Baughman *et al.*, 1994; Metersky and Catanzaro, 1991). The diagnostic yield is also best at institutions experienced in obtaining these specimens and examining the slides (Kovacs *et al.*, 1988; Ng *et al.*, 1993). Specimens recovered by suction or brushing of tracheobronchial secretions, such as through an endotracheal tube, or obtained during bronchoscopy without alveolar lavage can be positive for *Pneumocystis* in up to 80% of patients with proven PCP (Baughman *et al.*, 1994). Even in the rare patient who is spontaneously producing sputum, an induced specimen may be more likely to yield a diagnosis.

Bronchoalveolar lavage

Respiratory specimens obtained by bronchoalveolar lavage (BAL) will identify 90–99% of PCP cases (Baughman *et al.*, 1994). BAL is usually performed through a bronchoscope, although similar yields have been obtained by 'blind' alveolar lavage through endotracheal catheters. In the usual procedure, the bronchoscope is advanced as far as possible through the airways to a 'wedge' position in the area to be lavaged. The diagnostic yield is increased by performing the lavage in two areas of the lung. Because *Pneumocystis* has a predilection for the upper lobes and the yield of bronchoalveolar lavage might be reduced in patients receiving aerosolized pentamidine prophylaxis, the procedure should include a specimen from the upper lobe in most instances. After the bronchoscope is wedged, normal saline is instilled in 50 ml volumes and immediately withdrawn with suction or a hand-held syringe. Diagnostic yield increases with increased total lavage volume; the procedure usually employs 100–250 ml sterile non-bacteriostatic saline. The recovered specimen is centrifuged and studied for *Pneumocystis* as well as other pathogens and cellular elements (Meduri *et al.*, 1991; Baughman *et al.*, 1993).

Although the diagnostic sensitivity of bronchoscopy with bronchoalveolar lavage is better than that of induced sputum, bronchoscopy is more expensive, has some morbidity (especially in severely hypoxaemic patients) and fatalities have been reported rarely.

Lung biopsy

Transbronchial biopsy provides a high diagnostic yield for PCP, and some investigators have recommended that this procedure is done in patients undergoing bronchoscopy who are receiving aerosolized pentamidine for prophylaxis. However, lavage of more than one lobe, especially the upper lobes, also provides an excellent yield in these patients (Meduri *et al.*, 1991; Baughman *et al.*, 1993). Many bronchoscopists do not routinely perform transbronchial biopsy in this clinical setting because the risk of pneumothorax is as high as 10% (Huang *et al.*, 1995). Although the diagnosis of PCP can easily be made on an open-lung biopsy, this procedure is very rarely required to make the diagnosis in AIDS patients because of the large

number of organisms present in their lungs and the high diagnostic yield of induced sputum and bronchoalveolar lavage. Therefore, thoracotomy is only required when repeat bronchoscopies have not yielded a diagnosis. In one study of open-lung biopsies, information that could be used to guide therapy was found infrequently (Bonfils-Roberts *et al.*, 1990).

Laboratory examination of pulmonary secretions

Specimens obtained by expectoration–liquification, tracheal suction, and bronchoalveolar lavage are concentrated by centrifugation before staining. A cellular stain such as the Wright-Giemsa stain or its Diff-Quik modification will show the nuclei of all stages of *P. carinii* in 50–90% of cases when read by an experienced observer (Ng *et al.*, 1993). Some laboratories prefer the periodic acid-Schiff (PAS) stain for revealing *P. carinii*. Both of these stains are inexpensive, can be performed rapidly (in less than 1 h), and provide additional information about the cellular composition of endobronchial inflammatory response. Quantitation of *Pneumocystis* burden and assessment of neutrophil response provide some prognostic information (Mason *et al.*, 1989; Baughman *et al.*, 1990; Colangelo *et al.*, 1991). Since Wright-Giemsa and PAS stains are not 100% sensitive, specimens negative by these tests should be examined by silver staining or immunofluorescence (Baughman *et al.*, 1994).

Gomori's methenamine silver stain, originally developed to stain fungi, is the traditional pathological stain used to demonstrate *Pneumocystis* cysts (Figure 25.1). With this stain the cyst wall appears similar to a crushed table-tennis ball and is about the size of a red blood cell. Trophozoites are not stained, which occasionally leads to false-negative results. The original method requires overnight staining, although recent modifications require only 2 h. Papanicolaou's stain is the standard cytopathologist's stain and demonstrates *Pneumocystis* by staining the inflammatory cells and the amorphous material of the alveolar exudate but not *P. carinii* itself. Immunofluorescent stains that have greater sensitivity than the silver or Wright-Giemsa stain are available. Although they are expensive, these stains increase the sensitivity of induced sputum specimens for diagnosis of PCP (Kovacs *et al.*, 1988; Ng *et al.*, 1993).

Detection of *P. carinii* DNA in respiratory secretions following PCR amplification is the most sensitive diagnostic test available, but may be too sensitive for routine clinical use (Ribes *et al.*, 1997).

Overall diagnostic strategy for PCP

When both the clinic and the laboratory have experience in obtaining specimens and testing them for the presence of *P. carinii* and any results are rapidly available, induced sputum for PCP should be the first diagnostic test performed (Ng *et al.*, 1993). If the patient is in significant respiratory distress, if other diagnoses are considered, or the sputum examination is negative, a bronchoscopy with bronchoalveolar lavage should be performed as soon as possible (Huang *et al.*, 1995). Whether bronchoalveolar lavage or induced sputum is the first diagnostic test, the outcome can be improved by a rapid coordinated response by the clinic and laboratory leading to early diagnosis. Even in a centre with an efficient protocol for obtaining induced sputum, half of the patients with PCP will require bronchoalveolar lavage for diagnosis. If bronchoalveolar lavage is negative, empirical PCP therapy can be stopped without ill effects. A number of concomitant or alternative pathogens are diagnosed only by BAL (Huang *et al.*, 1995).

At the University of Cincinnati, we prefer bronchoalveolar lavage as the first diagnostic test because it identifies associated infections in up to 20% of cases (Mason *et al.*, 1989; Colangelo *et al.*, 1991; Baughman *et al.*, 1994). It also assesses factors such as endobronchial neutrophilia and organism density, which are measures of disease severity. If bronchoalveolar lavage is performed, the specimen should be processed for bacteria, fungi, and mycobacteria, as well as *Pneumocystis*. If there will be a delay in performing a specific diagnostic test for PCP, empirical therapy can be started, but a specific diagnosis must still be sought (preferably within a few days) because treatments are toxic, steroids are immunosuppressive, and concomitant infections are frequent. An analysis of empirically treated PCP compared to cytologically confirmed cases in patients from 56 hospitals suggested that the patients treated empirically had a significantly greater mortality despite adjustment for the severity of illness (Bennett *et al.*, 1995). Prior treatment is unlikely to render a bronchoalveolar lavage specimen falsely negative during the first several days of therapy.

Treatment of *P. carinii* infections

Antimicrobial chemotherapy

Trimethoprim-sulfamethoxazole

Trimethoprim-sulfamethoxazole (TMP-SMX) is the most useful agent for the treatment of PCP. It is equal to or more effective than other available agents, available for both intravenous and oral administration, and inexpensive. Thus, it remains the first choice of therapy for this infection (Table 25.2). The rate of treatment failure varies from 10 to 20%, depending on the severity of PCP (Sattler *et al.*, 1988; Sattler *et al.*, 1994; Safrin *et al.*, 1996). Because TMP-SMX is well absorbed, it can be given orally to patients with mild to moderately severe pneumonia and to patients with extrapulmonary pneumocystosis. For patients with malabsorption, those unable to take oral medications, and those who have severe pneumonia, TMP-SMX should be given intravenously.

The two components of this drug combination act by selectively interfering with successive steps of the folic-acid synthesis pathway and thus blocking *Pneumocystis* DNA synthesis. Trimethoprim is an inhibitor of dihydrofolate reductase, which has a much higher affinity for the *Pneumocystis* enzyme than the human one. Sulphamethoxazole is an inhibitor of dihydropteroate synthetase. Both trimethoprim and sulphamethoxazole are rapidly absorbed when given by mouth and are widely distributed throughout the body, penetrating into the cerebrospinal fluid (CSF), brain, and eye. In patients with normal renal and hepatic function, the half-life of each component is about 8–12 h, making an 8-h dosing schedule most reasonable. A regimen of TMP-SMX consisting of 20 mg of trimethoprim and 100 mg of sulphamethoxazole/kg/24 h was formerly recommended based on early treatment studies of PCP in both AIDS and non-AIDS patients. However, Sattler and colleagues (1988) showed that a dose of 15 mg trimethoprim and 75 mg sulphamethoxazole/kg/24 h achieved adequate blood levels of 5–8 µg trimethoprim/ml and that the doses could be reduced even further later in the course of therapy; this is now the recommended dosing regimen (Table 25.2). Lee *et al.* (1989) showed a bidirectional pharmacokinetic interaction between trimethoprim and sulphamethoxazole, documenting the mechanism by which adequate blood levels are achieved with the current dosing regimens. The oral dose for an average-sized adult male is two double-strength tablets every 8 h (Table 25.2).

Most authors recommend treating HIV-infected patients with PCP for 3 weeks. In HIV-uninfected patients with PCP, 2 weeks of therapy was found to be satisfactory. With the high recurrence rate of PCP seen in the early years of the AIDS epidemic, it became commonplace to extend the treatment period to 3 weeks in order to forestall relapse. Even though this strategy was unsuccessful, the 3-week

Table 25.2 Recommended drug dosages for treatment and prophylaxis of *P. carinii* pneumonia in adults

Treatment[a]	First choice agent	Alternative drugs
Intravenous	TMP-SMX, 5 mg trimethoprim and 25 mg sulfamethoxazole every 8 h[b]	Pentamidine, 3–4 mg/kg every 24 h
		Trimetrexate 45 mg/m^2 once daily plus leucovorin 0.8 mg/kg (for < 50 kg) or 0.5 mg/kg (for > 50 kg) every 6 h[b]
		Clindamycin, 900 mg every 8 h plus primaquine[c], 30 mg orally every 24 h
Oral	TMP-SMX, 5/25 mg T/S/kg every 8 h (two double-strength tablets every 8 h in a 70 kg patient)	Dapsone[c], 100 mg every 24 h plus trimethoprim, 4–5 mg/kg every 8 h
		Clindamycin, 600 mg every 6 h plus primaquine, 30 mg every 24 h
		Atovaquone, 750 mg every 12 h[e]
Prophylaxis[f]	TMP-SMX 160–180 mg T/S[g] (one double-strength tablet) or T/S 80–400 mg (one single-strength tablet) every 24 h	TMP-SMX 160–800 mg T/S three times a week
		Dapsone[c], 100 mg every 24 h
		Dapsone 50 mg every 24 h plus pyrimethamine 50 mg and leucovorin 25 mg once a week[g] or dapsone 200 mg plus pyrimethamine 75 mg plus leucovorin 25 mg once a week[g]
		Pentamidine 300 mg aerolized by Respirgard II nebulizer every 4 weeks or 60 mg aerosolized by a Fisoneb nebulizer every 2 weeks
		Atovaquone 750 mg every 12 h

TMP-SMX : trimethoprim-sulfamethoxazole; T/S:

[a]The recommended treatment duration is 3 weeks, although 2 weeks is adequate for those with good response who develop drug toxicity in the third week.
[b]The first dose of leucovorin must precede the first dose of trimetrexate and leucovorin should continue for 3 days after trimetrexate is discontinued.
[c]Should be avoided in patients with known glucose-6-phosphate dehydrogenase deficiency.
[d]Primaquine is unavailable in a parenteral form; 30 mg base = two 26.3 mg primaquine phosphate tablets.
[e]Should be avoided in patients with malabsorption or diarrhoea; must be taken with food to assure absorption.
[f]Should begin when the patient's peripheral blood CD4 lymphocyte count is less than 200 cells/μl.
[g]This regimen also provides prophylaxis for toxoplasmosis.

treatment period became standard practice. However, many AIDS patients who suffer adverse effects from their treatment regimen successfully clear their pneumonia when treatment is discontinued after 2 weeks.

TMP-SMX has numerous untoward effects, and the frequency is higher in HIV-infected than in uninfected patients (Table 25.3). In most large series, the frequency of untoward effects approaches or exceeds 50% in AIDS patients and up to 25% of patients will require a change in therapy due to drug toxicity (Sattler *et al.*, 1988; Medina *et al.*, 1990; Safrin *et al.*, 1996). Fever and rash are the most common side-effects of TMP-SMX therapy. The rash com-

monly occurs after around 10 days of treatment, suggesting an allergic basis. The reason(s) for the high incidence of rash in AIDS patients is not known, but there is an increased frequency of adverse reactions to many other drugs as well. The incidence of rash appears to be dose-related because it seems to occur relatively infrequently at the low doses used for prophylaxis. Van Der Ven and associates (1991) hypothesized that the hydroxylamine metabolite of sulphamethoxazole is responsible for the rash, with AIDS patients detoxifying it poorly. However, monitoring sulphamethoxazole levels and maintaining them in the range of 100–150 g/ml did not decrease the frequency

Table 25.3 Side-effects of trimethoprim-sulphamethoxazole therapy in patients with HIV-related *P. carinii* pneumonia

- Fever
- Rash, including Stevens–Johnson syndrome
- Haematologic toxicity
  Neutropenia
  Thrombocytopenia
- Hepatic toxicity
  Elevated serum transaminases
- Renal toxicity
  Elevated serum creatinine
- Gastrointestinal toxicity
  Nausea, vomiting, diarrhoea
- Neurologic toxicity
  Altered mental status (rare)

of side-effects (Joos *et al.*, 1995) and no relation between the development of rash and the plasma levels of either trimethoprim or sulphamethoxazole has been noted (Hughes *et al.*, 1995). Further, Lee *et al.* (1994) were unable to correlate hydroxylamine metabolic excretion and adverse reactions. Some patients with trimethoprim-sulpher-related rash are able to continue the drug, using symptomatic therapy for the control of fever and itching (Sattler *et al.*, 1988). However, most patients who develop fever or rash with the high doses of TMP-SMX required for treatment will have to discontinue the drug. In its most severe form, a Stevens–Johnson-like syndrome with high fever, mucosal involvement, and vesicle formation can occur. For that reason, finding oral lesions in a patient with suspected trimethoprim-sulpha rash is an absolute indication to discontinue the drug combination.

Hepatocellular disease and nephrotoxicity are also seen with high doses of TMP-SMX, and are usually seen in conjunction with fever and rash (Medina *et al.*, 1990; Safrin *et al.*, 1996). Hepatocellular enzymes (alanine aminotransferase and aspartate aminotransferase) and renal function should be monitored weekly during high-dose TMP-SMX therapy, and the drug discontinued if liver enzymes exceed 10 times normal or if serum creatinine exceeds twice normal levels (Sattler *et al.*, 1988).

Bone-marrow suppression, manifest predominantly as neutropenia with a lesser incidence of thrombocytopenia, can be seen with TMP-SMX therapy for PCP. In addition to the marrow-suppressive effects of this drug combination, AIDS patients frequently have cytopenias from HIV infec-

tion or the other marrow-suppressive agents that they commonly receive. Therefore, peripheral blood counts should be monitored frequently in patients being treated with TMP-SMX. Depending on marrow function at the start of TMP-SMX therapy, blood counts should be performed at least once or twice a week. Other marrow-suppressive agents may have to be discontinued during treatment of PCP with TMP-SMX. As trimethoprim decreases the renal clearance of zidovudine (ZDV, which in itself is bone-marrow suppressive) and increases ZDV blood levels, haematological toxicity should be anticipated in patients receiving both drugs (Lee *et al.*, 1996). Although the bone-marrow toxicity of TMP-SMX was thought to be due, at least in part, to drug-induced relative folate deficiency, folate supplementation of patients being treated with TMP-SMX for HIV-related PCP did not lessen the haematological toxicity and apparently markedly reduced therapeutic efficacy of this antimicrobial combination (Safrin *et al.*, 1994).

High-dose sulphonamides occasionally cause altered mental function with confusion, agitation, tremors, and seizures. Concomitant diseases such as toxoplasmosis and cryptococcosis should be excluded, but if neurological complications occur as a result of TMP-SMX therapy, the drug should be stopped.

Pentamidine

Pentamidine has been known to be effective against PCP since the 1950s (Wispelwey and Pearson, 1991). This once-standard therapy for PCP has been largely replaced by TMP-SMX, primarily because it cannot be given orally and also because of its daunting toxicity profile (see Table 25.2). Comparative studies suggest that the intravenous form of pentamidine is roughly equivalent to TMP-SMX in therapeutic efficacy for the treatment of PCP in AIDS, with some studies showing a slight advantage for one or the other (Sattler *et al.*, 1988).

Pentamidine is lipophilic and has an extremely large volume of distribution because it is highly bound to cell membranes. The half-life is approximately 1 week, and once daily therapy is the usual treatment regimen. Pentamidine can also be given intramuscularly, but injections are painful, may be difficult in HIV-infected patients with muscle wasting, and the incidence of sterile abscesses is high. This route of administration is not recommended. Hypotension is seen with both intramuscular therapy and with rapid intravenous infusion. A slow infusion over 60–120 min minimizes this problem (Wispelwey and Pearson, 1991).

Careful dose-ranging studies have not been performed with pentamidine. The most commonly recommended dose is 4 mg/kg/day, but some clinicians are comfortable with a regimen of 3 mg/kg/day, particularly in patients with mild disease or in the second and third week of treatment (Sattler *et al.*, 1988; Wispelwey and Pearson, 1991). Similar to the situation with TMP-SMX, the 21-day treatment duration is based on early attempts to prevent relapse of PCP in AIDS patients. Treatment studies in HIV-uninfected patients documented successful therapy with as little as 9 days of therapy, and thus the recommended course of treatment for these patients is 2 weeks. Therefore, pentamidine can be discontinued in AIDS patients who are responding to therapy after 2 weeks of intravenous pentamidine, especially in those with adverse drug effects. Therapeutic levels of pentamidine will be present in lung tissue for at least several additional days after the last dose because of the drug's long half-life.

The most common adverse effect of intravenous pentamidine is renal dysfunction; hypotension, hypoglycaemia, and cardiac arrhythmias are less common but more serious complications (Table 25.4; see also O'Brien *et al.*, 1997 for review). In addition, a number of bothersome side-effects such as metallic taste, nausea, and malaise are common. Pentamidine is toxic to renal tubular cells, and renal dysfunction, ranging from modest elevations of creatinine and potassium levels to acute tubular necrosis, has been described in up to two-thirds of patients. When carefully monitored and the drug dose is reduced or discontinued, these complications are generally reversible (Wispelwey and Pearson, 1991). Thus, patients receiving parenteral pentamidine for PCP should have renal function and electrolytes monitored frequently, at least twice weekly in the second and third week of therapy.

Selective pancreatic β-cell toxicity occurs in up to 47% of patients, most commonly in those who had a large total dose and pre-existing renal dysfunction. Hypoglycaemia is caused by excess insulin release, which can appear gradually or suddenly, either during or after a course of pentamidine. Fatalities due to unrecognized hypoglycaemia have been reported. Although the hypoglycaemic effect of pentamidine eventually clears, pentamidine-induced islet cell destruction may result in permanent insulin-dependent diabetes mellitus (Wispelwey and Pearson, 1991). Daily measurement of blood glucose level by a glucometer during the second and third week of therapy is an appropriate monitoring strategy and patients and their caregivers should be alerted to the symptoms, signs, and emergency management of hypoglycaemia.

Ventricular ectopy has been described with parenteral pentamidine therapy and usually occurs in the second or third week of treatment. Fatalities have occurred. The most common electrocardiographic manifestation is a *torsade de pointe* rhythm. Whether this phenomenon is a direct toxic effect of the drug or is related to electrolyte disturbances, such as hypomagnesaemia, is unclear. This rhythm is usually preceded by a prolongation of the QT interval on the electrocardiogram (Wispelwey and Pearson, 1991). Thus, regular monitoring of the QT interval with electrocardiograms is appropriate during the second and third week of therapy. A prolonged QT interval is sometimes corrected by the administration of magnesium. In the event that it cannot be corrected, pentamidine should be discontinued and cardiology consultation sought. Ventricular ectopy or *torsade de pointe* should not be treated with class 1 arrhythmic agents (such as lidocaine) because they may potentiate the arrhythmia. Administration of magnesium sulphate and overdrive pacing (by isoproterenol or a pacemaker) may be useful.

Like TMP-SMX, pentamidine can cause neutropenia and hepatitis, although these toxicities are infrequent with pentamidine. Because of its frequent and sometimes life-threatening toxicity when used intravenously, delivery of pentamidine by inhaled aerosol has been used for treatment

Table 25.4 Side-effects of pentamidine therapy in patients with HIV-related *P. carinii* pneumonia

- Renal dysfunction
  Elevation of serum creatinine
  Elevation of serum potassium
  Acute tubular necrosis
- Pancreatic toxicity
  Hypoglycaemia
  Hyperglycaemia
- Cardiovascular toxicity
  Arrhythmias
  Hypotension
- Hematologic toxicity
  Neutropenia
- Hepatotoxicity
  Elevation of serum transaminases
- Gastrointestinal
  Metallic taste
  Nausea

of active PCP. The observed failure rate (39–45%) in controlled trials has been substantially higher than for intravenous pentamidine or oral TMP-SMX, although there was less systemic toxicity (Conte *et al.*, 1990; Soo Hoo *et al.*, 1990; Montgomery *et al.*, 1995). Because a daily dose of 600 mg of aerosolized pentamidine is an extremely expensive regimen, this type of therapy should be reserved for patients with mild disease and no other treatment options.

Dapsone-trimethoprim

Dapsone is a sulphone derivative, which has a higher affinity for *Pneumocystis dihydropteroate* synthetase than sulphamethoxazole. When used as a single agent for treatment of PCP it had an unacceptably high failure rate of over 40% (Safrin *et al.*, 1991). Based on *in vitro* and animal studies, the combination of dapsone with trimethoprim was selected as a potential treatment option for PCP (Table 25.2). In a small, randomized but unblinded trial of 30 patients with mild-to-moderate PCP comparing dapsone-trimethoprim with TMP-SMX, the dapsone-trimethoprim combination appeared effective and well tolerated (Medina *et al.*, 1990). A larger multicentre comparative trial confirmed that dapsone-trimethoprim and TMP-SMX had similar efficacy and rates of dose-limiting toxicity in patients with mild-to-moderate PCP (Safrin *et al.*, 1996).

Dapsone has a half-life of approximately 36 h, so the drug can be given daily. In the small number of series that have been reported, dapsone has been administered at a dose of 100 mg in a single daily dose combined with trimethoprim, 12–20 mg/kg/day in divided doses (Table 25.2). As with trimethoprim and sulphamethoxazole, there is a bidirectional pharmacokinetic interaction between dapsone and sulphamethoxazole, such that levels of both drugs are increased when the combination is used. Thus, the recommended regimen is 15 mg trimethoprim/kg/day (in two or three divided doses) with 100 mg dapsone/day (Lee *et al.*, 1989).

The most common side-effects of dapsone therapy are fever and rash, similar to that seen with sulphamethoxazole. In the prospective comparative study of Medina and co-workers (1990), nearly half of each group (dapsone-trimethoprim or TMP-SMX) had rash, but only 10% of subjects in each arm of the study had to stop therapy for this reason. As with sulphamethoxazole, the Stevens–Johnson syndrome can be a complication of dapsone therapy. Dapsone causes haemolytical anaemia in patients with glucose-6-phosphate dehydrogenase deficiency, and

most authorities recommend screening for this disorder prior to initiating treatment. Methemoglobinaemia occurs in up to two-thirds of patients on dapsone, although it is usually not clinically significant (Medina *et al.*, 1990). However, if a patient receiving dapsone has persistent hypoxaemia, methemoglobinaemia should be considered as a cause.

Clindamycin-primaquine

The clindamycin-primaquine combination was shown to be effective treatment for experimental *P. carinii* infections in animals, and was thus evaluated as an alternative therapy for the treatment of PCP in humans in several small trials (Noskin *et al.*, 1992; Black *et al.*, 1994). Like dapsone-trimethoprim, this combination was compared with TMP-SMX in a blinded multicentre trial in the USA (ACTG 108), and found to be no different from the others in efficacy or tolerability (Safrin *et al.*, 1996).

Clindamycin is given intravenously in a dose of 900 mg every 8 h, with oral therapy at a dose of 600 mg every 6 h as an alternative. Primaquine is given as a single daily dose of 30 mg by mouth (Table 25.2).

Like the sulphur-containing combinations, the most common untoward effects from clindamycin-primaquine therapy are fever and rash in more than half of patients. In the series that have been reported to date, the rash is generally mild, and continued therapy has been reasonably well tolerated, with regression of the rash in some cases. Although the drug itself can cause diarrhoea, the development of diarrhoea during or after therapy might require an investigation for pseudomembranous colitis. This complication was very rarely seen in the series that have been reported (Safrin *et al.*, 1996).

Haematologic toxicities of primaquine-clindamycin, including neutropenia, anaemia and methemoglobinaemia occur commonly, but usually do not require discontinuing therapy (Black *et al.*, 1994; Safrin *et al.*, 1996). Primaquine also accelerates haemolysis of glucose-6-phosphate dehydrogenase-deficient red blood cells. Clinical trials to date have excluded patients with this deficiency and have also been limited to patients with mild-to-moderate PCP. Therefore, the wider applicability of this therapy is yet to be determined.

Atovaquone

Atovaquone is a hydroxynaphthoquinone recently licensed for the treatment of PCP. After early studies demonstrated efficacy for the treatment of mild PCP, a comparative study with TMP-SMX in 322 subjects with mild-to-moderate PCP (PA-aO$_2$ < 45 mmHg) revealed that although the drug was less toxic than TMP-SMX, it was also less effective (Hughes *et al.*, 1993). Patients who failed treatment had a higher incidence of diarrhoea and lower serum levels of atovaquone, suggesting that poor absorption may have been responsible for some of the treatment failures. In another comparison between pentamidine and atovaquone for mild-to-moderate PCP, only 4% of patients on atovaquone had treatment-limiting adverse effects versus one-third of patients on pentamidine, but almost twice as many patients on atovaquone were therapeutic failures (Dohn *et al.*, 1994).

The currently available formulation of atovaquone is an oral suspension given at a dose of 750 mg twice a day. It has a more predictable absorption than the original tablet form but patients must be able to eat to achieve adequate absorption of the drug (Rosenberg *et al.*, 2001). It should not be prescribed to patients with malabsorption or chronic diarrhoea. Because there is no parenteral form of atovaquone, its use also should be restricted to patients with mild-to-moderate PCP.

Atovaquone is a relatively non-toxic drug. The most common untoward effect is rash, which is usually mild and which patients can often tolerate while continuing the drug. If the rash becomes more severe or is associated with fever, the drug should be stopped. Gastrointestinal disturbances are also common. Mild hepatitis has also been seen occasionally with atovaquone therapy (Hughes, 1995).

Trimetrexate-leucovorin

Evaluation of compounds interfering with the folate pathway led to the identification of trimetrexate, an inhibitor of dihydrofolate reductase, which is 1500 times more potent than trimethoprim. The toxic effect of trimetrexate on mammalian cells, particularly bone-marrow cells, can be prevented by administration of folinic acid. Since *P. carinii* does not have an active transport mechanism for folinic acid, human cells are selectively protected by co-administration of folinic acid with trimetrexate. The addition of dapsone (100 mg/day) provides sequential blockade of folate synthesis, although this combination has not been studied clinically.

A multicentre study performed by the AIDS Clinical Trials Group compared trimetrexate and leucovorin (a folinic acid) with TMP-SMX in 303 patients with moderate-to-severe PCP (PA-aO$_2$ > 30 mmHg). This showed that trimetrexate-leucovorin was less effective (38% failure) than TMP-SMX (20% failure) but was also less toxic (Sattler *et al.*, 1994).

Trimetrexate is administered as a single intravenous daily dose calculated by weight (Table 25.2); leucovorin is co-administered intravenously or orally in four daily doses by weight (Table 25.2). The first dose of leucovorin must be given before trimetrexate and leucovorin should be continued for 3 days after stopping trimetrexate. The major toxicity of the trimetrexate-leucovorin regimen is bone marrow suppression, although this occurred less commonly than with TMP-SMX in the sole large comparative study (Sattler *et al.*, 1994). Neutropenia can be managed by increasing the dose of leucovorin or reducing the dose of trimetrexate.

Adjunctive therapy with corticosteroids

In the early-to-mid-1980s, empirical high-dose steroid therapy was used to treat the respiratory failure syndrome associated with PCP. This syndrome resembles the adult respiratory distress syndrome (ARDS) and usually develops during the first few days of treatment. However, comparative trial showed that patients with PCP who had already developed respiratory failure did not benefit from steriod therapy.

Because of the failure of therapeutic glucocorticoids in PCP-associated respiratory failure, a number of groups have investigated the utility of steroids for preventing ARDS in moderate-to-severe PCP, by initiating steroids with anti-*Pneumocystis* therapy (Bozzette *et al.*, 1990; Montaner *et al.*, 1990). These studies have consistently showed that the administration of steroids to such patients results in an improved outcome. Adjunctive corticosteroids at the onset of treatment for PCP reduced the incidence of respiratory failure measured by admission to intensive care units or by the incidence of endotracheal intubation. Some of the studies also showed improved survival. Glucocorticoid prophylaxis in patients with severe PCP appears to abrogate the progressive hypoxaemia that is seen during the first 3–4 days of treatment (Bozzette *et al.*, 1990; Montaner *et al.*, 1990).

A consensus committee convened by the National Institutes of Health and the University of California at Los Angeles formulated recommendations for the use of corticosteroids as adjunctive therapy for PCP. All patients with PA-aO$_2$ greater than 35 mmHg or PaO$_2$ less than

70 mmHg on room air should receive corticosteroids (National Institutes of Health–University of California Expert Panel for Corticosteroids as Adjunctive Therapy for *Pneumocystis carinii* Pneumonia, 1990). Although the committee recognized that complete dose-ranging studies had not been performed, they accepted the dose used in the largest of the clinical trials as reasonable. Thus, the recommended therapy is prednisone, 40 mg twice daily for 5 days, followed by 40 mg/day for 5 days, followed by 20 mg/day for the remainder of the course of PCP treatment (usually a further 10 days), at which time prednisone is stopped without further tapering of the dose. Equivalent doses of parenteral corticosteroids can be used for patients who cannot take oral prednisone. Whether different doses or treatment durations would be more useful is unknown. Steroids are not recommended for patients with mild PCP.

Reported complications of steroid therapy have been relatively few. In one study, the incidence of herpes simplex and Candida infections was increased with steroid therapy (Bozzette *et al.*, 1990), and clinicians have been concerned about activation of occult fungal, viral, or mycobacterial infections. In a large hospital in Spain, 7% of PCP patients treated with steroids developed disseminated tuberculosis within 1 year, compared with 12% of patients who had not received steroids, suggesting that short-term steroid use was without risk (Mantos *et al.*, 1995). However, careful monitoring of steroid-treated patients for the development of other opportunistic infections remains important, and the decision to use adjunctive steroid therapy for PCP requires the rapid confirmation of a PCP diagnosis and the exclusion of other infections, especially tuberculosis.

Clinical course of *P. carinii* pneumonia and management of complications

Prognostic features

Untreated PCP in the patient with unremitting immune dysfunction is probably 100% fatal. With current treatment strategies the average mortality in AIDS patients is about 15–20%, with a range from 0–90%, depending on a number of prognostic indicators. The degree of hypoxaemia, measured by arterial blood gas analysis while the patient breathes room air, is the best predictor of outcome (Bozzette *et al.*, 1990; Dohn *et al.*, 1992). In the large California Collaborative Treatment Group study of steroid therapy,

which represents the current standard of care, the mortality rates in the mild (PA-aO$_2$ > 35 mmHg), moderate (PA-aO$_2$ 35–45 mmHg), and severe (PA-aO$_2$ > 45 mmHg) steroid-treated groups were 0%, 10%, and 19%, respectively. Mortality rates in the non-steroid-treated groups were 3%, 21%, and 43%, figures that agree with studies conducted before the introduction of steroid therapy. As patients who presented for care with actual or incipient respiratory failure were excluded from that study, mortality rates in practice are somewhat higher (Dohn *et al.*, 1992).

As hypoxaemia may be more severe than the clinical appearance of the patient with PCP might suggest, arterial blood gases should always be analysed at the outset to assess prognosis and assist in management. Patients in the moderate or severe categories (PA-aO$_2$ > 35 mmHg) should be carefully monitored, and most should be hospitalized. Supplemental oxygen should be administered to those with dyspnoea or an arterial PO$_2$ of less than 60 mmHg. A number of studies have shown that treated PCP patients frequently become progressively hypoxic for the first 3–5 days of therapy, possibly as an accelerated host response to dead or dying organisms. If this deterioration occurs in patients with marginal oxygenation at the outset, they are more likely to develop respiratory failure. As Montaner and associates have demonstrated, steroid therapy reduces the severity of this early hypoxaemia, and thus reduces the incidence of respiratory failure (Montaner *et al.*, 1990). However, many patients continue to have fever, dyspnoea, and hypoxaemia during the first week of therapy, and persistent symptoms during the first 3–5 days of therapy are not necessarily an indication of treatment failure.

Although recurrent episodes of PCP were once thought to be associated with a poor outcome, Dohn and colleagues (1992) showed that this was not necessarily the case, and Bozzette and co-workers (1992) showed that an episode of PCP did not unfavourably alter the 1-year prognosis in AIDS patients with pneumonia.

A large number of *Pneumocystis* organisms in the initial lavage fluid and neutrophilia in bronchoalveolar lavage fluid indicate an increased risk of treatment failure and mortality (Mason, 1989; Colangelo *et al.*, 1991). Severity of radiographic abnormalities also correlates directly with severity of illness. The magnitude of serum lactate dehydrogenase elevations in AIDS patients with PCP can also be correlated with outcome, with higher levels associated with higher mortality. However, as a prognostic tool in the individual patient, serum lactate dehydrogenase levels must be used with caution, because the test is non-specific and it discriminates poorly between those who survive and those who do not.

Respiratory failure

Early in the course of the AIDS epidemic, a general pessimism about the outcome of *P. carinii*-induced respiratory failure led some clinicians to recommend that AIDS patients with PCP should not be admitted to intensive care units. This was particularly true for respiratory failure associated with a recurrent episode of PCP, with the reported mortality rate approaching 90%. More recently, however, the outcome of mechanical ventilatory support in AIDS patients with PCP has improved substantially and guidelines for care have broadened commensurately (Dohn *et al.*, 1992). Outcomes have improved because there has been a general improvement in the management of all types of respiratory failure in intensive care units, because of the increased experience of AIDS caregivers in management of PCP, and because of the introduction of adjunctive steroids for PCP-induced respiratory failure. Other possible factors that may have improved the outcome of PCP-related respiratory failure are the widespread use of antiretrovirals, the presence of milder disease in patients previously receiving prophylaxis, the availability of additional drugs and drug combinations for use in PCP treatment failures, and the better recognition and treatment of concomitant infections.

It is no longer appropriate to deny respiratory support to an AIDS patient with PCP on the basis of expected poor outcome, although patients with severe organ failure may have a very poor prognosis (Forrest *et al.*, 1998). The post-hospital survival of PCP patients who recover from respiratory failure now averages 80% at 1 year and aggressive treatment of these patients is appropriate (Franklin *et al.*, 1995). Management of respiratory failure in the context of HIV infection is discussed in Chapter 37.

Failure to respond to therapy

Most patients with PCP do not show improvement during the first few days of therapy, and it is usually unwarranted to change anti-*Pneumocystis* agents during this period, except in the case of severe adverse drug effects (which is very unusual). However, as most patients begin to improve after 7 days of treatment, if improvement does not occur by this time, the possibility of treatment failure should definitely be entertained. Failing treatment for PCP is only one reason

for lack of clinical improvement because concomitant respiratory pathogens can be present in up to 20% of patients (Baughman *et al.*, 1994). Therefore, in a patient suspected of failing therapy, many authorities suggest that other pathogens are excluded and *Pneumocystis* is confirmed as the offending agent by repeat bronchoscopy. If bronchoscopy has not previously been performed, a study at this time will confirm the diagnosis of PCP and will also identify any co-existing pathogens. If the patient has previously undergone bronchoscopy with bronchoalveolar lavage, a repeat study often provides information regarding the status of the *Pneumocystis* infection and may identify other pathogens not identified on the original procedure. Colangelo and colleagues (1991) showed that quantitation of *Pneumocystis* burden correlates with outcome and that a reduction of more than 50% in the number of *Pneumocystis* clusters found in a follow-up bronchoalveolar lavage specimen is associated with treatment success. They also showed that repeat bronchoscopy provides useful information regarding co-pathogens, either primary or hospital-acquired.

The decision to abandon first-line *Pneumocystis* therapy for a second agent is not easily made. Patients who fail treatment with TMP-SMX or pentamidine generally have a poor outcome when switched to alternate therapy. In addition, many patients have absolute or relative contraindications to one or more of these alternate drugs, which limits treatment options. Patients with PCP who are failing treatment are usually quite ill and unable to take oral medications; also, oral therapy is rarely appropriate in patients whose clinical condition is deteriorating. In addition, no oral regimen has been adequately studied in severely ill patients. For patients not responding to TMP-SMX, options include intravenous pentamidine, trimetrexate-leucovorin–possibly with dapsone, or intravenous clindamycin with oral primaquine; intravenous pentamidine is usually considered the drug of first choice.

Pneumothorax

The incidence of spontaneous pneumothorax in AIDS patients is 450 times the rate in the general population, and most cases of spontaneous pneumothorax in HIV-infected patients turn out to be early manifestations of PCP (Sepkowitz *et al.*, 1991). Pneumothorax can develop early or late in the course of PCP and appears to be more common in patients receiving aerosolized pentamidine for prophylaxis. This complication is probably due to destruction of lung by indolent peripheral *Pneumocystis* infection, with subpleural bullous formation and then rupture (Feuerstein *et al.*, 1990). Because lung damage is a prominent feature of PCP, management of a pneumothorax is particularly difficult. Most patients who undergo tube thoracostomy do not heal quickly, leading to long-term chest tube placement because of bronchopulmonary fistulae; attempts at sclerotherapy usually meet with limited success. Spontaneous or procedure-related pneumothorax increases morbidity but does not change in mortality. Patients who develop pneumothorax while receiving mechanical ventilation have a very bad prognosis, with almost 100% mortality (Pastores *et al.*, 1996). Since tension pneumothorax does not commonly develop in patients with pneumothorax unrelated to mechanical ventilation, conservative management without chest-tube placement is often the best strategy (see also Chapter 13).

Extrapulmonary *Pneumocystosis*

When it occurs, widespread dissemination of *P. carinii* usually develops concomitant with PCP and is often fatal. In contrast, isolated *P. carinii* infection of one or two extrapulmonary organs may occur with or without pneumonia and sometimes responds to systemic therapy with TMP-SMX, pentamidine, or in one case, trimetrexate. Of the 34 disseminated pneumocytosis cases reviewed by Raviglione (1990), only two of 15 survivors had concomitant pneumonia.

Epidemiology and prevention of *Pneumocystosis*

Epidemiology

Pneumocystis carinii is a globally-distributed ubiquitous organism to which most humans are exposed during childhood, and most children have developed antibodies by 4 years of age. People from all continents have similar frequency of antibodies to *P. carinii*, although there may be strain differences in different locations (Smulian *et al.*, 1993). However, *P. carinii* has not been identified outside of animal tissue, and the reservoir for this ubiquitous infection is unknown. Infection could arise by direct airborne transmission from other humans or from an environmental source in a fashion similar to the dimorphic fungi (e.g. *Histoplasma capsulatum*). Animal-to-human transmission probably does not occur because there is a distinct *Pneumocystis* strain specific for each mammalian species.

Most cases of PCP appear to be unconnected epidemiologically. However, there have been some reports suggesting common source or person-to-person transmission (Chave *et al.*, 1991). As none of these case clusters have had a definitive source for the infection identified, leaving open the possibility of human-to-human transmission, some experts have recommended respiratory isolation for patients with active PCP (Walzer, 1991). In any event, the possibility of concomitant tuberculosis (which required respiratory isolation) should always be kept in mind, and at the University of Cincinnati all new HIV-infected patients with lower respiratory syndromes are isolated until tuberculosis has been excluded, and PCP patients are separated from immunodeficient patients without PCP.

Because the source of infection is unknown, it is unclear whether recurrent episodes of PCP represent reactivation of the initial infection or are newly acquired infections. Recurrent pneumocystosis is uncommon in immunodeficient patients without HIV infection, although in many of these patients the immunosuppression predisposing to PCP is transient. However, among a group of AIDS patients who recovered from PCP and were subsequently treated with ZDV but not *Pneumocystis* prophylaxis, 66% developed a second episode of PCP during the following 12 months (Fischl *et al.*, 1990). A strategy of long-term secondary prophylaxis clearly seemed appropriate. The overall survival of patients who recovered from their first episode of PCP doubled if they received secondary prophylaxis (Fischl *et al.*, 1988; Bindels *et al.*, 1991; Graham *et al.*, 1991).

Chemoprophylaxis

Patients are selected for *Pneumocystis* prophylaxis based on a risk–benefit analysis. As those at the highest risk of developing PCP are those who have already recovered from an episode of PCP, these patients should be the first priority for prophylaxis (so-called 'secondary' prophylaxis). HIV-infected patients with other opportunistic diseases, indicating significant immunosuppression regardless of CD4 lymphocyte counts, should also be considered for PCP prophylaxis (Phair *et al.*, 1990). However, other than the occurrence of opportunistic infections, the CD4 lymphocyte count provides the best measure of immune function and risk of pneumocystosis, although adjunctive prognostic information can be derived from plasma HIV RNA concentration (viral load) (Lyles *et al.*, 1999).

The United States Public Health Service/Infectious Diseases Society of America (USPHS/IDSA) Prevention of

Opportunistic Infections Working Group (1999) recommended prophylaxis for HIV-infected patients who have a history of PCP or who had a CD4 lymphocyte count of less than 200 cells/μl, unexplained fever of greater than 37.7°C for 2 weeks, or a history of oropharyngeal candidiasis.

Patients who have responded to highly active antiretroviral (HAART) therapy with an increase in CD4 lymphocytes to well above 200 cells/μl can safely discontinue PCP prophylaxis. Numerous recent studies have clearly shown that risk of stopping either primary or secondary prophylaxis is virtually nil if the patients experience a sustained rise in CD4 lymphocyte counts to above 200 cell/μl (Furrer *et al.*, 1999, 2001; Weverling *et al.*, 1999; Ledergerber B *et al.*, 2001; Lopez Bernaldo de Quiros *et al.*, 2001). Patients enrolled in the Swiss Cohort Study who were receiving PCP prophylaxis for low CD4 counts (median nadir of 110) and who sustained a CD4 cell count above 200 cells/μl (median 325) for at least 12 weeks were eligible to stop prophylaxis. Of the 262 patients followed for 3–19 months, no cases of PCP were reported (Furrer *et al.*, 1999). However, additional questions about PCP prophylaxis in the context of HAART remain to be answered, including how long a CD4 response should be sustained before stopping prophylaxis and when to restart prophylaxis in relation to CD4 count or viral load changes.

Trimethoprim-sulfamethoxazole

Prophylaxis with TMP-SMX was first shown to prevent *Pneumocystis* in children with leukaemia in the 1970s, and was later shown to be effective in AIDS patients (Fischl *et al.*, 1988; Hardy *et al.*, 1992; Bozzette *et al.*, 1995). This drug is now the recommended prophylactic regimen for PCP (USPHS/IDSA Prevention of Opportunistic Infections Working Group, 1999). In addition to being the most effective agent, TMP-SMX has the advantages of low cost, ease of administration and excellent efficacy against systemic *Pneumocystis* infection. Both pulmonary and extrapulmonary pneumocystosis are extremely rare in patients receiving TMP-SMX prophylaxis. This combination has the added advantage of also preventing toxoplasmosis and some bacterial infections (Hardy *et al.*, 1992; Buskin *et al.*, 1999).

The optimum dose of TMP-SMX for prophylaxis is unclear. Most studies showing efficacy have used a double-strength tablet once daily (160 mg trimethoprim, 800 mg sulphamethoxazole). A large, multicentre American study using this regimen demonstrated a 3.2% incidence of recurrent disease over the subsequent 12 months in patients who had been successfully treated for their first episode of PCP (Hardy *et al.*, 1992). The expected recurrence rate in such a population would be in excess of 60% per year. In fact, nearly all patients with recurrent PCP in the TMP-SMX arm were not taking the prophylaxis at the time they developed the disease (Hardy *et al.*, 1992). Smaller studies have suggested that lower doses of TMP-SMX are effective. Two commonly administered lower-dose regimens are a single-strength tablet once daily or a double-strength tablet three times a week. A large meta-analysis of 35 randomized trials comparing different agents for PCP prophylaxis confirmed that TMP-SMX protected almost totally against PCP in patients able to tolerate it, and that using a lower dose apparently decreased the rate of adverse drug reactions without decreasing efficacy (Ioannidis *et al.*, 1996). The current first-line recommendation of the USPHS/IDSA Working Group (1999) is either one single-strength (80 mg trimethoprim, 400 mg sulphamethoxazole) tablet a day or one double-strength (160 mg trimethoprim, 800 mg sulphamethoxazole) a day. Unfortunately, 15–50% of HIV-infected patients develop intolerance to TMP-SMX. The most common treatment-limiting reactions are rash and fever (Table 25.3). Intolerance of TMP-SMX appears to be most common in patients with advanced HIV disease.

Aerosolized pentamidine

Because of the frequent toxicity of systemically administered TMP-SMX, pentamidine was studied as a prophylactic agent. Since pentamidine has considerable systemic toxicity, only a few small studies investigated the use of intermittent parenteral pentamidine for *Pneumocystis* prophylaxis. The efficacy of this approach was not high, and the expected systemic toxicities occurred frequently.

Delivery of pentamidine directly to the lung by aerosol was studied simultaneously in New York and California in the late 1980s. These early studies concentrated on delivery mechanisms and the generation of optimal particle size for deposition into the alveoli. A multicentre study in California, investigating different doses and intervals using a Respirgard II nebulizer, showed that 300 mg pentamidine inhaled every 4 weeks was more effective than 30 mg every 2 weeks (Leoung *et al.*, 1989). In patients with CD4 lymphocyte counts above 100 cells/μl, aerosolized pentamidine prophylaxis was as effective as TMP-SMX. However, patients with CD4 lymphocyte counts of less than 100 cells/μl (reflecting a greater degree of immunosuppression) receiving aerosol pentamidine prophylaxis had a 33% risk of PCP, compared to 20% in patients receiving systemic prophylaxis (Bozzette et al., 1995). In the largest randomized study of aerolized pentamidine compared with TMP-SMX for secondary prophylaxis of PCP, the incidence of secondary PCP was higher in the aerosol group (18.5%/year) than in the TMP-SMX group (3.2%/year) (Hardy et al., 1992). Aerosolized pentamidine, 300 mg/month by Respirgard II nebulizer, is therefore recommended only as an alternative PCP prophylactic agent for patients who are intolerant of TMP-SMX (USPHS/IDSA Working Group, 1999). Of course, aerosolised pentamidine does not prevent toxoplasmosis or bacterial infections, unlike TMP-SMX.

The only recommended delivery system for aerosolized pentamidine is the Respirgard II jet nebulizer, which requires a pressurized gas source to generate the aerosol. However, two ultrasonic nebulizers have also been shown to provide effective PCP prophylaxis. The Fisoneb nebulizer was studied in a placebo-controlled trial using 60 mg of pentamidine every 2 weeks in patients who had recovered from an episode of PCP. Although the placebo group had a 50% recurrence of disease in 6 months, the treated group had only a 9% recurrence rate (Montaner et al., 1991). In a randomized, controlled study of the Ultraneb 99 nebulizer, with 4 mg of pentamidine/kg every 4 weeks, a 9% relapse in 10 months of follow-up was compared with a 61% relapse rate in the untreated control group (Girard et al., 1993). Ultrasonic nebulizers are more expensive than the Respirgard II, but a compressed gas source is not required and, at least with the dose studied with the Fisoneb, the total monthly dose of pentamidine is lower. However, there have been no clinical studies comparing ultrasonically delivered aerosol pentamidine with that delivered by the Respirgard II nebulizer, or with systemic chemoprophylaxis.

Aerosolized pentamidine very rarely causes systemic toxicity. However, cough and bronchospasm are common, and many patients require administration of a short-acting agonist bronchodilator, such as metaproterenol, before receiving aerosolized pentamidine. For this purpose, a metered dose inhaler is a preferred delivery mechanism because the bronchodilator is intended for delivery to the airways, not the alveoli. Thus, the pentamidine nebulizer should not be used for delivery of the bronchodilator, and an appropriate waiting period of 10–15 min allows for maximum effect of the bronchodilator.

In the large, randomized open study (ACTG 021) comparing monthly aerosolized pentamidine to a double-strength TMP-SMX tablet daily for secondary prophylaxis of PCP, although TMP-SMX prevented PCP twice as well as aerosolized pentamidine, 27% of TMP-SMX-treated patients had to discontinue prophylaxis for toxicity, compared with only 4% of those given aerosolized pentamidine (Hardy et al., 1992).

Dapsone and dapsone combinations

Dapsone-containing regimens are also effective for PCP prophylaxis (Hughes, 1998). A large, multicentre randomized, open study of dapsone, 100 mg daily, versus TMP-SMX and aerosolized pentamidine for primary prophylaxis (subjects with no prior episodes of PCP) showed that dapsone was equivalent to TMP-SMX (Bozzette et al., 1995). The majority of patients who developed PCP were either on aerosolized pentamidine or a suboptimal dose of dapsone (50 mg/day).

The combination of dapsone and pyrimethamine has been studied in two small, randomized trials, which showed that this combination was as effective as aerosolized pentamidine but less effective than TMP-SMX three times weekly (Girard et al., 1993; Podzamczer et al., 1993). The combinations recommended by the USPHS/IDSA Working Group are dapsone 50 mg/day with pyrimethamine 50 mg and leucovorin 25 mg/week or dapsone 200 mg plus pyrimethamine 75 mg plus leucovorin 25 mg/week (USPHS/IDSA Prevention of Opportunistic Infections Working Group, 1999). The dapsone–pyrimethamine combination regimens provide protection against toxoplasmosis, in addition to PCP (Hughes, 1998). Twice-weekly pyrimethamine–sulfadoxine was also effective for preventing PCP and toxoplasmic encephalitis in one small study (Schurmann et al., 2001),

Summary recommendations for P. carinii prophylaxis

Trimethoprim-sulphamethoxazole in a dose of one single-strength or one double-strength tablet daily is the preferred strategy for preventing pneumocystosis, toxoplasmosis and some bacterial infections in patients with advanced HIV infection. Dapsone at 100 mg/day appears to be slightly less effective than conventional prophylaxis for preventing Pneumocystis and substantially less effective for toxoplasmosis or bacterial infections. Using dapsone in combination with pyrimethamine will also protect against toxoplasmosis. For patients unable to tolerate the systemic regimens, aerosolized pentamidine is the current third choice for PCP prevention.

Because of the high rate of drug intolerance with TMP-SMX and dapsone, and the inferior efficacy and lack of systemic activity with aerosolized pentamidine, other systemic prophylactic agents for *P. carinii* are needed. Atovaquone, licensed to treat PCP, is under evaluation as a prophylactic agent and appears promising. Two recent trials comparing atovaquone to either aerosolized pentamidine or dapsone have shown comparable efficacy, although complete analyses are not yet available (Chan *et al.*, 1997; El-Sadr *et al.*, 1997). Atovaquone (750 mg twice a day) can be used in patients intolerant of the other regimens. Clindamycin-containing regimens for prophylaxis are likely to have an unacceptable rate of treatment-limiting diarrhoea and rash (Jacobson *et al.*, 1992).

Because TMP-SMX is the preferred prophylactic therapy based on efficacy, cost, ease of administration and activity in preventing other infections, a number of uncontrolled studies have been performed evaluating desensitization procedures for patients who have had a previous reaction to the drug combination. A significant number of patients with a prior adverse reaction to TMP-SMX are able to tolerate the drug following densitization. In the ACTG 021 study, patients with a history of sulphonamide allergy were permitted to enter the study, as long as they had not had a dose-limiting adverse reaction. In the study, subjects who were given TMP-SMX, the incidence of untoward reaction was the same whether or not the patient had a past history of sulphonamide allergy (Hardy *et al.*, 1992), suggesting that a large number of adverse reactions to TMP-SMX may be a toxic effect, rather than true allergies. The reactions may be due to a drug metabolite (Van Der Ven *et al.*, 1991).

Future development in *Pneumocystosis*

The management and prevention of PCP has improved dramatically over the past decade. Many of these advances were the result of clinical studies based on existing knowledge. However, concurrently the tools of modern molecular biology have revealed many details of the basic biology and pathophysiology of *P. carinii* infection. In the next decade, application of these latter developments will also provide new clinical advances. Studies of the phylogenetic relationships of *P. carinii* and of its surface antigens will shed light on its natural history and epidemiology. The use of the polymerase chain reaction (PCR) to detect small numbers of *Pneumocystis* will allow us to unravel the epidemiology and transmission mechanism of this organism. Detection of *Pneumocystis* genetic material in respiratory secretions by PCR may become a sensitive diagnostic test for disease and may also shed light on the acquisition and transmission of the organism, particularly as this method may be adaptable for detection of strain or species differences. PCR technology could also be used for environmental sampling to search for potential reservoirs for infection. Ultimately, improved understanding of the natural history of the life cycle and transmission of *Pneumocystis* could lead to improved methods for prevention.

Our newly acquired knowledge of the biochemistry and metabolism of *P. carinii* may lead to improved drug therapies, targeted at specific metabolic pathways unique to this organism. Similarly, a better understanding of the life cycle of this organism may permit combination therapy to be targeted towards both the trophozoite and cyst stages, thus improving therapeutic and prophylactic efficacy. New drugs being studied include WR6026, an 8-aminoquinoline compound for which therapeutic efficacy has been demonstrated *in vitro*, and in animal models. Initial pharmacokinetic studies in humans have been completed, but early clinical trials have been delayed by the reduced incidence of PCP due to the widespread use of HAART. This drug and others in the class are similar to primaquine, but *in vitro* and in animal models they appear to be more active. These drugs may thus be useful as single drugs or as a more potent replacement for primaquine in combination therapies. Because the cell wall of *Pneumocystis* has β-1,3-glucan structures, inhibitors of glucan synthesis have been studied as potential therapeutic agents for *P. carinii*. The echinocandins are such agents but the pharmacokinetics of these drugs are unsatisfactory, and much more work needs to be done on drug formulation and delivery. The possibility of a new class of drugs active against both pathogenic fungi and *Pneumocystis* is exciting. Pentamidine analogues and pentamidine metabolism are also under study. The widespread clinical use of aerosol pentamidine may promote the development of resistance, and pentamidine resistance of *P. carinii* strains has been demonstrated in the laboratory. Development of molecular assays to detect pentamidine resistance is a high research priority.

Our knowledge of the host immune responses to *P. carinii* is growing rapidly. Although the alveolar macrophage appears to be the principal effector cell in host defense, the important role played by humoral and cellular immune mechanisms is becoming increasingly recognized. Some cytokines, such as interleukin-1, have been shown to have a direct inhibitory effect on *P. carinii*, and tumor necrosis factor-α may also play a role in host defense. For instance, tumor necrosis factor-α administration or induction by bacterial products improves the survival of *Pneumocystis*-infected animals. Other immune modulators, such as interferon-γ, may also have beneficial effects. Further studies on the natural immunity of immunologically intact humans should provide better understanding of strategies for selecting patients for preventive measures and might define immune modulators that could be used adjunctively with chemotherapeutic agents.

References

Baughman RP, Strohofer S, Colangelo G et al. (1990). Semiquantitative technique for estimating *Pneumocystis carinii* burden in the lung. *J Clin Microbiol* **28**: 1425–7.

Baughman RP, Dohn MN, Shipley R et al. (1993). Increased *Pneumocystis carinii* recovery from the upper lobes in pneumocystis pneumonia. The effect of aerosol pentamidine prophylaxis. *Chest* **103**: 426–32.

Baughman RP, Dohn MN, Frame PT. (1994). The continuing utility of bronchoalveolar lavage to diagnose opportunistic infection in AIDS patients. *Am J Med* **97**: 515–22.

Bennett C, Horner R, Weinstein R et al. (1995). Empirically treated *Pneumocystis carinii* pneumonia in Los Angeles, Chicago and Miami: 1987–1990. *J Infect Dis* **172**: 312–5.

Bindels PJ, Poos RMJ, Jong JT et al. (1991). Trends in mortality among AIDS patients in Amsterdam, 1982–1988. *AIDS* **5**: 853.

Black JR. Feinberg J, Murphy RL et al. (1994). Clindamycin and primaquine therapy for mild-to-moderate episodes of *Pneumocystis carinii* pneumonia in patients with AIDS: AIDS Clinical Trials Group 044. *Clin Infect Dis* **18**: 905–13.

Bonfils-Roberts EA, Nickodem A, Nealon TF. (1990). Retrospective analysis of the efficacy of open lung biopsy in acquired immunodeficiency syndrome. *Ann Thorac Surg* **49**: 115–7.

Bozzette SA, Sattler FR, Chiu J et al. (1990). A controlled trial of early adjunctive treatment with corticosteroids for *Pneumocystis carinii* pneumonia in the acquired immunodeficiency syndrome. *N Engl J Med* **323**: 1451–7.

Bozzette SA, Arcia J, Bartok AE et al. (1992). Impact of *Pneumocystis carinii* and cytomegalovirus on the course and outcome of atypical pneumonia in advanced human immunodeficiency virus disease. *J Infect Dis* **165**: 93–8.

Bozzette SA, Finkelstein DM, Spector SA et al. (1995). A randomized trial of three antipneumocystis agents in patients with advanced human immunodeficiency virus infection. *N Engl J Med* **332**: 693–9.

Buskin SE, Newcomer LM, Koutsky LA et al. (1999). Effect of trimethoprim-sulfamethoxazole as *Pneumocystis carinii* pneumonia prophylaxis on bacterial illness, *Pneumocystis carinii* pneumonia and death in persons with AIDS. *J Acquir Immune Defic Syndr Hum Retrovirol* **20**: 201–6.

Centers for Disease Control and Prevention. (1990). Guidelines for preventing the transmission of tuberculosis in health-care setting, with special focus on HIV-related issues. *MMWR* **39**: RR-17.

Chan C, Montaner J, Lefebvre G et al. (1997). Prophylaxis of *Pneumocystis carinii* pneumonia-comparison of Mepron suspension with aerosolized pentamidine. *IDSA Thirty-Fifth Annual Meeting*, San Francisco, CA, USA.

Chave J, David S, Wauters RA et al. (1989) Transmission of *Pneumocystis carinii* from AIDS patients to other immunosuppressed patients: a claster of *Pneumocystis carinii* pneumonia in renal transplant patients. *AIDS* **5**: 927–32.

Colangelo G, Baughman RP, Dohn MN et al. (1991). Follow-up bronchoalveolar lavage in AIDS patients with *Pneumocystis carinii* pneumonia. *Pneumocystis carinii* burden predicts early relapse. *Am Rev Respir Dis* **143**: 1067–71.

Conte JE, Chernoff D, Feigal DW et al. (1990). Intravenous or inhaled pentamidine for treating *Pneumocystis carinii* pneumonia in AIDS: a randomized trial. *Ann Intern Med* **113**: 203–9.

Dohn MN, Baughman RP, Vigdorth EM et al. (1992). Equal survival for first, second, and third episodes of *Pneumocystis carinii* pneumonia in AIDS patients. *Arch Intern Med* **152**: 2465–70.

Dohn MN, Weinberg WG, Torres RA et al. (1994). Oral atovaquone compared with intravenous pentamidine for *Pneumocystis carinii* pneumonia in patients with AIDS. *Ann Intern Med* **121**: 174–80.

El-Sadr W, Murphy R, Luskin-Hawk R et al. (1997). Atovaquone (ATV) versus dapsone (DAP) in patients intolerant to trimethoprim and/or sulfamethoxazole (TMP/SMX) CPCRA 034/ACTG 277. *IDSA Thirty fifth Annual Meeting*, San Francisco, CA, USA.

Feuerstein IM, Archer A, Pluda JM et al. (1990). Thin-walled cavities, cysts, and pneumothorax in *Pneumocystis carinii* pneumonia: further observations with histopathologic correlation. *Radiology* **174**: 697–702.

Fischl MA, Dickinson GM, La Voie L. (1988). Safety and efficacy of sulfamethoxazole and trimethoprim chemoprophylaxis for *Pneumocystis carinii* pneumonia in AIDS. *JAMA* **259**: 1185–9.

Fischl MA, Parker CB, Pettinelli C et al. (1990). A randomized controlled trial of reduced daily dose of zidovudine in patients with the acquired immunodeficiency syndrome. *N Engl J Med* **323**: 1009–14.

Forrest DM, Djurdjev O, Zala C et al. (1998). Validation of the modified multisystem organ failure score as a predictor of mortality in patients with AIDS-related *Pneumocystis carinii* pneumonia and respiratory failure. *Chest* **114**: 199–206.

Franklin C, Friedman Y, Wong T et al. (1995). Improving prognosis for survivors of mechanical ventilation in patients with PCP and acute respiratory failure. *Arch Intern Med* **155**: 91–5.

Furrer H, Egger M, Opravail M et al. (1999). Discontinuation of primary prophylaxis against *Pneumocystis carinii* pneumonia in HIV-1 infected adults treated with combination antiretroviral therapy. *New Engl J Med* **340**: 1301–6.

Furrer H, Opravil M, Rossi M et al. (2001). Discontinuation of primary prophylaxis in HIV-infected patients at high risk of *Pneumocystis carinii* pneumonia: prospective multicentre study. *AIDS* **15**: 501–7.

Girard PM, Landman R, Gaudebout C et al. (1993). Dapsone-pyrimethamine compared with aerosolized pentamidine as primary prophylaxis against *Pneumocystis carinii* pneumonia and toxoplasmosis in HIV infection. The PRIO Study Group. *N Engl J Med* **328**: 1514–20.

Graham NMH, Zeger SL, Park LB *et al.* (1991). Effect of zidovudine and *Pneumocystis carinii* prophylaxis on progression of HIV-1 infection to AIDS. *Lancet* **338**: 265–9.

Gruden J, Huang L, Turner J *et al.* (1997). High-resolution CT in the evaluation of clinically suspected *Pneumocystis carinii* pneumonia in AIDS patients with normal, equivocal, or non-specific radiographic findings. *Am J Roentgenology* **169**: 967–75.

Hardy WD, Feinberg J, Finkelstein DM *et al.* (1992). A controlled trial of trimethoprim-sulfamethoxazole or aerosolized pentamidine for secondary prophylaxis of *Pneumocystis carinii* pneumonia in patients with the acquired immunodeficiency syndrome: AIDS Clinical Trials Group Protocol 021. *N Engl J Med* **327**: 1842–8.

Huang L, Hecht F, Stansell J *et al.* (1995). Suspected *Pneumocystis carinii* pneumonia with a negative induced sputum examination. Is early bronchoscopy useful? *Am J Resp Crit Care Med* **151**: 1866–71.

Hughes WT. (1998). Use of dapsone in the prevention and treatment of *Pneumocystis carinii* pneumonia; a review. *Clin Infect Dis* **27**: 191–204.

Hughes WT, Leoung G, Kramer F *et al.* (1993). Comparison of atovaquone (566C80) and trimethoprim-sulfamethoxazole for the treatment of *Pneumocystis carinii* pneumonia in patients with the acquired immunodeficiency syndrome (AIDS). *N Engl J Med* **328**: 1521–7.

Hughes WT, LaFon SW, Scott JD *et al.* (1995). Adverse events associated with trimethoprim-sulfamethoxazole and atovaquone during treatment of AIDS-related *Pneumocystis carinii* pneumonia. *J Infect Dis* **171**: 1295–301.

Ioannidis JP, Cappelleri JC, Skolnik PR *et al.* (1996). A meta-analysis of the relative efficay and toxicity of *Pneumocystis carinii* prophylactic regimens. *Arch Intern Med* **156**: 177–88.

Jacobson MA, Child C, Matts JB *et al.* (1992). Toxicity of clindamycin as prophylaxis for AIDS-associated toxoplasmic encephalitis. *Lancet* **339**: 333–4.

Joos B, Blaser J, Opravail M *et al.* (1995). Monitoring of co-trimoxazole concerntrations in serum during treatment of *Pneumocystis carinii* pneumonia. *Antimicrob Agents Chemother* **39**: 2661–6.

Kovacs JA, Ng VL, Masur H *et al.* (1988). Diagnosis of *Pneumocystis carinii* pneumonia: improved detection in sputum with use of monoclonal antibodies. *New Engl J Med* **318**: 589–93.

Kuhlman JE, Kavuru M, Fishman E *et al.* (1990). *Pneumocystis carinii* pneumonia: spectrum of parenchymal CT findings. *Radiology* **175**: 711–4.

Ledergerber B, Mocroft A, Reiss P *et al.* (2001). Discontinuation of secondary prophylaxis against *Pneumocystis carinii* pneumonia in patients with HIV infection who have a response to antiretroviral therapy. Eight European Study Groups. *N Engl J Med* **344**: 168–74.

Lee BL, Medina I, Benowitz NL *et al.* (1989). Dapsone, trimethoprim, and sulfamethoxazole plasma levels during treatment of *Pneumocystis* pneumonia in patients with the acquired immunodeficiency syndrome. *Ann Intern Med* **110**: 606–11.

Lee BL, Delahunty T, Safrin S. (1994). The hydoxylamine of sulfamethoxazole and adverse reactions in patients with acquired immunodeficiency syndrome. *Clin Pharmacol Therapeut* **56**: 184–9.

Lee BS, Safrin S, Makrides V *et al.* (1996). Zidovudine, trimethoprim and dapsone pharmacokinetic interactions in patients with human immunodeficiency virus infection. *Antimicrob Agents Chemother* **40**: 1231–6.

Leoung GS, Feigal DW, Montgomery AB *et al.* (1989). Aerosolized pentamidine prophylaxis following *Pneumocystis carinii* pneumonia in AIDS patients: The San Francisco Community Prophylaxis Trial. *N Engl J Med* **323**: 769.

Lopez Bernaldo de Quiros JC, Miro JM, Pena JM *et al.* (2001). A randomized trial of the discontinuation of primary and secondary prophylaxis against *Pneumocystis carinii* pneumonia after highly active antiretroviral therapy in patients with HIV infection. Grupo de Estudio del SIDA 04/98. *N Engl J Med* **344**: 159–67.

Mantos A, Podzamcer D, Martinez-Lacosa J *et al.* (1995). Steroids do not enhance the risk of developing tuberculosis or other AIDS-related diseases in HIV-infected patients treated for *Pneumocystis carinii* pneumonia. *AIDS* **9**: 1037–41.

Mason GR, Hashimoto CH, Dickman PS *et al.* (1989). Prognostic implications of bronchoalveolar lavage neutrophilia in patients with *Pneumocystis carinii* pneumonia and AIDS. *Am Rev Respir Dis* **139**: 1336–42.

Medina I, Mills J, Leoung G *et al.* (1990). Oral therapy for *Pneumocystis carinii* pneumonia in the acquired immunodeficiency syndrome: a controlled trial of trimethoprim-sulfamethoxazole versus trimethoprim-dapsone. *N Engl J Med* **323**: 776–82.

Meduri GU, Stover DE, Greeno RA *et al.* (1991). Bilateral bronchoalveolar lavage in the diagnosis of opportunistic pulmonary infections. *Chest* **100**: 1272–6.

Metersky ML, Catanzaro A. (1991). Diagnostic approach to *Pneumocystis carinii* pneumonia in the setting of prophylactic aerosolized pentamidine. *Chest* **100**: 1345–9.

Montaner JSG, Lawson LM, Levitt N *et al.* (1990). Corticosteroids prevent early deterioration in patients with moderately severe *Pneumocystis carinii* pneumonia and the acquired immunodeficiency syndrome. *Ann Intern Med* **113**: 14–20.

Montaner JSG, Lawson LM, Gervais A *et al.* (1991). Aerosol pentamidine for secondary prophylaxis of AIDS-related *Pneumocystis carinii* pneumonia. *Ann Intern Med* **114**: 948–53.

Montgomery AB, Feigal DW, Sattler F *et al.* (1995). Pentamidine aerosol versus trimethoprim-sulfamethoxazole for *Pneumocystis carinii* in acquired immune deficiency syndrome. *Am J Respir Crit Care Med* **151**: 1068–74.

National Institutes of Health, University of California expert panel for corticosteroids as adjunctive therapy for *Pneumocystis carinii* pneumonia. (1990). Consensus statement on the use of corticosteriods as adjunctive therapy for *Pneumocystis* pneumonia in the acquired immunodeficiency syndrome. *N Engl J Med* **323**: 1500–04.

Ng V, Yajko D, Hadley WK *et al.* (1993). Update on laboratory tests for the diagnosis of pulmonary disease in HIV-1-infected individuals.

Ng VL, Yajko DM, Hadley WK. (1997). Extrapulmonary pneumocystosis. *Clin Microbiol Rev* **10**: 401–18.

Noskin GA, Murphy RL, Black JR *et al.* (1992). Salvage therapy with clindamycin/primaquine for *Pneumocystis carinii* pneumonia. *Clin Infect Dis* **14**: 183–8.

O'Brien JG, Dong BJ, Coleman RL *et al.* (1997). A 5 year retrospective review of adverse drug reactions and their risk factors in human immunodeficiency virus-infected patients who were receiving intravenous pentamidine therapy for *Pneumocystis carinii* pneumonia. *Clin Infect Dis* **24**: 854–9.

Opravail M, Marincek B, Fuchs W *et al.* (1994). Shortcomings of chest radiography in detecting *Pneumocystis carinii* pneumonia. *J AIDS* **7**: 39–45.

Palella F, Delaney K, Moorman A et al. (1998). Declining morbidity and mortality among patients with advanced human immunodeficiency virus infection. N Engl J Med 338: 853–60.

Pastores SM, Garay SM, Naidier DP et al. (1996). Review: Pneumothorax in patients with AIDS-related Pneumocystis carinii pneumonia. Am J Med Sci 312: 229–34.

Phair J, Munoz A, Detels R et al. (1990). The risk of Pneumocystis carinii pneumonia among men infected with human immunodeficiency virus type 1. N Engl J Med 322: 161–5.

Podzamczer D, Santin M, Jimenez J et al. (1993). Thrice weekly cotrimoxazole is better than weekly dapsone-pyrimethamine for the primary prevention of Pneumocystis carinii pneumonia in HIV-infected patients. AIDS 7: 501.

Raviglione MC. (1990). Extrapulmonary pneumocystosis: the first 50 cases. Rev Infect Dis 12: 1127–38.

Ribes JA, Limper AH, Espy MJ et al. (1997). PCR detection of Pneumocystis carinii in bronchoalveolar lavage specimens; analysis of sensitivity and specificity. J Clin Microbiol 35: 830–5.

Rosenberg DM, McCarthy W, Slavinsky J et al. (2001). Atovaquone suspension for treatment of Pneumocystis carinii pneumonia in HIV-infected patients. AIDS 15: 211–4.

Safrin S, Sattler FR, Lee BL et al. (1991). Dapsone as a single agent in suboptimal therapy for Pneumocystis carinii pneumonia. J Acquir Immune Defic Syndr 4: 244–9.

Safrin S, Lee BL, Sande MA. (1994). Adjunctive folinic acid with trimethoprim-sulfamethoxazole for Pneumocystis carinii pneumonia in AIDS patients is associated with an increased risk of therapeutic failure and death. J Infect Dis 170: 912–17.

Safrin S, Finkelstein DM, Feinberg J et al. (1996). Comparison of three regimens for treatment of mild to moderate Pneumocystis carinii pneumonia in patients with AIDS. Ann Intern Med 124: 792–802.

Sattler FR, Cowan R, Nielsen DM et al. (1988). Trimethoprim-sulfamethoxazole compared with pentamidine for treatment of Pneumocystis carinii pneumonia in the acquired immunodeficiency syndrome: a prospective, non-crossover study. Ann Intern Med 109: 280–7.

Sattler FR, Frame PT, Davis L et al. (1994). Trimetrexate with leucovorin versus trimethoprim-sulfamethoxazole for moderate to severe episodes of Pneumocystis carinii pneumonia in patients with AIDS: a prospective controlled multicenter investigation of the AIDS Clinical Trials Group, Protocol 029/031. J Infect Dis 170: 165–72.

Schurmann D, Bergmann F, Albrecht H et al. (2001). Twice-weekly pyimethamine-sulfadoxine effectively prevents Pneumocystis carinii pneumonia relapse and toxoplasmic encephalitis in patients with AIDS. J Infect Dis 42: 8–15.

Sepkowitz KA, Telzak EE, Gold JWM et al. (1991). Pneumothorax in AIDS. Ann Intern Med 114: 455–9.

Smulian AG, Sullivan DW, Linke MJ et al. (1993). Geographic variation in the humoral response to Pneumocystis carinii. J Infect Dis 167: 1243–7.

Soo Hoo GW, Mohsenifar Z, Meyer RD. (1990). Inhaled or intravenous pentamidine therapy for Pneumocystis carinii pneumonia in AIDS: a randomized trial. Ann Intern Med 113: 195–202.

Stansell J, Osmond D, Charlebois E. (1997). Predictors of Pneumocystis carinii pneumonia in HIV-infected persons. Am J Respir Crit Care Med 155: 60–6.

Stover DA, Greeno RA, Gagliardi AJ. (1989). The use of a simple exercise test for the diagnosis of Pneumocystis carinii pneumonia in patients with AIDS. Am Rev Respir Dis 139: 1343–6.

Telzak EE, Cote RJ, Gold JWM et al. (1990). Extrapulmonary Pneumocystis carinii infections. Rev Infect Dis 12: 380–6.

Travis WD, Pittaluga S, Lipschik GY et al. (1990). Atypical pathologic manifestations of Pneumocystis carinii pneumonia in the acquired immune deficiency syndrome. Review of 123 lung biopsies from 76 patients with emphasis on cysts, vascular invasion, vasculitis, and granulomas. Am J Surg Pathol 14: 615–25.

USPHS/IDSA Prevention of Opportunistic Infections Working Group. (1999). 1999 USPHS/IDSA guidelines for the prevention of opportunistic infections in persons infected with human immunodeficiency virus. MMWR 48: RR-10.

Van Der Ven AJAM, Koopmans PP, Vree TB et al. (1991). Adverse reactions to co-trimoxazole in HIV infection. Lancet 338: 431–3.

Walzer PD. (1991). Pneumocystis carinii – new clinical spectrum? N Engl J Med 324: 263.

Weverling GJ, Mocroft A, Ledergerber B et al. (1999). Discontinuation of Pneumocystis carinii pneumonia prophylaxis after start of highly active antiretroviral therapy in HIV-1 infection. Lancet 353: 1293–8.

Wispelwey B, Pearson RD. (1991). Pentamidine: a review. Infect Control Hosp Epidemiol 12: 375–82.

Yarchoan R, Venzon DJ, Pluda JM et al. (1991). CD4 count and the risk for death in patients infected with HIV receiving antiretroviral therapy. Ann Intern Med 115: 184–9

Zaman MK, White DA (1988). Serum lactate dehydrogenase levels and Pneumocystis carinii pneumonia. Am Rev Respir Dis 137: 796–800.

CHRISTINE KATLAMA

Infection with the parasite *Toxoplasma gondii* is widely distributed (Luft and Remington, 1992). It is commonly asymptomatic in children and young adults but may have potentially severe consequences during pregnancy, with a risk of fetal infection and congenital abnormalities. Immunodeficient individuals are at greater risk of severe infection with toxoplasma. The HIV epidemic has offered a unique opportunity to characterize the interactions between the immune system and infection with opportunistic pathogens such as *Toxoplasma gondii*. Before 1980, toxoplasma encephalitis was generally an autopsy diagnosis in patients with underlying immune deficiency. The AIDS epidemic has led to a marked increase in incidence of this disease. Active toxoplasmosis has been estimated to occur in 20 000–40 000 AIDS patients since the beginning of the 1990s in the USA alone, being the most common cause of encephalitis in the US population (Luft and Remington, 1988). Major advances in the treatment and chemoprophylaxis of toxoplasma infection have occurred between 1985 and 1995, making this infectious complication of HIV infection a preventable disease. Since 1996, the use of highly active antiretroviral therapy (HAART) to prevent the progressive decline in immunity or to partially restore immunity in HIV-infected patients, has modified the spectrum of opportunistic infection such as *Toxoplasma gondii*. However, this is true only for patients in Western countries who can afford the high costs of such antiretroviral therapy.

Epidemiology and pathogenesis

Toxoplasma gondii is an intracellular protozoon. Cats are the definitive hosts and excrete oocysts. Humans are infected through the ingestion of cysts from the faeces of cats or the ingestion of undercooked meat derived from muscles of animals containing *T. gondii* cysts. After acute infection, cysts persist in the central nervous system (CNS) or in extraneural tissues such as skeletal and cardiac muscle. In immunocompetent individuals, infection remains latent, since tachyzoites released by cyst rupture are contained by cellular immune response mechanisms. If the latter are defective, as occurs during HIV infection, reactivation of cysts and dissemination of tachyzoites result in the acute manifestations of toxoplasmosis (Luft and Remington, 1992).

The pathogenesis of *T. gondii* infection in AIDS remains unclear. It has been suggested that disease such as encephalitis, retinitis or pneumonitis results from haematogenous dissemination of parasites, rather than from a local reactivation of previous infection. Corroborating evidence for haematogenous dissemination of toxoplasma, rather than local reactivation of cysts, includes reports of parasitemia in patients with toxoplasma encephalitis (TE), retinitis and disseminated infection (Hofflin and Remington, 1985; Tirard *et al.*, 1991). In addition, the multifocal lesions observed during relapses of TE, in the absence of maintenance therapy, occur in areas of the brain not involved in the initial episode.

Latent toxoplasma infection is more prevalent in Africa and Europe (France, Germany, Switzerland and Spain), where 50–70% of the population have specific antibodies to *T. gondii* (Derouin *et al.*, 1991; Zangerle *et al.*, 1991; Renold *et al.*, 1992), than in the USA, where 10–40% of the adult population is latently infected (Remington and Desmonts, 1990; Zangerle *et al.*). Australia has an intermediate incidence of 30–40%. It has been shown that approximately one-third of HIV-infected patients with latent *T. gondii* infection (i.e. seropositive, asymptomatic patients) will develop toxoplasmosis at some time during the natural course of HIV disease (Grant *et al.*, 1990). The prevalence of TE in patients with AIDS therefore varies from 5 to 10% in areas such as the

USA (Luft and Remington, 1992), Northern Europe and the UK, 10–40% in European countries such as France, Germany, Belgium and Switzerland (J Lundgren, pers. comm.).

Data from two European cohort studies have recently reported the changing history regarding complications of HIV in the era of HAART, showing the falling incidence of opportunistic infections in patients receiving HAART. In the Swiss HIV cohort study, the incidence of new opportunistic infections fell from 22/100 person-years in 1990 to 5/100 person-years in 1997–98, an overall reduction of 86% in rates of opportunistic infections in this period. This decline was observed for all major complications of HIV infection, with the exception of non-Hodgkin's lymphoma (Egger, 1998). In a French study of 1700 HIV-infected patients, the incidence of toxoplasmosis increased from 0.7/100 person-years in 1992, and subsequently decreased to 0.2/100 person-years in 1995. This recent decline was attributed to the use of prophylaxis (Belanger *et al.*, 1999).

It has been suggested that the immune reconstitution that occurs following HAART may take several months to be functional, such that the risk of opportunistic infection may remain high in the weeks following commencement of antiretroviral therapy. In a study of 486 patients commencing HAART, 44% of whom had a CD4 lymphocyte count of less than 50 cells/μl, 50 clinical events were recorded during a mean follow-up of 6.1 months, of which 34 events (68%) were observed within the first 2 months of HAART (Michelet *et al.*, 1998).

Despite these important results in patients who are virologically and immunologically responding to HAART, there remain patients who are untreated or not adequately treated with antiretroviral drugs, even where resources are plentiful. In the Department of Infectious Diseases in Pitié-Salpêtrière Hospital, 141 new AIDS cases were registered between January 1997 and October 1998; 33 patients (23%) had TE as the first AIDS-defining event; in 60% of them the diagnosis of HIV infection was also unmasked (Katlama, unpubl. data).

Clinical presentation

Encephalitis is the most common manifestation of *T. gondii* infection in HIV-infected patients, occurring in up to 40% of patients with advanced HIV infection. Retinitis is less frequent (5–10%), and pneumonitis and myocarditis are uncommon. The timing of development of toxoplasmosis can be predicted since approximately 75% of patients with TE have a CD4 lymphocyte count of less than 100 cells/μl at the time of diagnosis. In 30–50% of the cases, toxoplasmosis is the index AIDS diagnosis (Dannemann *et al.*, 1992; Porter and Sande, 1992; Renold *et al.*, 1992).

Toxoplasma encephalitis

Toxoplasma encephalitis (TE) commonly presents as single or multiple intracerebral abscesses (Haverkos, 1987; Leport *et al.*, 1988). About three-quarters of patients present with focal neurological signs and symptoms, which progress over a few days or weeks. Constitutional symptoms are present in 70% of cases with fever (40–70%) and headaches (50–60%) being the most common. Focal neurological abnormalities include hemiplegia or hemiparesis, hemisensory deficit, aphasia, ataxia, cerebellar signs, cranial nerve palsies, and hemianopia. Other neurological findings include alteration of mental status, with confusion or lethargy (40–55%) and seizures (20–30%).

The constellation of fever, unusual headaches and mild neurological deficit should suggest the diagnosis of TE and prompt urgent computed tomographic (CT) scanning or magnetic resonance (MR) imaging. Delay in diagnosis and institution of therapy may result in rapid progression to a complete neurological deficit. Toxoplasmosis may also present as a diffuse encephalitis (Gray *et al.*, 1989) with fever and coma (10–20% of reported cases) and with diffuse necrosis and oedema on CT scan or MR imaging.

Neurological involvement outside of the brain is uncommon. Toxoplasma abscess of the spinal cord has been reported, as well as cases of transverse myelitis and the conus medullaris syndrome (Mehren *et al.*, 1988; Herskovitz *et al.*, 1989; Kayser *et al.*, 1990).

Retinitis

Retinitis is the second most frequent manifestation of toxoplasma infection and the second most frequent cause of retinitis in AIDS (Holland *et al.*, 1988; Cochereau-Massin *et al.*, 1992). A French retrospective study from January 1990 to September 1992 recorded 202 cases of extraneurological toxoplasma infection, which represents a risk of 1.5–2%. The retina was the most frequent extraneurological site of infection, with 111 cases (55%), and half the patients had associated cerebral involvement (May *et al.*, 1993).

Visual symptoms in toxoplasma retinitis include loss of visual acuity, 'floaters' and red eye. Ophthalmologic examination reveals yellow-white areas of full-thickness necrotizing retinitis, occasionally haemorrhagic with vascular sheathing and little overlying vitreal haze. Lesions are predominantly unilateral. The presence of inflammation in the anterior and/or posterior segment (hyalitis) is highly suggestive of toxoplasmic retinitis and occurs in 60–70% of cases. Fluorescein angiography reveals hyperfluorescence, starting from the periphery and progressing towards the centre of lesions. This distinguishes toxoplasma retinitis from cytomegalovirus (CMV) retinitis ((Holland *et al.*, 1988; Cochereau-Massin *et al.*, 1992). Toxoplasma retinitis should also be differentiated from retinitis due to varicella-zoster virus (VZV), syphilis and fungi and including *Pneumocystis carinii*.

Pneumonitis

In the French national survey, pulmonary manifestations of toxoplasmosis accounted for 35% of extraneurological toxoplasma disease (May *et al.*, 1993). Toxoplasma pneumonitis usually presents as a rapidly progressive interstitial pneumonia (Oksenhendler *et al.*, 1990; Pomeroy and Filice, 1992). Fever and dyspnoea are the most frequent symptoms, whereas cough and sputum may be absent. Chest radiographs usually show diffuse bilateral pulmonary infiltrates; multiple nodular densities have been reported. A rise in lactate dehydrogenase levels has been reported as suggestive of the diagnosis (Pugin *et al.*, 1992). Direct examination of bronchoalveolar lavage reveals *T. gondii* trophozoites (Derouin *et al.*, 1989).

Disseminated toxoplasma infection may manifest itself as acute respiratory distress syndrome (ARDS) associated with septic shock and thrombocytopenia (Lucet *et al.*, 1993). Diagnosis relies on the detection of *T. gondii* in the blood. The mortality rate is approximately 30% in toxoplasma pneumonitis and 50% in disseminated infection (Buhr *et al.*, 1992; Lucet *et al.*, 1993).

Other sites of toxoplasma infection

Toxoplasma infection may also be present in bone marrow, muscle, liver, heart, skin, pancreas, colon, pituitary, adrenal gland and testes (May *et al.*, 1993; Adair *et al.*, 1989; Hirschmann and Chugg, 1988). The diagnosis is made by histological examination of tissue. In these cases, the detection of *T. gondii* in blood should be considered as strong evidence to justify the initiation of treatment.

Diagnosis

Demonstration of the parasite in tissue or in culture provides the definitive diagnosis of toxoplasmosis. The AIDS epidemic and the consequent increase in prevalence of TE has led to a change in clinical practice. Because of the morbidity associated with brain biopsy, the difficulty in performing urgent biopsies or to access certain lesions, and the evidence that toxoplasma is the most frequent opportunistic pathogen in the brain, initiation of presumptive therapy in patients with characteristic findings by CT scan/or MRI is common practice (Cohn *et al.*, 1989). Brain biopsy is performed only after failure of specific antitoxoplasmic therapy.

Serology

Toxoplasma antibodies (IgG) are present in nearly all patients with established toxoplasma infection (Remington and Desmonts, 1990; Luft and Remington, 1992). Thus, the determination of a latent chronic infection with the presence of toxoplasma antibodies of IgG class detected by immunofluorescence assay or ELISA test is important in evaluating the risk of any HIV-infected patient for reactivation of toxoplasma infection. However, antibody titres are of little use in the diagnosis of toxoplasma: only approximately 20% of patients with TE have a significant rise in serial IgG levels, and such a rise is not very specific since it may be present in the absence of clinical toxoplasmosis (Luft and Remington, 1988; Remington and Desmonts, 1990; Luft and Remington, 1992). Furthermore, since disease is usually due to reactivation of a latent infection, IgM antibodies are commonly absent. When cerebrospinal fluid (CSF) is available, measurement of intrathecal production of specific antibodies may aid in the diagnosis of TE.

Other serological tests have been proposed: the measurement of IgG antibody titres to formalin-fixed toxoplasma antigens, Western blot testing, determination of specific IgE antibodies, or IgA by ELISA, agglutination or Western blot (Weiss *et al.*, 1988; Gross *et al.*, 1992; Lebech *et al.*, 1992; Pellax *et al.*, 1992). Results are conflicting and at this stage not sufficiently reliable for diagnosis of TE.

At the time of diagnosis, approximately 3% of patients have no detectable toxoplasma antibodies (Remington and Desmonts, 1990; Luft and Remington, 1992). There are several hypotheses to explain this observation. The serological test may lack the sensitivity to detect low-level antibodies in patients profoundly immunosuppressed.

(Therefore two different tests, including ELISA, are necessary to assess with certainty the absence of antibodies). Progression of HIV disease can result in a decline of antibody levels. Finally, TE may be a clinical manifestation of primary toxoplasma infection, with initially negative serology and a subsequent rise in toxoplasma antibodies during the following weeks.

In summary, determination of toxoplasma antibodies should be performed at least once during the course of HIV disease to evaluate the status of the patient regarding toxoplasma infection and plan the choice of dual *P. carinii*/toxoplasma prophylaxis. In the absence of antibodies, the diagnosis of toxoplasma infection is unlikely and prevention measures should be recommended.

Isolation of toxoplasma

The isolation of toxoplasma from body fluids or in tissue specimens indicates active infection. Because isolation of the organism from mouse inoculation takes several weeks, more practical techniques using inoculation of the fluid into tissue cultures of fibroblasts and detection by immunofluorescence have been developed. Parasitaemia has been reported in patients with cerebral toxoplasmosis. Isolation of *T. gondii* from bronchoalveolar fluid appears to be a sensitive test for pulmonary toxoplasmosis. Although results of laboratory investigations are often not available for the initial management of a patient with TE, the presence of circulating tachyzoites in blood is confirmatory evidence of toxoplasma dissemination.

Detection of toxoplasma in cerebrospinal fluid by polymerase chain reaction (PCR) has been investigated (Lebech *et al.*, 1992; Parmley *et al.*, 1992). This technique could be of use in clinical situations where diagnosis is difficult (e.g. the HIV-uninfected patient with primary infection).

Neuroradiology

Central nervous system imaging is of major importance for diagnosis and management of patients with neurological disorders. Every patient with signs or symptoms suggesting a CNS disorder or with unexplained fever and/or unusual headaches should be investigated with a brain CT or MRI scan. Lesions of TE are typically multiple, ring-enhancing and surrounded by oedema; a mass effect may be present, with displacement of ventricles in association with large lesions. MRI scans are more sensitive than CT scans and usually reveal multiple lesions. Because of its greater sensitivity (Porter and Sande, 1992), MRI scan is recommended as the initial investigation of patients with mild neurological symptoms or patients with non-specific symptoms. Furthermore, MRI scanning appears to be more sensitive in detecting lesions localized to the posterior fossa or near the cranial vault and is better at indicating the precise topography of lesions, which may help to distinguish toxoplasma lesions from lymphoma (Levy *et al.*, 1990). In addition, MRI scanning may reveal haemorrhages which are highly suggestive of toxoplasmic necrosis.

TE is most commonly located in the basal ganglia, frontal and parietal regions and at the cortico-medullary junction. However, lesions have been demonstrated in almost any site within the brain, including the cerebellum, the occipital region, and the thalamus. The mean size of lesions is 1–3 cm in diameter. Although no CT scan or MRI findings can be considered pathognomonic for TE, some neuroradiological findings, such as the presence of multiple contrast enhancing lesions, localization in basal ganglia and/or at the cortico-medullary junction and the presence of oedema and/or mass effect may help to distinguish TE from CNS lymphoma (Dina, 1991). Findings on CT scan or MRI scan consistent with TE should lead to the initiation of presumptive specific therapy. Changes on CT or MRI scans, together with clinical response, are used to evaluate the efficacy of therapy, and thus to confirm the diagnosis of TE. The size of lesions on CT or MRI scans typically diminish after 7–15 days of therapy. In a large, multicentre European study of 299 patients, complete resolution of lesions was achieved in 30% of the cases after completion of 6 weeks of therapy. Radiological sequelae (small hyperdensities) were persistent in 50% of the patients, despite complete clinical response (Katlama *et al.*, 1996a). Failure of therapy should be considered when there is an increase in size or number of lesions, appearance of new lesions or stability of size of initial lesions. When initial lesions are atypical or when the clinical situation is more suggestive of lymphoma (negative toxoplasma serology, compliance with effective primary prophylaxis), CT scan or MRI should be performed within 10 days of initiation of therapy for TE. This will enable the early performance of brain biopsy in cases of clinical and radiological failure of therapy.

Brain biopsy

Although the definitive diagnosis relies classically on the demonstration of *T. gondii* in brain tissue, there is now a consensus among physicians to perform a brain biopsy only as a second-line diagnostic procedure, after failure of 10–15 days of toxoplasma therapy.

Treatment

Acute therapy

Treatment is a major issue in the clinical management of toxoplasmosis, since response to therapy is the main criterion for TE diagnosis in the absence of specific laboratory biological diagnostic parameters. In addition, early treatment before the onset of major neurological dysfunction is associated with an improved prognosis. Treatment is usually divided into two stages; initial therapy, consisting of 4–6 weeks of maximal doses of the drugs used, followed by suppressive therapy (secondary prophylaxis) in which lower doses of drugs are used (Table 26.1).

Sulfadiazine-pyrimethamine combination

The combination of pyrimethamine (50–75 mg/day) and sulfadiazine (4–6 g/day) is the standard therapy for acute toxoplasmosis (Luft and Remington, 1988; Cohn *et al.*, 1989; Luft and Remington, 1992).

These drugs act synergistically by blocking the folic acid pathway of tachyzoites, but they have no effect on the cyst forms of the parasite. Dannemann and colleagues (1992) reported a 70% clinical response rate in 33 patients treated with 75 mg/day of pyrimethamine and 100 mg/per kg (up to 8 g/day) of sulfadiazine. In a European multicentre study, the clinical response rate was 76% in 147 patients receiving a combination of 50 mg/day of pyrimethamine and 4 g/day of sulfadiazine (P/S) for presumptive TE. Only three patients with proven TE failed to respond to P/S (Katlama *et al.*, 1996b).

The major limitation of this effective therapy is the high rate of side-effects (60%), leading to discontinuation of therapy in approximately 30% of patients. Fever and rash are the most frequent adverse events (20–25% of cases) (Renold *et al.*, 1992; Dannemann *et al.*, 1992; Porter and Sande, 1992; Katlama *et al.*, 1996b). Mild rash should not preclude the use of sulfadiazine because the rash may disappear spontaneously with continued therapy. Nevertheless, sulfadiazine should be avoided in patients with a previous history of severe cutaneous intolerance to sulphonamides. Haematological toxicity has been reported in up to 68% of cases (Dannemann *et al.*, 1992; Porter and Sande, 1992). In our experience, bone marrow toxicity occurs in 30% of cases but rarely leads to discontinuation of therapy (3% of cases). Although the optimal dosage of folinic acid to prevent haematological toxicity is unknown, a 20–25 mg/day dosage is recommended by the author. Good hydration, with alkalinization of urine is necessary to prevent crystalluria induced by sulfadiazine.

Clinical improvement occurs within 5–10 days. Neuroimaging is performed after 10–15 days of treatment. The diagnosis of TE is confirmed by a decrease in both clinical and radiological abnormalities after institution of presumptive therapy. Therapy is required for a minimum of 3 weeks in patients with an early complete clinical and radiological response and should be maintained for 6 weeks in patients with a slower initial response to therapy.

Concomitant therapies

Glucocorticoids may be used in patients with symptoms of raised intracranial pressure or moderately severe intracranial hypertension with displacement of median brain structures, although data supporting their use in this context are virtually non-existent. Patients with seizures at presentation should receive anticonvulsant therapy during the acute phase of antitoxoplasma therapy. Phenobarbital, phenytoin sodium, or diphenylhydantoin are not recommended because of potential drug interactions. Sodium valproate is preferred.

Pyrimethamine/clindamycin

Clindamycin has been investigated as an alternative therapy to sulphadiazine. Both *in vitro* and animal

Table 26.1 Treatment of toxoplasma encephalitis

Induction therapy (4–6 weeks)	
First line	
Sulphadiazine	2 g × 2/day
or	
Clindamycin	2.4 g/day
plus	
Pyrimethamine	100–200 mg loading dose, followed by 50–75 mg/day
Folinic acid	25 mg/day
Alternatives to sulphadiazine or clindamycin	
Azithromycin	1–1.5 g/day
Atovaquone	3 g/day (750 mg/day)
Dapsone	50–100 mg/day
Clarithromycin	2 g/day

models have suggested efficacy of clindamycin for the treatment of TE (Rolston and Hoy, 1987; Leport et al., 1989; Hofflin & Remington, 1997). It is well-absorbed with peak serum levels within 1–2 h, it achieves excellent tissue concentrations and it can be administered both orally and intravenously. In a retrospective study, the pyrimethamine-clindamycin (P/C) combination has been reported to be less toxic than the P/S combination (Renold et al., 1992).

Two prospective, controlled open studies that enrolled a total of nearly 400 patients (71 patients in the US study and 299 in the European [ENTA] study) have compared the combination of pyrimethamine-clindamycin (P/C) to the standard P/S therapy (P/S) (Porter and Sande, 1992; Katlama et al., 1996b). The dosage of clindamycin ranged from 2.4 g of oral clindamycin (Katlama et al., 1996b) to 4.8 g/day of intravenous administration in US studies (Porter and Sande, 1992). Efficacy rates based on an intent-to-treat analysis were similar: 65% and 68%, respectively in the USA (Porter and Sande, 1992) and the ENTA studies (Katlama et al., 1996b) and they were not statistically different from those of P/S. However, in the ENTA study, the number of patients who discontinued therapy because of lack of efficacy was higher in P/C-treated patients (13%) compared to those receiving P/S (0.3%). Toxicity of the P/C combination was unexpectedly high, similar to that of P/S (60–70% of cases): rash was present in 30% of the cases but less severe than the P/S combination, leading to discontinuation of therapy in 11% of the patients. Diarrhoea occurred more frequently with P/C (20% of cases) than with P/S. Because of the potential lethal risk, pseudomembranous colitis should be suspected and confirmed or ruled out by endoscopic examination, particularly in patients with pre-existing diarrhoea. *Clostridium difficile* toxin must be sought in the stool.

Given its efficacy (slightly less than P/S) and its less severe toxicity, P/C is a useful second-line therapy in acute therapy for *T. gondii* infection.

Atovaquone

Hydroxynapthoquinones are potent *in vitro* inhibitors of parasitic protozoa, including plasmodium and *T. gondii*. Atovaquone has been demonstrated to have a good protective activity against acute murine toxoplasmosis and appears to reduce the viability and the number of cysts in brains of chronically infected mice (Araujo et al., 1991). Atovaquone acts as an inhibitor of the mitochondrial electron transport chain of parasitic protozoa, resulting in inhibition of pyrimidine synthesis.

Several properties of atovaquone are attractive, particularly in patients with advanced HIV infection: a mechanism of action unrelated to folate antagonism activity against the two most frequent opportunistic agents (e.g. *P. carinii* and *T. gondii*); and a prolonged half-life (4–6 days) with a potential dosing advantage for long-term prophylaxis.

A phase I dose-ranging study of atovaquone in HIV-infected patients showed that highest plasma concentrations were achieved in patients receiving 750 mg three times a day. The plasma half-life of 51 h and absorption of atovaquone was enhanced by food. The most significant adverse event was a maculopapular rash with spontaneous resolution (Hughes et al., 1991). There have been few clinical studies to evaluate atovaquone in humans (Kovacs, 1992; Torres et al., 1997).

On a pilot study using atovaquone (750 mg sachets given four times daily) as a single therapy in patients with a first episode of TE and no previous treatment (Katlama et al., 1996a), 16 of the 24 evaluable patients (66%) responded to therapy; three remained clinically and radiologically stable and were dropped from the study after a mean period of 28 days; four patients failed to respond to therapy (all seven non-responders improved on P/S therapy). The mean plasma level of atovaquone after 2 weeks of therapy was 16–17 μg/ml (ranging from 4.5–34.9 μg/ml). The main side-effects were a slight increase in liver enzymes in 13 patients, cutaneous rash in six, and gastrointestinal disturbances in three. Only one patient had to stop therapy because of liver toxicity.

Atovaquone has been evaluated as salvage therapy in 93 patients with AIDS-related TE who were intolerant to or failing standard therapy with either P/S or P C (Torres et al., 1997). At the end of the 6-week acute therapy phase (750 mg four times a day), clinical improvement was noted in 52% of patients and radiological improvement noted in 37% of patients. Median survival for all patients was 189 days (Kaplan-Meier estimate). A *post-hoc* analysis revealed a correlation between clinical and radiological responses and median atovaquone plasma concentrations. These patients with higher plasma atovaquone concentrations were more likely to experience resolution of TE and to survive. Survival time among patients with high or medium median steady-state plasma concentrations (319 and 289 days, respectively) was significantly greater than among those with low median plasma concentration (114 days; $p = 0.003$ and $p = 0.006$, respectively) (Torres *et al.*, 1997).

Although some studies have suggested a clinical efficacy of atovaquone in acute TE therapy, there have been insufficient data to recommend atovaquone as first-line treatment for TE. Therefore, atovaquone should only be considered as salvage therapy in patients intolerant of standard regimens with pyrimethamine combined with sulfadiazine or clindamycin.

Macrolides

Macrolides at high concentrations are inhibitory for *T. gondii* tachyzoites *in vitro*. Clarithromycin and azithromycin have shown improved pharmacokinetic profiles with excellent bioavailability and higher and persistent serum and intracellular tissue concentrations, compared to earlier drugs of the same class.

Clarithromycin has shown activity against *T. gondii* both *in vitro* and in murine models. In a pilot study clarithromycin (2 g/day) combined with pyrimethamine (75 mg/day) was given to 13 AIDS patients with TE (Fernandez-Martin *et al.*, 1991). Complete clinical response was noted in six of eight evaluable patients and partial response in two patients. Five patients were withdrawn prematurely, mainly for toxicity. Major adverse events included significant liver toxicity in three (24%), haematological toxicity in four (31%), hearing loss in two (15%); nausea or vomiting and rash were also noted in two patients. Whether clarithromycin itself had a beneficial effect is questionable, since it was used in combination with higher doses of pyrimethamine than normally used in combination with sulfadiazine or clindamycin.

Azithromycin has been reported to be active both *in vitro* and in animal models. In a murine model of toxoplasmosis, prophylactic azithromycin administered alone at a high dosage was found to be only partly effective. Complete protection was not seen even at a dosage of 300 mg/kg day (Araujo *et al.*, 1988). In contrast, the combination of azithromycin with either sulfadiazine or pyrimethamine was synergistic, 100% and 93% survival respectively after 30 days. These findings are consistent with preliminary data in humans (Derouin *et al.*, 1992). Monotherapy at a dosage of 1200 mg/day, azithromycin was ineffective in two patients who developed progression of TE after 2 weeks of therapy (Kovacs *et al.*, 1992), whereas azithromycin (300 mg/day) in combination with 75 mg of pyrimethamine given to

10 patients (Saba *et al.*, 1993), led to a good clinical response after 4 weeks in five of eight evaluable patients (62%), and a partial response in one. Adverse events were observed in 60% of cases (leading to discontinuation of therapy in 50% of them) and consisted mainly of fever, rash and an increase in liver enzymes. In the absence of large, controlled studies comparing combination therapy with macrolides with standard therapy, macrolides should only be used in patients who do not respond to or are intolerant of conventional therapy with P/S, P/C or atovaquone.

Tetracyclines

Despite its activity in a murine model of toxoplasmosis, there are no data on the efficacy of minocycline in human acute toxoplasmosis (Chang *et al.*, 1991).

Maintenance (2° prophylaxis) therapy

The spontaneous rate of relapse of TE is high (50–80% of cases), due to the absence of effective antitoxoplasma agents on *T. gondii* cysts and to the progression of the underlying immune suppression in the absence of potent antiretroviral therapy. Thus, long-term suppressive therapy is necessary.

The ENTA study (Katlama *et al.*, 1996b) compared maintenance therapy comprising 25 mg of daily pyrimethamine with either 2 g of sulfadiazine daily or 1.2 g of oral clindamycin daily in 175 patients, with a mean follow-up of 13 months. The P/S combination appeared to be significantly more effective than the P/C combination, with a relapse rate of 7% and 28%, respectively. Toxicity of these two combinations was lower than in acute therapy, being 28% in the P/S treated patients and 20% in the P/C treated patients. Rash and fever were more frequent (12%) among P/S treated patients and diarrhoea more frequent (14%) in those receiving P/C. Of interest, haematological toxicity with both combinations was uncommon (< 5%). Other retrospective studies had found a lower efficacy of P/C combination than for maintenance therapy (Remington and Desmonts, 1990; Leport *et al.*, 1991; Porter and Sande, 1992).

Besides being the most effective antitoxoplasmic maintenance therapy, P/S is also effective as primary prophylaxis against PCP (Heald *et al.*, 1991). Intermittent maintenance therapy with twice weekly administration of pyrimethamine 50 mg and 4 g of sulfadiazine was shown to be effective in preventing relapses in all 15 patients treated over an

11-month period, whereas intermittent administration with twice weekly P/C was associated with a 40% relapse rate (Pedrol et al., 1990). Because of higher efficacy as suppressive therapy in patients with a prior diagnosis of TE with concomitant efficacy as primary prophylaxis against PCP, P/S is recommended as first-line maintenance therapy. Since toxicity appears partly dose-related, mild or moderate adverse reactions observed with high dosage of pyrimethamine or sulfonamides during acute therapy should not definitively preclude the use of this combination therapy. In a small retrospective study, it was suggested that pyrimethamine alone (50–100 mg/day) could also be effective in preventing TE relapse (De Gans et al., 1992). However, monotherapy is almost never used for this disease.

In 1998, with the common use of HAART in developed countries, the issue of discontinuing the maintenance of antitoxoplasma therapy in patients in whom CD4 lymphocytes have increased following the institution of HAART has been raised (Autran et al., 1997; Li et al., 1998). There is no formal recommendation in the absence of available data from prospective comparative studies. However, there are strong arguments to suggest that immune restoration resulting in an increase in CD4 lymphocytes above 200 cells/µl is effective in preventing breakthrough of toxoplasmosis in patients with a prior history of infection.

Primary prophylaxis

In the 1990s, the high incidence, morbidity and mortality of toxoplasmosis during HIV infection has justified the evaluation of primary prophylaxis in high-risk patients with a CD4 lymphocyte count below 200 cells/µl and positive toxoplasma (IgG) serology. The use of antimicrobial agents dually active against P. carinii and T. gondii has been a priority in order to enhance acceptance and compliance of such therapy (Table 26.2).

Table 26.2 Primary prophylaxis against toxoplasmosis[a]

First line	
Trimethoprim-sulphamethoxazole (TMP-SMX)	80–400 mg/day 200–800 mg/day
Alternative	
Dapsone	50 mg/day plus
Pyrimethamine	50–100 mg/day

[a]Also effective as prophylaxis against *Pneumocystis carinii* pneumonia.

Trimethoprim–sulfamethoxazole (TMP-SMX)

Although there has been no large, prospective, controlled study, based on available data there has been a consensus among physicians to accept TMP-SMX as effective prophylaxis against *T. gondii* disease.

In a retrospective analysis, Carr and colleagues first reported the effectiveness of a dose of TMP (160 mg) combined with SMX (800 mg) administered as one tablet twice daily, 2 days a week, as primary prophylaxis against toxoplasmosis. In 60 patients receiving TMP-SMX no cases of TE were compared to 12 cases in 95 patients (33%) receiving aerosolized pentamidine as secondary prophylaxis for PCP (Carr et al., 1992). Data from the ACTG 021 trial comparing TMP-SMX (one double-strength tablet daily) to aerosolized pentamidine as secondary prophylaxis against PCP are consistent with these findings, since of the 10 cases of TE observed in 310 patients, only one occurred in a patient receiving TMP-SMX (Hardy et al., 1992).

Prospective studies, although limited in terms of the number of patients studied, have confirmed the efficacy of TMP-SMX as dual PCP/toxoplasma prophylaxis (Girard et al., 1993; May et al., 1994). The minimal effective dosage is unknown. Regimens with TMP (160 mg) and SMX (800 mg) administered either once daily or every other day are commonly used. The reported toxicity of TMP-SMX in primary prophylaxis is highly variable among the different studies, mostly dependent on the selection criteria for enrolment in the trials. Adverse reactions leading to discontinuation of therapy are reported to be 5–29%. Dose-related toxicity is suggested, with a later occurrence of adverse reactions associated with lower dosage compared to higher dosage (Schneider et al., 1992).

At present, physicians should take into account the advantages of TMP-SMX, which has a high efficacy as dual PCP and *T. gondii* prevention, a reduction in the risk of bacterial infection and a lower cost compared to aerosolized pentamidine.

Dapsone/pyrimethamine

A multicentre randomized trial (Opravil et al., 1995) designed to compare 200 mg of dapsone and 75 mg of pyrimethamine weekly versus aerosolized pentamidine as primary prophylaxis against PCP and TE was interrupted when an interim analysis showed a significant protective effect of dapsone–pyrimethamine against toxoplasmosis: 29 cases of toxoplasmosis occurred in 176 patients receiving aerosolized pentamidine, compared with 15 cases in 173 patients with dapsone–pyrimethamine ($p = 0.016$). Furthermore, seven of the 15 toxoplasmosis cases occurred after discontinuation of dapsone–pyrimethamine therapy.

As expected with this class of compounds, side-effects were more frequent with dapsone–pyrimethamine than with aerosolized pentamidine. Discontinuation of prophylaxis due to side-effects occurred in 40 of 173 patients in the dapsone–pyrimethamine group compared to three of 173 in the aerosolized pentamidine group ($p < 0.001$).

In the multicentre Swiss study, a weekly regimen of 200 mg of dapsone plus 75 mg pyrimethamine showed similar results (Mallolas *et al.*, 1993). Lower doses of dapsone (100 mg/week) and pyrimethamine 25 mg/week had no antitoxoplasma effect (Salmon *et al.*, 1995). However, the tolerance of the pyrimethamine-dapsone combination offers no superiority compared to T/S, with approximately 25% of patients discontinuing the treatment due to toxicity. Main side-effects are rash, gastrointestinal intolerance and haematotological toxicity and occur mostly within 3 months of commencing therapy.

The weekly administration of high dosage of dapsone (200 mg) and pyrimethamine (75 mg) could be responsible for the higher rate of side-effects compared to daily administration of lower dosages (Mallolas *et al.*, 1993).

Dapsone

Dapsone used as monotherapy is poorly effective as prophylaxis against TE. In one prospective study, dapsone was associated with an excess mortality rate compared with aerosolized pentamidine, for reasons that are unclear. Furthermore, there was no significant difference between the two arms regarding antitoxoplasma efficacy (Leport *et al.*, 1996).

Dapsone-trimethoprim

A dapsone-trimethoprim combination is effective as PCP prophylaxis, and, based on *in vitro* and animal model data, should be effective for toxoplasmosis. Thus this regimen is a potential alternative for patients intolerant to T/S. No clinical data are available.

Pyrimethamine

The suggested efficacy of pyrimethamine alone in secondary TE prophylaxis has led to its evaluation in primary toxoplasmosis prophylaxis. A placebo-controlled study of 50 mg of pyrimethamine given three times a week showed

that there was no difference in the rate of occurrence of TE between the two groups in an intent-to-treat analysis. However, in the treatment analysis the incidence of TE was lower in the pyrimethamine group (4%) compared to placebo group (12%; $p = 0.006$) (Leport *et al.*, 1996). Interestingly, this study showed that patients with rash were at higher risk of developing TE (3.7 times higher risk) than those who did not experience rash, and thus dose monitoring is required (Rousseau *et al.*, 1997). Another study in the USA (CPCRA) was prematurely terminated because of an excess mortality rate in patients receiving 25 mg pyrimethamine twice weekly (Jacobson *et al.*, 1994).

Clindamycin

Due to high levels of toxicity, with rash (31%) and diarrhoea (21%), evaluation of clindamycin has been terminated in a double-blinded trial comparing clindamycin–pyrimethamine and placebo (Jacobson *et al.*, 1992).

Other antitoxoplasmic agents

Agents such as atovaquone or macrolides have not been investigated as long-term primary prophylaxis.

Summary of primary and secondary prophylaxis

The objective of prophylactic strategies is to provide long-term protection for HIV-infected patients against the two most frequent opportunistic infections, PCP and TE, with drugs that have low toxicity and at the best cost–benefit ratio.

TMP-SMX offers first-line prophylaxis against both PCP and TE and offers an excellent convenience/cost/efficacy rate. This regimen improves projected life expectancy, quality-adjusted life expectancy, reduces total lifetime medical costs and is cost-effective. In developing countries, where other infections due to *Salmonella* sp. or *Isospora belli* are prevalent, TMP-SMX has the advantage that it is also active against these pathogens.

In patients with minor/moderate toxicity resulting from TMP-SMX, dapsone plus pyrimethamine has been proposed as an alternative prophylactic regimen, since it is estimated that approximately 50% of patients intolerant to TMP-SMX can tolerate this combination. Desensitization to sulfonamides has been controversial. In the case of severe intolerance, only experimental or empirical prophylactic therapies are available, such as pyrimethamine with aerosolized pentamidine, macrolide or atovaquone.

The widespread use of potent combination antiretroviral therapy has raised the issue of the safety of discontinuation of prophylactic therapy against opportunistic pathogens in patients who experience an increase in their CD4 lymphocytes above 200 cells/μl. Although there is no official public health recommendation in the absence of a large, randomized, controlled study, physicians have started discontinuing PCP prophylaxis over the past year. The largest prospective study has been conducted by the Swiss HIV cohort study of 230 patients, of whom 196 were available for analysis; in 153 patients who discontinued a TPM-SMX prophylaxis regimen, no breakthrough of PCP or toxoplasmosis was observed over a median follow-up of 7 months (Furrer et al., 1999, 2000; Scheider et al., 1999). Athough these data are preliminary and larger cohort studies with a longer follow-up are necessary to firmly assess this issue, it seems reasonable to consider that immune restoration following HAART will be able to prevent initial episodes or relapse of opportunistic diseases such as toxoplasmosis. However, it is suggested that prophylaxis should not be discontinued during the first 2 months of HAART, despite significant reductions of viral load and increases in CD4 lymphocyte counts (Michelet et al., 1998).

In conclusion, toxoplasmosis remains a common opportunistic infection in patients with previously undiagnosed or untreated AIDS. It is a treatable and preventable disease, and early therapy is critical to obtain the best prognosis without sequelae.

References

Adair OV, Randive N, Krasnow N et al. (1989). Isolated toxoplasma myocarditis in acquired immune deficiency syndrome. Am Heart J 4: 856–7.

Araujo FG, Guptill DR, Remington JS. (1988). Azithromycin, a macrolide antibiotic with potent activity against Toxoplasma gondii. Antimicrob Agents Chemother 32: 755–7.

Araujo FG, Huskinson J, Remington JS. (1991). Remarkable in vitro and in vivo activities of the hydroxynaphthoquinone 566C80 against tachyzoites and tissue cysts of Toxoplasma gondii. Antimicrob Agents Chemother 35: 293–9.

Autran G, Carcelain T, Li S et al. (1997). Positive effects of combined antiretroviral therapy in advanced HIV disease. Science 277: 112–16.

Belanger F, Derouin F, Grangeot-Keros L et al. (1999). Incidence and risk factors of toxoplasmosis in a cohort of human immunodeficiency virus-infected patients; 1988–1995, HEMOCO and SEROCO Study Groups. Clin Infect Dis 28: 575–81.

Buhr M, Heise W, Aarsteh K et al. (1992). Disseminated toxoplasmosis with sepsis in AIDS. Clin Invest 70: 1079–81.

Carr A, Tindall B, Brew BJ et al. (1992). Low-dose trimethroprim-sulfamethoxazole prophylaxis for toxoplasmic encephalitis in patients with AIDS. Ann Intern Med 117: 106–11.

Chang HR, Comte R, Piguet PF et al. (1991). Activity of minocycline against Toxoplasma gondii infection in mice. J Antimicrob Chemother 27: 639–45.

Cochereau-Massin I, LeHoang P, Lautier-Frau M et al. (1992). Ocular toxoplasmosis in human immunodeficiency virus-infected patients. Am J Ophthalmol 114: 130–5.

Cohn J, McMeeking A, Cohen W et al. (1989). Evaluation of the policy of empiric treatment of suspected toxoplasma encephalitis in patients with the acquired immunodeficiency syndrome. Am J Med 86: 521–7.

Dannemann B, McCutchan JA, Israelski D et al. (1992). Treatment of toxoplasmic encephalitis in patients with AIDS: a randomized trial comparing pyrimethamine plus clindamycin to pyrimethamine plus sulfadiazine. Ann Intern Med 116: 33–43.

De Gans J, Portegies P, Rems P et al. (1992). Pyrimethamine alone in maintenance therapy for central neurosystem toxoplasmosis in 38 patients with AIDS. J Acquir Immune Defic Syndr 5: 137–42.

Derouin F, Sarfati CI, Beauvais B et al. (1989). Laboratory diagnosis of pulmonary toxoplasmosis in patients with acquired immunodeficiency syndrome. J Clin Microbiol 7: 1661–3.

Derouin F, Thuilliez P, Garin YJF. (1991). Value and limitations of toxoplasmosis serology in HIV patients. Pathol Biol 39: 255–9.

Derouin F, Almadany R, Chau F et al. (1992). Synergistic activity of azithromycin and pyrimethamine or sulfadiazine in acute experimental toxoplasmosis. Antimicrob Agents Chemother 36: 997–1001.

Dina TS. (1991). Primary central nervous system lymphoma versus toxoplasmosis in AIDS. Radiology 179: 823–8.

Egger M. (1998). Opportunistic infections in the era of HAART. Twelfth World AIDS Conference, Geneva, Switzerland.

Fernandez-Martin J, Leport C, Morlat P et al. (1991). Pyrimethamine-clarithromycin combination for therapy of acute toxoplasma encephalitis in patients with AIDS. Antimicrob Agents Chemother 10: 2049–52.

Furrer H, Egger M, Opravil M et al. (1999). Discontinuation of primary prophylaxis aginst Pneumocystis carinii pneumonia in HIV-infected adults heated with combination antiretroviral therapy. Swiss HIV Cohort Study. N Engl J Med 340: 1 301–6.

Furrer H, Opravil M, Bernasconi E et al. (2000). Stopping primary prophylaxis in HIV-1 infected patients at high risk of toxoplasma encephalitis: Swiss HIV Cohort Study. Lancet 355: 2217–18.

Girard PM, Landman R, Gaudebout C et al. (1993). Dapsone pyrimethamine compared with aerosolized pentamidine as primary prophylaxis against Pneumocystis carinii pneumonia and toxoplasmosis in HIV infection. N Engl J Med 328: 1514–20.

Grant IH, Gold JWM, Rosenblum M et al. (1990). Toxoplasma gondii serology in HIV-infected patients: the development of central nervous system toxoplasmosis in AIDS. AIDS 4: 519–21.

Gray F, Gherard R, Wingate E et al. (1989). Diffuse 'encephalitic' cerebral toxoplasmosis in AIDS. Report of four cases. J Neurol 236: 273–4.

Gross U, Roos T, Appoldt D et al. (1992). Improved serological diagnosis of Toxoplasma gondii infection by detention of immunoglobulin A (IgA) and IgM antibodies against P30 by using the immunoblot technique. J Clin Microbiol 30:1436–41.

Hardy WD, Feinberg J, Finkelstein D et al. (1992). A controlled trial of Trimethoprim-sulfamethoxazole or aerosolized pentamidine for secondary prophylaxis of Pneumocystis carinii pneumonia in patients with the acquired immunodeficiency syndrome – AIDS Clinical Trials Group Protocol 021. N Engl J Med 327: 1842–8.

Haverkos HW. (1987). Assessment of therapy for toxoplasma encephalitis. The TE Study Group. Am J Med 82: 907–14.

Heald A, Flepp M, Chave JP et al. (1991). Treatment for cerebral toxoplasmosis protects against *Pneumocytis carinii* pneumonia in patients with AIDS. *Ann Intern Med* **115**: 760–3.

Herskovitz S, Siegel SE, Schneider AT et al. (1989). Spinal cord toxoplasmosis in AIDS. *Neurology* **39**: 1552–3.

Hirschmann JV, Chugg AC. (1988). Skin lesions with disseminated toxoplasmosis in a patient with the acquired immunodeficiency syndrome. *Arch Dermatol* **124**: 1146–7.

Hofflin JM, Remington JS. (1985). Tissue culture isolation from blood of a patient with AIDS. *Arch Intern Med* **145**: 925–6.

Hofflin J, Remington JS. (1997). Effect of clindamycin on acute and chronic toxoplasmosis in mice. *Antimicrob Agents Chemother* **31**: 492–6.

Holland GN, Engstrom RE, Glasgow BJ et al. (1988). Ocular toxoplasmosis in patients with the acquired immunodeficiency syndrome. *Am J Ophthalmol* **106**: 653–67.

Hughes WT, Kennedy W, Shenep J et al. (1991). Safety and pharmacokinetics of 566C80, a hydroxynaphtoquinone with anti *Pneumocystis carinii* activity: a phase I study in HIV-infected men. *J Infect Dis* **163**: 843–8.

Jacobson MA, Besch CL, Child C et al. (1992). Toxicity of clindamycin as prophylaxis for AIDS-associated toxoplasmic encephalitis. *Lancet* **339**: 333–4.

Jacobson MA, Besch CL, Child C et al. (1994). Primary prophylaxis with pyrimethamine for toxoplasmic encephalitis in patients with advanced human immunodeficiency virus disease: results of a randomized trial. Terry Beirn Community. Programs for Clinical Research on AIDS. *J Infect Dis* **169**: 384–94.

Jouan M, Saves M, Tubiana R et al. (1999). A prospective multicentre study to evaluate the discontinuation of maintenance therapy MT for CMV retinitis (CMVR) in HIV-patients receiving HAART. *Sixth Conference on Retroviruses and Opportunistic Infections*, Chicago, IL USA.

Katlama C, Mouthon B, Gourdon D et al. (1996a). Atovaquone as long-term suppressive therapy for toxoplasmic encephalitis in patients with AIDS and multiple drug intolerance – *AIDS* **10**: 1107–12.

Katlama C, De Wit S, Guichard A et al. (1996b). ENTA Study Group: pyrimethamine-clindamycin vs pyrimethamine-sulfadiazine as acute and long-term therapy for toxoplasmic encephalitis in patients with AIDS. *Clin Infect Dis* **22**: 268–75.

Kayser C, Campbell R, Sartoriuous C et al. (1990). Toxoplasmosis of the conus medullaris in a patient with hemophilia A-associated AIDS. *J Neurosurg* **73**: 951–3.

Kovacs JA. (1992). Efficacy of atovaquone in treatment of toxoplasmosis in patients with AIDS. *Lancet* **340**: 637–8.

Kovacs JA, Polis MA, Baird B et al. (1992). Evaluation of azithromycin or the combination of 566C80 and pyrimethamine in the treatment of toxoplasmosis. *Eighth International Conference on AIDS*, Amsterdam, The Netherlands.

Lebech M, Lebech AM, Nelsing S et al. (1992). Detection of *Toxoplasma gondii* DNA by polymerase chain reaction in cerabrospinal fluid from AIDS patients with cerebral toxoplasmosis. *J Infect Dis* **165**: 982–3.

Leport C, Raffi F, Matheron S et al. (1988). Treatment of central nervous system toxoplasmosis with pyrimethamine/sulfadiazine combination in 35 patients with the acquired immunodeficiency syndrome: efficacy of long-term continuous therapy. *Am J Med* **84**: 94–100.

Leport C, Bastuji-Garin S, Perronne C et al. (1989). An open study of the pyrimethamine-clindamycin combination in AIDS patients with brain toxoplasmosis. *J Infect Dis* **160**: 577–8.

Leport C, Tournerie C, Raguin G et al. (1991). Long-term follow-up of patients with AIDS on maintenance therapy for toxoplasmosis. *Eur J Microbiol Infect Dis* **10**: 192–3.

Leport C, Chene G, Morlat P et al. (1996). Pyrimethamine for primary prophylaxis of toxoplasmic encephalitis in patients with human immunodeficiency virus infection: a double-blind, randomized trial. ANRS 005 ACTG 154 Group Members. Agence Nationale de Recherche sur le SIDA. AIDS Clinical Trial Group. *J Infect Dis* **173**: 91–7.

Levy RM, Mills CM, Posin JP et al. (1990). The efficacy and clinical impact of brain imaging in neurologically symptomatic AIDS patients: a prospective CT/MRI study. *J Acquire Immune Defic Synd* **3**: 461–71.

Li TS. Tubiana R, Katlama C et al. (1998). Long lasting recovery in CD4 T cell function mirrors viral load reduction after highly active anti-retroviral therapy in patients with advanced HIV disease. *Lancet* **351**.

Lucet JC, Baily MP, Bedos JP et al. (1993). Septic shock due to toxoplasmosis in patients infected with the human immunodeficiency virus. *Chest* **104**: 1054–8.

Luft BJ, Remington JS. (1988). Toxoplasmic encephalitis. *J Infect Dis* **157**: 1–6.

Luft BJ, Remington JS. (1992). Toxoplasmic encephalitis in AIDS. *Clin Infect Dis* **15**: 211–22.

Mallolas J, Zamora L, Gatell JM et al. (1993). Primary prophylaxis for *Pneumocystis carinii* pneumonia: a randomized trial comparing cotrimoxazole, aerosolized pentamidine and dapsone plus pyrimethamine. *AIDS* **7**: 59–64.

May T, Rabaud C, Katlama C et al. (1993). Toxoplasmose extracrcerbrale au cours du SIDA. Resultats d'une enquete nationale. *Med Mal Infect* **23**: 190–200.

May T, Beuscart C. Leclercq P. (1994). Trimethoprim-sulfamethoxazole (T-S) versus aerosolized pentamidine AP) for primary prophpylaxis of *Pneumocystis carinii* pneumonia (PCP): a prospective randomized controlled clinical trial. LFPMI study Group. *J Acquir Immune Defic Syndr* **7**: 457–62.

Mehren M, Burns PJ, Mamani MD et al. (1988). Toxoplasmic myelitis mimicking intramedullary cord tumor. *Neurology* **38**: 1648–50.

Michelet C, Arvieux C, Francois C et al. (1998). Opportunistic infections occurring during highly active antiretroviral treatment. *AIDS* **12**: 1815–22.

Oksenhendler E, Cadranel J, Sarfati C et al. (1990). *Toxoplasma gondii* pneumonia in patients with AIDS. *Am J Med* **88**: 18–21N.

Opravl M, Hirschel B, Lazzarini A et al. (1995). Once-weekly administration of dapsone/pyrimethamine vs aerosolized pentamidine as combined prophylaxis for *Pneumocystis carinii* pneumonia and toxoplasmic encephalitis in human immunodeficiency virus-infected patients. *Clin Infect Dis* **20**: 531–41.

Parmley SF, Goebel FD, Remington JS. (1992). Detection of *Toxoplasma gondii* in cerebrospinal fluid from AIDS patients by polymerase chain reaction. *J Clin Microbiol* **30**: 3000–2.

Pedrol E, Gonzalez-Clemente JM, Gatell JM et al. (1990). Central nervous system toxoplasmosis in AIDS patients: efficacy of an intermittent maintenance therapy. *AIDS* **4**: 511–17.

Pelloux H, Thelu J, Derouin F et al. (1992). Specific antitoxoplasmic immunoglobulin G detected by Western blot in AIDS patients; relationship to visceral localization. *AIDS* **6**: 885–6.

Pomeroy C, Filice GA. (1992). Pulmonary toxoplasmosis: a review. *Clin Infect Dis* **14**: 863–70.

Porter S, Sande MA. (1992). Toxoplasmosis of the central nervous system in the acquired immunodeficiency syndrome. *N Engl J Med* **327**: 1643–8.

Pugin J, Vanhems P, Hirschel B *et al.* (1992). Extreme elevations of serum lactic dehydrogenase differentiating pulmonary toxoplasmosis from pneumocystis pneumoniae. *N Engl J Med* **326**: 1226.

Remington JS, Desmonts G. (1990). Toxoplasmosis. In: JS Remington, JO Klein (eds.) *Infectious diseases of the foetus and newborn infant.* Philadelphia, PA: WB Saunders.

Renold C, Sugar A, Chave JP *et al.* (1992). Toxoplasma encephalitis. *Medicine* **71**: 224–38.

Rolston KV, Hoy J. (1987). Role of clindamycin in the treatment of central nervous system toxoplasmosis. *Am J Med* **83**: 551–4.

Rousseau F, Pueyo S, Morlat P *et al.* (1997). Increased risk of toxoplasmic encephalitis in human immunodeficiency virus-infected patients with pyrimethamine-related rash. ANRS 005-ACTG 154 Trial Group. Agence Nationale de Recherche sur le SIDA (ANRS-INSERM) and the NIAID-AIDS Clinical Trials Group. *Clin Infect Dis* **24**: 396–402.

Saba J, Leport C, Morlat P *et al.* (1993). Pyrimethamine plus azithromycin for treatment of acute toxoplasmic encephalitis in patients with AIDS. *Eur J Clin Microbiol Infect Dis* **12**: 853–6.

Salmon D, Saba J, Fontbonne A *et al.* (1995). Dapsone versus pentamidine aerosols for secondary prophylaxis on *Pneumocystis carinii* pneumonia in AIDS patients. Lower survival in AIDS patients receiving dapsone compared with aerosolized pentamidine for secondary prophylaxis of *Pneumocystis carinii* pneumonia. *J Infect Dis* **172**: 656–64.

Schneider M, Hoepelman A, Eeftinck-Schattenkerk JK *et al.* (1992). A controlled trial of aerosolized pentamidine or trimethoprim-sulfamethoxazole as primary prophylaxis against *Pneumocystis carinii* pneumonia in patients with human immunodeficiency virus infection. *N Engl J Med* **327**: 1836–41.

Schneider MM, Borleffs JC, Stolk RP *et al.* (1999). Discontinuation of prophylaxis for *Pneumocystis carinii* pneumonia in HIV-1-infected patients treated with highly active antiretroviral therapy. *Lancet* **353**: 201–3.

Tirard V, Niel G, Rosenheim M *et al.* (1991). Diagnosis of toxoplasmosis in patients with AIDS isolation of the parasite from the blood [letter]. *New Engl J Med* **324**: 634.

Torres RA, Weinberg W, Stansell J *et al.* (1997). Atovaquone for salvage treatment and suppression of toxoplasmic encephalitis in patients with AIDS. *Clin Infect Dis* **24**: 422–9.

Weiss LM, Udem SA, Tanowitz H *et al.* (1988). Western blot analysis of the antibody responses of patients with AIDS and toxoplasma encephalitis; antigenic diversity among toxoplasma strains. *J Infect Dis* **157**: 7–13.

Zangerle R, Allenberger F, Pohl P *et al.* (1991). High risk of developing toxoplasmic encephalitis in AIDS patients seropositive for *Toxoplasma gondii*. *Med Microbiol Immunol* **180**: 59–66.

STÉPHANE DE WIT AND NATHAN CLUMECK

Cryptococcus neoformans is the most common life-threatening fungal pathogen in patients with AIDS and mortality rates remain as high as 20% despite therapy. This yeast can infect normal hosts but has a predilection to infect patients with cellular immunodeficiency. Cryptococcal disease can be superficial or deep, localized or diffuse, and can selectively involve the brain or meninges. The infection is often limited to the lungs in immunocompetent hosts, whereas disseminated disease and meningitis are more common in immunocompromised hosts, particularly those with HIV infection.

Epidemiology

C. neoformans, an encapsulated yeast that is found worldwide, is responsible for almost all cases of human cryptococcosis, although a few cases of infection due to *C. albidus*, *C. laurentii* and *C. curvatus* have been described. Cryptococcosis is an uncommon sporadic disease that occurs in both immunocompetent and immunocompromised individuals. There is an increased incidence in patients with impaired cellular immunity caused by disease or corticosteroid therapy. The overall incidence of cryptococcosis has markedly increased over the past 15 years, due to its occurrence in patients with HIV infection (Levitz, 1991; Dromer *et al.*, 1995).

Between 1981 and 1987 the prevalence of cryptococcal infection in AIDS patients in the USA was found to be 7–8%, with rates as high as 15% in some states, e.g. Alabama, Mississippi, Tennessee and Kentucky (Diamond, 1991). The annual incidence of cryptococcosis among HIV-infected patients in New York City was estimated to be 6.1–8.5%. Ninety-six per cent of cases of cryptococcosis were thought to be related to HIV infection (Currie and Casadevall, 1994). Lower rates of HIV-related cryptococcosis have been reported in Europe, but data are available for only a few countries. In France, a national survey of cryptococcosis between 1985 and 1993 showed that 86% of cases involved patients with AIDS. The annual incidence of cryptococcosis varied around the country from 0.03 to 0.94 per 100 000 persons (Dromer *et al.*, 1996a). In the UK, cryptococcosis was reported in 3.2% of AIDS patients (Anon., 1988). In Belgium, 6% of AIDS patients who presented between 1983 and 1993 were diagnosed with cryptococcosis, either as their AIDS-defining illness or later during the course of their disease. Cryptococcosis was more common in African blacks living in Belgium (12%) than in Caucasians (3%). The prevalence of cryptococcosis in AIDS patients from developing countries appears to be higher than in patients from the USA, Europe or Australia. A prevalence of 13% in Haitian patients and approximately 30% in some areas of western Africa has also been noted (Holmberg and Meyer, 1986; Horsburgh and Selik, 1988).

The frequency of cryptococcosis in the USA and in Southern France has declined since fluconazole has become available. The decrease in incidence was demonstrated in the setting of declining or steady usage of other antifungal agents (Pradier *et al.*, 1992; McNeil and Kan, 1995). A marked decline in the incidence of cryptococcal disease has also been seen following the introduction of highly active antiretroviral therapies (HAART): for example, a 70% decline was seen in France between the first half of 1996 and the first half of 1997 (Costagliola, 1998; Sacktor *et al.*, 2001).

Two varieties of *C. neoformans* cause cryptococcosis: var. *neoformans* (serotypes A and D) and *var. gattii* (serotypes B and C). These two varieties differ strikingly in their geographical distribution. *C. neoformans* var. *gattii* is a biotrophic fungus, which shows a specific ecological association with its host tree, *Eucalyptus camaldulensis*. The geographical distribution of this tree corresponds to the distribution of C. *neoformans* var. *gattii* infections, namely Australia, Hawaii, California, Mexico, Brazil, parts of Africa and Southeast Asia (Bottone *et al.*, 1987). C. *neoformans* var. *neoformans* has been isolated from soil, pigeon excrement and sites contaminated by pigeon excrement in many regions of the world. It has also been isolated from the excrement of other avian species, including chickens, parrots and sparrows. It is occasionally found in non-avian sources including fruit, vegetable and dairy products (Levitz, 1991). Epidemiological surveys performed before the AIDS era showed that var. *neoformans* accounted for more than 90% of the clinical isolates in the USA, except in Southern California, where var. *gattii* accounted for 40% of the clinical isolates (Bennett *et al.*, 1984).

Presently, with only a few exceptions (Castanon-Olivares *et al.*, 1997), all the AIDS-associated cryptococcosis diagnosed in the USA as well as in Central Africa is due to var. *neoformans* (Swinne *et al.*, 1986; Bottone *et al.*, 1987; Kapenda *et al.*, 1987; St Germain *et al.*, 1988). A retrospective analysis of a population-based register of cases of cryptococcosis in Victoria, Australia, has shown a distinct association between immune status and C. *neoformans* variety: all C. *neoformans* var. *gattii* infections occurred in healthy hosts and led to no deaths, whereas var. *neoformans* was associated with immunosuppression in 90% of cases and had a high mortality rate. These findings appear to be related to variety-specific interactions between host and parasite (Speed and Dunt, 1995).

A retrospective survey performed in France has shown that some epidemiological differences between serotypes A and D could exist in cryptococcosis due to C. *neoformans* var. *neoformans*. In a multivariate analysis, serotype D infections (responsible for 21% of the infections) were significantly associated with patients receiving corticosteroid therapy, cutaneous cryptococcal skin lesions and residence in certain regions of France. Serotype D infections occurred less often in patients with meningitis, these coming from Africa and females, suggesting that individual and environmental factors could be associated with the serotype of C. *neoformans* (Dromer *et al.*, 1996b).

Pathogenesis

Cryptococcal infection is acquired by inhalation of the organism into the lungs. Neither animal-to-human nor human-to human transmission has been documented. After inhalation, the yeast remains localized in the lung or spreads to other organs, in particular the central nervous system (CNS). The risk of dissemination is markedly increased in immunocompromised subjects (Baker, 1976).

C. *neoformans* serotypes A and D have the ability to convert to a weakly encapsulated form in their natural habitat. This leads to the production of yeast cells smaller than $6\,\mu m$, which can be readily aerosolized and inhaled by humans. Once in the alveolar spaces, they regenerate their polysaccharide capsules (Dyktsra *et al.*, 1977), the organism's major virulence factor.

How the cryptococcal capsular polysaccharide functions as a virulence factor remains poorly understood, although in the host, encapsulation allows the organism to resist phagocytosis and limits the host inflammatory response. Production of a thick capsule and the release of large amounts of capsular polysaccharide and glycoproteins into the bloodstream serve as significant virulence factors. High titres of antigen are typically associated with poor outcome, both in AIDS and non-AIDS patients (Diamond and Bennett, 1974). Intravascular cryptococcal polysaccharide prevents leucocytes from migrating into sites of an acute inflammatory stimulus or into a delayed-type hypersensitivity (DTH) reaction site. Cryptococcal polysaccharide stimulates neutrophils to shed their surface L-selectin, a molecule required for leucocytes to attach to endothelial cells before moving from the blood vessels into tissues. This prevents leucocytes from entering the tissues and killing the organism. Moreover, melanin and mannitol produced by cryptococci may block components of the host's oxidative defensive mechanisms (Kozel and Mastroianni, 1976; Polak, 1989; Collins and Bancroft, 1991; Vecchiarelli *et al.*, 1994). The unencapsulated state favours growth and conversion to the sexual phase of the fungal life cycle. Clinical isolates are almost always encapsulated, although capsule-deficient variants have been found in AIDS patients (Bottone and Wormser, 1985). *Cryptoccocus neoformans* produces no toxins.

Humans have multiple host defenses against C. *neoformans* but the organism is able to counteract many of these. Cellular defences active against C. *neoformans* include phagocytic cells (neutrophils and monocytes–macrophages), and non-phagocytic effector cells such as natural killer (NK) cells and T lymphocytes. Phagocytic cells kill cryptococci either intracellularly or extracellularly by oxidative and non-oxidative mechanisms. As alveolar macrophages are minimally effective in eliminating encapsulated cryptococci in the lungs, other more effective natural effector cells (e.g. neutrophils) must be recruited from the bloodstream to the site of the infection before cryptococci can be eradicated.

Macrophages that ingest cryptococci can serve as antigen-presenting cells (APC), stimulating *C. neoformans*-specific T lymphocytes to differentiate and proliferate. Depending upon which population of cryptococcus-specific T lymphocytes expands, the T cells function either as helper (Th2) cells for antibody-producing B lymphocytes or as Th1 cells, which mediate cellular immune responses. In mice, a predominance of Th2 cytokines is associated with lethal cryptococcal infection. Administration of interleukin 12 and interleukin 18 synergistically induces nitric oxide-dependent anticryptococcal activity of murine peritoneal exudate cells by stimulating NK cells to produce interferon-γ (Kawakami *et al.*, 1997; Zhang *et al.*, 1997).

Antibodies to the cryptococcal polysaccharide opsonize cryptococci, triggering phagocytosis and antibody-dependent cellular cytotoxicity (ADCC). Unfortunately, as the capsular polysaccharide is not a good immunogen and some cryptococcal products may suppress humoral immune responses, the antibody response is usually weak or absent. However, the capsule also fixes complement by the alternative pathway, and opsonization may occur by this mechanism. The activated complement is also chemotactic.

Cell-mediated immune responses are the principal determinant of host resistance to *C. neoformans* infections. When stimulated by APCs bearing cryptococcal antigen, the cryptococcus-reactive T cells produce lymphokines, such as interferon-γ, that may activate natural effector cells, which then kill cryptococci. Activated T cells may also directly inhibit *C. neoformans* growth (Bulmer and Sans, 1967; Murphy, 1991; Murphy *et al.*, 1993; Buchanan and Murphy, 1994; Levitz *et al.*, 1994).

The neurotropism of cryptococci is partly explained by defects in host defense mechanisms. Normal cerebrospinal fluid (CSF) lacks immunoglobulins and complement and is a good growth media for the organism. As the CSF inflammatory response is delayed, peaking at 5–8 days after infection, significant unrestricted growth of the organism occurs beforehand. Moreover, although macrophages are an integral part of the CNS host defenses, their activation is insufficient for the elimination of cryptococci (Patterson and Andriole, 1989).

In AIDS patients, cryptococcal antigens have an additional mechanism for subverting host defenses. Crypto-coccal capsular polysaccharides may enhance binding of human immunodeficiency virus type 1 (HIV-1) gp120 to lymphocyte integral membrane proteins, thereby enhancing HIV infectivity. *C. neoformans* has also been shown to enhance HIV expression in monocytic cells through a TNF-α dependent mechanism. These findings suggest that in HIV-infected patients, cryptococcal disease might accelerate the course of HIV disease (Pettoello-Mantovani *et al.*, 1994; Harrison *et al.*, 1997).

Few studies have investigated the mechanisms of increased susceptibility of HIV-infected patients to *C. neoformans* infection. Natural-killer activity against *C. neoformans* has been shown to be impaired, and this may be related to defects in both oxidative and non-oxidative effector pathways that occur after the binding and internalization of the organism (Horn and Washburn, 1995; Harrison and Levitz, 1997).

Clinical presentation

The portal of entry for cryptococci is the lungs, and therefore pulmonary lesions are a prominent feature of primary infection. The disease may remain localized in the lung but it will disseminate to other tissues, notably the CNS, in immunocompromised patients, particularly those with HIV infection.

In AIDS patients, cryptococcal meningitis may present in an indolent manner or as an acute illness. The most common symptoms are fever and headache, which are present in 80–90% of patients. Meningismus and photophobia are less common (20–30% of patients). Alteration of mental status and non-specific symptoms, including nausea, vomiting and malaise, can also be present. Less common clinical findings include visual disturbances, papilloedema, cerebellar signs, seizures, dementia and aphasia. About 10% of patients are asymptomatic. The variable clinical presentation and the variety of symptoms associated with cryptococcal meningitis may explain why the duration of symptoms prior to diagnosis has been reported to range from 1 day to 4 months, with a mean of 1 month (Zuger *et al.*, 1988; Patterson, 1997).

Although the extent of extraneural disease has not been firmly established in AIDS patients, it has been documented in up to 66% in cases with meningitis (Table 27.1).

Lung involvement may present simultaneously with CNS disease. Symptoms include fever, cough and dyspnoea, and pleuritic chest pain may be present. Chest radiographs often

Table 27.1 Sites of extraneural cryptococcal infections

Common
  Lung
Unusual
  Skin (see Figure 27.1, in the colour plate section)
  Arthritis
  Cellulitis
  Pyomyositis
  Mediastinitis
  Myocarditis
  Pericarditis
  Intestinal infection
  Peritonitis
  Pancreatitis
  Hepatitis
  Placental infection

(Data derived from Brivet *et al.*, 1987; Lafont *et al.*, 1987; Torres, 1987; van Calck *et al.*, 1988; Ricciardi *et al.*, 1986; Kida *et al.*, 1989; Bonacini *et al.*, 1990; Adams *et al.*, 1992; Zimmerli *et al.*, 1992; Couiter *et al.*, 1993; Barber *et al.*, 1995; Finazzi *et al.*, 1996.)

show diffuse infiltrates, and rarely, isolated pleural effusions. Endobronchial abnormalities can been found at bronchoscopy. Severe lung involvement leading to adult respiratory distress syndrome (ARDS) may accompany disseminated cryptococcosis. Empyema has also been described (Mulanovich *et al.*, 1995; Perla *et al.*, 1985; Cameron *et al.*, 1991; Meyohas *et al.*, 1994). Numerous other extraneural sites have been described (Table 27.1).

Cutaneous lesions suggestive of molluscum contagiosum or herpes simplex infection may accompany disseminated disease (Borton and Wintroub, 1984; Ricchi *et al.*, 1991).

Cryptococcaemia, defined as positive blood cultures, is found in 20–50% of AIDS patients with cryptococcal CNS disease. This contrasts with the 5–20% incidence reported in other patients (Patterson and Andriole, 1989). Few data are available to establish the frequency of isolated cryptococcemia or antigenemia. In a retrospective study, nine out of 106 patients with cryptococcal disease had cryptococcaemia, although two of the nine had no lumbar puncture performed (Chuck and Sande, 1989). Isolated cryptococcal antigenaemia is frequently asymptomatic, although some patients have fever and malaise. Few studies have evaluated the prognostic significance of isolated cryptococcal antigenaemia. One prospective study performed in France suggests that isolated antigenaemia is an early stage of disease, recommends repeated attempts to isolate the fungus by culture and justifies the initiation of antifungal treatment (Debost *et al.*, 1992).

HIV-infected patients with cryptococcal infection have a much worse prognosis than HIV-uninfected patients, as 17–37% of patients die during the first 6 weeks after diagnosis. Clinical and laboratory findings may be useful to establish the prognosis of infection in both HIV- and non-HIV-infected hosts. In the pre-AIDS era, increased mortality was seen in patients with persistent immuno-suppression, elevated CSF opening pressures, low glucose, elevated CSF and serum cryptococcal antigen titres (> 1:32), the lack of a CSF white-cell response (< 20 cells), and cryptococci seen in the CSF by microscopy. In patients with AIDS, an abnormal mental status, elevated CSF or serum titres (> 1:1024), and CSF white blood lymphocyte count below 20 cells/μl predict mortality rates as high as 40% (Diamond and Bennett, 1974; Saag *et al.*, 1992).

Diagnosis

In view of the poorly characterized clinical presentation of cryptococcal disease in AIDS patients, the clinician should maintain a high index of suspicion and should initiate a search for cryptococcal organisms and antigen in the blood and CSF in all patients with symptoms of CNS disease and/or unexplained fever.

Cerebrospinal fluid

Lumbar puncture should be performed on all patients with suspected cryptococcal infection unless contraindicated, and the CSF fully investigated (Table 27.2). Elevated opening pressure is usual: in one series, two-thirds of the patients had levels higher than 200 mm H_2O (Chuck and Sande, 1989).

In contrast to other patients, HIV-infected patients often have a striking lack of inflammatory response to crypto-

Table 27.2 Investigations to be performed on cerebrospinal fluid of patients with suspected cryptococcal meningitis

- Opening pressure
- Protein concentration
- Glucose concentration (with simultaneous serum concentration)
- Leucocyte count and differential
- India-ink stain
- Cryptococcal antigen titre
- Fungal culture

coccal infection; abnormalities in routine CSF studies (protein, glucose and leucocyte count) are often minimal or absent. When present, abnormalities are invariably non-specific and are not helpful in differentiating cryptococcal infection from other CNS diseases, either infectious or malignant, found in AIDS patients.

Cryptococci are almost always found in CSF in patients with cryptococcal meningitis, whether using India-ink stains, cryptococcal antigen determination or culture. Cryptococci are frequently seen on direct examination (76%) and rates of positive cultures are as high as 95%. In most cases, large numbers of organisms are seen on India-ink smears and provide rapid diagnosis. Another area of contrast between AIDS and non-AIDS patients is in CSF cryptococcal antigen detection. In both groups, antigen detection using a commercial latex or enzyme-linked immunosorbent assay (ELISA) method is extremely sensitive, with well over 90% positive. However, AIDS patients often have extraordinarily high CSF antigen titres, with values at times over 1:1024 (Chuck and Sande, 1989; Patterson and Andriole, 1989; Perfect, 1989; Currie, 1993).

The isolation of cryptococcus by culture remains the gold standard for definitive diagnosis. Rare false-negative results may occur at a very early stage of the disease or in patients with a cryptococcoma (Patterson and Andriole, 1989; Diamond, 1991).

Blood and other fluids and tissues

Determination of cryptococcal antigen in the serum is a useful diagnostic test for cryptococcal disease in HIV-infected patients, with a sensitivity approaching 100%. As for CSF, the serum cryptococcal antigen titre in AIDS patients is generally much higher than that seen in patients without HIV infection, ranging up to 2×10^6 (Dismukes, 1988). False-negative results can be found with some of these high-titre samples when they are tested undiluted (prozone effect). Conversely, although unusual, false-positive tests should be considered, especially with titres of less than 1:8 (Diamond, 1991).

The value of cryptococcal serum antigen as a screening test for early diagnosis of cryptococcosis has been evaluated in several studies in different populations. In one study from Zaire, cryptococcal antigen was found in 12% of the screened sera, with a positive predictive value ranging from 66 to 92%, depending on the serum titres (Desmet et al., 1989). The low incidence of cryptococcosis in areas such as Scandinavia and the UK does not justify routine serum screening (Nelson et al., 1990; Hoffmann et al., 1991). However, systematic testing of HIV patients with fever for cryptococcal antigen could allow the diagnosis of early disease in a significant number of patients, leading to early therapeutic intervention and improved outcome (Debost et al., 1992; Wright et al., 1992).

Blood cultures for fungi should be obtained from all patients suspected of having cryptococcal infection. Moreover, in cases of suspected extracranial disease, culture and histopathological examination should be performed on specimens of potentially infected sites, such as skin, bone marrow, bronchial washings, urine or liver.

The value of serial cultures in the evaluation of the therapeutic response has not been extensively evaluated. The median length of time to the first negative CSF culture in one prospective study was 42 days with amphotericin B (range 28–71 days) and 64 days with fluconazole (range 53–67 days) (Saag et al., 1992). These periods were shorter among those patients who responded successfully to both treatments. However, given the wide range of values observed, repeated CSF cultures probably have no role in the management of patients during induction therapy (Saag et al., 1992).

The role of serial determination of serum antigen has been controversial till recently. The lack of standardization of commercial kits limits their usefulness for quantitative assessment. Characteristically, persistently high serum titres are often found in AIDS patients, contrasting with the progressive fall observed in HIV-uninfected patients during treatment. Increasing antigen titres may occur in patients with relapse of infection, although CSF antigen appears more reliable in this setting (Powderly et al., 1994). However, a recent study has demonstrated that there was no correlation between serum cryptococcal antigen titres and clinical evolution. Follow-up monitoring of the serum cryptococcal antigen is thus not useful in the management of patients with AIDS-related cryptococcal disease on treatment (Aberg et al., 2000).

Imaging studies

In HIV-infected patients with CNS cryptococcosis, especially meningitis, computed tomographic (CT) scan of the brain is usually normal or shows non-specific or unrelated alterations, such as diffuse cortical atrophy or ventricular enlargement. Occasionally, ring-enhancing lesions due to cryptococcomas are found (Clarck et al., 1990). There is a broad spectrum of changes seen on magnetic resonance (MRI) imaging of HIV-infected patients with proven CNS cryptococcosis. Normal scans have also been noted (Miszkiel *et al.*, 1996). Thus, at present the main value of brain imaging is to exclude other causes of CNS diseases.

Treatment

Treatment of cryptococcal disease in AIDS patients has been investigated in numerous prospective and retrospective studies. In general, therapy, is divided into two stages: initial (induction) therapy of the acutely ill patient lasting a few weeks, and then maintenance or suppressive therapy, which has generally been continued for the life of the patient (although the latter is being re-evaluated in patients with sustained responses to highly active antiretroviral therapy (HAART).

Induction therapy
Amphotericin B and flucytosine
Amphotericin B is a polyene antibiotic with antifungal activity dependent on binding to ergosterols present in the membrane of fungi (but not in mammalian cell membranes). Binding of the polyenes forms membrane pores, which allow the leakage of protons, monovalent cations and active oxygen from the cell, killing the fungus (Brajtburg *et al.*, 1990). Flucytosine is a fluorinated nucleoside analogue, orally bioavailable, with *in vitro* activity against many yeasts, including cryptococci.

Amphotericin B has been the cornerstone of therapy for cryptococcosis for more than 30 years. Studies performed by Bennett and colleagues (1979) in the pre-AIDS era established that combination therapy using low-dose amphotericin B with flucytosine was as effective as high-dose amphotericin B but less toxic. These studies also established that a 6-week period of treatment was superior to a 4-week period in patients with neurological symptoms (Bennett *et al.*, 1979; Dismukes *et al.*, 1987).

The use of flucytosine in AIDS patients has a checkered history. It is poorly tolerated because of the drug's haematological toxicity, which is augmented by bone-marrow involvement by HIV and opportunistic infections, and the cumulative effect of other bone marrow suppressive therapies such as zidovudine (ZDV). One retrospective study concluded that the addition of flucytosine to amphotericin B was of no therapeutic benefit in AIDS patients with

cryptococcal infections and led to a high rate of cytopenias (Chuck and Sande, 1989). However, as monotherapy with amphotericin B or fluconazole is associated with an unacceptably high mortality during the first 2 weeks of acute therapy, combination of amphotericin B with flucytosine for the first 2 weeks has been further evaluated (see below).

Intravenous amphotericin B is thus considered the mainstay of therapy in patients with AIDS. Dosages between 0.5 and 0.8 mg/kg/day have been the most effective. A minimum total dose of amphotericin B of 1 g has been recommended and is generally achieved after 6 weeks of therapy at 0.5–0.8 mg/kg/day. Continuation of therapy until cultures of CSF (or other fluids) are negative has been advocated, but the reliability of this end-point has been questioned (Polsky *et al.*, 1986; Dismukes, 1988).

Amphotericin B is a toxic drug with a low therapeutic ratio. The most frequent adverse reactions are fever and chills during and after infusion and impaired renal function. Patients should receive a 1 mg test dose over 1 hour, followed immediately by 50 mg if the test dose is tolerated. If the 1 mg dose is poorly tolerated, a smaller second dose (5–10 mg) is recommended. The large dose should be infused over 4–6 h, although no difference has been found in terms of incidence or severity of side-effects between a 1-h infusion rate and a 4-h infusion rate in one double-blind, randomized trial (Oldfield *et al.*, 1990). Premedication with diphenhydramine or acetaminophen can be used in order to prevent chills and fever. Intravenous meperedine can be used if chills or rigors are severe or last more than 5–10 min. Prehydration with normal saline (0.5–1 litre) may help to minimize renal toxicity.

Azole derivatives
Because of the toxicity associated with amphotericin B therapy, a number of azole derivatives have been tested for acute therapy of cryptococcal meningitis. Ketoconazole penetrates the CSF poorly and treatment failures have occurred when this drug has been used, even in cases where adequate CSF concentrations have been reached (Perfect *et al.*, 1982). Miconazole was also not very effective, and the drug required parenteral administration and was associated with serious side-effects.

Fluconazole is active against *C. neoformans in vitro* and has been shown to be effective in animal models. CSF levels are 50–100% of those found concomitantly in serum, and therapeutic levels can be achieved easily with oral administration. Fluconazole was first used successfully for treatment of cryptococcal meningitis when given at a dose of 400 mg/day intravenously in patients who failed or were intolerant to amphotericin B (Byrne and Wajszczuk, 1988; Stern et al., 1988; Rubin et al., 1989). Two prospective studies compared fluconazole 400 mg/day with amphotericin B (with or without flucytosine) for the acute treatment of cryptococcal meningitis in AIDS patients. The first study randomized a small number of patients but showed a statistically significant difference in favour of amphotericin B-flucytosine combination (Larsen et al., 1990). Response rates were 43% with fluconazole versus 100% with the combination ($p = 0.04$). During the first 10 weeks of therapy, 29% of the patients on fluconazole died versus none on the combination. A much larger second multicentre study showed no difference in overall outcome between fluconazole- and amphotericin B-treated patients; treatment was successful in 40% of amphotericin B-treated cases and 34% of those treated with fluconazole (Saag et al., 1992). Overall, mortality was also comparable (14% versus 18%). However, both studies demonstrated that the CSF was sterilized faster in those patients receiving amphotericin B (Saag et al., 1992). Although these data showed that fluconazole was as effective as amphotericin B for induction therapy of cryptococcal meningitis, many authorities feel that amphotericin B is preferred for initial therapy (first 1–2 weeks) of all but the mildest cases of cryptococcal meningitis, because of its rapid sterilization of CSF.

Current therapeutic recommendations

A large, double-blind multicentre trial (408 AIDS patients) was conducted between 1991 and 1994 by the US National Institutes of Health Mycoses Study Group and the AIDS Clinical Trials Group (van der Horst et al., 1997). This pivotal trial showed that for the initial treatment, the use of a relatively high dose of amphotericin B (0.7 mg/kg/day) plus flucytosine (100 mg/kg/day) for 2 weeks is associated with an increased rate of CSF sterilization and decreased mortality when compared to lower dose (0.4 mg/kg) amphotericin B alone or fluconazole (Table 27.3). Consolidation therapy with fluconazole for a further 8 weeks was associated with a higher rate of CSF sterilization compared with itraconazole in the study performed by Saag and colleagues (1992). Mortality rates of 5.5% with high-dose amphotericin B with or without flucytosine were much lower than the 14% noted with the lower dose, and the rate of CSF sterilization at 2 weeks was increased from 20 to 50%.

Table 27.3 Current recommendations for treatment of cryptococcal meningitis

Induction therapy
Amphotericin B, 0.7 mg/kg/day, i.v.
Flucytosine 100 mg/kg/day in divided doses for 2 weeks
Consolidation therapy
Fluconazole 400 mg/day for 8 weeks (alternatively itraconazole 400 mg/day)
Maintenance therapy
Fluconazole 200–400 mg/day (alternatively itraconazole 200–400 mg/day, amphotericin B 1 mg/per/kg week)

(Recommendations from van der Horst et al., 1997)

The addition of flucytosine to amphotericin B was not associated with an increased incidence of toxic effects (probably because of a short-term treatment of 2 weeks and a low daily dose of 100 mg/kg). The addition of flucytosine during the first 2 weeks also reduced the relapse rate over a period of 12 months during maintenance therapy (van der Horst et al., 1997). Current treatment recommendations are wholly based on this trial.

Other therapeutic modalities

Doses of amphotericin B higher than 0.7 mg/kg/day have been used by some investigators. In one prospective trial of amphotericin B, 1 mg/kg/day for 14 days (with or without flucytosine), the success rate was 93%; nephrotoxicity leading to reduction or discontinuation of dosing was seen in seven of the 31 patients (23%) (de Lalla et al., 1995).

Although intraventricular or intrathecal administration of amphotericin B appeared to be beneficial in the treatment of HIV-uninfected patients with severe cryptococcal meningitis in one study, these findings were not confirmed by a prospective randomized study in AIDS patients (Polsky et al., 1986; Holtom et al., 1990). Intraventricular or intrathecal amphotericin B therapy is also associated with serious complications, including bacterial meningitis and transverse myelitis.

Fluconazole has also been shown to be effective at dosages much higher than usual (800–1000 mg/day) as first-line or salvage therapy in patients who have failed other treatment regimens (Berry et al., 1992; Haubrich et al., 1994; Menichetti et al., 1996). However, such doses are not recommended routinely.

The combination of fluconazole and flucytosine was shown to be synergistic for 62% of cryptococci tested in vitro and was superior to either agent alone in a murine model of cryptococcal meningitis. A prospective non-comparative study evaluated this combination in 32 AIDS patients; CSF cultures were sterilized in 75% of cases after 10 weeks of therapy, and clinical success was achieved in 63%. Withdrawal of flucytosine due to toxicity occurred in nine subjects (28%) (Larsen et al., 1994; Nguyen et al., 1995; Nguyen et al., 1997).

In a randomized trial performed in Uganda, the addition of flucytosine 150 mg/kg/day to fluconazole 200 mg/day significantly increased survival at 2 and 6 months suggesting that this combination may be considered in patients unable to tolerate amphotericin B or in settings where its use is difficult, such as developing countries (Mayanja-Kizza et al., 1998).

Itraconazole has not been studied extensively for induction therapy of cryptococcal infections. Despite its poor CSF penetration, it has been shown in non-comparative studies to be effective at 400 mg day given orally. However, it was less effective than the combination of amphotericin B and flucytosine in one small, unblinded comparative trial (Denning et al., 1989; de Gans et al., 1992).

New amphotericin B formulations have shown some promising results. Liposomal amphotericin B (Ambisome; Vestar) has been the most extensively evaluated. A joint Dutch–Australian randomized prospective study of the initial therapy of HIV-related cryptococcal menigitis in 28 patients, comparing AmBisome (4 mg/kg/day) with conventional amphotericin B (0.7 mg/kg/day) (both given for 3 weeks, with subsequent fluconazole) showed that the two regimens had comparable clinical efficacy but the AmBisome-treated patients had accelerated sterilization of CSF (Leenders et al., 1997). The AmBisome-treated group also had fewer overall adverse events and less nephrotoxicity (Leenders et al., 1997) than those treated with conventional amphotericin B. Amphotericin B lipid complex (ABLC; the Liposome Company, London, UK) has been compared to amphotericin B in a randomized trial enrolling 55 patients. Clinical efficacy was reported in 86% of ABLC recipients versus 65% of amphotericin B recipients. Transfusion requirements, mean decreases in haemoglobin levels and mean increases in creatinine levels were also significantly lower with ABLC (Sharkey et al., 1996). Amphotericin B mixed with intralipid was evaluated as initial therapy in a small group (n = 15) of patients in France: neither tolerance nor efficacy were

improved compared to amphotericin B in 5% dextrose (Joly et al., 1996). Although AmBisome and ABLC appear to be slightly more effective and/or slightly less toxic than amphotericin B, they are also substantially more expensive. For this reason they have not generally been employed as first-line therapy, but instead have been reserved for patients with a poor response, or significant toxicity, to amphotericin B.

Management of raised intracranial pressure

Raised intracranial pressure is a frequent complication of cryptococcal meningitis in HIV-uninfected patients (30–40%). These patients usually present with papilloedema, frequently leading to visual impairment. Intracranial hypertension is not frequent in AIDS patients with cryptococcal meningitis, although a moderately elevated opening pressure (above 200 mm H_2O) is usual. The low incidence of raised intracranial pressure in AIDS patients is probably due to the reduced incidence of inflammatory arachnoiditis (which impairs CSF resorption) in AIDS patients compared to those without HIV infection. Raised intracranial pressure may contribute to early mortality in cryptococcal meningitis (death within the first 2 weeks despite adequate therapy), suggesting that CSF opening pressure should be measured in all patients (Van der Horst et al., 1997). Measures to reduce intracranial pressure, which have shown to be effective in HIV-infected patients, include frequent spinal taps, ventricular shunts and acetazolamide (Denning et al., 1991; Jonhston et al., 1992; Powderly, 1996; Fessler et al., 1998). In a retrospective analysis of the study published in 1997 by Van der Horst et al., patients with the highest baseline opening pressure ($\geq$ 250 mm H_2O) were distinguished by higher titres of cryptococcal antigen in CSF, more frequently positive India-ink smears of CSF, more severe neurological symptoms and lower survival at 2 weeks. Those whose CSF pressure was reduced by >10 mm or did not change, had more frequent clinical response at 2 weeks than those with pressure increased by more than 10 mm, leading to the recommendation that opening pressure above 250 mm H_2O should be treated with large-volume CSF drainage (Graybill et al., 2000).

Suppressive therapy

Retrospective studies have shown that AIDS patients with cryptococcal meningitis who do not receive chronic suppressive therapy following initial (induction) treatment have a very high risk of relapse (56%) and decreased survival (Zuger *et al.*, 1988; Chuck and Sande, 1989). The prostate gland may serve as a nidus for relapse of infection and persistence of microorganisms in prostatic secretions has been demonstrated after successful treatment of cryptococcal meningitis (Larsen *et al.*, 1989).

The retrospective study of Chuck and Sande showed that survival of the patients who received either ketoconazole (median survival: 238 days) or amphotericin B (median survival: 280 days) was significantly longer than in those who did not receive suppressive therapy (median survival: 141 days) (Chuck and Sande, 1989). A large, controlled trial comparing fluconazole 200 mg/day with placebo as maintenance therapy following acute treatment with amphotericin B showed that 37% of placebo-treated patients relapsed compared with only 3% of those receiving fluconazole (Bozette *et al.*, 1991). A further study compared fluconazole 200 mg/day with amphotericin B 1 mg/kg/weekly; prophylaxis was successful in 92% of patients receiving fluconazole, compared with only 67% of those receiving amphotericin B (Powderly *et al.*, 1992). Finally, fluconazole and itraconazole were compared for both consolidation therapy as well as for suppressive therapy in a large, randomized, blinded trial (van der Horst *et al.*, 1997). For consolidation therapy, fluconazole-treated patients (400 mg/day) had a higher rate of sterile CSF cultures at 10 weeks than the itraconazole-treated patients (400 mg/day); however, as the clinical outcomes were similar, itraconazole was felt to be a valuable alternative to fluconazole. For long-term suppressive therapy, fluconazole 200 mg/day was superior to itraconazole 200 mg/day (Saag *et al.*, 1999).

Whether life-long prophylaxis is required in patients who have had a dramatic rise in CD4 lymphocyte counts (e.g. to over 200–250 cells/μl) is unclear. It may be possible to discontinue prophylaxis if the rise in CD4 lymphocyte count is sustained. However, partial immune reconstitution in patients receiving HAART has unmasked latent cryptococcal meningitis (Woods *et al.*, 1998).

Prevention and primary prophylaxis

Because of the susceptibility of HIV-infected patients to cryptococcal infection and the high mortality and morbidity associated with the disease, any measure aimed at reducing the incidence of cryptococcosis would be valuable. Ideally, one would recommend avoiding situations likely to cause significant exposure to *C. neoformans* aerosols, such as any exposure to surfaces contaminated with pigeon droppings or being in the vicinity of flowering eucalyptus trees. Whether such precautions, whose practicability is highly questionable, would be beneficial, remains uncertain in view of the ubiquity of the microorganisms and the possibility that some cases of disease represents reactivation of a chronic latent focus. However, it would appear sensible to suggest that an AIDS patient contemplating breeding pigeons, for example, might want to reconsider this activity in the light of the potential hazards.

Primary cryptococcal prophylaxis with antifungal drugs has not been extensively evaluated. Cryptococcal disease has usually been diagnosed in AIDS patients whose mean CD4 lymphocyte count was between 44 and 97 cells/μl (Larsen *et al.*, 1990; Crowe *et al.*, 1991; Powderly *et al.*, 1992). This suggests that if primary prophylaxis is to be used it should be offered to patients with CD4 lymphocyte counts below 100 cells/μl. One non-comparative trial suggested that ketoconazole prophylaxis reduced the incidence of cryptococcal infection (Sprinz and Matias, 1992). In another trial comparing patients who received fluconazole 100 mg/day with historical controls who did not receive prophylaxis, the annual incidence was reduced from 7.5 to 1.8 cases/year (Nightingale *et al.*, 1992). These studies should be interpreted with caution because both studies were performed in an endemic area (Texas) and the data may therefore not be relevant for areas with low endemicity, although a retrospective case–control study has shown that fluconazole prophylaxis provides a 92% protective efficacy against cryptococcal disease in patients with less than 250 CD4 lymphocytes/μl (Quagliarello *et al.*, 1995). The risk of cryptococcal meningitis was reduced from 10 to 1.6% in 2 years in a prospective, randomized, controlled study of fluconazole 200 mg/day compared with clotrimazole troches 10 mg five times a day. The major benefit of primary fluconazole prophylaxis occurred in those with advanced disease (CD4 lymphocyte counts of less than 50 cells/μl) (Powderly *et al.*, 1995). Two other prospective studies using fluconazole at doses of 400 mg weekly or 200 mg three times weekly have also reported prophylactic efficacy (Havlir *et al.*, 1996; Singh *et al.*, 1996).

However, the use of primary fluconazole prophylaxis for all AIDS patients is not routinely recommended, due to cost of prophylaxis, and the possibility that the patient may develop resistant candidal infection or cryptococcal disease due to fluconazole-resistant strains in order to prevent a small number of infections (Clumeck, 1995; Viard *et al.*, 1995). The 1997 guidelines for the prevention of opportunistic infections in persons infected with HIV developed by the US Public Health Service (USPHS) and the Infectious Diseases Society of America (IDSA) do not recommend routine antifungal prophylaxis to prevent cryptococcal disease because of the low incidence of disease, the risks of toxicity, potential for drug interactions, development of resistance, and the cost of prophylaxis. In addition, no survival benefit has been demonstrated with the use of prophylaxis. However, in unusual occupational or other circumstances (e.g. bird breeder, excavation worker) primary prophylaxis with fluconazole 100–200 mg/day is recommended when the CD4 lymphocyte count falls below 50 cells/μl. An acceptable alternative is itraconazole 200 mg/day (USPHS/IDSA, 1999).

References

Adams JR, Mata JA, Culkin DJ *et al.* (1992). Acquired immunodeficiency syndrome manifesting as prostate nodule secondary to cryptococcal infection. *Urology* **39**: 289–91.

Aberg JA, Watson J, Segal M, Chang LW (2000). Clinical utility of monitoring serum cryptococcal antigen (sCRAG) titers in patients with AIDS-related cryptococcal disease. *HIV Clinical Trials* **1**: 1–6.

Anonymous. (1988). Cryptococcosis and AIDS. *Lancet* i: 1434–6.

Baker RD. (1976). The primary pulmonary lymph node complex of cryptococcosis. *Am J Clin Pathol* **65**: 83–92.

Barber BA, Crotty JM, Washburn RG *et al.* (1995). *Cryptococcus neoformans* myositis in a patient with AIDS. *Clin Infect Dis* **21**: 1510–11.

Bennett JE, Dismukes WE, Duma RJ *et al.* (1979). A comparison of amphotericin B alone and combined with flucytosine in the treatment of cryptococcal meningitis. *N Engl J Med* **301**: 126–1.

Bennett JE, Kwon-Chung KJ, Howard DH. (1984). Epidemiologic differences among serotypes of *Cryptococcus neoformans*. *Am J Epidemiol* **120**: 123–30.

Berry AJ, Rinaldi MG, Graybill JR. (1992). Use of high-dose fluconazole as salvage therapy for cryptococcal meningitis in patients with AIDS. *Antimicrob Agents Chemother* **36**: 690–2.

Bonacini M, Nussbaum J, Ahluwalia C. (1990). Gastrointestinal, hepatic and pancreatic involvement with *Cryptococcus neoformans* in AIDS. *J Clin Gastroenterol* **12**: 295–7.

Borton LK, Wintroub BU. (1984). Disseminated cryptococcosis presenting as herpetiform lesions in a homosexual man with acquired immunodeficiency syndrome. *J Am Acad Dermatol* **10**: 387–90.

Bottone EJ, Wormser GP. (1985). Capsule-deficient cryptococci in AIDS. *Lancet* i: 553.

Bottone EJ, Salkin IF, Hurd NJ *et al.* (1987). Serogroup distribution of *Cryptococcus neoformans* in patients with AIDS. *J Infect Dis* **156**: 242.

Bozette SA, Larsen RA, Chiu J *et al.* (1991). A placebo-controlled trial of maintenance therapy with fluconazole after treatment of cryptococcal meningitis in the acquired immunodeficiency syndrome. *N Engl J Med* **324**: 580–4.

Brajtburg J, Powderly WG, Kobayashi GS *et al.* (1990). Amphotericin B: current understanding of mechanisms of action. *Antimicrob Agents Chemother* **34**: 183–8.

Brivet F, Livartowski J, Herve P *et al.* (1987). Pericardial cryptococcal disease in acquired immune deficiency syndrome. *Am J Med* **82**: 1273.

Buchanan KL, Murphy JW. (1994). Regulation of cytokine production during the expression phase of the anticryptococcal delayed-type hypersensitivity response. *Infect Immunol* **62**: 2930–9.

Bulmer GS, Sans MD. (1967). *Cryptococcus neoformans*. II. Phagocytosis by human leukocytes. *J Bacteriol* **94**: 1480–3.

Byrne Wr, Wajszczuk CP. (1988). Cryptococcal meningitis in the acquired immunodeficiency syndrome (AIDS): successful treatment with fluconazole after failure of amphotericin B. *Ann Intern Med* **108**: 384–5.

Cameron ML, Barlett JA, Gallis HA *et al.* (1991). Manifestations of pulmonary cryptococcosis in patients with acquired immunodeficiency syndrome. *Rev Infect Dis* **13**: 64–7.

Castanon-Olivares LR, Lopez-Martinez R, Barriga-Angulo G *et al.* (1997). Crytococcus neoformans var. *gattii* in an AIDS patient. *J Med Virol Mycol* **35**: 57–9.

Chuck SL, Sande MA. (1989). Infections with *Cryptococcus neoformans* in the acquired immunodeficiency syndrome. *N Engl J Med* **321**: 794–9.

Clarck RA, Greer D, Atkinson W *et al.* (1990). Spectrum of *Cryptococcus neoformans* infections in 68 patients infected with human immunodeficiency virus. *Rev Infect Dis* **12**: 768–77.

Clumeck N. (1995). Primary prophylaxis against opportunistic infections in patients with AIDS [Editorial]. *N Engl J Med* **322**: 739–40.

Collins HL, Bancroft GJ. (1991). Encapsulation of *Cryptococcus neoformans* impairs antigen-specific T-cell responses. *Infect Immunol* **59**: 3883–8.

Costagliola D (for the Clinical Epidemiology Group from CISIH [INSERM SC41]). (1998). Trends in incidence of clinical manifestations of HIV infection and antiretroviral prescriptions in French University Hospitals. *Fifth Conference on Retroviruses and Opportunistic Infections*, Chicago, IL, USA.

Coulter C, Benson SM, Whitby M. (1993). Fluconazole for cryptococcal cellulitis. *Clin Infect Dis* **16**: 826–7.

Crowe SM, Carlin B, Stewart KI *et al.* (1991). Predictive value of CD4 lymphocyte numbers for the development of opportunistic infections and malignancies in HIV-infected persons. *J AIDS* **4**: 770–6.

Currie BP, Casadevall A. (1994). Estimation of the prevalence of cryptococcal infection among patients infected with the human immunodeficiency virus in New York City. *Clin Infect Dis* **19**: 1029–33.

Currie BP, Freundlich LF, Soto MA *et al.* (1993). False-negative cerebrospinal fluid cryptococcal latex agglutination tests for patients with culture-positive cryptococcal meningitis. *J Clin Microbiol* **31**: 2519–22.

de Gans J, Portegies P, Tiessens G *et al.* (1992). Itraconazole compared with amphotericin B plus flucytosine in AIDS patients with cryptococcal meningitis. *AIDS* **6**: 185–90.

de Lalla F, Pellizzer G, Vaglia A *et al.* (1995). Amphotericin B as primary therapy for cryptococcosis in patients with AIDS: reliability of relatively high doses administered over a relatively short period. *Clin Infect Dis* **20**: 263–6.

Debost I, Lecomte I, Roux P *et al.* (1992). Diagnostic and therapeutic implications of isolated seric soluble cryptococcal antigen (SSCA) in

AIDS patients. *East Paris CISIH Group. Eighth International Conference on AIDS*, Amsterdam, The Netherlands, Abst. POB3205, Vol. 2: B121.

Denning DW, Tucker RM, Hanson LH *et al.* (1989). Itraconazole therapy for cryptococcal meningitis and cryptococcosis. *Arch Intern Med* **149**: 2301–8.

Denning DW, Armstrong RW Lewis BH *et al.* (1991). Elevated cerebrospinal fluid pressures in patients with cryptococcal meningitis and acquired immunodeficiency syndrome. *Am J Med* **91**: 267–72.

Desmet P, Kayembe KD, De Vroey C. (1989). The value of cryptococcal serum antigen screening among HIV-positive/AIDS patients in Kinshasa, Zaire. *AIDS* **3**: 77–8.

Diamond RD. (1991). The growing problem of mycoses in patients infected with the human immunodeficiency virus. *Rev Infect Dis* **13**: 480–6.

Diamond RD, Bennett JE. (1974). Prognostic factors in cryptococcal meningitis: a study in 111 cases. *Ann Intern Med* **80**: 176–81.

Dismukes WE. (1988). Cryptococcal meningitis in patients with AIDS. *J Infect Dis* **157**: 624–8.

Dismukes WE, Cloud G, Gallis HA *et al.* (1987). Treatment of cryptococcal meningitis with combination amphotericin B and flucytosine for four as compared with six weeks. *N Engl J Med* **317**: 334–7.

Dromer F, Moulignier A, Dupont B *et al.* (1995). Myeloradiculitis due to *Cryptococcus curvatus* in AIDS. *AIDS* **9**: 395–408.

Dromer F, Mathoulin S, Dupont B *et al.* (1996a). Epidemiology of cryptococcosis in France: a 9-year survey (1985–1993). *Clin Infect Dis* **23**: 82–90.

Dromer F, Mathoulin S, Dupont B *et al.* (1996b). Individual and environmental factors associated with infection due to *Cryptococcus Neoformans* serotype D. *Clin Infect Dis* **23**: 91–6.

Dykstra MA, Friedman L, Murphy JW (1977). Capsule size of *Cryptococcus neoformans*: control and relationship to virulence. *Infect Immunol* **16**: 129–35.

Fessler RD, Sobel J, Guyot L. (1998). Management of elevated intracranial pressure in patients with cryptococcal meningitis. *J Acquir Immune Defic Syndr Hum Retrovirol* **17**: 137–42.

Finazzi R, Guffanti M Cernuschi M *et al.* (1996). Unusual presentation of cryptococcosis in a patient with AIDS. *Clin Infect Dis* **22**: 709–10.

Graybill JR, Sobel J, Saag M *et al.* and the NIAID Mycoses Study Group and AIDS Cooperative Treatment Groups. (2000). Diagnosis and management of increased intracranial pressure in patients with AIDS and cryptococcal meningitis. *Clinical Infectious Diseases* 2000; **30**: 47–54.

Harrison TS, Levitz SM. (1997). Mechanisms of impaired anticryptococcal activity of monocytes from donors infected with human immunodeficiency virus. *J Infect Dis* **176**: 537–40.

Harrison TS, Nong S, Levitz SM. (1997). Induction of human immunodeficiency virus type 1 expression in monocytic cells by *Cryptococcus neoformans* and *Candida albicans*. *J Infect Dis* **176**: 485–91.

Havlir DV, Bozette SA, McCutchan JA *et al.* (1996). A double blind randomized study of weekly versus daily fluconazole for the prevention of fungal infections in AIDS-patients. In: *Program and abstracts of the Third Conference on Retroviruses and Opportunistic Infections*, Washington, DC, USA, Abstr. 268, 158.

Haubrich RH, Haghighat D, Bozzette SA *et al.* (1994). High-dose fluconazole for treatment of cryptococcal disease in patients with human immunodeficiency virus infection. *J Infect Dis* **170**: 238–42.

Hoffmann S, Stenderup J, Mathiesen LR. (1991). Low yield of screening for cryptococcal antigen by latex agglutination assay on serum and cerebrospinal fluid from Danish patients with AIDS or ARC. *Scand J Infect Dis* **23**: 697–702.

Holmberg K, Meyer RD. (1986). Fungal infections in patients with AIDS and AIDS-related complex. *Sand J Infect Dis* **18**: 179–92.

Holtom PD, Leal M, Riley K *et al.* (1990). Lack of survival benefit and frequent neurologic complications of intrathecal amphotericin B for cryptococcal meningitis. *International Conference on AIDS*.

Horn CA, Washburn RG. (1995). Anticryptococcal activity of NK cell-enriched peripheral blood lymphocytes from human immunodeficiency virus-infected subjects: responses to interleukin-2, interferon-γ and interleukin-12. *J Infect Dis* **172**: 1023–7.

Horsburgh CR, Jr, Selik RM. (1988). Extrapulmonary cryptococcosis in AIDS patients: risk factors and association with decreased survival. In: *Proceedings of the Twenty-eighth Interscience Conference on Antimicrobial Agents and Chemotherapy*, American Society for Microbiology, Washington, DC, USA.

Johnston SRD, Corbett EL, Foster O *et al.* (1992). Raised intracranial pressure and visual complications in AIDS patients with cryptococcal meningitis. *J Infect Dis* **24**: 185–9.

Joly V, Geoffray C, Reynes J *et al.* (1996). Amphotericin B in a lipid emulsion for the treatment of cryptococcal meningitis in AIDS patients. *J Antimicrob Agents Chemother* **38**: 117–26.

Kapenda K, Komichelo K, Swinne D *et al.* (1987). Meningitis due to *Cryptococcus neoformans* biovar *gattii* in a Zairian AIDS patients. *Eur J Clin Microbiol* **6**: 320–1.

Kawakami K, Tohyama M, Qifeng X *et al.* (1997). Expression of cytokines and inducible nitric oxide synthase mRNA in the lungs of mice infected with *Cryptococcus neoformans*. Effects of interleukin-12. *Infect Immunal* **65**: 1307–12.

Kida M, Abramowsky CR, Santoscoy C. (1989). Cryptococcosis of the placenta in a woman with acquired immunodeficiency syndrome. *Hum Pathol* **20**: 920–1.

Kozel TR, Mastroianni RP. (1976). Inhibition of phagocytosis by cryptococcal polysaccharide: dissociation of the attachment and ingestion phases of phagocytosis. *Infect Immunol* **14**: 62–7.

Lafont A, Wolff M, Marche C *et al.* (1987). Overwhelming myocarditis due to *Cryptococcus neoformans* in an AIDS patients. *Lancet* **ii**: 1145–6.

Larsen RA, Bozette S, McCutchan A *et al.* (1989). Persistant *Cryptococcus neoformans* infection of the prostate after successful treatment of meningitis. *Ann Intern Med* **111**: 125–8.

Larsen RA, Leal MA, Chan LS. (1990). Fluconazole compared with amphotericin B plus flucytosine for cryptococcal meningitis in AIDS. A randomized trial. *Ann Intern Med* **113**: 183–7.

Larsen RA, Bozzette SA, Jone BE *et al.* (1994). Fluconazole combined with flucytosine for treatment of cryptococcal meningitis in patients with AIDS. *Clin Infect Dis* **19**: 741–5.

Leenders ACAP, Reiss P, Portegies P *et al.* (1997). Liposomal amphotericin B (AmBisome) compared with amphotericin B both followed by oral fluconazole in the treatment of AIDS-associated cryptococcal meningitis. *AIDS* **11**: 1463–71.

Levitz SM. (1991). The ecology of *Cryptococcus neoformans* and the epidemiology of cryptococcosis. *Rev Infect Dis* **13**: 1163–9

Levitz SM, Dupont MP, Smail EH. (1994). Direct activity of human T lymphocytes and natural killer cells against *Cryptococcus neoformans*. *Infect Immunal* **62**: 194–202.

Mayanja-Kizza H, Oishi K, Mitarai S et al. (1998). Combination therapy with fluconazole and flucytosine for cryptococcal meningitis in Uganda patients with AIDS. Clinical Infectious Diseases 26: 1362–6.

Mceil JI, Kan VL. (1995). Decline in the incidence of cryptococcosis among HIV-infected patients. J Acquir Immune Defic Syndr Hum Retroviral 9: 206–8.

Menichetti F, Fiorio M, Tosti A et al. (1996). High dose fluconazole therapy for cryptococcal meningitis in patients with AIDS. Clin Infect Dis 22: 838–40.

Meyohas MC, Roux P, Bollens D et al. (1994). Pulmonary cryptococcosis: localized and disseminated infections in 27 patients with AIDS. Clin Infect Dis 21: 628–33.

Miszkiel KA, Hall-Craggs MA, Miller RF et al. (1996). The spectrum of MRI findings in CNS cryptococcosis in AIDS. Clin Radiol 51: 842–50.

Mulanovich VE, Dismukes WE, Markowitz N. (1995). Cryptococcal empyema: case report and review. Clin Infect Dis 20: 1396–8.

Murphy JW. (1991). Mechanisms of natural resistance to human pathogenic fungi. Ann Rev Microbiol 45: 509–53.

Murphy JW, Wong SC, Hidore. (1993). Direct interactions of human lymphocytes with the yeast-like organism, Cryptococcus neoformans. J Clin Invest 91: 1553–66.

Nelson MR, Bower M, Smith D et al. (1990). The value of serum cryptococcal antigen in the diagnosis of cryptococcal infection in patients infected with the human immunodeficiency virus. J Infect Dis 21: 175–81.

Nguyen MH, Barchiesi F, McGough DA et al. (1995). In vitro evaluation of combination of fluconazole and flucytosine against cryptococcus neoformans var. neoformans. Antimicrob Agents Chemother 39: 1691–5.

Nguyen M, Najvar LK, Yu CK et al (1997). Combination therapy with fluconazole and flucytosine in the murine model of cryptococcal meningitis. Antimicrob Agents Chemother 41: 1120–3.

Nightingale SD, Cal SX, Peterson DM et al (1992). Primary prophylaxis with fluconazole against systemic fungal infections in HIV-positive patients. AIDS 6: 191–4.

Oldfield EC, Garst PD, Hostettler C et al. (1990). Randomized, double-blind trial of 1- versus 4-hour amphotericin B infusion durations. Antimicrob Agents Chemother 34: 1402–6.

Patterson TF. (1997). Cryptococcosis in HIV-infected and non-infected hosts. Int J Infect Dis 1: S64–9.

Patterson TF, Andriole VT. (1989). Current concepts in cryptococcosis. Euro J Clin Microbiol Infect Dis May: 457–65.

Perfect JD. (1989). Cryptococcosis. Infect Dis Clin Nor Am 3: 77–102.

Perfect JR, Durack DT, Hamilton JD et al. (1982). Failure of ketoconazole in cryptococcal meningitis. J Am Med Assoc 247: 3349.

Perla EN, Maayan S, Miller SN et al. (1985). Disseminated cryptococcosis presenting as the adult respiratory distress syndrome. NY State J Med 12: 704–6.

Pettoello-Mantovani M, Casadevall A, Smarnworawong P et al. (1994). Enhancement of HIV type 1 infectivity in vitro by capsular polysaccharide of Cryptococcus neoformans and Haemophilus influenzae. AIDS Res Hum Retrovir 10: 1079–87.

Polak A. (1989). Melanin as a virulence factor in pathogenic fungi. Mycoses 33: 215–24.

Polsky B, Depman MR, Gold JWM et al. (1986). Intraventricular therapy of cryptococcal meningitis via a subcutaneous reservoir. Am J Med 81: 24–8.

Powderly WG. (1996). Recent advances in the management of cryptococcal meningitis in patients with AIDS. Clin Infect Dis 22: S119–23.

Powderly WG, Saag MS, Cloud GA et al. (1992). The NIAID AIDS Clinical Trials Group and the NIAID Mycoses Study Group: a controlled trial of fluconazole or amphotericin B to prevent relapse of cryptococcal meningitis in patients with the acquired immunodeficiency syndrome. N Engl J Med 326: 793–8.

Powderly WG, Cloud GA, Dismukes WE et al. (1994). Measurement of cryptococcal antigen in serum and cerebrospinal fluid: value in the management of AIDS-associated cryptococcal meningitis. Clin Infect Dis 18: 789–92.

Powderly WG, Finkelstein DM, Feinberg J et al. (1995). A randomized trial comparing fluconazole with clotrimazole troches for the prevention of fungal infections in patients with advanced human immunodeficiency virus infection. N Engl J Med 332: 700–5.

Pradier C, Bernard E, Lubick C et al. (1992). Does fluconazole prevent cryptococcal meningitis in human immunodeficiency virus-infected patients? J Infect Dis 165: 787.

Quagliarello VJ, Viscoli C, Horwitz RI. (1995). Primary prevention of cryptococcal meningitis by fluconazole in HIV-infected patients. Lancet 345: 548–52.

Ricchi E, Manfredi R, Scarani P et al. (1991). Cutaneous cryptococcosis and AIDS. J Am Acad Dermatol 25: 335–6.

Ricciardi DD, Sepkowitz DV, Berkowitz LB et al. (1986). Cryptococcal arthritis in a patient with acquired immune deficiency syndrome. Case report and review of the literature. J Rheumotol 13: 455–8.

Rubin R, Robinson PA, Knirsch AK et al. (1989). Fluconazole therapy of patients with AIDS and cryptococcal meningitis and failed conventional antifugal therapy. International Conference on AIDS.

Saag MS, Powderly WG, Cloud GA et al. (1992). Comparison of amphotericin B with fluconazole in the treatment of acute AIDS-associated cryptococcal meningitis. N Engl J Med 326: 83–9.

Saag MS, Cloud GA, Graybill JR et al. and the National Institute of Allergy and Infectious Diseases Mycoses Study Group. (1999). A comparison of Itraconazole versus Fluconazole as maintenance therapy for AIDS-associated cryptococcal meningitis. Clinical Infectious Diseases 28: 291–6.

Sacktor N, Lyles RH, Skolasky R et al. (2001). HIV-associated neurologic disease incidence changes: Multicenter AIDS Cohort Study, 1990–1998. Neurology 56: 257–60.

Sharkey PK, Graybill JR, Johnson ES et al. (1996). Amphotericin B lipid complex compared with amphotericin B in the treatment of cryptococcal meningitis in patients with AIDS. Clin Infect Dis 22: 315–21.

Singh N, Barnish MJ, Berman S et al. (1996). Low-dose fluconazole as primary prophylaxis for cryptococcal infection in AIDS patients with CD4 cell counts of <100 mm^3: demonstration of efficacy in a prospective, multicenter trial. Clin Infect Dis 23: 1282–6.

Speed B, Dunt D. (1995). Clinical and host differences between infections with the two varieties of cryptococcus neoformans. Clin Infect Dis 21: 28–34.

Sprinz E, Matias K. (1992). Cryptococcal meningitis prophylaxis with ketoconazole in patients with AIDS. International Conference on AIDS.

St Germain G, Noel G, Kwon Chung KJ. (1988). Disseminated cryptococcosis due to Cryptococcus neoformans variety gattii in a Canadian patient with AIDS. Eur J Clin Microbiol Infect Dis 7: 587–8.

Stern JJ, Hartman BJ, Sharkey P et al. (1988). Oral fluconazole therapy for patients with acquired immunodeficiency syndrome and cryptococcosis: experience with 22 patients. Am J Med 85: 477–80.

Swinne D, Nkurikiyinfura JB, Muyembe TL. (1986). Clinical isolates of *Cryptococcus neoformans* from Zaire. *Euro J Clin Microbiol* **5**: 50–1.

Torres RA. (1987). Cryptococcal mediastinitis mimicking lymphoma in the acquired immune deficiency syndrome. *Am J Med* **83**: 1004–5.

USPHS/IDSA Prevention of Opportunistic Infections Working Group. (1999). 1999 USPHS/IDSA Guidelines for the prevention of opportunistic infections in persons infected with Human Immuno deficiency Virus. *Ann Intern Med* **131**: 873–908.

van Calck M, Motte S, Rickaert F *et al.*, (1988). Cryptococcal anal ulceration in a patient with AIDS. *Am J Gastroenterol* **83**: 1306–8.

van der Horst CM, Saag MS, Cloud GA *et al.* (1997). Treatment of cryptococcal meningitis associated with the acquired immunodeficiency syndrome. *N Engl J Med* **337**: 15–21.

Vecchiarelli A, Pietrella D, Dottorini M *et al.* (1994). Encapsulation of *Cryptococcus neoformans* regulates fungicidal activity and the antigen presentation process in human alveolar macrophages. *Clin Exp Immunol* **98**: 217–23.

Viard JP, Hennequin C, Fortineau N *et al.* (1995). Fulminant cryptococcal infections in HIV-infected patients on oral fluconazole. *Lancet* **345**: 118.

Woods ML, MacGinley R, Eisen DP *et al.* (1998). HIV combination therapy; partial immune restitution unmasking latent cryptococcal infection. *AIDS* **12**: 1491–4.

Wright E, Hoy JF, Street AC. (1992). Significance of cryptococcal antigenemia without CNS disease in HIV patients. *International Conference on AIDS*.

Zhang T, Kawakami K, Qureshi MH *et al.* (1997). Interleukin-12 (IL-12) and IL-18 synergistically induce the fungicidal activity of murine peritoneal exudate cells against *Cryptococcus neoformans* through production of gamma interferon by natural killer cells. *Infect Immunal* **65**: 3594–9.

Zimmerli W, Borer H, Rüttimann S. (1992). Pyomyositis and cryptococcal sepsis in an HIV-infected patient with severe granulocyte defect. *AIDS* **6**: 1399–1410.

Zuger A, Schuster M, Simberkoff MS. (1988). Maintenance amphotericin B for cryptococcal meningitis in the acquired immunodeficiency syndrome (AIDS). *Ann Intern Med* **109**: 592–3.

MITCHELL GOLDMAN AND JOE WHEAT

Candidiasis

Mucosal candidiasis has been noted to occur in up to 90% of HIV-infected persons during the course of HIV infection (Feigal *et al.*, 1991). While oropharyngeal and oesophageal candidiasis may develop during the transient severe immunosuppression associated with acute HIV infection, most often these mucosal infections occur years after HIV infection, following a significant decline in the CD4 lymphocyte count. Vaginal candidiasis may occur throughout the course of HIV infection in women and does not imply

significant immunosuppression. Candida oesophagitis most often occurs after a decline in the CD4 lymphocyte count to less than 100 cells/μl, while fluconazole-refractory mucosal candidiasis is usually restricted to patients with severe immunological dysfunction, as indicated by CD4 lymphocyte counts of less than 50 cells/μl (Figure 28.1). While patients benefiting from effective antiretroviral therapies appear to have a lower incidence of mucosal candidiasis compared to those unable to access such therapies, mucosal candidiasis remains a common infection and the vast majority of patients can be treated successfully with specific therapy.

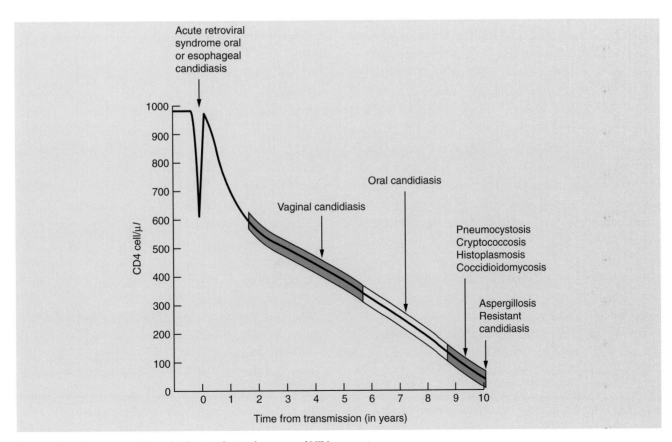

Figure 28.1 *Occurrence of fungal infections during the course of HIV progression.*

Microbiology

Candida yeast are 5–7 μm in diameter and form mycelia of varying lengths. *Torulopsis (Candida) glabrata* are smaller, 3–6 μm in diameter, and do not form mycelia. The most common species causing infection is *Candida albicans*, while infections with *Candida glabrata*, *Candida tropicalis*, *Candida parapsilosis*, *Candida kefyr*, *Candida krusei* and the recently described *Candida dublienses* (Sullivan and Coleman, 1998) occur less frequently. *Candida* are most often associated with local mucosal infections in the setting of HIV infection.

Epidemiology and transmission

Oropharyngeal candidiasis may occur in up to 90% of HIV-infected patients (Feigal *et al.*, 1991). This infection develops in most HIV-infected patients with CD4 lymphocyte counts below 200 cells/μl and recurrences are common in those with progressive immune suppression. Prior to the availability of potent antiretroviral therapy, the development of oral candidiasis was associated with significant risk for the development of subsequent opportunistic infections associated with AIDS (Katz *et al.*, 1992). Oesophageal candidiasis is an AIDS-defining illness that occurs in 10–20% of HIV-infected persons, most often when the CD4 lymphocyte count is less than 100 cells/μl. While populations unable to access antiretroviral combination therapies continue to have high rates of oropharyngeal candidiasis, recent studies have indicated that for patients treated with active antiretroviral therapies, the incidence of oral and oesophageal candidiasis appears to be declining (Hammer *et al.*, 1997; Martins *et al.*, 1997; Cameron *et al.*, 1998). Vaginal candidiasis occurs in 30–60% of women and may be diagnosed throughout the course of HIV infection. Of interest, vaginal candidiasis, unlike oropharyngeal candidiasis, does not appear to occur more frequently as the CD4 lymphocyte count declines (Schuman *et al.*, 1998).

Candida species are found throughout the environment and are part of the normal flora of the mouth, gastrointestinal tract and vagina. Infections presumably arise from colonizing organisms. Person-to-person transmission, though reported, is not believed to be a common route of transmission (Barchiesi *et al.*, 1995). Recurrent mucosal infections have occurred either due to repeated infection with the same strain or due to infection with different strain types (Powderly *et al.*, 1993).

Pathogenesis

Cellular immune mechanisms (e.g. activated macrophages) provide a defense against mucosal candida infections in healthy individuals. HIV infection is associated with a weakening of these cellular immune defenses, resulting in mucosal infections with colonizing candida organisms. Broad-spectrum antibiotics or corticosteroid therapy can also increase the risk for mucosal candidiasis in these patients. Bloodstream or disseminated infections with candida are uncommon in HIV-infected persons, as these forms of infection are chiefly controlled by granulocytes.

Clinical manifestations

Oropharyngeal candidiasis is a superficial infection of the oral mucosa. Although often asymptomatic, oral pain or alteration of taste can occur, and may result in inadequate oral nutrition. Examination most often reveals white plaques that may (if pseudomembranous) or may not (if hypertrophic) be removed by scraping (Figure 28.2, in the colour plate section). In about 25% of patients, oropharyngeal candidiasis may present as erythematous patches without plaques on the tongue, buccal mucosa or palate, which may therefore not be recognized as candidiasis. Angular cheilitis due to candida species may present as erythema and painful fissures at the corners of the mouth.

Oesophageal candidiasis occurs at a later stage of HIV infection and was noted to be an AIDS-defining illness in 14% of adult/adolescent patients in a recent surveillance study (Centers for Disease Control and Prevention, 1997). Common presenting symptoms of oesophageal candidiasis include odynophagia, dysphagia, or retrosternal pain. While one or more of these symptoms occurs in about 60% of those with endoscopically proven disease, some patients have relatively few symptoms, despite the presence of extensive oesophagitis at endoscopy (Porro *et al.*, 1989; Dupla-Lopez *et al.*, 1992). Oral thrush is present in 50%–90% of those with proven oesophagitis (Porro *et al.*, 1989; Dupla-Lopez *et al.*, 1992).

The clinical manifestations of vaginal candidiasis in HIV-infected women are similar to those described for immunocompetent women. Common complaints include vulvar itching and thick, white vaginal discharge, often accompanied by erythema of the vaginal mucosa and labia. Extension may occur to the vulva and perineum. Frequent recurrences of vaginal candidiasis have been described in HIV-infected women, though data showing that HIV-infected women are at greater risk for frequent recurrences compared to non-HIV-infected women are lacking (Shuman *et al.*, 1998).

Diagnosis

Oral candidiasis is most easily diagnosed upon examination when white pseudomembranes are visualized on the tongue, buccal mucosa, hard palate and gingivae (see Figure 28.2). Candidiasis should be distinguished from oral hairy leukoplakia, which characteristically presents as whitish-grey corrugated lesions on the lateral border of the tongue, which are not removed by scraping. Diagnosis of erythematous candidiasis by persons unfamiliar with this manifestation requires demonstration of fungal organisms by stains of mucosal scrapings using 10% KOH, Gram stain or calcofluor white staining. Fungal culture is not useful, as *candida* species are normal inhabitants of the mouth.

Candida species are the most common cause of oesophagitis in HIV-infected persons (Wilcox, 1992). In patients with advanced HIV infection, the symptoms of dysphagia and or odynophagia in the presence of oral thrush have a positive predictive value for oesophageal candidiasis from 71 to 100% (Porro *et al.*, 1989; Bonachi *et al.*, 1991). In patients with oesophageal symptoms accompanied by oral thrush, oesophageal candidiasis can be diagnosed presumptively. In these patients, the initiation of empirical antifungal therapy without endoscopic confirmation is appropriate. Endoscopy is preferred to barium oesophagography in the diagnostic evaluation of oesophageal complaints, and should be considered for patients with oesophageal symptoms in the absence of oral thrush or for those patients with persistent oesophageal symptoms despite antifungal therapy. Direct visualization of the oesophagus typically reveals whitish plaques characteristic of candida esophagitis, and the diagnosis is established by histopathological demonstration of yeasts in oesophageal brushings or biopsied material (see Figure 28.3, in the colour plate section). Oesophageal candidiasis may present as ulcerative lesions in about 25% of cases, and mucosal biopsies are preferred if ulcers or erythematous lesions are present, in order to provide material for evaluation for cytomegalovirus (CMV), herpes simplex virus (HSV) or idiopathic aphthous ulcers.

As a diagnosis of vaginal candidiasis cannot be made on the basis of vaginal symptoms alone, vaginal speculum examination and confirmation of the presence of typical pseudohyphae by 10% KOH or other fungal stains are required.

Treatment

Single episodes of mucosal candidiasis are easily treated with antifungals in the majority of patients. A variety of antifungals, including both topical and systemic agents are effective. Recurrent oropharyngeal or oesophageal candidiasis is common, particularly in those patients with CD4 lymphocyte counts of less than 100 cells/μl who have continued immunological decline. Chronic suppressive therapy may be required for patients with frequent recurrences of thrush and for patients with oesophagitis who are not expected to benefit from antiretroviral therapy. Vaginal candidiasis responds well (about 90%) to topical therapy with nystatin or azole creams (Imam *et al.*, 1990). Patients with oropharyngeal or vaginal candidiasis who do not respond to topical agents, as well as those with oesophagitis should be treated with oral azoles. Management of fluconazole-refractory candidiasis may be difficult and treatment options for this condition are discussed later in this chapter.

Oropharyngeal candidiasis

Commonly used treatments for oropharyngeal and oesophageal candidiasis are summarized in Tables 28.1 and 28.2. Topical non-absorbable clotrimazole 10 mg troches, used five times daily for 14 days resulted in a clinical response in about 85% of patients treated (Pons *et al.*, 1993). While this treatment is successful in most patients, clotrimazole is associated with a higher rate of early relapse and slower response rate when compared to fluconazole. Nystatin, a polyene used as a topical 'swish and swallow' suspension (5 ml [500 000 U] four times daily), is only effective in about 50% of patients with oropharyngeal candidiasis (Pons *et al.*, 1997) and is not recommended as first-line therapy.

A significant proportion of patients with oropharyngeal candidiasis will not respond to the topical therapies listed above. The inferior success rate associated with these topical therapies may be due to the need for frequent dosing, lack of palatability or reduced efficacy secondary to advanced immunosuppression in some patients. In patients with advanced HIV infection, treatment with the oral, systemically absorbed azole antifungals, ketoconazole, fluconazole or itraconazole (oral solution) has been quite useful.

In choosing a systemically-absorbed azole for the treatment of mucosal candidiasis in patients with HIV infection, the potential for drug interactions with the many

Table 28.1 Efficacy of therapy for candidiasis

Drug	Dose (mg/day)	% patients responding		Reference
		Oral thrush	Oesophageal candidiasis	
Clotrimazole	50	85%		Pons *et al.*, 1993
	300	100%		Lalor and Rabeneck, 1991
Ketoconazole	200	85%	65%	DeWit *et al.*, 1989
				Laine *et al.*, 1992
Fluconazole	100–200	90%	81–90%	Barbaro *et al.*, 1996
				Pons *et al.*, 1993
				Wilcox *et al.*, 1997
Itraconazole (oral solution)	100–200	90%	91%	Graybill *et al.*, 1998
				Murray *et al.*, 1997
				Wilcox *et al.*, 1997
				Phillips *et al.*, 1998

medications prescribed for HIV infection must be considered. One must also be aware that gastric acidity is required for the absorption of selected azole formulations.

Ketoconazole is an imidazole that requires gastric acidity for absorption. As it is metabolized by the cytochrome P450 enzyme system, ketoconazole may compete significantly with other drugs using this metabolic pathway. The effect of ketoconazole on medications sharing this enzyme system for metabolism is to increase the levels of the co-administered agent. On the other hand, drugs that induce this enzyme complex (e.g. rifampin, anticonvulsants) may reduce the plasma concentrations of ketoconazole.

Table 28.2 Recommendations for treatment of candidiasis

Type of infection		Drug	Induction dose (mg/day)	Duration (days)	Maintenance
Oropharyngeal	Mild	Clotrimazole	50	7–14	No
		Ketoconazole[a]	200	7–14	No
	Severe	Fluconazole	100–200	7–14	No
		Itraconazole[b] (solution)	100–200	7–14	No
	Frequently recurring	Fluconazole	100–200	14	Consider[c]
		Itraconazole[b] (solution)	100–200	14	Consider[d]
Vaginal		Clotrimazole or other azole	Topical	3–7	No
		Fluconazole	150	1–3	No
Oesophagitis		Fluconazole	100–200	21	Consider[c]
		Itraconazole[b] (solution)	100–200	21	Consider[d]

[a]Ketoconazole requires gastric acidity for absorption and has the potential for significant interactions with medications used in the care of HIV-infected persons.
[b]Itraconazole has the potential for significant interactions with medications used in the care of HIV-infected persons.
[c]For patients unlikely to have immunological improvement from antiretroviral therapy, consider maintenance fluconazole at a dose of 200 mg three times weekly or 100 mg daily.
[d]For patients unlikely to have immunological improvement, consider from antiretroviral therapy, maintenance itraconazole solution at a doses of 100–200 mg three times weekly or 100–200 mg daily.

Interference with the metabolism of the protease inhibitors (PIs) by ketoconazole may result in threefold increases in the ritonavir or saquinavir serum concentrations, with less effect seen upon the levels of indinavir or nelfinavir (Physicians' Desk Reference®, 1999). Ketoconazole is the least expensive systemically absorbed oral azole medication and is effective for oral thrush in about 80–85% of patients (DeWit et al., 1989). While ketoconazole is effective for the majority of cases of oropharyngeal candidiasis, it is less effective than fluconazole (DeWit et al., 1989).

Fluconazole is a triazole antifungal that does not require an acid environment for absorption. Additionally, fluconazole interferes less with the metabolism of other agents using the cytochrome P450 complex than ketoconazole or itraconazole, a property that may be of particular importance in the care of HIV-infected patients. Fluconazole in oral tablet or oral suspension formulations is considered more effective then ketoconazole for the treatment of oropharyngeal candidiasis (DeWit et al., 1989), though fluconazole is more expensive than ketoconazole.

Itraconazole is a triazole agent that is associated with effects on the cytochrome P450 enzyme system similar to ketoconazole. Itraconazole capsules require gastric acidity for absorption, whereas itraconazole solution does not. Itraconazole in the capsule preparation is no more effective than ketoconazole (de Repentigny and Ratelle, 1996), and is more costly than ketoconazole in the treatment of mucosal candidiasis. For these reasons the capsule preparation of itraconazole is generally not considered useful for the treatment of mucosal candidiasis. Itraconazole as an oral solution used as a 'swish and swallow' for treatment of oropharyngeal candidiasis has efficacy equal to fluconazole, is similar in cost to fluconazole, and efficacy is not dependent upon gastric acidity (Phillips et al., 1998). For the routine management of patients with mucosal candidiasis, itraconazole oral solution does not appear to have significant advantage over fluconazole and is associated with greater potential for drug interactions. However, for the treatment of mucosal candidiasis unresponsive to fluconazole, itraconazole oral solution has been shown to be quite useful (see section on treatment of refractory candidiasis).

Oesophageal candidiasis

Although high-dose topical clotrimazole (100 mg vaginal tablets three times daily) may be effective for the treatment of oesophageal candidiasis, the systemically absorbed azoles are preferred. Either fluconazole or itraconazole oral solution, when given for a 21-day course, are both highly effective in the treatment of oesophageal candidiasis with clinical response rates above 85% (Wilcox et al., 1997). The failure rates associated with the use of ketoconazole or itraconazole capsules are considered too high to support the routine use of these medications for patients with presumed or endoscopically proven oesophageal candidiasis. Of note is that following successful treatment of candida oesophagitis, relapse as evidenced by oral thrush or symptomatic oesophagitis may occur in as many as 80% of patients within 12 weeks of stopping antifungal therapy (Smith et al., 1991). It is therefore reasonable to consider oral maintenance antifungal therapy following resolution of Candida oesophagitis, particularly in those patients who are expected to experience a further decline in immune competence.

Vaginal candidiasis

Vaginal candidiasis may be successfully treated (90% success) with topical azoles or nystatin (Imam et al., 1990). Due to the lack of comparative studies of various antifungal agents for the treatment of vaginal candidiasis in HIV-infected women, treatment recommendations for vaginal infection should in general follow those suggested for women without HIV infection (Reef et al., 1995). As HIV-infected women may experience severe infections that are unlikely to respond to short courses of topical antifungal therapy, it has been suggested that 10–14 days of topical antifungal should be used (Sobel, 1997). Due to the prolonged vaginal tissue concentrations of the antifungal drug obtained after administration of fluconazole, single-dose treatment with fluconazole 150 mg taken orally has been used successfully for vaginal candidiasis in women without HIV infection. Although not adequately studied, the use of short courses of fluconazole (1–3 days) for HIV-infected women unlikely to comply with topical therapies may be a reasonable option. Treatment with the systemically absorbed azoles should be avoided during pregnancy.

Continuous antifungal prophylaxis

In patients with CD4 lymphocyte counts of less than 200 cells/μl, continuous prophylaxis with fluconazole at doses ranging from 50–200 mg/day has been associated with significant reductions in the rate of oropharyngeal and oesophageal candidiasis (Nubling-Just et al., 1991; Powderly et al., 1995). In women, a reduction in vaginal candidiasis episodes, as well as oropharyngeal candidiasis, was observed with maintenance fluconazole 200 mg given once weekly (Schuman et al., 1997). Fluconazole prophylaxis, 100 mg daily, every third week (Manfredi et al., 1997) 200 mg three times a week (Singh et al., 1996) or 200 mg given daily (Powderly et al., 1995) has also been shown to reduce the incidence of cryptococcal meningitis in persons with advanced HIV disease. Long-term prophylaxis with itraconazole (200 mg/day) in geographical areas with high rates of Histoplasma capsulatum infection was associated with reductions in the rate of histoplasmosis and crypto-coccosis in patients with CD4 lymphocyte counts of less than 100 cells/μl (McKinsey et al., 1999). Itraconazole in this formulation was associated with some reduction in the rate of mucosal candidiasis but did not appear to be as efficacious as fluconazole for the prevention of candidiasis.

While chronic systemic azole prophylaxis is efficacious for the prevention of superficial mucosal and invasive fungal infections, such prophylaxis has not been associated with reduction in overall mortality or improvement in quality of life. Furthermore, such therapies are expensive and, more importantly, may be associated with the development of infections resistant to this useful class of antifungal agents (Maenza et al., 1996; Vazquez et al., 1999). Therefore, the routine use of continuous systemic azoles for prevention of mucosal candidiasis should be discouraged. For patients with advanced HIV infection suffering from frequent infections or oesophageal candidiasis who are not expected to benefit from antiretroviral therapies, the use of continuous antifungals may be appropriate.

Treatment of refractory mucosal candidiasis

The majority of HIV-infected persons with mucosal candidiasis respond well to treatment with topical antifungals or systemic antifungal azoles. Mucosal candidiasis unresponsive to conventional doses of fluconazole or other antifungals may develop in patients with advanced HIV infection. The patients at highest risk for such infections are those with profound immunosuppression, as indicated by CD4 lymphocyte counts of less than 50 cells/μl, who have also been treated for multiple recurrent episodes of oropharyngeal candidiasis (Maenza et al., 1996). Fluconazole-refractory infections are estimated to occur in about 5% of patients with late-stage HIV disease (Fichtenbaum et al., 1996; Fichtenbaum, Powderly, 1998). As these infections often occur in individuals who are debilitated, a lack of response to antifungal therapy may result in inadequate

oral intake and considerable morbidity. Candida albicans remains the most common infecting organism recovered in cases of fluconazole-refractory mucosal candidiasis, though non-albicans candida species, inherently less susceptible to fluconazole, such as C. glabrata or C. krusei, are not infrequently recovered. In patients with refractory infections, clinical relapses are often attributed to persistence of the same infecting strain of candida species. Isolates of candida species recovered from the oropharynx in patients not responding to fluconazole therapy usually show reduced susceptibility to fluconazole in vitro (Ghannoum et al., 1996; Rex et al., 1997; Walmsley et al., 2001). The minimum inhibitory concentrations (MIC) of candida species recovered from infections failing to respond to fluconazole at doses of 100 mg daily have generally been greater than 16 μg/ml, while failures of treatment with fluconazole 400 mg daily have been associated with organisms with MICs of greater than 64 μg/ml (Ghannoum et al., 1996; Rex et al., 1997).

Although there has not been consensus regarding the diagnosis of treatment-refractory oropharyngeal candidiasis, a lack of response to 7 or 14 days of treatment with fluconazole 200 mg daily, oral itraconazole 200 mg twice daily, amphotericin B oral solution 500 mg four times daily or intravenous amphotericin B at a dose of 1 mg/kg/day has been proposed to define probable or definite failure of treatment with these antifungal agents (Fichtenbaum, Powderly et al., 1998). Prior to making a diagnosis of treatment-refractory candidiasis, one must ensure that there has been adequate compliance with the prescribed antifungal regimen and review the patient's medications for the use of agents with the potential for accelerating azole metabolism (e.g. rifampin). Although treatment-refractory candidiasis is a clinical diagnosis, fungal culture and susceptibility testing has the potential to assist in the choice of antifungal agents for therapy and should be considered in this setting.

Various agents have been used in the treatment of fluconazole-refractory mucosal candidiasis (Table 28.3). The best studied treatments for fluconazole-refractory thrush have been oral itraconazole solution and amphotericin B oral solution. Itraconazole oral solution is a cyclodextrin formulation of itraconazole that achieves serum levels of itraconazole approximately 50% higher than the capsule preparation. When used as a 'swish and swallow' treatment, itraconazole solution remains in prolonged contact with the oral mucosa, possibly exerting an additional topical effect.

Table 28.3 Treatment options for fluconazole-refractory mucosal candidiasis

Medication	Dose	Use supported by controlled study
Itraconazole solution	100–200 mg twice daily, 14–28 days swish and swallow	Yes
Amphotericin B oral solution	500 mg (5 ml) four times daily, 14–28 days swish and swallow	Yes
Melaleuca oral solution	15 ml four times daily, 14–28 days swish and expel	Yes
Fluconazole (high dose)	400–800 mg daily or twice daily	No
Flucytosine	100–50 mg/kg/day given four times daily	No
Clotrimazole (topical)	100/500 mg four to five times daily	No
Gentian violet	Apply to oropharynx once (may repeat weekly as needed)	No
Parenteral amphotericin B	0.3–1.0 mg/kg/day	No

At doses of 200–400 mg daily, this preparation has resulted in clinical response in 50–60% of patients with fluconazole-refractory thrush, and patients with fluconazole-refractory oesophageal disease have also responded to this medication (Cartledge *et al.*, 1994; Phillips *et al.*, 1996; Fessel *et al.*, 1997). Amphotericin B solution given in doses of 500 mg (5 ml, swish and swallow) four times daily has resulted in response rates of 44% and was tolerated reasonably well in the treatment of fluconazole-refractory thrush (Zingman *et al.*, 1997). Melaleuca (Breath-away®), an over-the-counter mouthwash preparation derived from an Australian tea leaf and having documented *in vitro* antifungal activity, was effective in seven of 12 patients with fluconazole-refractory thrush and may represent another potentially useful treatment option (Jandourek *et al.*, 1998). Other less well-studied oral preparations for the treatment of fluconazole-refractory infections have included higher doses of fluconazole (Ansari *et al.*, 1991; Revankar *et al.*, 1997) and the use of flucytosine alone, topical high-dose oral clotrimazole or topically applied gentian violet (anecdotal evidence only). For patients with infections unresponsive to oral therapies, amphotericin B given intravenously at a doses of 0.3–1.0 mg/kg may be useful. Unfortunately, relapse has been common following a successful treatment course and maintenance antifungal therapy is required for most patients who are not expected to benefit from any changes in their antiretroviral therapy.

Patients with fluconazole-refractory thrush. Therapies aimed at improving the immune system may also be effective. Granulocyte-macrophage colony-stimulating factor (GM-CSF), used as an adjunct to antifungal therapy, has been effective in a small number of patients with refractory candidiasis (Swindells *et al.*, 1997; Vazquez *et al.*, 1998).

Finally, the immunological improvement associated with use of combination antiretroviral therapy may result in resolution of treatment-refractory candidiasis (Zingman, 1996).

As treatment-refractory infections are associated with considerable morbidity, prevention of these infections is of importance. While exposure to fluconazole has been noted to be a risk factor for the development of mucosal candidiasis with *Candida* species resistant to fluconazole, in many patients, exposure to this agent has occurred as a result of experiencing frequent infections requiring intermittent courses of therapy. Whether intermittent treatment of episodes of mucosal candidiasis with fluconazole or continuous suppressive treatment with fluconazole results in a lower rate of fluconazole-refractory infections in patients at risk for refractory infections is unknown, and is presently an area of active study for the AIDS Clinical Trials Group and the Mycoses Study Group.

References

Ansari NM, Gould IM, Douglas JG. (1991). High dose oral fluconazole for oropharyngeal candidiasis in AIDS. *J Antimicrob Chemother* **288**: 720–1.

Barbaro G, Barbarini G, Calderon W *et al.* (1996). Fluconazole versus itraconazole for Candida esophagitis in acquired immunodeficiency syndrome. *Gastroenterology* **111**: 1169–77.

Barchiesi F, Hollis RJ, Del Poeta M *et al.* (1995). Transmission of fluconazole resistant *Candida albicans* between patients with AIDS and oropharyngeal candidiasis documented by pulsed-field gel electrophoresis. *Clin Infect Dis* **21**: 561–4.

Bonachi M, Young T, Laine L. (1991) The causes of esophageal symptoms in human immunodeficiency syndrome *Arch Intern Med* **151**: 1567–72.

Cameron WD, Heath-Chiozzi M, Danner S *et al.* (1998). Randomized placebo-controlled trial of ritonavir in advanced HIV-1 disease. *Lancet* **351**: 543–9.

Cartledge JD, Midgley J, Youle M et al. (1994). Itraconazole cyclodextrin solution effective treatment for HIV-related candidosis unresponsive to other azole therapy. J Antimicrob Chemother 33: 1071–3.

Centers for Disease Control and Prevention et al. (1997). HIV/AIDS Surveillance Report 9: 18.

de Repentigny L, Ratelle J, and the Human Immunodeficiency Virus Itraconazole Ketoconazole Project Group. (1996). Comparison of itraconazole and ketoconazole in HIV-positive patients with oropharyngeal or esophageal candidiasis. Chemotherapy 42: 374–83.

DeWit S, Weerts D, Goossens H et al. (1989). Comparison of fluconazole and ketoconazole for oropharyngeal candidiasis in AIDS. Lancet i: 746–8.

Dupla-Lopez M, Sanz PM, Garcia VP et al. (1992). Clinical endoscopic, immunologic, and therapeutic aspects of oropharyngeal and esophageal candidiasis in HIV-infected patients: a survey of 114 cases. Am J Gastroenterol 87: 1771–6.

Feigal DW, Katz MH, Greenspan D et al. (1991) The prevalence of oral lesions in HIV-infected homosexual and bisexual men: three San Francisco epidemiologic cohorts. AIDS 5: 519–25.

Fessel WJ, Merril KW, Ward D et al. (1997). Itraconazole oral solution for the treatment of fluconazole-refractory oropharyngeal candidiasis in HIV-positive patients. In: Programs and abstracts of the Fourth Conference on Retroviruses and Opportunistic Infections, Washington, DC, USA.

Fichtenbaum CJ, Powderly WG. (1998). Refractory mucosal candidiasis in patients with human immunodeficiency virus. Clin Infect Dis 26: 556–65.

Fichtenbaum CJ, Koletar S, Yiannoutsos C et al. (1996). Fluconazole-resistant mucosal candidiasis in advanced HIV infection. In: Program and abstracts of the Eleventh International Conference on AIDS, Vancouver, British Columbia, Canada.

Ghannoum MA, Rex JH, Galgiari JN (1996). Susceptibility terting of fungi: current status of correlation of in vitro data with clinical outcome. J Clin Microbiol 34: 488–95.

Graybill JR, Vazquez J, Darouiche RO et al. (1998). Randomized trial of itraconazole oral solution for oropharyngeal candidiasis in HIV/AIDS patients. Am J Med 104: 33–9.

Hammer JM, Squires KE, Hughes MD et al. (1997). A controlled trial of two nucleoside analogues plus indinavir in patients with HIV infection and CD4 cell counts of 250/mm³ or less. N Engl J Med 337: 725–33.

Imam N, Carpenter CCJ, Mayer KH et al. (1990). Hierarchical pattern of mucosal Candida infections in HIV-seropositive women. Am J Med 89: 142–6.

Jandourek A, Vaishampayan JK, Vazquez JA. (1998). Efficacy of melaleuca oral solution for the treatment of fluconazole refractory oral candidiasis in AIDS patients. AIDS 12: 1033–7.

Katz M, Greenspan D, Westenhouse J et al. (1992). Progression to AIDS in HIV-infected homosexual and bisexual men with hairy leukoplakia and oral candidiasis. AIDS 6: 95–100.

Laine L, Dretler RH, Conteas CN et al. (1992). Fluconazole compared with ketoconazole for treatment of candida esophagitis in AIDS. Ann Intern Med 117: 655–60.

Lalor E, Rabeneck L. (1991). Esophageal candidiasis in AIDS: successful therapy with clotrimazole vaginal tablets taken by mouth. Dig Dis Sci 36: 279–81.

Maenza JR, Keruly JC, Moore RD et al. (1996). Risk factors for fluconazole-resistant candidiasis in human immunodeficiency virus-infected patients. J Infect Dis 173: 219–25.

Manfredi R, Mastrianni A, Coronado OV et al. (1997). Fluconazole as prophylaxis against fungal infection in patients with advanced HIV infection. Arch Intern Med 167: 64–9.

Martins MD, Lozano-Chiu M, Rex JH. (1997). Declining rates of symptomatic oropharyngeal candidiasis, carriage of Candida albicans and fluconazole-resistance in HIV patients. In: Program and abstracts of the Infectious Diseases Society of America, Thirty-fifth Annual Meeting, San Francisco, CA, USA.

McKinsey DS, Wheat LJ, Cloud GA et al. (1999). Itraconazole prophylaxis for fungal infections in patients with advanced human immunodeficiency virus infection: randomized placebo-controlled double-blind study. Clin Infect Dis 28: 1049–56.

Murray PA, Koletar S, Mallegol I et al. (1997). Itraconazole oral solution versus clotrimazole troches for the treatment of oropharyngeal candidiasis in immunocompromised patients. Clin Ther 19: 471–80.

Nubling-Just K, Gentschew G, Meibner J et al. (1991). Fluconazole prophylaxis of recurrent oral candidiasis in HIV positive patients. Eur J Clin Microbiol Infect Dis 10: 917–21.

Phillips P, Zemcov J, Mahmood W et al. (1996). Itraconazole cyclodextrin solution for fluconazole-refractory oropharyngeal candidiasis in AIDS: correlation of clinical response with in vitro susceptibility. AIDS 10: 1369–76.

Phillips P, De Beule K, Frechette G et al. (1998). A double blind comparison of itraconazole oral solution and fluconazole capsules for the treatment of oropharyngeal candidiasis in patients with AIDS. Clin Infect Dis 26: 1368–73.

Physicians' Desk Reference® (1999). 53rd edition. Montvale, NJ: Medical Economics Co.

Pons V, Greenspan D, Debruin M et al. (1993). Therapy for oropharyngeal candidiasis in HIV-infected patients: a randomized, prospective multicenter study of oral fluconazole versus clotrimazole troches. J AIDS 6: 1311–16.

Pons V, Greenspan D, Lozada-Nur F et al. (1997). Oropharyngeal candidiasis in patients with AIDS: randomized comparison of fluconazole versus nystatin oral suspensions. Clin Infect Dis 24: 1204–7.

Porro GB, Parente F, Massimo C. (1989). The diagnosis of esophageal candidiasis in patients with acquired immune deficiency syndrome: is endoscopy always necessary? Am J Gastroenterol 84: 143–6.

Powderly WG, Robinson K, Keath EJ et al. (1993). Molecular epidemiology of recurrent oral candidiasis in human immunodeficiency virus-positive patients: evidence for two patterns of recurrence. J Infect Dis 168: 463–6.

Powderly WG, Finkelstein DM, Feinberg J et al. (1995) A randomized trial comparing fluconazole with clotrimazole troches for the prevention of fungal infections in patients with advanced human immunodeficiency virus infection. N Engl J Med 332: 700–5.

Reef SE, Levine WC, McNeil MM et al. (1995). Treatment options for vulvovaginal candidiasis, 1993. Clin Infect Dis 20: S80–90.

Revankar SG, Dib OP, Kirkpatrick WR et al. (1997). Clinical evaluation and microbiology of fluconazole-resistant oropharyngeal candidiasis. In: Programs and abstracts of the Fourth Conference on Retroviruses and Opportunistic Infections, Washington, DC, USA.

Rex JH, Pfaller MA, Galgiani JN et al. (1997). Development of interpretive breakpoints for antifungal susceptibility testing: conceptual framework and analysis of in vitro–in vivo correlation data for fluconazole, itraconazole, and candida infections. Clin Infect Dis 24: 235–47.

Schuman P, Capps L, Peng et al. (1997). Weekly fluconazole for the prevention of mucosal candidiasis in women with HIV infection. Ann Intern Med 126: 689–96.

Schuman P, Sobel JD, Ohmit SE et al. (1998). Factors associated with oral and vaginal candidiasis among Candida colonized HIV positive and at risk HIV negative women. In: Programs and abstracts of the Fifth Conference on Retroviruses and Opportunistic Infections, Chicago, IL, USA.

Singh N, Barnish MJ, Berman S et al. (1996). Low-dose fluconazole as primary prophylaxis for cryptococcal infection in AIDS patients with CD4 counts of ≤ 100/mm³: demonstration of efficacy in a positive multicenter trial. Clin Infect Dis 23: 1282–6.

Sobel JD. (1997). Current concepts: vaginitis. N Engl J Med 337: 1896–1903.

Smith DE, Midgley J, Allan M et al. (1991). Itraconazole versus ketoconazole in the treatment of oral and oesophageal candidosis in patients infected with HIV. AIDS 5: 1367–71.

Sullivan D, Coleman D. (1998). Candida dubliniensis: characteristics and identification. J Clin Microbiol 36: 329–34.

Swindells S, Kleinschmidt DR, Hayes FA. (1997). Pilot study of adjunctive GM-CSF (yeast derived) for fluconazole-resistant oral candidiasis in HIV-1 infection. Infect Dis Clin Pract 6: 278–9.

Vazquez JA, Gupta S, Villanueva A. (1998). Potential utility of recombinant human GM-CSF as adjunctive treatment of refractory oropharyngeal candidiasis in AIDS patients. Eur J Clin Microbiol Infect Dis 17: 781–3.

Vazquez JA, Sobel JD, Peng G et al. (1999). Evolution of vaginal Candida species recovered from human immunodeficiency virus-infected women receiving fluconazole prophylaxis: the emergence of Candida glabrata? Clin Infect Dis 28: 1025–31.

Walmsley S, King S, McGeer A, Ye Y, Richardson S (2001). Oropharyngeal candidiasis in patients with human immunodeficiency virus: correlation of clinical outcome with in vitro resistance, serum azole levels, and immunosuppression. Clin Infect Dis 32: 1554–61.

Wilcox CM. (1992). Esophageal disease in the acquired immunodeficiency syndrome: etiology, diagnosis, and management. Am J Med 92: 412–21.

Wilcox CM, Darouiche RO, Laine L et al. (1997). A randomized, double-blind comparison of itraconazole oral solution and fluconazole tablets in the treatment of esophageal candidiasis. J Infect Dis 176: 227–32.

Zingman BS. (1996). Resolution of refractory AIDS-related mucosal candidiasis after initiation of didanosine plus saquinavir. N Engl J Med 334: 1674–5.

Zingman BS, Zackin R, Wheat J et al. (1997). Amphotericin B oral suspension for fluconazole-resistant oral candidiasis in HIV-infected patients. In: Program and abstracts of the Thirty-Seventh Interscience Conference on Antimicrobial Agents and Chemotherapy, Toronto, Canada.

Histoplasmosis, aspergillosis and miscellaneous mycoses, and AIDS

29

MITCHELL GOLDMAN AND JOE WHEAT

Opportunistic fungal infections are common in patients with AIDS (see Figure 29.1). Mucocutaneous candidiasis occurs in up to 90% of these individuals during the course of HIV infection. Cryptococcal meningitis occurs in 5–10% of patients in most areas of the world and 30% of patients in parts of Africa. Histoplasmosis has been reported in 2–5% of patients with AIDS in endemic areas of the USA and Latin America, and over 20% in selected cites. Coccidioidomycosis may be seen in patients from the southwest USA and penicilliosis (caused by *Penicillium marneffei*) in those from parts of Southeast Asia and China. Other less common or rare systemic mycoses include infections with *Blastomyces dermatitidis*, *Paracoccidioides brasiliensis*, and *Sporothrix schenckii*. Aspergillosis is becoming more prevalent as a consequence of drug-induced neutropenia or corticosteroid use, and infection with a variety of moulds have been reported.

Histoplasmosis

Histoplasmosis is a serious opportunistic infection in patients with HIV infection and is the first manifestation of AIDS in most cases in endemic areas. *Histoplasma capsulatum* grows as a mould in the soil and on appropriate culture media at temperatures of less than 35°C. Hyphae bear tuberculate macroconidia, which are 8–14 μm in diameter and smaller (2–5 μm) microconidia, which are the infectious form of the organism. At temperatures above 35°C and in patients, *H. capsulatum* grows as a yeast, measuring 2–4 μm in diameter. Growth on fungal media is relatively slow, requiring incubation for 1–4 weeks before growth is visible.

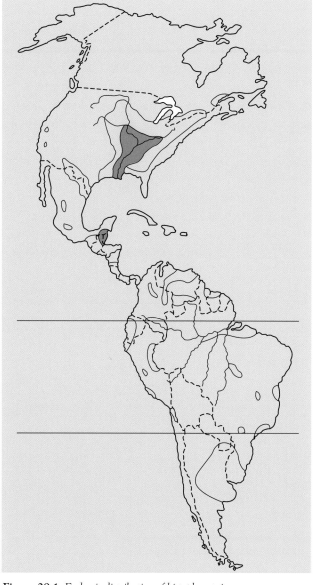

Figure 29.1 *Endemic distribution of histoplasmosis.*

Epidemiology, transmission and geographical distribution

H. capsulatum var. *capsulatum* is endemic in areas of North and Latin America (Figure 29.1) but infections occur more widely. Most cases arise in patients who live in the Ohio and Mississippi River valleys of the USA. Histoplasmosis afflicts 2–5% of patients with AIDS from endemic areas but less than 1% of those from non-endemic areas. Rates up to 25% have been observed in Indianapolis, Kansas City and Memphis (Wheat and Small, 1984). *H. capsulatum* var. *capsulatum* is localized to microfoci contaminated with bird or bat droppings. Infection occurs when aerosols contaminated with microconidia are inhaled, or when dormant infection is reactivated. Person-to-person or animal-to-person transmission does not occur.

In endemic areas, histoplasmosis is the first AIDS-defining illness in up to 85% of cases in most reports (Wheat *et al.*, 1990; McKinsey *et al.*, 1997). Risk factors for histoplasmosis in those residing in an endemic area include CD4 lymphocyte counts below 150 cells/μl, positive serological tests for antibodies to *H. capsulatum*, and a history of exposure to contaminated sites such as chicken coops (Hajjeh *et al.*, 2001). Skin-test reactivity to histoplasmin and pulmonary calcifications are not risk factors (McKinsey *et al.*, 1997).

H. capsulatum var. *duboisii* is the cause of African histoplasmosis and has been reported in patients with AIDS in that continent (Carme *et al.*, 1992). A few cases have been reported in Europe, Africa and Australia.

Many patients who have been diagnosed with histoplasmosis in non-endemic areas had previously visited or resided in areas of the world where histoplasmosis is endemic.

Pathogenesis

Infection with *H. capsulatum* develops when microconidia are inhaled and germinate into yeasts in the lungs. Cell-mediated immunity is the main defence against *H. capsulatum*; progressive haematogenous dissemination develops only in immunodeficient patients. *H. capsulatum* parasitizes macrophages, which may assist in dissemination throughout the reticulo-endothelial system. With development of specific cell-mediated immunity, cytokines arm macrophages and other cellular defense mechanisms to kill the fungus and halt progression of the disease. Infection progresses unchecked in patients with AIDS because of their profound cellular immunodeficiency. Cases of histoplasmosis occurring in AIDS patients from non-endemic areas represent reactivation of latent infection (Wheat and Small, 1984).

Clinical manifestations

H. capsulatum behaves as an opportunistic pathogen, causing disseminated disease in patients with AIDS. CD4 lymphocyte counts are below 100 cells/μl in most patients (Wheat *et al.*, 1990b). Occasionally, self-limited pulmonary histoplasmosis is recognized in patients with CD4 lymphocyte counts of more than 200 cells/μl.

Table 29.1 Clinical and laboratory findings in histoplasmosis

Finding	Percentage of patients	Finding	Percentage of patients
Fever	95	Antigen positive	95
Weight loss	95	Urine	95
Pneumonia	50	Serum/plasma	86
Hepatosplenomegaly	25	CSF	70
Lymphadenitis	20	Alveolar lavage	70
Meningitis	15	Culture positive	85
Septicaemia syndrome	10	Serology positive	67
Cerebritis	5	Immunodiffusion	62
Skin lesions	5	Complement fixation	63
Mucosal lesions	5	Fungal stain	41
		Alveolar lavage	70
		Bone marrow	40
		Blood	30

CSF: cerebrospinal fluid.
(From Wheat *et al.*, 1990b; Wheat, 1996, with permission).

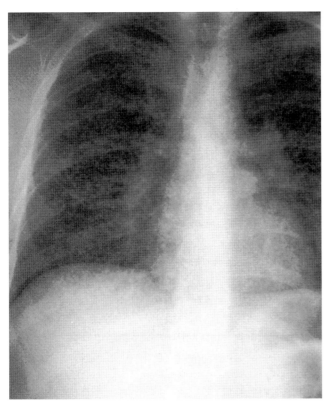

Figure 29.2 *Chest X-ray showing diffuse reticulonodular infiltrate characteristic of histoplasmosis.*

Clinical findings of disseminated histoplasmosis are non-specific and most commonly include fever and weight loss of a few months' duration (Table 29.1) (Wheat *et al.*, 1990b; Wheat, 1996). Respiratory complaints occur in half of patients and chest X-rays show diffuse infiltrates in 60% (Conces *et al.*, 1993) (Figure 29.2). A septicaemic presentation with hypotension, respiratory, renal and hepatic failure, rhabdomyolysis and coagulopathy is seen in 10% of patients. Skin manifestations, including pustular, follicular, maculopapular, and papulonecrotic lesions may be seen. Central nervous system (CNS) manifestations of meningitis, encephalitis or cerebral granulomas occur in 5–20% of cases. Unusual manifestations include pericarditis, pleuritis, chorioretinitis, pancreatitis, colonic ulcers or masses, mesenteric and omental nodules, cholecystitis, and prostatitis.

Anaemia, leucopenia and thrombocytopenia suggest bone marrow involvement in patients with histoplasmosis. Elevation of hepatic enzymes and bilirubin may be a clue to histoplasma hepatitis. Marked elevation of the lactic acid dehydrogenase (Kurtin *et al.*, 1990; Corcoran *et al.*, 1997) has been a useful but non-specific clue to the presence of histoplasmosis in patients with AIDS. Elevation of serum ferritin has also been observed in patients with disseminated histoplasmosis (Kirn *et al.*, 1995) but is not specific for histoplasmosis. Haemophagocytic syndrome has also been reported in patients with histoplasmosis (Koduri *et al.*, 1995).

Diagnosis

H. capsulatum has been isolated from blood, bone marrow and respiratory secretions in over 85% of cases. Less frequently, it also has been isolated from cerebrospinal fluid (CSF), liver, lymph nodes, skin, colonic lesions, and peritoneal fluid. However, recovery of *H. capsulatum* by culture may take up to 4 weeks.

Detection of a glycoprotein antigen in body fluids is an extremely useful method for rapid diagnosis of disseminated histoplasmosis (Figure 29.3) (Wheat *et al.*, 1990b; Wheat, 1996). Antigen detection allows diagnosis within 1 working day and permits prompt treatment. Antigen has been detected in the urine of 95% and blood of 86% of cases, and the bronchoalveolar lavage fluid and CSF of 70% of patients with pulmonary or meningeal involvement (Wheat *et al.*, 1996). Cross-reactions occur in patients with paracoccidioidomycosis, blastomycosis, penicilliosis and African histoplasmosis (*H. capsulatum* var. *duboisii*) (Wheat *et al.*, 1997b). Antigen testing is available at the Histoplasmosis Reference Laboratory in Indianapolis, IN (website: www.iupui.edu/it/histodgn; or call 1-800-HIS-TODGN in the USA, 317-630-2525 overseas or facsimile to the USA, 317 630 8605). For specimens sent by express mail, results are available within 24 h of receipt.

Histopathological staining of tissue sections or peripheral blood smears also permits rapid diagnosis (Figure 29.4, in the colour plate section). Fungal stains of tissues were positive in 41% of histoplasmosis cases in Indianapolis (Wheat *et al.*, 1990b; Williams *et al.*, 1994). *H. capsulatum* may be seen in peripheral blood smears in over one-quarter of patients with severe disease. Demonstration of high levels of anti-*H. capsulatum* antibodies may provide a clue to the diagnosis and a basis for further investigation. Antibodies are detected by immunodiffusion or complement fixation in about 70% of cases (Wheat *et al.*, 1990b).

Use of antigen detection for diagnosis of relapse

When monitoring patients for response to therapy, *Histoplasma* antigen levels should be measured in both urine and serum at 3–6 month intervals, and the current and the last prior specimen should be compared in the same assay.

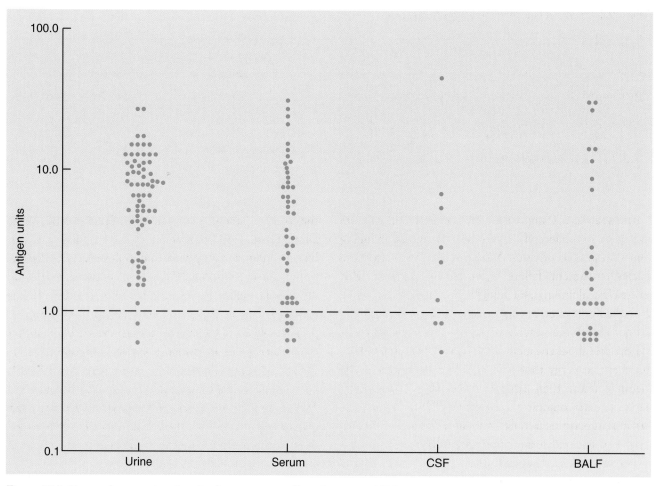

Figure 29.3 H. capsulatum *antigen detection for management of histoplasmosis in AIDS.*

Antigen concentrations in blood or urine fall with successful therapy and increase with relapse (Wheat *et al.*, 1990b, 1991, 1992, 1993, 1997a; Hecht *et al.*, 1997). Increases in antigen concentrations of more than two units suggest recurrence and support further laboratory evaluation and consideration for resumption of induction therapy. Antigen increases of more than four units are even more concerning and warrants resumption of induction therapy while waiting for the results of laboratory tests to confirm the diagnosis.

Treatment

Induction therapy

Treatment for histoplasmosis in patients with AIDS includes an induction phase to attain a clinical remission and a life-long maintenance phase to prevent relapse.

Amphotericin B is highly effective for induction treatment of histoplasmosis in patients with AIDS, inducing remission in 80% of patients (Table 29.2) (Wheat *et al.*,

1990b). Most failures occur in patients who are severely ill or have meningitis (Wheat, 1996). In patients with severe disease, mortality approaches 50%, despite amphotericin B treatment. Often renal impairment caused by histoplasmosis or amphotericin B therapy prevents administration of daily doses of 0.7 mg/kg during the critical early phase of the illness (Wheat, 1996). The newer lipid formulations of amphotericin B should be useful in such cases, allowing aggressive therapy despite renal compromise. Amphotericin B or one of its lipid formulations is the treatment of choice in patients with severe manifestations of histoplasmosis (hypotension, hypoxia pO_2 of less than 60 torr, meningitis, or high-grade laboratory abnormalities [neutrophils of fewer than 750 cells/μl, platelets of fewer than 50 000 cells/μl, hepatic enzymes more than five times normal]). Amphotericin B, 0.7–1 mg/kg/day or 3 mg/kg/day of the lipid formulations of amphotericin B should be given for 1–2 weeks, followed by treatment with itraconazole (Table 29.3).

Table 29.2 Efficacy of induction therapy for histoplasmosis

Drug	Dose	(Months)	Duration response	Reference
Amphotericin B	50 mg every second day	3	80%[a]	Wheat et al., 1990b; Wheat, 1996
Itraconazole	400 mg/day	3	85%	Wheat et al., 1995
Fluconazole	800 mg/day	3	74%	Wheat et al., 1997b

[a]Includes severe cases ineligible for azole therapy.

Itraconazole 200 mg twice daily is effective in patients with mild to moderately severe histoplasmosis, inducing remission in 85% of cases (Wheat et al., 1995). In these studies, treatment failures occurred in patients with severe clinical findings, including high-grade pancytopenia or markedly elevated hepatic enzymes and in patients who did not absorb the itraconazole. Blood concentrations of itraconazole should be measured during the second week of treatment to verify that itraconazole concentrations are adequate (more than $2 \mu g/ml$ by bioassay). The clinical response to itraconazole may be slower than it is to amphotericin B, supporting initial treatment with amphotericin B or one of its lipid formulations in patients with severe disease who require hospitalization.

Drug interactions may interfere with itraconazole's effectiveness in therapy of patients with histoplasmosis (Table 29.4). As itraconazole requires an acidic gastric pH for absorption, it should be administered with food or an acidic beverage, such as cola (Chin et al., 1995). Itraconazole blood levels were reduced about 20% by co-administration of H-2 antagonists (Stein et al., 1989), and the proton pump inhibitor omeprazole is likely to lower itraconazole concentrations as well. Omeprazole lowered ketoconazole concentrations by 80% (Chin et al., 1995) but has not been studied with itraconazole. Sucralfate had only a minimal impact on ketoconazole absorption (30% reduction with sucralfate versus 90% with H-2 antagonists) (Piscitelli et al., 1991) and would be a better choice in patients who require treatment for gastritis or ulcer disease. If patients must receive H-2 blockers or omeprazole, the cyclodextran formulation of itraconazole should be used and blood concentrations should be measured.

Itraconazole is eliminated by hepatic metabolism. Hepatic cytochrome P450 inducers (rifampin, rifabutin, phenytoin, phenobarbital) reduce intraconazole blood concentrations (Table 29.4). Itraconazole was undetectable in the blood of patients taking rifampin (Tucker et al., 1992; Drayton et al., 1994), so rifampin should be strictly avoided. Enzyme induction may persist up to 2 weeks after discontinuing the cytochrome P450 inducer, potentially delaying response to treatment or causing treatment failure. Lesser cytochrome P450 induction may occur with other agents; they should be avoided, if possible, particularly during induction therapy. If they must be given concurrently, itraconazole levels should be measured during the second week of combined therapy. Drugs that inhibit cytochrome P450 3A4, such as the protease inhibitors (PIs), may increase the blood concentrations of itraconazole. Blood concentrations of itraconazole should be measured in patients receiving concurrent treatment with PIs.

Itraconazole inhibits hepatic cytochrome P450 3A4 enzymes, and thus slows metabolism of many other drugs. This interaction increases blood concentrations of terfenadine (Seldane®), astemizole (Hismanal®), and cisapride (Propulsid®), potentially causing serious ventricular arrhythmias, and even death. Such combinations should be

Table 29.3 Recommendations for treatment of histoplasmosis

Severity	Drug	Dose	Duration
Induction phase			
Mild	Itraconazole[a]	400 mg/day	12 weeks
Severe	Amphotericin B then	50 mg/day	1–2 weeks
	Itraconazole	400 mg/day	10 weeks
Maintenance phase	Itraconazole[a]	200 mg/day	Life
		400 mg/day[2]	Life

[a]Fluconazole alternative if cannot take itraconazole, 800 mg/day induction and 400 mg/day maintenance (if itraconazole concentration is less than $4 \mu g/ml$ on 400 mg/day induction dose).

Table 29.4 Important drug interactions with azole antifungals

Cytochrome P450 enzyme inducers, which reduce ittraconazole concentration	**Reference**
Rifampin	Drayton et al., 1994
Rifabutin	Tucker et al., 1992; Blum et al., 1991
Phenytoin	Tucker et al., 1992; Ducharme et al., 1995
Carbamazepine (Tegretrol)	Tucker et al., 1992
Phenobarbital	Narang et al., 1994
Azole inhibition of cytochrome P450 enzymes delays clearance of:	
Terfenadine (Seldane)[a]	Honig et al., 1993a, b; Ahonen et al., 1995
Astemizole (Hismanal)	
Cisapride (Propulsid)	Bran et al., 1995
Triazolam (Halcion)	Varhe et al., 1994; Neuvonen et al., 1996
Midazolam (Versed)	Olkkola et al., 1994
Simvastatin (Zocor)	Horn, 1996
Lovastatin (Mevacor)	Lees and Lees, 1995; Neuvonen and Jalava, 1996
Oral hypoglycaemics	
Phenytoin	
Coumadin	Crussell-Porter et al., 1993
Digitalis	McClean and Sheehan, 1994; Sachs et al., 1993
Quinidine	
Cyclosporine	Sorenson et al., 1994; Kramer et al. 1997
Tacrolimus	Kramer et al., 1997
Rifabutin (Mycobutin)	Jalava et al., 1997
Calcium channel blockers	Tailor et al., 1996
Busulfan	Buggia et al., 1996
Vincristine	Bohme et al., 1995
Oxybutynin	Lukkari et al., 1997
Medications that impair itraconazole absorption Histamine receptor antagonists	
Cimetidine (Tagament)	Stein et al., 1989; Piscitelli et al., 1991
Ranitidine(Zantact)	Stein et al., 1989; Piscitelli et al., 1991
Famotidine (Pepcid)	Stein et al., 1989; Piscitelli et al., 1991
Nizatidine (Axid)	Stein et al., 1989; Piscitelli et al., 1991
Proton pump inhibitors	
Omeprazole (Prilosec)	Chin et al., 1995
Sucralfate (Carafate)	Piscitelli et al., 1991; Hoeschele et al., 1994

PI: protease inhibitors.
[a]These combinations must be strictly avoided because of potential for life-threatening complications.

strictly avoided. Other drugs that must be strictly avoided because of the potential for life-threatening complications include midazolam (Versed®), triazolam (Halcion®), simvastatin (Zocor®) and lovastatin (Mevacor®).

Itraconazole interactions also increase blood concentrations and toxicities of phenytoin, coumadin, oral hypoglycaemics, digitalis, tacrolimus and cyclosporin. As itraconazole also elevates the blood concentrations of some of the PIs, the dose of co-administered indinavir and riton-

avir probably should be reduced to avoid toxicities. Dose reduction is not recommended with nelfinavir or saquinavir (see also Chapters 5 and 6).

Fluconazole 800 mg daily induced remission in 74% of AIDS patients with mild to moderately severe manifestations of disseminated histoplasmosis, but nearly one-third relapsed during maintenance treatment with 400 mg daily (Wheat et al., 1997a). The poor response to fluconazole may be caused by the relatively poor in vitro activity of fluconazole for *H. capsulatum* (Wheat *et al.*, 1997a). Also, although resistance to fluconazole absorption is predictable and drug interactions that significantly reduce fluconazole concentrations are rare, fatal hepatotoxicity has been noted in a patient with markedly elevated blood concentrations (Bronstein *et al.*, 1997), supporting a recommendation to monitor blood concentrations and hepatic enzymes in patients receiving high doses of fluconazole, especially if renal function is impaired.

Ketoconazole is not an acceptable treatment for histoplasmosis in patients with AIDS. Reports from several institutions indicate that fewer than 10% of such patients respond to ketoconazole (Wheat *et al.*, 1990a; Sarosi and Johnson, 1992). Reasons for ketoconazole's ineffectiveness may include poor absorption caused by reduced gastric acidity (Lake-Bakaar *et al.*, 1988) or non-compliance due to gastrointestinal side-effects.

Treatment of meningitis

The treatment of *Histoplasma* meningitis poses special problems, and the outcome of treatment is inferior to that in patients without meningitis (Wheat *et al.*, 1990b; Wheat 1996). Itraconazole is not recommended for induction or maintenance therapy in patients with meningitis because it does not achieve adequate concentrations in the CSF. Although fluconazole is not as effective as itraconazole for treatment of histoplasmosis, its excellent penetration into CSF makes it a better choice in meningitis. Amphotericin B, 0.7–1 mg/kg/day, is recommended for induction therapy, followed by fluconazole 800 mg/day for chronic maintenance therapy. Liposomal amphotericin B (e.g. AmBisome® 3–5 mg/kg/day or every other day given over a 3–4 month period) might be considered in patients who have failed therapy with conventional amphotericin B followed by fluconazole. In animal studies, AmBisome® achieved higher concentrations in the blood and brain than did amphotericin B itself or the other lipid formulations of amphotericin B (Groll *et al.*, 1997), providing a theoretical basis for its use in meningitis. However, neither the amphotericin B lipid preparations nor conventional amphotericin B achieve detectable concentrations in CSF (Dugoni *et al.*, 1989; Groll *et al.*, 1997; Leenders *et al.*, 1997) and none have been evaluated in cases of *Histoplasma* meningitis. However, AmBisome® sterilized the CSF more rapidly than did conventional amphotericin B in patients with cryptococcal meningitis (Leenders *et al.*, 1997).

Maintenance therapy

Suppressive maintenance treatment is indicated in all patients with AIDS-related histoplasmosis who have responded to induction therapy. Relapse has occurred in 35% (Sarosi and Johnson, 1992) to 80% (Wheat *et al.*, 1990b) of patients not receiving maintenance therapy. Weekly or biweekly amphotericin B (50–100 mg) (Wheat *et al.*, 1990; McKinsey *et al.*, 1992) and itraconazole (200–400 mg/day) (Wheat *et al.*, 1993; Hecht *et al.*, 1997) are more than 90% effective as maintenance therapy (Table 29.3). Fluconazole, however, is less effective. Relapse occurred in 12% of patients receiving 100–400 mg of fluconazole for maintenance after completing induction therapy with amphotericin B in a retrospective trial (Norris *et al.*, 1992) and in 31% of those in a prospective trial receiving fluconazole 400 mg/day after successful induction therapy (Wheat *et al.*, 1997a). Itraconazole is therefore the maintenance therapy of choice (Table 29.5), with weekly amphotericin B or fluconazole 600–800 mg/day being acceptable alternatives. In patients with AIDS who have achieved a good immunological response (CD4 lymphocyte count above 150 cells/μl) to combination antiretroviral therapy, life-long maintenance therapy may not be essential, a hypothesis that requires investigation before implementation.

Prophylaxis

Patients with CD4 lymphocyte counts below 100 cells/μl should be advised to avoid activities that expose them to microfoci, which are likely to harbour *Histoplasma*, such as chicken coops, caves or bird roosts (Hajjeh, 1995; McKinsey *et al.*, 1997). Prophylaxis against histoplasmosis in people with AIDS warrants consideration in endemic regions. A trial comparing itraconazole 200 mg/day versus placebo in patients with HIV infection and CD4 lymphocyte counts below 150 cells/μl showed a two-fold reduction in the incidence of histoplasmosis in the itraconazole group (2.7% of 149 patients), compared to the placebo group (6.8% of 146 patients) after a median follow-up of 13 months (McKinsey *et al.*, 1996). All cases occurred in persons with CD4 lymphocyte counts below 100 cells/μl. Seropositivity may be a risk factor for development of histoplasmosis (McKinsey *et al.*, 1997), supporting a recommendation to measure antibodies to *H. capsulatum* in those with CD4 lymphocyte counts below 100 cells/μl and to initiate itraconazole 200 mg daily prophylactically in those with H or M bands by immunodiffusion or with complement fixation titres of 1:8 or greater.

Table 29.5 Recommendations for treatment of fungal infections in AIDS

Infection	Induction		Maintenance
	Severe	Mild	
Histoplasmosis	Amphotericin B	Itraconazole	Itraconazole
Blastomycosis	Amphotericin B	Itraconazole	Itraconazole
Coccidioidomycosis	Amphotericin B	Fluconazole or itraconazole	Fluconazole
Sporotrichosis	Amphotericin B	Itraconazole	Itraconazole
Aspergillosis	Amphotericin B	Itraconazole or voriconazole	Itraconazole
Mucormycosis	Amphotericin B	Amphotericin B	Amphotericin B
Penicilliosis	Amphotericin B	Itraconazole	Itraconazole

Histoplasmosis prophylaxis in patients with AIDS had no impact on survival, however, probably because of the excellent outcome of treatment in patients who are followed closely during clinical trials. Itraconazole failed to prevent recurrent oral candidiasis or oesophagitis, which occurred in about 15% of patients in both groups, presumably because of its inability to achieve detectable concentrations in saliva (see Chapter 28). Use of the oral solution formulation of itraconazole, which is more effective than the capsule formulation for treatment of oral and oesophageal candidiasis, should overcome this limitation. Prophylaxis should be considered in patients with CD4 lymphocyte counts below 100 cells/μl in areas with rates of histoplasmosis above five cases/100 patient-years.

Coccidioidomycosis

Coccidioidomycosis is caused by the pathogenic fungus, *Coccidioides immitis*. It is a dimorphic fungus, which grows as a mould with septate hyphae in the soil and on culture media and as an endosporulating spherule in the tissues of patients. Its growth in the soil is enhanced by bat and rodent droppings. Exposure is heaviest in the late summer and autumn, when dusty conditions exist, especially after rainy winters. Its arrow shaped arthroconidia are 2.5–4 × 6 μm in size. *C. immitis* converts to an endosporulating spherule at 37–40°C. Spherules measure 30–60 μm in diameter and contain endospores that are 2–5 μm in diameter. Growth on fungal media occurs by the fourth day and identification may be possible by the tenth day.

Epidemiology

Although infrequent, coccidioidomycosis is a serious opportunistic infection in patients with AIDS. Occurring in about 0.3% of patients with AIDS in the USA, it is 10 times more common in those who reside in the endemic regions of the arid southwestern states of the USA (Jones et al., 1995). Endemic areas of the USA include certain parts of California, Arizona, New Mexico, Texas and Utah (Jones et al., 1995). The highest rate was in Arizona (8.2%).

Of coccidioidomycosis cases occurring in patients with AIDS in the USA between 1987 and 1992, two-thirds were diagnosed in residents of endemic states while one-third occurred outside the endemic states and nearly half developed outside endemic countries (Jones et al., 1995). The surprising finding that nearly half of cases occurred in patients outside of the endemic areas emphasizes the importance of considering coccidioidomycosis in the differential diagnosis of diffuse lung disease and meningitis in any patient with AIDS and of careful documentation of prior residence or travel to endemic areas. Interestingly, black race was not found to be a risk factor for disseminated coccidioidomycosis in patients with AIDS (Jones et al., 1995), in sharp contrast to the experience in those without AIDS. Coccidioidomycosis occurs more commonly in persons with occupations or hobbies associated with exposure to soil.

Pathogenesis

Following inhalation *C. immitis* causes asymptomatic or mild respiratory illness in most healthy individuals, but severe, often fatal disease occurs regularly in patients with AIDS. Spherules rupture, releasing endospores, that cause further local spread and extrapulmonary dissemination. Cellular immunity is the key defense mechanism in coccidioidomycosis, serving to arm macrophages to halt the progression of the infection. Lacking intact cellular immunity, patients with AIDS experience severe progressive forms of the infection. While reactivation of latent disease may occur in patients with AIDS and prior coccidioidomycosis, most clinically evident infections are due to recent exogenous exposure (Ampel et al., 1993).

Clinical presentation

The mortality of disseminated coccidioidomycosis in persons with AIDS is above 60% and even higher in those with diffuse pulmonary disease or meningitis (Singh et al., 1996). A CD4 lymphocyte count below 50 cells/μl is also a poor prognosis indicator (Singh et al., 1996). Seventy per cent of patients experience pulmonary and 30% extrapulmonary illnesses (Fish et al., 1990). Common clinical findings include fatigue, fever, weight loss, night sweats, chest pain, cough, and dyspnoea. Patients may manifest CNS findings of headache and confusion or symptoms of pain at sites of bone or joint involvement. Diffuse pulmonary involvement with reticulonodular infiltrates is most common, but focal pulmonary disease occurs in one-quarter of cases. Diffuse pulmonary disease may mimic that seen in Pneumocystis carinii pneumonia (PCP).

Meningitis or other manifestations of disseminated disease may be identified in up to one-quarter of cases. CSF leucocytosis is characteristic of coccidioidal meningitis. The other most common sites of involvement include lymph nodes, liver, skin, peritoneum, kidneys, thyroid, adrenal, heart, pituitary, oesophagus and pancreas, occurring in less than 10% of cases. Cutaneous, bone and joint involvement are less common in patients with AIDS than in other individuals (Bronnimann et al., 1987).

Diagnosis

Coccidioidomycosis is diagnosed by fungal staining or culture of body fluids or tissues, and by serological testing. Examination of sputum is appropriate in patients who can produce samples (Ampel, 1992). Organisms are seen in bronchoalveolar lavage fluid in less than half to two-thirds of cases (Galgiani and Ampel, 1990; Singh et al., 1996). Blood cultures are infrequently positive (Galgiani and Ampel, 1990). Serological tests, positive in over two-thirds of cases, may give an early clue to the diagnosis (Fish et al., 1990; Singh et al., 1996). The complement fixation test is positive in 75% and the tube precipitin test in 40% of patients (Fish et al., 1990), but coccidioidin skin tests are positive in less than 20% of cases (Galgiani and Ampel, 1990; Singh et al., 1996). A positive skin test is not associated with a higher risk for development of coccidioidomycosis (Ampel et al., 1993).

Treatment

Response to treatment has been disappointing. The mortality in those with diffuse pulmonary involvement was 70% (Fish et al., 1990; Singh et al., 1996), and it was 90% in those with meningitis (Singh et al., 1996). Patients have developed coccidioidomycosis while receiving ketoconazole therapy, underscoring its lack of efficacy for this serious infection (Galgiani and Ampel, 1990). Amphotericin B 0.7–1 mg/kg/day is recommended for patients with serious, life-threatening manifestations, especially diffuse interstitial infiltrates. Fluconazole or itraconazole, at doses of at least 400 mg/day, are alternatives in those with milder illnesses (Table 29.5) (Ampel, 1992; McNeil and Ampel, 1995). Azoles would appear to be most appropriate for patients with mild illnesses and for completion of induction therapy in patients who responded to amphotericin B. Fluconazole (Galgiani et al., 1993) and itraconazole (Graybill et al., 1990; Tucker et al., 1990) are the best-studied alternatives to amphotericin B.

Chronic maintenance treatment to prevent recurrence is indicated in patients who respond to induction treatment (McNeil and Ampel, 1995). Recurrence or demonstration of active infection at autopsy in patients who have discontinued treatment supports this approach. Fluconazole or itraconazole 200–400 mg/day or amphotericin B administered weekly is recommended (Ampel, 1992; McNeil and Ampel, 1995).

Prevention

Individuals with advanced HIV infection (CD4 lymphocyte counts below 100 cells/μl) residing within the endemic area should avoid exposure to dust and soil (McNeil and Ampel, 1995). Authorities do not, however, recommend against residence within the endemic area or propose use of antifungal prophylaxis (McNeil and Ampel, 1995). A suggestion has been made to periodically monitor serological tests for antibodies to C. immitis and consider antifungal prophylaxis in those with positive results (McNeil and Ampel, 1995), based on the observation that 38% of such cases exhibited active coccidiodomycosis within the following 5 years (Arguinchona et al., 1995), but no data yet supports this approach.

Blastomycosis

Introduction

Blastomyces dermatitidis is a thermally dimorphic fungus producing mycelia with 2–10 μm dumbbell-shaped conidia at 25°C and broad-based budding yeasts varying in size from 8 to 15 μm up to 30 μm in diameter at 37°C. Although not widely recognized as an opportunistic pathogen, the cases that have been described in patients with AIDS and illnesses have been unusually severe (Pappas *et al.*, 1992).

Epidemiology

The geographical distribution of blastomycosis overlaps that of histoplasmosis. Cases primarily occur in the midwestern and southeastern USA, and the parts of New York State and Canada bordering the St Lawrence River. The natural habitat of *B. dermatitidis* has not been established, but the organism may be found in soil enriched with animal excreta. Decaying organic matter is needed to support the growth of the organism in the soil. Rare isolations from soil have occurred in samples from areas inhabited by farm animals and from beaver lodges or dams.

Pathogenesis

Disease is acquired by inhaling conidia, which cause local pulmonary infection, often accompanied by extrapulmonary dissemination. Neutrophils are recruited first to sites of infection but lymphocytes arrive later, leading to pyogranuloma formation. Cellular immunity is less important for defence against *B. dermatitidis* than other endemic mycoses but does play a role in recovery from blastomycosis. The importance of cellular immunity has also been established in animal models, which demonstrates that suppression of cellular immunity leads to progressive infection (Bradsher, 1988).

Clinical manifestations

Most cases of blastomycosis have occurred in patients with CD4 lymphocyte counts below 200 cells/μl. Clinical findings are more severe in patients with AIDS than in non-immunocompromized individuals. Patients may present with localized pulmonary involvement or with disseminated disease, each occurring in about half of patients. Patients with pulmonary blastomycosis have focal or diffuse infiltrates on chest X-rays. Bilateral nodules, cavities and pleural effusions may also be seen. CNS involvement occurs in nearly half of patients.

Widespread disseminated disease typically involves multiple organs. Sites of dissemination have included the adrenal glands, gastrointestinal tract, brain, epididymis, gall bladder, heart, kidneys, liver, lymph nodes, lungs, pituitary gland, pancreas, prostate, skin, spleen, testis and thyroid. Patients have presented with clinical findings of septicaemia, as seen with histoplasmosis. Cutaneous lesions are less common in patients with AIDS than in normal hosts, occurring in about 25% of cases (Pappas *et al.*, 1992). Meningitis or brain lesions are common (approximately 40%).

Diagnosis

Diagnosis is based on demonstration of organisms by culture or examination of tissues by fungal stains. Cultures are positive in over 90% of patients (Pappas *et al.*, 1992). *B. dermatitidis* is isolated most frequently from bronchoscopy specimens, CSF or brain, skin, and blood. Fungal stains have been positive in most cases, thus providing a more rapid diagnosis than culture. *B. dermatitides* antibodies are rarely positive and thus are not useful for diagnosis of blastomycosis (Pappas *et al.*, 1992). A cross-reacting antigen may be detected in the *H. capsulatum* antigen assay, which also provides a method for rapid diagnosis (Wheat *et al.*, 1997b). Specimens of urine, blood, or other body fluids may be submitted for testing to the Histoplasmosis Reference Laboratory in Indianapolis, Indiana (see contact details in section on diagnosis of histoplasmosis).

Treatment

Amphotericin B is a moderately effective treatment for blastomycosis in patients with AIDS. In one report, nine of 11 patients (82%) with AIDS complicated by blastomycosis responded to amphotericin B (Pappas *et al.*, 1992). Itraconazole is effective treatment for blastomycosis in the normal host (approximately 95% response) (Dismukes *et al.*, 1992) and should be useful in patients with AIDS. Fluconazole 400–800 mg/day was also moderately effective (87% response) for treatment of blastomycosis in non-immunosuppressed patients and could be used in patients who cannot be treated with itraconazole (Pappas *et al.*, 1997). The 800 mg/day dose was less well tolerated than the 400 mg/day dose and not clearly more effective; 85%, versus 89%, respectively.

These findings support the use of amphotericin B for induction treatment in patients with moderate-to-severe clinical manifestations (Table 29.5) oral itraconazole is a reasonable alternative for patients with mild disease. Relapse is common, supporting the need for chronic maintenance treatment to prevent recurrence. Itraconazole is the best choice for maintenance therapy (200–400 mg/day).

The prevalence of blastomycosis in patients with HIV infection is too low to justify prophylaxis. Persons with advanced HIV disease with CD4 lymphocyte counts below 200 cells/μl might be advised to avoid occupations or hobbies that expose them to soil in endemic areas for blastomycosis.

Sporotrichosis

Sporotrichosis is caused by the dimorphic fungus *Sporothrix schenckii*, which is found worldwide and grows as a mould in association with dead plant matter such as roses, thorns, sphagnum moss, hay, straw and wood. Cases are more common in tropical and subtropical regions, including Mexico and parts of Central and South America. Occupational or avocational exposures occur in farmers, florists, gardeners, nursery and forest workers or others who experience traumatic contact with soil or plant matter. Sporotrichosis has been reported in several patients with AIDS. Patients should be advised to use gloves when working with soil or plant matter.

Disease occurs when the mould enters the body through breaks in the skin or by inhalation. The mould then transforms into budding yeasts. Clinical findings include local ulcerations with lymphocutaneous extension, pneumonitis, and disseminated infection. Bone, joint, sinus, eye, brain and meninges have been involved with disseminated disease (Matter *et al.*, 1984; Lipstein-Kresch *et al.*, 1985; Bibler *et al.*, 1986; Fitzpatrick and Eubanks, 1988; Kurosawa *et al.*, 1988; Shaw *et al.*, 1989; Heller and Fuhrer, 1991; Keiser and Whittle, 1991; Oscherwitz and Rinaldi, 1992; Penn *et al.*, 1992; Donabedian *et al.*, 1994; Morgan and Reves, 1996; Rotz *et al.*, 1996). Meningitis appears to be an especially common complication of spororichosis in patients with AIDS (Penn *et al.*, 1992; Rotz *et al.*, 1996).

Response to treatment is variable. In patients without AIDS, itraconazole was effective in 83%, but nearly 30% of responders relapsed after treatment was stopped (Sharkey-Mathis *et al.*, 1993). Fluconazole appears to be less effective than itraconazole or amphotericin B for the treatment of sporotrichosis, including a response in 71% of

cases with lymphocutaneous disease but only 31% with osteoarticular manifestations (Kauffman *et al.*, 1996). Lymphocutaneous manifestations respond well to amphotericin B (Lipstein-Kresch *et al.*, 1985; Bibler *et al.*, 1986; Fitzpatrick and Eubanks 1988; Shaw *et al.*, 1989; Heller and Fuhrer, 1991) or itraconazole (Oscherwitz and Rinaldi, 1992; Bolao *et al.*, 1994; Morgan and Reves, 1996), but disseminated disease is often fatal, especially in those with meningitis or brain involvement (Heller and Fuhrer, 1991; Penn *et al.*, 1992; Donabedian *et al.*, 1994; Rotz *et al.*, 1996). Interestingly, skin lesions may clear despite progression of meningitis (Penn *et al.*, 1992; Rotz *et al.*, 1996). Amphotericin B is recommended for patients with severe disease and itraconazole for those with mild disease and for maintenance treatment (Table 29.5).

Paracoccidioidomycosis

Paracoccidioidomycosis, caused by the thermally dimorphic fungus, *Paracoccidioides brasilienis*, is the most prevalent systemic mycosis in Latin America. Endemic to Central and South America, its distribution is patchy. Most cases have been reported from Brazil (Goldani and Sugar, 1995). *P. brasiliensis* grows as a mould in soil that is humid and rich in protein in areas with little temperature variation, such as tropical and subtropical forests, and infection occurs when airborne spores are inhaled. Depression of cell-mediated immunity leads to progressive disseminated forms of the infection. Reactivation is also thought to occur in paracoccidioidomycosis.

Twenty-seven cases of paracoccidioidomycosis have been reported in patients with AIDS (Goldani and Sugar, 1995), and in 59%, paracoccidioidomycosis was the AIDS-defining illness. Illnesses may be indolent or rapidly progressive. Pneumonitis was present in 63% of cases, with involvement of skin in half, followed by lymph nodes in 37%. Hepatosplenomegaly and skin lesions were also common. Chest radiograms show a diffuse infiltrate in most cases. In rare cases, meningitis may complicate the course.

Paracoccidioidomycosis was diagnosed by direct microscopic examination or culture of tissues in most cases. Recently, detection of a cross-reactive antigen in urine specimens tested in the *Histoplasma* antigen assay in nearly 90% of cases illustrates the potential role of this approach for rapid diagnosis of paracoccidioidomycosis (Wheat *et al.*,

1997b). Serologic tests can also be useful for diagnosis of paracoccidioidoymcosis.

Treatment with amphotericin B was effective in two-thirds of cases of paracoccidioidomycosis (Goldani and Sugar, 1995). Trimethoprim-sulfamethoxazole (TMP–SMV), sulfonamides, or ketaconazole have also been used successfully. Itraconazole was effective in 90% of cases in patients without AIDS (Restrepo et al., 1987; Naranjo et al., 1990). Aggressive induction therapy with amphotericin B is recommended, followed by life-long maintenance therapy with itraconazole (Table 29.5).

Penicilliosis

Penicilliosis, caused by the thermally dimorphic fungus *Penicillium marneffei*, is common in those with AIDS from Southeast Asia (Thailand, and southern China, Vietnam, Indonesia, Hong Kong, Cambodia, Laos, Malaysia and Burma) (Supparatpinyo et al., 1992; Cooper, 1998; Sirisanthana and Supparatpinyo, 1998) (see also Chapter 36). While the exact environmental site of contamination is unknown, infection is associated with soil exposure and is linked to the presence of bamboo rats. Patients often live in rural areas. Delay in diagnosis may occur in cases outside the endemic areas (Jones, 1992).

Infection is acquired by inhalation and characterized by widespread dissemination (Deng et al., 1988; Supparatpinyo et al., 1992; Supparatpinyo et al., 1994; Duong, 1996; Cooper, 1998). Clinical manifestations include fever, weight loss, lymphadenopathy, hepatomegaly and anaemia (see Chapter 36). Pulmonary involvement is very common (approximately 85%), including local or diffuse infiltrates and abscesses. Cutaneous lesions occur in about 70% of cases and include papules, pustules and nodules; lesions may be mistaken for molluscum contagiosum. Bony lesions and arthritis also may occur.

Penicilliosis is diagnosed by fungal stains showing sausage-shaped yeasts or recovery of the fungus by culture of blood, bone marrow or skin lesions (Cooper 1998; Deng et al., 1988). Stains of tissues show intracellular yeasts, which may be confused with *H. capsulatum var capsulatum*. The arthroconidia of *P. marneffei* seen in the tissues of infected patients by fungal stain, however, has a central septum, which distinguishes it from the yeast phase of *H. capsulatum*. Recent studies have shown a cross-reacting urinary antigen in 94% of cases tested with the *Histoplasma* antigen assay, supporting the use of this test for rapid diagnosis

(Wheat et al., 1997b). Other methods for antigen detection (Kauffman et al., 1996) are not available for general clinical use.

Treatment with amphotericin B or itraconazole is highly effective in cases of penicilliosis (Supparatpinyo et al., 1993; Sirisanthana et al., 1998). Amphotericin B given for 2 weeks, followed by itraconazole for 10 weeks was successful in 97% of cases (Sirisanthana et al., 1998a). Relapse is common without maintenance therapy (Supparatpinyo et al., 1993). In a recent controlled trial, none of the 36 patients receiving itraconazole prophylaxis (200 mg/day) relapsed, versus nearly 60% relapsing of those given placebo (Supparatpinyo et al., 1998). Amphotericin B may be used in severely ill patients or those requiring parenteral therapy until they are well enough to receive itraconazole. Fluconazole is less active than itraconazole (Supparatpinyo et al., 1993) and is not recommended.

Aspergillosis

Aspergillus hyphae range from 2.5 to 4.5 μm in diameter, demonstrate multiple septations, and branch at 45° angles. *Aspergilli* are ubiquitous fungi, found in air, soil, decaying vegetation and food, and commonly contaminate hospital air and surfaces. Most human infections are caused by A. *fumigates* or *flavus*. No geographical pattern is recognized. Although exposure to *Aspergillus* is common, disease is rare; less than 1% of AIDS patients develop aspergillosis (Klapholz et al., 1991; Minamoto et al., 1992; Pursell et al., 1992).

Aspergillosis is typically acquired by inhaling spores and rarely by cutaneous inoculation. Mycelia invade blood vessels, causing thrombosis and ischaemic necrosis. Histoplathologically, the infection is characterized by a neutrophilic inflammatory response. Neutropenia or neutrophil dysfunction caused by myelosuppressive medications or corticosteroids contributes to the increased risk for aspergillosis in patients with AIDS.

Invasive pulmonary disease is most common, occurring in 75% of cases (Minamoto et al., 1992; Khoo and Denning, 1994; Miller et al., 1994; Nash et al., 1997; Shetty et al., 1997). Concurrent sino-orbital infection occurs in half and disseminated disease in one-third of patients (Teh et al., 1995; Mylonakis et al., 1997). Common sites of dissemination include the brain, heart and kidney, but any tissue may be involved. Chest X-rays show diffuse reticulonodular, patchy or lobar infiltrates, occasionally with cavities, pneumothorax, pleural effusion or pleural thickening.

The diagnosis can be suspected by visualization of septate hyphae in tissue by fungal stains but must be established by cultures since other moulds may resemble *Aspergillus* morphologically. Culture of respiratory secretions is not a useful diagnostic test for aspergillosis, as *Aspergillus* may colonize the airways or contaminate laboratory cultures. In one study in which *Aspergillus* was isolated from respiratory secretions of 5% of patients with AIDS, it was a mere colonizer in 90% (Pursell *et al.*, 1992). Polymerase chain reation (PCR) methods (Einsele *et al.*, 1997) and antigen detection (Verweij *et al.*, 1996) have been described but have not been validated and are not available for clinical diagnosis.

Antifungal treatment for aspergillosis is unsatisfactory (Holding *et al.*, 2000). Only 38% of AIDS patients with invasive aspergillosis responded to amphotericin B (Minamoto *et al.*, 1992). A few patients improved or stabilized during therapy, with itraconazole at doses of 400–600 mg/day (Denning *et al.*, 1991, 1994). A new azole–voriconazole–is also active against *Aspergillus*, and may prove to be an alternative to amphotericin B (Murphy *et al.*, 1997; Schwartz *et al.*, 1997). Currently, amphotericin B is the best choice for all but mild cases (Table 29.5). Itraconazole or voriconazole are alternative choices for mild cases and for chronic maintenance therapy. Of note, resistance has developed to itraconazole during therapy (Denning *et al.*, 1997), emphasizing the need to observe patients for relapse. High doses of itraconazole (800 mg/day) may be required to induce a response in some cases (Sanches *et al.*, 1995; Verweij *et al.*, 1996). Ketoconazole and fluconazole are ineffective in aspergillosis.

Mucormycosis (Zygomycosis) and other rare fungal infections

Mucormycosis, more appropriately termed zygomycosis, is caused by several different fungi belonging to the class Zygomycetes. These organisms are widely present in nature, growing as saprophytes on plant debris and in soil. They are rarely pathogenic, except in immunocompromized hosts and diabetics. Infection most commonly occurs following inhalation of spores but may result from cutaneous inoculation or ingestion. Mucor invades blood vessels, causing tissue necrosis similar to that seen in aspergillosis. The mortality is high and the typical course of the infection is rapidly progressive in immunocompromized hosts.

Over 20 cases of mucormycosis have been reported in patients with AIDS (Micozzi and Wetli, 1985; Bronnimann *et al.*, 1987; Mostaza *et al.*, 1989; Smith *et al.*, 1989; Blatt *et al.*, 1991; Ampel, 1992; Hopwood *et al.*, 1992; Vesa *et al.*, 1992; Santos *et al.*, 1994; Margolis and Epstein, 1994; Nagy-Agren *et al.*, 1995; Abril *et al.*, 1996; Blazquez *et al.*, 1996; Lee *et al.*, 1996; Pastor-Pons *et al.*, 1996; Carvalhal *et al.*, 1997; Weinberg *et al.*, 1997). Most cases have occurred in injecting drug users. Clinical manifestations have included rhinocerebral disease involving the sinuses, eye and brain, disseminated disease, oesophagitis, and localized renal infection. Although fungal stains of tissues showed broad non-septate hyphae with right-angle branching, cases were often not diagnosed until autopsy. Successful treatment requires aggressive antifungal therapy with amphotericin B and either surgical débridement of necrotic tissue or removal of the infected organ in the case of isolated renal mucormycosis. The prognosis is poor; about half of cases do not survive the infection.

Almost any fungus can cause disease in patients with AIDS. Reports of rare mycoses were reviewed by Cunliffe and Denning in 1995. These included infections with *Alternaria*, *Aureobasidium*, *Chrysosporium*, *Cryptococcus cuvatus*, *Exophiala*, *Fusarium*, *Geotrichum*, *Hanseniaspora*, *Rhinocladiella*, *Rhodotorula*, *Saccharamyces*, *Scedosporium*, *Schizophyllum*, *Sporobolomyces*, and *Trichosporon* (Cunliffe and Denning, 1995). Others have reported infection with *Penicillium chrysogenum* (Hoffman *et al.*, 1992), *Pseudallescheria* (Raffanti *et al.*, 1990), *Cladosporium* (Drabick *et al.*, 1990), *Trichophyton* (Lowinger-Seoane *et al.*, 1992; Tsang *et al.*, 1996), *Microsporum* (Lowinger-Seoane *et al.*, 1992) and *Cladophilalophora* (Brenner *et al.*, 1996).

References

Abril V, Ortega E, Segarra P *et al.* (1996). Rhinocerebral mucormycosis in a patient with AIDS: a complication of diabetic ketoacidosis following pentamidine therapy. *Clin Infect Dis* **23**: 845–6.

Ahonen J, Olkkola KT, Neuvonen PJ. (1995). Effect of itraconazole and terbinafine on the pharmacokinetics and pharmacodynamics of midazolam in healthy volunteers. *Br J Clin Pharmacol* **40**: 270–2.

Ampel NM. (1992). Coccidioidomycosis in the HIV-infected patient: diagnosis and treatment. *AIDS Reader* **Jan/Feb**: 12–16.

Ampel NM, Dols CL, Galgiani JN. (1993). Coccidioidomycosis during human immunodeficiency virus infection: results of a prospective study in a coccidioidal endemic area. *Am J Med* **94**: 235–40.

Arguinchona HL, Ampel NM, Dols CL *et al.* (1995). Persistent coccidioidal seropositivity without clinical evidence of active coccidioidomycosis in patients infected with human immunodeficiency virus. *Clin Infect Dis* **20**: 1281–5.

Bibler MR, Luber HJ, Glueck HI et al. (1986). Disseminated sporotrichosis in a patient with HIV infection after treatment for acquired factor VIII inhibitor. J Am Med Assoc 256: 3125–6.

Blatt SP, Lucey DR, DeHoff D et al. (1991). Rhinocerebral zygomycosis in a patient with AIDS. J Infect Dis 164: 215–6.

Blazquez R, Pinedo A, Cosin J et al. (1996). Nonsurgical cure of isolated cerebral mucormycosis in an intravenous drug user. Eur J Clin Microbiol Infect Dis 15: 598–9.

Blum RA, Wilton JH, Hilligoss DM et al. (1991). Effect of fluconazole on the disposition of phenytoin. Clin Pharmacol Ther 49: 420–5.

Bolao F, Podzamczer D, Ventin M et al. (1994). Efficacy of acute phase and maintenance therapy with itraconazole in an AIDS patient with sporotrichosis. Eur J Clin Microbiol Infect Dis 13: 609–12.

Bohme A, Ganser A, Hoelzer D. (1995). Aggravation of vincristine-induced nrutotoxicity by itraconazole in the treatment of adult ALL. Ann Hematol 71: 311–12.

Bradsher RW. (1988). Blastomycosis. Infect Dis Clin N Am 2: 877–98.

Bran S, Murray WA, Hirsch IB et al. (1995). Long QT syndrome during high-dose cisapride. Arch Intern Med 155: 765–8.

Brenner S, Morgan J, Rickert P et al. (1996). Cladophialophora bantiana isolated from an AIDS patient with pulmonary infiltrates. J Med Vet Mycol 34: 427–9.

Bronnimann MD, Rodney D, Adam MD et al. (1987). Coccidioidomycosis in the acquired immunodeficiency syndrome. Ann Intern Med 106: 372–9.

Bronstein JA, Gros P, Hernandez E et al. (1997). Fatal acute hepatic necrosis due to dose-dependent fluconazole hepatotoxicity. Clin Infect Dis 25: 1266–7.

Buggia I, Zecca M, Alessandrino EP et al. (1996). Itraconazole can increase systemic exposure to busulfan in patients given bone marrow transplantation. Anticancer Res 16: 2083–8.

Carme B, Itoua Ngaporo A, Ngolet A et al. (1992). Disseminated African histoplasmosis in a congolese patient with AIDS. J Med Vet Mycol 30: 245–8.

Carvalhal GF, Machado MG, Pompeo A et al. (1997). Mucormycosis presenting as a renal mass in a patient with the human immunodeficiency virus. J Urol 158: 2230–1.

Chin TWF, Loeb M, Fong IW. (1995). Effects of an acidic beverage (Coca-Cola) on absorption of ketoconazole. Antimicrob Agents Chemother 39: 1671–5.

Conces DJ, Stockberger SM, Tarver RD et al. (1993). Disseminated histoplasmosis in AIDS: findings on chest radiographs. Am J Roentgenol 160: 15–19.

Cooper CR. (1998). From bamboo rats to humans; the odyssey of Penicillium marneffei. ASM News 64: 390–7.

Corcoran GR, Al-Abdely H, Flanders CD et al. (1997). Markedly elevated serum lactate dehydrogenase levels are a clue to the diagnosis of disseminated histoplasmosis in patients with AIDS. Clin Infect Dis 24: 942–4.

Crussell-Porter LL, Rindone JP, Ford MA et al. (1993). Low-dose fluconazole therapy potentiates the hypoprothrombinemic response of warfarin sodium. Arch Intern Med 153: 102–4.

Cunliffe NA, Denning DW. (1995). Uncommon invasive mycoces in AIDS. AIDS 9: 411–20.

Deng Z, Ribas JL, Gibson DW et al. (1988). Infection caused by Penicillium marneffei in China and Southeast Asia: review of eighteen published cases and report of our more Chinese cases. Rev Infect Dis 10: 640–52.

Denning DW, Follansbee SE, Scolaro M et al. (1991). Pulmonary aspergillosis in the acquired immunodeficiency syndrome. N Engl J Med 324: 654–62.

Denning DW. Lee JY, Hostetler JS et al. (1994). NIAID Mycoses Study Group multicenter trial of oral itraconazole therapy for invasive aspergillosis. Am J Med 97: 135–44.

Denning DW, Venkateswarlu K, Oakley KL et al. (1997). Itraconazole resistance in Aspergillus fumigatus. Antimicrob Agents Chemother 41: 1364–8.

Dismukes WE, Bradsher RW, Cloud GC et al. (1992). Itraconazole therapy for blastomycosis and histoplasmosis. Am J Med 93: 489–97.

Donabedian H, O'Donnell E, Olszewski C et al. (1994). Disseminated cutaneous and meningeal sporotrichosis in an AIDS patient. Diag Microbiol Infect Dis 18: 111–15.

Drabick JJ, Gomatos PJ, Solis JB. (1990). Cutaneous cladosporiosis as a complication of skin testing in a man positive for human immunodeficiency virus. J Am Acad Dermatol 22: 135–6.

Drayton J, Dickinson G, Rinaldi MG. (1994). Co-administration of rifampin and itraconazole leads to undetectable levels of serum itraconazole. Clin Infect Dis 18: 266.

Ducharme MP, Slaughter RL, Warbasse LH et al. (1995). Itraconazole and hydroxyitraconazole serum concentrations are reduced more than tenfold by phenytoin. Clin Pharmacol Ther 58: 617–24.

Dugoni B, Guglielmo BJ, Hollander H. (1989). Amphotericin B concentration in cerebrospinal fluid of patients with AIDS and cryptococcal meningitis. Clin Pharm 8: 220–1.

Duong TA. (1996). Infection due to Penicillium marneffei, an emerging pathogen: review of 155 reported cases. Clin Infect Dis 23: 125–30.

Einsele H, Hebart H, Roller G et al. (1997). Detection and identification of fungal pathogens in blood by using molecular probes. J Clin Microbiol 35: 1353–60.

Fish DG, Ampel NM, Galgiani JN et al. (1990). Coccidioidomycosis during human immunodeficiency virus infection: a review of 77 patients. Medicine 69: 384–91.

Fitzpatrick JE, Eubanks S. (1988). Acquired immunodeficiency syndrome presenting as disseminated cutaneous sporotrichosis. Int J Dermatol 27: 406–7.

Galgiani JN, Ampel NM. (1990). Coccidiodomycosis in human immunodeficiency virus-infected patients. J Infect Dis 162: 1165–9.

Galgiani JN, Catanzero A, Cloud GA et al. (1993). Fluconazole therapy for coccidioidal meningitis. Am Intern Med 119: 28–35.

Goldani LZ, Sugar AM (1995). Paracoccidioidomycosis and AIDS: an overview. Clin Infect Dis 21: 1275–81.

Graybill JR, Stevens DA, Galgiani N et al. (1990). Itraconazole treatment of coccidioidoymcosis. Am J Med 89: 282–90.

Groll A, Giri N, Gonzalez C et al. (1997). Penetration of lipid formulations of amphotericin B into cerebrospinal fluid and brain tissue. Program and abstracts of the Thirty-seventh Interscience Conference on Antimicrobial Agents and Chemotherapy, Toronto, Canada.

Hajjeh RA (1995). Disseminated histoplasmosis in persons infected with human immunodeficiency virus. Clin Infect Dis 21: S108–10.

Hajjeh RA, Pappas PG, Henderson H et al. (2001). Multicenter case-control study of risk-factors for histoplasmosis in HIV-infected persons. Clin Infect Dis 32: 1215–20.

Hecht FM, Wheat J, Korzun AH et al. (1997). Itraconazole maintenance treatment for histoplasmosis in AIDS. A prospective, multicenter trial. J Acquir Immune Defic Syndr Hum Retrovirol 16: 100–7.

Heller HM, Fuhrer J. (1991). Disseminated sporotrichosis in patients with AIDS: case report and review of the literature. *AIDS* **5**: 1243–6.

Hoeschele JD, Roy AK, Pecoraro VL et al. (1994). *In vitro* analysis of the interaction between sucralfate and ketoconazole. *Antimicrob Agents Chemother* **38**: 319–25.

Hoffman M, Bash E, Berger SA et al. (1992). Fatal necrotizing esophagitis due to *Penicillium chrysogenum* in a patient with acquired immunodeficiency syndrome. *Eur J Clin Microbiol Infect Dis* **11**: 1158–60.

Holding KJ, Dworkin MS, Way PC et al. (2000). Aspergillosis among people infected with human immunodeficiency virus: incidence and survival. Adult and Adolescent Spectrum of HIV Disease Project. *Clin Infect Dis* **31**: 1253–7.

Honig PK, Wortham DC, Hull R et al. (1993a). Itraconazole affects single-dose terfenadine pharmacokinetics and cardiac repolarization pharmacodynamics. *J Clin Pharmacol* **33**: 1201–6.

Honig PK, Wortham DC, Zamani K et al. (1993b). The effect of fluconazole on the steady-state pharmacokinetics and electrocardiographic pharmacodynamics of terfenadine in humans. *Clin Pharmacol Ther* **53**: 630–6.

Hopwood V, Hicks DA, Thomas S et al. (1992). Primary cutaneous zygomycosis due to *Absidia corymbifera* in a patient with AIDS. *J Med Vet Mycol* **30**: 399–402.

Horn M. (1996). Co-administration of itraconazole with hypolipidemic agents may induce rhabdomyolysis in healthy individuals. *Arch Dermatol* **132**: 1254.

Jalava KM, Olkkola KT, Neuvonen PJ. (1997). Itraconazole greatly increases plasma concentrations and effects of felodipine. *Clin Pharacol Ther* **61**: 410–15.

Jones PD. (1992). *Penicillium marneffei* infection in patients infected with human immunodeficiency virus; late presentation in an area of non-endemicity. *Clin Infect Dis* **15**: 744–6.

Jones JL, Fleming PL, Ciesielski CA et al. (1995). Coccidioidomycosis among persons with AIDS in the United States. *J Infect Dis* **171**: 961–6.

Kauffman CA, Pappas PG, McKinsey DS et al. (1996). Treatment of lymphocutaneous and visceral sporotrichosis with fluconazole. *Clin Infect Dis* **22**: 46–50.

Keiser P, Whittle D. (1991). Sporotrichosis in human immunodeficiency virus-infected patients. Report of a case. *Rev Infect Dis* **13**: 1027–8.

Khoo SH, Denning DW. (1994). Invasive aspergillosis in patients with AIDS. *Clin Infect Dis* **19**: S41–8.

Kirn DH, Fredericks D, McCutchan JA et al. (1995). Marked elevation of the serum ferritin is highly specific for disseminated histoplasmosis in AIDS. *AIDS* **9**: 1204–5.

Klapholz A, Salomon N, Perlman DC et al. (1991). Aspergillosis in the acquired immunodeficiency syndrome. *Chest* **100**: 1614–18.

Koduri PR, Chundi V, Demarais P et al. (1995). Reactive hemophagocytic syndrome. A new presentation of disseminated histoplasmosis in patients with AIDS. *Clin Infect Dis* **21**: 1463–5.

Kramer MR, Merin G, Rudis E et al. (1997). Dose adjustment and cost of itraconazole prophylaxis in lung transplant recipients receiving cyclosporine and tacrolimus (FK 506). *Transplant Proc* **29**: 2657—9.

Kurosawa A, Pollock SC, Collins MP et al. (1988). *Sporothrix schenckii* endeophthalmitis in a patient with human immunodeficiency virus infection. *Arch Ophthalmol* **106**: 376–80.

Kurtin PJ, McKinsey DS, Gupta MR et al. (1990). Histoplasmosis in patients with acquired immunodeficiency syndrome; hematologic and bone marrow manifestations. *Am J Clin Pathol* **93**: 367–72.

Lake-Bakaar G, Tom W, Lake-Bakaar D et al. (1988). Gastropathy and ketoconazole malabsorption in the acquired immunodeficiency syndrome (AIDS). *Ann Intern Med* **15**: 471–3.

Lee BL, Holland GN, Glasgow BJ. (1996). Chiasmal infarction and sudden blindness caused by mucormycosis in AIDS and diabetes mellitus. *Am J Ophthalmol* **122**: 895–6.

Leenders A, Reiss P, Portegies P et al. (1997). Liposomal amphotericin B (AmBisome®) compared with amphotericin B both followed by oral fluconazole in the treatment of AIDS-associated cryptococcal meningitis. *AIDS* **11**: 1463–71.

Lees RS, Lees AM. (1995). Rhabdomyolysis from the co-administration of lovastatin and the antifungal agent itraconazole. *N Engl J Med* **333**: 664–5.

Lipstein-Kresch E, Isenberg HD, Singer C et al. (1985). Disseminated *Sporothrix schenckii* infection with arthritis in a patient with acquired immunodeficiency syndrome. *J Rheumatol* **12**: 805–8.

Lowinger-Seoane M, Torres-Rodriquez JM, Madrenys-Brunet N et al. (1992). Extensive dermatophytoses caused by *Trichophyton mentagrophytes* and *Microsporum canis* in a patient with AIDS. *Mycopathologia* **120**: 143–6.

Lukkari E. Juhakoski A, Aranko K et al. (1997). Itraconazole moderately increases serum concentrations of oxybutynin but does not affect those of the active metabolite. *Eur J Clin Pharmacol* **52**: 402–6.

Margolis PS, Epstein A. (1994). Mucormycosis esophagitis in a patient with the acquired immunodeficiency syndrome. *Am J Gastroenterol* **89**: 1990–2.

Matter SE, Bailey DM, Sexton DJ. (1984). Immune deficiency presenting as disseminated sporotrichosis. *J Okla State Med Assoc* **77**:114–17.

McClean KL, Sheehan GJ. (1994). Interaction between itraconazole and digoxin. *Clin Infect Dis* **18**: 259–60.

McKinsey DS, Gupta MR, Driks MR et al. (1992). Histoplasmosis in patients with AIDS: efficacy of maintenance amphotericin B therapy. *Am J Med* **92**: 225–7.

McKinsey D, Wheat J, Cloud G et al. (1996). Itraconazole is effective primary prophylaxis against systemic fungal infections in patients with advanced HIV infection. Program and abstracts of the Thirty-sixth Interscience Conference on Antimicrobial Agents and Chemotherapy, New Orleans, LA, USA.

McKinsey DS, Spregel RA, Hurtwager L et al. (1997). Prospective study of histoplasmosis in patients infected with human immunodefiency virus; prevention issues and management. *Clin Intect Dis* **21** (Suppl. 1): S111–13.

McNeil MM, Ampel NM. (1995). Opportunistic coccidioidomycosis in patients infected with human immunodeficiency virus, prevention issues and priorities. *Clin Infect Dis* **21**: S111–13.

Micozzi MS, Wetli CV. (1985). Intravenous amphetamine abuse, primary cerebral mucormycosis, and acquired immunodeficiency. *J Forensic Sci* **30**: 504–10.

Miller WT, Sais GJ, Frank I et al. (1994). Pulmonary aspergillosis in patients with AIDS; clinical and radiographic correlations. *Chest* **105**: 37–44.

Minamoto GY, Barlam TF, Vander Els NJ. (1992). Invasive aspergillosis in patients with AIDS. *Clin Infect Dis* **14**: 66–74.

Morgan M, Reves R. (1996). Invasive sinusitis due to *Sporothrix schenckii* in a patient with AIDS. *Clin Infect Dis* **23**: 1319–20.

Mostaza JM, Barbado FJ, Fernandez-Martin J. (1989). Cutaneoarticular mucormycosis due to *Cunninghamella bertholletiae* in a patient with AIDS. *Rev Infect Dis* **11**: 316–18.

Murphy M, Bernard EM, Ishimaru T et al. (1997). Activity of viriconazole (UK-109, 496) against clinical isolates of Aspergillus species and its effectiveness in an experimental model of invasive pulmonary aspergillosis. Antimicrob Agents Chemother 41: 696–8.

Mylonakis E, Rich J, Skolnik PR et al. (1997). Invasive Aspergillus sinusitis in patients with human immunodeficiency virus infection. Report of two cases and review. Medicine 76: 249–55.

Nagy-Agren SE, Chu P, Smith GJW et al. (1995). Zygomycosis (mucormycosis) and HIV infection, report of three cases and review. J Acquir Immune Defic Syndr Hum Retrovirol 10: 441–9.

Narang PK, Trapnell CB, Schoenfelder JR et al. (1994). Fluconazole and enhanced effect of rifabutin prophylaxis. N Engl J Med 330: 1316–17.

Naranjo MS, Trujillo M, Munera MI et al. (1990). Treatment of paracoccidioidomycosis with itraconazole. J Med Vet Mycol 28: 67–76.

Nash G, Irvine R, Kerschmann RL et al. (1997). Pulmonary aspergillosis in acquired immune deficiency syndrome. Autopsy study of an emerging pulmonary complication of human immunodeficiency virus infection. Hum Pathol 28: 1268–75.

Neuvonen PJ, Jalava KM. (1996). Itraconazole drastically increases plasma concentrations of lovastatin and lovastatin acid. Clin Pharmacol Ther 60: 54–61.

Neuvonen PJ, Varhe A, Olkkola KT. (1996). The effect of ingestion time interval on the interaction between itraconazole and triazolam. Clin Pharmacol Ther 60: 326–31.

Norris S, McKinsey D, Lancaster D et al. (1992). Retrospective evaluation of fluconazole maintenance therapy for disseminated histoplasmosis in AIDS. Program and abstracts of the Thirty-second Interscience Conference on Antimicrobial Agents and Chemotherapy, Anaheim, CA, USA.

Olkkola KT, Backman JT, Neuvonen PJ. (1994). Midazolam should be avoided in patients receiving the systemic antimycotics ketoconazole or itraconazole. Clin Pharmacol Ther 55: 481–5.

Oscherwitz S, Rinaldi MG. (1992). Disseminated sporotrichosis in a patient infected with human immunodeficiency virus. Clin Infect Dis 15: 568–9.

Pappas PG, Pottage JC, Powderly WG et al. (1992). Blastomycosis in patients with the acquired immunodeficiency syndrome. Ann Intern Med 116: 847–53.

Pappas PG, Bradsher RW, Kauffman CA et al. (1997). Treatment of blastomycosis with higher doses of fluconazole. Clin Infect Dis 25: 200–5.

Pastor-Pons E, Martinez-Leon MI, Alvarez-Bustos G et al. (1996). Isolated renal mucormycosis in two patients with AIDS. Am J Roentgenol 166: 1282–4.

Penn C, Goldstein E, Bartholomew W. (1992). Sporothrix schenckii meningitis in a patient with AIDS. Clin Infect Dis 15: 741–3.

Piscitelli SC, Goss TF, Wilton JH et al. (1991). Effects of ranitidine and sucralfate on ketoconazole bioavailability. Antimicrob Agents Chemother 35: 1765–71.

Pursell KJ, Talzak EE, Armstrong D. (1992). Aspergillus species colonization and invasive disease in patients with AIDS. Clin Infect Dis 14: 141–8.

Raffanti SP, Fyfe B, Carreiro S et al. (1990). Native valve endocarditis due to Pseudallescheria boydii in a patient with AIDS: case report and review. Rev Infect Dis 12: 993–6.

Restrepo A, Gomez I, Robledo J et al. (1987). Itraconazole in the treatment of Paracoccidioidomycosis: a preliminary report. Rev Infect Dis 9: S51–6.

Rotz L. Slater L, Scott EN et al. (1996). Disseminated sporotrichosis with meningitis in a patient with AIDS. Infect Dis Clin Pract 5: 566–8.

Sachs MK, Blanchard LM, Green PJ. (1993). Interaction of intraconazole and digoxin. Clin Infect Dis 16: 400–3.

Sanches C, Mauri E, Dalmau D et al. (1995). Treatment of cerebral aspergillosis with itraconazole; do high doses improve the prognosis? Clin Infect Dis 21: 1485–7.

Santos J, Espigado P, Romero C et al. (1994). Isolated renal mucormycosis in two AIDS patients. Eur J Clin Microbiol Infect Dis 13: 430–2.

Sarosi GA, Johnson PC. (1992). Disseminated histoplasmosis in patients infected with human immunodeficiency virus. Clin Infect Dis 14: S60–7.

Schwartz S, Milatovic D, Thiel E. (1997). Successful treatment of cerebral aspergillosis with a novel triazole (voriconazole) in a patient with acute leukaemia. Br J Hematol 97: 663–5.

Sharkey-Mathis PK, Kauffman CA, Graybill JR et al. (1993). Treatment of sporotrichosis with itraconazole. Am J Med 95: 279–85.

Shaw JC, Levinson W, Montanaro A. (1989). Sporotrichosis in the acquired immunodeficiency syndrome. J Am Acad Dermatol 21: 1145–7.

Shetty D, Giri N, Gonzalez CE et al. (1997). Invasive aspergillosis in human immunodeficiency virus infected children. Pediatr Infect Dis J 16: 216–21.

Singh VR, Smith DK, Lawrence J et al. (1996). Coccidioidomycosis in patients infected with human immunodeficiency virus: review of 91 cases at a single institution. Clin Infect Dis 23: 563–8.

Sirisanthana T, Supparatpinyo K. (1998). Epidemiology and management of penicilliosis in human immunodeficiency virus-infected patients. J Infect Dis 3: 48–53.

Sirisanthana T, Supparatpinyo K, Perriens J et al. (1998). Amphotericin B and itraconazole for treatment of disseminated Penicillium marneffei infection in human immunodeficiency virus-infected patients. Clin Infect Dis 26: 1107–10.

Smith AG, Bustamante C, Gilmor GD. (1989). Zygomycosis (absidiomycosis) in an AIDS patient. Mycopathologia 105: 7–10.

Sorenson AL, Lovdahl M, Hewitt JM et al. (1994). Effects of ketoconazole on cyclosporine metabolism in renal allograft recipients. Transplant Proc 26: 2822.

Stein AG, Daneshmend TK, Warnock D et al. (1989). The effects of H2-receptor antagonists on the pharmacokinetics of itraconazole, a new oral antifungal. Br J Clin Pharmacol 27: 105–6P.

Supparatpinyo K, Chiewchanvit S, Hirunsri P et al. (1992). Penicillium marneffei infection in patients infected with human immunodeficiency virus. Clin Infect Dis 14: 871–4.

Supparatpinyo K, Neilson KE, Merz WG et al. (1993). Response to antifungal therapy by human immunodeficiency virus-infected patients with disseminated Penicillium marneffei infections and in vitro susceptibilities of isolates from clinical specimens. Antimicrob Agents Chemother 37: 2407–11.

Supparatpinyo K, Khamwan C, Baosoung V et al. (1994). Disseminated Penicillium marneffei infection in Southeast Asia. Lancet 334: 110–13.

Supparatpinyo K, Perriens J, Nelson KE et al. (1998). A controlled trial of itraconazole to prevent relapse of Penicillium marneffei infection in patients infected with the human immunodeficiency virus. N Engl J Med 339: 1739–43.

Tailor SAN, Gupta AK, Walker SE et al. (1996). Peripheral edema dye to nifedipine–itraconazole interaction: a case report. Arch Dermatol 132: 350–2.

Teh W, Matti BS, Marisiddaiah H *et al.* (1995). Aspergillus sinusitis in patients with AIDS. Report of three cases and review. *Clin Infect Dis* **21**: 529–35.

Tsang P, Hopkins T, Jimenez-Lucho V. (1996). Deep dermatophytosis caused by *Trichophyton rubrum* in a patient with AIDS. *J Am Acad Dermatol* **34**: 1090–1.

Tucker RM, Denning DW, Dupont B *et al.* (1990). Itraconazole therapy for chronic coccidioidal meningitis. *Ann Intern Med* **112**: 108–12.

Tucker RM, Denning DW, Hanson LH *et al.* (1992). Interaction of azoles with rifampin, phenytoin, and carbamazepine: *in vitro* and clinical observations. *Clin Infect Dis* **14**: 165–74.

Varhe A, Olkkola KT, Neuvonen PJ. (1994). Oral triazolam is potentially hazardous to patients receiving systemic antimycotics ketoconazole or itraconazole. *Clin Pharmacol Ther* **56**: 601–7.

Verweij PE, Donnelly JP, Meis JFGM. (1996). High-dose itraconazole for the treatment of cerebral aspergillosis. *Clin Infect Dis* **23**: 1196–7.

Vesa J, Bielsa O, Arango O *et al.* (1992). Massive renal infarction due to mucormycosis in an AIDS patient. *Infection* **20**: 234–6.

Weinberg JM, Baxt RD, Egan CL *et al.* (1997). Mucormycosis in a patient with acquired immunodeficiency syndrome. *Arch Dermatol* **133**: 249–51.

Wheat LJ. (1996). Histoplasmosis in the acquired immunodeficiency syndrome. *Curr Top Med Mycol* **7**: 7–18.

Wheat LJ, Small CB. (1984). Disseminated histoplasmosis in the acquired immune deficiency syndrome. *Arch Intern Med* **144**: 2147–9.

Wheat LJ, Batteiger BE, Sathapatayavongs B. (1990a). Histoplasma capsulatum infections of the central nervous system. A clinical review. *Medicine* **69**: 244–60.

Wheat LJ, Connolly-Stringfield P, Baker RL *et al.* (1990b). Disseminated histoplasmosis in the acquired immune deficiency syndrome: Clinical findings, diagnosis and treatment, and review of the literature. *Medicine* **69**: 361–74.

Wheat LJ, Connolly-Stringfield P, Blair R *et al.* (1991). Histoplasmosis relapse in patients with AIDS: detection using *Histoplasma capsulatum* variety *capsulatum* antigen levels. *Ann Intern Med* **115**: 936–41.

Wheat LJ, Connolly-Stringfield P, Blair R *et al.* (1992). Effect of successful treatment with amphotericin B on *Histoplasma capsulatum* variety *capsulatum* polysaccharide antigen levels in patients with AIDS and histoplasmosis. *Am J Med* **92**: 153–60.

Wheat LJ, Hafner R, Wulfsohn M *et al.* (1993). Prevention of relapse of histoplasmosis with itraconazole in patients with the acquired immunodeficiency syndrome. *Ann Intern Med* **118**: 610–16.

Wheat LJ, Hafner R, Korzun AH *et al.* (1995). Itraconazole treatment of disseminated histoplasmosis in patients with the acquired immunodeficiency syndrome. *Am J Med* **98**: 336–42.

Wheat LJ, MaWhinney S, Hafner R *et al.* (1997a). Treatment of histoplasmosis with fluconazole in patients with acquired immunodeficiency syndrome. *Am J Med* **103**: 223–32.

Wheat LJ, Wheat H, Connolly P *et al.* (1997b). Cross-reactivity in Histoplasma capsulatum variety capsulatum antigen assays of urine samples from patients with endemic mycoses. *Clin Infect Dis* **24**: 1169–71.

Williams B, Fojtasek M, Connolly-Stringfield P *et al.* (1994). Diagnosis of histoplasmosis by antigen detection during an outbreak in Indianapolis, *In Arch Pathol Lab Med* **118**: 1205–8.

30

Cryptosporidium, Cyclospora, Isospora and microsporidial infections and AIDS

CAROLYN PETERSEN

Cryptosporidium parvum, Cyclospora cayentenensis, Isospora belli, Enterocytozoon bieneusi and *Encephalitizoon intestinalis* are oocyst or spore-producing protozoa, which cause clinically indistinguishable syndromes of mild-to-severe gastroenteritis in AIDS patients (Goodgame, 1996). These organisms are known as *Cryptosporidium* and *Cyclospora* and are suspected to be major causes of food and waterborne disease in immunocompetent as well as immunocompromised people. They have also been associated with biliary tree disease in AIDS patients (Beaugerie *et al.*, 1992; Farman *et al.*, 1994; French *et al.*, 1995; Leiva *et al.*, 1997).

In one series, *Cryptosporidium* was the most common organism identified and *coccidia* or *microsporidia* was the second most prevalent pathogen (Table 30.1) (French *et al.*, 1995). A second series of 26 AIDS patients with cholangeographic and pancreatographic changes associated with cholangitis (Farman *et al.*, 1994) found opportunistic infections with *Cryptosporidium*, *microsporidian* species or *Isospora* in 21 of them.

Table 30.1 Detection of enteric parasites and other pathogens in a histopathology examination of cholecystectomy specimens from 107 patients during 1987–1993

Pathogen(s)	No. of specimens positive
Enterocytozoon bieneusi	6
Encephalitozoon intestinalis	2
Cryptosporidium and CMV	15
Cryptosporidium only	8
Isospora belli	2
Total	33

CMV: cytomegalovirus.
(Adapted from French *et al.*, 1995.)

Cryptosporidium

Cryptosporidium is a zoonotic pathogen that infects the gastrointestinal or respiratory tracts of fish, birds, reptiles and mammals (Fayer and Ungar, 1986). Chronic cryptosporidiosis in an HIV-infected person is an AIDS-defining opportunistic infection when symptoms persist for longer than 1 month.

Epidemiology, transmission and geographical variability

Human cryptosporidiosis was first reported in 1976, but it wasn't until 1982 that *Cryptosporidium* was recognized as a major human pathogen in both immunocompetent and immunocompromised individuals (Anon., 1982a, 1982b). Infection has been reported in health-care workers and hospitalized patients, day-care centre staff and their charges, animal care workers, elderly patients in institutions, travellers and immunocompromised patients (Current *et al.*, 1983; Koch *et al.*, 1985; Combee *et al.*, 1986; Sterling *et al.*, 1986; Ravn *et al.*, 1991; Neill *et al.*, 1996).

Transmission of *Cryptosporidium* appears to be primarily by the faecal–oral route. Water- and foodborne, person-to-person and animal-to-person transmission have been described (Juranek, 1995). Only a low innoculum is required for infection (human ID_{50} of approximately 132 oocysts) (DuPont *et al.*, 1995), and some infections appear to be established with a single oocyst (Haas and Rose, 1994). Infected persons and animals may excrete large numbers of organisms, for example over $\times 10^9$ organisms/day. Oocysts may survive in the environment for months (Current, 1986), are difficult to remove from water by filtration due to their small size (4–6 μm), and are resistant to many household and institutional disinfectants, as well as the usual levels of chlorine and ozone used in water purification plants (Sundermann et al., 1987; Korich et al., 1990; Current and Garcia, 1991).

Waterborne outbreaks have been reported with increasing frequency over the past few years (D'Antonio et al., 1985; Hayes et al., 1989) culminating in the largest known outbreak, which occurred in 1993 in Madison, Wisconsin and in which over 400 000 persons acquired disease from municipal water (MacKenzie et al., 1994). In 1994, an outbreak in Las Vegas occurred in a state-of-the-art municipal system which, met all US Environmental Protection Agency standards, yet failed to detect oocysts (Goldstein et al., 1996). This outbreak indicates that transmission of C. parvum from water supplies may frequently go unrecognized. The Las Vegas outbreak was only detected due to the presence of a large AIDS population and an active surveillance system for cryptosporidiosis in Clark County, Nevada. Active surveillance systems are being established in many communities through the support of federal, state and municipal agencies.

Recreational waterborne outbreaks have been associated with chlorinated swimming pools and with commercial water recreational facilities, such as water slides and freshwater lakes (MacKenzie et al., 1995; Steiner et al., 1997; Kramer et al., 1998). Infectious C. parvum oocysts have been recovered from Eastern oysters in the Chesapeake Bay, but outbreaks of C. parvum with raw oysters identified as the vector have not yet been reported (Fayer et al., 1998). In the USA, foodborne epidemics (Anon., 1996a) have been associated with fresh apple cider made from contaminated apples (Millard et al., 1994) and milk products. Recent isolation of Cryptosporidium from vegetables from markets in Peru and Costa Rica indicate that contamination of imported fruits and vegetables is a risk (Monge and Arias, 1996; Ortega et al., 1997b).

In the USA, it has been estimated that over the course of HIV infection 10–15% of patients will develop cryptosporidiosis and 3–5% will have it as an AIDS-defining diagnosis (Soave and Johnson, 1988; Colford et al., 1996). In other countries, AIDS patients with persistent diarrhoea have an incidence of cryptosporidiosis that varies from 6 to 48%, depending on the level of development of the country (Colebunders et al., 1988; Conlon et al., 1990; Edwards et al., 1990; Dieng et al., 1994; Pape et al., 1994; Adal et al., 1996). Anecdotally, Cryptosporidium parvum isolates have been reported to vary in virulence, but very little is understood about the biological basis for this vari-

ation and its effect on disease in AIDS patients (Fayer and Ungar, 1986). Two-dimensional gel electrophoresis studies of sporozoite protein patterns from five geographically different isolates of C. parvum revealed that their protein patterns were varied, but quite similar (Mead et al., 1990).

Pathogenesis

Cryptosporidium infection is initiated when oocysts are ingested and excyst in the small bowel, just as occurs with members of the related genera Toxoplasma, Isospora, Cyclospora and Sarcocystis. Four Cryptosporidium sporozoites are released from each oocyst and initiate the asexual cycle by invading the microvillous border of gut epithelial cells. Intracellularly, sporozoites develop into meronts which release eight merozoites, the second form of Cryptosporidium, which invades gut epithelial cells. Both sexual and asexual cycles occur in the intestine, resulting in the production of fully sporulated, infectious oocysts. Human disease is primarily localized to the jejunum, but in immunocompromised patients organisms may be found throughout the epithelium of the gastrointestinal and respiratory tracts from the pharynx, sinuses and lungs to the rectum (Ungar, 1990). Histological changes in the gastrointestinal tract include villus atrophy and blunting, epithelial flattening, and inflammation of the lamina propria, characterized by infiltration of plasma cells, lymphocytes and macrophages (Godwin, 1991). When infected, the pancreatic ducts, biliary tree and gall bladder exhibit moderate-to-severe epithelial hyperplasia and mural thickening.

The mechanism by which Cryptosporidium causes diarrhoea has not been defined. As malabsorption is characteristic of cryptosporidiosis, it has been suggested that Cryptosporidium primarily causes an osmotic diarrhoea (Gillin et al., 1985). However, voluminous watery diarrhoeal stools are also a feature of cryptosporidiosis in many patients. Some have speculated that cholera-like secretion of fluids and electrolytes might be triggered by a cryptosporidial toxin (Navin and Juranek, 1984; Guarino et al., 1995). Although a toxin has not been identified, recent reports have described an increase in production of the proinflammatory cytokines tumor necrosis factor-α, interleukin-8 and GRO-α (Laurent et al., 1997; Seydel et al., 1998), as well as prostaglandins E2 and F2α (Laurent et al., 1998) by intestinal epithelial cells in the presence of C. parvum infection. Interferon-γ, intraepithelial CD4 lymphocytes, and secretory IgA appear to be important factors mediating resistance to and resolution of cryptosporidiosis (McDonald *et al.*, 1996; Culshaw, 1997; Theodos *et al.*, 1997). IL-12 prevents or mitigates the effects of *C. parvum* infection in animals when given before *C. parvum* challenge by increasing IFN-γ (Urban *et al.*, 1996).

Clinical presentation

Cryptosporidium infection in immunocompetent hosts produces diarrhoea, abdominal cramping, nausea, vomiting, low-grade fever, and anorexia after an incubation period of 2–14 days, which remits spontaneously in 4–20 days in most instances (Navin and Juranek, 1984; Wolfson *et al.*, 1985).

In AIDS patients, cryptosporidiosis may be asymptomatic or, or more usually, presents as profuse watery diarrhoea (Pitlik *et al.*, 1983a; Zar *et al.*, 1985; McGowan *et al.*, 1993). Stool volume and frequency are variable, but stool output may reach 17 litres/day. Nausea, vomiting, abdominal pain, cramping, anorexia, weight loss and marked wasting commonly accompany the diarrhoea of cryptosporidiosis in AIDS patients. Although low-grade fever may be present, high fever is unusual and suggests the presence of another infectious disease. Abnormal D-xylose and abnormalities of the 72-h faecal fat are common (Soave *et al.*, 1984; Whiteside *et al.*, 1984; Modigliani *et al.*, 1985).

In HIV-infected patients, cryptosporidiosis may resolve spontaneously (Saltzberg *et al.*, 1991), may improve with antiretroviral therapy (Greenberg *et al.*, 1989; Flanigan *et al.*, 1992; Carr *et al.*, 1998; Foudraine *et al.*, 1998), or progress rapidly (Navin and Juranek, 1984). CD4 lymphocyte numbers, B-cell mucosal immunity, and other host factors, as well as differences in virulence of *Cryptosporidium* isolates, may account for this marked variability in outcome.

The most serious extraintestinal complications of cryptosporidiosis are secondary to involvement of the gall bladder, biliary tree and pancreatic ducts (Pitlik *et al.*, 1983b; Blumberg *et al.*, 1984). At a New York Hospital it has been estimated that 15% of AIDS patients have biliary involvement (Gellin and Soave, 1992). Right upper quadrant pain, nausea, vomiting and elevated alkaline phosphatase and gamma glutamyl transpeptidase levels in the absence of elevated bilirubin and transaminase levels are features of ths complication (Gellin and Soave, 1992). Imaging studies often reveal intrahepatic strictures and irregular beading of the ducts. The common bile duct may be dilated with or without stenosis of the papilla of Vater (Teixidor *et al.*, 1991). Acalculous cholecystitis may be present. Biliary cryptosporidiosis is diagnosed by finding the organism in bile or on histological examination of tissue from the biliary tree (Blumberg *et al.*, 1984). Papillotomy may relieve pain (Cello, 1989; Teixidor *et al.*, 1991). Pulmonary cryptosporidiosis with cough has been reported, but is rare (Forgacs *et al.*, 1983; Weber *et al.*, 1992b).

Diagnosis

The modified Kinyoun iron haematoxylin staining procedure is increasingly used for the detection of gastrointestinal parasites, as it has the advantage of detecting the traditional ova and parasites (amoeba, giardia, helminth ova), as well as the *Apicomplexa* (*Cryptosporidium, Cyclospora* and *Isospora*) (Figures 30.1–30.3, all the figures appear in the colour plate section). However, specific screening for *Cryptosporidium* must be requested in many laboratories that do not use this staining procedure; it is important to know which tests are currently employed in your own institution. The 4–6 μm oocyst is easily mistaken for yeast on routine stool examination. The modified, acid-fast stains, including cold Kinyoun and modified Ziehl-Neelsen, compare well with a wide variety of detection methods that have been evaluated for *C. parvum* (Garcia *et al.*, 1983). Sensitive and specific fluorescein-labelled IgG monoclonal antibodies are commercially available (Merifluor, Meridian Diagnostics; Crypto-CEL IF, Bradsure Biologicals) as are enzyme immunoassays (Prospect, Alexon; Color Vue, LMD Laboratories) (Marshall *et al.*, 1997). Acid-fast stain and indirect immunofluorescence are more sensitive than the enzyme immunoassays and represent the preferred methods for diagnosis (Ignatius *et al.*, 1997).

Haematoxylin and eosin staining of intestinal biopsy specimens may still be necessary for diagnosis of cryptosporidiosis in some cases (Soave *et al.*, 1984; Whiteside *et al.*, 1984), although increased clinical expertise and improvement in stool diagnostics have reduced the need substantially.

An acute rise in serum IgG titre to the oocyst occurs during the transmissive stage and falls off after 3 months in normal individuals. Serum IgG is not generally useful for acute diagnosis because the symptoms are resolving by the time the antibody response occurs; however, as it detects both symptomatic and asymptomatic infection, it may prove very useful for seroepidemiological studies of disease prevalence and transmission patterns.

Treatment and prevention

There is no effective specific chemotherapy for cryptosporidiosis. A wide variety of drugs including quinine, chloroquine, efluornithine, pyrimethamine, diclazuril, spiramycin, (TMP-SMX) and octreotide have been tried without success for cryptosporidiosis. Clinical trials of paromomycin, azithromycin, and nitazoxanide have been disappointing. Bovine hyperimmune globulin is not available. Data supporting FDA approval of any therapeutic agent for cryptosporidiosis have not been generated, although there are anecdotal reports of efficacy (Tzipori et al., 1996; Nord et al., 1990; Ungar et al., 1990; Rehg, 1991; Armitage et al., 1992; Marshall and Flanigan, 1992; Fichtenbaum et al., 1993). The clinical trial for paromomycin showed that 20–25% of patients improved when placed on placebo, indicating the variable history of chronic cryptosporidiosis.

Standard antidiarrhoeal medications (opiates, diphenoxylate and loperamide) and judicious fluid and nutrition management have been helpful in the treatment of cryptosporidiosis in AIDS patients, particularly when the symptoms are mild. However, institution of highly active antiretroviral therapy (HAART) currently appears to be the single most effective way of managing the symptoms of cryptosporidiosis in this patient population. In the HAART era, there has been a marked decrease in newly reported cases of cryptosporidiosis and an improvement in the symptoms of those who had previously had symptomatic infection. Both effects have been ascribed to the improvement in immune parameters of patients on HAART. HAART should be offered to any HIV-infected patient and who has been diagnosed with cryptosporidiosis and who is not already taking it (Grube et al., 1997; Carr et al., 1998; Foudraine et al., 1998; Le Moing et al., 1998; Maggi et al., 2000).

In the absence of effective therapies for cryptosporidiosis, prevention depends on intervening in transmission. All persons infected with or exposed to the infection should be educated about the risk of transmission and the need for hygienic precautions. Immunocompromised persons should be counselled to avoid contaminated water, food and infected persons. Unfortunately, these risks are rarely apparent. At this time it would be seem wise for HIV-infected persons to avoid drinking water from lakes or rivers, including accidental ingestion associated with recreation, to avoid swimming pools used by others, and to drink distilled, properly filtered or boiled water and cooked foods where the risk of cryptosporidiosis in the water and fresh fruits and vegetables is significant (for example, in developing countries). The risk of developing cryptosporidiosis from municipal water in the USA is not known; however, some risk is thought to be present (Perz et al., 1998), even in areas where the water is filtered, and patients with severe immunodeficiency should be so advised. Boiling water for 1 min or the use of absolute 1 μm or submicron filters, preferably reverse osmosis filters, which meet the National Sanitation Foundation standard no. 53 for cyst removal (Juranek, 1995), will eliminate the risk of cryptosporidiosis. Bottled water is not regulated by industry standards and may not be free of Cryptosporidium.

Epidemiologic data suggesting that pets transmit cryptosporidiosis to humans is weak, but the evidence for transmission from calves is very strong (Juranek, 1995; Glaser et al., 1998). It is prudent for immunosuppressed patients to avoid contact with pet faeces, especially those of animals with diarrhoea or less than 6 months of age, with farm animals, with soiled nappies from children and with persons known to have diarrhoea secondary to Cryptosporidium or diarrhoea for which an aetiological agent has not been established. Enteric precautions should be implemented routinely for infected individuals with Cryptosporidium or unexplained diarrhoea, especially in a hospital setting.

Cyclospora

Cyclospora cayetanensis is an emerging cause of diarrhoea in immunocompetent persons and AIDS patients worldwide (Ortega et al., 1993; Wurtz, 1994).

Epidemiology, transmission and pathogenesis

The natural ecology, infective dose, and host range of Cyclospora cayetanensis are unknown. Epidemics of cyclosporiasis in the USA have been associated with faecal–oral transmission through contaminated water and food (Anon. 1996b, 1997; Herwaldt and Ackers, 1997; Marshall et al., 1997; Meng and Doyle, 1997; Steiner et al., 1997). A large outbreak of 1465 cases of cyclosporiasis in 1996 in 20 states, the district of Columbia and two provinces of Canada was associated with contaminated raspberries from Guatemala, stressing the importance of point source contamination of perishable foodstuffs in widespread epidemics of cyclosporiasis (Herwaldt and Ackers, 1997). Cyclospora has also been identified in vegetables from markets in Peru (Ortega et al., 1997b).

Cyclospora infections have been identified in otherwise healthy travellers to developing countries, infants and children in developing countries, children in child-care centres in the USA and AIDS patients (Ortega *et al.*, 1993; Pape *et al.*, 1994; Gascon *et al.*, 1995; Crowley *et al.*, 1996; Fryauff *et al.*, 1996; Petry *et al.*, 1997; Soave *et al.*, 1998). The relative importance of cyclosporiasis as a cause of community-acquired diarrhoea in the USA is unknown (Ooi *et al.*, 1995). Like *Cryptosporidium*, *Cyclospora* is resistant to chlorine.

Cyclospora is a common cause of diarrhoea in AIDS patients in the USA. Reasons cited for the low prevalence relative to developing countries include a lower prevalence in the population at large; confusion of *Cyclospora* on microscopy between the better-known *Cryptosporidium* and widespread use of sulfamethoxazole-trimethoprim (TMP-SMX) prophylaxis for *Pneumocystis carinii* pneumonia (PCP). In Haiti, the prevalence of *Cyclospora cayetanensis* (11%) in stools of AIDS patients with diarrhoea approximates the incidence of *Isospora belli* (12%).

Jejunal biopsies from Peruvian patients with cyclosporiasis showed an altered mucosal architecture, with shortening and widening of the intestinal villi due to diffuse oedema and infiltration by a mixed inflammatory cell infiltrate. Dilation and congestion of villous capillaries was present (Ortega *et al.*, 1997a).

Clinical presentation

Illness caused by Cyclospora is characterized by watery diarrhoea, abdominal cramping, flatulence, nausea and weight loss (Wurtz, 1994; Huang *et al.*, 1995; Ortega *et al.*, 1997a). Symptoms typically wax and wane for several weeks and may persist for several months (Huang *et al.*, 1995). *Cyclospora* may be associated with prolonged diarrhoea in both immunocompetent as well as immunocompromised populations (Berlin *et al.*, 1994).

In the Haitian study of AIDS patients, symptoms were indistinguishable from those reported in AIDS patients with isosporiasis or cryptosporidiosis. *Cyclospora*, like *Cryptosporidium*, *Isospora* and microsporidial species, may cause biliary tract disease in AIDS patients (Sifuentes-Osornio *et al.*, 1995; Goodgame, 1996).

Diagnosis

Cyclospora were recognized as a separate coccidian species in 1993 (Ortega *et al.*, 1993; Wurtz, 1994). Previously, they had been designated 'big *Cryptosporidium*' in AIDS patients and had been associated with waterborne outbreaks as 'cyanobacterium-like bodies' thought to be a form of blue–green algae. Although the morphology of the *Cyclospora* oocyst resembles *C. parvum*, the morphology of intracellular intestinal forms is similar to *Isospora* (Sun *et al.*, 1996). *Cyclospora* belongs within the *Eimeria* clade phylogenetically and may be a mammalian *Eimeria* species (Relman *et al.*, 1996; Pieniazek and Herwaldt, 1997).

Microscopic examination of stool specimens using a modified Ziehl-Neelsen technique, for example the modified Kinyoun iron haematoxylin stain, reveals spherical oocysts 8–10 μm in diameter, which are morphologically similar to, but larger than *Cryptosporidium* oocysts (Wurtz, 1994) (Figure 30.2). However, modified Ziehl-Neelson stains *Cyclospora* variably (Clark and McIntyre, 1996). Recent assessment of six different procedures that included Giemsa, trichrome, chromotrope, Gram-chromotrope, acid-fast and safranin stains indicated that heating of faecal smears prior to safranin-based staining yielded a uniform, fast, reliable and simple procedure, which was superior to acid-fast staining (Visvesvara *et al.*, 1997). *Cyclospora* oocysts autofluoresce, rendering fluorescent microscopy a rapid, sensitive and inexpensive method of diagnosis (Eberhard *et al.*, 1997).

The tissue stages of *Cyclospora* may be detected in biopsy specimens by light rather than electron microscopy using haematoxylin stain alone for 15 min (Nhieu *et al.*, 1996).

Treatment

Immunocompetent adult patients have been successfully treated with TMP-SMX (160 mg and 800 mg [one double-strength tablet] orally twice a day for 7 days) (Wurtz, 1994; Hoge *et al.*, 1995; Fryauff *et al.*, 1996; Goodgame, 1996). A three-day course of TMP-SMX in immunocompetent children resulted in a significant decrease in the duration of oocyst excretion from 12 to 5 days (Madico *et al.*, 1997). Patients with AIDS should be treated with higher doses of TMP-SMX (160 mg and 800 mg orally four times a day for 10 days), followed by TMP-SMX prophylaxis three times a week to prevent relapse (Pape *et al.*, 1994).

Isospora

Isospora belli is an uncommon cause of watery diarrhoea in travellers, immigrants from endemic areas and immunocompromised persons, especially AIDS patients in the USA. In developing nations, it is much more prevalent in both the general population and AIDS patients. Chronic

Isospora diarrhoea, like cryptosporidiosis, is an indicator disease for the diagnosis of AIDS in HIV-infected persons. As is the case with *Cyclospora* and *Cryptosporidium*, the diagnosis is usually made by examination of modified acid-fast or modified acid-fast iron haematoxylin-stained slides of stool or duodenal contents. However, intestinal biopsy may be required for diagnosis in some patients. The disease usually responds to TMP-SMX or pyrimethamine sulfadiazine, but relapse is frequent without long-term suppressive therapy.

Epidemiology and transmission

Isosporiasis was rarely reported as a cause of human disease in the USA prior to the AIDS epidemic, but it is endemic in Indochina, South America, and islands of the southwestern Pacific. Human disease is caused by *Isospora belli*, a coccidian parasite phylogenetically related to *Toxoplasma*, *Cryptosporidium*, *Cyclospora* and *Sarcocystis*. All life-cycle stages of *Isospora* and *Cryptosporidium*, unlike toxoplasma or malaria, develop in the individual host.

Isospora belli infection has been reported in less than 0.2% of AIDS patients in the USA (Forthal and Guest, 1984; Whiteside et al., 1984; Modigliani et al., 1985; Soave and Johnson, 1988) and in 15% of AIDS patients in Haiti (DeHovitz et al., 1986). Isospora was found in 12–16% of AIDS patients with chronic diarrhoea in Zaire (now the Democratic Republic of the Congo), Senegal and Zambia (Colebunders et al., 1988; Conlon et al., 1990; Dieng et al., 1994). Rates of infection in the USA may be high in groups immigrating from endemic areas (Sorvillo et al., 1990). In Los Angeles, Hispanic patients, who accounted for 17% of AIDS patients, represented 81% of AIDS patients with isosporiasis (Sorvillo et al., 1990).

Prevalence of infection was highest among patients from El Salvador and Mexico and lowest among persons with a prior history of PCP, suggesting that TMP-SMX may prevent primary infection with, or expression of, latent isosporiasis (Sorvillo et al., 1995). Chronic *Isospora* diarrhoea may occur in immunocompetent travellers, but its relative importance as a cause of chronic traveller's diarrhoea is unknown (Godiwala and Yaeger, 1987). Nonetheless, *Isospora* should be considered a hazard to the HIV-infected traveller, particularly those travelling to developing countries and who are not receiving TMP-SMX prophylaxis (Sorvillo et al., 1995).

It has been suggested that person-to-person transmission might occur via oral–anal contact (Forthal and Guest,

1984). Several lines of evidence indicate that sexual contact or direct faecal–oral contact are not the usual routes of transmission. *I. belli* oocysts, unlike *Cryptosporidium* oocysts, are released unsporulated and usually require a period of 2 days or more in the environment for the oocyst to sporulate and become infectious (Lumb and Hardiman, 1991; Wolf, 1991). Heterosexual partners of Haitian bisexual men with AIDS and isosporiasis did not have an increased prevalence of isosporiasis (DeHovitz et al., 1986). Faecal contamination of food, water or the environment is probably the usual source of transmission, but the exact modes of transmission remain unknown.

Pathogenesis

Sporulated oocysts of *Isospora* that are ingested release sporozoites, which invade the villus epithelium of the gastrointestinal tract, initiating the asexual replication cycle. The sexual cycle also occurs in humans and culminates when the unsporulated oocyst is shed into the gut lumen and released into the environment. Intracellular *Isospora* are seen deep within the cytoplasm of the villus epithelium when stained with haematoxylin and eosin. In contrast, intracellular *cryptosporidia* lie adjacent to the host cell membrane and give the appearance of being extracellular by light microscopy. Electron microscopy shows that all phases of the sexual and asexual life cycle of *Isospora* occur within gut epithelial cells.

The immune defences against *Isospora*, and the mechanism by which this parasite produces diarrhoea, are unknown. Mucosal alterations, including shortened villi and eosinophilic infiltration of the lamina propria, particularly in the proximal small intestine, are seen by electron microscopy (Trier et al., 1974). Villus architecture may return to normal with treatment.

Clinical presentation

Clinical features of isosporiasis are very similar to those of cryptosporidiosis. Infection may be asymptomatic or it may cause profuse watery diarrhoea (between eight and 10 stools a day), abdominal cramping, anorexia, nausea and vomiting, weight loss, weakness and occasionally low-grade fever (Whiteside et al., 1984). Immunocompetent patients clear the infection in several weeks. If left untreated, immunocompromised patients experience chronic diarrhoea, which results in malnutrition and dehydration (Pape et al., 1989). Malabsorption has been well described (Trier et al., 1974; Whiteside et al., 1984; Modigliani et al., 1985).

Red blood cells or faecal leukcocytes are not seen on stained stool specimens, but peripheral blood eosinophilia as high as 15% has been observed.

Isospora can infect the biliary tree, as do *Cyclospora*, *Cryptosporidium* and *Enterocytozoon bieneusi*, a microsporidian described in the next section (Benator *et al.*, 1994) Disseminated extraintestinal isosporiasis has been described in a few patients with AIDS (Restrepo *et al.*, 1987; Michiels *et al.*, 1994; Bernard *et al.*, 1997).

Diagnosis

Isospora oocysts are about five times larger than *Cryptosporidium* oocysts, and are elliptical rather than round shape. A stool sample may be stained with modified Kinyoun iron haematoxylin or a modified Kinyoun stain (an acid-fast stain using carbolfuchsin and a bright-green counterstain), which stain *Isospora*, *Cyclospora* and *Cryptosporidium* oocysts bright red.

Biopsy of the villus epithelium, particularly of the small bowel, has a high diagnostic sensitivity, but has the obvious disadvantages of cost and adverse reactions. Electron microscopy of biopsy material may be required for a definitive diagnosis (Whiteside *et al.*, 1984). There are no serological tests for diagnosis of active *Isospora* infection.

Treatment

The largest treatment trial of *Isospora* infection in AIDS was conducted in Haiti. Symptomatic *Isospora belli*-infected AIDS patients were treated with TMP-SMX (160 and 800 mg [one double-strength tablet] orally four times a day for 10 days) and then randomized to TMP-SMX (160 and 800 mg three times a week) or sulfadoxine (500 mg) and pyrimethamine (25 mg) or placebo once a week. All patients responded clinically to the initial TMP-SMX therapy and *Isospora* was eradicated in all. Recurrent disease was prevented by ongoing treatment with either TMP-SMX or sulfadoxine-pyrimethamine. Of the patients given placebo after the initial course of intensive therapy, 50% relapsed by 2 months (Pape *et al.*, 1989).

Patients who failed to respond to multiple forms of therapy have responded to pyrimethamine (50 mg/day) and sulfadiazine (4.5 g/day) (Modigliani *et al.*, 1985; Ebrahimzadeh and Bottone, 1996). Two patients with hypersensitivity reactions to sulfa drugs were treated successfully with pyrimethamine alone (75 mg/day). Recurrences were prevented with daily pyrimethamine (25 mg/day) (Weiss *et al.*, 1988).

Genera of the order *Microsporidia*

Introduction

Protozoan parasites of the phylum *Microspora*, called collectively *Microsporidia*, infect insects and a wide range of wild and domesticated animals including fish, rodents, rabbits and primates. They are small, spore-forming, obligate intracellular parasites, which are found in the intestine, liver, kidney, cornea, brain, nerves and muscles of their animal hosts (Bryan *et al.*, 1991). Recently, microsporidiosis has been recognized as a cause of gastrointestinal disease, keratitis, sinusitis, and, with some genera of *Microsporidia*, disseminated disease in those with AIDS (Shadduck, 1989; Weber *et al.*, 1994; Bryan, 1995).

Microsporidia multiply in the cytoplasm of host cells. Four genera of the order *Microsporida* (*Nosema*, *Enterocytozoon*, *Encephalitozoon*, and *Pleistophora*) have been associated with human disease. A fifth genera of *Microsporidium* is sometimes described and is composed of *microsporidia* that have not yet been fully characterized. Members of these genera have variable and complex structural relationships with the host cell cytoplasm, but all are released into a cell from a spore by ejection from a long, coiled polar tubule, a characteristic feature of members of the phylum *Microspora*. The organism develops into intracellularly schizonts (meronts), sporonts, sporoblasts and spores (Bryan *et al.*, 1991).

Epidemiology, transmission and geographical variability

The source of human infections with microsporidia is unknown, but both vertebrates and invertebrates are considered potential reservoirs of infection by virtue of the broad host range of these parasites. For example, species of three genera that infect man – *Encephalitozoon*, *Nosema* and *Pleistophora* – also infect birds, mammals, insects and insects/fish, respectively. *Enterocytozoon* has only been identified in humans. Spores, ingested after passage from the gastrointestinal or urinary tract of infected animals appear to initiate infection. Spores are stable in the environment and may be infective up to 4 months after being shed (Waller, 1979). Serological studies suggest that antibodies to *Encephalitozoon cuniculi* are widespread in animals and humans and are more frequently found in persons who have travelled to the tropics, especially homosexual men at risk for AIDS (Berquist *et al.*, 1984). One group has reported that *E. bieneusi* is present in intestinal biopsy specimens in asymptomatic HIV-infected individuals as frequently as in those with diarrhoea (Rabeneck *et al.*, 1993), a finding which suggests that microsporidiosis in immunocompromised patients reflects activation of a latent infection (Shadduck, 1989). Geographical variation in the incidence of *microsporidia* has not been studied.

Pathogenesis

Microsporidia have not been studied extensively as agents of disease because they are small, stain poorly, and require electron microscopy for definitive classification and, until recently, for diagnosis (Shadduck, 1989). These parasites may evoke an inflammatory response in tissues, especially in immunocompromised patients, or may elicit moderate granulomatous inflammation with a mononuclear cell infiltrate.

E. bienusi infection of the intestinal epithelium is confined to enterocytes covering the villi, especially those at the tip of the villus, and is associated with villous atrophy, cell degeneration, necrosis and sloughing (Modigliani *et al.*, 1985; Orenstein *et al.*, 1990). The jejunum appears to be the preferred site of infection; the duodenum is less commmonly infected; and the large intestine is relatively spared (Orenstein *et al.*, 1990). Parasites may not evoke an inflammatory response in tissues, especially in immunocompromised patients, or may elicit moderate granulomatous inflammation with a mononuclear cell infiltrate. *Encephalitozoon* spp. (*E. cuniculi*, *E. intestinalis*, *E. hellem*) infection may disseminate. Animals may be latently infected with microsporidia, although latent infection has not been documented in man (Shadduck, 1989).

Clinical presentation

Although there are occasional reports of microsporidiosis in immunocompetent patients (Bryan *et al.*, 1991), disease caused by *microsporidia* is much more widespread in immunocompromised hosts, especially those with AIDS. Interpretation of clinical findings in AIDS patients is complicated by the high rates of concurrent infections and other diseases (Leder *et al.*, 1998). *Enterocytozoon bieneusi* infection of the intestinal epithelium, first reported in 1985, is by far the most common manifestation of microsporidiosis in AIDS (Desportes *et al.*, 1985; Dobbins and Weinstein, 1985; Modigliani *et al.*, 1985; Riijpstra *et al.*, 1988; Shadduck, 1989; Canning and Hollister, 1990; Orenstein *et al.*, 1990; Leder *et al.*, 1998). *E. bieneusi* was found to be the cause of unexplained diarrhoea in 27–30% of HIV-infect-

ed patients (Orenstein *et al.*, 1990; van Gool *et al.*, 1990; Eeftinck Schattenkerk *et al.*, 1991; Peacock *et al.*, 1991; Weber, 1992a). It has been estimated that *microsporidial* diarrhoea occurs in up to 15% of HIV-infected persons in the USA, approximately the same prevalence as reported for *Cryptosporidium* (Orenstein *et al.*, 1990). Clinical manifestations of disease include wasting and chronic diarrhoea, and are indistinguishable from the the manifestations of isosporiasis, cyclosporiasis and cryptosporidioisis in AIDS patients (Leder *et al.*, 1998). Diarrhoeal stools are watery, are not accompanied by blood or fever and are exacerbated by food intake (Orenstein *et al.*, 1990). Routine laboratory tests are generally normal in patients with intestinal microsporidiosis, although hypokalaemia and hypomagnesaemia may occur if the diarrhoea is severe (Leder *et al.*, 1998). Carbohydrate and fat malabsorption may be present as well as vitamin B_{12} deficiency (Molina *et al.*, 1993; Leder *et al.*, 1998).

A second intestinal *microsporidia*n, first called *Septata intestinalis* but now classified as *Enterocytozoon intestinalis*, causes severe enteritis and may disseminate. In the large retrospective series Leder *et al.* (1998), disseminated infection was seen in eight of 11 patients with *E. intestinalis* infection where evidence of dissemination was sought. Renal infection may result in granulomatous tubulointerstitial nephritis with associated haematuria and renal failure. Occasionally, cystitis or bowel perforation may occur (Orenstein *et al.*, 1992; Croft *et al.*, 1997; Soule *et al.*, 1997; Leder *et al.*, 1998). *E. intestinalis* may also spread to the sinus and lower respiratory tract (Leder *et al.*, 1998). This organism, like *Encephalitozoon cuniculi*, which can disseminate widely in animals, was also found in gut mucosal macrophages. Spores have been identified in the portal vein, suggesting that the parasite may disseminate directly. Urine samples may contain free or intracellular spores.

Biliary tract disease, including cholangitis and acalculous cholecystitis, has been described in microsporidiosis and attributed to *E. bieneusi* on the basis of histological changes in the lamina propria associated with parasites in the bile duct epithelium (McWhinney *et al.*, 1991; Beaugerie *et al.*, 1992; Pol *et al.*, 1992, 1993; Leder *et al.*, 1998). Symptoms include abdominal pain and low-grade fever. Alkaline phosphatase, gamma-glutamyl transferase, and serum aminotransferases were more than two times normal in most patients (Pol *et al.*, 1993), but none of the patients reported had jaundice. *Microsporidial* infection of bile ducts appears to be common, as does co-infection of the bile duct with *Cryptosporidium*. *Cryptosporidium* was detected in the bile of three of eight patients with *E. bieneusi* infection of the biliary tree (Pol *et al.*, 1993). Morphological abnormalities in patients with *microsporidial* cholangitis include luminal irregularities of the intrahepatic bile ducts, dilation of the common bile duct, gallbladder wall thickening, distension or sludge and papillary stenosis (McWhinney *et al.*, 1991; Beaugerie *et al.*, 1992; Pol *et al.*, 1992, 1993). Hepatitis in an AIDS patient due to *Encephalitozoon cuniculi* has also been reported (Terada *et al.*, 1987).

Two distinct types of *microsporidial* ocular infections have been reported. The first, corneal stromal infection, usually occurs in immunocompetent persons following trauma, may progress to corneal perforation and blindness and appears to be caused by organisms of the genus *Vittaforma cornea*, previously catalogued as *Nosema* (Lowder *et al.*, 1990; Cali *et al.*, 1991). The second type of eye infection is a keratoconjunctivitis seen in patients with AIDS. Disease presents as conjunctivitis, is characterized by punctate epithelial keratopathy, and is caused by a newly described organism, *Encephalitozoon hellem*. *E. hellem* infection should be suspected in HIV-infected persons having persistent epithelial keratopathy with negative cultures (Friedberg *et al.*, 1990; Didier *et al.*, 1991). Like other *Enterocytozoon* species *E. hellem* may disseminate, and members of this genus have been isolated from peritoneum (Zender *et al.*, 1989) and liver (Terada *et al.*, 1987) of AIDS patients. *Pleistophora* was found in skeletal muscle of one patient with AIDS, and in one patient with acquired immunodeficiency without HIV infection (Ledford *et al.*, 1985; Chupp *et al.*, 1993). A further AIDS patient with chronic diarrhoea, chronic cough, dyspnoea and an infiltrate and pleural effusion on chest radiograph was found to have *E. bieneusi* in transbronchial lung and ileal biopsies, as well as in the stools (Weber *et al.*, 1992b). However, an association between pulmonary *microsporidia* and symptoms has not been established and *Microsporidium* in the lung may represent colonization (Weber *et al.*, 1992b; Lanzafame *et al.*, 1997). *Microsporidia* in pulmonary specimens cannot be readily distinguished from Gram-positive bacteria. Sinusitis and otitis associated with microsporidiosis have also been reported; in the large series of Leder *et al.* (1998) five of 29 patients with *E. bieneusi* infection had sinusitis (four also had bronchitis), but nasopharyngeal and sputum specimens were negative for the organism. One additional patient had *E. bieneusi* in a nasopharyngeal aspirate but no symptoms of sinusitis. In contrast, of seven patients with *E. intestinalis*

infection and symptoms of sinusitis, five had the organism demonstrated in nasal secretions. Ten of 13 patients with *E. intestinalis* infection complained of bronchitis and sputum was positive for *E. intestinalis* in four of six patients examined (Leder *et al.*, 1998).

Diagnosis

Encephalitozoon spores are Gram-positive and some are acid-fast, but spores of other genera stain unpredictably with these stains, electron microscopy may be required for identification. *Enterocytozoon bieneusi* may be identified on light microscopy of plastic- or paraffin-embedded sections of intestinal biopsies material stained with methylene blue-azure II basic fuchsin stain, haematoxylin and eosin or Giemsa (Orenstein *et al.*, 1990; Peacock *et al.*, 1991). Pol suggested that the optimal stain for light microscopic examination of resin-embedded material is toluidine blue, which gives good contrast between the spores and background and allows detection at lower magnification (Pol *et al.*, 1993). Small-bowel touch preps containing microsporida may be Giemsa stained, but many authors have noted the unpredictable staining pattern of *E. bieneusi* with this stain (Riijpstra *et al.*, 1988; Orenstein *et al.*, 1990). Spores appear as refractile bodies in haematoxylin and eosin stain, Brown-Brenn and acid-fast stains (Orenstein *et al.*, 1990). Spores also have a PAS-positive polar inclusion.

Several groups have reported success with the use of Giemsa and the Ryan modification of the trichrome stains of stool smears for the diagnosis of *Enterocytozoon bieneusi* diarrhoea (van Gool *et al.*, 1990; Weber, 1992a; Didier *et al.*, 1995; Leder *et al.*, 1998). The modified trichrome stain (Figure 30.4) has come into common usage, as it stains the spore wall a bright pinkish red (Weber *et al.*, 1992a), rendering the extremely small oval organisms ($1.5 \times 0.9 \mu$m) more easily visible. Leder *et al.* (1998) found the Ryan-modified trichrome stain to be the best diagnostic test (Leder *et al.*, 1998, and Didier *et al.*, 1995) found a sensitivity of 100% compared to transmission on electron microscopy and a specificity of 83–100%. Giemsa-stained oocysts in the stool exhibit light grey–blue cytoplasm and an intensely purple nucleus (van Gool *et al.*, 1990). Various methods of stool concentration (Ritchie formalin–ethyl acetate stool concentration, Sheather's sucrose flotation, sodium chloride flotation, sucrose and Percoll gradients) did not improve the rate of detection when compared to unconcentrated faecal smears (Weber *et al.*, 1992a).

Detection of the polar filament of *microsporidia*, its characteristic feature, and speciation of this phylum, requires electron microscopy (Orenstein *et al.*, 1990; Pol *et al.*, 1993). *Enterocytozoon bieneusi* is characterized by intranuclear development in enterocytes as a large, multinucleate plasmodia in direct contact with the cell cytoplasm, which divides into individual spores as polar filaments surround individual nuuclei. It exhibits several unique structures called electron lucent inclusions and electron-dense discs. Spores of *E. bieneusi* also have a thin endospore, an electronlucent vacuole and between six and eight turns of the polar tubule (Cali and Owen, 1990; Orenstein *et al.*, 1990).

Treatment and prevention (Table 30.2)

Treatment of intestinal microsporidiosis currently includes the empirical use of antidiarrhoeals, hydration and total parenteral nutrition. Blanshard and associates (1992) reported that albendazole, an inhibitor of tubulin polymerization with activity against *Giardia*, *Echinococcus* and nematodes, was a useful palliative treatment for *microsporidial* diarrhoea in the six HIV-infected patients they studied. Subsequent reports suggest that albendazole is more useful for the treatment of *Encephalitozoon intestinalis* than *Enterocytozoon bieneusi* diarrhoea (Dieterich *et al.*, 1994; Goodgame, 1996). Of the eight *E. bieneusi*-infected patients treated with albendazole by Leder *et al.* (1998), the best response was a transient decrease in stool frequency and volume, with 100% relapsing in 6–8 weeks. In contrast, symptoms (sinusitis or diarrhoea) resolved completely in all

eight patients with *E. intestinalis* treated with albendazole, and none of the treated patients relapsed (Leder *et al.*, 1998). Albendazole was administered at a dose of 400 mg twice daily for 4 weeks. The three patients who relapsed were treated with a further 400 mg twice daily for 6 weeks. Severe pancytopenia and *C. difficile*-induced pseudomembranus colitis have been reported in patients receiving albendazole (Blanshard *et al.*, 1992; Shah *et al.*, 1996). Albendazole may also be of use for *Enterocytozoon hellem* infection. Further controlled studies of the efficacy of albendazole in microsporidiosis in HIV-infected persons are underway. Metronidazole has also been used with variable results for *microsporidial* diarrhoea and cholangitis (Eeftinck Schattenkerk *et al.*, 1991; Beaugerie *et al.*, 1992; Weber *et al.*, 1992a; Pol *et al.*, 1993). Like albendazole, metronidazole does not eradicate *microsporidia* infection.

Fumagillin, a water-insoluble antibiotic derivative from *Aspergillus fumigatus*, is effective for the topical treatment of *Enterocytozoon hellem* keratoconjunctivitis (Diesenhouse *et al.*, 1993), but oral therapy, although effective for *E. bieneusi* diarrhoea, has been associated with thrombocytopenia (Molina *et al.*, 1997, 2000). A more highly absorbed semisynthetic analogue of fumagillin, TNP-470, is 10 times more active than the parent compound against *Encephalitozoon cuniculi* and *E. hellem in vitro* and *E. cuniculi* in athymic mice (Coyle *et al.*, 1998). TNP-470 also has activity against *E. intestinalis* and *Vittaforma cornea in vitro* (Didier, 1997) and is a prime candidate for further evaluation for *microsporidial* diarrhoea.

Table 30.2 Treatment of *Cryptosporidium*, *Cyclospora*, *Isospora* and *Microsporidial* infections in AIDS patients

Species	Suggested treatment
Cryptosporidium parvum	No specific therapy proven efficacious; HAART therapy may relieve symptoms in AIDS patients with symptomatic cryptosporidiosis
Cyclospora cayetanensis	Trimethoprim (160 mg) and sulfamethoxazole (800 mg) four times daily for 10 days; continue trimethoprim and sulfamethoxazole suppressive therapy three times a week indefinitely to prevent relapse
Isospora belli	Trimethoprim (160 mg) and sulfamethoxazole (800 mg) q.i.d. for 10 days, followed by suppressive therapy to prevent relapse; pyrimethamine may be substituted for trimethoprim Sulfa-allergic patients: pyrimethamine alone at 50–75 mg/day

Microsporidial species
  Enterocytozoon bieneusi
  Encephalitizoon intestinalis
	HAART therapy may relieve symptoms in AIDS patients with symptomatic microsporidiosis; albendazole 400 mg orally twice daily appears to be more efficacious for *Encephalitizoon intestinalis* than for *Enterocytozoon bieneusi*; no controlled trials have been completed

HAART: highly-active antiretroviral therapy.

Summary

Diarrhoea may occur in as many as 80% of AIDS patients from developed countries. The usual diagnostic approach is to obtain stool for diagnostic studies, followed by treatment of identified pathogens or empirical antidiarrhoeal therapy. If diarrhoea persists, then lower and/or upper endoscopy may be performed. With an aggressive diagnostic approach including stool examination for ova and parasites (including *Apicomplexan* organisms and *Microsporidium*), tests for *C. difficile* toxin, routine culture, histology, electron microscopy and endoscopy, a potential pathogen may be identified in as many as 85% of patients (Smith *et al.*, 1988; Blanshard *et al.*, 1996; Brown *et al.*, 1996). Although examination of duodenal biopsies or aspirate specimens by light and electron microscopy will establish a microbiological diagnosis in about one-quarter of AIDS patients with chronic diarrhoea and negative routine studies, the value of these procedures is arguable, as there is no effective therapy for the most commonly identified protozoan pathogens, *Cryptosporidum* and *microsporidial* species (Brown *et al.*, 1996). Reconstitution of the immune system with combination antiretroviral therapy appears to offer the best opportunity for relief of symptomatology due to infections with these agents. The prevalence of clinical cryptosporidiosis and microsporidiosis in AIDS patients appears to be decreasing in the era of highly effective antiretroviral therapy (Carr *et al.*, 1998; Foudraine *et al.*, 1998); however, recurrent disease has occurred with declining CD4 lymphocyte counts in patients on such therapy (Carr *et al.*, 1998). Prudent recommendations for avoidance of cryptosporidiosis by HIV-infected individuals have been defined (Juranek, 1995). These recommendations may be expected to prevent infection with *Isospora* and *Cyclospora*, but recommendations for *Microsporidium* have not been formulated, due to uncertainty about the modes of transmission and the small size of spores. *Isospora* and *Cyclospora* appear to be less common causes of disease in AIDS patients in developed countries than in undeveloped countries, at least partially due to the widespread use of TMP-SMX (which is effective against both parasites), for *Pneumocystis carinii* prophylaxis in developed countries.

References

Anon. (1982a). Cryptosporidiosis: assessment of chemotherapy of males with acquired immune deficiency syndrome (AIDS). *MMWR* **31**: 589–92.

Anon. (1982b). Human cryptosporidiosis–Alabama. *MMWR* **31**: 252–4.

Anon. (1996a). Foodborne outbreak of diarrhoeal illness associated with *Cryptosporidium parvum* – Minnesota, 1995. *MMWR* **45**: 783–4.

Anon. (1996b). Outbreaks of *Cyclospora cayetanensis* infection – United States, 1996. *MMWR* **45**: 549–51.

Anon. (1997). Outbreaks of cyclosporiasis – United States, 1997. *MMWR* **46**: 451–2.

Adal KA, Sterling CR, Guerrant RL. (1996). *Cryptosporidium* and related species. In: MJ Blaser, PD Smith, JI Ravdin, HB Greenberg and RL Guerrant (eds.) *Infections of the gastrointestinal tract*. New York: Raven Press, 1107–28.

Armitage K, Flanigan T, Carey J *et al.* (1992). Treatment of cryptosporidiosis with paromomycin. A report of five cases. *Arch Intern Med* **152**: 2497–9.

Beaugerie L, Teilhac MF, Deluol AM *et al.* (1992). Cholangiopathy associated with *Microsporidia* infection of the common bile duct mucosa in a patient with HIV. *Ann Intern Med* **117**: 401–2.

Benator DA, French AL, Beaudet LM *et al.* (1994). *Isospora belli* infection associated with acalculous cholecystitis in a patient with AIDS. *Ann Intern Med* **121**: 663–4.

Berlin OG, Novak SM, Porschen RK *et al.* (1994). Recovery of *Cyclospora* organisms from patients with prolonged diarrhoea. *Clin Infect Dis* **18**: 606–9.

Bernard E, Delgiudice P, Carles M *et al.* (1997). Disseminated isosporiasis in an AIDS patient. *Eur J Clin Micro ID* **19**: 699–701.

Berquist R, Morfeldt-Mansson L, Pehrson PO *et al.* (1984). Antibody against *Encephalitozoon cuniculi* in Swedish homosexual men. *Scand J infect Dis* **16**: 389–91.

Blanshard C, Ellis DS, Tovey G *et al.* (1992). Treatment of intestinal microsporidiosis with albendazole in patients with AIDS. *AIDS* **6**: 311–13.

Blanshard C, Francis N, Gazzard BG. (1996). Investigation of chronic diarrhoea in acquire immunodeficiency syndrome. A prospective study of 155 patients. *Gut* **39**: 824–32.

Blumberg RS, Kelsey P, Perrone T *et al.* (1984). Cytomegalovirus- and *Cryptosporidium*-associated acalculous gangrenous cholecystitis. *Am J Med* **76**: 1118–23.

Brown JW, Savides TJ, Mathews C *et al.* (1996). Diagnostic yield of duodenal biopsy and aspirate in AIDS-associated diarrhoea. *Am J Gastroenterol* **91**: 2289–92.

Bryan RT. (1995). Microsporidiosis as an AIDS-related opportunistic infection. *Clin Infect Dis* **21**: S62–5.

Bryan RT, Cali A, Owen RL *et al.* (1991). *Microsporidia*: opportunistic pathogens in patients with AIDS. In: Sun T. (ed.) *Progress in Clinical Parasitology*. New York: Field and Wood Medical Publishers. II: 1–26.

Cali A, Owen RL. (1990). Intracellular development of *Enterocytozoon*, a unique *microsporidian* found in the intestine of AIDS patients. *J Protozool* **37**: 145–55.

Cali A, Meisler D, Lowder CY *et al.* (1991). Corneal microsporidiosis, characterization and identification. *J Protozool* **38**: 215–17.

Canning EU, Hollister WS. (1990). *Enterocytozoon bieneusi* (Microspora): prevalence and pathogenicity in AIDS patients. *Trans R Soc Trop Med* **84**: 181–6.

Carr A, Marriott D, Field A *et al.* (1998). Treatment of HIV-1 associated microsporidiosis and cryptosporidiosis with combination antiretroviral therapy. *Lancet* **351**: 256–61.

Cello JP. (1989). Acquired immunodeficiency syndrome cholangiopathy: spectrum of disease. *Am J Med* **86**: 539–46.

Chupp GL, Alroy J, Adelman LS et al. (1993). Myositis due to Pleistophora (Microsporidia) in a patients with AIDS. Clin Infect Dis 16: 15–21.

Clark SC, McIntyre M. (1996). Modified detergent Ziehl-Neelsen technique for the staining of Cyclospora cayetanensis. J Clin Path 49: 511–12.

Colebunders R, Lusakumuni K, Nelson AM et al. (1988). Persistent diarrhoea in Zairian AIDS patients: an endoscopic and histological study. Gut 29: 1687–91.

Colford JM, Tager IB, Hirozawa AM et al. (1996). Cryptosporidiosis among patients infected with human immunodeficiency virus factors related to symptomatic infection and survival. Am J Epidemiol 144: 807–16.

Combee CL, Collinge ML, Britt EM. (1986). Cryptosporidiosis in a hospital-associated day care center. Pediatr Infect Dis 5: 528–32.

Conlon CP, Pinching AJ, Perera CU et al. (1990). HIV-related enteropathy in Zambia: a clinical, microbiological, and histological study. Am J Trop Med Hyg 42: 83–8.

Coyle C, Kent M, Tanowitz HB et al. (1998). TNP-470 is an effective antimicrosporidial agent. J Infect Dis 177: 515–18.

Crowley B, Path C, Moloney C et al. (1996). Cyclospora species – a cause of diarrhoea among Irish travellers to Asia. Irish Med J 89: 110–12.

Croft SL, Williams J, McGowan I. (1997). Intestinal microsporidiosis. Sem Gastro Dis 8: 45–55.

Culshaw RJ, Bancroft GJ, McDonald V. (1997). Gut intraepithelial lymphocytes induce immunity against Cryptosporidium infection through a mechanism involving gamma interferon production. Infect Immun 65: 3074–79.

Current WL. (1986). Cryptosporidium: its biology and potential for environmental transmission. CRC Crit Rev Environ Control 17: 21.

Current WL, Garcia LS. (1991). Cryptosporidiosis. Clin Lab Med 11: 873–97.

Current WL, Reese NC, Ernst JV et al. (1983). Human cryptosporidiosis in immunocompetent and immunodeficient persons. Studies of an outbreak and experimental transmission. N Engl J Med 308: 1252–7.

D'Antonio RG, Winn RE, Taylor JP et al. (1985). A waterborne outbreak of cryptosporidiosis in normal hosts. Ann Intern Med 103: 886–8.

DeHovitz JA, Pape JW, Boncy M et al. (1986). Clinical manifestations and therapy of Isospora belli infection in patients with the acquired immunodeficiency syndrome. N Engl J Med 315: 87–90.

Desportes I, Le-Charpentier Y, Galian A et al. (1985). Occurrence of a new microsporidian: Enterocytozoon bieneusi n. g., n. sp., in the enterocytes of a human patient with AIDS. J Protozool 32: 250–4.

Didier ES. (1997). Effects of albendazole, fumagillin, and TNP-470 and microsporidial replication in vitro. Antimicrob Agents Chemother 41: 1541–6.

Didier ES, Shadduck JA, Didier PJ et al. (1991). Studies on ocular microsporidia. J Protozool 38: 635–6.

Didier ES, Orenstein JM, Aldras A et al. (1995). Comparison of three staining methods for detection of microsporidia in fluids. J Clin Microbiol 33: 3138–45.

Dieng T, Ndir O, Diallo S et al. (1994). Prevalence of Cryptosporidium sp. and Isospora belli in patients with acquired immunodeficiency syndrome (AIDS) in Dakar (Senegal). Dakar Med 39: 121–4.

Diesenhouse MC, Wilson LA, Corrent GF et al. (1993). Treatment of microsporidioal keratoconjunctivitis with topical fumagillin. Am J Opthalmol 115: 293–8.

Dieterich DT, Lew EA, Kotler DP et al. (1994). Treatment with albendazole for intestinal disease due to Enterocytozoon bieneusi in patients with AIDS. J Infect Dis 169: 178–83.

Dobbins WO, Weinstein WM. (1985). Electron microscopy of the intestine and rectum in acquired immunodeficiency syndrome. Gastroenterology 88: 738–49.

DuPont HL, Chappell CL, Sterling C et al. (1995). The infectivity of Cryptosporidium parvum in healthy volunteers. N Eng J Med 332: 855–9.

Eberhard ML, Pieniazek NJ, Arrowood MJ. (1997). Laboratory diagnosis of Cyclospora infections. Arch Path Lab Med 121: 792–7.

Ebrahimzadeh A, Bottone EJ. (1996). Persistent diarrhoea caused by Isospora belli: therapeutic response to pyrimethamine and sulfadiazine. Diag Micro Infect Dis 26: 87–9.

Edwards P, Wodak A, Cooper DA et al. (1990). The gastrointestinal manifestations of AIDS. Aust NZ J Med 20: 141–8.

Eeftinck Schattenkerk JKM, van Gool T, van Ketel RJ et al. (1991). Clinical significance of small-intestinal microsporidiosis in HIV-1-infected individuals. Lancet 337: 895–8.

Farman J, Brunetti J, Baer JW et al. (1994). AIDS-related cholangio-pancreatographic changes. Abdom Imaging 19: 417–22.

Fayer R, Ungar BL. (1986). Cryptosporidium spp. and cryptosporidiosis. Microbiol Rev 50: 458–83.

Fayer R, Graczyk TK, Lewis EJ et al. (1998). Survival of infectious Cryptosporidium parvum oocysts in seawater and eastern oysters (Crassostrea virginica) in the Cheasapeake Bay. App Environ Micro 64: 1070–4.

Fichtenbaum CJ, Ritchie DJ, Powderly WG. (1993). Use of paromomycin in patients with AIDS. Clin Infect Dis 16: 298.

Flanigan T, Whalen C, Turner J et al. (1992). Cryptosporidium infection and CD4 counts. Ann Intern Med 116: 840–2.

Forgacs P, Tarshis A, Ma P et al. (1983). Intestinal and bronchial cryptosporidiosis in an immunodeficient homosexual man. Ann Intern Med 99: 793–4.

Forthal DN, Guest SS. (1984). Isospora belli enteritis in three homosexual men. Am J Trop Med Hyg 33: 1060–4.

Foudraine NA, Weverling GJ, van Gool T et al. (1998). Improvement of chronic diarrhoea in patients with advanced HIV-1 infection during potent antiretroviral therapy. AIDS 12: 35–41.

French AL, Beaudet LM, Benator DA et al. (1995). Cholecystectomy in patients with AIDS: clinicopathologic correlations in 107 cases. Clin Infect Dis 21: 852–8.

Friedberg DN, Stenson SM, Orenstein JM et al. (1990). Microsporidial keratoconjnctivitis in acquired immunodeficiency syndrome. Arch Opthal 108: 504–8.

Fryauff DJ, Krippner R, Purnomo et al. (1996). Short report: case report of Cyclospora infection acquired in Indonesia and treated with cotrimoxazole. Am J Trop Med Hyg 55: 584–5.

Garcia LS, Bruckner DA, Brewer TC et al. (1983). Techniques for the recovery and identification of Cryptosporidium oocysts from stool specimens. J Clin Microbiol 18: 185–90.

Gascon J, Corachan M, Bombi JA et al. (1995). Cyclospora in patients with traveller's diarrhoea. Scan J Infect Dis 27: 511–4.

Gellin BG, Soave R. (1992). Coccidian infections in AIDS. Toxoplasmosis, cryptosporidiosis, and isosporiasis. Med Clin N Am 76: 205–34.

Gillin JS, Shike M, Alcock N et al. (1985). Malabsorption and mucosal abnormalities of the small intestine in the aquired immunodeficiency syndrome. Ann Intern Med 102: 903–9.

Glaser CA, Safrin S, Reingold A et al. (1998). Association between Cryptosporidium infection and animal exposure in HIV-infected individuals. J AIDS HR 17: 79–82.

Godiwala T, Yaeger R. (1987). *Isospora* and traveller's diarrhoea. *Ann Intern Med* **106**: 908–9.

Godwin TA. (1991). Cryptosporidiosis in the acquired immunodeficiency syndrome: a study of 15 autopsy cases. *Hum Pathol* **22**: 1215–24.

Goldstein ST, Juranek DD, Ravenholt O *et al.* (1996). Cryptosporidiosis: an outbreak associated with drinking water despite state-of-the-art water treatment. *Ann Intern Med* **124**: 459–68.

Goodgame R. (1996). Understanding intestinal spore-froming protozoa: Cryptosporidia, Microsporidia, Isospora and Cyclospora. *Ann Intern Med* **124**: 429–41.

Greenberg RE, Mir R, Bank S *et al.* (1989). Resolution of intestinal cryptosporidiosis after treatment of AIDS with AZT. *Gastroenterol* **97**: 1327–30.

Grube H, Ramratnam B, Ley C *et al.* (1997). Resolution of AIDS associated cryptosporidiosis after treatment with indinavir. *Am J Gastroenterol* **92**: 726.

Guarino A, Canani RB, Casola A *et al.* (1995). Human intestinal cryptosporidiosis: secretory diarrhoea and enterotoxic activity in Caco-2 cells. *J Infect Dis* **171**: 976–83.

Haas CN, Rose JB. (1994). Reconciliation of microbial risk models and outbreak epidemiology: the case of the Milwaukee outbreak. *Proc Am Water Works Assoc* 517–23.

Hayes EB, Matte TD, OBrien TR *et al.* (1989). Large community outbreak of cryptosporidiosis due to contamination of a filtered public water supply. *N Engl J Med* **320**: 1372–6.

Herwaldt BL, Ackers ML. (1997). An outbreak in 1996 of cyclosporiasis associated with imported raspberries The *Cyclospora* Working Group. *N Engl J Med* **336**: 1548–56.

Hoge CW, Shlim DR, Ghimire M *et al.* (1995). Placebo-controlled trial of co-trimoxazole for *Cyclospora* infections among travellers and foreign residents of Nepal. *Lancet* **345**: 691–3.

Huang P, Weber JT, Sosin DM *et al.* (1995). The first reported outbreak of diarrhoeal illness associated with *Cyclospora* in the United States. *Ann Intern Med* **123**: 409–14.

Ignatius R, Eisenblatter M, Regnath T *et al.* (1997). Efficacy of different methods for detection of low *Cryptosporidium parvum* oocyst numbers or antigen concentration in stool samples. *Eur J Clin Micro ID* **16**: 732–6.

Juranek DD. (1995). Cryptosporidiosis: sources of infection and guidelines for prevention. *Clin Infect Dis* **21**: S57–61.

Koch KL, Phillips DJ, Aber RC *et al.* (1985). Cryptosporidiosis in hospital personnel. Evidence for person-to-person transmission. *Ann Intern Med* **102**: 593–6.

Korich DG, Mead JR, Madore, MS *et al.* (1990). Effects of ozone, chlorine dioxide, chlorine, and monochloramine on *Cryptosporidium parvum* oocyst viability. *Appl Environ Microbiol* **56**: 1423–8.

Kramer MH, Sorhage FE, Goldstein ST *et al.* (1998). First reported outbreak in the United States of cryptosporidiosis associated with a recreational lake. *Clin Infect Dis* **26**: 27–33.

Lanzafame M, Bonora S, DiPerri G *et al.* (1997). Microsporidium species in pulmonary cavitary lesions of AIDS patients infected with *Rhodococcus equi*. *Clin Infect Dis* **25**: 926–7.

Laurent F, Eckmann L, Savidge TC *et al.* (1997). *Cryptosporidium parvum* infection of human intestinal epithelial cellsinduces the polarized secretion of C-X-C chemokines. *Infect Immun* **65**: 5067–73

Laurent F, Kagnoff MF, Savidge TC *et al.* (1998). Human intestinal epithelial cells respond to *Cryptosporidium parvum* infection with increased prostaglandin H synthase 2 expression and prostaglandin E2 and F2 alpha production. *Infect Immun* **66**: 1787–90.

Leder K, Ryan N, Spelman D *et al.* (1998). Microsporidial disease in HIV-infected patients: a report of 42 patients and review of the literature. *Scand J Infect Dis* **30**: 331–8.

Le Moing V, Bissuel F, Costagliola D *et al.* (1998). Decreased prevalence of intestinal cryptosporidiosis in HIV-infected patients concomitant to the widespread use of protease inhibitors. *AIDS* **12**: 1395–7.

Ledford DK, Overman MK, Gonzaleo A *et al.* (1985). Microsporidiosis myositis in a patient with the acquired immunodeficiency syndrome. *Ann Intern Med* **102**: 628–30.

Leiva JI, Etter EL, Gathe JJ *et al.* (1997). Surgical therapy for 101 patients with acquired immunodeficiency syndrome and symptomatic cholecystitis. *Am J Sur* **174**: 414–16.

Lowder CY, Meisler DM, McMahon JT *et al.* (1990). Microsporidia infection of the cornea in an HIV-positive man. *Am J Opthalmol* **109**: 242–4.

Lumb R, Hardiman R. (1991). *Isospora belli* infection. A report of two cases in patients with AIDS. *Med J Aust* **155**: 194–6.

MacKenzie WR, Hoxie NJ, Proctor ME *et al.* (1994). A massive outbreak in Milwaukee of *Cryptosporidium* infection transmitted through the public water supply. *N Engl J Med* **331**: 161–7.

MacKenzie WR, Kazmierczak JJ, Davis JP. (1995). An outbreak of cryptosporidiosis associated with a resort swimming pool. *Epidem Infect* **115**: 545–53.

Madico G, McDonald J, Gilman RH *et al.* (1997). Epidemiology and treatment of *Cyclospora cayetanensis* in Peruvian children. *Clin Infect Dis* **24**: 977–81.

Maggi P, Larocca AM, Quarto M *et al.* (2000). Effect of antiretroviral therapy on cryptosporidiosis and microsporidiosis in patients infected with human immunodeficiency virus type 1. *Eur J Clin Microbiol Infect Dis* **19**: 213–17.

Marshall MM, Naumovitz D, Ortega Y *et al.* (1997). Waterborne protozoan pathogens. *Clin Micro Rev* **10**: 67–85.

Marshall RJ, Flanigan TP. (1992). Paromomycin inhibits *Cryptosporidium* infection of a human enterocyte line. *J Infect Dis* **165**: 772–4.

McDonald V, Robinson HA, Kelly JP *et al.* (1996). Immunity to *Cryptosporidium* muris infection in mice is expressed through gut CD4+ intraepithelial lymphocytes. *Infect Immun* **64**: 2556–62.

McGowan I, Hawkins AS, Weller IV. (1993). The natural history of cryptosporidial diarrhoea in HIV-infected patients. *AIDS* **7**: 349–54.

McWhinney PHM, Nathwani D, Green ST *et al.* (1991). Microsporidiosis detected in association with AIDS-related sclerosing cholangitis. *AIDS* **5**: 1394–5.

Mead JR, Humphreys RC, Sammons DW *et al.* (1990). Identification of isolate-specific sporozoite proteins of *Cryptosporidium parvum* by two-dimensional gel electrophoresis. *Infect Immun* **58**: 2071–5.

Meng J, Doyle MP. (1997). Emerging issues in microbiological food safety. *Ann Rev Nutr* **17**: 255–75.

Michiels JF, Hofman P, Bernard E *et al.* (1994). Intestinal and extraintestinal *Isospora belli* infection in an AIDS patient: A second case report. *Path Res Pract* **190**: 1089–93.

Millard PS, Gensheimer KF, Addiss DG *et al.* (1994). An outbreak of cryptosporidiosis from fresh-pressed apple cider. *J Am Med Assoc* **272**: 1592–6.

Modigliani R, Bories C, Le CY *et al.* (1985). Diarrhoea and malabsorption in acquired immune deficiency syndrome: a study of four cases with special emphasis on opportunistic protozoan infestations. *Gut* **26**: 179–87.

Molina JM, Sarfati C Beauvais B *et al.* (1993). Intestinal microsporidiosis in human immunodeficiency virus-infected patients with chronic unexplained diarrhoea: prevalence and clinical and biological features. *J Infect Dis* **167**: 217–21.

Molina JM, Goguel J, Sarfati C et al. (1997). Drug screening for the treatment of *Enterocytozoon bieneusi* infections in patients with HIV Infection (ANRS 034). In: *Program and abstracts of the Fourth Conference on Retroviruses and Opportunistic Infections*, Washington, DC. Alexandria, VA: Infectious Diseases Society of America, 191.

Molina JM, Goguel J, Sarfati C et al. (2000). Trial of oral fumagillin for the treatment of intestinal microsporidiosis in patients with HIV infection: ANRS 054 Study Group. *AIDS* **14**: 1341–8.

Monge R, Arias ML. (1996). Presence of various pathogenic microorganisms in fresh vegetable in Costa Rica. *Archi Latinamericanos de Nutricion* **46**: 292–4.

Navin TR, Juranek DD. (1984). Cryptosporidiosis: clinical, epidemiologic, and parasitologic review. *Rev Infect Dis* **6**: 313–27.

Neill MA, Rice SK, Ahmad NV et al. (1996). Cryptosporidiosis – an unrecognized cause of diarrhoea in elderly hospitalized patients. *Clin Infect Dis* **22**: 168–70.

Nhieu JT, Nin F, Fleury-Feith J et al. (1996). Identification of intracellular stages of *Cyclospora* species by light microscopy of thick sections using haematoxylin. *Hum Path* **27**: 1107–9.

Nord, J, Ma P, DiJohn D et al. (1990). Treatment with bovine hyperimmune colostrum of cryptosporidial diarrhoea in AIDS patients. *AIDS* **4**: 581–4.

Ooi WW, Zimmerman SK, Needham CA. (1995). *Cyclospora* species as a gastrointestinal pathogen in immunocompetent hosts. *J Clin Micro* **33**: 1267–9.

Orenstein JM, Chiang J, Steinberg W et al. (1990). Intestinal microsporidiosis as a cause of diarrhoea in human immunodeficiency virus-infected patients: a report of 20 cases. *Hum Path* **21**: 475–81.

Orenstein JM, Dieterich DT, Kotler DP. (1992). Systemic dissemination by a newly recognized intestinal *microsporidia* species in AIDS. *AIDS* **6**: 1143–50.

Ortega YR, Sterling CR, Gilman RH et al. (1993). *Cyclospora* species – a new protozoan pathogen of humans. *N Engl J Med* **328**: 1308–12.

Ortega YR, Nagle R, Gilman RH et al. (1997a). Pathological and clinical findings in patients with cyclosporiasis and a description of intracellular parasite life-cycle stages. *J Infect Dis* **176**: 1584–9.

Ortega YR, Roxas CR, Gilman RH et al. (1997b). Isolation of *Cryptosporidium parvum* and *Cyclospora cayentanensis* from vegetables collected in markets of an endemic region in Peru. *Am J Trop Med* **57**: 683–6.

Pape JW, Verdier RI, Boncy M et al. (1994). *Cyclospora* infection in adults infected with HIV. Clinical manifestations, treatment, and prophylaxis. *Ann Intern Med* **121**: 654–7.

Pape JW, Verdier RI, Johnson WD. (1989). Treatment and prophylaxis of *Isospora belli* infection in patients with the acquired immunodeficiency syndrome. *N Engl J Med* **320**: 1044–7.

Peacock CS, Blanchard C, Tovey DG et al. (1991). Histological diagnosis of intestinal microsporidiosis in patients with AIDS. *J Clin Pathol* **44**: 558–63.

Perz JF, Ennever FK, LeBlancq SM. (1998). *Cryptosporidium* in tap water Comparison of predicted risks with observed levels of disease. *Am J Epid emiol* **147**: 289–301.

Petry F, Hofstatter J, Schultz BK et al. (1997). *Cyclospora cayetanensis*: first imported infections in Germany. *Infect* **25**: 167–70.

Pieniazek NJ, Herwaldt BL. (1997). Reevaluating the molecular taxonomy: is human associated *Cyclospora* a mammalian *Eimeria* species? *Emerg Infect Dis* **3**: 381–3.

Pitlik SD, Fainstein V, Garza D et al. (1983a). Human cryptosporidiosis: spectrum of disease. Report of six cases and review of the literature. *Arch Intern Med* **143**: 2269–75.

Pitlik SD, Fainstein V, Rios A et al. (1983a). Cryptosporidial cholecystitis. *N Engl J Med* **308**: 967.

Pol S, Romana C, Richard S et al. (1992). *Enterocytozoon bieneusi* infection in acquired immunodeficiency syndrome-related sclerosing cholangitis. *Gastroenterology* **102**: 1778–81.

Pol S, Romana CA, Richard S et al. (1993). *Microsporidia* infection in patients with the human immunodeficiency virus and unexplained cholangitis. *N Engl J Med* **328**: 95–9.

Rabeneck L, Gyorkey F, Genta RM et al. (1993). The role of *Microsporidia* in the pathogenesis of HIV-related chronic diarrhoea. *Ann Intern Med* **119**: 895–9.

Ravn P, Lundgren JD, Kjaeldgaard P et al. (1991). Nosocomial outbreak of cryptosporidiosis in AIDS patients. *Br Med J* **302**: 277–80.

Rehg JE. (1991). Activity of azithromycin against cryptosporidia in immunosuppressed rats. *J Infect Dis* **163**: 1293–6.

Relman DA, Schmidt TM, Gajadhar A et al. (1996). Molecular phylogenetic analysis of *Cyclospora*, the human intestinal pathogen, suggests that it is closely related to *Eimeria* species. *J Infect Dis* **173**: 440–5.

Restrepo C, Macher AM, Radany EH. (1987). Disseminated extraintestinal isosporiasis in a patient with acquired immune deficiency syndrome. *Am J Clin Pathol* **87**: 536–42.

Riijpstra AC, Canning EU, Van Ketel RJ et al. (1988). Use of light microscopy to diagnose small-intestinal microsporidiosis in patients with AIDS. *J Infect Dis* **156**: 827–31.

Saltzberg DM, Kotloff KL, Newman JL et al. (1991). *Cryptosporidium* infection in acquired immunodeficiency syndrome: not always a poor prognosis. *J Clin Gastroenterol* **13**: 94–7.

Seydel KB, Zhang T, Champion GA et al. (1998). *Cryptosporidium parvum* infection of human intestinal xenografts in SCID mice induces production of human tumor necrosis factor alpha and interleukin-8. *Infect Immun* **66**: 2379–82.

Shadduck JA. (1989). Human microsporidiosis and AIDS. *Rev Infect Dis* **11**: 203–7.

Shah V, Marins C, Altice FL. (1996). Albendazole-induced pseudomembranous colitis. *Am J Gastroenterol* **91**: 1453–4.

Sifuentes-Osornio J, Porras-Cortes G, Bendall RP et al. (1995). *Cyclospora cayetanensis* infection in patients with and without AIDS: biliary disease as another clinical manifestation. *Clin Infect Dis* **21**: 1092–7.

Smith PD, Lane HC, Gill VJ et al. (1988). Intestinal infections in patients with the acquired immunodeficiency syndrome: etiology and response to therapy. *Ann Intern Med* **108**: 328–33.

Soave R, Johnson WD. (1988). *Cryptosporidium* and *Isospora belli* infections. *J Infect Dis* **157**: 225–9.

Soave R, Danner RL, Honig CL et al. (1984). Cryptosporidiosis in homosexual men. *Ann Intern Med* **100**: 504–11.

Soave R, Herwaldt BL, Relman DA. (1998). *Cyclospora*. *Infect Dis Clin Nor Am* **12**: 1–12.

Sorvillo F, Lieb L, Iwakoshi K et al. (1990). *Isospora belli* and the acquired immunodeficiency syndrome. *N Eng J Med* **322**: 131–2.

Sorvillo FJ, Lieb LE, Kerndt P et al. (1995). Epidemiology of isosporiasis among persons with acquired immunodeficiency syndrome in Los Angeles County. *Am J Trop Med Hyg* **53**: 656–9.

Soule JB, Halverson AL, Becker RB et al. (1997). A patient with acquired immunodeficiency syndrome and untreated *Encephalitozoon (Septata) intestinalis* microsporidiosis leading to small bowel perforation. *Arch Path Lab Med* **121**: 880–7.

Steiner TS, Thielman NM, Guerrant RL. (1997). Protozoal agents: what are the dangers for the public water supply? *Ann Rev Med* **48**: 329–40.

Sterling CR, Seegar K, Sinclair NA. (1986). *Cryptosporidium* as a causative agent of traveller's diarrhoea. *J Infect Dis* **153**: 380–1.

Sun T, Ilardi CF, Asnis D *et al.* (1996). Light and electron microscopic identification of *Cyclospora* species in the small intestine. Evidence of the presence of asexual life cycle in human host. *Am J Clin Path* **105**: 216–20.

Sundermann CA, Linsay DS, Blagburn BL. (1987). Evaluation of disinfectants for ability to kill avian *Cryptosporidium* oocysts. *Companion Animal Pract* **2**: 36.

Teixidor HS, Godwin TA, Ramirez EA. (1991). Cryptosporidiosis of the biliary tract in AIDS. *Radiology* **180**: 51–56.

Terada S, Reddy R, Jeffers LJ *et al.* (1987). *Microsporidian* hepatitis in the acquired immunodeficiency syndrome. *Ann Intern Med* **107**: 61–2.

Theodos CM, Sullivan KL, Griffiths JK *et al.* (1997). Profiles of healing and nonhealing *Cryptosporidium parvum* infection in C57BL/6 mice with functional B and T lymphocytes: the extent of gamma interferon modulation determines the outcome of infection. *Infect Immun* **65**: 4761–9.

Trier JS, Moxey PC, Schimmel EM *et al.* (1974). Chronic intestinal coccidiosis in man: intestinal morphology and response to treatment. *Gastroenterology* **66**: 923–35.

Tzipori S, Roberton D, Chapman C. (1986). Remission of diarrhoea due to cryptosporidiosis in an immunodeficient child treated with hyperimmune bovine colostrum. *Br Med J* **293**: 1276–7.

Ungar BLP. (1990). Cryptosporidiosis in humans (*Homo sapiens*). In: JP Dubey, CA Speer, R Fayer, FL Boca Raton, (eds.) *Cryptosporidiosis of man and animals*. CRC Press. 59–82.

Ungar BLP, Ward DJ, Fayer R *et al.* (1990). Cessation of *Cryptosporidium*-associated diarrhoea in an acquired immunodeficiency syndrome patient after treatment with hyperimmune bovine colostrum. *Gastroenterology* **98**: 486–9.

Urban JF, Fayer R, Chen SJ. (1996). IL-12 protects immunocompetent and immunodeficient neonatal mice against infection with *Cryptosporidium parvum*. *J Immunol* **156**: 263–8.

van Gool T, Hollister WS, Eefinck Schattenkerk JKM *et al.* (1990). Diagnosis of *Enterocytozoon bieneusi* microsporidiosis in AIDS patients by recovery of spores from feces. *Lancet* **336**: 697–8.

Visvesvara GS, Moura H, Kovacs-Nace E *et al.* (1997). Unifrom staining of *Cyclospora* oocysts in fecal smears by a modified safranin technique with microwave heating. *J Clin Micro* **35**: 730–3.

Waller T. (1979). Sensitivity of *Encephalitozoon cuniculi* to various temperatures, disinfectants and drugs. *Lab Animal* **13**: 227–30.

Weber R, Bryan RT, Owen RL *et al.* (1992a). Improved light-microscopical detection of *microsporidia* spores in stool and duodenal aspirates. *N Engl J Med* **326**: 161–6.

Weber R, Kuster H, Keller R *et al.* (1992b). Pulmonary and intestinal microsporidiosis in a patient with the acquired immunodeficiency syndrome. *Am Rev Resp Dis* **146**: 1603–5.

Weber R, Bryan RT, Schwartz DA *et al.* (1994). Human *microsporidial* infections. *Clin Micro Rev* **7**: 426–61.

Weiss LM, Perlman DC, Sherman J *et al.* (1988). *Isospora belli* infection: treatment with pyrimethamine. *Ann Intern Med* **109**: 474–5.

Whiteside ME, Barkin JS, May RG *et al.* (1984). Enteric coccidiosis among patients with the acquired immunodeficiency syndrome. *Am J Trop Med Hyg* **33**: 1065–72.

Wolf MS. (1991). Miscellaneous intestinal protozoa. In: GT Strickland (ed.) *Hunters's tropical medicine*. Philadelphia, PA: Saunders, 578.

Wolfson JS, Richter JM, Waldron MA *et al.* (1985). Cryptosporidiosis in immunocompetent patients. *N Engl J Med* **312**: 1278–82.

Wurtz R. (1994). *Cyclospora*: a newly identified intestinal pathogen of humans. *Clin Infect Dis* **18**: 620–3.

Zar F, Geiseler PJ, Brown VA. (1985). Asymptomatic carriage of *Cryptosporidium* in the stool of a patient with acquired immunodeficiency syndrome. *J Infect Dis* **151**: 95.

Zender HO, Arrigoni E, Eckert J *et al.* (1989). A case of *Encephalitozoon cuniculi* peritonitis in a patient with AIDS. *Am J Clin Pathol* **92**: 352–6.

PEDRO CAHN, ROBERTO BADARÓ AND HECTOR FREILIJ

In the developing countries of the world, co-infection with multiple pathogenic microorganisms is the rule, rather than the exception. With the rapidly increasing prevalence of HIV infection, co-infection of HIV with the pathogens commonly found in these countries is being seen with increasing frequency. This effect is most striking with M. tuberculosis (see Chapter 23), but it also applies to Plasmodium sp. and many other bacterial and parasitic infections.

Parasitic infections are a major cause of morbidity and mortality in patients with HIV infection. Although parasitic infections such as toxoplasmosis and cryptosporidiosis are well recognized in regions with a temperate climate, there are a number of serious and prevalent parasitic infections that are predominantly confined to tropical regions, also often developing countries. These infections include the protozoan infections trypanosomiasis and leishmaniasis; and infestation with the multicellular parasitic worm, Strongyloides stercoralis, which although predominantly localized to the intestine of immunocompetent patients, often disseminates in those with HIV-related immunodeficiency. Due to international travel and immigration, these infections, although acquired in tropical areas, may present anywhere in the world. Because of their importance in the tropical areas of the world, American trypanosomiasis, leishmaniasis and probably other regional diseases should be included in the list of AIDS-defining conditions.

American trypanosomiasis (Chagas' disease)

American trypanosomiasis or Chagas' disease is an anthropozoonosis caused by Trypanosoma cruzi, a flagellated protozoan transmitted to humans and mammals by a group of haematophagus reduviid insects (Figure 31.1, all the figures appear in the colour plate section) and discovered in 1909 by the brilliant Brazilian physician and parasitologist Carlos Chagas. T. cruzi causes a lifelong chronic bloodstream infection in vertebrate hosts, including humans.

Epidemiology and pathogenesis

Chagas' disease vectors have been reported in the Americas from 42°N to 46°S and the disease is therefore distributed from the southern USA to the southern regions of Argentina and Chile (UNDP et al., 1991). When reduviid insects ('kissing bugs') bite the vertebrate host's skin to take a blood meal, Trypanosoma cruzi parasites are deposited with the bug's faeces and penetrate through the skin defect into the host. Reduviid bugs live in the interstices of primitive rural houses, and the bugs leave their shelters during the night to feed by biting domestic animals and man. Humans may also acquire trypanosomiasis by blood transfusion (Grant et al., 1989; Villalba et al., 1992; Kirchof, 1993; Schmunis et al., 1998), transplacentally (Freilij and Altcheh 1995; Bittencourt et al., 1976), from an infected transplanted organ (Gonzalez Cappa et al., 1992) or from laboratory accidents.

Chagas' disease affects 16–18 million people, and a total of about 100 million (about 25% of the population of Latin America) are at risk of becoming infected (Pan American Health Organization, 1990). About 45 000 deaths annually are attributed to Chagas' disease in the Americas (Moncayo, 1993). It is estimated that 7.2% of the population of Argentina is chronically infected, 22% of that of Bolivia, 4.3% in Brazil and 10% in Chile (Anon. 1990; Hayes and Schofield 1990). In the USA, there are about 370 000 people infected. The situation in Europe, Japan and Australia is unknown, but there are at least 150 000 Brazilians in Japan, 80 000 Latin Americans live in Australia and there are at least 300 000 living in Europe (Wendel et al., 1992).

From a global perspective the tropical disease burden of American trypanosomiasis is the third largest after malaria and schistosomiasis. According to the UNDP Human Development Report (Kirchof, 1993), the estimated economic loss for the continent due to early mortality and disability from this disease in young adults (the economically most productive sector of the population) currently amounts to US$8 156 million, which is equivalent to 2.5% of the external debt of the whole continent in 1995.

Trypanosoma cruzi is a flagellate of the *Kinetoplastida* Order, Family *Tripanosomatidae*, characterized by the presence of one flagellum and a single, large mitochondrion (Figure 31.2). *T. cruzi* is not a genetically homogeneous population, but is composed of a pool of strains (a concept similar to the HIV quasispecies), which circulate in the insect vectors and in their hosts, humans and over 100 wild and domestic mammals (Brener, 1985).

T. cruzi is able to invade a large range of vertebrate cells including macrophages, fibroblasts, epithelial cells, muscle cells and neurons (Figure 31.3). As *T. cruzi* is an obligate intracellular parasite, it must enter cells to multiply; the intracellular form is a small (2 µm in diameter), rounded parasite without a flagellum. The blood stage is enlarged (25 µm × 2 µm), extracellular and has a flagellum.

In humans, *T. cruzi* infection is followed by an acute illness with high-level parasitaemia which, after a period of a few months is followed by a lifelong chronic infection, characterized by low-grade and intermittent parasitaemia and in which tissue parasites are scarce and difficult to demonstrate. All patients with chronic infection are potentially able to transmit Chagas' disease to others, via triatomid bug bites, pregnancy, blood transfusion or organ donation.

Clinical aspects

General clinical features
Chagas' disease can be divided into two stages: acute infection and chronic infection. The acute phase of Chagas' disease, usually seen in children, begins shortly after infection with *T. cruzi* and lasts for 1 or 2 months. This stage of the disease is often asymptomatic, although fever, malaise, anorexia, induration and lymphadenitis around the inoculation site (chagoma) or periocular oedema (Romaña sign) may be seen. Generalized lymphadenopathy and splenomegaly may also occur. Very young children and, rarely, adults may develop myocarditis or meningoencephalitis during acute Chagas' disease; the latter has a fatality rate

of 30–50% in infants (Jorg *et al.*, 1980; Prata, 1994). Acute *T. cruzi* infection is characterized by high-grade parasitaemia and can usually be diagnosed easily by direct parasitological testing (see section on diagnosis, below).

The acute illness of Chagas' disease usually resolves spontaneously, and the patient enters the asymptomatic 'indeterminate' phase of the illness. After one or two decades 10–15% of infected patients develop cardiac and/or digestive tract disease (Rezende, 1975; Marin-Neto *et al.*, 1992; Storino *et al.*, 1992). Chronic Chagas' cardiopathy has three main clinical presentations: arrhythmias, cardiac failure (especially right heart failure) and thromboembolic disease. These syndromes may be present alone or in varying combinations in the same patient. Megaesophagus and megacolon are the main gastrointestinal manifestations of chronic Chagas' disease; they are caused by a loss of autonomic nervous system ganglion cells in the gut. The symptoms of megaesophagus include dysphagia, chest pain, regurgitation and cough (from aspiration). Megacolon causes constipation and belly pain.

Clinical features of Chagas' disease in patients with HIV infection
Reactivation of chronic, latent *T. cruzi* infection can be triggered by immunosuppression, whether caused by HIV infection, other diseases, or chemotherapy (Monteverde *et al.*, 1976; Kohl *et al.*, 1982; Leiguarda *et al.*, 1990). The clinical features of immunosuppression-induced reactivation of Chagas' disease differ from that of chronic infection in immunocompetent patients, with the most overt difference being the high frequency of central nervous system (CNS) involvement, with attendant high morbidity and mortality. The first reports of Chagas' disease causing a brain mass in patients with HIV infection and AIDS came from Argentina and the USA (Gluckstein *et al.*, 1992).

Neurological signs and symptoms are therefore the main clinical findings in HIV-infected patients with reactivation of *T. cruzi* infection (Oddo *et al.*, 1992; Rosemberg *et al.*, 1992; Solari *et al.*, 1993; Di Lorenzo *et al.*, 1996; Pimentel *et al.*, 1996; Cohen *et al.*, 1998; Rocha *et al.*, 1993). In a review of 23 patients with HIV and Chagas' disease, most of whom came from Brazil, Chile and Argentina, 20 (87%) had severe multifocal or diffuse acute meningoencephalitis with necrosis and haemorrhage associated with a large number of amastigotes (Rocha *et al.*, 1994). Co-infection with *T. gondii*, cytomegalovirus (CMV) and herpes simplex virus (HSV) was identified by brain biopsy in one patient. Cerebrospinal fluid (CSF) was analyzed in only nine of these cases, and usually showed a lymphocytic pleocytosis, although a few patients had neutrophilic and eosinophilic granulocytosis. The CSF protein concentration was increased in eight of nine cases.

Pagano *et al.* (1998) evaluated 10 patients with AIDS and CNS involvement due to *T. cruzi* infection. All had clinical findings of a cerebral tumor (chagoma) (Figure 31.4). Initially, nine patients received therapy for toxoplasmosis, based upon the results of computerized homography (CT) or magnetic resonance imaging (MRI) studies. Chagas' disease was diagnosed when initial treatment failed, at which point all patients received specific treatment for Chagas' disease (nifurtimox or benznidazol – see section on treatment below). Eight cases survived less than 7 months, three died of causes unrelated to *T. cruzi* infection; one survived for more than 12 months. Six of the patients underwent brain decompression with total or partial resection of the masses. Most of these patients (8–10) had a single supratentorial lesion and one had multiple lesions in both supratentorial and infratentorial regions. Histological examination of the intracerebral masses was performed in eight cases. The inflammatory pattern varied from case to case, but all had *T. cruzi* amastigotes. Some tissue samples showed predominantly granulomatous inflammatory cell infiltration, while others showed chiefly necrotic tissue with macrophage infiltration. In the two patients in whom biopsy was not performed, the parasite was present in CSF.

The imaging pattern of brain chagoma is similar to that of cerebral toxoplasmosis. In the series of Rocha *et al.* (1994), pseudotumor lesions were seen in 15 of the 16 patients who had CT scans performed; eight of them had multiple lesions and the remaining seven only one. Di Lorenzo *et al.* (1996) described two patients with HIV infection and neurological symptoms in whom the diagnosis of Chagas' disease was established by brain biopsy. MRI imaging showed hypodense lesions which enhanced with gadolinium.

In patients with HIV infection, Chagas' heart disease is infrequently associated with clinical manifestations; however, pathological examinations often demonstrate acute myocarditis with an intense inflammatory infiltrate, cardiac myofibre necrosis, and *T. cruzi* amastigote forms. Reactivation of *T. cruzi* infection clinically manifest as myocarditis is rare in HIV infection (Labarca *et al.*, 1992). In the series of Rocha *et al.* (1994), histopathological evidence of myocarditis was present in all seven patients who came to

autopsy. Four of these seven patients had acute chagasic myocarditis, two had focal lesions similar to that found in patients with chronic Chagas' disease, and one had both acute and chronic features in different areas of the myocardium.

Sartori *et al.* (1998) followed 18 patients with HIV infection and chronic *T. cruzi* infection for 2–66 months, with serological and parasitological tests every 3 months. Exacerbation of *T. cruzi* infection causing cardiac disease occurred in three of the 18 patients. All 18 patients had two serological tests reactive for Chagas' disease, and HIV infection was confirmed by western blotting. Reactivation of Chagas' disease was defined by finding *T. cruzi* by direct parasitological testing. The manifestations of cardiac disease were typical of that caused by Chagas' disease in immunocompetent patients. One patient presented with arrhythmias and cardiogenic shock, another with severe congestive heart failure and the third had worsening of a previous cardiac disease. Myocarditis was observed by histological examination in two out of three cases. Treatment with beznidazol was effective for controlling the clinical manifestations attributed to *T. cruzi*, and for reducing the level of parasitaemia in these patients (see section on treatment below). The only other reported adult case of Chagas' cardiomyopathy in a patient with HIV infection is that of Labarca *et al.* (1992).

The clinical manifestations of perinatally acquired combined infection with HIV and *T. cruzi* have not been well studied. Freilij *et al.* (1995) studied six infants born from mothers infected with both HIV and *T. cruzi*; four of the infants became dually infected. Three of these (all under 3 months of age) presented with serious clinical manifestations, primarily meningoencephalitis. Although the symptomatic infants had a good response to nifurtimox, they died of other causes. The fourth patient was 17 months old and was asymptomatic.

Diagnosis

Chagas' disease should be considered in any patient from an endemic area, and in anyone who has been transfused or was born to an infected mother. At present, the diagnosis of *T. cruzi* infection depends upon identifying the parasite (or its products) in blood or tissue, or detecting the serological response to infection; preliminary results of tests to identify *T. cruzi* DNA in clinical specimens after polymerase chain reaction (PCR) amplification are promising (Ribeiro dos Santos *et al.*, 1999; Schijman *et al.*, 2000).

Direct tests for identifying *T. cruzi* depend upon detecting this parasite by microscopy. They are useful during the acute stage and in reactivation of chronic infection (e.g. in the setting of HIV infection) because in these phases large numbers of parasites circulate in the bloodstream. These tests may also be employed in CSF in patients with suspected CNS Chagas' disease. The diagnosis can be made in half an hour, and is simple and cheap. Examples of this test are the microhematocrit test (so called 'MH' test) in which the parasite is detected by microscopy of a blood smear (Freilij *et al.*, 1983; Strout, 1962). Parasites may also be seen in lymph nodes, bone marrow, pericardial fluid and CNS mass lesions.

Indirect tests such as xenodiagnosis (recovering the organism after inoculation of laboratory-raised insect vectors) (Schenone *et al.*, 1974) or haemoculture (culture in liquid medium) are somewhat more sensitive than the direct methods, but may take 2–8 weeks to become positive. They are very useful in the chronic stages of *T. cruzi* infection, when the level of parasitaemia is low.

Tests are being developed to detect *T. cruzi* nucleic acids in body fluids (especially blood) following PCR amplification; these tests appear to be substantially more sensitive than current parasitological or serological tests for detecting *T. cruzi*, but are not yet widely available (Russomando *et al.*, 1992).

Serological tests, to detect the IgG antibody response to *T. cruzi* infection, are useful for diagnosis of chronically infected patients, to screen blood donors, to evaluate the effect of drug treatment and for seroepidemiological studies. The techniques used are indirect haemagglutination, direct agglutination reactions, complement fixation, indirect immunofluorescence and ELISA (Ferreira, 1992). Few of the commercially available tests now use recombinant antigens, which would provide more specific tests than those that depend on purified protozoal antigens. Detection of IgM antibodies is not useful, even during the acute stage of infection.

Chagas' disease should not be diagnosed serologically unless at least two different types of serological tests for *T. cruzi* antibodies are positive. Although all these tests are reasonably sensitive and specific, both false-positive and false-negative reactions have been reported. For that reason, the diagnosis of Chagas' disease should not be discarded based on negative serological tests if the patient comes from an endemic region and has clinical findings compatible with Chagas' disease. In this instance, direct parasitological testing (e.g. microscopic examination of brain tissue and for parasitaemia) is the best diagnostic strategy. Not surprisingly, neonates born to mothers with chronic *T. cruzi* infection will have positive antibody tests, yet may not be infected; parasitological tests are recommended in this instance as well (Freilis *et al.*, 1995).

In the series of 23 patients reported by Rocha *et al.* (1994) who were co-infected with *T. cruzi* and HIV, 17 of 23 patients had serum antibody assays performed, and 15 of 17 were reactive. In contrast, only two of five CSF antibody studies were positive. Parasitological tests were performed in 12 patients, eight of whom were positive, four by direct methods indicating high-grade parasitaemia. *T. cruzi* were also found in nine of ten CSF investigated.

Treatment

There is no really satisfactory treatment for Chagas' disease in the chronic stage, and as the available agents are also toxic, specialty consultation should be sought. Benznidazol (Radanil®), 5–8 mg/kg/day for 30–60 days is the drug commonly used for treatment; nifurtimox (Lampit®) production was discontinued from the year 2000. Although there are no data available specifically to address this question, it is likely that the earlier treatment is begun, the more effective it will be (that is, treatment of acute Chagas' disease is likely to be much more effective than treatment of patients with late-stage complications, such as myocarditis). There is also little data regarding the efficacy of these agents in HIV-infected patients with Chagas' disease. These drugs are only partially effective in chronic stages, are suppressive rather than curative, and probably require lifelong secondary prophylaxis. Both drugs are quite toxic, nifurtimox causing anorexia, nausea, vomiting, belly pain and weight loss, restlessness, seizures and peripheral neuropathy; and benznidazol causing peripheral neuropathy, rash and granulocytopenia. The adverse effects of both drugs wane when the drugs are discontinued.

The possibility of primary Chagas' disease prophylaxis should also be considered in patients known to be co-infected with HIV and *T. cruzi*, particularly in patients with CD4 lymphocyte counts below 200 cells/μl. Although no clinical data on relative efficacy are currently available, primary prophylaxis needs to be explored in clinical trials. The interest of the pharmaceutical industry in drug development for Chagas' disease needs to be stimulated, as the economic constraints of the countries involved in the endemic is such that a highly profitable market is unlikely.

The potential impact of immune reconstitution due to highly active antirtroviral therapy (HAART) on HIV-related Chagas' disease remains to be established; however, it seems likely that maintaining normal immune function will decrease the frequency of reactiviation of *T. cruzi*, as it has other opportunistic infections.

Conclusions

Chagas' disease should be considered in the differential diagnosis of CNS mass lesions and cardiac disease (arrhythmias or heart failure) in patients with HIV infection. Although the patients at highest risk are current or former residents of Central and South America, there is some risk for any patient who has received blood transfusions or organ transplants anywhere in the world, given that millions of Central and South Americans have emigrated over the past two decades.

Strongyloidiasis

Epidemiology and pathogenesis

Strongyloidiasis is caused by the nematode *Strongyloides stercoralis*, whose natural host range includes humans, primates and dogs (Berk and Vergnese, 1988; Kramer *et al.*, 1990; Liu and Weller, 1993). The parasite is most commonly found in tropical climates but can survive in colder regions, and thus is considered to have a cosmopolitan distribution (García *et al.*, 1997). Primary infection usually occurs through penetration of the skin by infective third-stage larvae present in the soil; thus, the usual human host is a barefoot child. After penetrating the skin, the larvae disseminate systemically, with some migrating through the vascular system into pulmonary vessels and some migrating to peritoneal organs (Schad *et al.*, 1989). Larvae entering the lungs via the pulmonary arteries reach the alveolar capillaries, where they break into the alveoli, ascend the respiratory tree and are swallowed. In the small intestine the swallowed larvae develop into mature adult females. Female worms reproduce by parthenogenesis and produce eggs that hatch in the host intestine, releasing first-stage larvae in the stool. Autoinfection of the host occurs when larval development is accelerated, and the third-stage larvae within the gastrointestinal tract invade the gastrointestinal mucosa. *S. stercoralis* is also transmitted by the faecal–oral route (including sexual activity involving anal contact) and by contaminated food and water.

Clinical features and diagnosis

Penetration of the skin by larvae may cause an itchy papular erythematous rash. Pulmonary symptoms, which are due to larvae exiting the pulmonary capillaries and migrating up the respiratory tract from the alveoli, can result from either primary skin infection or autoinfection (Grove, 1989). During migration through the lungs, larvae cause an inflammatory foreign-body response, producing symptoms of coughing and wheezing, as well as pulmonary infiltrates on chest radiographs. The predominant manifestation of intestinal strongyloidiasis is diarrhoea.

Of particular importance to AIDS patients are two systemic forms of strongyloidiasis: the hyperinfection syndrome, in which a disturbance in the host and parasite equilibrium leads to massive autoinfection and overwhelming gastrointestinal and pulmonary disease; and disseminated infection, in which autoinfection disseminates from the gastrointestinal tract, and adult female worms and massive numbers of larvae are found in the brain, lungs, bladder and other sites. In addition to tissue damage resulting directly from larval migration, the patient may die of sepsis, primarily as a result of the intestinal flora that are dragged along by larvae during the migration process. The larvae in tissue may cause localized findings not customarily associated with strongyloidiasis; for example, neurological signs and symptoms, gastrointestinal bleeding from *S. stercoralis* ulceration and severe pneumonitis with respiratory failure.

Both forms of invasive strongyloidiasis can arise from chronic infection or from acute, overwhelming initial infection, but the mechanism is largely unknown. Both types of invasive strongyloidiasis have also been documented in patients immunocompromized as the result of malnutrition, and in patients on glucocorticoid therapy (Grove, 1989).

Although several cases of hyperinfection have been documented in patients with AIDS, disseminated strongyloidiasis is actually very rare considering the number of AIDS patients infected with *S. stercoralis*, particularly in certain parts of Africa, where HIV-associated immunodeficiency is prevalent (Gompels *et al.*, 1991). Although disseminated strongyloidiasis or the hyperinfection syndrome had previously been an AIDS-defining illness, it has been removed from the list. The relative rarity of hyperinfection in patients with AIDS suggests that cell-mediated immunity may not be as important in the defence against multicellular helminths as it is for unicellular protozoa (Maayan *et al.*, 1987).

Strongyloidiasis should be included in the differential diagnosis of any febrile illness in AIDS patients, especially when pulmonary or gastrointestinal symptoms are present, and particularly if there is polymicrobial bacteraemia, or unexpected bacteraemia due to enteric coliform bacteria (Levi *et al.*, 1997). A combination of these findings in an HIV-infected patient with late-stage disease who has been to an endemic area should prompt the clinician to search for *S. stercoralis*.

Strongyloides stercoralis larval worms can be found in the gastrointestinal and respiratory tracts. Although the traditional method of diagnosing strongyloidiasis is to search for larvae in stool, the larvae may be infrequent and examination of multiple fresh stool specimens may be required. Duodenal aspirates are the preferred, and most rewarding, source of larvae. If there are pulmonary symptoms, sputum specimens (again, fresh are preferred) should be scrutinized for the presence of larvae, and bronchoscopy with lavage or brushings may improve the diagnostic yield. Again, even in the setting of a severe hyperinfection syndrome, it may require multiple sputum specimens before the larvae are found.

Treatment and prevention

There is no really satisfactory therapy for disseminated strongyloidiasis or the strongyloides hyperinfection syndrome. The antiparasitic agents thiabendazole (25 mg/kg twice daily for 2–3 weeks), albendazole (10 mg/kg/day) and cambendazole (360 mg/day) had been used to treat hyperinfection and disseminated strongyloidiasis (Gompels *et al.*, 1991). Some reports have suggested that ivermectin may be effective in AIDS patients with invasive strongyloidiasis (Mansfield and Schad, 1989; Torres *et al.*, 1993; Heath *et al.*, 1996).

The mainstay of prevention is to practice good personal and food hygiene, to avoid unprotected sexual practices that involve anal contact, and to avoid walking barefoot when outdoors in tropical areas harburing the parasite.

Malaria

HIV infection is either already prevalent or spreading rapidly in many areas of the world with pre-existing high levels of malaria endemnicity, and as a consequence, malaria is already very common among HIV-infected subjects in malaria-endemic regions. Early serological surveys appeared to support the existence of an association

between HIV-1 and malaria. A study in Burundi found malaria in 57% of 120 AIDS patients, and controversial studies in Kinshasa, Zaire, showed higher levels of parasitaemia in HIV-infected subjects than in those who were uninfected. A recent large prospective study from Uganda had suggested that HIV immunosuppression increases parasite densities, increases the incidence of clinical malaria in infected subjects, and makes severe disease more likely (Whitworth *et al.*, 2000). In an animal model, malaria infection also augmented HIV replication (Freitag *et al.*, 2001).

However, subsequent, well-controlled studies have failed to establish a pathophysiological relationship between HIV infection and malaria (Chandramohan and Greenwood, 1998). Several cross-sectional studies in Zaire and Zambia showed that HIV seroprevalence was similar in individuals with and without *Plasmodium falciparum* parasitaemia. Other prospective studies found no difference in mean parasite densities between HIV-infected and uninfected patients. Similarly, no differences were found in the rates of malaria-related hospitalization, death and severity of cerebral malaria among HIV-infected and uninfected Zairians; a study of Ugandan infants came to the same conclusion (Kalyesubula *et al.*, 1997). Furthermore, many *P. falciparum* immune responses are well-maintained in HIV-infected subjects (Migot *et al.*, 1996). Although current evidence has consistently failed to demonstrate a direct biological association between HIV-1 and *P. falciparum* malaria, the studies are not powered to detect small differences in outcome between HIV-infected and uninfected subjects, and larger, carefully designed studies are needed to provide a definitive answer to this question (Chandramohan and Greenwood, 1998). In particular, these studies should examine a possible role for the HIV-infected placenta in facilitating HIV transmission, whether the mortality in severe malaria (especially cerebral malaria) is increased in HIV-infected subjects, and whether malaria infection accelerates progression of HIV infection (Chandramohan and Greenwood, 1998; Xiao *et al.*, 1998). Another association between HIV and malaria which is likely, albeit not clearly established by epidemiological studies, is that HIV may be transmitted to patients with malaria being treated with parenteral therapy with unsterile needles, or with transfusion of HIV-infected untested blood or blood products.

At present, it can be assumed that for the most part the clinical presentation, diagnosis and management of suspected malaria is the same in HIV-infected patients as in those who are uninfected. If the patient with malaria is taking antiretrovirals or drugs for opportunistic infections, the possibility of drug interactions should be considered before treatment is implemented; it may be safer to simply stop antiretrovirals until the course of antimalarials is complete. If parenteral antimalarial therapy or supportive care (e.g. blood or fluid transfusions) are required for the HIV-uninfected patient with malaria in a region where HIV infection is prevalent, care must be taken to use sterile infusion equipment and to ensure that the blood or blood products have been tested to exclude HIV-infected donations. Malarial placentitis in HIV-infected pregnant women should be avoided, as it may facilitate vertical transmission of HIV, and vigorous chemotherapy may be required to achieve this outcome (Parise *et al.*, 1998).

Leishmaniasis

Leishmaniasis is a heterogenous group of clinical conditions due to tissue invasion by unicellular parasites of the genus *Leishmania*. This condition is distributed globally, but the clinical manifestations vary widely, depending upon the individual infected and the species of *Leishmania* causing the disease. There are two generally recognized disease categories, visceral (disseminated) leishmaniasis, also known as kala-azar or Dumdum fever, and generally caused by *L. donovani* or *infantum*; and cutaneous leishmaniasis, caused by a large number of different *Leishmania* sp. Leishmaniasis is a major problem among HIV-infected patients living in endemic regions.

Epidemiology and pathogenesis

Leishmania are obligate intracellular parasites, which survive and replicate in parasitophorous vacuoles in tissue macrophages. The numerous species of *Leishmania* have traditionally been differentiated epidemiologically and on *in vivo* growth patterns, as they cannot be differentiated morphologically. More recently, isoenzyme patterns, and monoclonal antibodies have been used for speciation (e.g. Pratlong *et al.*, 1995). The taxonomy of *Leishmania* sp. will doubtless undergo substantial revision as molecular tools are applied to speciation.

Visceral leishmaniasis is generally caused by *Leishmania donovani* or *L. infantum*. However, the immunosuppression associated with HIV infection has resulted in some *Leishmania* species, usually associated with only localized cutaneous disease in immunocompetent patients, causing mucosal or diffuse cutaneous leishmaniasis in HIV-infect-

ed patients (Gradoni and Gramiccia, 1990; Jimenez *et al.*, 1991; Gramiccia *et al.*, 1992; Gradoni *et al.*, 1994; Ndiaye *et al.*, 1996; Morsy *et al.*, 1997). Likewise, *L. donovani* or *L. infantum* may cause infections localized to the skin in occasional patients. Cutaneous leishmaniasis is caused by a wide range of *Leishmania* species, including *L. major, tropica, mexicana, amazonensis*, and *braziliensis*, with the most prevalent species being region-specific.

Leishmaniasis is spread virtually exclusively by insect vectors. *L. donovani* and *L. infantum* are not known to have any animal reservoirs (and are therefore assumed to be spread exclusively between humans), whereas the species of *Leishmania* causing cutaneous leishmaniasis are all zoonoses, with small mammals (species varying with the geographical region) being the principal host.

Although *L. donovani* and *L. infantum*, the principal aetiological agents of visceral leishmaniasis, are globally distributed (Asia, Mediterranean basin, East Africa and Latin America), over 93% of cases of visceral leishmaniasis in HIV-infected patients have been reported from southern Europe and the Mediterranean basin (WHO, 1997; Alvar, 1994). Co-infection of HIV and *Leishmania* sp. has been reported predominantly in males and is associated with intravenous drug use, suggesting that *Leishmania* and HIV infection might both be acquired by needle sharing (Alvar *et al.*, 1997; Pineda *et al.*, 1998). In one study from southern Spain, 11% of a random sample of asymptomatic HIV-infected subjects had *Leishmania* infection, and the infection was completely asymptomatic in over one-third of them (Pineda *et al.*, 1998). Cutaneous leishmaniasis is found in Asia, North Africa and the Middle East ('Old-World' cutaneous leishmaniasis) and in Latin America ('New World' cutaneous leishmaniasis), and a few patients with HIV infection and cutaneous leishmaniasis have been reported from Latin America, primarily Brazil (Porro *et al.*, 1994).

The *Leishmania* species and strains causing disease in HIV-infected patients are the same as those infecting immunocompetent subjects in the same geographical region. For example, isoenzyme and genotyping of 100 isolates of the *Leishmania infantum* complex revealed that the dominant clonal genotype (MOM 1) was the most common isolate from both HIV-infected and uninfected patients with visceral leishmaniasis (Pratlong *et al.*, 1995).

As would be expected of an obligate intracellular parasite of macrophages, *Leishmania* infections are controlled predominantly by cellular immune responses. Immunocompetent patients with cutaneous leishmaniasis invariably have preserved delayed-type hypersensitivity to *Leishmania*. However, local immune responses are still deficient, as shown by the persistence of the infection and reduced phagocytic capacity of macrophages and altered cytokine secretion by mononuclear cells at the site of inflammation (Pirmez *et al.*, 1990; Da Cruz *et al.*, 1992; Da Cruz *et al.*, 1994; Pirmez *et al.*, 1993). In contrast, patients with visceral leishmaniasis lack delayed-type hypersensitivity reactions and protective Th1-type immune reactions to *Leishmania*, even if they were immunocompetent prior to becoming ill. *Leishmania* are rarely eradicated, either by host immune responses or chemotherapy, and thus reactivation of latent *Leishmania* is always a possibility if the subject becomes immunosuppressed.

Although the mechanisms by which *Leishmania* persists in macrophages despite a host immune response are unknown, the cytokine pattern of impaired macrophage activation has been well established in murine models of, and human infection with, *Leismania* sp. (Reed and Scott, 1993; Scott, 1993). High levels of Th2-type cytokines such as IL-10, IL-4 and TGF-β, which down regulate Thl responses, inhibit macrophage activation and consequently abrogate production of the protective Th1-type cytokines that activate macrophages to kill *Leishmania*, such as interferon-γ and IL-12 (Murray *et al.*, 1983; Mooci and Coffman, 1995).

In patients co-infected with *Leishmania* and HIV, T-cell blastogenesis responses are impaired, even with the cutaneous form of the disease (Da Cruz *et al.*, 1992). A dominant Th2 cytokine profile, with high levels of IL-4, IL-6 and IL-10 was seen in patients co-infected with HIV and *Leishmania*, compared to a dominant Th1 pattern in those with only HIV infection (Preiser *et al.*, 1996). In one report, the HIV viral load was higher in patients co-infected with *Leishmania* and HIV than in those infected with HIV alone, suggesting that *Leishmania* infection could accelerate the rate of HIV disease progression (Preiser *et al.*, 1996).

Clinical features and diagnosis (Table 31.1)

The interactions between *Leishmania* and HIV infection are such that co-infected patients should be considered to have a new disease entity, not resembling either HIV infection or leishmaniasis alone.

Visceral leishmaniasis

Visceral leishmaniasis (VL) is the most common disease presentation in patients with HIV infection, comprising 70% of the 672 cases reported to WHO (WHO, 1997). The clinical picture of VL in HIV-infected patients resembles the

Table 31.1 Clinical, epidemiological and general laboratory features highly suggestive of leishmaniasis as an AIDS-defining disease

Visceral leishmaniasis (VL)
- VL in an adult living outside of leishmaniasis endemic area
- VL in an adult injecting drug user with no previous exposure to leishmaniasis
- Any exotic clinical manifestation associated with a classic picture of VL
- Peripheral lymphopenia in an adult VL patient
- Clinical VL with negative tests for leishmania antibodies
- Recurrence of VL after 1 year in a patient previously treated successfully
- Grade 3 or higher index of leishmania parasitism on a peripheral blood smear in VL
- Multiple visceral localizations of leishmania outside the reticuloendothelial system in blood, skin, gastrointestinal tract, lung or central nervous system
- VL in a patient with a previous history of any AIDS-related opportunistic infections

Cutaneous or mucosal leishmaniasis
- Disseminated or diffuse leishmaniasis in an adult with a past history of exposure in endemic areas of leishmaniasis
- DCL caused strains different from *L. amazonensis*, *L. aethiopia* and *L. mexicana*
- Cutaneous leishmaniasis caused by non-pathogenic strains of *Leishmania* (as determined by enzyme isotyping)
- A negative leishmanian (Montenegro) skin test in a patient with mucosal leishmaniasis
- *Leishmania* organisms documented in a Kaposi's sarcoma lesion

classic description of adult kala-azar (Badaró *et al.*, 1986; Montalban *et al.*, 1990; Pintado *et al.*, 2001; Rosenthal *et al.*, 2000), with patients generally experiencing the gradual onset of fever, malaise, weight loss and abdominal enlargement as the result of progressive hepatosplenomegaly. Common laboratory abnormalities include anaemia, leucopenia and hypergammaglobulinaemia. In patients with HIV infection and VL, exotic mucocutaneous lesions, interstitial pneumonia, and diarrhoea occurred relatively frequently (Montalban *et al.*, 1990; Peters *et al.*, 1990; Belda Mira *et al.*, 1994) (Figure 31.5). The cutaneous lesions tend to be acrally located and are very pleomorphic; biopsy invariably shows *Leishmania* amstigotes. Although granulocytopenia and anaemia are the most common haematological manifestations of kala-azar in HIV-uninfected subjects (Badaró *et al.*, 1994), in HIV co-infected patients lymphopenia or pancytopenia are common. CD4 lymphocyte counts were below 200 cells/μl in 90% of the patients and below 100 cells/μl in

79%. As in immunocompetent patients with kala-azar, platelet counts in the HIV-infected patients with VL were between three and five times lower than normal. In Europe, where the majority of cases of leishmaniasis in HIV-infected patients have been seen, mucosal involvement is rarely reported in patients with infection caused by *L. infantum* (Gradoni and Gramiccia, 1994).

HIV infection markedly alters the course and clinical presentation of leishmania infection, and is a major cause of reactivation of latent infection. Among 850 patients recently reviewed who were co-infected with *Leishmania* and HIV, 7–17% of the HIV-infected individuals with fever had amastigotes in blood without clinical findings of leishmaniasis. A full-blown clinical picture of visceral leishmaniasis was seen as soon as the HIV infection had progressed to AIDS (Alvar *et al.*, 1997; WHO, 1997). About 4% of unselected, asymptomatic HIV-infected subjects from southern Spain had asymptomatic infection with strains of *Leishmania* capable of causing VL (Pineda *et al.*, 1998); presumably these would reactivate to cause VL as HIV-induced immunosuppression progressed. The profound impact of HIV-induced immunosuppression on immunity to *Leishmania* is illustrated by a report of insect tripanosomatids, not known to be pathogenic for humans, causing leishmaniasis in patients with AIDS (Jimenez *et al.*, 1996).

A diagnosis of VL requires demonstration of *Leishmania* parasites in tissue, or on culture of blood, bone marrow or other body fluids. In immunocompetent patients with kala-azar, *Leishmania* amastigotes are rarely found in peripheral blood leukocytes, but can usually be demonstrated easily in bone marrow or splenic aspirates (Chulay and Bruceson, 1983). In contrast, *Leishmania* sp. can readily be seen in buffy coat blood films in the majority of HIV-infected patients with VL (Martinez *et al.*, 1993; Alvar *et al.*, 1997; WHO, 1997) (Figure 31.6). In one series, every patient with HIV infection and VL had *Leishmania* amastigotes seen in leucocytes from peripheral blood smears using a leucocyte concentration technique (Izri *et al.*, 1996). In contrast, the peripheral blood smear is not a sensitive method for detecting subclinical (asymptomatic) infection with strains of *Leishmania* causing VL in patients with HIV infection; in this situation, microscopic examination of bone marrow aspirates increases sensitivity (Pineda *et al.*, 1998). Culture of blood and/or bone marrow is also a highly sensitive test for diagnosis of VL and detection of asymptomatic *Leishmania* infection in HIV-infected patients (Laguna *et al.*, 1997).

Other methods shown to be useful for demonstrating *Leishmania* in the blood of co-infected patients include detection of *Leishmania* nucleic acids after PCR amplification and xenodiagnosis using colonized sand flies (Ravel *et al.*, 1986; Molina *et al.*, 1994; Piarroux *et al.*, 1994; Pizzuto *et al.*, 2001; Salotra *et al.*, 2001). In one study from Spain, 90% of sand flies fed on patients co-infected with HIV and *Leishmania* became infected with the parasite in 3–7 days (Alvar *et al.*, 1997).

Immunocompetent patients who develop VL usually have high titres of leishmania antibodies easily detected by any one of several serodiagnostic tests (Badaró *et al.*, 1994). In contrast, serological tests are virtually useless in HIV-infected patients. A large proportion (50–80%) of patients with HIV infection and a clinical picture of VL have negative serological tests using immunofluorescence (IFAT) or enzyme immunoassays (ELISA) (Montalban *et al.*, 1990; Alvar *et al.*, 1997; WHO, 1997). Use of a recombinant *Leishmania* antigen (rK39) improved antibody detection by ELISA, but false negatives still remain a major problem (Houghton *et al.*, 1998). In one study, immunoblotting (Western blotting) was the best serological test, but over 20% of patients still had false-negative results.

Cutaneous leishmaniasis

The first reported case of cutaneous leishmaniasis in an HIV-infected patient was disseminated cutaneous leishmaniasis due to *L. brasiliensis* in a Brazilian (Coura *et al.*, 1987). The patient had dermal erythematous papules and nodules and non-ulcerated lesions on the thorax, face and lower limbs. To date, 17 cases of disseminated cutaneous leishmaniasis have been reported in abstracts from the Brazilian Society of Infectious Diseases meetings (Cunha *et al.*, 1991; Carnaúba *et al.*, 1992; Sousa *et al.*, 1993; Osaki *et al.*, 1994; Porro *et al.*, 1994), and an additional 20 or so have been published elsewhere. Cases of cutaneous leishmaniasis in HIV-infected subjects usually have multiple cutaneous lesions and mucosal involvement, features that are rare in immunocompetent patients with this disease, and the granulomatous and invasive aspects of the lesions are often dominant clinical manifestations (Figure 31.7). Of interest, in four cases in which mucosal involvement was reported, all had negative Montenegro skin test reactions, a test measuring delayed-type hypersensitivity to *Leishmania* sp. Virtually 100% of immunocompetent patients with cutaneous leishmaniasis will have delayed-type hypersensitivity reactions to this parasite (Cuba *et al.*, 1985).

Another rare condition, diffuse cutaneous leishmaniasis (DCL) caused by *L. mexicana amazonensis* in Brazil and *L. aethiopia* in Africa has been reported with other leishmania, such as *L. brasiliensis*, *L major* and *L. infantum* in HIV co-infected patients (Coura *et al.*, 1987; Gradoni *et al.*, 1990; Ndiaye *et al.*, 1996; Morsy *et al.*, 1997).

The diagnosis of cutaneous *leishmaniasis* is made by demonstrating *Leishmania* amastigotes in tissue or tissue swabs, or by recovering the organism by culture of the lesions. Specimens should preferably be taken from the edge of the lesions, not from the necrotic centre. The sensitivity of diagnostic tests depends on the species of *Leishmania* causing the infection (e.g. *L. brasiliensis* is present in only small numbers in tissue and is also difficult to recover on culture). As with visceral leishmaniasis, serological testing is unreliable in most cases.

Treatment and prevention

Pentavalent antimonials remain the mainstay of treatment for visceral leishmaniasis. The therapeutic ratio of these drugs was never good, and the increasing prevalence of drug resistance has further diminished their efficacy (Herwaldt and Berman, 1992). Antimonials suppress *Leishmania* infection but do not eradicate it, and relapses are therefore common following cessation of therapy, especially in patients with HIV-induced immunosuppression (Montalban *et al.*, 1990; Peters *et al.*, 1990).

The two drugs used for treatment of VL are stibogluconate (Pentostam®) or meglumine antimoniate (Glucantime®), and they are generally given in doses of 20 mg (of Sb) per kg/day for 1 month. However, because of the toxicity of these drugs, specialty consultation should be sought before initiating treatment. Amphotericin B has been used successfully to treat some HIV-uninfected patients failing therapy with antimonials (Davidson *et al.*, 1991), as has pentamidine isethionate (Thakur *et al.*, 1991). Other agents that have been used, often adjunctively, in a small number of patients include allopurinol, ketoconazole, itraconazole and immunotherapy with interferon-γ; insufficient data are available to comment on the efficacy of these drugs. The response of HIV-infected patients to any treatment is poor, and relapses are very common (Montalban *et al.*, 1990; Peters *et al.*, 1990), although one study suggested that increasing the antimony dose might improve treatment efficacy (Laguna *et al.*, 1997). This latter study also showed that monthly pentamidine was not effective for preventing relapses of visceral leishmaniasis (Laguna *et al.*, 1997).

Cutaneous leishmaniasis can be treated with antimonials, pentamidine or amphotericin B, as with visceral leishmaniasis, although the responses are highly variable, depending on the infecting species of *Leishmania*. Virtually no data are available on treatment specifically in HIV-infected subjects. Ketoconazole and itraconazole have been reported to be effective in some cases.

Although highly active antiretroviral therapy has reduced or eliminated the risk of relapse with many opportunistic infections, preliminary indications are that visceral leishmaniasis still has a high risk of relapse (Casado *et al.*, 2001).

References

Alvar J. (1994). *Leishmaniasis* and AIDS co-infection: the Spanish example. *Parasitol Today* **10**: 160–3.

Alvar J, Canacate C, Gutierrez-Solar B *et al.* (1997). *Leishmania* and human immunodeficiency virus co-infection: the first 10 years. *Clin Microbiol Rev* **10**: 298–319.

Anon. (1990). Chagas' disease: frequency and geographical distribution. *Wkly Epidemiol Rec* **65**: 257–64.

Badaró R, Jones TC, Carvalho EM *et al.* (1986). New perspectives on a subclinical form of visceral leishmaniasis. *J Infect Dis* **154**: 1003–11.

Badaró R, Nascimento C, Carvalho JS *et al.* (1994). Recombinant human granulocyte-macrophage colony-stimulating factor reverses neutropenia and reduces secondary infections in visceral leishmaniasis. *J Infect Dis* **170**: 413–18.

Belda Mira A, Diaz Sanchez F, Martines Garcia B *et al.* (1994). Visceral leishmaniasis and AIDS. Report of 2 cases with cutaneous dissemination. *Ann Intern Med* **11**: 398–400.

Berk SL, Verghese A. (1988). Parasitic pneumonia. *Semin Respir Infect* **3**: 172–8.

Bittencourt AL. (1976). Congenital chagas' disease. *Am J Dis Child* **130**: 97–103.

Brener Z. (1985). General review of *Trypanosoma cruzi* classification and taxonomy. *Rev Soc Bras Med Trop* **18**: 1–8.

Carnaúba D. Guimaráes MRAS, Correira VMSC *et al.* (1992). Leishmaniose cutáneo-mucosa em paciente com a Síndrome da Imunodeficiência Adquirida. A propósito de um caso. VII *Congresso Brasileiro de Infectologia.*

Casado JL, Lopez-Velez R, Pintado V *et al.* (2001). Relapsing visceral leishmaniasis in HIV-infected patients undergoing successful protease inhibitor therapy. *Eur J Clin Microbiol Infect Dis* **20**: 202–5

Chulay JD, Bruceson ADM. (1983). Quantitation of amastigotes of *Leishmania* donovani in smears of splenic aspirates from patients with visceral leishmaniasis. *Am J Trop Med Hyg* **32**: 475–9.

Chandramohan D, Greenwood BM. (1998). Is there an interaction between human immunodeficiency virus and *Plasmodium falciparum?* *Int J Epidemiol* **27**: 296–301.

Cohen JE, Tsai EC, Ginsberg HJ *et al.* (1998). Pseudotumoral chagasic meningoencephalitis as the first manifestation of AIDS. *Surg Neurol* **49**: 324–7.

Coura JR, Galv·o-Castro B, Grimaldo G. (1987). Disseminated American cutaneous leishmaniasis in a patient with AIDS. *Mem Inst Oswaldo Cruz* **8**: 581–2.

Cuba CA, Marsden PD, Barreto AC et al. (1985). The use of different concentrations of leishmanial antigen in skin testing to evaluate delayed hypersensítivity in American cutaneous leishmaniasis. Rev Soc Bras Med Trop **8**: 231–6.

Cunha RMC, Hafiack HA, Castañon MCMN. (1991). Leishmaniose tegumentar difusa em paciente infectado pelo HIV: relato de um caso. Rev Soc Bras Med Trop **24**: 109–10.

Da Cruz AM, Machado ES, Menczes JA et al. (1992). Cellular and humoral immune responses of patients with American cutaneous leishmaniasis and AIDS. Trans R Soc Trop Med Hyg **86**: 417–23.

Da Cruz AM, Conceição-Silva F, Bertho AL (1994). Leishmania-reactive CD4+ and CD8+ T cells associated with cure of human cutaneous leishmaniasis. Infec Immun **62**: 2614–18.

Davidson RN, Croft SL, Scott A et al. (1991). Liposomal amphotericin B in drug-resistant visceral leishmaniasis. Lancet **337**: 1061.

Di Lorenzo GA, Pagano MA, Taratuto AL et al. (1996). Chagasic granulomatous encephalitis in immunodepressed patients. Computed tomography and magnetic resonance imaging findings. J Neuroimaging **6**: 94–7.

Ferreira AW. (1992). Serological diagnosis. In: S Wendel (ed.) Chagas disease: its impact on transfusion and clinical medicine. Sao Paulo: ISBT Brazil, 179–93.

Freilij H, Altcheh J. (1995). Congenital Chagas' disease: diagnostic and clinical aspects. Clin Infect Dis **21**: 551–5.

Freilij H, Muller L, Gonzalez Cappa SM. (1983). Direct micromethod for diagnosis of acute and congenital Chagas' disease. J Clin Microbiol **18**: 327–30.

Freilij H, Altcheh J, Muchinik G. (1995). Perinatal HIV infection and congenital Chagas' disease. Pediatr Infect Dis J **14**: 161–2.

Frietag C, Chaougnet C, Schito M et al. (2001). Malaria infection induces virus expression in human immunodeficiency virus transgenic mice by CD4-cell-dependent immune activation. J Infect Dis **183**: 1260–8.

García L, Bruckner D. (1997). Diagnostic medical parasitology. Washington DC: ASM Press, 430–1.

Gluckstein D, Ciferri F, Ruskin J. (1992). Chagas' disease: another cause of cerebral mass in the acquired immunodeficiency syndrome. Am J Med **92**: 429–32.

Gompels MM, Todd J, Peters BS et al. (1991). Disseminated strongyloidiasis in AIDS: uncommon but important. AIDS **5**: 329–32.

Gonzalez Cappa SM, Lopez-Blanco OA, Muller LA et al. (1992). Chronic intracellular protozoan infections and kidney transplantation. Transplantation **52**: 2377–80.

Gradoni L, Gramiccia M. (1990). Fatal visceral disease caused by a dermotropic Leishmania in patient with human immunodeficiency virus infection. J Infect **20**: 169–84.

Gradoni L, Gramiccia M. (1994). Leishmania infantum tropism: strain genotype or host immune status? Parasitol Today **10**: 264–7.

Gramiccia M, Gradoni L, Troiani M. (1992). HIV-Leishmania co-infections in Italy. Isoenzyme characterization of Leishmania causing visceral leishmaniasis in HIV patients. Trans R Soc Trop Med Hyg **86**: 161–3.

Grant IH, Gold JW, Wittener M et al. (1989). Transfusion-associated acute Chagas' disease acquired in the United States. Ann Intern Med **111**: 849–51.

Grove DI. (1989). Strongyloidiasis: a major roundworm infection of man. Philadelphia, PA: Taylor & Francis, 1–336.

Hayes R, Schofield CY. (1990). Estimacion de las tasas de incidencia de infecciones y parasitosis cronicas a partir de la prevalencia: la Enf. de Chagas en America Latina. Bol Of Sanit Panam **108**: 308.

Heath T, Riminton S, Garsia R et al. (1996). Systemic strongyloidiasis complicating HIV: a promising response to ivermectin. Int J STD AIDS **7**: 294–6.

Herwaldt BL, Berman, JD. (1992). Recommendations for treating leishmaniasis with sodium stibogluconate (Pentostam®) and review of pertinent clinical studies. Am J Trop Med Hyg **46**: 296–306.

Houghton RL, Petrescu M, Benson DR et al. (1998). A cloned antigen (rK39) of L. chagasi diagnostic for visceral leishmaniasis in HIV-1 patients and a prognostic indicator for monitoring patients undergoing drug therapy. J Infect Dis **177**: 1339–44.

lzri MA, Deniau M, Briere C et al. (1996). Leishmaniasis in AIDS patients: results of leukoconcentration, a fast biological method of diagnosis. WHO **74**: 91–3.

Jimenez MI, Gutierrez-Solar B, Benito A et al. (1991). Cutaneous leishmania L. Infantum zymodemes isolated from bone marrow in AIDS patients. Res Rev Parasitol **51**: 95–9.

Jimenez MI, Lopez-Velez R Molina R et al. (1996). HIV co-infection with a currently non-pathogenic flagellate. Lancet **347**: 264–5.

Jorg ME, Zalazar Rovira J, Oliva R. (1980). Encefalitis aguda por Trypanosoma cruzi. Prensa Med Arg **67**: 5–14.

Kalyesubula I, Musoke-Mudido P, Marum L et al. (1997). Effects of malaria infection in human immunodeficiency virus type 1-infected Ugandan children. Pediatr Infect Dis J **16**: 876–81.

Kirchof LV. (1993). American trypanosomiasis (Chagas' disease). A tropical disease now in the United States. N Engl J Med **9**: 632–4.

Kohl S, Pickering LK, Frankel LS et al. (1982). Reactivation of Chagas' disease during therapy of acute lymphocytic leukemia. Cancer **50**: 827–8.

Kramer MR, Gregg PA, Goldstein M et al. (1990). Disseminated strongyloidiasis in AIDS and non-AIDS immunocompromised hosts: diagnosis by sputum and bronchoalveolar lavage. South Med J **83**: 1226–9.

Labarca J, Acuña G, Saavedra C et al. (1992). Enfermedad de Chagas en el sindrome inmunodeficiencia adquirida. asos clinicos. Rev Med Chile **120**: 174–9.

Leiguarda R, Roncoroni A, Taratuto AL et al. (1990). Acute CNS infection by Trypanosoma cruzi in immunosuppressed patients. Neurology **40**: 850–1.

Levi G, Kalla E, Ramos Moreira K. (1997). Disseminated Strongyloides stercoralis infection in an AIDS patient: the role of suppressive therapy. Braz J Infect Dis **1**: 49–53.

Liu XL, Weller PF. (1993). Strongyloidiasis and other intestinal nematode infections. Infect Dis Clin N Am **7**: 655–82.

Maayan S, Worsmer GP, Widerhorn J et al. (1987). Strongyloides stercoralis hyperinfection in a patient with the acquired immune deficiency syndrome. Am J Med **83**: 945–8.

Mansfield LS, Schad GA. (1989) Ivermectin treatment of naturally acquired and experimentally induced Strongyloides stercoralis infection in dogs. J Am Vet Med Assoc **201**: 726–30.

Marin-Neto JA, Marzullo P, Marcassa C et al. (1992). Myocardial perfusion abnormalities in chronic Chagas' disease as detected by thallium 201. Am J Cardiol **69**: 780–4.

Martinez P, de la Vega E, Laguna F et al. (1993). Diagnosis of visceral leishmaniasis in HIV-infected individuals using peripheral blood smears. AIDS **7**: 227–30.

Migot F, Ouedraogo JB, Diallo J et al. (1996). Selected P. falciparum specific immune responses are maintained in AIDS adults in Burkina Faso. Parasite Immunol **18**: 333–9.

Molina R, Cañavate C, Cercenado E et al. (1994). Indirect xenodiagnosis of visceral leishmaniasis in 10 HIV-infected patients using colonized Phlebotomus pernicious. AIDS **8**: 277.

Moncayo A. (1993). Chagas' disease. In: *Tropical disease research: progress 1991–92. Eleventh programme report of the UNDP/WORLD BANK/WHO, Special Programme for Research and Training in Tropical Disease*. Geneva: World Health Organization, 67–75.

Montalban C, Calleja JL, Erice A et al. (1990). Visceral leishmaniasis in patients infected with human immunodeficiency virus. *J Infect* **21**: 261–70.

Monteverde DA, Taratuto AL, Lucatelli N. (1976). Meningoencefalitis chagásica en paeientes inmunosuprimidos. *Rev Neurol Arg* **2**: 260–6.

Mooci S, Coffman RL. (1995). Induction of Th2 population from a polarized leishmania -specific Th1 population by *in vitro* culture with IL-4. *J Immunol* **54**: 379–87.

Morsy TA, Inrahim BB, Lashin AH. (1997). *Leishmania major* in an Egyptian patient manifested as diffuse cutaneous leishmaniasis. *J Egypt Soc Parasitol* **27**: 205–10.

Murray HW, Rubin BY, Rothermel CD. (1983) Killing of intracellular *Leishmania donovani* by lymphokine-stimulated human mononuclear phagocytes. Evidence that interferon-γ is the activating cytokine. *J Clin Invest* **72**: 1506–10.

Ndiaye PB, Develoux M, Dieng MT. (1996). Diffuse cutaneous leishmaniasis and acquired immunodeficiency syndrome in a Senegalese patient. *Bun Soc Pathol Exot* **89**: 282–6.

Oddo D, Casanova M, Acuna G et al. (1992). Acute Chagas' disease in AIDS. *Hum Pathol* **23**: 41–4.

Osaki KS, Cruz MA, Hueb M et al. (1994). Leishmaniose tegumentar americana em paciente com SIDA: relato de caso. *Rev Soc Bras Med Trop* **27**: 1.

Pagano MA, Segura MJ, Di Lorenzo GA et al. (1998). Cerebral tumour-like American trypanosomiasis in AIDS. *Am Neurol* **45**: 403–406.

Pan American Health Organization. (1990). Health conditions in the Americas. *Sci Pub* **524**: 211.

Parise ME, Ayisi JG, Nahlen BL et al. (1998). Efficacy of suldfadoxine-pyrimethamine for prevention of placental malaria in an area of Kenya with a high prevalence of malaria and human immunodeficiency virus infection. *Am J Trop Med Hygiene* **59**: 813–22.

Peters BS, Fish D, Golden R et al. (1990). Visceral leishmaniasis in HIV infection and clinical features and response to therapy. *Q J Med* **77**: 1101–11.

Piarroux R, Gambarelli F, Dumon H et al. (1994). Comparison of PCR with direct examination of bone marrow aspiration, myeloculture, and serology for diagnosis of visceral leishmaniasis in immunocompromised patients. *J Clin Microbiol* **32**: 746–9.

Pimentel PC, Handfas BW. (1996). *Trypanosoma cruzi* meningoencephalitis in AIDS mimicking cerebral metastases: case report. *Arq Neuropsiquiatr* **54**: 102–6.

Pintado V, Martin-Rabadan P, Rivera ML et al. (2001). Visceral leishmaniasis in HIV-infected and non-HIV-infected patients. A comparative study. *Medicine* (*Baltimore*) **80**: 54–73.

Pirmez C, Cooper C, Paes-Oliveira M et al. (1990). Immunologic responsiveness in American cutaneous leishmaniasis lesions. *J Immunol* **3**: 100–4.

Pirmez C, Yamamura M, Uyemura K et al. (1993). Cytokine patterns in the pathogenesis of human leishmaniasis. *J Clin Invest* **91**: 1390–6.

Porro AN, Pozzan G, Duarte MI et al. (1994). Leishmaniose cutâneomucosa em paciente HIV-positivo: relato de três casos. *Rev Soc Bras Med Trop* **27**: 1.

Prata A. (1994). Chagas' disease. *Infect Dis Clin No Am* **8**: 61–76.

Pratlong F, Dedet JP, Marty P et al. (1995). Leishmania-human immunodeficiency virus co-infection in the Mediterranean basin: isoenzymatic characterization of 100 isolates of the *Leishmania infantum* complex. *J Infect Dis* **172**: 323–6.

Preiser W, Cacopardo B, Nigro L et al. (1996). Immunological findings in HIV-Leishmana co-infection. *Intervirology* **39**: 285–8.

Pizzuto M, Piazza M, Senese D et al. (2001). Role of PCR in diagnosis and prognosis of visceral leishmaniasis in patients co-infected with HIV-1. *J Clin Microbiol* **39**: 357–61.Ravel S, Cuny G, Reynes J et al. (1986). A highly sensitive and rapid procedure for direct PCR detection of *Leishmania infantum* within human peripheral blood mononuclear cells. *Acta Trop Med Hyg* **35**: 79–85.

Reed SG, Scott P. (1993). T cells and cytokine response in *Leishmania*. *Curr Opin Immunol* **5**: 524–3.

Rezende JM. (1975). Chagasic mega-syndromes and regional differences. In: *New approaches in American* Trypanosomiasis. *Research. Washington PAHO, Sc Publ* 318: 195–205.

Ribeiro dos Santos G, Nishiya AS, Sabino EC et al. (1999). An improved, PCR-based strategy for the detection of *Trypanosoma cruzi* in human blood samples. *Ann Trop Med Parasitol* **93**: 689–94.

Rocha A, Ferreira M, Nishioka S et al. (1993). *Trypanosoma cruzi* meningoencephalitis and myocarditis in a patient with acquired immunodeficiency syndrome. *Rev Inst Med Trop S. Paulo* **35**: 2205–8.

Rocha A, Oliveira de Meneses AC, Moreira da Silva A et al. (1994). Pathology of patients with Chagas' disease and AIDS. *Am J Trop Med Hyg* **50**: 261–8.

Rosemberg S, Chaves CJ, Higuchi ML et al. (1992). Fatal meningoencephalitis caused by reactivation of *Trypanosoma cruzi* infection in a patient with AIDS. *Neurology* **42**: 640–2.

Rosenthal E, Marty P, del Guidice P et al. (2000). HIV and Leishmania co-infection: a review of 91 cases with focus on atypical locations of Leishmania. *Clin Infect Dis* **31**: 1093–5.

Russomando G, Figueredo A, Almiron M et al. (1992). Polymerase chain reaction-based detection of *Trypanosoma cruzi*i DNA in serum. *J Clin Microbiol* **30**: 2864–8.

Salotra P, Sreenivas G, Pogue GP et al. (2001). Development of a species-specific PCR assay for detection of *Leishmania donovani* in clinical samples from patients with kala-azar and post-kala-azar dermal leishmaniasis. *J Clin Microbiol* **39**: 849–54.

Sartori A, Shikanai Yasuda MA, Amato Neto V et al. (1998). Follow up of 18 patients with HIV infection and chronic Chagas' disease, with reactivation of Chagas' disease causing cardiac disease in three patients. *Clin Infect Dis* **26**: 177–9.

Schad GA, Aikens LM, Smith G. (1989). *Strongyloides stercoralis*: is there a canonical migratory route through the host? *J Parasitol* **75**: 740–9.

Schenone H, Alfaro E, Rojas A. (1974). Bases y rendimiento del Xenodiagnóstico en la infectión chagásica humana. *Bol Chil Parasit* **29**: 24–6.

Schijman AG, Vigliano C, Burgos J et al. (2000). Early diagnosis of recurrence of *Trypanosoma cruzi* infection by PCR after heart transplantation of a chronic Chagas' heart disease patient. *J Heart Lung Transplant* **19**: 1114–7.

Schmunis GA, Zicker F, Pinheirio F et al. (1998). Risk for transmitted infectious diseases in Central and South America. In: *Emerg Infect Dis* **4**: 5–11.

Scott P. (1993). IL-12: initiation cytokine for cell mediated immunity. *Science* **260**: 496–7.

Solari A, Saavedra H, Sepulveda C et al. (1993). Successful treatment of *Trypanosoma cruzi* encephalitis in a patient with hemophilia and AIDS. *Clin Infect Dis* **16**: 255–9.

Sousa AQ, Queiroz TBS, Pompeu MML *et al.* (1993). Leishmaniose cut,nea difusa (LCD) por *Leishmania braziliensis* mimetizendo sarcoma de Kaposi em um paciente com AIDS [Suppl]. *XXIX Congresso da Sociedade Brasileira de Medicina Tropical.*

Storino R, Millei J, Beigelman R. (1992). Enfermedad de Chagas :12 años de seguimiento en area urbana. *Rev Arg Cardiol* **60**: 205.

Strout RG. (1962). A method for concentrating hemoflagellates. *J Parasitol* **48**: 100.

Thakur CP, Kumar M, Pandey AK *et al.* (1991). Comparison of regimens of treatment of antiomony-resistant patients [with visceral leishmaniasis]: a randomized study. *Am J Trop Med Hyg* **45**: 435–41.

Torres JR, Isturiz R, Murillo J *et al.* (1993). Efficacy of ivermectin in the treatment of strongyloidiasis complicating AIDS. *Clin Infect Dis* **17**: 900–2.

UNDP/World Bank/WHO Special Programme for Research and Training in Tropical Diseases, (1991). *Tenth Programme Report: Chagas' disease.* Geneva: WHO, 69.

USA (1992). *Statistical abstract.* Washington DC; 42.

Villalba R, Fornes G, Alvarez M *et al.* (1992). Acute Chagas' disease in a recipient of a bone marrow transplant in Spain. *Clin Infect Dis* **14**: 594–5.

Wendel S, Pinto Dias JC. (1992). Transfusion transmitted Chagas disease. In: S Wendel, Z Brener (eds.) *Chagas disease: its impact on transfusion and clinical medicine.* Sao Paulo: ISBT Brazil, 49–81.

Whitworth J, Morgan D, Quigley M *et al.* (2000). Effect of HIV-1 and increasing immunosuppression on malaria parasitaemia and clinical episodes in adults in rural Uganda: a cohort study. *Lancet* **356**: 1051–6.

World Health Organization (WHO). (1997). *Leishmania*/HIV co-infection. *Wkly Epidemiol Rec* **72**: 49–56.

Xiao L, Owen SM, Rudolph DL *et al.* (1998) *Plasmodium falciparum* antigen-induced human immunodeficiency virus type 1 replication is mediated through induction of tumor necrosis factor-α. *J Infect Dis* **177**: 437–45.

Herpes simplex and varicella-zoster virus infections in HIV-infected individuals

CLAUDIA ESTCOURT AND ADRIAN MINDEL

Herpes simplex virus infection

Epidemiology

Herpes simplex virus (HSV) infection has troubled mankind for millenia. It was first described in the fifth century BC by ancient Greek and Roman physicians, and remains highly prevalent in the general population today. The recent introduction of type-specific serological assays for HSV antibodies has facilitated a large number of seroprevalence studies, which have altered perceptions about HSV epidemiology. These studies have reported considerable geographical variation in the prevalence of HSV-2 antibodies and in many areas the prevalence appears to be increasing (Nahmias et al., 1990; Mertz, 1993). In the USA, a population survey in 1978 reported a sero-prevalence of 16.4% in people over 16 years of age (Johnson et al., 1989). Twelve years later, a similar survey demonstrated a 32% increase in seroprevalence to 21.7% (Fleming et al., 1997). Rates of HSV-2 infection differ around the world and in different communities, being as low as 0.4% in first-year university students and up to 96% in female sex workers. Data from developing countries are limited, although there is some information suggesting an upward trend in HSV-2 prevalence.

HSV-2 infection behaves as a classical sexually transmitted disease, with acquisition related to age. Prevalence rises only after puberty and is linked to number of sexual partners (Cowan et al., 1994) and gender (women greater than men). HSV-2 antibodies are particularly prevalent in homosexual or bisexual men with HIV infection (68–77%) (Holmberg et al., 1988; Safrin et al., 1991a). Rates of detection of HSV-2 infection in other HIV-infected populations have not been as well studied, though data from a Baltimore sexually transmitted disease (STD) clinic showed an HSV-2 seroprevalence of 63% in HIV-infected heterosexual men, as compared to 81% in HIV-infected homo- or bisexual men (Hook et al., 1992). A recent study in male factory workers in Zimbabwe reported a sero-prevalence of 35.7% in HIV-uninfected men, as compared with 82.7% in HIV-infected men (Gwanzura et al., 1998).

Overall, about 62–70% of the general population have antibodies to HSV-1. The seroprevalence increases with age, reflecting acquisition of orolabial herpes. However, recently there has been a decrease in the age-specific seroprevalence (Schomogyi, 1998) parallelled by a relative increase in HSV-1-associated genital herpes (Ross et al., 1993). Possible reasons for this decrease include decreased acquisition of HSV-1 in childhood due to improved living standards, decrease in age at first orogenital contact (Schomogyi, 1998), or an overall increase in the practice of orogenital sex, perhaps in response to safer sex messages (Bourne et al., 1995).

Pathogenesis and transmission

HSV is transmitted by direct inoculation through skin or mucous membrane contact. The virus is then transported intra-axonally along sensory nerves to the nerve cell bodies in the corresponding dorsal nerve root or trigeminal ganglia, where latency is established. Upon reactivation, triggered by incompletely understood stimuli, initiation of virus replication is followed by virus transport to mucocutaneous surfaces via efferent nerves, with the subsequent appearance of clinically apparent lesions or subclinical virus replication. In contrast to varicella-zoster virus (VZV) infection (see below), viraemic dissemination of HSV is rare, even in immunocompromised hosts.

It is well recognized that people may shed HSV at times when no clinical lesions are apparent and that most people do so at some stage in their infection (Wald *et al.*, 1997). This has been termed asymptomatic shedding or subclinical recurrence. Viruses may be isolated from sites of previous lesions, seemingly uninvolved parts of the genital tract and other cutaneous areas within the same dermatome, in particular the thighs and buttocks. Rates of shedding depend on virus type, as HSV-2 is associated with higher rates of asymptomatic shedding (as well as higher symptomatic recurrence rates) than HSV-1.

Published studies using culture to detect HSV have reported shedding on 2–3% of days for most patients (Brock *et al.*, 1992; Wald *et al.*, 1995), while polymerase chain reaction (PCR) studies have reported shedding on 28% of days (Wald *et al.*, 1997). Genital shedding of HSV is increased in HIV-infected individuals. A cross-sectional study of HIV-infected and HIV-uninfected women in the USA reported significantly more days of predominately asymptomatic virus shedding for the infected women: 13.2% as compared with 3.6% for uninfected women (Augenbaum *et al.*, 1995). These observations have important implications for both horizontal (i.e. sexual) (Koutsky *et al.*, 1990, 1992; Mertz *et al.*, 1992), as well as vertical transmission of HSV infection (Brown *et al.*, 1991).

Disruption of mucosal or cutaneous integrity almost certainly facilitates HIV transmission. The increased numbers of activated CD4 lymphocytes present in HSV-associated ulcers may act as a reservoir of target cells for HIV, thereby increasing the likelihood of infection following exposure. In addition, T-cell activation facilitates HIV replication and may mean that an HIV-infected person co-infected with HSV is a more effective HIV transmitter. The frequent detection of HIV RNA in genital ulcers caused by HSV-2 in HIV-infected patients at different stages of disease supports this theory (Schacker *et al.*, 1997).

There is an increased risk of acquisition of HIV in the presence of genital ulcer disease *per se* (Greenblatt *et al.*, 1988; Simonsen *et al.*, 1988), and herpes simplex infection is the most common cause of genital ulceration, at least in developed countries. People with pre-existing genital HSV have a two- to three-fold increased risk for acquisition of HIV in most studies (Dickerson *et al.*, 1996).

The factors modulating the frequency and duration of clinical recurrences of genital HSV are not well understood, although both cell-mediated and humoral immune defenses may be involved. Immunosuppressed patients, particularly those with impaired cell-mediated immunity, tend to manifest a greater frequency and severity of HSV infec-

tion. In an attempt to define the role of cellular responses in the reactivation process, cytotoxic T-cell responses have been compared in HIV-infected and HIV-uninfected individuals infected with HSV-2, and in HIV-infected individuals with different HSV-2 recurrence rates (Posavad *et al.*, 1997). Patients co-infected with HSV and HIV had fewer HSV-2-specific cytotoxic lymphocyte precursors (pCTL) than those infected only with HSV, and in those co-infected, lesion severity correlated with HSV-2 pCTL frequency.

Other factors may also affect the HSV recurrence rate. After an episode of primary genital herpes, for example, recurrences were found to be more frequent in men than in women, in those infected by HSV-2 rather than HSV-1, and in those acquiring HSV-% infection without serological evidence of prior infection with HSV-1 (Reeves *et al.*, 1981; Koelle *et al.*, 1992).

It is generally felt that mucocutaneous lesions due to HSV are less prone to resolve spontaneously in HIV-infected individuals than in immunocompetent patients. A case series in 1981 (prior to the availability of aciclovir) described chronic perianal ulcerations in four patients with HIV infection (Siegal *et al.*, 1981), consistent with the speculation that tendency for chronicity increases as the severity of HIV-associated impairment of immune defences progresses. The case definition of AIDS was revised by the Centers for Disease Control and Prevention in 1987 to include chronic mucocutaneous HSV lesions persisting for longer than 1 month, in the absence of other causes of immunodeficiency or in the presence of serum antibody against HIV. However, a retrospective study at San Francisco General Hospital found that neither frequency of herpetic recurrence nor duration of herpetic lesions was prolonged in the majority of patients with AIDS (Safrin *et al.*, 1991a).

The relationship between active HSV infection and the plasma HIV-1 viral load has been studied in a group of 16 subjects (Mole *et al.*, 1997). Plasma HIV-1 viral load increased for most, but not all, patients during acute HSV infection (median of rise 3.4 times), despite concurrent oral aciclovir. Levels of plasma viral load remained above baseline in some subjects 30–45 days after the appearance of lesions, when patients were still taking oral aciclovir. The significance of these results in terms of HIV progression is unclear.

Clinical presentation

Clinically apparent primary or recurrent lesions caused by HSV present as vesiculo-ulcerative lesions on an erythematous base, occurring at any mucocutaneous site. Although

HSV-1 most commonly causes lesions in the mouth or on the lips, and HSV-2 in genital and perianal areas, either virus may cause lesions at any location, according to the site of primarym mucocutaneous inoculation. Primary episodes have a longer duration of clinical symptoms and of virus shedding than recurrent outbreaks; in the case of persons with genital herpes, a primary episode averages 16–19 days while a recurrent episode lasts approximately 6–7 days. In general, as most HIV-infected people acquired HSV infection before acquiring HIV, they principally have recurrent HSV disease. The typical clinical presentation of herpes simplex virus infection has been challenged by the recent recognition that up to 87% of people with serum antibody to HSV-2 have no history of genital outbreaks (Koutsky et al., 1992; Siegel et al., 1992). The presence of atypical lesions may also contribute to underdiagnosis.

Orolabial HSV

Although orolabial infection in HIV-infected adults tends to be recurrent HSV-1 disease, in children primary infection is more likely. If primary infection does occur in HIV-infected adults, there are reports that a severe illness may result, with widespread blistering lesions involving much of the buccal mucosa, lips and tongue, accompanied by fever (Straus, 1982). Orolabial HSV-1 in many HIV-infected adults will be similar to that in immunocompetent hosts, but frequency of recurrences and time taken for healing of lesions may increase with advancing immunosuppression.

Anogenital HSV

Anogenital outbreaks of HSV in patients with HIV infection are common, perhaps due to the high prevalence of HSV-2 infection (Holmberg et al., 1988; Safrin et al., 1991a) and the inability of host defenses to prevent reactivation. Several authors have expressed the view that anogenital herpetic recurrences are more frequent in HIV-infected patients, particularly as immunosuppression advances. To date, however, this has not been demonstrated in observational studies. In a retrospective study of patients with AIDS at San Francisco General Hospital, no evidence of an increased frequency or severity of recurrences was demonstrated (Safrin et al., 1991a). A recent report showed that mucocutaneous ulcerative lesions in HIV-infected persons were most commonly due to HSV, particularly as the CD4 lymphocyte count decreased; however, this study did not address the issues of frequency or severity of recurrence (Bagdades et al., 1992). Although chronic herpetic ulcer-

ation has been reported in patients with AIDS, it is frequently associated with resistance to aciclovir (see below).

Lesions in the perianal area may cause pain and/or itching and may coalesce and extend up the gluteal cleft to the sacral area. The distal rectum may be involved, resulting in severe anorectal pain, tenesmus, constipation and fever (Goodell et al., 1983). Sigmoidoscopic findings include friable mucosa with vesicular or pustular lesions and/or diffuse ulceration. Cervical involvement may lead to mucopurulent cervicitis. Neurological symptoms such as difficulty in initiating micturition and sacral paresthesiae may also be present.

There is no evidence that patients with HIV infection have more frequent complications of HSV infection than HIV-uninfected individuals.

Disseminated HSV

Extragenital HSV disease does appear to be more common in HIV-infected patients than in the uninfected. Oesophagitis may occur in HIV-infected as in other immunocompromised hosts, causing dysphagia and/or odynophagia (Connolly et al., 1989). In such patients, concomitant perioral HSV lesions may be absent, so that differentiation from other causes of oesophagitis (such as candida or cytomegalovirus [CMV]) requires endoscopic visualization and sampling of the lesion for culture and histopathology. Haemorrhagic cystitis, ocular keratitis, aseptic meningitis and ascending myelitis have also been reported to occur rarely in patients with HIV infection.

HSV encephalitis

Herpes simplex encephalitis is a rare but serious complication of both HSV-1 and HSV-2 infection in HIV-infected individuals (Chrétien et al., 1996). In adults, it often follows reactivation of orolabial HSV, although in HIV-infected neonates, encephalitis may complicate a primary infection. The clinical diagnosis of HSV encephalitis is difficult as the symptoms and signs are variable, and may mimic other more common central nervous system (CNS) opportunistic infections due to Cryptococcus neoformans or Toxoplasma gondii. An insidious onset with headache, meningismus and personality change has been described, as has an abrupt onset of fever, headache, confusion, cranial nerve involvement, seizures and coma. Death or severe permanent disability are common outcomes if prompt aciclovir therapy is not initiated.

Diagnosis

Virus culture remains the gold standard for the diagnosis of active HSV infection. The specimen, obtained by un-roofing the vesicular or crusted lesion and/or swabbing the base of the ulcer with a cotton-tipped or dacron swab, should be forwarded to the clinical virology laboratory in appropriate transport media, where it is inoculated onto continuous or semi-continuous cell culture lines (e.g. Vero or foreskin fibroblast cells). Upon detection of character-istic changes in cell morphology (cytopathic effect), gen-erally within 24–72 h, HSV is confirmed (i.e. HSV-1 versus HSV-2), with specific fluorescein-conjugated monoclonal antibodies. Common causes of false-negative cultures include sampling late in the clinical episode, when viral shedding is diminishing, and using inappropriate culture techniques or patients in whom HSV is cleared rapidly from the genital tract (Schomogyi et al., 1998). The overall sen-sitivity of HSV culture is around 50% (Lafferty et al., 1987), though may be increased to around 60% in women if mul-tiple sites are swabbed (Koutsky et al., 1992).

Alternatives to virus culture include direct antigen detection (by immunofluorescent, immunoperoxidase, or enzyme-linked immunoassay techniques) and the Tzanck smear. Antigen detection requires the presence of infected cells obtained directly from the clinical lesion. The main advantages of this method are the rapidity of results and increased availability to office-based physicians. However, sensitivity and specificity depend on the adequacy of the specimen obtained, and the stage of the lesion (early vesic-ular lesions have the highest yield). Therefore, several slides should be prepared to maximize diagnostic accuracy. In the Tzanck smear, multinucleated giant cells are visualized on a Giemsa or Wright's stain of scrapings from the base of an herpetic ulcer; however, this examination has a sensitivity of approximately 50% when compared with tissue culture and is also unable to differentiate between HSV and VZV infection.

Detection of HSV DNA following amplification by the PCR has increased sensitivity when compared with tissue culture, and has therefore been applied both to the exam-ination of cerebrospinal fluid in patients with suspected her-pes simplex encephalitis and for improved detection of cutaneous virus shedding (Safrin et al., 1997). The sensi-tivity and specificity of cerebrospinal fluid (CSF) exami-nation in patients with HSV encephalitis approaches 100% (Lakeman et al., 1995), and HSV DNA remains present in genital lesions for twice as long as replication-competent virus (Cone et al., 1991), which would favour PCR as a diagnostic tool when sampling lesions relatively late in the clinical episode. This assay is not commercially available, but it may supersede culture as the preferred diagnostic test in the future.

The development of type-specific serological techniques for HSV-1 and HSV-2 has dramatically facilitated assessment of the prevalence of these infections. However, the detection of serum antibody to HSV-1 or HSV-2 has limited clinical value given the high prevalence rates in HIV-infected pop-ulations and the inherent difficulties in interpreting an indi-vidual result (e.g. determining the presence of active infection). The tests rely on the identification of type-specific glycoproteins on the virus surface, denoted gG1 and gG2. Accurate type-specific antibody testing can be accomplished with use of enzyme immunoassay, or immunoblotting (Levi et al., 1996; Ashley et al., 1998). A direct comparison of these techniques in immunocompetent individuals failed to detect any differences in overall sensitivity (Ashley et al., 1988); however, in patients with HIV infection the glyco-protein assay was less sensitive than immunoblot for detec-tion of HSV-2 antibody (Safrin et al., 1992a).

Treatment

Antiviral therapy decreases the duration of HSV episodes and decreases both the symptoms and duration of virus shedding. However, current treatments fail to eradicate latent virus in the paraspinous ganglia. As HSV infections have a propensity for reactivation, our current management options represent control of disease, rather than a cure.

Antiviral drugs active against HSV were first developed in the 1950s, and included 5-iododeoxyuridine (IUdR), tri-fluorothymidine (TFT), and cytosine arabinoside (ara-C). Although they were found to be too toxic for systemic use, topical IUdR and TFT remain first-line topical therapies for herpes keratitis. Adenine arabinoside (vidarabine, ara-A), a parenteral agent licensed in the mid-1970s, was shown to be effective for the treatment of neonatal HSV infection and for HSV encephalitis. However, newer therapies have taken its place in first-line management and this drug is no longer available.

HSV genes involved in antiviral drug activity are shown in Figure 32.1.

Aciclovir

The advent of aciclovir in the early 1980s revolutionized the management of HSV infections. Over recent years, two

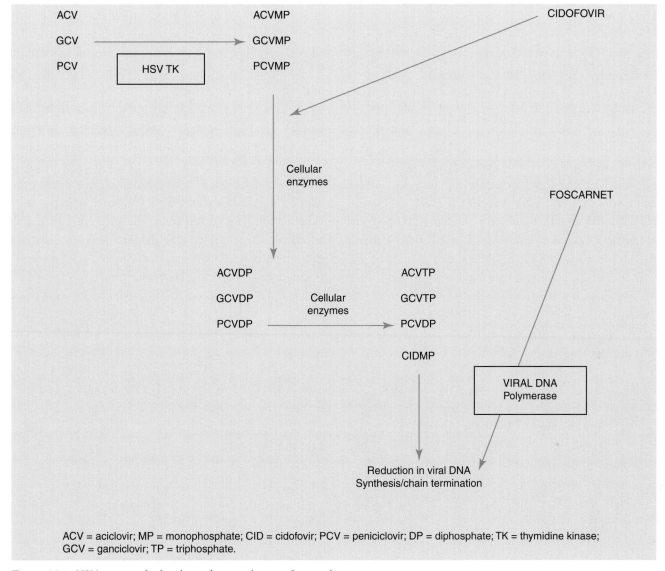

ACV = aciclovir; MP = monophosphate; CID = cidofovir; PCV = penciclovir; DP = diphosphate; TK = thymidine kinase; GCV = ganciclovir; TP = triphosphate.

Figure 32.1 *HSV genes involved in the mechanism of action of antivirals.*

related compounds, valaciclovir and famciclovir (penciclovir), have added to the available therapeutic options. Although the newer compounds have better bioavailability and simpler dosing schedules than aciclovir, they have similar clinical efficacy.

Aciclovir is an acyclic guanosine analogue formulated in intravenous, oral and topical preparations. Aciclovir, like all nucleoside analogs, is a prodrug which requires activation by a phosphorylation step catalysed by a virus-specified thymidine kinase. The exquisite specificity of aciclovir, the result-selective activation of the drug by virion thymidine kinase in HSV-infected cells, and its lack of cellular toxicity (due to the drug inactivity toward cellular DNA polymerases), makes aciclovir a particularly useful antiviral

agent for the treatment of HSV infection. Following monophosphorylation by the virus-specified thymidine kinase, di- and tri-phosphorylation is accomplished by cellular enzymes, such that the triphosphorylated form of aciclovir is available to compete with the natural substrate, dGTP, for the virus DNA polymerase. Due to its high affinity for the virion enzyme, aciclovir is preferentially incorporated into virion DNA, causing termination of DNA synthesis due to the lack of a 3'-hydroxyl on the incorporated aciclovir molecule (Elion, 1986).

Both HSV-1 and HSV-2 are highly susceptible to aciclovir, requiring *in vitro* concentrations of approximately 0.1 and 1.6 μM, respectively, for inhibition of virus replication by 50% (ID$_{50}$) (Dorsky and Crumpacker,

1987). Intravenous dosing of aciclovir results in serum levels of the drug that are well above the ID_{50} of HSV-1 and HSV-2. Despite the relatively poor (15–25%) bioavailability of the oral formulation of aciclovir, steady-state serum concentrations following dosing of 200 mg five times daily range from 1.4 to $4.0 \mu M$ (mean, 2.5), such that the ID_{50} of the virus is generally exceeded (Dorsky and Crumpacker, 1987). For the reasons outlined above, aciclovir has a high therapeutic:toxic ratio. When given in high doses intravenously, however, aciclovir has been associated with a reversible azotaemia due to crystallization and deposition of the drug in the renal tubules, particularly in patients with pre-existing renal insufficiency or dehydration, or those in whom the drug is infused rapidly and in high doses (Dorsky and Crumpacker, 1987). Oral aciclovir has not been associated with renal dysfunction. A neurological syndrome consisting of lethargy, confusion, and/or acute psychiatric disturbances has also been described in patients receiving high-dose intravenous therapy (Dorsky and Crumpacker, 1987). Despite the concentration of aciclovir in semen, a prospective study of men receiving long-term daily chemosuppressive aciclovir therapy for recurrent genital herpes failed to demonstrate a clinically significant effect of the drug on sperm count, motility, or morphology (Douglas et al., 1988). A survey of 312 aciclovir-exposed pregnancies found no evidence of an increase in birth defects over that expected in the general population (Andrews et al., 1992).

Orolabial HSV. Aciclovir treatment of herpes labialis in the immunocompetent host provides only modest benefit. Oral aciclovir (400 mg five times daily for 5 days), begun within 1 h of the first sign or symptom of recurrent herpes simplex labialis, did not prevent the occurrence of lesions but did decrease the mean duration of pain and the total time to healing when compared with placebo in one study (Spruance et al., 1990). Results from treatment trials using topical formulations of aciclovir have demonstrated minimal effect. Oral aciclovir (400 mg twice daily) has recently been shown to prevent reactivation in persons with frequently recurring herpes labialis in a placebo-controlled trial (Rooney et al., 1993), as it did in UV-exposed skiers (Spruance et al., 1988). Although not directly compared, oral aciclovir appears to be more effective than topical sun screen for preventing exposure-induced recurrences of orofacial HSV (Mills et al., 1987).

Chronic orofacial HSV infections in both HIV-infected and uninfected immunocompromised individuals respond to aciclovir, providing it is administered in adequate doses during an early stage of the infection (Cohen and Greenberg, 1985). Thus, evidence of HSV infection should be sought in any immunocompromised patient with multiple ulcers of the palate, alveolar ridge, or oral mucosa, particularly since such lesions may become resistant to aciclovir once chronic (Safrin et al., 1991c).

Anogenital HSV. Placebo-controlled trials have established the clinical and virological efficacy of both intravenous (5 mg/kg every 8 h) and oral (200 mg five times daily) aciclovir for treatment of primary and recurrent genital herpes (Mindel and Adler, 1982; Nilsen et al., 1982). Treatment shortened the duration of virus shedding by about 50% and accelerated healing by about 30%. A recent trial showed that a 5-day regimen of 800 mg twice daily may also be effective for the treatment of recurrent genital herpes. Both intravenous and oral aciclovir are far more effective for the treatment of primary genital infections than recurrent HSV infection. Topical aciclovir (5%) has a slight beneficial effect on the clinical course of primary genital herpes, but did not prevent new lesion formation and had only minimal clinical impact on recurrent lesions (Corey et al., 1982). There is no evidence that treatment with aciclovir prevents establishment of latency or decreases the frequency of subsequent recurrences.

In a placebo-controlled study, oral aciclovir therapy for first-episode HSV proctitis (400 mg five times daily for 10 days) reduced the duration of rectal lesions and of virus shedding, but surprisingly had no effect on symptoms (Rompalo et al., 1988).

Recurrent anogenital herpes can be prevented by chronic aciclovir administration, so called 'chemosuppression'. In one study, 227 of 519 (44%) immunocompetent patients chemosuppressed with aciclovir, 400 mg twice daily, were free of recurrence after 1 year, compared to seven of 431 (2%) placebo-treated patients. Aciclovir also decreased the mean number of recurrences per year (11.4 versus 1.8) (Mertz et al., 1988; Straus et al., 1988a). However, aciclovir chemosuppression does not prevent all recurrent episodes, even in immunocompetent patients (Mertz et al., 1988), and asymptomatic virus shedding may also continue (Straus et al.,1989). Dose-ranging studies in immunocompetent individuals have established that the most effective dose for chemosuppression is 200 mg four times daily (Mindel et al., 1988). However, more convenient doses, such as 400 mg twice daily and 200 mg three times daily, have been shown to be nearly as effective in placebo-controlled trials (Mertz et al., 1988; Straus et al., 1989). Aciclovir chemosuppression remains effective and safe, for even up to 9 years of continuous use (Baker et al., 1995).

Standard doses of aciclovir (e.g. 200 mg five times daily orally or 5 mg/kg every 8 h intravenously) are generally administered to patients with mucocutaneous HSV infection who are immunosuppressed due to haematological malignancy or organ transplantation, and a prompt response usually follows. Although some clinicians believe that higher doses of aciclovir are necessary in HIV-infected patients, this has never been formally evaluated. As chronic herpetic ulcerative lesions have been sporadically reported in both HIV-infected and uninfected immunosuppressed patients, it is unclear whether this is a more frequent occurrence in one group of patients than the other. HIV-infected patients whose HSV lesions do not respond within 5–7 days while receiving standard doses of aciclovir should be treated with maximum oral doses (e.g. 800 mg five times daily) without delay. Some authors also recommend the addition of topical to oral aciclovir in these circumstances. While this approach has not been validated in clinical trials, it seems appropriate to avoid continued subtherapeutic dosing of aciclovir in immunocompromised patients, which may in turn select aciclovir-resistant mutants. Many authorities consider that it is preferable to manage HIV-infected patients with recurrent herpes by chemosuppression, rather than episodic treatment, to prevent the development of resistance.

Valaciclovir and famciclovir

Two aciclovir-related compounds have recently become available for the treatment of primary and recurrent HSV disease. Valaciclovir is the 1-valine ester of aciclovir, which has an oral bioavailability between three and five times that of aciclovir (Weller et al., 1993). It is a pro-drug, converted to aciclovir and valine in the liver, and has the same mechanism of action as aciclovir. A large, randomized, controlled trial of episodic valaciclovir treatment of recurrent genital herpes in immunocompetent patients shortened the duration of lesions, pain and virus shedding compared to placebo (Spruance et al., 1996). Valaciclovir is effective as treatment for first episodes and secondary recurrences and also as chemosuppression (Patel et al., 1997). The simple dosing schedule (once or twice daily) and excellent oral availability make valaciclovir an appealing choice of therapy, but clear clinical benefits over

aciclovir have not been demonstrated. Treatment regimens are summarized in Table 32.1.

Famciclovir, the oral pro-drug of penciclovir, is another acyclic nucleoside, which is activated selectively via viral thymidine kinase (Earnshaw et al., 1992). The intracellular half-life of penciclovir triphosphate is longer than that of aciclovir triphosphate. Famciclovir is effective for acute therapy for recurrent HSV episodes and for chronic suppression and is well tolerated (Sacks et al., 1996; Mertz et al., 1997). It is likely that famciclovir will also be approved shortly for the treatment of primary episodes. Patient acceptability rather than any superior clinical efficacy would favour famciclovir over aciclovir or valaciclovir.

Famciclovir chemosuppression was evaluated in a double-blind, placebo-controlled trial in HIV-infected subjects (Schacker et al., 1998). Compared with placebo, famciclovir shortened the clinical findings due to HSV infection, and both symptomatic and asymptomatic virus shedding. Treatment regimens are illustrated in Table 32.1.

Antiviral resistance

Up to 11% of HSV isolates from mucocutaneous lesions from immunocompetent and immunosuppressed populations have been shown to have reduced susceptibility to aciclovir (Dekker et al., 1983; Englund et al., 1990). Initially, this finding was not believed to be of clinical significance in immunocompetent patients, but a report of aciclovir resistant refractory vulval HSV in an HIV-uninfected immunocompetent woman suggests otherwise (Swetter et al., 1998). In contrast, aciclovir-resistant HSV disease is well recognized in HIV-infected individuals. The reported cases have usually occurred in patients with severe immunosuppression (Safrin et al., 1991c), but the chronicity of the lesion also appears to be important (Safrin et al., 1992b). Aciclovir-resistance has been described most frequently with HSV-2, although aciclovir-resistant lesions caused by HSV-1 also occur (Norris et al., 1987; Erlich et al., 1989a; Gateley et al., 1990; Safrin et al., 1990; Safrin et al., 1991c). In a recent postal survey of UK HIV physicians, 70% had cared for at least one case of resistant HSV infection (Scoular et al., 1997). Since both valaciclovir and famciclovir act via viral thymidine kinase-dependent mechanisms, resistance to aciclovir is synonymous with resistance to valaciclovir and famciclovir.

Resistance to aciclovir is readily induced in the laboratory by serial passage of the virus in the presence of the drug (Field et al., 1980). However, resistance can occur in the

Table 32.1 Management of HSV infections in HIV-infected patients

Clinical presentation	First line (preferred)	Alternative
Orogenital, perianal		
1. Mild	Aciclovir 200 mg/five times per day p.o. for 5–10 days or Aciclovir 400 mg/three times per day p.o. for 5–10 days	Valaciclovir 1 g/three times per day p.o. for 5–10 days or [a]Famciclovir 250 mg/three times per day p.o. for 5–10 days
2. Severe	Aciclovir 5 mg/kg/three times per day i.v. for 5–10 days	Foscarnet 40 mg/kg/three times per day i.v. for 21 days
Extensive disease **Encephalitis**	Acylovir 10 mg/kg/three times per day i.v. for 10 days	Foscarnet 40 mg/kg/three times per day i.v. for 21 days
Chemosuppression	Aciclovir 200 mg/four times per day PO or [b]Aciclovir 400 mg/two times per day PO	Valaciclovir 500 mg/two times per day p.o. or famciclovir 500 mg/two times per day p.o. or foscarnet 40 mg/kg/three times per day i.v.
Aciclovir-resistant HSV	Foscarnet 40 mg/kg/three times per day i.v.	[c]Foscarnet 1% cream five times per day or cidofovir 0.3% gel once per day or trifluridine 1% solution three times per day

HSV: Herpes simplex virus.
[a]Not yet licensed for acute therapy.
[b]More convenient dosing schedule.
[c]May be used as adjunct to i.v. therapy or as sole agent.

(Adapted from Sanford et al., 1999.)

absence of exposure to aciclovir: in one study, six of 97 isolates of HSV-2 from aciclovir naïve patients were resistant *in vitro* (McLaren *et al.*, 1983a). Evidence has accumulated to suggest that in the majority of clinical HSV lesions, at least some of the virions present are resistant to aciclovir *in vitro* (Parris and Harrington, 1982). Spontaneous mutations to the resistant phenotype in the thymidine kinase gene occur at a rate of approximately 1 in every 10 000–100 000 virus replications. HSV replication is likely to be accelerated in the immunocompromised host, which may predispose to greater emergence of resistant strains in HIV-infected patients, as well as in uninfected immunocompromised persons (Vinckier *et al.*, 1987; Sacks *et al.*, 1989).

Three mechanisms of resistance have been described (Balfour, 1983): marked deficiency or absence of the virus-specified thymidine kinase; alteration in substrate specificity of the thymidine kinase; and alteration in the substrate specificity of the viral DNA polymerase. Presumably, intact host defences in immunocompetent individuals are usually able to eradicate the subpopulation of aciclovir-resistant strains present in a given mucocutaneous lesion. With or

without aciclovir, HSV recurrences in these patients are usually self-limited. In the severely immunocompromised patient who lacks immune defences against HSV, aciclovir eradicates the aciclovir-susceptible strains, allowing the resistant strains, uncontrolled by the normal host defence mechanisms, to predominate within the lesion.

Although animal studies have typically demonstrated diminished virulence in thymidine kinase-deficient mutants of HSV, both the ability to establish latency and neurovirulence (Erlich *et al.*, 1989a) have now been clearly demonstrated in some of these strains. In addition, Gateley *et al.* (1990) showed that a thymidine kinase-deficient HSV strain from the CSF of a patient with AIDS who developed fatal meningoencephalitis caused cutaneous lesions and fatal CNS infection in mice. Therefore, it seems that in the setting of severe immunosuppression, thymidine kinase-deficient strains of HSV may cause considerable morbidity and even occasional mortality.

Susceptibility testing. There are a variety of HSV susceptibility testing methods that have not been standardized by reference laboratories. The neutral red dye uptake (McLaren et al., 1983b), plaque reduction (McLaren et al., 1983b) and DNA hybridization (Swierkosz et al., 1987) assays are the most commonly utilized; direct comparison of the techniques using clinical correlation has not been performed. In addition, the thymidine kinase phenotype of an HSV isolate can be determined using plaque auto-radiography (Martin et al., 1985), and the specific mutations in the thymidine kinase or DNA polymerase genes by sequencing. Virtually all aciclovir-resistant mutants derived from clinical lesions are thymidine kinase-deficient. However, both thymidine kinase altered and DNA polymerase mutants have been isolated from clinical lesions on rare occasions (Ellis et al., 1987; Parker et al., 1987).

Management of aciclovir-resistant HSV

Although a number of drugs have been tested for treatment of aciclovir-resistant HSV, foscarnet is the drug of choice. Patients suspected of having thymidine kinase-resistant HSV should stop aciclovir, famciclovir or valaciclovir and commence alternative treatment with foscarnet within 7–10 days (Balfour et al., 1994).

Foscarnet, a pyrophosphate analogue, acts by direct inhibition of the virus DNA polymerase and so retains in vitro activity against thymidine kinase-deficient strains of aciclovir-resistant HSV. Its clinical efficacy for the treatment of aciclovir-resistant HSV infection was initially suggested by several uncontrolled studies and case reports (Vinckier et al., 1987; Erlich et al., 1989b; Safrin et al., 1990), and subsequently confirmed in a randomized, multicentre trial sponsored by the AIDS Clinical Trials Group of the National Institutes for Allergy and Infectious Diseases (Safrin et al., 1991c). In this study, patients randomized to receive foscarnet (40 mg/kg every 8 h) experienced accelerated healing of their lesions and a lower incidence of serious toxicity compared with patients receiving vidarabine (15 mg/kg/day) (Safrin et al., 1991c). Superior efficacy was manifested both by significant reduction in the median time to complete healing (13.5 versus 38.5 days) and median time to cessation of viral shedding (6 versus 17 days) in foscarnet-treated patients, as compared with the vidarabine treated group ($p = 0.001$, $p = 0.006$, respectively).

Administration of foscarnet requires close and frequent monitoring for potential toxicities, which include nephrotoxicity (often with proteinuria), hypocalcaemia, hyperphosphataemia, anaemia, neurotoxicity, gastrointestinal intolerance, neutropenia, penile and scrotal ulcerative drug

eruptions, and the concomitant bacterial complications of central venous catheterization. Nephrotoxicity can be minimized by pre-hydration with saline, and by avoiding concomitant administration of other nephrotoxic agents. Adjustment of the dosage of foscarnet according to changes in body weight and/or serum creatinine will help to prevent serious toxicity (see Chapter 21 for full prescribing information on foscarnet).

One case report showed that topical foscarnet (1% cream) induced rapid healing, starting within 24 h of chronic non-healing vulvar lesions in an immunocompetent woman, in whom high-dose oral aciclovir, valaciclovir and topical triflurothymidine had no effect (Swetter et al., 1998). The cream formulation may have a particular role in HIV-infected individuals (Hardy et al., 1996).

Scattered reports of foscarnet-resistant HSV infection in patients with AIDS have appeared (Sacks et al., 1989; Birch et al., 1990). These rare reports suggest that emergence of resistance to foscarnet may increase as this drug is used more widely. Indeed, a series of six patients with foscarnet-resistant HSV infection has been collated by one group (Safrin et al., 1994). Five of the six patients had received foscarnet intermittently for the treatment of aciclovir-resistant HSV infection prior to the development of foscarnet resistance; three of the five had received foscarnet chronically to suppress reactivation of aciclovir-resistant HSV. The sixth patient was receiving daily foscarnet for the suppression of CMV retinitis. These reports underscore the importance of continuing to evaluate other therapeutic alternatives for patients with resistant infection.

Erlich et al. (1989a) described 12 patients with AIDS and clinically significant resistance to aciclovir following intermittent or chronic exposure to aciclovir. All HSV isolates were thymidine kinase deficient, resistant to aciclovir, and fully cross-resistant to ganciclovir (Erlich et al., 1989a). Thus, despite the potency of ganciclovir against HSV, as well as the achievement of higher intracellular levels of the ganciclovir-triphosphate (tenfold higher than aciclovir triphosphate in HSV-infected cells (Elion, 1986), ganciclovir is unlikely to be effective in the therapy of aciclovir-resistant HSV infection, and should not be administered as an alternative to aciclovir in patients who are showing poor response.

In contrast to ganciclovir, strains of thymidine kinase-deficient, aciclovir-resistant HSV isolates are invariably susceptible to vidarabine in vitro. As vidarabine is triphosphorylated entirely by cellular enzymes and thus circumvents the need for activation by virion thymidine kinase, it would be expected to be active against thymidine kinase-deficient strains of HSV. However, vidarabine therapy failed in at least five patients with aciclovir-resistant HSV infection (Norris *et al.*, 1987; Vinckier *et al.*, 1987; Safrin *et al.*, 1990), and in a randomized, prospective trial, vidarabine treatment of HIV-infected patients with aciclovir-resistant HSV resulted in no clinical or virological benefit, and caused significant toxicity, compared to foscarnet (Safrin *et al.*, 1991c). Frequent and severe neurological toxicity from vidarabine resulted in premature termination of the study (Safrin *et al.*, 1991c). The lack of efficacy of vidarabine in treatment of aciclovir-resistant infection, despite *in vitro* susceptibility, is not well understood.

Occasionally, administration of aciclovir by continuous infusion will heal HSV lesions in patients with AIDS who were unresponsive to aciclovir at standard dosages (Engel *et al.*, 1990). Monitoring of serum levels of aciclovir is helpful in patients receiving aciclovir by continuous infusion, to avoid toxicity and ascertain sufficiently high concentrations for efficacy.

TFT, a nucleoside analogue currently licensed in the USA as an ophthalmic solution for the treatment of herpes keratitis, has been applied topically in several patients with aciclovir-resistant HSV infection, resulting in full healing (Kessler *et al.*, 1992; Murphy *et al.*, 1992; Kessler *et al.*, 1996). Also, *in vitro* synergism of interferon-α with TFT has been described by one group of investigators, and topical application of the combination resulted in healing in three patients with aciclovir-resistant HSV infection (Birch *et al.*, 1992). A more recent open-label, pilot study of topical TFT in aciclovir-resistant mucocutaneous HSV in patients with AIDS, reported complete healing in seven of 24 patients with a median time of 7 weeks, and lesion healing in a further seven patients (Kessler *et al.*, 1996). Topical TFT, with or without added interferon, may therefore be an option in certain individuals.

Ribonucleotide reductase is an enzyme crucial to the synthesis of deoxyribonucleotides in both herpes virus and mammalian cells. Specific inhibitors of the HSV ribonucleotide reductase have been shown to potentiate the *in vitro* antiviral activity of aciclovir by increasing intracellular pools of aciclovir triphosphate while reducing dGTP levels in HSV-infected cells. The combination of ribonucleotide reductase inhibitors with aciclovir is synergistic and has been shown to have activity against both aciclovir-sus-

ceptible and aciclovir-resistant viruses *in vitro* (Lobe *et al.*, 1991). However, a recent study of topical application of the ribonucleotide reductase inhibitor 348U87 (3%) in combination with 5% aciclovir cream was not effective in AIDS patients with aciclovir-resistant HSV infection (Safrin *et al.*, 1993b). The reason for this disappointing result is unclear, and it remains possible that alternative ribonucleotide reductase inhibitors will be effective clinically.

Cidofovir ((S)-1-[3-hydroxy-2-phosphonylmethoxy)propyl]cytosine) is a nucleotide with potent activity against both HSV and CMV (Naesens *et al.*, 1997). Due to the presence of a phosphonate moiety, activation by the virus-specific thymidine kinase is unnecessary. Cidofovir is active *in vitro* against aciclovir-resistant HSV strains and in animal studies (DeClercq and Holy, 1991), and a recent study showed topical application of a gel formulation-induced healing in two patients with mucocutaneous HSV infection due to aciclovir-resistant virus (Snoeck *et al.*, 1993). A randomized, double-blind, placebo-controlled trial of 0.3% or 1% cidofovir gel in the treatment of aciclovir-unresponsive HSV in HIV-infected patients reported complete or more than 50% lesion healing in half of the cidofovir-treated patients, in addition to reduced viral shedding and significant pain reduction (Lalezari *et al.*, 1997).

Virend is a naturally occurring multihydroxylated heteropolymer with activity against both aciclovir-resistant and foscarnet-resistant mutants of HSV in the laboratory (Safrin *et al.*, 1993a). A multicentre, double-blind, placebo-controlled trial of virend 15% ointment applied topically three times a day for recurrent genital HSV in patients with AIDS found that nine of 22 (41%) patients using virend for 21 days, compared with three of 21 (14%) of patients in the placebo group experienced complete healing of lesions ($p = 0.09$, Fisher exact test) (Orozco-Topete *et al.*, 1997).

Adefovir dipivoxil is a pro-drug that is converted to the active antiviral nucleotide (adenine) analogue, adefovir (PMEA) *in vivo* (Naesens *et al.*, 1997). Adefovir dipivoxil is currently under development as an antiretroviral for HIV infection, but it is also active *in vitro* against other viruses, including herpesviruses (specifically, CMV, FBV and HHV-8) and hepatitis B virus. However, at present the manufacturer (Gilead) is not pursuing a herpesvirus indication for this drug (Barditch-Crovo *et al.*, 1997).

Agents in development. Several other agents are being considered as therapies for patients with aciclovir-resistant

HSV infection. These include cyclobut-G (racemic SQ 33,054), and aphidicolin. Cyclobut-G has *in vitro* activity against thymidine kinase-deficient mutants of HSV; whether or not this activity will be sufficient to effect a response clinically remains to be studied. Aphidicolin is a tetracyclic diterpenoid, which inhibits DNA polymerase and has activity against both thymidine kinase and DNA polymerase mutants of HSV *in vitro*, but has not been studied clinically to date.

Vaccines. Clinical trials with genetically engineered HSV glycoprotein vaccines have demonstrated minimal efficacy in reducing the frequency of recurrence in immuno-competent individuals with frequently recurring genital herpes (Straus *et al.*, 1994), and it seems unlikely that this form of immunotherapy will be of much benefit in patients with defective cell-mediated immunity, due to HIV infection or those with aciclovir-resistant herpes infection.

Management of recurrences of aciclovir-resistant HSV. Patients in whom healing of aciclovir-resistant HSV lesions is successful are at risk of recurrences also due to aci-clovir-resistant HSV strains. In one series (Safrin *et al.*, 1991c), the first recurrences following healing of resistant lesions were susceptible to aciclovir in 10 of 17 patients, suggesting that virus latent within the paraspinous ganglion retained the wild-type (i.e. thymidine kinase intact) phenotype. However, all 17 patients ultimately went on to have recurrences of aciclovir-resistant HSV infection within the 3-month follow-up period in that study, at a median of 41 days, following discontinuation of foscarnet therapy (Safrin *et al.*, 1991c). Current guidelines suggest retreatment with foscarnet in these patients (Balfour *et al.*, 1994).

Varicella-zoster virus infection

Varicella-zoster virus (VZV) is responsible for two different clinical presentations; chicken pox or varicella, which results from primary infection and shingles or zoster, which largely develops during reactivation of the virus.

Seroepidemiological studies demonstrate that more than 90% of individuals in the USA have been exposed to varicella (Straus *et al.*, 1988b) and similar seroprevalence has been demonstrated in other Western countries. Infection tends to occur in children between the ages of 1 and 15 years, most often in the late winter and early spring. The infection is highly communicable, with a secondary attack rate of up to 90% after a median incubation period of 14 days (Straus *et al.*, 1988b). In immunosuppressed patients, the incubation period for varicella may be shortened.

The epidemiology of zoster (reactivation of VZV), differs from that of varicella. Zoster disease is generally limited to elderly and immunosuppressed patients. Between 10 and 20% of people will develop zoster in their lifetime (Cunningham and Dwyer, 1996). The estimated annual incidence of cases of varicella in the USA is 3.5 million; that of zoster 1.5 million. The latter estimate, however, is derived from the years preceding the AIDS epidemic. The higher incidence of zoster in patients with HIV infection has been recognized since 1986, and age-adjusted relative risk estimates have ranged from 7 to 17 (Friedman-Kien *et al.*, 1986; Coen *et al.*, 1989; Fessel, 1995). Zoster may occur either early or late in the course of HIV infection (Van de Perre *et al.*, 1988; Buchbinder *et al.*, 1992). Recently published data from two large European studies suggest that there is an increased incidence of first episode VZV infection with advancing stage of HIV infection (Veenstra *et al.*, 1995; Alliegro *et al.*, 1996). This association is dependent on the CD4 lymphocyte count and corresponding level of immunosuppression, and once the CD4 lymphocyte count is adjusted for, there is no link between the incidence of zoster and risk of AIDS *per se* (Veenstra *et al.*, 1995; Alliegro *et al.*, 1996). About 25% of HIV-infected individuals experience zoster (Buchbinder *et al.*, 1992; Veenstra *et al.*, 1995). There is no evidence that zoster is predictive of a more rapid progression to AIDS (Buchbinder *et al.*, 1992; Veenstra *et al.*, 1995; Alliegro *et al.*, 1996).

A recent study presented in abstract suggested a higher than expected incidence of zoster shortly after initiation of protease inhibitor (PI) therapy (Martinez *et al.*, 1998). These episodes of zoster were milder than previously reported, and the long-term significance of these observations remains to be clarified.

Pathogenesis

Varicella is spread from person to person by either mucous membrane contact or droplet transmission in pharyngeal and respiratory secretions. A period of asymptomatic viraemia of 1–11 days precedes the appearance of the typical rash in both immunocompetent and immunocompromised hosts (Friedman-Kien *et al.*, 1986). In one study, VZV DNA was detected in the oropharyngeal epithelium of 62% of patients early in the course of varicella and in less than one-quarter of patients after the sixth day of disease. These data support the clinical observation that infectivity is typically limited to the first few days after the onset of rash. The early presence of T-lymphocyte proliferation to VZV antigen appears to correlate with milder illness and rapid termination of viraemia. In contrast, the early production of VZV-specific IgG or IgM antibodies does not correlate with the clinical course of the infection.

Zoster or shingles is an acute infection of the dorsal root ganglia and skin, caused mostly by reactivation of latent VZV. Exogenous acquisition of zoster is possible but unusual. Recent documentation of airborne spread of nosocomial infection from patients with either disseminated or localized zoster has prompted the recommendation that strict isolation precautions be instituted for all hospitalized patients with zoster, regardless of the extent of the lesions. In contrast to HSV (see above), there is no evidence for cutaneous shedding of VZV from asymptomatic hosts.

The ability to recover VZV DNA from the trigeminal or thoracic ganglia of persons sero-positive for VZV suggests strongly that viral latency is established in such ganglia. Latency appears to be lifelong. Cell-mediated immune mechanisms appear to be important in maintaining this latent state, as well as in limiting the clinical course of infection. Impaired cell-mediated immune responses of any cause are believed to facilitate virus reactivation and production of disease. In HIV-uninfected individuals, the incidence of zoster is increased in patients with haematological malignancies or those receiving immunosuppressive therapies (Arvin et al., 1980). The increased incidence of zoster with increasing age has been proposed to be due to senescence of the immune system (Berger et al., 1981). The role of humoral immunity in VZV infection is unclear but it is unlikely to be the dominant mechanism for viral control. Zoster infection is not more severe or frequent in agammaglobulinaemic patients (Straus et al., 1988b) and has been described in patients with high titres of VZV-specific antibody.

Clinical manifestations

Varicella

Varicella infection in immunocompetent children is manifest by a generalized pruritic skin eruption, composed of macular, papular, vesicular and crusted lesions, which follow a 2–3-day prodrome of fever and malaise. New lesions generally form for approximately 4 days and most lesions are fully crusted by day 6 (Straus et al., 1988b).

In immunocompromised children and in immunocompetent adults, varicella is often severe. The systemic prodrome may be more pronounced, the course more prolonged, and the incidence of pulmonary, neurological and haematological complications higher than in immunocompetent patients. Case studies of varicella in eight children with perinatal HIV infection reported a severe and prolonged course of disease, which tended to be complicated by bacterial superinfection (bacteraemia, osteomyelitis) and led to death in one case (Jura et al., 1989). However, a recent prospective cohort study of HIV-infected children in the USA reported that varicella, although common, was not usually a serious clinical problem and did not appear to herald clinical deterioration (Gershon et al., 1997).

Zoster

Herpes zoster is generally heralded by unilateral pain or dysesthesiae, which precedes the appearance of a rash by 1–4 days. Clusters of vesicles on an erythematous base ('dewdrop on a rose petal') subsequently erupt in a dermatomal distribution, evolving from a maculopapular appearance to vesicles, pustules and then scabbed ulcers over the course of 4–14 days. The thoracic dermatome is most frequently involved. Full healing generally occurs within 4 weeks, although cutaneous scarring is common. Rarely, pain and dysesthesiae are not accompanied by the rash ('zoster sine herpete').

Cutaneous zoster. Cutaneous VZV infection in HIV-infected individuals is more frequent, severe, prolonged and more likely to be associated with complications than in immunocompetent individuals (Colebunders et al., 1988; Janier et al., 1988; Gilson et al., 1989; Hoppenjans et al., 1990; Tronnier et al., 1994; Glesby et al., 1995; Veenstra et al., 1996). The morphology of the skin lesions may be atypical (Lokke-Jensen et al., 1993), manifesting as hyperkeratotic, 'verrucous' (Hoppenjans et al., 1990; Jacobson et al., 1990) or necrotic (Cohen et al., 1988) lesions. Complications include persistent hyperkeratotic or necrotic skin lesions; post-herpetic neuralgia; neurological or ocular complications, pneumonitis; disseminated skin lesions and rarely, visceral involvement (Cohen et al., 1989). The complication rate has been linked to the degree of immunosuppression, multidermatomal distribution and trigeminal localization (Veenstra et al., 1996). Recurrent zoster has been described in up to 19% of cases (Colebunders et al., 1988; Veenstra et al., 1996).

Zoster infection of the ophthalmic branch of the trigeminal cranial nerve may give rise to ocular complications. Corneal involvement occurs in approximately 50% of patients and may be complicated by uveitis and scleritis. This syndrome occurs more frequently in patients with HIV infection (Cobo, 1988).

Retinal involvement by VZV is uncommon. Two forms of necrotizing retinitis may occur: acute retinal necrosis (ARN) and progressive outer retinal necrosis (PORN). PORN is rarely seen in HIV-uninfected individuals. These conditions are bilateral in approximately one-third of patients and result in retinal detachment in up to three-quarters. Zoster-associated optic neuritis has also been described.

Neurological complications of zoster include myelitis and meningoencephaloid segmental motor paralysis. Encephalitis of delayed or chronic onset has also been described in patients with HIV infection (Ryder et al., 1986; Gilden et al., 1988). Contralateral hemiplegia may develop due to a cerebral arteritis. An uncommon specific motor neuropathy associated with cephalic zoster, known as the Ramsey-Hunt syndrome, occurs in both HIV-infected and uninfected patients. Affected patients have cutaneous lesions in the external auditory canal, hearing loss and vertigo due to involvement of the seventh and eighth cranial nerves. A less serious but more common complication of zoster is post-herpetic neuralgia, or pain persisting for more than 1 month following the onset of zoster. Post-herpetic neuralgia occurs in approximately 17% of immunocompetent adults; the incidence increases with age. The incidence of post-herpetic neuralgia is similar in immunosuppressed patients, such as those with HIV infection. Necrotizing retinitis, meningoencephaltis and myelitis have all been described in HIV-infected individuals in the absence of skin lesions (Veenstra, 1996) and may result in diagnostic difficulty.

Laboratory diagnosis

VZV may be identified by virus culture or detection of zoster antigen in vesicle fluid cells by immunofluorescence. In CSF VZV is best recognized by PCR amplification of virion DNA. Detection of VZV IgG and IgM antibodies is useful in selected circumstances.

The yield of virus culture for VZV is much lower than that for HSV, and the cultures must often be observed for 2 weeks or more before viral cytopathology is observed, in contrast to the 2–5 days required for HSV.

Some authors suggest aspiration of vesicles with a tuberculin syringe, as well as rubbing of the base of the lesion with the bevel of the syringe, with rapid inoculation of the specimen onto cell monolayers, to increase the yield of virus culture.

Direct fluorescent antigen staining of cells swabbed from the base of the lesion is more sensitive than virus culture and is nearly equally specific. A recent study comparing virus isolation, and direct immunofluorescence as methods of detection of VZV reported sensitivities of 65% and 92%, respectively (Dahl et al., 1997). The Tzanck smears have also been used for diagnosis of VZV but it has suboptimal sensitivity and is unable to distinguish between VZV and HSV.

PCR has been used to detect VZV in CSF samples from HIV-infected and uninfected individuals with neurological disease and suspected VZV infection (PuchhammerStöckl et al., 1991; Fox et al., 1995; Cinque et al., 1996). Only a small quantity of CSF is required, storage and sample preparation are not onerous and the technique is rapid to perform. Two recent studies (Cinque et al., 1996; Burke et al., 1997) using samples from HIV-infected patients with neurological symptoms have detected VZV in the CSF of 3% and 7% of patients, respectively. It is unknown whether patients with non-neurological presentations of VZV will have detectable virus in the CSF, but it is probably unlikely.

The presence of IgG antibodies to VZV indicate past VZV infection, and their abscence indicates susceptibility to infection. The appearance of IgM, or changes in IgG titres, are unreliable means of diagnosing VZV infection. In one recent study of HIV-infected individuals with zoster, only 65% of patients had significant VZV IgG rises and only 28% had detectable IgM (Dahl et al., 1997).

Treatment

Nucleoside analogues are the mainstay of treatment for VZV infection. Although vidarabine was used extensively in the past for treatment of VZV infection in immunosuppressed hosts, it is now of historical interest only. As with HSV, aciclovir is selectively activated by VZV thymidine kinase, and the triphosphate is a selective and irreversible inhibitor of the virion DNA polymerase. However, inhibitory concentrations of aciclovir against VZV are approximately ten-fold higher than against HSV, so that higher doses are required.

Varicella

Aciclovir is an effective treatment for varicella in both immunocompromised and immunocompetent children

(Dunkle et al., 1991) as it decreases morbidity from visceral dissemination in the former group and limits the duration of clinical illness in the latter. In addition, aciclovir accelerates healing in adults with varicella (Wallace et al., 1992). Initiation of therapy within 24 h of the onset of rash appears to be necessary for optimal efficacy. Recommended doses are shown in Table 32.2.

In the HIV-infected patient with varicella, it would seem prudent to treat all but very mild episodes in order to limit morbidity and/or mortality. The choice of oral or intravenous therapy will depend on the extent of the lesions, whether there is ocular involvement, the presence of complications, and the degree of immunosuppression of the patient.

Treatment of zoster in the HIV-infected patient has three main aims, to hasten resolution of mucocutaneous lesions, to prevent visceral or neurological involvement and to reduce the incidence and severity of post-herpetic neuralgia.

Aciclovir has been shown in placebo-controlled trials to shorten the period of virus shedding and to accelerate the time to healing, in both immunocompetent (McKendrick et al., 1986; Peterslund et al., 1992) and immunocompromised (Balfour et al., 1983) patients. A meta-analysis of placebo-controlled trials of oral aciclovir designed to assess its value in reducing zoster-associated pain, with a total of almost 700 patients, showed a clear benefit for the aciclovir group (Wood et al., 1996).

In the treatment of zoster, valaciclovir and famciclovir offer potential benefits of increased oral bioavailability and simpler dosing regimens (Degreef, 1994; Beutner et al., 1995). Valaciclovir was compared with aciclovir in a randomized, double-blind, study in immunocompetent adults with zoster (Beutner et al., 1995). Valaciclovir accelerated the resolution of zoster-associated pain and reduced the duration of post-herpetic neuralgia compared to aciclovir, but these differences were not reflected in improved quality-of-life scores. Likewise, when famciclovir was compared with aciclovir for the treatment of zoster in immunocompetent adults, famciclovir was not found to be any more effective than aciclovir but was effective in decreasing the duration of post-herpetic neuralgia when administered in acute zoster (Boon, 1996; Tyring et al., 1995; Tyring, 1996).

There have been numerous case reports of aciclovir-resistant VZV infection in HIV-infected adults and children (Janier et al., 1988; Pahwa et al., 1988; Safrin et al., 1991b; Smith et al., 1991; Fillet et al., 1995). All the patients described have had advanced HIV disease with either an AIDS-defining condition prior to the onset of resistant zoster infection or a markedly depressed CD4 lymphocyte count. Although most of these patients had been treated previously with aciclovir, at least two patients developing aciclovir-resistant VZV during the first course of therapy (Janier et al., 1988; Safrin et al., 1991b). Aciclovir-resistant zoster lesions are usually hyperkeratotic or 'poxlike' in appearance. However, some patients have typical vesiculoulcerative lesions that are resistant to aciclovir (Safrin et al., 1991b), while others manifest hyperkeratotic lesions which are aciclovir responsive (Linnemann et al., 1990; Safrin et al., 1991b). Thus, while the presence of hyperk-

Table 32.2 Treatment of VZV infections in HIV-infected patients

Clinical presentation	First line (preferred)	Alternative
Varicella (chicken pox)	Aciclovir 800 mg/five times per day p.o. or [a]Aciclovir 10 mg/kg/three times per day i.v.	
Zoster	[b]Aciclovir 10 mg/kg/five times per day i.v. Famciclovir 500 mg/three times per day p.o. or Valaciclovir 1 g/three times per day p.o. Aciclovir 800 mg/three times per day p.o.	Foscarnet 60 mg/kg/twice per day i.v.
Aciclovir-resistant zoster	Foscarnet 60 mg/kg twice per day i.v.	

Treatment should be commenced as soon as possible and continued until all external lesions are crusted or for at least 7 days.
[a]Adjuste dose in renal impairment.
[b]Severe: >1 dermatome, trigeminal nerve involvement or disseminated.

(Adapted from Sanford et al., 1999.)

eratotic lesions in the context of a suboptimal aciclovir response may prompt evaluation for aciclovir resistance, it is not possible to determine susceptibility phenotype from the appearance of the lesion alone. It is likely that the 'heaped-up' or verrucous appearance results from lesion chronicity, rather than decreased susceptibility to aciclovir.

As with aciclovir resistance in HSV, the most common mechanism of resistance to aciclovir noted in VZV isolates collected from unresponsive lesions is thymidine kinase deficiency (Hoppenjans et al., 1990; Safrin et al., 1991b; Talarico et al., 1993). Genotypic analysis of 12 such strains has demonstrated either nucleotide deletions in the thymidine kinase gene producing a premature termination codon with a truncated protein, or a nucleotide substitution in the thymidine kinase gene resulting in an altered protein (Safrin et al., 1991b). In contrast to aciclovir-resistant HSV, isolated instances of VZV resistant to aciclovir on the basis of mutations in both thymidine kinase (Jacobson et al., 1990; Safrin et al., 1991b) and DNA polymerase (Safrin et al., 1991b) have also been reported.

Treatment. Clinical trials of therapeutic agents for the relatively rare condition of aciclovir-resistant VZV infection have been limited. Clinical isolates of zoster have shown susceptibility *in vitro* to vidarabine (Pahwa et al., 1988; Hoppenjans et al., 1990; Jacobson et al., 1990) and to foscarnet (Linnemann et al., 1990; Safrin et al., 1991b; Smith et al., 1991). However, treatment with vidarabine has been unsuccessful in at least four patients (Pahwa et al., 1988; Hoppenjans et al., 1990; Jacobson et al., 1990), and failure with foscarnet has been described by a number of authors (Safrin et al., 1991b; Fillet et al., 1995). Foscarnet remains the first-line therapeutic alternative for patients with aciclovir-resistant VZV infection.

A separate problem is that of recurrence of zoster following successful healing of aciclovir-resistant infection. Two of four patients who demonstrated healing in one series (Safrin et al., 1991b) had recurrent episodes of zoster 7 and 14 days after discontinuation of foscarnet. Fortunately, *in vitro* testing demonstrated susceptibility to aciclovir in both, suggesting that the virus latent in the ganglion may not have undergone mutation to the resistant phenotype. Nevertheless, recurrence of aciclovir-resistant zoster after healing has been reported (Bernhard et al., 1995). Intravenous foscarnet was used successfully to treat a recurrence of aciclovir-resistant chronic cutaneous ulcerative VZV lesions in one patient. The utility of chronic suppressive

therapy with foscarnet in patients who have responded well during acute therapy has not been evaluated.

It is possible that TFT, by virtue of its *in vitro* activity against VZV, as well as preliminary reports of effectiveness against aciclovir-resistant HSV infection (Kessler et al., 1992; Murphy et al., 1992), may prove useful for aciclovir-resistant VZV infection. However, no reports of therapeutic attempts for this indication have been published to date.

Sorivudine is a pyrimidine nucleoside analogue, which has 2000–5000 times the *in vitro* potency of aciclovir towards VZV (Machida, 1986). It has good oral bioavailability and it can be administered once daily. In a multicentre, randomized, double-blind trial of sorivudine versus aciclovir in the treatment of localized zoster in HIV-infected patients, sorivudine significantly shortened the median period of new vesicle formation and the time to complete crusting of lesions. The sorivudine-treated patients also had a significantly reduced rate of first VZV recurrence during the 12 months of follow-up (Bodsworth et al., 1997). However, this drug has now been withdrawn due to several deaths in Japan.

Adefovir is a nucleotide analog that has *in vitro* activity toward VZV. However, as with its use in HSV infection, no clinical data are available for adefovir in VZV infections.

VZV: prevention and immunity

In the immunocompetent host, an episode of varicella appears to confer lifelong immunity, and episodes of reactivation manifesting as zoster, if they occur, are almost always single, rather than multiple. In the HIV-infected patient, it is unclear whether reinfection occurs; however, recurrences of zoster do appear to be more common.

Varicella-zoster immune globulin (VZIG) should be administered to susceptible individuals who are at high risk of complicated infection following close contact with patients with varicella or zoster. Susceptible individuals are those lacking IgG antibodies to VZV. In the individual in whom a prior history of varicella is unknown, it should be borne in mind that at least 85–90% of adults in the USA and other industrialized countries are immune. In the immunosuppressed patient with unknown VZV immune status, however, administration of VZIG should be considered if respiratory or cutaneous contact with active VZV infection was significant. The administration of VZIG needs to be as early as possible after exposure in order to be effective. This may mean that decisions are made without the benefit of serological tests to determine susceptibility.

A live attenuated varicella (Oka strain) vaccine was developed by Takahashi and colleagues in 1974 (Straus *et al.*, 1988b) and is now available in many countries, including the USA, as part of routine childhood vaccination programmes. It is currently contraindicated in HIV-infected children, though has been used in children with leukaemia and was found to cause less reactivation than wild-type VZV (Hardy *et al.*, 1991). Although vaccination of high-risk immunosuppressed individuals confers protection, there is a small risk of severe adverse reactions, which resemble natural varicella. As varicella does not seem to accelerate the course of HIV infection, some authorities have called for varicella vaccination in HIV-infected children (Gershon *et al.*, 1997), suggesting vaccination at a time when CD4 lymphocyte counts are well preserved, when a good response to the vaccine could be anticipated.

Conclusion

Diseases caused by members of the *Herpesviridae* continue to be a problem in both immunocompetent and immunocompromised individuals. Serology-based prevalence studies have highlighted the widespread penetration of HSV into the general community, and high rates of asymptomatic virus shedding contribute significantly to the spread of infection. The interplay between HIV and HSV occurs on a number of levels: herpes-associated ulcers may facilitate virus transmission and acquisition; HIV and HSV frequently coexist and anogenital HSV is very common in HIV-infected individuals; and aciclovir resistance is well recognized. New compounds are in development for the treatment of HSV infections, but to date none can prevent nor eradicate viral latency. Despite the availability of several drugs with some clinical efficacy against VZV, this virus continues to cause morbidity in HIV-infected individuals. Challenges for the future include containment of HSV transmission, reduction in HSV-associated morbidity and abolition of viral latency.

References

Alliegro MB, Dorrucci M, Pezzotti P *et al.* (1996). Herpes zoster and progression to AIDS in a cohort of individuals who seroconverted to human immunodeficiency virus. *Clin Infect Dis* **23**: 990–5 .

Andrews EB, Yankaskas BC, Cordero JF *et al.* (1992). Aciclovir in pregnancy registry: six years' experience. *Obstet Gynecol* **79**: 7–13.

Arvin AM, Pollard RB, Rasmussen LE *et al.* (1980). Cellular and humoral immunity in the pathogenesis of recurrent herpes viral infections in patients with lymphoma. *J Clin Investig* **65**: 869–78.

Ashley RL. (1998). Type-specific antibodies to herpes simplex virus types 1 and 2: a review of methodology. *Sex Trans Infect* (in press).

Ashley RL (1988). Genital herpes. Type-specific antibodies for diagnosis and management. *Dermatol Clin* **16**: 789–93, xiii–xiv.

Augenbaum M, Feldman J, Chirgwin K *et al.* (1995). Increased genital shedding of herpes simplex virus type 2 in HIV-seropositive women. *Ann Intern Med* **123**: 845–7.

Bagdades EK, Pillay D, Squire SB *et al.* (1992). Relationship between herpes simplex virus ulceration and CD4+ cell counts in patients with HIV infection. *AIDS* **6**: 1317–20.

Baker DA, Safrin S, Deeter RG *et al.* (1995). Nine year effectiveness of continuous suppressive therapy with aciclovir (ACV) in patients with recurrent genital herpes (RGH). *J Eur Acad Dermatol Venereol* **5**: S169.

Balfour HH. (1983). Resistance of herpes simplex to aciclovir. *Ann Intern Med* **98**: 404–6.

Balfour HH, Bean B, Laskin OL *et al.* (1983). Aciclovir halts progression of herpes zoster in immunocompromised patients. *N Engl J Med* **308**: 1448–53.

Balfour HH, Benson C, Braun J *et al.* (1994). Management of aciclovir resistant herpes simplex and varicella zoster virus infections. *J Acquir Immune Defic Syndrom Retrovir* **7**: 254–60.

Barditch-Crovo P, Toole J, Hendrix CW *et al.* (1997). Anti-human immunodeficiency virus (HIV) activity, safety, and pharmacokinetics of adefovir dipivoxil (9-[2-(bis-pivaloyloxymethyl)-phosphonylmethoxyethyl]adenine) in HIV-infected patients. *J Infect Dis* **176**: 406–13.

Berger R, Florent G, Just M. (1981). Decrease of the lymphoproliferative response to varicella zoster antigen in the aged. *Int Immunology* **32**: 24–7.

Bernhard P, Obel N. (1995). Chronic ulcerating aciclovir-resistant varicella zoster lesions in an AIDS patient. *Scand J Infect Dis* **27**: 623–5.

Beutner KR, Friedman DJ, Forszpaniak C *et al.* (1995). Valaciclovir compared with aciclovir for improved therapy for herpes zoster in immunocompetent adults. *Antimicrob Agents Chemother* **39**: 1546–53.

Birch CJ, Tachedjian G, Doherty RR *et al.* (1990). Altered sensitivity to antiviral drugs of herpes simplex virus isolates from a patient with the acquired immunodeficiency syndrome. *J Infect Dis* **162**: 731–4.

Birch CJ, Tyssen DP, Tachedjian G *et al.* (1992). Clinical effects and *in vitro* studies of trifluorothymidine combined with interferon- for treatment of drug-resistant and -sensitive herpes simplex virus infections. *J Infect Dis* **166**: 108–12.

Bodsworth NJ, Boag F, Burdge D *et al.* (1997). Evaluation of sorivudine (BV-araU) versus aciclovir in the treatment of acute localised herpes zoster in human immunodeficiency virus-infected adults. *J Infect Dis* **176**: 103–7.

Boon RJ, Griffin DRJ. (1996). Famciclovir: efficacy in zoster and issues in the assessment of pain. In: J Mills *et al.* (ed.) *Antiviral chemotherapy*. New York: Plenum Press **4**: 17–31.

Bourne C, Mills J, Mindel A. (1995). Genital herpes and genital human papilloma virus infection. *Curr Opin Infect Dis* **8**: 10–5.

Brock BV, Selke S, Benedetti J *et al.* (1992). Frequency of asymptomatic shedding of herpes simplex virus in women with genital herpes. *J Am Med Assoc* **263**: 418–20.

Brown ZA, Benedetti J, Ashley R *et al.* (1991). Neonatal herpes simplex virus infection in relation to asymptomatic maternal infection at the time of labor. *N Engl J Med* **324**: 1247–52.

Buchbinder SP, Katz MH, Hessol NA et al. (1992). Herpes zoster and human immunodeficiency virus infection. J Infect Dis 166: 1153–6.

Burke DG, Kalayjian RC, Vann VR et al. (1997). Polymerase chain reaction detection and clinical significance of varicella zoster virus in cerebrospinal fluid from human immunodeficiency virus infected patients. J Infect Dis 176: 1080–4.

Chrétien F, Belec L, Hilton DA et al. (1996). Herpes simplex virus type-1 encephalitis in acquired immune deficiency syndrome. Neuropathol App Neurobiol 22: 394–404.

Cinque P, Vago L, Dahl H et al. (1996). Polymerase chain reaction on cerebrospinal fluid for diagnosis of virus-associated opportunistic diseases of the central nervous system in HIV-infected patients. AIDS 10: 951–8.

Cobo M. (1988). Reduction of the ocular complications of herpes zoster ophthalmicus by oral aciclovir. Am J Med 85: 90.

Coen DM, Goldstein DJ, Weller SK. (1989). Herpes simplex virus ribonucleotide reductase mutants are hypersensitive to aciclovir. Antimicrob Agents Chemother 3: 1395–9.

Cohen PR, Grossman ME. (1989). Clincal features of human immunodeficiency virus-asssociated disseminated herpes zoster infection – a review of the literature. Clin Exp Dermatol 14: 73–276.

Cohen PR, Beltrani VP, Grossman ME. (1988). Disseminated herpes zoster in patients with human immunodeficiency virus infection. Am J Med 84: 1076–80.

Cohen SG, Greenberg MS. (1985). Chronic oral herpes simplex virus infection in immunocompromised patients. Oral Surg 59: 465–71.

Colebunders R, Mann JM, Francis H et al. (1988). Herpes zoster in African patients: a clinical predictor of human immunodeficiency virus infection. J Infect Dis 157: 314–8.

Cone RW, Hobson AC, Palmer J et al. (1991). Extended duration of herpes simplex virus DNA in genital lesions detected by the polymerase chain reaction. J Infect Dis 164: 757–8.

Connolly GM, Hawkins D, Harcourt-Webster JN et al. (1989). Oesophageal symptoms, their causes, treatment, and prognosis in patients with the acquired immunodeficiency syndrome. Gut 30: 1033–9.

Corey L, Nahmias AJ, Guinan ME et al. (1982). A trial of topical aciclovir in genital herpes simplex virus infection. N Engl J Med 306: 1312–9.

Cowan F, Johnson AM, Ashley R et al. (1994). Antibodies to herpes simplex virus type 2 as a serological marker of sexual lifestyle in populations. Br Med J 309: 791–7.

Cunningham AL, Dwyer DE. (1996). Advances and controversies in the antiviral therapy of herpes zoster. Eur J Clin Microbiol Infect Dis 15: 272–5.

Dahl H, Marcoccia J, Linde A. (1997). Antigendetection: the method of choice in comparison with virus isolation and serology for the laboratory diagnosis of herpes zoster in human immunodeficiency virus-infected patients. J Clin Microbiol 35: 347–9.

DeClercq E, Holy A. (1991). Efficacy of (S)-1-(3-hydroxy-2-phosphonylmethoxypropyl)-cytosine in various models of herpes simplex virus infection in mice. Antimicrob Agents Chemother 35: 701–6.

Degreef H. (1994). Famciclovir herpes Zoster Clinical Studies Group: Famciclovir, a new oral antiherpes drug: results of the first controlled clinical study demonstrating its efficacy and safety in the treatment of uncomplicated herpes zoster in immunocompetent patients. Int J Antimicrob Agents 4: 241–6.

Dekker C, Ellis MN, McLaren C et al. (1983). Virus resistance in clinical practice. J Antimicrob Chemother 12: 137–52.

Dickerson MC, Johnston J, Delea TE et al. (1996). The causal role for genital ulcer disease as a risk factor for transmission of human immunodeficiency virus. Sex Trans Dis 9: 429–40.

Dorsky DI, Crumpacker CS. (1987). Drugs five years later: aciclovir. Ann Intern Med 107: 859–74.

Douglas JM, Davis LG, Remington ML et al. (1988). A double-blind, placebo-controlled trial of the effect of chronically administered oral aciclovir on sperm production in men with frequently recurrent genital herpes. J Infect Dis 157: 588–93.

Dunkle LM, Arvin AM, Whitley RJ et al. (1991). A controlled trial of aciclovir for chickenpox in normal children. N Engl J Med 325: 1539–44.

Earnshaw DL, Bacon TH, Darlinson SJ et al. (1992). Mode of action of penciclovir in MRC-5 cells infected with herpes simplex type 1 (HSV 1), HSV 2 and varicella-zoster virus. Antimicrob Agents Chemother 36: 2747–57.

Elion GB. (1986). Mechanism of action, spectrum and selectivity of nucleoside analogs. In: J Mills, L Corey (eds.) Directions for clinical application and research. New York: Elsevier, 118–37.

Ellis MN, Keller PM, Fyfe JA et al. (1987). Clinical isolate of herpes simplex virus type 2 that induces a thymidine kinase with altered substrate specificity. Antimicrob Agents Chemother 31: 1117–25.

Engel JP, Englund JA, Fletcher CV et al. (1990). Treatment of resistant herpes simplex virus with continuous-infusion aciclovir. J Am Med Assoc 263: 1662–4.

Englund JA, Zimmerman ME, Swierkosz EM et al. (1990). Herpes simplex virus resistant to aciclovir: a study in a tertiary care center. Ann Intern Med 112: 416–22.

Erlich KS, Mills J, Chatis P et al. (1989a). Aciclovir-resistant herpes simplex virus infections in patients with the acquired immunodeficiency syndrome. N Engl J Med 320: 293–6.

Erlich KS, Jacobson MA, Koehler JE et al. (1989b). Foscarnet therapy for severe aciclovir-resistant herpes simplex virus type-2 infections in patients with the acquired immunodeficiency syndrome (AIDS): an uncontrolled trial. Ann Intern Med 110: 710–3.

Fessel WJ. (1995). Early symptoms of human innunodeficiency virus infection (invited commentary). Am J Epidemiol 141: 405–6.

Field HJ, Darby G, Wildy P. (1980). Isolation and characterization of aciclovir-resistant mutants of herpes simplex virus. J Gen Virol 49: 115–24.

Fillet AM, Visse B, Caumes E et al. (1995). Foscarnet resistant multidermatomal zoster in a patient with AIDS. Clin Infect Dis 21: 1348–9.

Fleming DT, McQuillan GM, Johnson RE et al. (1997). Herpes simplex virus type 2 in the United States, 1976 to 1994. N Engl J Med 337: 1105–11.

Fox JD, Brink NS, Zuckerman MA et al. (1995). Detection of herpesvirus DNA by nested polymerase chain reaction in cerebrospinal fluid of human immunodeficiency virus-infected persons with neurologic disease: a prospective evaluation. J Infect Dis 172: 1087–90.

Friedman-Kien AE, Lafleur FL, Gendler E et al. (1986). Herpes zoster: a possible early clinical sign for development of acquired immunodeficiency syndrome in high-risk individuals. J Am Acad Dermatol 14: 1023–8.

Gateley A, Gander RM, Johnson PC et al. (1990). Herpes simplex virus 2 meningoencephalitis resistant to aciclovir in a patient with AIDS. J Infect Dis 161: 711–5.

Gershon AA, Mervish N, LaRussa P et al. (1997). Varicella-zoster virus infection in children with underlying human immunodeficiency virus infection. J Infect Dis 176: 1496–500.

Gilden DH, Murray RS, Wellish M et al. (1988). Chronic progressive varicella-zoster virus encephalitis in an AIDS patient. Neurology 38: 1150–3.

Gilson IH, Barnett JH, Conant MA et al. (1989). Disseminated ecthymatous herpes varicella-zoster virus infection in patients with acquired immunodeficiency syndrome. *J Am Acad Dermatol* **20**: 637–42.

Glesby MJ, Moore RD, Chaisson RE. (1995). Clinical spectrum of herpes zoster in adults infected with human immunodeficiency virus. *Clin Infect Dis* **21**: 370–5.

Goodell SE, Quinn TC, Mkrtichian E et al. (1983). Herpes simplex virus proctitis in homosexual men: clinical, sigmoidoscopic and histolopathological features. *N Engl J Med* **308**: 868–71.

Greenblatt RM, Lukehart SA, Plummer FA et al. (1988). Genital ulceration as a risk factor for human immunodeficiency virus infection. *AIDS* **2**: 47–59.

Gwanzura L, McFarlane W, Alexander D et al. (1998). Association between human immunodeficiency virus and herpes simplex virus type 2 seropositivity among male factory workers in Zimbabwe. *J Infect Dis* **177**: 481–4.

Hardy D, Javaly K, Wohlfeiler M et al. (1996). Pilot study of the safety and efficacy of foscarnet (PFA) cream for the treatment of aciclovir-unresponsive (ACV-R) herpes simplex (HSV) In: *Program and abstracts of Third Conference on Retroviruses and Opportunistic Infections* (Washington DC). Alexandria, VA: Infectious Diseases Society of America, 167.

Hardy IB, Gershon A, Steinberg S et al. (1991). The incidence of zoster after immunisation with live attenuated varicella vaccine. A study in children with leukaemia. *N Engl J Med* **325**: 1545–50.

Holmberg SD, Stewart JA, Gerber R et al. (1988). Prior herpes simplex virus type 2 infection as a risk factor for HIV infection. *J Am Med Assoc* **259**: 1048–50.

Hook EW, Cannon RO, Nahmias AJ. (1992). Herpes simplex virus infection as a risk factor for human immunodeficiency virus infection in heterosexuals. *J Infect Dis* **165**: 251–5.

Hoppenjans WB, Bibler MR, Orme RL et al. (1990). Prolonged cutaneous herpes zoster in acquired immunodeficiency syndrome. *Arch Dermatol* 1048–50.

Jacobson MA, Berger TG, Fikrig S et al. (1990). Aciclovir-resistant varicella zoster virus infection after chronic oral aciclovir therapy in patients with the acquired immunodeficiency syndrome (AIDS). *Ann Intern Med* **112**: 187–91.

Janier M, Hillion B, Baccard M et al. (1988). Chronic varicella zoster infection in acquired immunodeficiency syndrome. *J Am Acad Dermatol* **18**: 584–5.

Johnson RE, Nahmias AJ, Magder LS et al. (1989). A seroepidemiologic survey of the prevalence of herpes simplex virus type 2 infection in the United States. *N Engl J Med* **321**: 7–12.

Jura E, Chadwick EG, Josephs SH et al. (1989). Varicella-zoster virus infections in children infected with human immunodeficiency virus. *Ped Infect Dis J* **8**: 586–90.

Kessler HA, Hurwitz S, Farthing C et al. (1996). A pilot study of topical trifluridine for the treatment of aciclovir-resistant mucocutaneous herpes simplex diseases in patients with AIDS (ACTG 172). AIDS clinical Trials Group. *J Acquir Immune Defic Syndr Hum Retrovirol* **12**: 147–52.

Koelle DM, Benedetti J, Langenberg A et al. (1992). Asymptomatic reactivation of herpes simplex virus in women after the first episode of genital herpes. *Ann Intern Med* **116**: 433–7.

Koutsky LA, Ashley RL, Holmes KK et al. (1990). The frequency of unrecognised type 2 herpes simplex virus infection among women: implications for the control of genital herpes. *Sex Trans Dis* **17**: 90–5.

Koutsky LA, Stevens CE, Holmes KK et al. (1992). Underdiagnosis of genital herpes by current clinical and viral-isolation procedures. *N Engl J Med* **326**: 1533–9.

Lafferty WE, Coombs RW, Benedetti J et al. (1987). Recurrences after oral and genital herpes simplex infection: influence of the site of infection and viral type. *N Engl J Med* **316**: 1444–9.

Lakeman FD, Whitely RJ. (1995). Diagnosis of herpes simplex encephalitis: application of polymerase chain reaction to cerebral spinal fluid from brain biopsied patients and correlation with disease. *J Infect Dis* **171**: 857–63.

Lalezari J, Schaker T, Feinberg J et al. (1997). A randomised, double-blind, placebo-controlled trial of cidofovir gel for the treatment of aciclovir-unresponsive mucocutaneous herpes simplex virus infection in patients with AIDS. *J Infect Dis* **176**: 892–8.

Levi M, Ruden U, Wahren B. (1996). Peptide sequences of glycoprotein G-2 discriminate between herpes simplex virus type 2 (HSV-2) and HSV-1 antibodies. *Clin Diag Lab Immunol* **3**: 265–9.

Linnemann CC, Biron KK, Hoppenjans WG et al. (1990). Emergence of aciclovir-resistant varicella zoster virus in an AIDS patient on prolonged aciclovir therapy. *AIDS* **4**: 577–9.

Lobe DC, Spector T, Ellis MN. (1991). Synergistic topical therapy by aciclovir and A1110U for herpes simplex virus induced zosteriform rash in mice. *Antivir Res* **15**: 87–100.

Lokke-Jensen B, Weismann K, Mathiesen L et al. (1993). Atypical varicella-zoster infection in AIDS. *Acta Dermatol Venereol* **73**: 123–5.

Machida H. (1986). Comparison of susceptibilities of varicella-zoster virus and herpes simplex virus to nucleoside analogues. *Antimicrob Agents Chemother* **29**: 524–6.

Martin JL, Ellis MN, Keller PM et al. (1985). Plaque autoradiography assay for the detection and quantitation of thymidine kinase-deficient and thymidine kinase-altered mutants of herpes simplex virus in clinical isolates. *Antimicrob Agents Chemother* **28**: 181–7.

Martinez E, Gatell JM, Moran Y et al. (1998). High incidence of herpes zoster early after starting antiretroviral therapy with a protease inhibitor. *Fifth Conference on Retroviruses and Opportunistic Infections*, Chicago, IL, USA.

McKendrick MW, McGill JI, White JE et al. (1986). Oral aciclovir in acute herpes zoster. *Br Med J* **293**: 1529–32.

McLaren C, Corey L, Dekket C et al. (1983a). *In vitro* sensitivity to aciclovir in genital herpes simplex viruses from aciclovir-treated patients. *J Infect Dis* **148**: 868–75.

McLaren C, Ellis MN, Hunter GA. (1983b). A colorimetric assay for the measurement of the sensitivity of herpes simplex viruses to antiviral agents. *Antivir Res* **3**: 223–34.

Mertz GJ. (1993). Epidemiology of genital Herpes infection. *Infect Dis Clin N A* **7**: 825–39.

Mertz GJ, Jones CC, Mills J et al. (1988). Long-term aciclovir suppression of frequently recurring genital herpes simplex virus infection. *J Am Med Assoc* **260**: 201–6.

Mertz GJ, Benedetti J, Ashley R et al. (1992). Risk factors for the sexual transmission of genital herpes. *Ann Intern Med* **116**: 197–202.

Mertz GJ, Loveless MO, Levin MJ et al. (1997). Oral famciclovir for suppression of recurrent genital herpes simplex infection in women. *Arch Intern Med* **157**: 343–9.

Mills J, Hauer L et al. (1987). Recurrent herpes labialis in skiers: clinical observations and effect of sunscreen. *Am J Sports Med* **15**: 76–8.

Mindel A, Adler MW. (1982). Intravenous aciclovir treatment for primary genital herpes. *Lancet* i: 697–700.

Mindel A, Faherty A, Carey O et al. (1988). Dosage and safety of long-term suppressive aciclovir therapy for recurrent genital herpes. Lancet 23: 926–8.

Mole L, Ripich S, Margolis D et al. (1997). The impact of active herpes simplex virus infection on human immunodeficiency virus load. J Infect Dis 176: 766–70.

Murphy M, Morley A, Eglin RP et al. (1992). Topical trifluridine for mucocutaneous aciclovir-resistant herpes simplex II in AIDS patient. Lancet 340: 1040.

Naesens L, Snoeck R, Andrei G et al. (1997). HPMPC (cidofovir), PMEA (adefovir) and related acyclic-nucleoside phosphonate analogues: a review of their pharmacology and clinical potential in the treatment of vital infections. Antivir Chem Chemother 8: 1–23.

Nilsen AE, Aasen T, Halsos AM et al. (1982). Efficacy of oral aciclovir in the treatment of initial and recurrent genital herpes. Lancet 2: 571–3.

Nahmias AJ, Lee FK, Beckman-Nahmias S. (1990). Sero-epidemiological and sociological patterns of herpes simplex virus infection in the world. Scand J Infect Dis 69: 19–36.

Norris SA, Kessler HA, Fife KH. (1987). Severe progressive herpetic whitlow caused by an aciclovir-resistant virus in a patient with AIDS. J Infect Dis 157: 209–10.

Orozco-Topete R, Sierra-Madero J, Cano-Dominguez C et al. (1997). Safety and efficacy of Virend for topical treatment of genital and anal herpes simplex in patients with AIDS. Antivir Res 35: 91–103.

Pahwa S, Biron K, Lim W et al. (1988). Continuous varicella-zoster infection associated with aciclovir resistance in a child with AIDS. J Am Med Assoc 260: 2879–82.

Parker AC, Craig JIO, Collins P et al. (1987). Aciclovir-resistant herpes simplex virus infection due to altered DNA polymerase. Lancet 2: 1461.

Parris DS, Harrington JE. (1982). Herpes simplex virus variants resistant to high concentrations of aciclovir exist in clinical isolates. Antimicrob Ag Chemother 22: 71–7.

Patel R, Bodsworth NJ, Woolley P. (1997). Valaciclovir for the suppression of recurrent genital HSV infection: a placebo controlled study of once daily therapy. International Valaciclovir HSV Study Group Genitourinary Med 73: 105–9.

Peterslund NA, Ipsen J, Schonheyder H et al. (1992). Aciclovir in herpes zoster. Lancet 1: 827–30.

Posavad CM, Koelle DM, Shaughnessy MF et al. (1997). Severe genital herpes infections in HIV-infected individuals with impaired herpes simplex virus-specific CD8+ cytotoxic T lymphocyte precursors. Proc Natl Acad Sci USA 94: 10289–94.

Puchhammer-Stöckl E, Popow-Kraupp T, Heinz FX et al. (1991). Detection of varicella zoster virus DNA by polymerase chain reaction in the cerebrospinal fluid of patients suffering from neurological complications associated with chicken pox or herpes zoster. J Clin Microbiol 29: 1513–6.

Reeves WC, Corey L, Adams HG et al. (1981). Risk of recurrence after first episodes of genital herpes: relation to HSV type and antibody response. N Engl J Med 305: 315–9.

Rompalo AM, Mertz GJ, Davis LG et al. (1988). Oral aciclovir for treatment of first-episode herpes simplex virus proctitis. J Am Med Assoc 259: 2879–81.

Rooney JF, Straus SE, Mannix ML et al. (1993). Oral aciclovir to suppress frequently recurrent herpes labialis: a double-blind, placebo-controlled trial. Ann Intern Med 118: 268–72.

Ryder JW, Croen K, Kleinschmidt-DeMasters BK et al. (1986). Progressive encephalitis three months after resolution of cutaneous zoster in a patient with AIDS. Ann Neurol 19: 182–8.

Ross JDC, Smith IW, Elton RA. (1993). The epidemiology of herpes simplex types 1 and 2 infection of the genital tract in Edinburgh 1978–1991. Genitourin Med 69: 381–3.

Sacks SL, Wanklin RJ, Reece DE et al. (1989). Progressive esophagitis from aciclovir-resistant herpes simplex. Clinical roles for DNA polymerase mutants and viral heterogeneity. Ann Intern Med 111: 893–9.

Sacks S, Aoki F, Diaz-Mitoma F et al. (1996). Patient-initiated, twice daily oral femciclovir for early recurrent genital herpes. A randomised, double-blind multicentre trial. Canadian Famciclovir Study Group. J Am Med Assoc 276: 44–9.

Safrin S, Assaykeen T, Follansbee S et al. (1990). Foscarnet therapy for aciclovir-resistant mucocutaneous herpes simplex virus infection in 26 AIDS patients: preliminary data. J Infect Dis 161: 1078–84.

Safrin S, Ashley R, Houlihan C et al. (1991a). Clinical and serologic features of herpes simplex virus infection in patients with AIDS. AIDS 5: 1107–10.

Safrin S, Berger TG, Gilson I et al. (1991b). Foscarnet therapy in five patients with AIDS and aciclovir-resistant varicella-zoster virus infection. Ann Intern Med 115: 19–21.

Safrin S, Crumpacker C, Chatis P et al. (1991c). A controlled trial comparing foscarnet with vidarabine for aciclovir-resistant mucocutaneous herpes simplex in the acquired immunodeficiency syndrome. N Engl J Med 325: 551–5.

Safrin S, Arvin A, Mills J et al. (1992a). Comparison of the western immunoblot assay and a glycoprotein G enzyme immunoassay for detection of serum antibodies to herpes simplex virus type 2 in patients with AIDS. J Clin Microbiol 30: 1312–4.

Safrin S, Elbaggari A, Elbeik T. (1992b). Risk factors for the development of aciclovir-resistant herpes simplex virus (HSV) infection. Seventh International AIDS Conference, Florence, Italy, 1548.

Safrin S, Phan L, Elbeik T. (1993a). Evaluation of the in vitro activity of SP-303 against clinical isolates of aciclovir-resistant and foscarnet-resistant herpes simplex virus (HSV). Antivir Res 20: 117.

Safrin S, Schacker T, Delehanty J et al. (1993b). Topical treatment of infection with aciclovir-resistant mucocutaneous herpes simplex virus with the ribonucleotide reductase inhibitor 348U87 in combination with aciclovir. Antimicrob Agents Chemother 37: 975–9.

Safrin S, Kemmerly S, Plothin B et al. (1994). Foscarnet-resistant herpes simplex virus infection in patients with AIDS. J Infect Dis 169: 193–6.

Safrin S, Shaw H, Bolan G et al. (1997). Comparison of virus culture and the polymerase chain reaction for diagnosis of mucocutaneous herpes simplex. Sex Trans Dis 24: 176–80.

Sanford JP, Gilbert DN, Moellering RC et al. (1999). The Sanford guide to antimicrobial therapy. New York: Antimicrobial therapy Inc., 102–3.

Schacker T, Ryncarz A, Goddard J et al. (1997). Frequent recovery of replication competent HIV from genital herpes simplex virus lesions in HIV-infected persons. Fourth Conference on Retroviruses and Opportunistic Infections, Washington DC, USA.

Schacker T, Hu H, Koelle DM et al. (1998). Famciclovir for the suppression of symptomatic and asymptomatic herpes simplex virus reactivation in HIV-infected persons. Ann Intern Med 128: 21–8.

Schomogyi M, Wald A, Corey L. (1998). Herpes simplex virus-2 infection: an emerging disease. Infect Dis Clin N Am 12: 47–61.

Scoular A, Barton S, On Behalf of the Herpes Simplex Advisory Panel. (1997). Therapy for genital herpes in immunocompromised patients: a national survey. Genitourin Med 73: 391–3.

Siegal FP, Lopez C, Hammer GS et al. (1981). Severe acquired immuno-deficiency in male homosexuals, manifested by chronic perianal ulcerative herpes simplex lesions. N Engl J Med **305**: 1439–44.

Siegel D, Golden E, Washington AE et al. (1992). Prevalence and correlates of herpes simplex infections: the population-based AIDS in multiethnic neighborhoods study. J Am Med Assoc **268**: 1702–8.

Simonsen JN, Cameron W, Gakinya MN et al. (1988). Human immun-odeficiency virus infection among men with sexually transmitted diseases: experience from a center in Africa. N Engl J Med **319**: 274–7.

Smith KJ, Kahlter DC, Davis C et al. (1991). Aciclovir-resistant varicella zoster responsive to foscarnet. Arch Dermatol **127**: 1069–71.

Snoeck R, Andrei G, Balzarini J et al. (1993). (S)-1-(3-Hydroxy-2-phos-phonylmethoxypropyl)cytosine (HPMPC): successful topical treat-ment of aciclovir-resistant HSV-2 perineal lesions in an AIDS patient. Antivir Res **20**: 133.

Spruance SL, Hamill ML et al. (1988). Aciclovir prevents reactivation of herpes simplex labialis in skiers. JAMA **260**: 1597–9.

Spruance SL, Stewart JCB, Rowe NH et al. (1990b). Treatment of recur-rent herpes simplex labialis with oral aciclovir. J Infect Dis **161**: 185–90.

Spruance SL, Tyring SK, De Gregorio B et al. (1996). A large scale place-bo-controlled, dose ranging trial of peroral valaciclovir for episodic treatment of recurrent herpes genitalis. Arch Intern Med **156**: 1729–35.

Straus SE, Smith HA, Brickman C et al. (1982). Aciclovir for chronic mucocutaneous herpes simplex virus infection in immunosuppressed patients. Ann Intern Med **96**: 270–7.

Straus SE, Croen KD, Sawyer MH et al. (1988a). Aciclovir suppression of frequently recurring genital herpes: efficacy and diminishing need during successive years of treatment. J Am Med Assoc **260**: 2227–30.

Straus SE, Ostrove JM, Inchauspe G et al. (1988b). Varicella-zoster virus infections. Ann Intern Med **108**: 221–37.

Straus SE, Seidlin M, Takiff HE et al. (1989). Effect of oral aciclovir treat-ment on symptomatic and asymptomatic virus shedding in recurrent genital herpes. Sex Trans Dis **16**: 107–13.

Straus SE, Corey L, Burke RL et al. (1994). Placebo-controlled trial of vaccination with recombinant glycoprotein D of herpes simplex virus type 2 for immunotherapy of genital herpes. Lancet **304**: 1460–3.

Swetter SM, Hill EL, Kern ER et al. (1998). Chronic vulvar ulceration in an immunocompetent woman due to aciclovir resistant, thymidine kinase-deficient herpes simplex virus. J Infect Dis **177**: 543–50.

Swierkosz EM, Scholl DR, Brown JL et al. (1987). Improved DNA hybridisation method for detection of aciclovir-resistant herpes sim-plex virus. Antimicrob Agents Chemother **31**: 1465–9.

Talarico CL, Phelps WC, Biron KK. (1993). Analysis of the thymidine kinase genes from aciclovir-resistant mutants of varicella-zoster virus isolated from patients with AIDS. J Virol **67**: 1024–33.

Tronnier M, Plettenberg A, Miegel WN. (1994). Recurrent verrucous herpes zoster in an HIV patient. Demonstration of the virus by immunofluorescence and electron microscopy. Eur J Dermatol **4**: 604–7.

Tyring SK. (1996). Efficacy of famciclovir in the treatment of herpes zoster. Semin Dermatol **15**: 27–31.

Tyring S, Barbarash R, Nahik J et al. (1995). Famciclovir for the treat-ment of acute herpes zoster: effects on acute disease and postherpetic neuralgia. Ann Intern Med **123**: 89–96.

Van de Perre P, Bakkers E, Batungwanayo J et al. (1988). Herpes zoster in African patients: an early manifestation of HIV infection. J Scand Infect Dis **20**: 277–82.

Veenstra J, Krol A, van Praag RME et al. (1995). Herpes zoster, immuno-logical deterioration and disease progression in HIV-1 infection. AIDS **9**: 1153–8.

Veenstra J, Van Praag RME, Krol A et al. (1996). Complications of vari-cella zoster virus reactivation in HIV-infected homosexual men. AIDS **10**: 393–9.

Vinckier F, Boogaerts M, De Clerck D et al. (1987). Chronic herpetic infection in an immunocompromised patient: report of a case. J Oral Maxillofacial Surg **45**: 723–8.

Wald A, Zeh J, Selke S et al. (1995). Virologic characteristics of sub-clinical and symptomatic genital herpes infections. N Engl J Med **333**: 770–5.

Wald A, Corey L, Cone R et al. (1997). Frequent genital herpes simplex virus 2 shedding in immunocompetent women. Effect of aciclovir treatment. J Clin Investig **99**: 1092–7.

Wallace MR, Bowler WA, Murray NB et al. (1992). Treatment of adult varicella with oral aciclovir: a randomised, placebo-controlled trial. Ann Intern Med **117**: 358–63.

Weller S, Blum MR, Doucette M et al. (1993). Pharmacokinetics of the aciclovir pro-drug, valaciclovir after single and multiple-dose administration in normal volunteers. Clin Pharmacol Exp Ther **54**: 595–606.

Wood MJ, Kay R, Dworkin RH et al. (1996). Oral aciclovir accelerates pain resolution in patients with herpes zoster: a meta-analysis of placebo-controlled trials. Clin Infect Dis **22**: 341–7.

ALICE REIER AND RONALD MITSUYASU

Research sparked by the AIDS epidemic has led to our present understanding of the pathogenesis of HIV infection and of HIV-related immune dysregulation. In recent years, there have been dramatic scientific advances in the areas of antiretroviral and immune therapies. Better control of HIV viral replication has been associated with a decline in the incidence of some AIDS-associated malignancies. There is also evidence that suppression of HIV replication may result in partial immune reconstitution. With prophylactic antibiotics, higher CD4 lymphocyte counts and the availability of growth factors, patients with AIDS-related malignancies can now tolerate more aggressive chemotherapy regimens and may soon have tumour remission rates approaching those of more immunocompetent patients.

In addition to new and highly effective HIV therapy, novel cancer treatment strategies, such as antibody therapy, angiogenesis inhibition, cytokine therapy and gene therapy are being evaluated and may prove useful in the treatment and prevention of these tumours.

The increased incidence of cancers in HIV-infected patients is understood to be associated with underlying immunodeficiency. Some of these cancers have been strongly associated with viruses, such as Epstein–Barr virus (EBV) and human papilloma virus (HPV). Kaposi's sarcoma (KS) and non-Hodgkin's lymphoma (NHL) are the most frequent tumours encountered in HIV-infected persons. The recently discovered human herpes virus-8 (HHV-8), also called Kaposi's sarcoma virus (KSHV), has been implicated, not only in KS, but also in primary effusion NHL and multicentric Castleman's disease (Boshoff et al., 1997; Brook et al., 1997; Chang, 1997; O'Leary et al., 1997; Said, 1997). Its role in multiple myeloma remains controversial (Rettig et al., 1997).

According to US reference data, women with AIDS have a relative risk (RR) for invasive cervical cancer of 2.9 (Goedert et al., 1998). Patients with AIDS have also been shown to be at increased risk for other cancers not included in the Centers for Disease Control (CDC) list of AIDS-defining cancers (Schultz et al., 1996; Johnson et al., 1997; Goedert et al., 1998; Jacobson, 1998; Jones et al., 1998; Speck et al., 1998). These cancers include anal cancer (RR = 31.7), leukaemias other than lymphoid and myeloid (RR = 11.0), Hodgkin's disease (RR = 7.6), soft tissue sarcomas (RR = 7.2), multiple myeloma (RR = 4.5), primary brain cancers other than primary central nervous system (CNS) lymphoma (RR = 3.5), testicular cancer (RR = 2.9) and lung adenocarcinomas (RR = 2.5) (Goedert et al., 1998; Ricaurte et al., 2001).

Recent medical advances in the management of HIV disease, especially the widespread use of protease inhibitor-containing multidrug 'cocktails' in conjunction with changing sexual practices, have led to longer and healthier lives for patients infected with HIV. Improved control of opportunistic infections has also had a positive impact on the incidence and natural history of KS and on the incidence of primary CNS lymphoma (Figure 33.1). Based on CDC data of nearly 18 000 cases, comparing January–June, 1994 with July–December, 1996, the incidence of KS decreased from 53.4 to 10.3/1000 patient-years ($p < 0.001$) and primary CNS lymphoma decreased from 8.5 to 0.9/1000 patient-years ($p < 0.04$). The incidence of NHLs decreased by one-third, although this was not a significant decline, and the incidence of invasive cervical cancer among HIV-infected women showed no significant change (Johnson et al., 1997). Patients in the Multicenter AIDS Cohort Study (MACS) showed a similar decline in the incidence of KS during 1996–1997, but no change in the incidence of NHL (Jones et al., 1998).

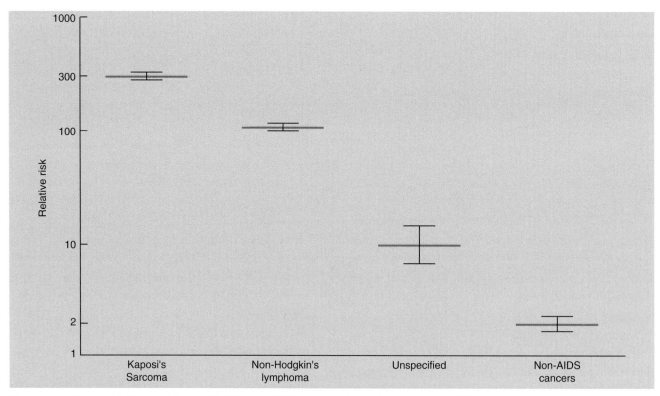

Figure 33.1 *Relative risk (log$_{10}$ scale) and 95% CI of post-AIDS cancer incidence (Goedert et al., 1998).*

Kaposi's sarcoma

Kaposi's sarcoma, first described by Moritz Kaposi Kohn in 1872, is a multifocal, cytokine-regulated, vascular tumour.

Epidemiology

KS is the most common malignancy in the HIV-infected patient, affecting 10–30% of all HIV-infected males and 1% of all HIV-infected females at some time in the course of their disease (Mitsuyasu, 1987; Friedman-Kien and Saltzman, 1990; Haverkos *et al.*, 1990; Biggar and Rabkin, 1996; Miles, 1994; Cooley *et al.*, 1996; Dezube, 1996). When initially described, it was thought to be a rare tumour, mainly affecting elderly males of Eastern European Jewish or Mediterranean descent. In this population, it commonly presents with vascular plaques and nodules limited to the lower extremities and adjacent lymph nodes and rarely, mucous membranes and visceral organs. This presentation is now referred to as 'classic' KS. KS is also an endemic malignancy of equatorial Africa, more common in males and sometimes affecting prepubescent boys. This 'endemic' form can be seen in four distinct variations: a benign,

nodular presentation, similar to 'classic' KS, a more aggressive local fungating and invasive presentation, a widely disseminated invasive type affecting visceral organs and a very virulent lymphadenopathic type. During the 1960s and 1970s, KS was identified in renal allograft and other immunocompromised patients (Friedman-Kien and Saltzman, 1990; Boshoff and Moore, 1997). As early as 1977, an excess of cases of KS was reported in New York and California. Several years later, this 'epidemic' form was recognized as a major manifestation of AIDS, heralding the start of the AIDS epidemic (Friedman-Kien and Saltzman, 1990; Biggar and Rabkin, 1996; Miles, 1996; Schultz *et al.*, 1996). The AIDS-associated or 'epidemic' form of KS is also more common in men than in women, with a ratio of approximately 4:1 in the USA. It is more common in homosexual and bisexual men than in men who contracted HIV through blood products, and it is more common in women who have bisexual partners than in women who contracted HIV through injecting drug use.

Reference data from the pre-AIDS epidemic (1975–79) AIDS-Cancer Match Registry indicated a relative risk (RR) of patients with AIDS being diagnosed with KS to be 100 000, compared to the general population and with

NHL to be 280. US reference data of these patients from 1985 to 1989, compared to the general population, have indicated lower relative risks of 310 and 113 for KS and NHL, respectively (Goedert *et al.*, 1998). Other studies have estimated the relative risk of KS in HIV-infected males to be 1000–73 000 (Schultz *et al.*, 1996; Johnson *et al.*, 1997; Goedert *et al.*, 1998; Speck *et al.*, 1998).

Aetiology

Because of the epidemiology of KS, this malignancy has long been suspected to be due to an infectious agent transmitted sexually. Although candidate viruses were identified in KS tissue, including cytomegalovirus (CMV), human papilloma virus (HPV), human herpes virus (HHV)-6, herpes simplex virus (HSV) type-1 and type-2 and human polyoma virus (BK virus), none adequately fitted the epidemiology of KS (Kempf *et al.*, 1995; Boshoff and Moore, 1997). In 1994, Chang *et al.* identified a previously undescribed herpes-like virus in KS tissue, now referred to as human herpes virus (HHV)-8 or the Kaposi's sarcoma herpes virus (KSHV) (Chang *et al.*, 1994). It is now known that this is a gamma II herpes virus (genus Rhadinovirus). HHV-8 genomes are found in virtually all KS spindle and endothelial cells, including tissue from all subtypes of the disease (classic, endemic and epidemic) and in the tumour tissue of HIV-uninfected immunocompromised patients who have KS (Boshoff *et al.*, 1995; Moore and Chang, 1995; Gillison and Ambinder, 1997; O'Leary *et al.*, 1997). KSHV has also been identified in primary effusion lymphomas (PEL), in the lymph nodes, associated with multicentric Castleman's disease and in the dendritic cells of patients with multiple myeloma (Moore and Chang, 1995; Oksenhendler *et al.*, 1996; O'Leary *et al.*, 1997; Rettig *et al.*, 1997; Said, 1997). Current data strongly support a causative role for HHV-8 in the development of KS, although the mechanism of oncogenesis is incompletely understood. It has been proposed that activated G-protein-coupled receptor genes and other HHV-8 genes may act as oncogenes by encoding proteins that stimulate the production of angiogenic growth factors (Boshoff and Moore, 1997; Guo *et al.*, 1997; Bais *et al.*, 1998; Boshoff, 1998).

Pathology

Although KS is now thought to be primarily a spindle cell cancer, this mesenchymal tumour is also characterized pathologically by inflammatory lymphocytes, extravasated red blood cells and a proliferation of endothelial cells.

These endothelial cells may be the origin of the tumour spindle cells (Ganem, 1997; Cornali *et al.*, 1998). The proliferation of endothelial and spindle cells leads to thin-walled microvascular proliferation, a histological hallmark of this tumour (Ganem, 1997; Rabkin *et al.*, 1997).

HIV infection is not necessary for the development of KS, but it does facilitate its growth. By infecting CD4 lymphocytes, HIV leads to suppression of immune function and decreased tumour surveillance. Multiple cytokines, including interleukin (IL)-1β, transforming growth factor (TGF)-β, tumour necrosis factor (TNF)-α and IL-6 are increased in advanced HIV disease and have been closely associated with the development of KS (Miles *et al.*, 1990a; Boshoff and Moore, 1997; Ganem, 1997; Cornali *et al.*, 1998; Neipal *et al.*, 1997). Other cytokines thought to regulate KS growth are angiogenic factors, such as platelet-derived growth factor (PDGF), IL-8, vascular endothelial growth factor (VEGF), basic fibroblast growth factor (bFGF) and oncostatin-M (Karp *et al.*, 1996; Miles, 1996; Cai *et al.*, 1997; Nakamura *et al.*, 1997; Neipal *et al.*, 1997; Rabkin *et al.*, 1997; Cornali *et al.*, 1998). VEGF is also thought to be responsible for the vascular permeability and oedema seen in advanced KS disease. This factor is the target of several angiogenesis inhibitors currently in clinical trials for the treatment of KS. HIV also makes a protein – Tat – which is essential for HIV replication. Ensoli and colleagues have reported that HIV-infected CD4 lymphocytes and monocytes may release biologically active Tat, which stimulates the proliferation of spindle cells and may be involved in endothelial cell migration, thereby playing an integral role in the pathogenesis of AIDS-KS (Ensoli *et al.*, 1993; Ensoli *et al.*, 1994). Corticosteroid treatment has also been associated with the development of KS in immunocompromised patients with or without HIV and with exacerbation of KS in patients' established tumours. This association is thought to be due to a synergistic effect between glucocorticoids and various growth factors (Dezube, 1996; Cai *et al.*, 1997).

In the early stages of KS, lesions can be confused with other diseases. Bacillary angiomatosis, caused by the *Bartonella* sp. bacteria can result in raised red papules or nodules, which can be confused with KS clinically or histologically (see Chapter 17). Angiomas, naevi and dermatofibromas can also be mistaken for KS. Although a clinical diagnosis can often be made by physical examination, a small punch biopsy of the lesion for pathologic diagnosis should always be performed.

Disease course and prognosis

Clinical manifestations

In patients with AIDS, KS can present with single or multiple cutaneous lesions on the face, extremities or trunk, with or without clinically obvious lymph node involvement. Mucocutaneous lesions of the oral cavity are common, occurring in 30% of patients (Dezube, 1996). Involvement of the eyelid and conjunctival lesions, which may be mistaken for chronic conjunctival haemorrhages, are also seen in this patient population and can lead to ocular irritation, infection, trichiasis and visual obstruction (Mitsuyasu and Miles, 1987; Shuler et al., 1989). Visceral organs, such as the gastrointestinal (GI) tract and lung, and less commonly, the kidneys, adrenal gland, spleen, testes, bone marrow and heart can be affected (Mitsuyasu and Miles, 1987, Friedman-Kien and Saltzman, 1990; Dezube, 1996; Chyu et al., 1998). Cutaneous lesions may be plaque-like, nodular or pedunculated. They can appear as violaceous nodules, clear fluid-filled papules or fungating lesions. Facial lesions can be cosmetically disturbing, and lesions on the extremities can be accompanied by mild or severe, and sometimes debilitating oedema. Visceral disease may be present in the absence of cutaneous lesions. Patients who present with clinically extensive disease should have a chest X-ray, and bronchoscopy or endoscopy should be performed in those patients who have clinical or radiographic evidence of pulmonary or gastrointestinal disease.

KS can present at any stage of HIV infection and may be seen in patients with normal CD4 lymphocyte counts, although extensive disease is more frequently seen in severely immunocompromised patients. Commonly, KS presents after the development of an opportunistic infection; likewise, the development of an opportunistic infection or an increase in HIV viral replication in established KS can result in more rapid tumour progression. Successful treatment of the opportunistic infection or antiretroviral treatment, which decreases HIV RNA, often results in tumour regression and sometimes disappearance of the KS (Murphy et al., 1997). When patients present with progressive, unresponsive KS, therefore, clinicians should rule out concurrent opportunistic infections and high HIV viral load.

Large population studies have shown that survival of patients with KS generally parallels survival of patients after the diagnosis of any AIDS-defining illness. Prior to the widespread use of protease inhibitors (PIs), survival of patients with AIDS-associated KS generally ranged from 3 months to 3 years, with better survival in patients with CD4 lymphocyte counts of greater than 300 cells/μl, no prior opportunistic infection and no systemic symptoms (Chachoua et al., 1989). In a retrospective study of 688 patients with AIDS-associated KS seen at a single institution from 1981 to 1990, four variables predicted survival, including baseline CD4 lymphocyte count, haematocrit, number of KS lesions and body mass index. In this study, the overall median survival was 412 days (13 months), with a 65% reduction in mortality across all prognostic categories in those patients presenting after 1987 (Miles et al., 1994). It has been proposed that this decrease in mortality could have been attributable to the 1987 commercial availability of zidovudine (ZDV) and the widespread use of Pneumocystis carinii pneumonia (PCP) prophylaxis, the mainstays of HIV therapy at that time. Today, more effective and less toxic KS therapy in combination with highly active antiretroviral therapy (HAART), routine PCP prophylaxis and improved treatments for CMV and other opportunistic infections, are believed to have greatly improved the survival of all HIV-infected patients. While death directly related to KS is unusual, there is presently no cure for this malignancy. Goals of KS management, therefore, are to improve the appearance of cosmetically unappealing lesions, to decrease lymphatic obstruction and extremity oedema and to relieve the symptoms of visceral disease.

Management

A greater understanding of the viral and immune pathogenesis of KS over the past few years has led to advances in the development of effective and minimally toxic KS therapy. The control of HIV viral replication and the prevention and treatment of opportunistic infections are fundamental to the successful treatment of KS (Levine and Pieters, 1998). Acute progression of KS should always signal an aggressive search for a new or inadequately treated opportunistic infection or high viral load measurements. It is presently understood that KS is a systemic disease and should be treated with systemic therapy, except in those cases of disease limited to a few small cutaneous lesions (Table 33.1). Proven effective systemic therapies include liposomal anthracyclines, paclitaxel and interferon (IFN)-α. Other promising systemic agents include angiogenesis inhibitors, systemic retinoids and other biomodulators.

Table 33.1 Management of HIV-associated Kaposi's sarcoma

Treatment	Indications	Side-effects
Local therapy	Patients who have a few cutaneous lesions, including on the eyelid, conjuctiva, sclera, oral mucous membranes, glans penis or perirectal area	KS lesions may regrow in the field of treatment or in perimeter
Cryotherapy 20–60 min freeze time, may be divided and given every 2 weeks	Treatment of choice	Hypopigmentation
Vinblastine intralesional injection 0.01 mg/0.1 sterile water	Small, cosmetically-disfiguring lesions	Painful Repeated injections often needed Hyperpigmentation
Lasers		Infections Scarring Hyperpigmentation
Radiotherapy 700–2200 cGy in divided divided doses for periorbital and oral lesions	Cosmetically-disfiguring lesions which are too large for effective cryotherapy KS-involved lymph nodes to relieve obstruction of lymphatic drainage	Tissue necrosis in overlapping fields, 'Radiation recall' Sclerosis of the lymphatics; fibrosis of muscle, connective tissue
Topical retinoids	May replace cryotherapy as treatment of choice	Hypersensitivity to sunlight
Systemic therapy	Treatment of choice for patients with more than a few small cutaneous lesions	
Liposomal doxorubicin 20 mg/m^2 i.v. every 2–4 weeks		Mild hair thinning, occasional nausea, mild myelosuppression, hand–foot syndrome
Liposomal daunorubicin 40 mg/m^2 i.v. every 2–4 weeks		Same as liposomal doxorubicin, except no reported hand–foot syndrome
Paclitaxel 135–175 mg/m^2 i.v. over 3–96 h every 2–4 weeks	Liposomal anthracycline-resistant KS	Alopecia, myelosuppression, neuropathy
Interferon-α 3–9 MIU sq every day or t.i.v.	As an adjunct to liposomal anthracyclines. Will also decrease Kaposi's sarcoma pigmentation	Hair-thinning, mild myelosuppression, headache, flu-like symptoms, mucositis

Local therapy

Local therapy is often done for cosmetic reasons, and the benefits are confined to the locally treated area. Tumour regrowth can occur within the treated area or at the perimeter. Risks of local treatment include infection at the treatment site, pain, pigmentation changes, scarring and tissue fibrosis. In considering local therapy, it is important to remember that local treatments can sometimes cause a worse cosmetic result than the original KS lesion. Local therapies include cryotherapy with liquid nitrogen, intralesional chemotherapy with vinblastine, laser therapy, topical retinoid creams and radiation therapy.

Cryotherapy with liquid nitrogen is the treatment of choice for small cutaneous lesions anywhere on the body, including the eyelid, conjunctiva, sclera, oral mucous membranes, glans penis or perirectal area. Freeze time is approximately 20–60 and can be divided and given at 2-week intervals until the lesion is adequately treated (Tappero et al., 1991). Post-treatment hypopigmentation can result, however, and should be considered before using this method to treat dark-skinned patients.

Intralesional injection of vinblastine, 0.01 mg in 0.1 ml sterile water has been used successfully to treat small, cosmetically disfiguring KS lesions (Newman, 1988).

Vinblastine intralesional injections can be painful, however, and repeated injections are often required. In addition, hyperpigmentation usually remains.

Various lasers have been used to destroy small KS lesions (Wheeland et al., 1985; Webster, 1995; Marchell and Alster, 1997). Side-effects include post-treatment infections due to prolonged tissue healing. Scarring and hyperpigmentation can also result. Pulsed dye laser treatment may have minimal associated side-effects compared with other laser therapies, although large population studies have not been done (Marchell and Alster, 1997).

KS lesions are exquisitely sensitive to radiation, and radiotherapy has been used successfully to treat muco-cutaneous and cutaneous lesions presenting in any area of the body. This treatment modality is palliative only and is best used to treat cosmetically disfiguring lesions in areas not easily treated with or too large for effective cryotherapy. Patients with periorbital and oral lesions may be treated with doses of 700–2200 cGy in divided doses (Nisce and Safai, 1985; Nobler et al., 1987; Kirova et al., 1998). Radiation can also be used to treat enlarged, KS-involved lymph nodes to relieve obstruction of lymphatic drainage. As with other local therapies, radiation therapy can cause severe and long-lasting side-effects. Avoiding overlap of radiation ports can be extremely difficult and overlapping radiation fields can cause tissue necrosis. Irradiation of lymph nodes can also cause sclerosis of the lymphatics, resulting in further drainage obstruction or fibrosis of muscle and connective tissue and leading to joint immobility and muscle disuse contractures and atrophy. KS tumours can regrow in previously treated areas or around the perimeter of a previously treated tumour. In addition, a phenomenon termed 'radiation recall' has been documented in patients treated with systemic anthracyclines after having been treated with radiation therapy. Although the mechanism is unknown, severe tissue damage can occur in previously irradiated sites and can result in full thickness ulcers.

Systemic cytotoxic therapy

For patients with more than a few small cutaneous lesions and for patients with progressive cutaneous or visceral KS, systemic therapy is the treatment of choice. Until 1996, combination cytotoxic chemotherapy with bleomycin and vincristine (BV) or adriamycin, bleomycin and vincristine (ABV) were considered to be the most effective chemotherapy for KS, with reported response rates of 23–80% (Gompels et al., 1992; Gill et al., 1994b). Etoposide

was used as a single agent as salvage therapy, administered intravenously or orally, with a reported response rate of 32% (Schwartsmann et al., 1997). These regimens had a high incidence of severe adverse reactions. In addition to dose-limiting bone marrow suppression, there were often pulmonary, cardiac and neurological toxicities, which made it difficult to treat these patients with effective doses for extended periods of time.

In 1996, two liposomal anthracyclines were approved by the US Food and Drug Administration (FDA) for the treatment of AIDS-related KS. Liposomal doxorubicin (Doxil®) and liposomal daunorubicin (DaunoXome®) are anthracyclines encapsulated in liposomes, microscopic vesicles composed of one or more lipid bilayers enclosing an aqueous phase containing the drug. Liposome encapsulation prolongs the plasma half-life of the anthracycline, increases drug concentrations in KS tissue and diminishes organ toxicity (Amantea et al., 1997; Stewart et al., 1998). Phase II studies using liposomal doxorubicin, $20\,mg/m^2$ administered intravenously every 2–3 weeks in patients with AIDS-related KS showed response rates of 66–90%. In a multicentre phase III trial, 241 patients with AIDS-related KS, were randomized to receive liposomal doxorubicin, ($20\,mg/m^2$ given intravenously over 30 min) or bleomycin and vincristine (at standard doses of bleomycin, 15 units/m^2 given intravenously over 30 min and vincristine, $1.4\,mg/m^2$ [maximum 2 mg] given as an intravenous bolus every 3 weeks for six cycles). Of the 218 evaluable patients, 58.7% responded to liposomal doxorubicin, compared with only 23.3% responding to bleomycin and vincristine (Stewart et al., 1998).

Over the past 3 years, since the widespread use of PIs and more experience with liposomal anthracyclines for AIDS-related KS, some investigators are reporting greater than 90% response rates and increased survival in patients with pulmonary KS (Grunaug et al., 1998). Because of the modest side-effect profile and excellent efficacy, liposomal anthracyclines are now considered to be first-line therapy for AIDS-related KS.

Side-effects of liposomal doxorubicin given at a dose of $20\,mg/m^2$ in 2–3-week cycles include mild myelosuppression, hand–foot syndrome and rarely, hair thinning and mild nausea. Some patients have had hypersensitivity reactions during the infusion, resulting in dyspnoea, hypotension, flushing and a mild choking sensation. Slowing the standard liposomal doxorubicin infusion to a 90 min duration (rather than the conventional duration of

60 min) usually prevents this infusional reaction. For subsequent infusions, patients should also be premedicated with hydrocortisone, 25 mg and diphenhydramine, 25 mg intravenously. Prochlorperazine, 10 mg orally prior to infusion usually prevents nausea. Hand–foot syndrome, which is painful erythema of the hands or plantar surfaces of the feet, may occur with repetitive 2-week dosing cycles. Severe hand–foot syndrome can result in desquamation of the palmar or plantar surfaces. Increasing the dosing interval to 3 or 4 weeks and decreasing the dose to 15 mg/m^2 normally allows hand–foot syndrome to resolve without a break in KS treatment. Often, after resolution of hand–foot syndrome, chemotherapy can be resumed at 20 mg/m^2 at the increased dosing interval. Pyridoxine, 50 mg orally twice daily on the day of chemotherapy and for the next 2 or 3 days, may be of some benefit in preventing or decreasing the severity of hand–foot syndrome.

Liposomal daunorubicin is given at a dose of 40 mg/m^2 in 2-week dosing intervals, has slightly lower reported response rates than liposomal doxorubicin and has not been reported to cause hand–foot syndrome. In a phase II study, liposomal daunorubicin (60 mg/m^2 every 2 weeks) was given to 53 patients who had a median CD4 lymphocyte count of less than 20 cells/μl and symptomatic pulmonary KS. Median survival for the treated patients was 7.1 months as compared to 1–4 months for historical controls. Of the treated patients, reversible grade 3 or 4 neutropenia, severe anaemia or thrombocytopenia were reported in 85%, 32% and 17% of patients, respectively. Non-haematologic toxicities, such as alopecia and mucositis, occurred in 11% and 6% of patients, respectively (Tulpule et al., 1998). Anthracycline-induced cardiotoxicity due to liposomal anthracyclines has not been documented, and there is as yet no established cumulative dose limit.

In 1997, paclitaxel (Taxol®) was approved as a single agent for AIDS-related KS treatment. A phase II study demonstrated that when given in the recommended dose of 135 mg/m^2 infused over 3 h in 3-week cycles, there was a major response in more than 70% of patients, even in those patients who had failed other agents (Welles et al., 1998). Response rates over 80% were reported when the paclitaxel infusion was given over 96 h (Welles et al., 1998). Paclitaxel causes significant myelosuppression and alopecia, more severe than that seen with liposomal anthracyclines. Prolonged paclitaxel therapy can also cause peripheral neuropathy. In addition, paclitaxel is delivered in Cremophor®. This excipient causes hypersensitivity reactions characterized by dyspnoea, chest pain, hypotension, flushing, angiooedema and generalized urticaria in some patients. These reactions can be eliminated or diminished by pretreatment with prednisone 10–20 mg orally 12 h and 6 h prior to each paclitaxel treatment, in addition to decadron, 10 mg administered intravenously with an H2 blocker, such as famotidine or ranitidine and diphenhydramine, 25–50 mg intravenously within an hour prior to the paclitaxel infusion. Because of the more severe side-effect profile for paclitaxel, this drug is presently considered to be second-line systemic therapy for AIDS-related KS. To date, there are no large studies documenting response rates in KS patients treated with liposomal anthracyclines or paclitaxel who are also receiving HAART regimens and prophylactic antibiotics; however, there have been anecdotal reports of nearly 100% response rates in such patients.

Immunomodulators

Interferon-α (IFN-α), long recognized for its antiproliferative and antiretroviral effects, has been used for the treatment of AIDS-related KS since the beginning of the epidemic (Krown et al., 1983; Volberding and Mitsuyasu, 1985; Mitsuyasu and Miles, 1987; Frissen et al., 1997; Shepherd et al., 1998). Initial studies involved doses as high as 50 million IU/m^2/day and although response rates of 32–40% were reported, side-effects such as the flu-like symptoms of chills, headaches, myalgias, anorexia, diarrhoea and fever, as well as thrombocytopenia, neutropenia and hepatic enzyme abnormalities, precluded long-term therapy. It has recently been observed that for patients with AIDS-related KS taking effective antiretroviral chemotherapy, lower doses of IFN-α given alone or after induction chemotherapy with anthracyclines or paclitaxel, appear to extend the benefit of the chemotherapy. This benefit has been seen with doses of IFN-α2a or IFN-α2b, 2–6 million IU/m^2/day and with consensus IFN at equivalent doses.

The mechanism of action of IFN-α as an effective AIDS-related KS therapy is unclear. Given in the lower doses, it may act by indirectly inhibiting the activity of tumour necrosis factor (TNF)-α and IL-1 and by inhibition of angiogenesis by downregulation of basic fibroblast growth factor (bFGF) (Fidler et al., 1994). In the higher doses, it may have additional antiretroviral and/or antitumour properties.

Subjective toxicities can be experienced even with the lower doses of IFN-α and can be mitigated by taking anti-inflammatory agents, such as naproxen, 250 mg orally 1 h before and 4 h after each IFN dose. IFN-β and IFN-γ have not been shown to be active against KS (Mitsuyasu, 1988; Miles *et al.*, 1990b).

Other immunomodulators, such as IL-4, which is known to inhibit IL-6 production, and specific inhibitors of tumour necrosis factor (TNF)-α have not as yet proven to be effective therapeutic agents for patients with AIDS-related KS (Aboulafia *et al.*, 1989; Tulpule *et al.*, 1997). Although an IL-1 antagonist has been observed to competitively inhibit KS cell proliferation in a dose-dependent manner *in vitro*, it was not shown to be effective clinically when given to KS patients in a phase I/II trial as soluble recombinant human IL-1 receptor (Krown *et al.*, 1995).

Hormones

Although AIDS-associated KS is seen primarily in men, it is not clear whether sex hormones play a significant role in this disease. Investigators have found that human chorionic gonadotropin (hCG) can induce apoptosis of KS cell lines *in vitro* by a mechanism that is not yet understood. Small clinical trials using hCG administered by local intralesional injections and by parenteral injection have yielded conflicting results (Gill *et al.*, 1996; Krown, 1996; Bouscarat *et al.*, 1997; Gill *et al.*, 1997; Harris, 1997; Lang *et al.*, 1997). There have also been a few anecdotal reports of worsening KS with androgen therapy, but there have been no large, controlled studies of androgen deprivation or of hCG therapy for AIDS-associated KS.

New treatment approaches

Retinoids are known to regulate proliferation and differentiation in many types of normal cells and tumour cells. Cultured KS cells express abundant retinoic acid receptors, and both all-trans retinoic acid and 13-cis-retinoic acid inhibit growth of KS cells *in vitro* cells and *in vivo* in a dose-dependent manner (Guo *et al.*, 1995). In small, clinical trials, retinoids given both topically and orally have been shown to produce some tumour response (Corbeil *et al.*, 1994; Gill *et al.*, 1994a). In a phase-II trial treating 24 patients with oral all-trans retinoic acid at a target dose of 150 mg/m^2, there was a 17% partial response, 13% minor response and 29% stable disease for 4 or more months. Headache was the most frequent adverse side-effect, followed by nausea and vomiting, skin dryness, hypertriglyceridaemia, anaemia and neutropenia (Gill *et al.*, 1994a). It is thought that the mechanism of action of the

retinoids is through downregulation of IL-6 by way of ligand-dependent receptor transcription interactions, as well as by downregulation of bFGF and inhibition of growth-promoting effects of oncostatin-M and TNF-α (Corbeil *et al.*, 1994; Guo *et al.*, 1995; Nagpal *et al.*, 1997).

Angiogenesis inhibition is currently an area of great interest in the treatment of KS. It is now understood that KS is a vascular tumour and that angiogenic factors are largely responsible for the growth and proliferation of KS cells. Both vascular endothelial growth factor (VEGF) and basic fibroblast growth factor (bFGF) have been found to be present in great abundance in KS tissue. VEGF is thought to be associated with the vascular permeability found in KS tumour tissue, as well as being an important angiogenesis growth factor. When VEGF binds to growth factor receptors on endothelial and spindle cells (receptor tyrosine kinases), the receptors dimerize, causing tyrosine kinase activation, which leads to autophosphorylation of the receptors. This causes a cascade of signalling events within the cells, resulting in proliferation and differentiation of the endothelial and spindle cells and thus in new blood vessel formation (Nakamura *et al.*, 1997). SU5416, a twice-weekly, intravenously-administered VEGF inhibitor, is a promising new treatment for KS. It acts by inhibiting autophosphorylation of the VEGF-mediated receptor. Preliminary data from an ongoing phase I study and from an ongoing phase I/II study show SU5416 to be well tolerated and effective in treating AIDS-related KS at doses of 17–65 mg/m^2, decreasing tumour growth as well as the extremity oedema associated with KS.

IM862, an angiogenesis inhibitor that is self-administered intranasally, is currently being studied in a phase I/II clinical trial of AIDS-related KS. Preliminary results reveal that it is well tolerated and eight of 15 evaluable patients have had a partial response lasting a median of 7.4 months when given 5 mg intranasally in regimens of 5 days on and 5 days off, or on alternate days. The mechanism of action of IM862 is not fully understood.

TNP-420, an analogue of fumagillin, inhibits bFGF-induced endothelial cell proliferation. In a small phase I clinical trial within the ACTG-215 trial, doses of 10–70 mg/m^2 given weekly as a 1-h intravenous infusion, were shown to be safe. Out of 38 patients with KS, seven (18%) had some tumour response (Dezube *et al.*, 1997).

Thalidomide, well known for its teratogenic effects, has been shown to inhibit production of TNF-α, as well as intracellular adhesion molecules and has been shown to interfere with basement membrane formation. It has also recently been shown to inhibit blood vessel formation and is currently being studied for possible use in the treatment of KS.

As discussed above, the HIV Tat protein is capable of stimulating the growth of KS cells, and controlling HIV viral replication (which would also reduce Tat protein synthesis) facilitates treatment of KS. Specifically inhibiting HIV Tat production or blocking the Tat receptor on KS cells is a possible new approach to the treatment of AIDS-related KS.

The HHV-8 (KSHV) found in KS tumour tissue is primarily in the latent (episomal) stage, with only small numbers of cells infected with replicating virus (Zhong et al., 1996). Since episomal-phase virus is not generally sensitive to antiviral drugs, it has been suggested that HHV-8 could be controlled by inducing replication of the virus in latently-infected cells followed by antiviral therapy. It may also be possible to prevent HHV-8 induction of KS by prophylaxis with antivirals. HHV-8 is susceptible to foscarnet, ganciclovir, cidofovir, adefovir and lobucavir (Medveczky et al., 1997; Panyutich et al., 1998).

Non-Hodgkin's lymphoma

Epidemiology

In the early 1980s, an increase in the incidence of NHL among relatively young, homosexual men was observed. The average age of these cases was between 30 and 39 years old, in contrast to the average age of about 55 years in the general population. Also, in contrast to the general population, where high-grade lymphomas of the large cell, immunoblastic type and small, non-cleaved Burkitt's-like cell type are rare, in HIV-infected patients these cell types comprised approximately 60% of all reported NHL. In the USA, Burkitt's-like lymphoma was found to be 1000 times more common in HIV-infected patients than in the general population (Beral et al., 1991). Most of the other cell types were diffuse large cell histologies, considered 'intermediate grade'. In 1987, the CDC revised its list of AIDS-defining illnesses to include HIV-infected individuals diagnosed with NHL of intermediate or high-grade B-cell histologies (CDC, 1987a). T-cell lymphomas and low-grade B-cell lymphomas have been reported in the HIV-infected population at rates higher than the general population, but are not included in the CDC's AIDS definition (Anon, 1987; Lust et al., 1989; Crane et al., 1991).

Prior to the widespread use of HAART regimens, the risk of HIV-infected patients developing aggressive B-cell NHL at some time in the course of their disease was approximately 60–200 times that of the general population, with a prevalence of 5–10% among all HIV-infected patients (Beral et al., 1991; Levine, 1992; Cote et al., 1997). Today, because of more effective antiretroviral therapy and effective prophylaxis against opportunistic infections, HIV-infected patients are living longer. Although some predict that this will bring a higher incidence of AIDS-related NHL in the years to come, it is not yet fully understood how the current HAART medication will affect the development of NHL in HIV-infected patients over the long term.

Patients with HIV-related NHL present more often with extranodal disease than their HIV-uninfected counterparts, with approximately 60% of these patients having extranodal disease at the time of diagnosis (Kaplan et al., 1989; Vaccher et al., 1996; Cote et al., 1997; Davis et al., 1998). Common extranodal sites include bone marrow, leptomeninges and the gastrointestinal tract. Primary brain lymphomas will be discussed separately.

Small, non-cleaved-cell lymphomas in HIV-infected individuals are associated with EBV in 10–40% of cases, c-myc rearrangements in approximately 75% of cases and p53 mutations in approximately 60% of cases, most resembling sporadic Burkitt's lymphoma. African (endemic) Burkitt's lymphoma is associated with both EBV and c-myc rearrangements in 100% of cases and with p53 mutations in about 30% of cases. HIV-related diffuse large cell lymphomas are associated with EBV in about 70% of cases and c-myc rearrangements occur in approximately 20% of cases (Knowles, 1993; Shibata et al., 1993; Gaidano and Dalla-Favera, 1997). This is in contrast to diffuse large-cell lymphomas in immunocompetent hosts, where neither EBV nor c-myc translocations are normally found (Shiramizu et al., 1992; Shibata et al., 1993).

PEL, also called body cavity-based lymphoma, is a disease of lymphomatous body cavity effusions, such as of the pericardium, pleura, and peritoneum, has been observed to occur mainly in HIV-infected male homosexuals and is extremely rare in HIV-uninfected patients. It is the first neoplasm shown to be dually infected with two herpes viruses. Lymphomatous cells from these effusions contain HHV-8 and EBV in the majority of cases (Horenstein et al., 1997). Unlike most other HIV-associated NHLs, PEL

B-cells lack the c-myc oncogene rearrangement. Morphologically, PEL is a large-cell lymphoma with immunoblastic and anaplastic features (Nador et al., 1996).

Diagnosis and staging

HIV-infected patients with mass lesions, asymmetric or rapidly progressive lymphadenopathy, with or without constitutional 'B' symptoms of fever, night sweats or weight loss, should be suspected of having NHL. Moreover, since extranodal presentation in the GI tract is found in 10–25% of cases at diagnosis, patients who complain of changing GI habits, obstructive symptoms or GI bleeding should have a complete bowel evaluation, including endoscopy with biopsies (Straus, 1997a,b). Diagnostic core biopsies are preferred over fine-needle aspirations and should be done whenever possible. Immunophenotyping of the tumour should always be done to aid in planning the treatment regimen.

Once NHL is diagnosed by tissue biopsy, a standard staging work-up should be done including computerized tomography (CT) of the chest, abdomen and pelvis, CT or magnetic resonance imaging (MRI) of the brain, cerebrospinal fluid analysis and bone marrow biopsy with aspirate sent for immunophenotyping and gene rearrangement studies. Approximately 10–20% of patients will have leptomeningeal involvement at presentation and approximately 30% will have bone marrow involvement. In addition, a complete peripheral blood count should be done, as well as complete blood chemistries, including electrolytes, liver function tests and blood urea and creatinine. Serum lactate dehydrogenase should be measured to help assess tumour burden and uric acid to help assess cell turnover. Prior to starting chemotherapy, all patients should have electrocardiograms, and patients over the age of 40 years or those patients suspected of having cardiac dysfunction should undergo a baseline multiple gated acquisition (MUGA) scan or echocardiogram for estimation of ejection fraction.

Prognosis

Although NHL can present at any stage of HIV disease, it is more common in patients who are more immunocompromised, with CD4 lymphocyte counts of less than 200 cells/µl (Northfelt et al., 1992; Pluda et al., 1993; Cote et al., 1997). The lymphomas tend to behave more aggressively than those seen in HIV-uninfected patients. Combination chemotherapy regimens have also been less successful in HIV-infected patients than in their HIV-uninfected counterparts. Reported response rates for HIV-infected patients with NHL are 17–56% and the median survival after diagnosis is 4–8 months; whereas, the median survival of non-HIV-infected patients with intermediate or high-grade NHL is about 12–36 months (Levine, 1992; Grogan and Miller, 1995; Hermans et al., 1995; Kaplan et al., 1997).

Indicators of poor prognosis in HIV-infected patients diagnosed with NHL include CD4 lymphocyte counts of less than 100 cells/µl, a history of opportunistic infections, age greater than 35 years, Karnofsky performance status of less than 70, elevated serum lactate dehydrogenase and the presence of extranodal disease (Oksenhendler et al., 1994; Vaccher et al., 1996; Straus, 1997b).

Treatment

Early in the AIDS epidemic, treatment strategies for AIDS-related NHL were similar to those used to treat aggressive lymphomas in HIV-uninfected patients. They involved dose-intensive combination chemotherapy regimens, including M-BACOD, CHOP, CHOMP, ProMACE-MOPP, MACOP-B and ProMACE-CytaBOM (Goldie et al., 1982; Fisher et al., 1983; Skarin et al., 1983; Fisher et al., 1984; Klimo and Connors, 1985; Gordon et al., 1989; Weick et al., 1989). A retrospective analysis of HIV-infected patients treated with these regimens showed that while complete response rates were similar to those of immunocompetent patients, HIV-infected patients had shorter response durations, higher rates of central nervous system (CNS) relapse, significantly lower median survivals and a high rate of death due to opportunistic infections (Levine et al., 1991). It was also observed that patients who received more intensive chemotherapy regimens had a shorter survival than patients who received less intensive regimens (Kaplan et al., 1989). Because of these observations, the AIDS Clinical Trials Group (ACTG) began studying the efficacy of modified regimens of M-BACOD and CHOP, with and without the use of haematopoietic growth factors and including intrathecal prophylaxis with Ara-C and methotrexate (Kaplan et al., 1991; Levine et al., 1991; Straus, et al., 1995). These regimens include methotrexate, bleomycin, doxorubicin, cyclophosphamide, vincristine, dexamethasone and cyclophosphamide, doxorubicin, vincristine and prednisone, respectively. The results of these early trials demonstrated that intrathecal prophylaxis was effective in preventing CNS disease, median survival increased from approximately 5.2 to approximately 6.5 months and patients who received growth factors experienced fewer neutropenic episodes and fewer days hospitalized with neutropenic fever than those patients who did not receive growth factors. Although patients who received GM-CSF had a transient increase in HIV p24 antigen, there was no clear clinical significance to this finding (Kaplan *et al.*, 1991).

In the ACTG protocol 142 study, 198 patients were randomized to receive 3-week cycles of standard-dose m-BACOD (methotrexate, 200 mg/m^2 day 15, bleomycin, 4 unit/m^2 day 1, doxorubicin, 45 mg/m^2 day 1, cyclophosphamide, 600 mg/m^2 day 1, vincristine, 1.4 mg/m^2 day 1 and dexamethasone, 6 mg/m^2 days 1–5) versus reduced-dose m-BACOD (methotrexate, 200 mg/m^2 day 15, cyclophosphamide, 300 mg/m^2 day 1, doxorubicin, 25 mg/m^2 day 1, bleomycin, 4 unit/m^2 day 1, vincristine, 1.4 mg/m^2 and dexamethasone, 3 mg/m^2 days 1–5) (Kaplan *et al.*, 1997). The results of this study confirmed equivalent overall survival for both groups; however, when the groups were pooled and the patients stratified by the number of adverse prognostic factors, median survival varied from 11 months for those patients with no or one adverse prognostic factor to 4 months for those patients with three or more adverse factors (Straus, 1997a).

More recently, HIV-infected patients presenting with NHL and CD4 lymphocyte counts of more than 200 cells/µl have been treated with standard-dose and intensive-dose chemotherapy in various regimens with prophylaxis for PCP, growth factor support and continuous antiretroviral therapy (Gisselbrecht *et al.*, 1993; Sparano *et al.*, 1993; Vaccher *et al.*, 1996). They have been shown to tolerate standard and intensive regimens with marginally better overall survival than severely immunocompromised HIV-infected patients, but less well than HIV-uninfected counterparts. Specifically, the duration of the response to chemotherapy and the length of survival have been considerably shorter in HIV-infected patients than in uninfected patients.

Despite numerous attempts to find an NHL combination chemotherapy regimen that is more effective than the CHOP regimen without more toxicity, CHOP is still the standard first-line chemotherapy treatment for immunocompetent patients with NHL. Whether or not other combination regimens may be more effective for patients with HIV-related NHL is still unknown. Moreover, it is also unknown at this time how HAART will affect the natural history of HIV-related NHL, although improved survival has been reported (Chow *et al.*, 2001).

Refractory and relapsing disease

Response rates in HIV-related lymphoma are poor, with only 30–50% of patients having complete responses, and nearly all responses being of short duration. Treating refractory and relapsing NHL is always difficult and with HIV-infected patients there is the added difficulty of treating patients with even greater myelosuppression and immune compromise than normally encountered. There is no salvage regimen that has proven to be ideal.

Just as with immunocompetent patients who are refractory to first-line treatment or who relapse, regimens such as ESHAP and various other etoposide-containing regimens have been used and have been reported in several small series of patients, with median survivals of 2.2–3.5 months (Tirelli *et al.*, 1996; Kaplan *et al.*, 1998). In a study of 26 patients, mitoguazone was given to patients for treatment of refractory or relapsing HIV-related NHL (Levine *et al.*, 1997). Mitoguazone, a polyamine biosynthesis inhibitor, was studied because of its relative lack of bone marrow suppression, its ability to cross the blood–brain barrier and initial reports of reasonably good response rates in HIV-uninfected patients with relapsed or refractory NHL. Of the 26 patients, however, median survival was only 2.6 months for the group as a whole. There have also been a few small single-institution studies and anecdotal reports of patients with AIDS-related NHL who have undergone high-dose chemotherapy with peripheral stem cell rescue. While most of these patients were able to tolerate the conditioning regimens, survival was not increased significantly, with the more immunocompromised patients mainly dying of opportunistic infections and less immunocompromised patients dying of complications from refractory lymphoma (pers. comm., Dr Steven Miles, Ronald Mitsuyasu and Michael Lill, UCLA, 1996).

Immunomodulators

IL-2 is a cytokine produced by activated T cells, which has been shown to increase proliferation of T cells, B cells and natural killer (NK) cells, which can then generate lymphokine-activated killer (LAK) cells. When given to HIV-infected patients who have baseline CD4 lymphocyte counts of 200 cells/µl or greater, either by subcutaneous injection or by continuous intravenous infusion, it has been shown to increase CD4 lymphocyte counts by twofold or more and to increase circulating NK cells (Mazza *et al.*, 1992; Teppler *et al.*, 1993; Wood *et al.*, 1993; Kovacs *et al.*, 1996; Davey *et al.*, 1997). Although some of the early patients have tolerated doses up to 18 million IU/day, toxicities, mainly attributable to TNF-α release, such as fatigue, fever, chills, malaise, rash, nausea, vomiting, diarrhoea, gastritis and hypotension, and life-threatening toxicities, such as myocardial infarction, vascular leak syndrome and pancytopenias, can occur. More recent studies use IL-2 doses of up to 12 million IU/day. There have been several small series reports of IL-2 given to patients with HIV-associated lymphoma, some of whom having had CD4 lymphocyte counts of less than 200 cells/μl, at doses of 0.4–6.0 million/m^2/day for varying lengths of time (Mazza et al., 1992; Bernstein et al., 1995). Of 12 patients with HIV-related NHL given IL-2, 6 million IU/m^2/day by continuous intravenous infusion over 5 days with ZDV in an Italian trial, six patients (50%) had a complete or partial response after four cycles. The Eastern Co-operative Oncology Group (ECOG) and the AIDS Malignancies Consortium (AMC) are currently studying the efficacy and safety of giving IL-2 to HIV-infected patients with NHL in remission. The AMC is also conducting a phase II trial for HIV-infected patients who have refractory or relapsed NHL, where patients will be treated with ifosfamide/mesna, 2 gm/m^2/day for 2 days by continuous intravenous infusion and etoposide, 150 mg/m^2/day for 2 days administered intravenously over 2 h every 21 days for a minimum of four cycles. All patients will continue to take combination antiretroviral therapy. Patients who have a complete or partial response will be randomized to receive a maintenance regimen of IL-2, 4.5 million IU subcutaneously twice per day for 5 days every four weeks, IL-12, 300 ng/kg subcutaneously twice per week continuously or no maintenance therapy.

IL-12 is a cytokine produced by monocytes and macrophages. It can induce both T cells and NK cells to produce cytokines, such as IFN-γ and to enhance lymphocyte-mediated cytotoxicity (Kobayashi et al., 1989). In vitro it can induce LAK cell proliferation, possibly in concert with TNF-α (Gately et al., 1992; Naume et al., 1992; Chehimi et al., 1993). IL-12 enhances in vitro cytotoxicity mediated by NK cells from healthy donors against colon cancer and neuroblastoma cell lines and NK-mediated cytotoxicity against autologous hairy cell leukaemia. IL-12 also enhances cytotoxic activity by tumour-infiltrating lymphocytes in various types of tumours (Lieberman et al., 1991; Andrews et al., 1993; Bigda et al., 1993). IL-12 has also been shown to downregulate and to suppress HIV replication in macrophage cultures and to enhance HIV-

specific cytotoxic T-lymphocyte activity (Akridge and Reed, 1996; McFarland et al., 1996). HIV-infected patients with baseline CD4 lymphocyte counts of less than 100 cells/μl and with CD4 lymphocyte counts of 100–500 cells/μl have been given IL-12 in randomized, placebo-controlled, dose-escalating trials. The 300 ng/kg twice-weekly dose was reasonably well tolerated, with side-effects being asthenia, headache, fever, nausea, vomiting, pharyngitis, rhinitis, sweating, pain, chills and arthralgias.

One of the more exciting new immune-based therapies to be used for the treatment of NHL is the CD20 antibody. CD20 is a protein expressed on the surface of most B-cell lymphoma cells and has been found on B cells in 95% of cases of HIV-related NHL (Tedder, 1985). CD20 appears to act by regulating the B cell as it progresses through its cell cycle, controlling cycle initiation and differentiation (Golay et al., 1985; Tedder et al., 1985). CD20 may also regulate signal transduction (Tedder et al., 1990). CD20 seems to be a good target for the treatment of lymphoma because it does not circulate in the plasma as a free protein, it is not shed from the surface of cells after antibody binding to antibody, nor does it internalize after binding (Reff et al., 1994; Press et al., 1997).

A chimeric mouse/human monoclonal CD20 antibody has been developed, which fixes complement, mediates antibody-dependent cellular cytotoxicity (ADCC) and induces apoptosis of CD20-expressing cells (Nadler et al., 1994; Demidem et al., 1995). This antibody can also sensitize drug-resistant human B-cell lymphoma cell lines to the cytotoxic effects of cisplatin, etoposide and ricin (Demidem et al., 1995). The pivotal clinical trial used for registration of the CD20 antibody (rituximab) was a multicentre, open-label, single-arm, phase III trial in non-HIV patients who presented with relapsed low-grade or follicular NHL. The patients received 375 mg/m^2 of rituximab by intravenous infusion weekly for four doses. The overall response was 48%, with a median duration of response not reached after a median follow-up of 11.2 months. Other smaller trials of rituximab have been performed in patients with refractory or relapsed intermediate and high-grade NHL. In these trials, overall response rates were 32–46%, with a time to progression for responders of 10.2 months. The most common toxicities of rituximab reported were low-grade episodes of fever, chills, hypotension, rash, nausea, headache, asthenia and thrombocytopenia.

The standard dose of rituximab is 375 mg/m^2/ week. It is infused intravenously, starting at 50 ml/h (50 mg/h). The rate of infusion is increased by 50 mg/h every 30 min to a maximum rate of 400 mg/h. Patients should be premedicated 30–60 min prior to each infusion with acetaminophen, 650 mg orally, diphenhydramine, 50 mg and an H2 blocker, such as ranitidine or famotidine. Patients should be monitored carefully, and if they develop a transient infusion-related toxicity, the infusion can be temporarily discontinued and then restarted at a lower rate after the patient has been given another dose of diphenhydramine and intravenous fluids.

There have been anecdotal reports of treating patients who have HIV-related NHL with rituximab alone or in combination with chemotherapy, with encouraging results. The AMC has recently begun a randomized trial of standard-dose CHOP chemotherapy with or without rituximab for the treatment of newly-diagnosed HIV-related NHL. Two-thirds of the patients will receive rituximab on day 1 with each 21-day cycle of CHOP (the CHOP chemotherapy starting on day 3 in the rituximab arm) for a minimum of four cycles. This will be followed by a maintenance phase, where responders will be given rituximab every 28 days for three more doses. All patients will be monitored closely and will be followed for 1 year after the completion of their chemotherapy.

A radiolabelled CD20 antibody (linked to ^{131}I) is currently in clinical trials for patients with refractory and relapsed low-grade and follicular NHL. However, because of the potential for severe myelosuppression caused by radioactive antibodies, this may not be a reasonable treatment option for HIV-infected patients.

Another area of investigation is the use of intensive chemotherapy with peripheral stem cell support. As in non-HIV-infected individuals, relapse of lymphoma carries a very poor prognosis and long-term results with salvage chemotherapy have been poor. Studies are in progress to assess the effects of high-dose marrow ablative therapy with peripheral stem cell support in chemotherapy-sensitive relapsed lymphoma. HIV-directed gene therapies are also incorporated into several of these stem cell protocols.

Most HIV-infected patients presenting with NHL can be treated safely with standard-dose chemotherapy. Antiretroviral therapy, as well as opportunistic infection prophylaxis medications, should be continued throughout the course of chemotherapy. Patients who are taking ZDV should be switched to another reverse transcriptase inhibitor for the duration of chemotherapy because of the potential myelosuppressive effects of ZDV. Leptomeningeal prophylaxis with intrathecal methotrexate, 12 mg or cytosine arabinoside, 50 mg is suggested for all patients with HIV-related lymphomas and is considered standard in patients with small non-cleaved and immunoblastic lymphomas and in patients who present with bone marrow involvement.

Primary central nervous system lymphoma

Primary central nervous system lymphoma (PCNSL) is NHL limited to the CNS and which at the time of diagnosis has often spread to the leptomeninges, eye or spinal cord. PCNSL is 1000–3000 times more common in HIV-infected patients than in their non-HIV-infected counterparts. It is seen most often in severely immunocompromised patients with CD4 lymphocyte counts of less than 50 cells/μl (Beral et al., 1991). In the HIV-infected patient, all PCNSLs are high grade, either immunoblastic or small, non-cleaved cell types, and all are associated with EBV. This is in contrast to those seen in non-HIV-infected individuals, where only about 22% are high grade and EBV is uncommonly found. Without treatment, the median survival of PCNSL is less than 1 month. With treatment, the median survival is 2–4 months. This is in contrast to treated non-HIV-infected patients, where median survival is 12–18 months (Levine, 1992; Straus, 1997b). New diagnoses of primary CNS lymphoma in HIV-infected patients have declined ten-fold between 1994 and 1996, perhaps due to improvements in antiretroviral chemotherapy.

Presenting symptoms of PCNSL may be subtle and can be confused with CNS infections such as toxoplasmosis, herpes encephalitis, tuberculosis or cryptococcosis. These symptoms include personality changes, headache, unsteadiness, nausea and weakness. More pronounced manifestations include seizure, hemiplegia, difficulty with speech or language or visual changes. Because it can be confused with treatable infectious diseases, a diagnosis should be made as soon as possible.

The diagnostic evaluation should include a contrast MRI or CT scan, thallium scan, lumbar puncture with cerebrospinal fluid (CSF) cytology, ophthalmologic examination and toxoplasma serology. Patients with masses on imaging scan and who are sero-negative for toxoplasmosis in the CSF should have a stereotactic biopsy. False sero-negativity for toxoplasmosis reported to be only about 5% CSF cytology can establish the diagnosis of PCNSL in 30% of patients (Grant *et al.*, 1990; Forsyth *et al.*, 1994). Unlike immunocompetent patients who have PCNSLs, which are almost never ring enhancing, 52% of HIV-infected patients with PCNSL have ring-enhancing lesions on CT or MRI. Additionally, whereas 75% of immunocompetent patients have solitary lesions, only 48% of HIV-infected patients have solitary lesions. Recently, detection of EBV DNA in CSF using Polymerase chain reaction (PCR) has been shown to have good sensitivity and specificity for PCNSL in HIV. Early brain biopsy is warranted if the patient has negative toxoplasmosis antibody titres and if the patient deteriorates clinically within the first week of treatment for toxoplasmosis (DeAngelis, 1995). Patients with PCNSL should also have CT scans of the chest, abdomen and pelvis, as well as a bone marrow biopsy to completely exclude systemic NHL (DeAngelis, 1995).

Treatment

All HIV-infected patients with brain mass lesion(s) should be treated empirically for toxoplasmosis encephalitis until a diagnosis of toxoplasmosis has been excluded (see Chapter 26). After a diagnosis of PCNSL has been made, patients with CD4 lymphocyte counts of greater than 200 cells/μl, a good performance status and a life expectancy of more than 2 months should be treated with chemotherapy and whole-brain irradiation (Chamberlain, 1994). There have been several small series reports of patients with HIV-associated PCNSL who have survived 11 months or longer who were treated with radiation followed by PCV (CCNU, 110 mg/m^2 orally day 1, procarbazine, 60 mg/m^2 orally days 1–21 and vincristine, 1.4 mg/m^2 intravenously days 8, 29) or other chemotherapy regimens (Gill *et al.*, 1985; Formenti *et al.*, 1989; Chamberlain, 1994). For patients whose life expectancy is less than 2 months because of poor performance status or concurrent infections, palliative radiation with 3000 cGy in 10 fractions may be the most appropriate treatment (DeAngelis, 1995).

Anogenital cancer

Epidemiology

Invasive cervical cancer

In 1993, the CDC expanded the AIDS definition to include HIV-infected women with invasive cervical cancer (Table 33.2). It has long been recognized that HIV-infected women are at increased risk for cervical intraepithelial neoplasia (CIN) and the CDC's expanded definition was based

Table 33.2 CDC recommendations for Papanicolaou smear screening of HIV-infected women

- Women who are HIV-infected should be advised to have a comprehensive gynaecological examination, including a Papanicolaou smear, as part of their initial medical evaluation
- If initial Papanicolaou smear results are within normal limits, at least one additional Papanicolaou smear should be obtained in approximately 6 months to rule out the possibility of false-negative results on the initial Papanicolaou smear
- If the repeat Papanicolaou smear is normal, HIV-infected women should be advised to have a Papanicolaou smear obtained annually
- If the initial or subsequent Papanicolaou smear shows severe inflammation with reactive squamous cellular changes, another Papanicolaou smear should be collected within 3 months.
- If the initial or follow-up Papanicolaou smear shows SIL (or equivalent) or ASCUS, the woman should be referred for colposcopic examination of the lower genital tract and, if indicated, colposcopically directed biopsies

SIL: squamous infraepithelial lesion; ASCUS: atypical squamous cells of uncertain significance.
(From Center for Disease Central and Prevention, 1993)

on the fact that CIN can progress to cervical cancer. Although a few small studies supported an increase in invasive cervical cancer among HIV-infected women, many questioned the validity of the expanded definition, since most cases of CIN do not progress to cervical cancer (Maiman *et al.*, 1990). Chin and colleagues at the CDC reviewed hospital records and analysed serum samples of 40 524 women, aged 20–54 years, from 1 January 1994 to 31 December 1995, at 14 'surveillance' hospitals designated in 1988 to serve a population at high risk for HIV disease (Chin *et al.*, 1998). During this 2-year period, there were 264 new cases of invasive cervical cancer reported, representing 0.7% of the women studied. The prevalence of invasive cervical cancer in HIV-infected women was 10.4/1000, compared to the prevalence in HIV-uninfected women of 6.7/1000 (relative risk of 1.7). When HIV-infected women were stratified by race, African-American women had a relative risk of 1.8 and Latino women had a relative risk of 4.8 (Chin *et al.*, 1998). Interestingly, the prevalence of cervical cancer was higher in women known to be HIV infected prior to their cancer diagnosis than those whose HIV status had not previously been known, possibly explained by more intensive screening in the known HIV-infected population (Chin et al., 1998). In addition to the increased prevalence of invasive cervical cancer in HIV-infected women, there was also a higher prevalence of extensive and multifocal disease (Maiman et al., 1990).

Anal cancer

Epidemiological studies have confirmed that the risk factors for anal cancer are homosexuality, receptive anal intercourse, presence of anal condylomata and smoking. In recent years, there has also been an increase in reported cases of anal cancer in the general population, including among women and unmarried men (Palefsky et al., 1990; Melbye et al., 1994a,b; Frisch et al., 1997; Palefsky et al., 1998). While HPV has long been recognized to have a causal relationship with cervical cancer, it is only recently that HPV has been studied as a possible cause of anal cancer. It is now known that HPV serotypes 16, 18, 31, 33 and 35, those associated with CIN and invasive cervical cancer, are also commonly associated with anal epithelial neoplasia and anal cancer (Palefsky et al., 1990; Melbye et al., 1994a, b; Frisch et al., 1997; Shah, 1997; Sun et al., 1997; Palefsky et al., 1998).

Cervical cancer

Independent variables found to be associated with CIN are cervicovaginal HPV infection, HIV infection, CD4 lymphocyte counts of less than 200 cells/μl and age greater than 34 years (Wright et al., 1994; Cappiello et al., 1997). Papanicolaou smears appear to be effective in detecting early squamous intraepithelial lesions in HIV-infected women (Maiman et al., 1991; Fink et al., 1994; Korn et al., 1994; Wright et al., 1994). The CDC now recommends that HIV-infected women be monitored for cervical disease with Papanicolaou smears every 6–12 months (Wright and Sun, 1996).

Treatment of cervical neoplastic disease is primarily determined by the stage of disease, and standard treatment strategies should be used; however, approximately 50–78% of HIV-infected women with CIN stages 2 or 3 have recurrent disease after treatment, and HIV-infected women more commonly present with extensive and multifocal disease than uninfected women (Maiman et al., 1993; Fink et al., 1994). Patients with stage Ia disease can be treated with cervical conization. Patients with stage Ib have a 15–25% risk of having pelvic lymph node involvement and therefore, patients with stage Ib, II or III should be treated

with radical hysterectomy and pelvic lymphadenectomy, with radiation or with both surgery and radiation. Patients with tumour extending into the bladder or rectum – stage IV disease – should be treated with external beam radiation and possibly with pelvic exenteration.

Chemotherapy has not proven to be very effective, although several agents have resulted in 15–25% response rates. The recurrence rate for HIV-infected women who have extensive cervical cancer has been reported to be 100%, compared to a recurrence rate of 49% in HIV-uninfected women (Maiman et al., 1993).

Anal cancer

Anal cancer is a squamous cell cancer arising anywhere along the anal canal, including the transitional zone (cloacogenic) and the anal margin. Anal cancers arising from the transitional zone have been found to be preceded by multicentric areas of dysplasia. Long recognized to be a risk factor for cervical cancer, smoking may also confer an additional risk for anal cancer. One study documented a fivefold increased risk for anal cancer among women and a fourteenfold increased risk among men who currently smoke compared with non-smokers (Daling et al., 1992). At this time, however, despite the prevalence of AIN of 15% in men with advanced AIDS, the incidence of anal cancer in the general population is low, with Surveillance, Epidemiology and End Results (SEER) cancer registries reporting new diagnoses of anal cancer in only 806 men and 1642 women in the years between 1973 and 1989 (Palefsky et al., 1990). At present, there is not a clear role for screening anal Pap smears.

Anal pain, pruritus and bleeding are the most common symptoms of anal carcinoma in situ, and the most common physical finding of invasive cancer is an intraluminal mass. The use of transrectal ultrasound may be useful to help determine the depth of penetration (Goldman et al., 1988). Any suspicious lesion should be biopsied. Prognostic factors include size of lesion, depth of penetration, location at the anal margin and lymph node involvement (Place et al., 2000). Recommended treatment for anal carcinoma in situ is local application of 5-fluorouracil (5-FU). Invasive disease should be treated with combination chemotherapy and radiation with 5-FU, 1000 mg/m^2/day by continuous intravenous infusion over 4 days on days 1–4, in weeks 1 and 4, mitomycin-C, 10 mg/m^2 by intravenous bolus on days 1 and 29 and external beam radiation with 4500 cGy, with radiation boosts to larger tumours (Flam et al., 1995).

Summary

The widespread use of opportunistic infection prophylaxis and HAART has led not only to an increased life expectancy for HIV-infected individuals, but also an apparent partial immune reconstitution. As a result, fewer patients are presenting with KS and primary CNS lymphoma and possibly systemic NHL as well. We do not know, however, whether the partial immune reconstitution gained by patients who are taking HAART medication will persist or whether there will again be a surge of new HIV-associated malignancy diagnoses in those patients who finally become resistant to the HAART medication.

In recent years, there has also been a greater understanding of the aetiology and pathology of KS, with the discovery and characterization of the KS herpesvirus. Treatment of KS with liposomal anthracyclines and with paclitaxel has proven to be more effective and less toxic than previous treatments. In the future, treatments with angiogenesis inhibitors and other immune modulators may replace chemotherapy agents completely.

Treatment for HIV-infected patients with lymphoma has also changed over recent years, largely because of HAART therapy. HIV-infected patients who are diagnosed with NHL are now nearly always able to tolerate standard doses of chemotherapy, and recent developments in antibody therapy and cytokine therapy may increase duration of response and survival in these patients. For HIV-infected women with CIN, there is evidence that more frequent screening Papanicolaou smears may reduce the incidence of HIV-associated cervical cancer.

References

Aboulafia D, Miles SA, Saks SR et al. (1989). Intravenous recombinant tumor necrosis factor in the treatment of AIDS-related Kaposi's sarcoma. J Acquir Immune Defic Synd Hum Aetiovirol 2: 54–8.

Akridge RE, Reed SG. (1996). Interleukin-12 decreases human immunodeficiency virus type 1 replication in human macrophage cultures reconstituted with autologous reconstituted peripheral blood mononuclear cells. J Infect Dis 173: 559–64.

Amantea MA, Forrest A, Northfelt DW et al. (1997). Population pharmacokinetics and pharmacokinetics of pegylated-liposomal doxorubicin in patients with AIDS-related Kaposi's sarcoma. Clin Pharmacol Ther 61: 301–11.

Andrews JV, Schoof DD, Bertagnolli MM et al. (1993). Immunomodulatory effects of interleukin-12 on human tumor-infiltrating lymphocytes. J Immunother 14: 1–10.

Anonymous. Centers for Disease Control and Prevention (CDC). (1987). Revision of the CDC surveillance case definition of acquired immunodeficiency syndrome. CDC Surveillance Summary. MMWR 36: 3–15.

Anon. (1987). Revision of the CDC surveillance case definition for acquired immunodeficiency syndrome. JAMA 258: 1143–54.

Bais C, Santomasso B, Coso O et al. (1998). G-protein-coupled receptor of Kaposi's sarcoma-associated herpes virus is a viral oncogene and angiogenesis activator. Nature 391: 86-9.

Beral V, Peterman T, Berkelman R et al. (1991). AIDS-associated non-Hodgkin's lymphoma. Lancet 337: 805–9.

Bernstein ZP, Porter MM, Gould M et al. (1995). Prolonged administration of low-dose interleukin-2 in human immunodeficiency virus-associated malignancy results in selective expansion of innate immune effectors without significant clinical toxicity. Blood 86: 3287–94.

Bigda J, Mysliwska J, Dziadziuszko R et al. (1993). Interleukin-12 augments natural killer cell-mediated cytotoxicity in hairy-cell leukemia. Leuk Lymphoma 10: 121–5.

Biggar RJ, Rabkin CS. (1996). The epidemiology of AIDS-associated neoplasms. Hematol Oncol Clin N Am 10: 997–1010.

Boshoff C. (1998). Coupling herpesvirus to angiogenesis. Nature 391: 24–5.

Boshoff C, Moore PS. (1997). Kaposi's sarcoma-associated herpesvirus: a newly recognized pathogen. AIDS Clin Review 98: 323–49.

Boshoff C, Whitby D, Hatziioannou T et al. (1995). Kaposi's sarcoma-associated herpes virus in HIV-negative Kaposi's sarcoma. Lancet 345: 1043–4.

Boshoff C, Endo Y, Collins PD et al. (1997). Angiogenic and HIV-inhibitory functions of KSHV-encoded chemokines. Science 278: 290–3.

Bouscarat F, Dazza MC, Melchior JC et al. (1997). Kaposi's sarcoma and sex hormones. AIDS 11: 687–8.

Brooks LA, Wilson AJ, Crook T. (1997). Kaposi's sarcoma-associated herpesvirus (KSHV)/human herpesvirus 8 (HHV8) a new human tumor virus. J Pathol 182: 262–5.

Cai J, Zheng T, Lotz M et al. (1997). Glucocorticoids induce Kaposi's sarcoma cell proliferation through the regulation of transforming growth factor-β. Blood 5: 1491–500.

Cappiello G, Garbuglia AR, Salvi R et al. (1997). HIV infection increases the risk of squamous cell intra-epithelial lesions in women with HPV infection: an analysis of HPV genotypes. Int J Cancer 72: 982–6.

Center for Disease Control and Prevention (CDC). (1993). Sexually transmitted diseases treatment guidelines. MMWR 42: RR–14.

Chachoua A, Kriegel R, Lafleur F et al. (1989). Prognostic factors and staging classifications of patients with epidemic Kaposi's sarcoma. J Clin Oncol 7: 774–80.

Chamberlain MC. (1994). Long survival in patients with acquired immune deficiency syndrome-related primary central nervous system lymphoma. Cancer 73: 1728–30.

Chang Y. (1997). Kaposi's sarcoma and Kaposi's sarcoma-associated herpesvirus (human herpesvirus 8): where are we now? J Natl Cancer Inst 89: 1829–31.

Chang Y, Cesarman E, Pessin MS et al. (1994). Identification of herpes-like DNA sequences in AIDS-associated Kaposi's sarcoma. Science 266: 1865–9.

Chehimi J, Valiante NM, D'Andrea A et al. (1993). Enhancing effect of natural killer cell stimulatory factor (NSKSF/interleukin-12) on cell-mediated cytotoxicity against tumor-derived and virus-infected cells. Eur J Immunol 23: 1826–30.

Chin KM, Sidhu JS, Janssen RS et al. (1998). Invasive cervical cancer in human immunodeficiency virus-infected and uninfected hospital patients. Obstet Gynecol 92: 83–7.

Chow KU, Mitrou PS, Gedulolig K et al. (2001). Changing incidence and survival in patients with AIDS-related Non-Hodgkin's lymphoma in the era of Highly Active Antiretroviral Therapy (HAART). Leuk Lymphoma 41: 105–16.

Chyu K-Y, Birnbaum Y, Naqvi T et al. (1998). Echocardiographic detection of Kaposi's sarcoma causing cardiac tamponade in a patient with acquired immunodeficiency syndrome. Clin Cardiol 21: 131–3.

Cooley TP, Hirschhorn LR, O'Keane JC. (1996). Kaposi's sarcoma in women with AIDS. AIDS 10: 1221–5.

Corbeil J, Rapaport E, Richman DD et al. (1994). Antiproliferative effect of retinoid compounds on Kaposi's sarcoma cells. J Clin Invest 93: 1981–6.

Cornali E, Zietz C, Benelli R et al. (1998). Vascular endothelial growth factor regulates angiogenesis and vascular permeability. Am J Pathol 149: 1851–69.

Cote TR, Biggar RJ, Rosenberg PS et al. (1997). Non-Hodgkin's lymphoma among people with AIDS: Incidence, presentation and public health burden. Int J Cancer 73: 645–50.

Crane CA, Variakojis D, Rosen ST et al. (1991). Cutaneous T-cell lymphoma in patients with human immunodeficiency virus infection. Arch Dermatol 127: 989–94.

Daling JR, Sherman KJ, Hislop TG et al. (1992). Cigarette smoking and the risk of anogenital cancer. Am J Epidemiol 135: 180–9.

Davey RT, Chaitt DG, Piscitelli SC et al. (1997). Subcutaneous administration of interleukin-2 in human immunodeficiency virus type-1 infected persons. J Infect Dis 175: 781–9.

Davis AJ, Goldstein D, Millikin S. (1998). Long term follow-up of CEOP in the treatment of HIV related non-Hodgkin's lymphoma (NHL). Aust NZ J Med 28: 28–32.

DeAngelis LM. (1995). Current management of primary central nervous system lymphoma. Oncology 9: 63–71.

Demidem A, Hanna N, Hariharan H et al. (1995). Chimeric anti-CD20 antibody (IDEC rituximab) is apoptotic and sensitizes drug-resistant human B-cell lymphomas and AIDS-related lymphomas to the cytotoxic effect of CDDP, VP-16 and toxins. FASEB J 9: A206.

Dezube BJ. (1996). Clinical presentation and natural history of AIDS-related Kaposi's sarcoma. Hematol Oncol Clin N Am 10: 1023–9.

Dezube BJ, Von Roenn JH, Holden-Wiltse J et al. (1997). Fumagillin analog (TNP-420) in the treatment of Kaposi's sarcoma: a Phase 1 AIDS Clinical Trial Group Study. J Acquir Immune Defic Syndr Hum Retrovirol 14: A35.

Ensoli B, Buonaguro L, Barillari G et al. (1993). Release, uptake, and effects of extracellular human immunodeficiency virus type 1 Tat protein on cell growth and transactivation. J Virol 67: 277.

Ensoli B, Gendelman R, Markham P et al. (1994). Synergy between basic fibroblast growth factor and HIV-1 Tat protein in induction of Kaposi's sarcoma. Nature 371: 674.

Fidler IJ, Singh RK, Gutman M et al. (1994). Interferons alpha and beta down regulate the expression of basic fibroblast growth factor (bFGF) in human carcinomas. Proc Am Assoc Cancer Res 35: 47.

Fink MJ, Fruchter RG, Maiman et al. (1994). The adequacy of cytology and colposcopy in diagnosing cervical neoplasia in HIV-seropositive women. Gynecol Oncol 55: 133–7.

Fisher RI, DeVita VT Jr, Hubbard SM. (1983). Diffuse aggressive lymphomas: increased survival after alternating flexible sequence of Pro-MACE and MOPP chemotherapy. Ann Intern Med 98: 304.

Fisher RI, DeVita VT, Hubbard SM et al. (1984). Randomized trial of ProMACE-MOPP versus ProMACE-CytaBOM in previously untreated, advanced stage, diffuse aggressive lymphomas. Proc ASCO 3: 242.

Flam MS, John M, Pajak T et al. (1995). Radiation (RT) and 5-fluorouracil (5-FU) vs radiation, 5-FU and mitomycin-C (MMC) in the treatment of anal carcinoma: results of a phase III randomized RTOG/ECOG intergroup trial. Proc Am Soc Clin Oncol 14: 191.

Formenti SC, Gill PS, Lean E et al. (1989). Primary central nervous system lymphoma in AIDS: results of radiation therapy. Cancer 63: 1101–7.

Forsyth PA, Yahalom J, DeAngelis LM. (1994). Combined modality therapy in the treatment of primary central nervous system lymphoma in AIDS. Neurology 44: 1473–9.

Friedman-Kien AE, Saltzman BR. (1990). Clinical manifestations of classical, endemic African, and epidemic AIDS-associated Kaposi's sarcoma. J Am Acad Dermatol 22: 1237–50.

Frisch M, Glimelius B, Vanden Brule ASC et al. (1997). Sexually transmitted infection as a cause of anal cancer. N Engl J Med 337: 1350–8.

Frissen PH, deWolf F, Reiss P et al. (1997). High-dose interferon-2a exerts potent activity against human immunodeficiency virus type 1 not associated with antitumor activity in subjects with Kaposi's sarcoma. J Infect Dis 176: 811–14.

Gaidano G, Dalla-Favera R. (1997). Molecular biology of lymphomas. In: VT DeVita, S Heilman, SA Rosenberg (eds.) Cancer: principles and practice of oncology. Fifth edition. Lippencott-Raven, Philadelphia, PA: 2131–45.

Ganem D. (1997). KSHV and Kaposi's sarcoma: the end of the beginning? Cell 91: 157–60.

Gately MK, Wolitzky AG, Quinn PM et al. (1992). Regulation of human cytolytic lymphocyte responses by interleukin-12. Cell Immunol 143: 127–42.

Gill PS, Levine AM, Meyer PR et al. (1985). Primary central nervous system lymphoma in homosexual men: Clinical, immunologic, and pathologic features. Am J Med 78: 742–8.

Gill PS, Espina BM, Moudgil T et al. (1994a). All-trans retinoic acid for the treatment of AIDS-related Kaposi's sarcoma: results of a pilot phase II study. Leukemia 8: 26–32.

Gill PS, Miles SA, Mitsuyasu RT et al. (1994b). Phase I AIDS Clinical Trials Group (075) study of adriamycin, bleomycin and vincristine chemotherapy with zidovudine in the treatment of AIDS-related Kaposi's sarcoma. AIDS 8: 1695–9.

Gill PS, Lunardi-Iskandar Y, Louie S et al. (1996). The effects of preparations of human chorionic gonadotropin on AIDS-related Kaposi's sarcoma. N Engl J Med 335: 1261–9.

Gill PS, McLaughlin T, Espina BM et al. (1997). Phase I study of human chorionic gonadotropin given subcutaneously to patients with acquired immunodeficiency syndrome-related mucocutaneous Kaposi's sarcoma. J Natl Cancer Inst 89: 1797–802.

Gillison ML, Ambinder RF. (1997). Human herpesvirus-8. Curr Opin Oncol 9: 440–9.

Gisselbrecht C, Oksenhendler E, Tirelli U et al. (1993). Human immunodeficiency virus-related lymphoma treated with intensive combination chemotherapy. Am J Med 95: 188–96.

Goedert JJ, Cote TR, Virgo P et al. (1998). Spectrum of AIDS-associated malignant disorders. Lancet 351: 1833–9.

Golay JT, Clark EA, Beverly PCL. (1985). The CD20 (Bp35) antigen is involved in activation of B cells from the Go to the G1 phase of the cell cycle. J Immunol 135: 3795–801.

Goldie JH, Coldman AJ, Gudauskas GA. (1982). Rationale for the use of alternating non-cross resistant chemotherapy. Cancer Treat Rep 66: 439–49.

Goldman S, Glimelius B, Norming U et al. (1988). Transanorectal ultrasonography in anal carcinoma: A prospective study of 21 patients. Acta Radiol 29: 337–41.

Gompels MM, Hill A, Jenkins P et al. (1992). Kaposi's sarcoma in HIV infection treated with vincristine and bleomycin. AIDS 6: 1175–80.

Gordon LI, Harrington D, Glick JH et al. (1989). Randomized phase III comparison of CHOP versus m-BACOD in diffuse large cell and diffuse mixed lymphoma: equivalent complete response rates and time to treatment failure but greater toxicity with m-BACOD. Proc Am Soc Clin Oncol 8: 255.

Grant IH, Gold JWM, Rosenblum M et al. (1990). Toxoplasma gondii serology in HIV-infected patients: the development of central nervous system toxoplasmosis in AIDS. AIDS 4: 519–21.

Grogan TM, Miller TP. (1995). Natural history and pretreatment evaluation of non-Hodgkin's lymphomas. In: Cancer Treatment. Fourth edition. Philadelphia, PA: WB Saunders, 979–1005.

Grunaug M, Bogner JR, Loch O et al. (1998). Liposomal doxorubicin in pulmonary Kaposi's sarcoma: improved survival as compared to patients without liposomal doxorubicin. Eur J Med Res 3: 13–19.

Guo W, Gill PS, Antakly T. (1995). Inhibition of AIDS – Kaposi's sarcoma cell proliferation following retinoic acid receptor activation. Cancer Res 55: 823–9.

Guo HG, Browning P, Nichols J et al. (1997). Characterization of a chemokine receptor-related gene in human herpes virus 8 and its expression in Kaposi's Sarcoma. Virology 228: 371–8.

Harris PJ. (1997). Intralesional human chorionic gonadotropin for Kaposi's sarcoma. N Engl J Med 336: 1187–9.

Haverkos HW, Friedman-Kien AE, Drotman AE et al. (1990). The changing incidence of Kaposi's sarcoma among patients with AIDS. J Am Acad Dermatol 22: 1250–3.

Hermans J, Krol ADG, van Groningen K et al. (1995). International prognostic index for aggressive non-Hodgkin's lymphoma is valid for all malignancy grades. Blood 86: 1460–3.

Horenstein MG, Nador RG, Chadburn A et al. (1997). Epstein–Barr virus latent gene expression in primary effusion lymphomas containing Kaposi's sarcoma-associated herpesvirus/human herpesvirus-8. Blood 90: 1186–91

Jacobson LP. (1998). Impact of highly effective antiretroviral therapy on the incidence of malignancies among HIV-infected individuals. Second National AIDS Malignancy Conference, Bethesda, MD, USA.

Johnson CC, Wilcosky T, Kvale P et al. (1997). Cancer incidence among an HIV-infected cohort. Am J Epidemiol 146: 470–5.

Jones JL, Hanson DL, Dworkin MS et al. (2000). Incidence and trends in Kaposi's sarcoma in the era of effective antiretroviral therapy. J Acquir Immun Defic Syndr 24: 270–4.

Kaplan LD, Abrams DI, Feigal E et al. (1989). AIDS-associated non-Hodgkin's lymphoma in San Francisco. JAMA 261: 719–24.

Kaplan LD, Kahn JO, Crowe S et al. (1991). Clinical and virologic effects of recombinant human granulocyte-macrophage colony-stimulating factor in patients receiving chemotherapy for human immunodeficiency virus-associated non-Hodgkin's lymphoma: results of a randomized trial. J Clin Oncol 9: 929–40.

Kaplan LD, Straus DJ, Testa MA et al. (1997). Low-dose compared with standard-dose m-BACOD chemotherapy for non-Hodgkin's lymphoma associated with human immunodefiency virus infection. N Engl J Med 336: 1641–8.

Kaplan LD, Moran T, Song L et al. (1998). Continuous infusion ifosfamide/Mesna with etoposide for refractory HIV-associated non-Hodgkin's lymphoma (NHL). Thirty-Fourth Annual Meeting of the American Society of Clinical Oncology, Bethesda, MD, USA.

Karp JE, Pluda JM, Yarchoan R. (1996). AIDS-related Kaposi's sarcoma: a template for the translation of molecular pathogenesis into targeted therapeutic approaches. Hematol Oncol Clin N Am 10: 1031–49.

Kempf W, Adams V, Pfaltz M et al. (1995). Human herpes virus type 6 and cytomegalovirus in AIDS-associated Kaposi's sarcoma. No evidence for an etiologic association. Hum Pathol 26: 914–19.

Kirova YM, Belembaogo E, Frikha et al. (1998). Radiotherapy in the management of epidemic Kaposi's sarcoma: a retrospective study of 643 cases. Radiother Oncol 46: 19–22.

Klimo P, Connors JM. (1985). MACOP-B chemotherapy for the treatment of diffuse large cell lymphoma. Ann Intern Med 102: 596–602.

Knowles DM. (1993). Biologic aspects of AIDS-associated non-Hodgkin's lymphoma. Curr Opin Oncol 5: 845–51.

Kobayashi M, Fitz L, Ryan M et al. (1989). Identification and purification of natural killer cell stimulatory factor (NKSF), a cytokine with multiple biologic effects on human lymphocytes. J Exp Med 170: 827–45.

Korn A, Autry M, DeRemer P et al. (1994). Sensitivity of the Papanicolaou smear in human immunodeficiency virus-infected women. Obstet Gynecol 83: 401–4.

Kovacs JA, Vogel S, Albert JM et al. (1996). Controlled trial of interleukin-2 infusions in patients infected with the human immunodeficiency virus. N Engl J Med 335: 1350–6.

Krown SE. (1996). Kaposi's sarcoma – what's human chorionic gonadotropin got to do with it? N Eng J Med 335: 1309–10.

Krown SE, Real FX, Cunningham-Rundles S et al. (1983). Preliminary observations on the effect of recombinant leukocyte A interferon in homosexual men with Kaposi's sarcoma. N Engl J Med 308: 1071–6.

Krown SE, Paredes J, Polsky B et al. (1995). Phase I/II trial of soluble recombinant human interleukin-1 receptor (rhu IL-1R) in patients with human immunodeficiency virus-1 (HIV-1) infection. Proc Am Soc Clin Oncol 14: 292.

Lang ME, Lottersberger C, Roth B et al. (1997). Induction of apoptosis in Kaposi's sarcoma spindle cell cultures by the subunits of human chorionic gonadatropin. AIDS 11: 1333–40.

Levine AM. (1992). Acquired immunodeficiency syndrome-related lymphoma. Blood 80: 8–20.

Levine AM, Pieters AS. (1998). Lymphoma and KS: the impact of HAART. Second National AIDS Malignancy Conference, Bethesda, MD, USA. Summaries, 3–4.

Levine AM, Wernz JC Kaplan L et al. (1991). Low dose chemotherapy with central nervous system prophylaxis and azidothymidine maintenance in AIDS-related lymphoma: a prospective multi-institutional trial. JAMA 266: 84.

Levine AM, Tulpule A, Tessman, D et al. (1997). Mitoguazone therapy in patients with refractory or relapsed AIDS-related lymphoma: Results from a multicenter phase II trial. J Clin Oncol 15: 1094–103.

Lieberman MD, Sigal RK, Williams II NN et al. (1991). Natural killer cell stimulatory factor (NKSF) augments natural killer cell and antibody-dependent tumoricidal response against colon cancer cell lines. J Surg Res 50: 410–15.

Lust JA, Banks PM, Hooper WC et al. (1989). T-cell non-Hodgkin lymphoma in human immunodeficiency virus-1 infected individuals. Am J Hematol 31: 181–7.

Maiman M, Fruchter RG, Serur E et al. (1990). Human immunodeficiency virus infection and cervical neoplasia. Gynecol Oncol 38: 377–82.

Maiman M, Tarricone N, Vieira J et al. (1991). Colposcopic evaluation of human immunodeficiency virus seropositive women. Obstet Gynecol 78: 84–8.

Maiman M, Fruchter RG, Guy L et al. (1993). Human immunodeficiency virus infection and invasive cervical carcinoma. *Cancer* **71**: 402–6.

Marchell N, Alster TS. (1997). Successful treatment of cutaneous Kaposi's sarcoma by the 585-nm pulsed dye laser. *Dermatol Surg* **23**: 973–5.

Mazza P, Bocchia M, Tumietto F et al. (1992). Recombinant interleukin-2 (rIL-2) in acquired immune deficiency syndrome (AIDS): Preliminary report in patients with lymphoma associated with HIV infection. *Eur J Haematol* **49**: 1–6.

McFarland EJ, Harding PA, Schooley RT et al. (1996). Interleukin-12 (IL-12) enhances HIV-specific cytotoxic T-lymphocyte (CYL) activity. *Third Conference on Retroviruses and Opportunistic Infections*, Washington, DC, USA, 95.

Medveczky MM, Horvath E, Lund T et al. (1997). In vitro antiviral drug sensitivity of the Kaposi's sarcoma-associated herpesvirus. *AIDS* **11**: 1327–32.

Melbye M, Cote TR, Kessler L et al. (1994a). High incidence of anal cancer among AIDS patients. *Lancet* **343**: 636–9.

Melbye M, Rabkin C, Frisch M et al. (1994b). Changing patterns of anal cancer incidence in the United States, 1940-89. *Am J Epidemiol* **139**: 772–80.

Miles SA. (1994). Pathogenesis of HIV-related Kaposi's sarcoma. *Curr Opin Oncol* **6**: 497–502.

Miles SA. (1996). Pathogenesis of AIDS-related Kaposi's sarcoma: evidence of a viral etiology. *Hematol Oncol Clin North Am* **10**: 1011–21.

Miles SA, Rezai AR, Salazar-Gonzalez FJ et al. (1990a). AIDS Kaposi sarcoma-derived cells produce and respond to interleukine 6. *Proc Natl Acad Sci* **87**: 4068–72.

Miles SA, Wang H, Cortes E et al. (1990b). Beta interferon therapy in patients with poor-prognosis Kaposi sarcoma related to the acquired immunodeficiency syndrome (AIDS). *Ann Intern Med* **112**: 582–9.

Miles SA, Wang H, Elashoff R et al. (1994). Improved survival for patients with AIDS-related Kaposi's sarcoma. *J Clin Oncol* **12**: 1910–16.

Mitsuyasu RT. (1987). Clinical variants and staging of Kaposi's sarcoma. *Semin Oncol* **14**: 13–18.

Mitsuyasu RT. (1988). Treatment of AIDS-associated Kaposi's sarcoma with interferons. *Biotherapy* **2**: 1–7.

Mitsuyasu RT, Miles SA. (1987). Biotherapy with interferon in AIDS-related Kaposi's sarcoma. *Oncol Nurs Forum* **14**: 27–31.

Mitsuyasu RA. (1998). Clinical care options for HIV. From *Second National AIDS Malignancy Conference*, Summaries, 22–7.

Moore PS, Chang Y. (1995). Detection of Herpesvirus-like DNA sequences in Kaposi's sarcoma in patients with and without HIV infection. *N Engl J Med* **332**: 1181–5.

Murphy M, Armstrong KA, Sepkowitz RN et al. (1997). Regression of AIDS-related Kaposi's sarcoma following treatment with an HIV-1 protease inhibitor. *AIDS* **11**: 261–2.

Nadler L, Botnik L, Finberg R et al. (1994). Anti-B1 monoclonal antibody and complement treatment in autologous bone marrow transplantation for relapsed B-cell non-Hodgkin's lymphoma. *Lancet* **2**: 427–31.

Nador RG, Cesarman E, Chadburn A et al. (1996). Primary effusion lymphoma: A distinct clinopathologic entity associated with the Kaposi's sarcoma-associated herpes virus. *Blood* **88**: 645–56.

Nagpal S, Cai J, Zheng T et al. (1997). Retinoid antagonism of NF-IL6: insight into the mechanism of antiproliferative effects of retinoids in Kaposi's sarcoma. *Mol Cell Biol* **17**: 4159–68.

Nakamura S, Murakami-Mori K, Rao N et al. (1997). Vascular endothelial growth factor is a potent angiogenic factor in AIDS-associated Kaposi's sarcoma-derived spindle cells. *J Immuol* **158**: 4992–5001.

Naume B, Gately M, Espevik T et al. (1992). A comparative study of IL-12 (cytotoxic lymphocyte maturation factor)-, IL-2-and IL-7-induced effects on immunomagnetically purified CD+ NK cells. *J Immunol* **148**: 2429–36.

Neipal F, Albrecht JC, Ensser A et al. (1997). Human herpesvirus 8 encodes a homolog of interleukin-6. *J Virol* **71**: 839–42.

Newman SB. (1988). *Treatment of epidemic Kaposi's sarcoma in patients with intralesional vinblastine injection (IL-VLB)*.New Orleans: American Society Clinical Oncology.

Nisce LZ, Safai B. (1985). Radiation therapy of Kaposi's sarcoma in AIDS. Memorial Soan Kettering experience. *Front Radiat Ther Oncol* **19**: 133–7.

Nobler MP, Leddy ME, Huh SH. (1987). The impact of palliative irradiation on the management of patients with acquired immune deficiency syndrome. *J Clin Oncol* **5**: 107–12.

Northfelt D, Volberding P, Kaplan L. (1992). Degree of immunodeficiency at diagnosis of AIDS-associated non-Hodgkin's lymphoma. *Proc Am Soc Clin Oncol* **11**: 45

Oksenhendler E, Dubrueil ML, Gerard V et al. (1994). Intensive chemotherapy and G-CSF in HIV-associated non-Hodgkin's lymphoma. *Tenth International Conference on AIDS*, Yokohama, USA.

Oksenhendler E, Duarte M, Soulier J et al. (1996). Multicentric Castleman's disease in HIV infection: a clinical and pathological study of 20 patients. *AIDS* **10**: 61–7.

O'Leary JJ, Kennedy MM, McGee J. (1997). Kaposi's sarcoma associated herpes virus (KSHV/HHV 8: epidemiology, molecular biology and tissue distribution. *Mol Pathol* **50**: 4–8.

Palefsky JM, Gonzales J, Greenblatt RM et al. (1990). Anal intraepithelial neoplasia and anal papillomavirus infection among homosexual males with group IV HIV disease. *JAMA* **263**: 2911–16.

Palefsky JM, Holly EA, Ralston ML et al. (1998). Prevalence and risk factors for human papillomavirus of the anal canal in human immunodeficiency virus (HIV)-positive and HIV-negative homosexual men. *J Infect Dis* **177**: 361–7.

Panyutich EA, Said JW, Miles SA. (1998). Infection of primary dermal microvascular endothelial cells by Kaposi's sarcoma-associated herpesvirus. *AIDS* **12**: 467–72.

Place RJ, Gregorcyk SG, Huber PJ, Simmang CL (2001). Outcome analysis of HIV-positive patients with anal squamous cell carcinoma. *Dis Colon Rectum* **44**: 506–12.

Pluda JM, Venzon DJ, Tosato G et al. (1993). Parameters affecting the development of non-Hodgkin's lymphoma in patients with severe human immunodeficiency virus infection receiving antiretroviral therapy. *J Clin Oncol* **11**: 1099–107.

Press OW, Appelbaum F, Ledbetter JA et al. (1997). Monoclonal antibody 1FA (anti-CD20) serotherapy of human B cell lymphomas. *Blood* **69**: 584–91.

Rabkin CS, Janz S, Lash A et al. (1997). Monoclonal origin of multicentric Kaposi's sarcoma lesions. *N Engl J Med* **336**: 988–93.

Reff ME, Carner K, Chambers KS et al. (1994). Depletion of B cells in vivo by a chimeric mouse-human monoclonal antibody to CD20. *Blood* **83**: 435–45.

Rettig M, Ma H, Vescio RA et al. (1997). Kaposi's sarcoma-associated herpes virus infection of bone marrow dendritic cells from multiple myeloma patients. *Science* **276**: 1851–5.

Ricaurte JC, Hoerman MF, Nord JA, Tietjen PA (2001). Lung cancer in HIV-infected patients: a one-year experience. *Int J STD AIDS* **12**: 100–2.

Said J. (1997). Kaposi's sarcoma-associated herpesvirus (KSHV): a new viral pathogen associated with Kaposi's sarcoma, primary effusion lymphoma, and multicentric Castleman's disease. *West J Med* **167**: 37–8.

Schultz TF, Boshoff CH, Weiss RA. (1996). HIV infection and neoplasia. *Lancet* **348**: 587–91.

Schwartsmann G, Sprinz E, Kromfield M et al. (1997). Clinical and pharmacokinetic study of oral etoposide in patients with AIDS-related Kaposi's sarcoma with no prior exposure to cytotoxic therapy. *J Clin Oncol* **15**: 2118–24.

Shah KV. (1997). Human papillomaviruses and anogenital cancers. *N Engl J Med* **337**: 1386–8.

Shepherd FA, Beaulieu R, Gelmon K et al. (1998). Prospective randomized trial of two dose levels of interferon alfa with zidovudine for the treatment of Kaposi's sarcoma associated with human immunodeficiency virus infection: a Canadian HIV clinical trials network study. *J Clin Oncol* **16**: 1736–42.

Shibata D, Weiss LM, Hernandez AM et al. (1993). Epstein–Barr virus-associated non-Hodgkin's lymphoma in patients infected with the human immunodeficiency virus. *Blood* **81**: 2102–9.

Shiramizu B, Herndier B, Meeker T et al. (1992). Molecular and immunophenotypic characterization of AIDS-associated, Epstein–Barr virus-negative, polyclonal lymphoma. *J Clin Oncol* **10**: 383–9.

Shuler JD, Holland GN, Miles Sa et al. (1989). Kaposi Sarcoma of the conjunctiva and eyelids associated with the acquired immunodeficiency syndrome. *Arch Opthalmol* **107**: 858–62.

Skarin AT, Canellos GP, Rosenthal DS et al. (1983). Improved prognosis of diffuse histiocytic and undifferenciated lymphoma by use of high dose methotrexate alternating with standard agents (M-BACOD), *J Clin Oncol* **1**: 91–8.

Sparano JA, Wiernik PH, Strack M et al. (1993). Infusional cyclophosphamide, doxorubicin and etoposide in human immunodeficiency virus-and human T-cell leukemia virus type 1-related non-Hodgkin's lymphoma: a highly active regimen. *Blood* **81**: 2810–15.

Speck CE, Levine AM, Carter N et al. (1998). Non-AIDS-defining malignancies among 5,574 HIV seropositive members of a large managed care-based cohort. *Second National AIDS Malignancy Conference*, Bethesda, MD, USA.

Straus DJ. (1997a). HIV-associated lymphomas. *Curr Opin Oncol* **9**: 450–4.

Straus DJ. (1997b). Human immunodeficiency virus-associated lymphomas. *Med Clin N Am* **81**: 495–511.

Straus DJ, Huang J, Testa M et al. (1995). Prognostic factors in the treatment of HIV-associated non-Hodgkin's lymphoma: analysis of ACTG 142 (low-dose vs standard-dose mBACOD + GM-CSF). *ASH*, Seattle WA, **2404**: 604.

Stewart S. Jablonowski H, Goebel FD et al. (1998). Randomized comparative trial of pegylated liposomal doxorubicin versus bleomycin and vincristine in the treatment of AIDS-related Kaposi's sarcoma. *J Clin Oncol* **16**: 683–91.

Sun X-W, Kuhn L, Ellerbrock TV et al. (1997). Human papillomavirus infection in women infected with the human immunodeficiency virus. *N Engl J Med* **337**: 1343–9.

Tappero JW, Berger TG, Kaplan LD et al. (1991). Cryotherapy for cutaneous Kaposi's sarcoma (KS) associated with acquired immune deficiency syndrome (AIDS): a phase II trial. *J Acquir Immune Defic Syndr Hum Retrovirol* **4**: 839–46.

Tedder TF, Bubien JK, Ahou LS, Bell PD et al. (1993). Transfection of the CD20 cell surface molecule into ectopic cell types generates a Ca^{2+} conductance found constitutively in B cells. *J Cell Biochem* **21**: 1121–32.

Tedder TF, Zhou LJ, Bell PD et al. (1990). The CD20 surface molecule of B lymphocytes functions as a calcium channel. *J Cell Biochem* **14**: 195.

Teppler H, Kaplan G, Smith K et al. (1993). Efficacy of the low doses of the polyethylene-glycol derivative of interleukin-2 in modulating the immune response of patients with immunodeficiency virus type-1 infection. *J Infect Dis* **167**: 291–8.

Tirelli U, Errante D, Spina M et al. (1996). Second-line chemotherapy in human immunodeficiency virus-related non-Hodgkin's lymphoma: evidence of activity of a combination of etoposide, mitoxantrone and prednimustine in relapsed patients. *Cancer* **77**: 2127–31.

Tulpule A, Joshi B, DeGuzman N et al. (1997). Interleukin-4 in the treatment of AIDS-related Kaposi's Sarcoma. *Ann Oncol* **8**: 79–83.

Tulpule A, Yung RC, Wernz J et al. (1998). Phase II trial of liposomal daunorubicin in the treatment of AIDS-related pulmonary Kaposi's sarcoma. *J Clin Oncol* **16**: 3369–74.

Vaccher E, Tirelli U, Spina M et al. (1996). Age and serum lactate dehydrogenase level are independent prognostic factors in human immunodeficiency virus-related nonHodgkin's lymphomas: a single-institute study of 96 patients. *J Clin Oncol* **14**: 2217–23.

Volberding PA, Mitsuyasu R. (1985). Recombinant interferon Alpha in the treatment of acquired immune deficiency syndrome-related Kaposi's sarcoma. *Semin Oncol* **12**: 2–6.

Webster G. (1995). Local therapy for mucocutaneous Kaposi's sarcoma in patients with acquired immunodeficiency syndrome. *Dermatol Surg* **21**: 205–8.

Weick J, Dahlberg S, Miller T. (1989). The treatment of non-Hodgkin's lymphoma with m-BACOD, ProMACE-CytaBOM and MACOP-B: The Southwest Oncology Group (SWOG) experience. *Proc Am Soc Clin Oncol* **8**: 254.

Welles L, Saville W, Lietzau J et al. (1998). Phase II trial with dose titration of paclitaxel for the therapy of human immunodeficiency virus-associated Kaposi's sarcoma. *J Clin Oncol* **16**: 1112–21.

Wheeland RG, Bailin PL, Norris MJ. (1985). Argon laser photocoagulative therapy of Kaposi's sarcoma: a clinical and histologic evaluation. *J Dermatol Surg Oncol* **11**: 1180–5.

Wood R, Montoya JG, Kundu SK et al. (1993). Safety and efficacy of polyethylene glycol-modified interleukin-2 and zidovudine in human immunodeficiency virus type 1 infection: a phase I/II study. *J Infect Dis* **167**: 519–25.

Wright TC, Sun XW. (1996). Anogenital papilloma virus infection and neoplasia in immunodeficient women. *Obstet Gyn Clin N Am* **23**: 861–93.

Wright TC, Ellerbrock TV, Chiasson MA et al. (1994). Cervical intraepithelial neoplasia in women infected with human immunodeficiency virus: prevalence, risk factors, and validity of Papanicolau smears. *Obstet Gynecol* **84**: 591–7.

Zhong W, Wang H, Herndier B et al. (1996). Restricted expression of Kaposi's sarcoma-associated herpesvirus (human herpesvirus 8) genes in Kaposi's sarcoma. *Proc Natl Acad Sci USA* **93**: 6641–6.

JULIE LOUISE GERBERDING AND ANNE MIJCH

Occupational HIV issues for health-care providers

Epidemiology of occupationally acquired HIV infection

The infection risk associated with occupational exposure to HIV has been measured in several prospective studies of health-care personnel tested for HIV antibody soon after exposure (baseline) and then retested for at least 6 months to detect seroconversion (Gerberding *et al.*, 1987; Beekmann *et al.*, 1990; Henderson *et al.*, 1990; Cavalcante *et al.*, 1991; Centers for Disease Control and Prevention [DCD], 1992; Tokars *et al.*, 1993; Gerberding, 1995). Pooled data indicate that the average transmission risk associated with needle punctures or similar percutaneous injuries involving HIV is about 0.3% (95% CI 0.2–0.5%) (Gerberding 1995, CDC, 1998). The risk from mucous membrane exposure is reported to be 0.09% (95% CI, 0.006–0.5%). (This estimate may be biased because it is based on a single infection that occurred before prospective data collection was initiated.) The magnitude of risk associated with non-skin contamination is too small for reliable estimation.

Although measuring the incidence of infection among populations of exposed health-care providers is useful in evaluating the average infection risk, it is more difficult to determine the risk associated with a specific HIV exposure event. In a retrospective case–control study of HIV sero-conversion among health–care workers exposed to HIV through percutaneous injuries, four factors were associated with increased infection risk (CDC, 1995; Cardo *et al.*, 1997). These included deep injuries (odds ratio [OR] = 15; 95% C.I. 6.0–41), visible blood on the device

before exposure (OR 6.2; 95% C.I. 2.2–21), device previously used in an artery or vein (OR 4.3; 95% C.I. 1.7–12), and terminal illness in the source patient (defined as death within 2 months of the exposure) (OR 5.6; 95% C.I. 2.0–16).

The titre of virus in the source material is likely to be an important factor predictive of the infection risk. The total amount of HIV in blood includes both cell-free virus (measured by standard viral load assays) and the cell-associated virus in circulating lymphocytes and monocytes. Patients with seroconversion illness or with advanced stages of HIV infection usually have HIV RNA titres in the plasma that are 100–10 000 times greater than those typically found in asymptomatic patients, and relatively large numbers of infected circulating lymphocytes and monocytes (Ho *et al.*, 1989; Daar *et al.*, 1991). The association of terminal HIV infection with transmission risk observed in the case–control study of occupational transmission risk factors (Cardo *et al.*, 1997) might be related to the high plasma viral load levels typically found in patients with advanced infection not responding to combination antiretroviral therapy. However, genotypical (e.g. multiple quasi-species) and phenotypical (e.g. syncytium induction) characteristics also typify patients with advanced disease. Little data are available to assess the importance of these factors in predicting transmissibility. For this reason, exposures to asymptomatic source patients with low viral loads should not be assumed to be low risk. In fact, transmission of HIV from a source with undetectable viral load has been observed in one health care worker and in two instances of maternal–foetal transmission (Sperling *et al.*, 1996; Cao *et al.*, 1997; CDC, 1998).

Post-exposure decontamination procedures (e.g. cleaning the puncture site with antiseptics) could reduce the effective inoculum and therefore the risk of subsequent infection. However, data are still lacking on the value of any physical or chemical intervention at the exposure site. In at least one case, transmission occurred despite prompt application of 100% bleach to the entry wound (Henderson et al., 1990).

The vast majority (99.7%) of percutaneous HIV exposures do not transmit HIV infection. Data from a small series of patients exposed to HIV but with no evidence of infection indicate that cellular immune responses develop in some subjects, including health-care workers, who sustain low inoculum exposures to HIV (Clerici et al., 1992, 1994; Pinto et al., 1997). These patients do not develop serum HIV antibodies and have no other evidence of infection. The relevance of this finding to occupational transmission has not yet been evaluated in controlled clinical studies.

Descriptive epidemiology of occupational HIV

The true number of health-care workers infected with HIV as the result of occupational exposure is unknown because detection and reporting are incomplete. The most rigorous criteria for occupational infection requires documentation of HIV antibody seroconversion temporally associated with a discrete exposure to HIV. In some cases, genetic sequence analysis has been used to demonstrate the similarity of virus strains obtained from the source patient and the infected recipient, but this technique is not widely available. Concerns about continued employment and loss of confidentiality may discourage those with documented occupational infection to report their experience to health authorities. Health-care providers who do not recognize or report their exposure will not be detected.

As of December 1997, the Centers for Disease Control and Prevention (CDC) received reports of 59 US health-care workers with documented HIV seroconverison temporally associated with an occupational HIV exposure (CDC, 1998). Another 132 HIV infections among health-care workers are considered possible occupational transmission. These workers recalled one or more occupational exposure to HIV and had no other exposure risks, but did not have a baseline test to demonstrate the temporal association of exposure with infection. Percutaneous injuries by needles or other sharp instruments caused transmission in 52 of these cases, while infection occurred through mucous membranes or non-intact skin in five individuals. One person was exposed via percutaneous and mucosal routes, and in one the exposure route was not established. Transmission as the result of HIV contamination of intact skin, inhalation of blood aerosols, or close patient contact has not been reported.

The majority of occupationally infected health-care providers in the USA are nurses and laboratory personnel. The high frequency of exposure to blood from patients with HIV infection probably accounts for this distribution. Although surgeons, dentists, emergency personnel and labour and delivery staff are at high risk for blood exposure, the number of HIV-infected patients they encounter is relatively low in most institutions. The cumulative risk associated with health-care occupations is not yet known. To date, there is no evidence that the risk is higher than that experienced by the general population. No HIV infections attributable to occupational exposure were detected in a study of 3407 orthopaedic surgeons practicing in the US (Tokars et al., 1992). Among USA Army personnel categorized as health-care providers, an excess risk for HIV infection was detected only among never-married white male nurses, a risk possibly attributable to non-occupational behaviours (Cowan et al., 1990; Cowan et al., 1991).

Preventing occupational HIV infection
Preventing occupational exposure to HIV

Preventing percutaneous injuries is the highest priority for protecting health-care workers because such exposures account for the majority of occupational infections. Universal precautions are designed to prevent exposure to blood and other body fluids that may confer a risk of HIV and hepatitis B or C virus transmission (CDC, 1987, 1988). Implementation of this system of infection control has been associated with a 40–60% reduction in the frequency of cutaneous blood contacts, but less impact on needle puncture rates has been documented (Krasinski et al., 1987; Fahey et al., 1991; Linnemann et al., 1991; Wong et al., 1991; Kirstensen et al., 1992; Saghafi et al., 1992).

The failure of universal precautions to prevent percutaneous injuries has stimulated interest in improving the safety of sharp medical devices. Examples include syringes with sheaths that can be passed over the needle after use, devices with retracting needles, and needleless infusion systems. These new products have been implemented in many institutions, but their efficacy has not been completely evaluated. However, in one multicentered study, introduction of needle safety devices for phlebotomy was associated with a significant reduction in the number of percutaneous injuries among health-care personnel (CDC, 1997). Safer devices are usually more expensive than the traditional devices they are designed to replace, and training is needed to ensure that they are properly used. These new devices represent an important advance in needle-stick prevention efforts and some are likely to become standard in many health-care settings.

Many needle punctures occur while the needle is being used for its intended purpose. For example, the majority of suture needles injuries are associated with manual palpation of the needle tip or manual retraction of tissue at the site of suturing (Wright *et al.*, 1991; Tokars *et al.*, 1992). These injuries are more difficult to prevent with engineered controls, although substituting blunt suture needles for sharp needles has been successful in certain types of surgical procedures, such as abdominal fascial closures and gynaecological surgery (Montz, 1991). 'No touch' surgical techniques, where instruments instead of fingers are used to manipulate tissue and suture needles, are also advocated to prevent intraoperative exposures (Gerberding, 1993).

Post-exposure prophylaxis for exposed health-care workers

Experimental studies. Understanding the pathogenesis of initial HIV infection following exposure is a critical prerequisite to identifying potential targets for prophylactic interventions. Although the biology of transcutaneous and transmucosal infection has not been completely elucidated, a growing body of evidence suggests that Langerhans cells or dermal dendritic cells could play an important role during the first stages of HIV infection (Blauvelt, 1997). These cells are derived from the bone marrow and express CD4 and chemokine receptors on their surface. They are found in the epidermis and mucosal tissues of the vagina, cervix, and oral cavity. They interact with T-lymphocytes, particularly in lymphoid tissues, to provide immune surveillance against invading microorganisms and tumor cells. Dendritic cells present antigen to T-lymphocytes either locally or after migration to regional lymph nodes. When the vaginal mucosa of rhesus macaques is inoculated with simian immunodeficiency virus (SIV), SIV is associated with mucosal dendritic cells for the first 24 h, but no evidence of local virus replication can be detected (Spira

et al., 1996). After 48 h, active SIV replication is evident in association with T-lymphocytes in the germinal centres of the regional lymph nodes. By 5 days after inoculation, SIV can be detected in the peripheral blood of these animals. The relevance of this animal model to HIV infection has not been proven, but it does suggest that a 'window of opportunity' for effective prophylaxis may exist.

Early studies in primate models of retrovirus infection, which typically employed high viral inocula compared to the levels involved in most occupational exposures, administered via the intravenous route, failed to demonstrate the efficacy of post-exposure treatments with zidovudine (ZDV) (McClure *et al.*, 1990; Fazely *et al.*, 1991; Gerberding *et al.*, 1991; Lundgren *et al.*, 1991). However, more recent animal studies, in which low viral inocula were used, have shown that nucleoside analogues and other agents can prevent some infections (Van Rompay *et al.*, 1992; Black, 1997). Three factors affected the efficacy of prophylactic treatment in these models: inoculum size, time until treatment was started, and treatment duration. Animals exposed to relatively low titres of virus who are treated with one or more antiviral agent within 24 h of the exposure for several days were most likely to be protected. Current treatment standards for post-exposure therapy among health-care workers are based on similar characteristics: a presumed low inoculum exposure, institution of two or more drugs within hours (not days) of the exposure, and treatment for 4 weeks.

Zidovudine efficacy and toxicity in health-care providers. In 1988, Burroughs Wellcome began a double-blinded, placebo-controlled, randomized trial to evaluate the efficacy and toxicity of post-exposure ZDV prophylaxis. The trial was discontinued a year later because too few subjects agreed to participate (LaFon *et al.*, 1988, 1990). No subsequent randomized trials have been attempted, because of the difficulties imposed by the need for a large sample size to demonstrate efficacy and the accruing data to show that post-exposure prophylaxis is effective.

In 1988, investigators at the National Institutes of Health Clinical Centers and San Francisco General Hospital independently developed protocols for administering ZDV to exposed employees and evaluating its safety (Gerberding and Henderson, 1992; Beekmann *et al.*, 1997). With the support of Burroughs Wellcome (Research Triangle Park, NC), these protocols were merged in 1991 and were used to form the basis for a multicentre open-label study of ZDV toxicity among health-care providers. This consortium of 19 participating medical centres enrolled more than 170 subjects and demonstrated the feasibility of initiating treatment within 4 h of exposure (Beekmann et al., 1997). No haematological or other objective toxicity requiring treatment modification were observed in study subjects. However, drug-related symptoms (including nausea, fatigue, insomnia, and headache) required dose reduction or treatment discontinuation in approximately one-third of recipients. This experience is similar to the frequency of premature treatment discontinuation related to adverse symptoms reported by others (Puro et al., 1992; Tokars et al., 1993).

Because it was not feasible to conduct a randomized, prospective, placebo-controlled clinical trial for the evaluation of antiviral prophylaxis to prevent HIV infection, other study designs were needed. In the CDC's retrospective case–control study, treatment with ZDV after percutaneous exposure was associated with an 81% (OR 0.19; 95% CI 0.6–0.53) reduction in the odds of occupational HIV infection (Cardo et al., 1997). This finding prompted the US Public Health Service (USPHS) to revise its position on post-exposure prophylaxis and to disseminate new guidelines, which recommend treatment after high-risk exposures to HIV (CDC, 1998a).

Post-exposure treatment is not 100% efficacious; at least 13 failures among occupationally exposed people from several countries have been detected (Jochimsen, 1997). Drug-resistant strains of virus could have contributed to failure in some, but in at least one instance, transmission of HIV lacking mutations associated with ZDV resistance occurred (Jochimsen, 1997).

Antiretroviral post-exposure prophylaxis: new recommendations. Post-exposure antiretroviral treatment is an option that should be offered to health-care providers suffering occupational accidents that expose them to a risk of HIV infection. Exposed health-care workers should be fully informed of the potential benefits and risks associated with therapy, and told that the vast majority of HIV exposures do not cause infection even without treatment, that only ZDV has been shown to prevent HIV infection in humans, and that there are no data that prove that other drugs or drug combinations are more effective than ZDV alone.

Several approaches to assessing the transmission risk from individual exposures have been developed to help guide treatment decisions, but none have been validated (Ger-

berding, 1996; CDC, 1998a). Factors weighing in favour of antiretroviral prophylaxis include parenteral exposures, in which either the viral titre in the source material is likely to be high or the exposure characteristics are suggestive of a relatively large volume of blood transfer (deep punctures, visibly bloody device, obvious blood injection). Thus, prophylaxis is appropriate for most needle-stick injuries. There are also many cases when the exposure risk is so low that treatment should not be provided. These cases include most instances of contamination of intact skin with infected material and mucocutaneous exposures to non-bloody body fluids such as stool, urine, and sweat. The risk of treatment might also outweigh the benefits for many very low-risk exposures, such as mucocutaneous and non-intact skin exposures involving a few drops of infectious material for brief periods before decontamination.

Choosing the best post-exposure prophylaxis regimen is now complicated by emerging antiviral drug resistance among infected patients on complex treatment regimens. Although a study completed well before 1997 showed that treatment with ZDV alone was associated with an 81% reduction in infection risk (Cardo et al., 1997), the prevalence of ZDV resistance is increasing in most communities. For this reason, ZDV monotherapy is no longer recommended for the prophylaxis of exposed health-care workers. Instead, a minimum of two drugs, usually ZDV and lamivudine (3TC) ('basic regimen'), are recommended by the USPHS when treatment is elected (Gerberding, 1996; CDC, 1998a). A third drug, usually indinavir or nelfinavir, is added ('expanded regimen') when drug resistance is suspected, or in cases where the exposure is of especially high risk (Table 34.1).

In settings such as San Francisco General Hospital, where the prevalence of HIV infection among adult medical patients usually exceeds 20% and drug resistance is of great concern, more complex algorithms for selecting the prophylactic drug regimen are used (Gerberding, 1996). Antiretroviral treatment is offered to all personnel who sustain parenteral HIV exposures, but treatment advice is modified according to the severity of the exposure. Even though the distinction between exposure categories is often subjective, this approach has proved to be of practical value in treating clinicians. To facilitate timely implementation, exposures are reported to a 'Needle-stick Hotline', staffed by clinicians with expertise in exposure management. The clinician can initiate treatment by calling to instruct the hospital pharmacist to provide the first few doses of drug as soon as possible. The health-care provider is then seen in the

Table 34.1 The estimated probability of HIV transmission by type of HIV exposure

Exposure type	Estimated risk of HIV transmission per exposure		Reference
Receptive anal intercourse	0.008–0.032	1:125–1:31	DeGruttola *et al.*, 1989
Receptive vaginal intercourse	0.0005–0.0015	1:2000–1:667	Wiley *et al.*, 1985
	0.0003–0.0009	1:3333–1:1111	Peterman *et al.*, 1989
Puncture of HCW by contaminated needle	0.0032	1:313	Henderson *et al.*, 1990
Use of contaminated injecting drug equipment	0.0067	1:149	Kaplan and Heimer, 1992

employee health clinic the next business day, where exposure risks and the pros and cons of treatment can be reviewed in detail. Allowing the exposed health-care worker to discontinue treatment at any time eliminates the pressure to commit to an experimental therapy when he or she is preoccupied with the exposure crisis. Those who elect to continue therapy are seen every 2 weeks for the duration of treatment. A targeted history to identify symptoms of drug intolerance and a complete blood count and other blood chemistries are checked at each visit.

Follow-up for occupational exposures. Testing for HIV antibody at the time of exposure and periodically for at least 6 months (e.g. 1, 2, 3 and 6 months) is recommended to detect infection. Seroconversion is usually evident within the first 6 weeks–3 months following exposure, but delayed seroconversion (after 6 months) may occur rarely (Busch and Satten, 1997; Ciesielski and Metler, 1997). The majority of occupationally infected health-care providers will develop the acute retroviral syndrome (Jochimsen, 1997). If the HIV ELISA antibody test (ELISA plus Western blot) is negative or indeterminate in a health care worker who presents with clinical evidence of HIV infection, then a quantitative HIV viral load test should be performed to detect primary infection. The quantitative HIV viral load tests are not licensed for diagnosis of HIV infection, and false-positive results may occur, especially with the ultra-sensitive assays. There is currently no role for the routine use of virus cultures or plasma viral load tests in the follow-up of most occupational exposures, unless symptoms of acute infection appear.

Worrisome anecdotal reports suggest that when the source patient is infected with both HIV and hepatitis C virus (HCV), and the health-care worker acquires early HCV infection, HIV seroconversion may be delayed for more than 6 months and the clinical course of HCV infection may be rapid and severe (CDC, 1998a). Hepatitis C

virus appears to be more transmissible through needle punctures than HIV, and many health-care workers are at risk for both these viruses (Gerberding, 1995). Occupational exposure follow-up should always include assessment of the HCV status of the source patient, and serological follow-up for 6–9 months among those exposed to detect HCV seroconversion. If a health-care worker exposed to both viruses does acquire HCV, then HIV testing should probably continue 12–18 months post-exposure, to detect late HIV seroconversion.

Access to supportive counselling is an important component of post-exposure care. Even though the statistical risk of infection is low, most exposed health-care providers experience considerable stress during the post-exposure follow-up period, and some require crisis intervention in the first few weeks.

Post-exposure prophylaxis (PEP) in individuals with exposure to HIV via sexual intercourse or injecting drug use (IDU)

Background
Prevention of HIV transmission is of major public health importance worldwide. Education and prevention programmes based on behaviour modification have been implemented in many countries and remain the foundation of risk reduction. These programmes have been variably successful. In Australia, substantial reductions in newly diagnosed HIV infections have been documented, both in homosexual men and in injecting drug users (IDUs). The continuing adherence to safe sex and safe injecting drug-use practices in Australia has maintained a low prevalence (estimated to be less than 0.6–3% among heterosexual IDUs) and a low incidence of HIV infection in the population.

Nevertheless, despite adoption of safer behaviours, inadvertent exposure to HIV does occur in a number of circumstances. These include sexual contact (broken condoms, sexual assault victim) or via injecting drug use, as well as in the health-care setting (needle-stick injury). The latter is discussed earlier in this chapter.

Estimated average risks of transmission per exposure by differing exposure type are shown in Table 34.1. Factors such as amount of blood involved (Seidlin et al., 1993), associated trauma, concurrent sexually transmitted diseases (Wasserheit, 1992) or ulcerative genital disease (Kreiss and Hopkins, 1993), the level of HIV plasma RNA (viral load) in the infected individual (Lee et al., 1996) and chemokine receptor status of the recipient (Liu et al., 1996) are all likely to influence the individual risk of HIV transmission following exposure.

Post-exposure prophylaxis using ZDV has been reported as being effective for health-care workers with occupational exposure to HIV, reducing transmission by 79% (60–90%) (CDC, 1995; Cardo et al., 1997), and post-exposure prophylaxis with antiretroviral drugs is now the standard of practice for health-care workers parenterally exposed to HIV (CDC, 1997). Maternal–foetal transmission of HIV is reduced by 69% through prenatal maternal ZDV therapy combined with 6 weeks of therapy in the infant (Cao et al., 1997) and antiretroviral therapy has also become standard practice in this setting (CDC, 1996).

The long-term safety of the antiretroviral drugs used for post-exposure prophylaxis is not known among HIV-uninfected individuals. Even with short-term treatment, triple antiretroviral regimens are not well tolerated and induce significant objective toxicity. Among health-care workers receiving post-exposure prophylaxis with ZDV, one-third discontinued therapy because of intolerance (Tokars et al., 1992). In pregnant women there is a special risk because of potential teratogenicity.

There are no data available to indicate that post-exposure prophylaxis is effective in any situation other than in HIV-exposed health-care workers and newborns, although it seems reasonable to postulate that it may be so. There are no current prospective randomized, placebo-controlled studies of this issue and it is not likely that such a trial could be performed in individuals with exposure to HIV via sexual intercourse or injecting drug use. In the absence of controlled data, it seems reasonable to offer post-exposure prophylaxis in these settings, provided both the practitioner and the patient are aware of the potential risks and that data are accumulated to give some measure of the efficacy and toxicity of such interventions.

Recommendations

Individuals with a sexual or needle exposure to HIV should be assessed as soon as practicable (preferably within 72 h). Following assessment, all individuals with high-risk exposures should be offered post-exposure prophylaxis. The highest risk is sexual exposure to an HIV-infected individual via insertive intercourse (without condom) or IDU exposure via injecting equipment, where percutaneous exposure has occurred with a used, hollow needle.

The post-exposure prophylaxis regimen should be one of those recommended by the CDC following parenteral blood exposure of health-care workers to HIV, with some modifications (CDC 1998a,b).

Follow-up HIV antibody testing should be performed at 3–6 weeks, 3 months, and 6 months. Follow-up appropriate to other exposures to hepatitis B and C viruses (other sexually transmitted diseases and tetanus) should be undertaken as indicated. Assessment of physical and emotional responses, as well as monitoring for toxicity, should be performed as needed during this treatment phase. In the event of HIV transmission, consideration should be given to ongoing antiretroviral therapy, as recommended in primary HIV infection treatment protocols (see Chapter 1).

Costs

Recent studies have shown that strategies of post-exposure prophylaxis for health-care workers and ZDV therapy for pregnant women are cost-effective (Pinkerton et al., 1997). In the absence of data proving the efficacy of post-exposure prophylaxis following inadvertent exposure through sexual intercourse or injecting drug use, assessment of such benefits can not easily be made. The cost of 4 weeks of triple therapy is approximately US$500. Thus, on the conservative assumption that the lifetime cost of a single case of HIV infection is about US$100 000, one would only have to prevent one case of HIV infection for every 200 individuals treated for post-exposure prophylaxis to be cost-neutral. Although some exposed individuals may be able to afford such therapy, mechanisms to provide such treatment for those unable to do so should be established.

Conclusions

Public health strategies of universal safe sexual practices and safe needle use behaviour among injecting drug users remain the major strategies for reducing HIV transmission. Individuals at ongoing HIV exposure risk should be counselled to change behaviour. Post-exposure prophylaxis should be used cautiously in settings of known exposure and data should be collected prospectively in order to provide evidence to guide future therapeutic strategies. Post-exposure prophylaxis should be provided by practitioners experienced in the management of HIV-infected individuals and should be available in a timely manner (preferably within 2–4 h of exposure). It may be appropriate to designate specific sites (e.g. emergency departments) that provide this service.

References

Beekmann SE, Fahey BJ, Gerberding JL et al. (1990). Risky business: using necessarily imprecise casualty counts to estimate occupational risks for HIV infection. Infect Control Hosp Epidemiol 11: 371–9.

Beekmann SE, Fahrner R, Henderson DK et al. (1997). Zidovudine safety and tolerance among uninfected health care workers: a brief update. Am J Med 102: 63–4.

Black RJ. (1997). Animal studies of prophylaxis. Am J Med 102: 39–44.

Blauvelt A. (1997). The roles of skin dendritic cells in the initiation of human immunodeficiency virus infection. Am J Med 102: 16–20.

Busch MP, Satten GA. (1997). Time course of viremia and antibody seroconversion following human immunodeficiency virus exposure. Am J Med 102: 117–24.

Cao Y, Krogstad P, Korber BT et al. (1997). Maternal HIV-1 viral load, zidovudine treatment, and the risk of transmission of human immunodeficiency virus type 1 from mother to infant. N Engl J Med 3: 549–52.

Cardo DM, Culver DH, Ciesielski CA et al. (1997). A case–control study of HIV seroconversion in health care workers after perccutaneous exposures. N Engl J Med 337: 1485–90.

Cavalcante NJ, Abreu ES, Fernandes ME et al. (1991). Risk of health care professionals acquiring HIV infection in Latin America. AIDS Care 3: 311–16.

Centres for Disease Control and Prevention (CDC). (1987). Recommendations for prevention of HIV transmission in health-care settings. MMWR 36: 2S.

CDC. (1988). Update: universal precautions for prevention of transmission of human immunodeficiency virus, hepatitis B virus, and other blood borne pathogens in health-care settings. MMWR 37: 377–91.

CDC. (1992). Surveillance for occupationally acquired HIV infection – United States, 1981–1992. MMWR 41: 823–5.

CDC. (1994). Recommendations for the use of zidovudine to reduce perinatal transmission of human immunodeficiency virus. MMWR 43: 1–20.

CDC. (1995): Case-control study of HIV seroconversion in health care workers after percutaneous exposure to HIV-infected blood – France, United Kingdom, United States, January 1988–August 1994. MMWR 44: 929.

CDC. (1996). Update: provisional Public Health Service recommendations for chemoprophylaxis after occupational exposure to HIV. MMWR 45: 468–72.

CDC. (1997). Evaluation of safety devices for preventing percutaneous injuries during phlebotomy procedures. MMWR 46: 21–5.

CDC. (1998a). Public Health Service Guidelines for the management of health-care worker exposures to HIV and recommendations for post-exposure prophylaxis. MMWR 47: 1–33.

CDC. (1998b). Management of possible sexual, injecting-drug-use, or other non-occupational exposure to HIV including considerations related to antiretroviral therapy. MMWR 47: No. RR–17.

Ciesielski CA, Metler RP. (1997). Duration of time between exposure and seroconversion in health care workers with occupationally acquired infection with human immunodeficiency virus. Am J Med 102: 115–16.

Clerici M, Berzofsky JA, Shearer GM et al. (1992). Exposure to HIV-1 indicated by HIV-specific T helper cell responses before detection of infection by polymerase chain reaction and serum antibodies. J Infect Dis 165: 1012–19.

Clerici M, Levin J, Kessler HA et al. (1994). HIV-specific T-helper activity in seronegative health care workers exposed to contaminated blood. J Am Med Soc 271: 42–6.

Cowan DN, Pomerantz RS, Wann ZF et al. (1990). Human immunodeficiency virus infection among members of the reserve components of the US Army: prevalence, incidence, and demographic characteristics. The Walter Reed Retrovirus Research Group. J Infect Dis 162: 827–36.

Cowan DN, Brundage JF, Pomerantz RS et al. (1991). HIV infection among members of the US Army Reserve Components with medical and health occupations. J Am Med Assoc 265: 2826–30.

Daar ES, Moudgil T, Meyer RD et al. (1991). Transient high levels of viremia in patients with primary human immunodeficiency virus type 1 infection. N Engl J Med 25: 733–5.

DeGruttola V, Seage GR, Mayer KH et al. (1989). Infectiousness of HIV between male homosexual partners. J Clin Epidemiol 42: 849–56.

Fahey BJ, Koziol DE, Banks SM et al. (1991). Frequency of nonparenteral occupational exposures to blood and body fluids before and after universal precautions training. Am J Med 90: 145–53.

Fazely F, Haseltine WA, Rodger RF et al. (1991). Post-exposure chemoprophylaxis with ZDV or ZDV combined with interferon-alfa: failure after inoculating rhesus monkeys with high dose of SIV. J Acquir Immune Defic Syndr Hum Retrovirol 4: 1093–7.

Gerberding JL. (1993). Is antiretroviral treatment after percutaneous HIV exposure justified? Ann Intern Med 118: 979–80.

Gerberding JL. (1995). Management of occupational exposures to bloodborne viruses. N Engl J Med 332: 444–51.

Gerberding JL. (1996). Prophylaxis for occupational exposures to HIV. Ann Intern Med 125: 497–501.

Gerberding JL, Henderson DK. (1992). Management of occupational exposures to bloodborne pathogens: hepatitis B virus, hepatitis C virus, and human immunodeficiency virus. Clin Infect Dis 14: 1179–85.

Gerberding JL, Bryant-LeBlanc CE, Nelson KN et al. (1987). Risk of human immunodeficiency virus, cytomegalovirus, and hepatitis B virus transmission to health care workers with exposure to patients with AIDS and AIDS-related conditions (ARC). J Infect Dis 156: 1–8.

Gerberding JL, Marx P, Gould R et al. (1991). Simian model of retrovirus chemoprophylaxis with constant infusion zidovudine with or without interferon-alpha. Program and abstracts of the Thirty-first Interscience Congress on Antimicrobial Agents and Chemotherapy, Washington DC. Am Soc Microbiol.

Henderson DK, Fahey BJ, Willy M et al. (1990). Risk for occupational transmission of human immunodeficiency virus type-1 (HIV-1) associated with clinical exposures. A prospective evaluation. Ann Intern Med 113: 740–6.

Ho DD, Moudgil T, Alam M. (1989). Quantitation of human immunodeficiency virus type 1 in the blood of infected persons. *N Engl J Med* **321**: 1622–5.

Jochimsen EM. (1997). Failures of zidovudine post exposure prophylaxis. *Am J Med* **102**: 52–5.

Kaplan EH, Heimer R. (1992) A model-based estimate of HIV infectivity via needle sharing. *J Acquir Immune Defic Syndr Hum Retrovirol* **5**: 1116–18.

Katz MH, Gerberding JL. (1997). Postexposure treatment of people exposed to the human immunodeficiency virus through sexual contact or injection-drug use. [Comment in *N Engl J Med* **337**: 499–500.] *N Engl J Med* **336**: 1097–100.

Katz MH, Gerberding JL. (1998). The care of persons with recent sexual exposure to HIV. [*Comment in: Ann Intern Med* **129**: 671–2.] *Ann Intern Med* **128**: 306–12.

Krasinski K, LaCouture R, Holzman RS. (1987). Effect of changing needle disposal systems on needle puncture injuries. *Infect Control* **8**: 59–62.

Kreiss J, Hopkins SG. (1993). The association between circumcision status and human immunodeficiency virus infection among homosexual men. *J Infect Dis* **168**: 1404–8.

Kristensen MS, Wernberg NM, Anker-Moller E. (1992). Health care workers' ris of contact with body fluids in a hospital: effect of complying with universal precautions policy. *Infect Control Hosp Epidemiol* **13**: 719–24.

LaFon SW, Lehrman SN, Barry DW. (1988). Prophylactically administered Retrovir in health care workers potentially exposed to the human immunodeficiency virus. *J Infect Dis* **158**: 503.

LaFon SW, Mooney BD, McMullen JP et al. (1990). A double-blind, placebo-controlled study of the safety and efficacy of Retrovir (zidovudine, ZDV) as a chemoprophylactic agent in health care workers. In: *Program and abstracts of the Thirtieth Interscience Conference on Antimicrobial Agents and Chemotherapy*, Washington, DC, American Society for Microbiology.

Linnemann CC, Cannon C, DeRonde M et al. (1991). Effect of educational programs, rigid sharps containers, and universal precautions on reported needlestick injuries in healthcare workers. *Infect Control Hospital Epidemiol* **12**: 214–19.

Lee TH, Sakahara N, Fiebig E et al. (1996). Correlation of HIV-1 RNA levels in plasma and heterosexual transmission of HIV-1 from infected transfusion recipients. *J Acquir Immune Defic Syndr Hum Retrovirol* **12**: 427–8.

Liu R, Paxton WA, Choe S et al. (1996). Homozygous defect in HIV-1 coreceptor accounts for resistance of some multiply-exposed individuals to HIV-1 infection. *Cell* **86**: 367–77.

Lundgren B, Bottinger D, Ljungdahl-Stahle E et al. (1991). Antiviral effects of 3′-fluorothymidine and 3′-azidothymidine in cynomologous monkeys infected with simian immunodeficiency virus. *J Acquir Immune Defic Syndr Hum Retrovirol* **4**: 489–98.

McClure HM, Anderson DC, Ansari AA et al. (1990). Non-human primate models for evaluation of AIDS therapy. *Ann NY Acad Sci* **616**: 287–98.

Montz FJ, Fowler JM, Farias-Eisner R et al. (1991). Blunt needles in fascial closure. *Surg Gynecol Obstetr* **173**: 147–8.

Peterman TA, Stoneburner RL, Allen JR et al. (1989). Risk of human immunodeficiency virus transmission from heterosexual adults with transfusion-associated infections. *JAMA* **259**: 55–8.

Pinkerton SD, Holtgrave DR, Pinkerton HJ. (1997). Cost-effectiveness of chemoprophylaxis after occupational exposure to HIV. *Arch Intern Med* **157**: 1972–80.

Pinto LA, Landay AL, Berzofsky JA et al. (1997). Immune response to human immunodeficiency virus (HIV) in health care workers occupationally exposed to HIV-contaminated blood. *Am J Med* **102**: 21–4.

Puro V, Ippolito G, Guzzanti E et al. (1992). Zidovudine prophylaxis after accidental exposure to HIV: the Italian experience. The Italian Study Group on Occupational Risk of HIV Infection. *AIDS* **6**: 963–9.

Saghafi L, Raselli P, Francillon C et al. (1992). Exposure to blood during various procedures: results of two surveys before and after the implementation of universal precautions. *Am J Infect Control* **20**: 53–7.

Seidlin M, Vogler M, Lee E et al. (1993). Heterosexual transmission of HIV in a cohort of couples in New York City. *AIDS* **7**: 1247–54.

Spira AI, Marz PA, Patterson BK et al. (1996). Cellular targets of infection and route of vital dissemination after an intravaginal inoculation of simian immunodeficiency virus into rhesus macaques. *J Exp Med* **183**: 215–25.

Sperling RS, Shapiro DE, Coombs RW et al. (1996). Maternal viral load, zidovudine treatment, and the risk of transmission of human immunodeficiency virus type 1 from mother to infant. *N Engl J Med* **335**: 1621–9.

Tokars JI, Chamberland ME, Schable C et al. (1992). A survey of occupational blood contact and HIV infection among orthopedic surgeons. *J Am Med Assoc* **268**: 489–94.

Tokars JI, Marcus R, Culver DH et al. (1993). Surveillance of human immunodeficiency virus (HIV) infection and zidovudine use among health care workers with occupational exposure to HIV-infected blood. *Ann Intern Med* **118**: 913–19.

Van Rompay KKA, Marthas ML, Ramos RA et al. (1992). Simian immunodeficiency virus (SIV) infection of infant rhesus macaques as a model to test antiretroviral drug prophylaxis and therapy: oral 3′-azido-3′-deoxythymidine prevents SIV infection. *Antimicrob Agents Chemother* **36**: 2381–6.

Wasserheit JN. (1992). Epidemiological synergy: interrelationships between human immunodeficiency virus infection and other sexually transmitted diseases. *Sex Transm Dis* **19**: 61–77.

Wiley JA, Herschkorn SJ, Padian NS. (1989). Heterogeneity in the probability of HIV transmission per sexual contact: the case of male-to-female transmission in penile-vaginal intercourse. *Stat Med* **8**: 93–102.

Wong ES, Stotka JL, Chincilli VM et al. (1991). Are universal precautions effective in reducing the number of occupational exposures among health care workers? *J Am Med Assoc* **265**: 1123–8.

Wright JG, McGeer AJ, Chyatte D et al. (1991). Mechanisms of glove tears and sharp injuries among surgical personnel. *J Am Med Assoc* **266**: 1668–71.

HIV infection and injecting drug use

35

ALEX WODAK AND JENNIFER HOY

Injecting drug use as a growing problem globally, especially in developing countries

HIV has spread with astonishing speed in many injecting drug user populations around the world. Within a few years, large numbers of injecting drug users (IDUs) have presented to health-care workers seeking assistance for complications of HIV infection. Mortality rates among HIV-infected IDUs are higher than in uninfected users even before the onset of AIDS, and they increase even further following the onset of AIDS. As IDUs are generally still quite fertile, large numbers of HIV-infected children are an important consequence of poorly controlled HIV epidemics in this population. HIV has spread rapidly from IDUs to the general population heterosexually in most countries, where the infection has become established among IDUs. The health, social and economic cost of an uncontrolled epidemic of HIV among IDUs is possibly greater than for any other risk group.

Worldwide use of illicit drugs expanded rapidly over the last quarter of the twentieth century (UN Commission on Narcotic Drugs, 1995). The consequences of illicit drug use have become an important public health concern in many countries. Drug overdose deaths and bloodborne viral infections associated with sharing of injection equipment are at present the major causes of mortality and morbidity among IDUs. HIV-infected drug users have been reported in an increasing number of countries (Stimson et al., 1996) and the variety of illicit drugs available continues to expand. It is estimated that there are now over 8 million drug injectors in more than 120 countries around the world. Global production of heroin alone is estimated to be approximately 400 tons/year. This figure is believed to have doubled and global cocaine production to have trebled during the past decade. The global illicit drug industry is estimated to have an annual turnover of US$400 billion; this represents 8% of the value of all international trade.

A decade ago injecting drug use was thought to be uncommon in developing countries. Now, developing countries where injecting drug use is not a problem are the exception rather than the rule. The pattern of drug use around the world is also changing rapidly. One or two generations ago, opium smoking was prevalent in many countries in Asia. Anti-opium policies inadvertently resulted in opium smoking among elderly men being replaced by heroin injecting among young and sexually active men (Westermeyer, 1976).

It is easier to evade law enforcement with the more compact and almost odourless heroin compared to bulky opium. Similarly, the smaller utensils used for injecting are easier to conceal than the large pipes used for smoking opium. The change in preferred drug and preferred route of administration has had a profound public health impact by creating the fertile conditions for an explosive spread of HIV infection. This epidemic began among IDUs in Thailand (about the same time as an HIV epidemic among commercial sex workers) and then spread rapidly to the general Thai population (Weniger et al., 1991). HIV also spread rapidly from IDUs in Thailand to other drug users in neighbouring countries including Burma, China, India, Vietnam and Malaysia.

The most commonly injected drug in the world is heroin, followed by cocaine. Cocaine injecting is now seen increasingly in countries where only heroin injection was previously known. Heroin injecting has recently been reported for the first time in South America, where only cocaine injecting was known previously. Plant-derived drugs are increasingly being replaced by chemically synthesized drugs, as they are easier to conceal from law enforcement authorities. The illicit drug industry has become more dynamic and volatile during recent decades, although almost all countries have intensified law enforcement in response to illicit drugs. Nevertheless, illicit drug supplies have expanded relentlessly, despite the huge amounts of money being spent on law enforcement. It has been difficult to reconcile supply restriction approaches to illicit drugs with the more flexible and pragmatic approach required to control epidemics of HIV among and from IDUs.

Great efforts have been made in recent decades to ease the global movement of capital, labour, goods and services. Inevitably, mood altering substances in high demand can also now move readily from producer to consumer countries, especially if the price increases several thousand times during transit. When law enforcement has been strengthened, street drug prices have often increased and purity fallen, thereby increasing profit margins to offset the 'business risks' of an increased likelihood of detection and more severe punishment.

In Australia, heroin dependence in the first half of the twentieth century was uncommon (Manderson, 1993). It was managed by heroin prescription approved by health authorities if all other measures to achieve abstinence had failed. In 1953, the production and importation of heroin was banned in Australia following international pressure. Significant heroin injecting only became evident in Australia in the late 1960s, when US soldiers on rest and recreation leave from the Vietnam War introduced young Australians to the drug and the practice of injecting. The number of drug users in Australia has increased steadily over the past three decades. It was estimated that in 1997 there were 100 000 regular IDUs and an additional 175 000 injecting occasionally (Australian National Council on AIDS and Related Diseases, 1998). The rate of increase was estimated to be 7% per annum, equivalent to a doubling every 10 years. As illicit drug use is an illegal and highly stigmatized behaviour, estimates of the number of IDUs are inevitably only approximations. These estimates do, however, provide an indication of the likely size and growth of the population at risk. The illicit drug industry in Australia is estimated to have an annual turnover of $A7 billion. Heroin is the most commonly injected drug in Australia, followed by amphetamine and then cocaine, and the number of new heroin injectors appears to be increasing in Australia, judging by multiple indicators, including size and number of heroin seizures, drug overdose deaths, declining age of initiation, first presentation for treatment, presentation at needle exchange and person arrested for

drug-related crimes. Cocaine injecting is also increasing but is mainly restricted to Sydney at present.

Injecting drug use is present throughout Australia and is found in all socio-economic groups; however, it is more common in lower socio-economic groups. About two-thirds of IDUs are male. Although IDUs often have a background of limited education, long periods of unemployment and a history of criminal activity preceding any illicit drug use, there are many IDUs with a long history of stable partnerships, residence, employment and no history of criminal activity. Indeed, a US study based on health insurance records estimated that in New York State there are more apparently stable and functioning IDUs than those known to health or law enforcement authorities, who are usually considered more stereotypical (Eisenhandler and Drucker, 1993). Many IDUs consume a wide variety of legal drugs as well as heroin, amphetamine and cocaine. Alcohol, tobacco and benzodiazepines all contribute to the excess morbidity and mortality observed in the IDU population (as they do in the population at large). Poly-drug use is also replacing single-drug use in Australia and most other countries. IDUs are often intoxicated with a variety of drugs before even beginning to inject heroin or other drugs, which complicates the problems of controlling the spread of bloodborne pathogens in this population.

Epidemiology of HIV infection among injecting drug users

History of the injecting drug use epidemic

Some of the earliest cases of AIDS detected in the USA had a history of injecting drug use. Soon after the AIDS epidemic was first recognized in 1981, injecting drug use was identified as a risk behaviour associated with transmission of the presumed bloodborne pathogen. Following the identification of HIV and development of an antibody test in late 1984, it was recognized that half the IDUs in New York City were already infected with HIV. Retrospective studies of stored blood samples indicated that HIV had entered the IDU population in New York City in the mid-1970s and slowly spread to the majority of IDUs in that city and beyond (Des Jarlais et al., 1989).

The population of HIV-infected IDUs in the northeastern states of New York, Connecticut and New Jersey is the oldest and largest such population in the world. HIV infection spread from IDUs in this region to the general population by sexual transmission. Many heterosexual male

IDUs find non-drug using female sexual partners. Consequently, one of the key features of HIV epidemics involving IDUs is the rapid spread to the general population. In fact, IDUs have been described as the 'bridge' between marginalized groups and the population at large. HIV prevalence and incidence is now declining among IDUs in New York city (Des Jarlais *et al.*, 1996). However, HIV is already well established among non-drug using heterosexual men and women in the north east of the USA. Drug injecting is estimated to account for about half of the 40 000 new cases of HIV infection in the USA each year.

A large HIV-infected injecting drug user population stretches along the northern Mediterranean shores from Spain through southern France and on into Italy and Croatia. This pool of HIV infection was recognized soon after the similar population in the north east of the USA. HIV spread from the Mediterranean focus to IDUs north of the Alps and to non-drug using heterosexual men and women in Southern Europe. Two-thirds of AIDS cases in Spain and Italy are attributed directly to HIV infection associated with the sharing of injection equipment.

In 1987, HIV infection was detected among IDUs in Thailand (Weniger *et al.*, 1991). Prevalence increased from 1% to over 40% in less than 1 year. Prostitutes in Thailand were infected at about the same time. Within 5 years, one in six male military recruits and one in eight pregnant women from northwest Thailand were HIV-infected. HIV then spread to IDUs in neighbouring countries including Burma, China, Vietnam and Malaysia. From IDUs in Burma, it spread to IDUs in the state of Manipur in northeast India. Within a few years, HIV prevalence among IDUs reached 80% in some parts of Burma and in Manipur, where IDUs comprise 2% of the total population.

The fourth major concentration of HIV-infected IDUs is in Brazil. The geographical centre of the AIDS epidemic in Brazil has followed the trafficking route of cocaine in that country. HIV has spread rapidly to the general population of Brazil and has also spread to IDUs in other countries in South America.

The future of the injecting drug use HIV epidemic

In the last years of the twentieth century, HIV linked to injecting drug use spread rapidly around the world. Injecting drug use in many developed countries is now stable, or only increasing gradually. But injecting drug use continues to spread alarmingly in the developing world. Uncontrolled epidemics of HIV have been detected among IDUs in several former Soviet block countries in eastern Europe and central Asia only a few years after injecting drug use was first recognized.

HIV incidence now appears to be declining in New York City. The HIV epidemic has probably peaked in much of Western Europe. At least half the new cases of HIV infection following heterosexual transmission in the USA are believed to have followed sexual contact with an IDU. In western Europe, the countries with the highest incidence of AIDS cases attributed to injecting drug use generally have the highest incidence of total AIDS cases and AIDS cases attributed to heterosexual contact.

Alarming as the situation is in north eastern USA and southern Europe, it cannot be compared with the dangerous situation in the developing countries of Asia and South America. A high prevalence of HIV-infected IDUs has now been detected in numerous cities in China and a number of major cities in India. IDUs are now contributing substantially to the HIV epidemics in several South American countries, in addition to Brazil.

Lessons from the Australian experience

In Australia, the prevalence of HIV among IDUs without other risk factors remains under 5% and has been reported at 2% or less in most surveys. Data is abundant and consistent. Prevalence of HIV in Australian prisons, where IDUs comprise at least 50% of male and 80% of female inmates, is less than 1%.

Reassuring as the situation is in Australia, there are some very disturbing indicators that all may not be well. Many of these 'early warning signals' may be applicable to HIV control programmes in other countries. Australia has relied heavily on bipartisan cross-political support to implement controversial HIV prevention and control measures. This support is now starting to unravel. Success has become a problem as controversial prevention measures were easier to justify at a time when an uncontrolled epidemic appeared imminent. After more than a decade of good control, complacency has set in.

There are also increasing indications that HIV spread among prison inmates has been underestimated. Few HIV prevention strategies have yet been implemented in Australian prisons (Dolan *et al.*, 1995). Many prisons in Australia are now privatized. Some owners reject HIV surveillance and control measures arbitrarily, claiming 'commercial in confidence'. Increasing cocaine injection in Australia is alarming because it is far more difficult to control HIV infection among cocaine injectors than among heroin injectors. Cocaine users often inject the drug 10–15 times a day compared to two or three times a day for heroin injectors. Supplying sufficient sterile injecting equipment to control HIV in this situation is very difficult. While methadone is very effective in reducing the spread of HIV among heroin injectors, there is no equivalent to methadone treatment for cocaine injectors. Some of the increase in prevalence of HIV injection among IDUs in Canada – a country similar to Australia with an established and extensive needle exchange programme – has been attributed to cocaine use. Injecting drug use among Aboriginal Australians is also believed to be already in extensive and to be increasing in some areas. It has been difficult to implement HIV prevention strategies in some Aboriginal communities because these populations are often under great stress and elders are understandably apprehensive about prevention measures, which they fear may exacerbate the difficulties of their already troubled communities. Similar difficulties have been experienced in other disadvantaged minority and indigenous populations in other countries.

In New South Wales in 1998, needle exchange programmes stopped supplying wide-bore syringes. This threatened an HIV epidemic, because the risk of HIV transmission increases directly with increasing needle-bore size.

Some populations overlapping with IDUs are of particular relevance to controlling the HIV epidemic. These populations include homosexually active male IDUs, prisoners and prostitutes. The largest concentration of IDUs in Australia is in eastern Sydney. This area is also identified as having a large population of HIV-infected homosexually active males. HIV prevalence among homosexually active male IDUs in eastern Sydney is more than 10 times higher than among female and heterosexual male IDUs, suggesting that HIV is spreading among homosexually active male IDUs predominantly by sexual, rather than injecting drug use contacts. Comparison between Australia and the USA suggests that the most likely explanation for the very different course of the HIV epidemics in the two countries is the very different policies implemented in response to illicit drugs (Wodak and Lurie, 1997).

Risk behaviour

Sharing of needles and syringes is responsible for the spread of HIV among IDUs. The risk of HIV following a single instance of sharing a needle and syringe between an HIV-discordant couple is estimated to be 0.67%. Sharing of other injecting paraphernalia, spoons, filters, swabs, tourniquets, and contact between fingers of IDUs probably plays a minor role in HIV transmission, but may be more important in the transmission of other bloodborne infections, such as hepatitis C virus.

Almost 50 behavioural studies of IDUs were published in Australia between 1985 and 1994. The proportion reporting sharing in the month preceding interview declined from over 90% to less than 20% during that decade (Feacham, 1995). However, self-reported sexual behaviour among heterosexual IDUs has scarcely changed.

Hepatitis C prevalence among IDUs in Australia has been estimated in most reports to be between 50 and 70% (Crofts et al., 1997). Annual incidence is about 15%, but may be declining. It is estimated that 190 000 Australians have been exposed to hepatitis C (Australian National Council on AIDS and Related Diseases, 1998). At least 80% of prevalent cases and more than 90% of the estimated 11 000 incident cases per annum are IDUs.

Retrospective studies of stored blood samples suggest that hepatitis C had already entered the IDU population in Australia by the early 1970s. Although HIV among IDUs is well controlled in Australia, hepatitis C spread continues among the same population because of the far more infectious nature of the hepatitis C virus following bloodborne contact and the far higher baseline prevalence when prevention measures were introduced.

Strategies to prevent HIV spread among injecting drug users

Education

In most countries where news of HIV arrived before HIV itself, spread appeared to be slower than in locations where HIV arrived first. While some information appeared to be beneficial, extensive education seldom improved on these results. A little knowledge of HIV among IDUs has turned out to be a very good thing. Transmission of information about HIV/AIDS between IDUs appears to be very important, but should be facilitated by government-funded educational campaigns. These are more likely to be effective if the educational intervention is explicit, non-judgmental, credible and intelligible to the target population. Many of the most successful educational campaigns for IDUs in Australia have actively involved IDUs in their design and implementation ('peer-group educators'). It is now accepted that knowledge of HIV among IDUs does not predict attitudes and that attitudes do not predict future risk behaviour.

Reducing the circulation time of HIV-contaminated injecting equipment

Increasing the availability of sterile injecting equipment and decreasing the availability of unsterile injecting equipment reduces HIV spread among IDUs. This conclusion is supported by abundant and consistent evidence (Lurie et al., 1993; National Research Council/Institute of Medicine, 1995). The proposition also has an inherent plausibility. HIV prevalence and risk behaviour is generally lower among IDUs who attend needle exchange programmes. However, this finding can also be explained by selection bias. Lower HIV incidence has also been found among needle and syringe exchange programme attenders. IDUs who do not attend needle exchange programmes were found in one (as yet unreplicated) study to have between seven and eight times the incidence of hepatitis B and hepatitis C infection (Hagan et al., 1995). Mathematical modeling was used to produce estimates of a reduction in HIV incidence by at least one-third following introduction of a needle exchange programme (Kaplan and Heimer, 1994). An ecological study showed that HIV prevalence in 21 cities without needle exchange increased by 21% from about 3%, compared to an increase of 6% from 3% in eight cities with needle exchange programmes (Hurley et al., 1997). In Australia, the US$6.5 million expenditure on needle exchange programmes in 1991 was estimated to have prevented 2900 HIV infections in the same year, saving an estimated US$176 million at an estimated cost/life-year saved of US$228 (Feacham, 1995).

There is no convincing evidence that needle exchange programmes increase illicit drug use. In Sydney, Australia, the extent of drug use measured by urine analysis did not alter between patients of two methadone units, one of which was adjacent to a needle exchange programme. At least six major reports commissioned or completed by the US government or its agencies concluded that needle exchange programmes reduced the spread of HIV without increasing illicit drug use. Recent outbreaks of HIV among IDUs in the Canadian cities of Montreal and Vancouver, despite the presence of needle exchange programmes in both cities, have highlighted a number of important additional issues (Bruneau et al., 1997). In both cities, researchers have found that attendance at needle exchange programmes was associated with greater likelihood of HIV infection. Ideological opponents of harm reduction have misrepresented this finding in their campaigns to obstruct or even close down needle exchange programmes. It now appears that the finding of an association between needle exchange programme attendance and HIV infection is explained by the fact that high-risk IDUs were much more likely to attend these programmes in the first place. These outbreaks have also highlighted the importance of the 'dose' and coverage of interventions. Cocaine injecting dominates both of these Canadian cities. It is now clear that the scale of the needle exchange programme in Montreal was clearly inadequate. The Vancouver needle exchange programme was far larger, but ancillary services for IDUs in that city were very limited. Needle exchange programmes have been proposed as a harm reduction, rather than a harm elimination intervention. No claim has ever been made that needle exchange programmes prevent all HIV infections, rather that they are an important component of a comprehensive strategy, which is very effective in aggregate (Wodak and Des Jarlais, 1993).

In Italy, needles and syringes have always been available for sale in supermarkets, but little attempt was made by authorities to encourage IDUs to inject only with sterile needles and syringes. The continuing spread of HIV among IDUs in Italy, despite the availability of sterile injecting equipment, emphasizes the need for educational interventions to encourage IDUs to reduce the risk of HIV by using sterile injection equipment.

Drug treatment

Enrolment in methadone treatment has been consistently found to be strongly protective against HIV infection for heroin injectors (Caplehorn and Ross, 1995; Ward et al., 1998). This effect relies on an overall decrease in the frequency of heroin injections, rather than a change in the proportion of shared injections. Methadone treatment is generally the most commonly preferred form of treatment for heroin injectors. It attracts and retains many more heroin injectors then other treatment modalities. The notion that one form of drug dependence (heroin) is being treated with another from of drug dependence (methadone) is regarded by some as a criticism of this treatment yet the same concerns are not levelled against nicotine replacement, therapy used to promote cessation or reduction of smoking. In most countries, demand for methadone treatment far outstrips supply.

Effective organization of drug users

In many countries that responded successfully to the threat of an uncontrolled epidemic of HIV infection among IDUs, organizations of drug users have been established. Government-funded organizations of drug users are found in all states and territories in Australia. These organizations play an important role in the development and implementation of prevention policies, especially community-sensitive targeted educational interventions (Friedman et al., 1993).

Harm reduction

The philosophy of harm reduction has been an important component of effective public health responses to HIV infection among IDUs. This approach emphasizes the paramount need to reduce the individual and societal adverse complications of illicit drug use; a decrease in consumption of illicit drugs is regarded as only one of many possible means of achieving this objective. The more conventional response to illicit drug use at the time HIV/AIDS was first recognized relied heavily on law enforcement measures to reduce consumption.

Implementation of effective harm reduction and prevention measures in many countries initially resulted in some degree of conflict between the health and law enforcement arms of government. In contrast, in Australia there has been increasing collaboration between health and law enforcement sectors. Health authorities realized that effective implementation of needle exchange and methadone treatment required cooperation with law enforcement. Otherwise, IDUs attending harm reduction facilities might be arrested, deterring others from attending.

Harm reduction emphasizes the importance of intermediate, achievable goals, rather than the utopian and unachievable objectives promoted by conventional abstinence-based approaches. Attempting to achieve a drug-free nation has been the paramount drug policy goal of the USA. Not only has this goal not been reached, but the USA has failed to reach the achievable goal of HIV control among IDUs. Opponents of harm reduction fear that it may just be the thin edge of the wedge of drug policy

reform. In some cases, advocates for harm reduction have also supported drug policy reform as the self-evident gains achieved with more modest reforms have spurred them on to consider the bigger picture. In other cases, supporters of harm reduction do not support drug policy reform, which they regard as a luxury for possible discussion when the epidemic of HIV infection among IDUs has been safely brought under control.

Clinical aspects of HIV infection in the injecting drug user

There is an important need to address both clinical and psychosocial issues related to both HIV infection and drug use. A non-judgemental approach is important to engage the HIV-infected individual and gain sufficient trust to obtain an accurate history of the type and amount of substances used, as well as the duration and routes of administration. A comprehensive review of medical complications of drug use unrelated to HIV infection should be sought.

Epidemiology

Disease progression is determined by host factors (genetic markers, CD4 lymphocyte numbers) and viral factors (viral load and phenotype) (Vlahor et al., 1998). It does not appear to be influenced by route of transmission of HIV. Baseline viral load has been used to predict progression to AIDS and survival in several cohorts. It is evident that the predictive value of viral load on clinical progression does not vary by risk group (homosexual male, IDU) (Lyles et al., 1999). The longer time from seroconversion to progression to AIDS in IDUs compared with homosexual men found by Spijkerman is probably related to the indicator conditions used for the definition of AIDS, which do not include the common infections experienced by IDUs (Spijkerman et al., 1996). The AIDS surveillance definition has probably greatly underestimated HIV-related morbidity and mortality in IDUs over time (Stoneburner et al., 1988).

Clinical manifestations

Bacterial infections are more common in IDUs, especially bacterial pneumonia, endocarditis and bloodstream infections, and this group have up to a four times higher risk of these complications compared with HIV-seronegative drug users (Selwyn et al., 1988). A retrospective study in Switzerland revealed markedly increased risk ratios for pneumonia, tuberculosis, soft-tissue infections, osteo-articular infections and endocarditis for HIV-infected IDUs, compared with their non-HIV-infected counterparts (Scheidegger and Zimmerli, 1996). Bacterial pneumonia (usually due to *Streptococcus pneumoniae*, and less commonly to *Haemophilus influenzae*) is more common than *Pneumocystis carinii* pneumonia (PCP) in IDUs and can occur at higher CD4 lymphocyte counts (Selwyn *et al.*, 1992a).

An increased incidence of infective endocarditis in drug users has been noted since recognition of the HIV epidemic. Differing opinions concerning the influence of HIV infection and degree of immunodeficiency on the incidence and outcome of endocarditis prevail. Weisse and colleagues determined that there was no effect of HIV on the risk of endocarditis or response to treatment (Weisse *et al.*, 1993), but others have noted an increased incidence of bacterial infections, including endocarditis in HIV-infected drug users (Selwyn *et al.*, 1992a) (see Chapter 15). Manoff and colleagues estimated the risk of infective endocarditis to be greater for those with lower CD4 lymphocyte counts (adjusted odds ratio of endocarditis was 2.31 for those HIV-infected individuals with greater than 350 CD4 lymphocytes/μl, and 8.31 for those with less than 350 CD4 lymphocytes/μl) (Manoff *et al.*, 1996). The clinical presentation of infective endocarditis appears to be similar in both HIV-uninfected and HIV-infected individuals, but there does seem to be increased mortality from endocarditis in the HIV-infected drug user. This mortality varies according to the immune status of the individual. Survival was greater for asymptomatic HIV-infected individuals compared with those with advanced disease, with mortality inversely associated with the CD4 cell count (Pulvirenti *et al.*, 1996). The most common infecting organism was *Staphylococcus aureus* in 75% of cases in one series, with viridans streptococci and Gram-negative bacilli also causing endocarditis in HIV-infected drug users. The tricuspid valve was affected in 43% of cases. There was no difference in response to therapy between the two groups, but complications occurred more frequently in the HIV-infected group (Nahass *et al.*, 1990, Pulvirenti *et al.*, 1996).

The febrile IDU should be investigated for the possibility of infective endocarditis with serial blood cultures and echocardiography. In a study by Weisse, only 8% of IDUs admitted to hospital with fever for investigation were given a final diagnosis of endocarditis (Weisse and Noble, 1986). In a later study of a similar population, 42% of hospitalized febrile drug users had bacteraemia, and of those with bacteraemia, one-third had infective endocarditis, with vege-

tations identified by echocardiography in 94% (Weisse *et al.*, 1993). Presumptive antibiotic therapy should cover penicillin-resistant, methicillin-sensitive *Staphylococcus aureus* while blood cultures are incubating. Some clinicians would add gentamicin and/or rifampicin to the antistaphylococcal penicillin.

Prophylaxis with trimethoprim-sulfamethoxazole (TMP-SMX) for the common opportunistic infections (PCP, toxoplasmosis) will also provide some protection against recurrent bacterial infections experienced by the drug users. It may be worth considering the introduction of (TMP-SMX) at CD4 lymphocyte counts of less than 350 cells/μl in the IDU, instead of the conventional recommendation of 200 CD4 lymphocytes/μl. Prevention of infection with *Streptococcus pneumoniae* and *Haemophilus influenzae* by vaccination at CD4 lymphocyte counts of greater than 350 cells/μl has been demonstrated in other HIV-infected risk groups and should be recommended for all HIV-infected drug users.

Tuberculosis is also more common in drug users, and the increase in HIV-related tuberculosis in the USA is associated with the drug-user population. Pulmonary disease is more common in those without significant immunodeficiency, and extrapulmonary disease occurs with advancing HIV disease. HIV-infected IDUs with a positive Mantoux test should receive 12 months of isoniazid prophylaxis (Selwyn *et al.*, 1992b). Isoniazid prophylaxis should also be considered for anergic individuals in high endemic areas for tuberculosis. Recently, an 8-week course of pyrazinamide and rifampin was shown to be as effective as isoniazid for the prevention of active tuberculosis (see Chapter 23).

Serological evidence of both hepatitis B and C can be found in over 65% of HIV-infected IDUs. Whether HIV infection worsens the course of concurrent hepatitis B or C remains controversial, as does the effect of hepatitis C on the course of HIV disease (see Chapter 16). There was no evidence of a negative impact on HIV disease by HCV co-infection in one study of 240 IDUs, although there may be an associated reduction in survival in the co-infected group (Haydon *et al.*, 1998). The interpretation of abnormal liver function tests becomes a challenge in those individuals with underlying liver disease and superimposed hepatotoxicity from HIV-related medications.

Female IDUs with HIV infection who become sex workers to sustain their drug habit, have a higher incidence of sexually transmitted disease and are at increased risk of cervical dysplasia and cancer.

The differentiation of mental state changes in the HIV-infected drug user due to HIV dementia, central nervous system (CNS) opportunistic complications of AIDS, from the acute or chronic intoxication of various substances such as alcohol, cocaine or other drugs, or withdrawal of opioids, is important.

Antiretroviral therapy

Drug users often have poor access to health care, using the emergency room rather than a single health clinic providing consistent primary care. They are less likely to access antiretroviral therapy, but rates of compliance with therapy are good when care is delivered through hospital-based specialized clinics or drug treatment centres. Two surveys of antiretroviral use in drug users revealed that only 40–50% were receiving antiretroviral therapy, but only 14–17% were receiving potent antiretroviral combination therapy as recommended by the US Public Health guidelines (Celentano et al., 1998; Strathdee et al., 1998). IDUs were more likely to be receiving antiretroviral therapy if they were in a substance-abuse programme or had a regular source of primary health care or health insurance. Recent incarceration and active drug use appeared to be obstacles for the receipt of appropriate therapy. Adherence to treatment regimens declines in the setting of active drug use, underscoring the importance of combined programmes of treatment for drug abuse and review of HIV infection (Palepu et al., 2001).

Important drug interactions

Methadone is a long-acting opiate, and is one of the agents used for the treatment of heroin dependence. It is metabolised by the hepatic cytochrome P450 enzymes, primarily 3A4 and 2D6. It is important to recognize the known and potential interactions of methadone with antiretroviral agents, which can result in symptoms of withdrawal or excess (see Chapter 6). The protease inhibitors (PIs) are both inhibitors and substrates for the cytochrome P450 3A4 enzymes and ritonavir is also an inducer of this system. There have been no results published from formal human studies to date of the interaction between methadone and the PIs in HIV-infected subjects. In vitro studies have shown significant inhibition of methadone metabolism, underscoring the importance of predicted clinical interactions and resultant increased methadone concentrations (Iribarne et al., 1998). The non-nucleoside reverse transcriptase inhibitors (NNRTIs) as a class of agent have more complex interactions with the P450 enzymes. Nevirapine induces the P450 3A4 enzymes and has been shown to cause withdrawal symptoms when introduced to individuals stabilized on methadone. Doubling of the methadone dose was required to restabilize these individuals (Altice et al., 1999). Delavirdine is a potent inhibitor of the hepatic cytochrome P450 3A4 enzymes and is predicted to cause an increase in methadone levels. Efavirenz is both an inducer and inhibitor of the P450 3A4 system, and the interactions with methadone are currently under investigation. The nucleoside analogue reverse transcriptase inhibitors (NRTIs) are not metabolized by the hepatic cytochromes so that interactions with methadone were not anticipated. The interaction between zidovudine (ZDV) and methadone has been formally studied and results in a 40% increase in exposure to ZDV without any effect on the methadone concentration. The effects are due to inhibition of glucuronidation of ZDV as well as reduced renal clearance. Individuals may experience greater ZDV toxicity, and a reduction in dose of ZDV may be warranted (Schwartz et al., 1992; McCance-Katz et al., 1998). Exposure to didanosine was decreased by 60% and stavudine by 20%, with concomitant methadone administration (Rainey et al., 1999). There are currently no recommendations concerning dose adjustment for didanosine in combination with methadone. The pharmacokinetic interaction with stavudine is not thought to be clinically significant.

Rifampicin, an important component of combination treatment for tuberculosis, causes a significant reduction in plasma methadone concentration and results in opioid withdrawal symptoms when administered to drug users stabilized on methadone (Kreek et al., 1976). Unlike rifampicin, rifabutin does not appear to alter the pharmacokinetics of methadone (Brown et al., 1996).

Aspects of management specific to narcotic drug users

Concurrent psychiatric disorders are common in drug users, including personality disorders, depression, psychosis, and anxiety (see Chapter 11). Recognition and management of psychiatric disorders, in the setting of opioid, alcohol, or other drug dependence, and the potential neuropsychiatric complications of HIV infection, is a challenge. Responses to psychoactive medication may be exaggerated in HIV infection, with reduced doses of medication providing a therapeutic effect compared with non-HIV-infected individuals (see Chapter 11). Both counselling and pharmacotherapy are important aspects of care for the drug user, to enable adherence to antiretroviral treatment, monitoring HIV infection and general health.

Conclusion

After more than a decade of global experience in implementing harm-reduction responses to HIV spread among IDUs, it is now abundantly clear that these measures are generally effective, relatively inexpensive and free of serious unintended negative consequences. In the case of Australia (Wodak and Lurie, 1997) and the UK (Stimson, 1996), a strong case can be argued that an HIV epidemic has so far actually been averted. This seems far more likely than alternative explanations, such as the failure of surveillance to detect an existing epidemic. Perhaps the most convincing evidence that an epidemic has been averted is the high prevalence of HIV infection among homosexual IDUs in eastern Sydney, who were presumably infected through sexual contact, and the low HIV prevalence among heterosexual IDUs from the same areas.

References

Altice FL, Friedland GH, Cooney EL. (1999). Nevirapine induced opiate withdrawal among injection drug users with HIV infection receiving methadone. *AIDS* **13**: 957–62.

Australian National Council on AIDS and Related Diseases. Hepatitis C Subcommittee. (1998a). *Hepatitis C Virus Projections Working Group: estimates and projections of the hepatitis C virus epidemic in Australia.* Sydney: National Centre in HIV Epidemiology and Clinical Research.

Australian National Council on AIDS and Related Diseases. (1998b). Projections Working Party on the Epidemiology of Hepatitis C infection in Australia. Sydney: National Centre for HIV Epidemiology and Clinical Research.

Brown LS, Sawyer RC, Li R et al. (1996). Lack of pharmacologic interaction between rifabutin and methadone in HIV-infected former IDUs. *Drug Alcohol Depend* **43**: 71–7

Bruneau J, Lamothe F, Franco E et al. (1997). High rates of HIV infection among IDUs participating in needle exchange programs in Montreal: results of a cohort study. *Am J Epidemiol* **146**: 994–1002.

Caplehorn JRM, MW Ross. (1995). Methadone maintenance and the likelihood of risky needle sharing. *J Addict* **30**: 685–98.

Celentano DD, Vlahov D, Cohn S et al. (1998). Self-reported antiretroviral therapy in injection drug users *J Am Med Assoc* **280**: 544–6.

Crofts N, Jolly D, Kaldor J et al. (1997). The epidemiology of hepatitis C virus infection among injecting drug users in Australia. *J Epi Comm Health* **51**: 692–7.

Des Jarlais DC, Friedman SR, Novick D et al. (1989). HIV-1 infection among intravenous drug users in Manhattan, from 1977 through 1987. *J Am Med Assoc* **261**: 1008–12.

Des Jarlais DC, Marmour M, Paone D et al. (1996). HIV incidence among injecting drug users in New York City syringe-exchange programs. *Lancet* **348**: 987–91.

Dolan K, Wodak A, Penny R. (1995). AIDS behind bars: preventing HIV spread among incarcerated drug injectors. *AIDS* **9**: 825–32.

Eisenhandler J, Drucker E. (1993). Opiate dependency among the prescribers of a New York area private insurance plan. *JAMA* **269**: 2890–1.

Feacham RGA. (1995). *Valuing the past ... investing in the future. Evaluation of the National HIV/AIDS Strategy 1993-94 to 1995–96.* Canberra: Australian Government Publishing Service, Commonwealth Department of Human Services and Health.

Friedman SR, de Jong W, Wodak A. (1993). Community development as a response to HIV among drug injectors. *AIDS* **7**: S263–9.

Hagan H, DC Des Jarlais, SR Friedman et al. (1995). Reduced risk of hepatitis B and hepatitis C among injection drug users in the Tacoma syringe exchange program. *Am J Pub Health* **85**: 1531–7.

Haydon GH, Flegg PJ, Blair CS et al. (1998). The impact of chronic hepatitis C virus infection on HIV disease and progression in intravenous drug users. *Eur J Gastroenterol Hepatol* **10**: 485–9.

Hurley SF, Jolley DJ, Kaldor JM. (1997). Effectiveness of needle exchange programs for prevention of HIV infection. *Lancet* **349**: 1797–1800.

Iribarne C, Berthou F, Carlhant D et al. (1998). Inhibition of methadone and buprenorphine N-dealkylations by three HIV-1 protease inhibitors. *Drug Metab Dispos* **26**: 257–60.

Kaplan EH, Heimer R. (1994). HIV incidence among needle exchange participants: estimates from syringe tracking and testing data. *J Acquir Immune Defic Syndr Hum Retrovirol* **7**: 182–9.

Kreek MJ, Garfield JW, Gutjarh CL et al. (1976) Rifampin induced methadone withdrawal. *N Engl J Med* **294**: 1104–6.

Lurie P, Reingold AL, Bowser B et al. (1993). *The public health impact of needle exchange programs in the United States and abroad.* Volume I. San Francisco, CA: University of California.

Lyles CM, Graham NMH, Astemborski J et al. (1999). Cell-associated infectious HIV-1 viral load as a predictor of clinical progression and survival among HIV-1 infected injection drug users and homosexual men. *Eur J Epidemiol* **15**: 99–108.

Manderson D. (1993). *From Mr Sin to Mr Big. A history of Australian drug laws.* Oxford: Oxford University Press.

Manoff SB, Vlahov D, Herskovitz A et al. (1996). Human immunodeficiency virus infection and infective endocarditis among injecting drug users. *Epidemiology* **7**: 566–70.

McCance-Katz E, Rainey PM, Jatlow P et al. (1998). Methadone effects on zidovudine disposition (AIDS Clinical Trial Group 262). *J Acquir Immune Defic Syndr Hum Retrovirol* **18**: 435–43.

Nahass RG, Weinstein MP, Bartels J et al. (1990) Infective endocarditis in intravenous drug users: a comparison of human immunodeficiency virus type-1 negative and -positive patients. *J Infect Dis* **162**: 967–70.

National Research Council/Institute of Medicine. (1995). J Normand, D Vlahos, LE Moses (eds.) (Panel on Needle Exchange and Bleach Distribution Programs) *reventing HIV transmission: the role of sterile needles and bleach.* Washington, DC: National Academy Press.

Palepu A, Yip B, Miller C et al. (2001). Factors associated with the response to antiretroviral therapy among HIV-infected patients with and without a history of injection drug use. *AIDS* **15**: 423–4.

Pulvirenti JJ, Kerns E, Benson C et al. (1996). Infective endocarditis in injection drug users: Importance of human immunodeficiency virus serostatus and degree of immunosuppression. *Clin Infect Dis* **22**: 40–5.

Rainey PM, McCance EF, Mitchell SM et al. (1999). Interaction of methadone with didanosine (ddI) and stavudine (d4T). *Program and abstracts of the Sixth Conference on Retroviruses and Opportunistic Infections*, Chicago, IL, USA.

Scheidegger C, Zimmerli W. (1996). Incidence and spectrum of severe medical complications among hospitalized HIV-seronegative and HIV-seropositive narcotic drug users. *AIDS* **10**: 1407–14.

Schwartz EL, Brechbuhl AB, Kahl P et al. (1992). Pharmacokinetic interactions of zidovudine and methadone in intravenous drug-using patients with HIV infections. *J Acquir Immune Defic Syndr Hum Retrovirol* **5**: 619–26.

Selwyn PA, Feingold AR, Hartel D et al. (1988) Increased risk of bacterial pneumonia in HIV-infected intravenous drug users without AIDS. *AIDS* **2**: 267–72.

Selwyn PA, Alcabes P, Hartel D et al. (1992a). Clinical manifestations and predictors of disease progression in drug users with human immunodeficiency virus infection. *N Engl J Med* **327**: 1697–703.

Selwyn PA, Sckell BM, Alcabes P et al. (1992b). High risk of active tuberculosis in HIV-infected drug users with cutaneous anergy. *JAMA* **268**: 504–9.

Spijkerman IJB, Langen MW, Veugelers PJ et al. (1996). Differences in progression to AIDS between injection drug users and homosexual men with documented dates of seroconversion. *Epidemiology* **7**:571–7.

Stimson GV. (1996). Has the United Kingdom averted an epidemic of HIV-1 infection amongst drug injectors? [Editorial]. *Addiction* **91**: 1085–8.

Stimson GV, Adelekan M, Rhodes T. (1996). The diffusion of drug injecting in developing countries. *Int J Drug Policy* **7**: 245–55.

Stoneburner RL, Des Jarlais DC, Benezra D et al. (1988). A larger spectrum of severe HIV-1-related disease in intravenous drug users in New York City. *Science* **242**: 916–19.

Strathdee SA, Palepu A, Cornelisse PGA et al. (1998). Barriers to use of free antiretroviral therapy in injection drug users *J Am Med Assoc* **280**: 547–9.

UN Commission on Narcotic Drugs. (1995). *Economic and social Consequences of drug abuse and illicit trafficking: an interim report*. Vienna: United Nations Economic and Social Council.

Vlahov D, Graham N, Hoover D et al. (1998). Prognostic indicators for AIDS and Infectious Disease death in HIV-infected injection drug users: viral load and CD4+ cell count. *JAMA* **279**: 35–40.

Ward J, Mattick R, Hall W. (1998). *Methadone maintenance treatment and other opioid replacement therapies*. Amsterdam: Harwood Academic Publishers.

Weisse AB, Noble MC. (1986). Echocardiographic screening for acute infectious endocarditis in drug abusers. *New Jersey Med* **83**:239–41.

Weisse AB, Heller DR, Schimenti RJ et al. (1993). The febrile parenteral drug user: a prospective study in 121 patients. *Am J Med* **94**: 274–80.

Weniger BG, Limpakarnjanarat K, Ungchusak K et al. (1991). The epidemiology of HIV infection and AIDS in Thailand. *AIDS* **5**: S71–85.

Westermeyer J. (1976). The pro-heroin effects of anti-opium laws in Asia. *Arch Gen Psychiatr* **33**: 1135–9.

Wodak A, Des Jarlais DC. (1993). Strategies for the prevention of HIV infection among and from injecting drug users. *Bull Narc* **45**: 47–60.

Wodak A, Lurie P. (1997). A tale of two countries: attempts to control HIV among injecting drug users in Australia and the United States. *J Drug Issues* **27**: 117–34.

36

Management of the HIV-infected patient in a developing country

KIAT RUXRUNGTHAM, N. KUMARASAMY, SUNITI SOLOMON AND MARK NEWELL

Recent advances in management of the HIV-infected patient in developed countries have led to an improved length and quality of life in these patients (Palella *et al.*, 1998). However, these advances have had little impact on patients in the developing world, where the vast majority of infected individuals have no access to these new therapies. In addition, the impact of the AIDS epidemic in the developing world continues to increase at a rate estimated by UNAIDS at over 16 000 new infections per day, representing 90% of all new infections worldwide (Piot, 1998). Provision of these new 'standard of care' therapies described in Chapter 7 are well beyond the available health resources of much of the developing world. Therefore, the approach to the management of the HIV-infected patient in developing countries should be based on a holistic, cost-effective approach. This should take into account the number of infected people, the spectrum of HIV disease and the available resources available in each individual country.

In the absence of an effective vaccine, prevention of new HIV infections through education and condom use remains the most cost-effective way to control the HIV epidemic, especially in the developing world (Nelson *et al.*, 1996). A specific method of HIV prevention with proven efficacy is the treatment of pregnant HIV-infected women around the time of late pregnancy, labour and delivery with antiretroviral therapy (Connor *et al.*, 1994) (see also Chapter 9). Early screening, diagnosis and treatment of sexually transmitted diseases (STDs) has also been shown to reduce transmission (Centers for Disease Control and Prevention, 1998).

Priorities for managing established HIV infection for an individual in a developing country include encouragement of earlier diagnosis and access to medical care; the prevention, early diagnosis and treatment of the more preva-lent opportunistic infections in that country; appropriate antiretroviral therapy; palliative care; and encouragement of a healthier lifestyle for those infected. Since AIDS remains a highly stigmatized disease in most countries, the HIV-infected patient also needs considerable psychosocial support.

Crucial to the success of clinical management guidelines is the integration of services at all levels, including teaching hospitals, community hospitals, day-care services, community-based care services and home care. This involves coordination between doctors and other health-care community-based services and non-government organizations. In this regard, HIV is providing a model for the optimal care of severe chronic illness with the best utilization of resources. Care based principally in the home, or with low-cost facilities close to home, can still provide many aspects of basic medical care and considerable relief of suffering. If it is supported by intermittent or occasional referral to more specialist services and access to more expensive drugs, then the quality of life can be improved and length of life extended. Issues of fear of contagion, confidentiality and discrimination impact directly on medical care and need to be addressed at all levels within society.

Clinical presentation of HIV infection in developing countries

Natural history of HIV infection

The clinical manifestations and course of HIV infection among patients in developing countries differs from that observed in developed countries (Deschamps *et al.*, 2000). The time to progression to AIDS varies from 6.5 to 13 years in developed world cohorts (Munoz *et al.*, 1997). In Africa, the median time to AIDS diagnosis varies from 2.0 to 7.5 years across several cohorts (Grant *et al.*, 1997; Morgan and Whitworth, 2001). Factors that may affect the natural history of HIV in the developing world are the HIV subtype, genetic differences, concurrent infections such as tuberculosis, cultural and socio-economic backgrounds and differences in access to health care.

A retrospective study of 757 Thai HIV-infected patients showed that the rate of progression to AIDS according to CD4 lymphocyte count at baseline was comparable with Western cohorts (Wannamethee *et al.*, 1998). In this study, individuals with CD4 lymphocyte counts of less than 200 cells/μl at baseline showed a greater than ninefold increase in the risk of developing AIDS compared to subjects with CD4 lymphocyte counts of 500 cells/μl or more (RR = 9.1, 95% CI, 5.4–16.0). The slope of CD4 lymphocyte decline in Thai patients is approximately 50–100 cells/year, which is also comparable to studies performed in the USA. The annual rate of clinical progression from asymptomatic to symptomatic HIV infection in Thai patients was 6.8% (Sirivichyakul *et al.*, 1992). A study of AIDS patients in the early phase of the epidemic in Bangkok reported a much shorter survival time of only 7 months following AIDS diagnosis compared to patients in developed countries (Kitayaporn *et al.*, 1996). This short survival time was attributed to the fact that in the developing world, AIDS is often diagnosed late in the course of HIV infection.

There is no clear evidence either *in vitro* or *in vivo* to support the notion that individuals infected with subtype E (predominant in Thailand) progress more rapidly than those infected with subtype B. A report that HIV-1 subtype E displays a preferential tropism for Langerhans cells (epidermal dendritic cells) compared to subtype B strains provides a possible explanation for the rapid heterosexual spread of subtype E strains in Thailand (Soto-Ramirez *et al.*, 1996). However, this observation has not been confirmed by other investigators (Pope *et al.*, 1997). A cross-sectional study of 1241 patients suggested that the infecting HIV-1 subtype may independently influence the course of immune suppression and clinical disease (Limpakarnjanarat *et al.*, 1996). In multivariate analyses (adjusted for gender, age, and risk category), HIV-1 subtype E was associated with lower lymphocyte counts (OR = 1.9; 95% CI, 1.1–3.3) and increased risk of cryptococcal meningitis (OR 2.7; 95% CI, 1.2 – 6.5). In contrast, a retrospective study reported that the rate of CD4 lymphocyte decline was comparable among patients infected with either subtype E or B (Ubolyam *et al.*, 1998). An observation from a hospital-based cohort has found that individuals with heterosexually acquired HIV infection had a significantly higher rate of progression compared to a group with homosexually acquired HIV infection (Wannamethee *et al.*, 1998). In the same cohort, the rate of progression of AIDS in Thai women, presumably infected with mostly subtype E, was comparable to men. Until more evidence is obtained from a larger prospective cohort, the natural history of individuals infected with subtype E and whether it differs from the natural history of other subtype infections remains inconclusive. A number of studies involving prospective cohorts of recent HIV seroconvertors has recently been initiated, the results of which will provide more understanding of the natural history of HIV infection in Thailand and will be of relevance to other countries in the developing world.

Clinical course of HIV infection

The clinical manifestations of HIV infection are classified into four clinical stages (Fauci and Lane, 1998). These are acute (primary) HIV infection, asymptomatic HIV infection, early symptomatic HIV infection (formerly termed AIDS-related complex or ARC) and advanced HIV disease or AIDS.

Acute HIV infection

In Australian cohorts (Carr and Cooper, 1997), 50–90% of individuals infected with HIV-1 developed a symptomatic primary HIV infection syndrome (see Chapter 1). However, this clinical syndrome has not been observed to the same extent among Thai patients. One retrospective study reported symptomatic acute HIV infection in less than 1% of 446 patients (Ruxrungtham *et al.*, 1996 and unpubl. data). This marked difference in the prevalence of the primary HIV infection syndrome in the Thai population compared to western cohorts may be due to various factors, such as different HIV-1 subtypes, host factors and failure to diagnose the syndrome, as it can clinically resemble malaria, typhoid fever or flu-like illness frequently self-treated by patients with over-the-counter medications. Further study of primary HIV infection in the developing world is required.

Early symptomatic HIV infection

Herpes zoster (shingles) is one of the most common first presentations of immune deficiency in HIV-infected persons in developing countries. Among 446 HIV-1 infected Thais attending an HIV clinic at Chulalongkorn hospital in Bangkok, shingles was reported in 16–17% (Sivayathorn *et al.*, 1995; Ruxrungtham *et al.*, 1996) and in 7.3% of an Indian cohort (Kumarasamy *et al.*, 1995). Most patients developed lesions that were distributed in more than one dermatome. The average CD4 lymphocyte count in these patients was approximately 300 cells/μl and the time to progression to AIDS after the appearance of shingles was approximately 2–3 years (Sivayathorn *et al.*, 1995; Ruxrungtham *et al.*, 1996). A hospital study in Zaïre found that at presentation 11% of patients with HIV had a recent history of herpes zoster (Tyndall *et al.*, 1995).

Oral hairy leukoplakia (OHL) was found in 15–45% of Thai HIV-infected patients with a mean CD4 lymphocyte count at presentation of 350 cells/μl (Sivayathorn *et al.*, 1995; Ruxrungtham *et al.*, 1996). In a series of 1010 HIV-infected patients from India, the prevalence of OHL was low at 1.2% (Kumarasamy *et al.*, 1995).

Oral candidiasis is also a common finding, with a prevalence of 26–34 % in Thailand (Sivayathorn *et al.*, 1995; Ruxrungtham *et al.*, 1996), 42% in India (Kumarasamy *et al.*, 1995) and 69% in Papua New Guinea (Seaton *et al.*, 1996) . Patients with oral candidiasis usually have a CD4 lymphocyte count of below 300 cells/μl.

Persistent generalized lymphadenopathy was found in 39% of asymptomatic HIV-infected Thai patients in one study (Ruxrungtham *et al.*, 1996).

Approximately 10% of HIV-infected patients attending an HIV clinic at Chulalongkorn Hospital, Bangkok had symptoms of chronic fever, weight loss and/or chronic diarrhoea, with no other obvious aetiology (Ruxrungtham *et al.*, 1996). In a series of 323 HIV-infected patients from Papua New Guinea, chronic diarrhoea was found in 48% and wasting in 94% (Seaton *et al.*, 1996).

The most common and characteristic skin manifestation among HIV-infected patients is pruritic papular eruptions (PPE), with a reported prevalence of 27–33% in two Thai cohorts (Sivayathorn *et al.*, 1995; Ruxrungtham *et al.*, 1996) and 7.9% in an Indian cohort. These eruptions were seen in patients with mean CD4 lymphocyte counts of 151 cells/μl (Kumarasamy *et al.*, 2000). The pathogenesis of PPE is not well understood and no known causative microorganism has been identified. The lesions have the appearance of insect bites, but with intense itching and a widespread distribution (Figure 36.1, all the figures appear in the colour plate section). The extremities are the most

common location of PPE; however, when the disease becomes more advanced, trunk involvement is not uncommon. PPE rarely involves the face, which is in contrast to the papulo-necrotic lesions of penicilliosis or other systemic fungal infections, where facial presentations are more common. The most common pathological finding is an eosinophilic infiltration.

Herpes simplex, onychomycosis, cutaneous ringworm, psoriasis and folliculitis are other commonly reported skin diseases in Thai HIV-infected patients; with a prevalence of 6–11%, this is similar to that reported in western cohorts (Sivayathorn *et al.*, 1995). An Indian study reported cutaneous tinea in 13.4%, scabies in 1.6% and molluscum contagiosum in 1.3% of patients (Kumarasamy *et al.*, 1998a).

Advanced symptomatic HIV infection (AIDS)

The clinical spectrum of AIDS-defining illnesses varies across countries in the developing world (Table 36.1). However, there are limitations to the interpretation of data concerning their relative prevalence in different countries for several reasons. Most data are derived from hospital-based clinics, the diagnosis is often presumptive due to limited diagnostic resources and generally the data only include initial, rather than subsequent, AIDS-defining illnesses, so that opportunistic infections that occur at very advanced levels of immunodeficiency will be under-represented (Hira *et al.*, 1998).

However, data derived from routine AIDS surveillance are available in Thailand. In a large Thai survey of 47 218 patients, the four most common presentations of AIDS were HIV wasting syndrome, tuberculosis, *Pneumocystis carinii* pneumonia (PCP) and cryptococcosis. In Northern Thailand only, penicilliosis was the fifth most common presentation (Chariyalertsak *et al.*, 1997). In a cohort of 183 children infected by vertical transmission, the most common AIDS-defining conditions were PCP (32%) salmonellosis (usually septicaemia, 16%), cytomegalovirus (CMV); (11%) and bacterial pneumonia (11%) (Sirisanthana *et al.*, 1995). In another series of 754 HIV-infected individuals in India, pulmonary tuberculosis was the most common opportunistic infection (42.8%), followed by extrapulmonary tuberculosis (7.7%) and PCP (4.6%). However, in this cohort, idiopathic diarrhoea was detected in 25.7% and bacterial respiratory infections in 20.7% (Kumarasamy *et al.*, 1998a). In a series of 86 African-born patients living in the UK, the most frequent diagnoses

Table 36.1 Spectrum (%) of AIDS-defining illnesses in selected developing countries

AIDS-defining illness	Thailand (North)	Thailand (Total)	India (Madras) (n = 754)	Indonesia	Papua New Guinea	Cote d'Ivoire	Kenya	Africans in UK
Tuberculosis	32.0	34.0	42.8	44.2	68.6	13.0	18.0	20
MAC	–	0.2	–	–	–	–	–	–
Osophageal candidiasis	3.5	6.4	–	83.7[a]	68.7[a]	3.0	–	13
Cryptococcosis	17.4	20.3	0.5	–	8.6	3.0	1.0	11
PCP	13.0	13.4	4.6	–	8.6	[b]	30.0[c]	21
Toxoplasmosis	5.4	4.0	2.5	18.6	–	7.0	–	–
Cryptosporidosis	2.5	1.1	2.5	–	–	–	–	0.8
Penicilliosis	14.0	4.5	–	–	–	–	–	–
CMV disease	–	0.1	3.3	37.2	–	–	–	–
AIDS dementia complex	–	2.5	–	4.6	4.3	–	–	–
KS	–	0.1	0.1	11.6	–	1.0	2.0	5.0
Lymphoma	–	0.7	1.6	2.3	–	–	–	0.8
Salmonella septicemia	8.2	–	–	–	–	–	–	–

MAC: *Mycobacterium avium* complex; PCP: *Pneumocystis carinii* pneumonia; CMV: cytomegalovirus; KS: Kaposi's sarcoma.
[a]Includes oral candidiasis.
[b]Patients with respiratory disease were under-represented.
[c]Non-specific 'pneumonia'.
(Modified from O'Farrell *et al.*, 1995; Grant, 1996; Kumarasamy *et al.*, 1998a; Hira *et al.*, 1998).

were PCP (21%), tuberculosis (20%), toxoplasmosis (14%), oesophageal candidiasis (13%) and cryptococcal meningitis (11%) (O'Farrell *et al.*, 1995).

Tuberculosis. The HIV epidemic has had a major effect on the incidence and prevalence of tuberculosis in the developing world and has challenged tuberculosis control programmes. In Thailand, the prevalence of tuberculosis started to decline from a peak of 58 cases per 100 000 people in 1983 to 28 cases per 100 000 people in 1991. However, with the onset of the HIV epidemic it has increased back up to 50 cases per 100 000 people in 1993. The increase in prevalence in northern Thailand was from 30 to 43.4 cases per 100 000 people between 1987 and 1995, corresponding to the rise in the HIV epidemic. In India, pulmonary tuberculosis is the most common opportunistic infection among HIV-infected persons (Kumarasamy *et al.*, 1995). Conversely, there has been a sharp rise of prevalence of HIV infection among patients with tuberculosis, particularly in northern Thailand, where HIV seroprevalence rose from 5.4% in 1989 to 41% in 1994 (Paliphat *et al.*, 1997a). This increase in HIV-related tuberculosis has also been observed in Africa (Raviglione *et al.*, 1997). The proportion of HIV-infected patients with a tuberculin skin test reaction greater than 5 mm varies from 20 to 80% (Suwanagool *et al.*, 1995; Yanai *et al.*, 1997). Whether this is due to the differences in antigen, the technique being used or a population bias is not known. The benefits of tuberculin skin tests to identify latent TB infection and implement TB chemoprophylaxis in HIV-infected patients in Thailand and India requires further investigation.

Among Thai HIV-infected patients extrapulmonary TB, in particular lymphadenitis, is much more common than pulmonary tuberculosis (Ruxrungtham *et al.*, 1996). Although TB can occur at any stage during the course of HIV infection, it is more common in patients with advanced HIV disease. In one cohort, 81.6% of patients co-infected with TB and HIV-1 had CD4 lymphocyte counts of less than 400 cells/μl, and 60.5% had CD4 lymphocyte counts of less than 200 cells/μl (Uthaivoravit *et al.*, 1994). Other studies have found tuberculosis predominantly in more advanced HIV-infected patients, CD4 lymphocyte counts of below 200 cells/μl (median of 64 cells/μl) (Ruxrungtham *et al.*, 1996; Saenghirunvattana, 1996). In a case–control study of pulmonary tuberculosis, there was no difference in the frequency of pyrexia, dyspnoea, cough or haemoptysis. However cavitating lesions and upper zone infiltrates were observed significantly less often in the HIV-infected group (Hongthiamthong et al., 1994). Middle- and lower-lobe infiltrate and mediastinal lymphadenitis were observed in the chest radiographs of 72.3% of pulmonary TB patients (Kumarasamy et al., 1995). Direct smear positivity is comparable between both HIV-infected and HIV-uninfected patients. Cutaneous hypersensitivity reactions and drug-induced hepatitis tend to occur more often in treated HIV-infected patients than in uninfected persons. The culture conversion rate was satisfactory among patients who complete treatment. Table 36.2 compares the clinical features of tuberculosis in non-HIV and HIV-infected persons (Chuchottharworn, 1996).

Pneumocystis carinii *pneumonia.* Although the incidence of PCP as an AIDS-defining illness in Australia and the USA is approximately 50%, the reported incidence in developing countries in Asia and Africa is much lower, ranging from 3 to 13.4%. The very low incidence rates in Africa probably reflect a lack of diagnostic services, although geographical variation in prevalence may be a contributing factor (Grant et al., 1997; Hira et al., 1998; Kumarasamy et al., 1998b).

Cryptococcosis. Cryptococcal meningitis has been reported in 18.7% of patients in a Thai cohort (Chariyalertsak et al., 1997) but in only 1.9% of 1820 patients in India (Hira et al., 1998) and 1–3% of two African hospital studies of HIV-related admissions (Grant et al., 1997). This wide variation may represent geographical differences in distribution of the fungus.

Penicilliosis. Penicilliosis is a unique disseminated infection, caused by the dimorphic fungus *Penicillium marneffei* and is the fifth most common opportunistic infection in Thai HIV-infected adults. This infection is endemic in Southeast Asia, (mainly northern Thailand and southern China) (Supparatpinyo et al., 1994) but is rare in India. *Rhizomys sumatrensis* and *Cannomys badius,* both bamboo rats, may be important animal hosts for this fungus (Chariyalertsak et al., 1996a). Penicilliosis is rarely found in HIV-uninfected individuals but has been occasionally reported in non-HIV immunocompromised patients. It is considered an AIDS-defining illness according to the guidelines of the Thai Department of Communicable Disease Control (CDC) (Ministry of Public Health, Thailand, 1997). With the increasing incidence of HIV infection in Thailand, *Penicillium marneffei* emerged as an important HIV-associated opportunistic infection in HIV-infected patients residing in northern Thailand (Supparatpinyo, 1992b; Imwidthaya, 1994). *P. marneffei* infections appear to be more frequent in the rainy season than in the dry season (Chariyalertsak et al., 1996b).

The most common symptoms and signs at presentation (Table 36.3) are fever (99%), anaemia (78%), weight loss (76%), and skin lesions (71%). Lymphadenopathy (58%) and hepatomegaly (51%) are also common findings. Most patients (up to 90%) present with generalized skin lesions, consisting of papules with central umbilication, (described as molluscum contagiosum-like or papulonecrotic lesions), as illustrated in Figure 36.1 (Sirisanthana, 1997).

In HIV-1 infected children, common clinical and laboratory features of penicilliosis include generalized

Table 36.2 Comparison of clinical features of tuberculosis in non-HIV and HIV-infected patients

Comparison	TB alone	TB in early HIV disease	TB in late HIV disease
Clinical	Non-specific	Weight loss and fever more prominent	Other stigmata of late HIV infection
Extrapulmonary	Uncommon	20%	More than 50%
Chest X-ray	Apical disease with cavities common	Apical disease with cavities, adenopathy	Hilar adenopathy, lower lobe infiltrates, diffuse interstitial, milliary, pleural effusion
Tuberculin test	Positive > 95%	Positive 80%	Positive 20%
Bacteriology	Positive > 85%; bacteraemia very rare	Positive > 95%; bacteraemia 25–42%	Positive 60%; bacteraemia common; bone marrow culture positive, stool culture positive

(Modified from Chuchottharworn, 1996.)

lymphadenopathy (90%), hepatomegaly (90%), fever of higher than 38.5°C (81%), papular skin lesions with central umbilication (67%), splenomegaly (67%), failure to thrive (52%), severe anaemia (haemoglobin of less than 60 g/litre) (43%) and thrombocytopenia (platelet count of less than 0.5×10^{11}/litre) (21%) (Sirisanthana *et al.*, 1995b).

As the skin lesions of penicilliosis may not be easily distinguished from other systemic fungal infections such as cryptococcosis or histoplasmosis, diagnosis is based on the demonstration of the organism in clinical specimens. Presumptive diagnosis can be made by microscopic examination of Wright's-stained touch smears of skin biopsy (Figure 36.2) and/or bone marrow aspirate or lymph node biopsy specimens (Imwidthaya 1994; Supparatpinyo and Sirisanthana, 1994). Presumptive diagnosis can also be made by microscopic examination of a Wright's-stained peripheral blood smear, which may show many yeast cells present within neutrophils, some with clear central septation (Supparatpinyo *et al.*, 1994). These diagnostic approaches may allow the commencement of antifungal therapy prior to the availability of culture results and may reduce morbidity and mortality. Cultures from clinical specimens (Figure 36.3) will commonly yield a definitive diag-

nosis of *Penicillium marneffei*. Bone marrow culture is found to be the most sensitive (100%) diagnostic method, followed by skin biopsy (90%) and blood culture (76%) (Sirisanthana, 1997).

A few cases of penicilliosis acquired in Thailand among European HIV-infected persons have been noted. Therefore, HIV-infected patients having travelled to Southeast Asia (especially northern Thailand and southern China) and presenting with fever, skin lesions (Figure 36.4), hepatomegaly, lymphadenopathy, productive cough or lung disease should be investigated for *Penicillium marneffei* infection (Hilmarsdottir *et al.*, 1993; Viviani *et al.*, 1993; Julander and Petrini, 1997).

Non-typhoidal salmonella septicemia. This has been reported in 8.2% of 866 Thai patients (Hira *et al.*, 1998) and in 6–12% of five cohorts comprising 809 African hospital admissions (Grant *et al.*, 1997).

Mycobacterium avium complex. Mycobacterium avium complex (MAC) is an uncommon opportunistic infection among Thai patients with AIDS, possibly due to shorter survival of most patients with advanced HIV infection, lack of appropriate diagnostic techniques and because tubercu-

Table 36.3 Characteristic features and management of penicilliosis

Causative organism	*Penicillium marneffei*, a dimorphic fungus
Endemic area	South East Asia, especially northern Thailand, southern China
Reservoir	Bamboo rats, soil
Clinical features	Adults: fever (99%), papulonecrotic skin lesions (71%), weight loss (76%), anaemia (77%), lymphadenopathy (58%), hepatomegaly (51%), productive cough, lung disease
	Children: generalized lymphadenopathy (90%), hepatomegaly (90%) fever higher than 38.5°C (81%) papular skin lesions with central umbilication (67%), splenomegaly (67%) failure to thrive (52%), severe anaemia (Hb < 60 g) (43%), thrombocytopenia (21%)
Diagnosis	Presumptive: Wright's staining of skin scraping or biopsy, bone marrow or lymph node aspiration or biopsy, shows oval organism (size 3–5 μm), some with septum (see Figure 36.3); role of immunodiagnosis under investigation
	Definitive: bone marrow culture most sensitive (100%), followed by culture from skin biopsy (90%) and blood culture (76%)
Treatment	Amphotericin B 0.5 mg/kg/day for 6–8 weeks or amphotericin B 0.5 mg/kg/day for 2 weeks followed by itraconazole 400 mg oral daily for 10 weeks. Mild cases. Itraconazole 400 mg/day for 8 weeks, Ketoconazole anecdotally comparable to itraconazole in efficacy, more controlled data required
	Fluconazole: despite a report of successful treatment (Liu *et al.*, 1994), a study showed low susceptibility with high failure rate of up to 64%
Prognosis	High mortality if diagnosis and treatment delayed
Secondary prophylaxis	Itraconazole 100–200 mg/day for life to prevent high rate of relapse

(Modified from Imwidthaya, 1994; Supparatpinyo *et al.*, 1994; Chariyalertsak *et al.*, 1996b; Kantipong, 1996; Kaufman *et al.*, 1996; Sirisanthana, 1997; Ungsedhaphan, 1998.)

losis is endemic in Thailand. Recently, however, with more awareness and better culture technique, 22 cases of MAC in AIDS patients have been reported. Additionally, 22% of blood or bone-marrow specimens from HIV-infected patients with chronic fever and/or weight loss were found to be positive on culture for MAC (Sathapatayakul and Tansupsawasdikul, 1996). Clinical features of MAC in HIV-infected Thai patients are similar to those of western patients. The incidence of MAC may rise in certain developing countries with improving early diagnosis, treatment and prophylaxis of opportunistic infections and access to antiretroviral therapy.

Rhodococcus. Rhodococcosis is caused by the coccobacillus *Rhodococcus equi* (Verville *et al.*, 1994; Golub *et al.*, 1967). It was not reported in Thailand until 1993–1995, during which time 29 cases, mostly in HIV-infected patients, were found in Chiang Mai (Sirisanthana , 1996). Almost all cases had pulmonary involvement, except one patient with a pyopericardium. Common clinical features were subacute onset of high fever, malaise and cough, which is usually productive; some patients had pleurisy and haemoptysis. Most patients also had oral candidiasis and few had either concurrent PCP or salmonella septicaemia. Chest X-ray findings commonly showed dense pulmonary infiltration, sometimes with cavitation. Differential diagnosis includes TB, other causes of pneumonia and lung abscess. It is important for physicians in the developing world to be aware of rhodococcosis as it may be an emerging opportunistic infection in the near future, if the more common opportunistic infections become amenable to early treatment and prophylaxis.

Toxoplasmosis. In several studies of patients in southeast Asia, toxoplasmosis accounted for 4–18.6% of AIDS-defining illness (Hira, 1998).

Cryptosporidium. In one study of 45 Thai AIDS patients, cryptosporidium was the most common cause of chronic diarrhoea (20%). Of note, other pathogens were TB (intestine and colon) (18%), *Salmonella* sp. (16%), CMV (11%), *Mycobacterium avium intracellulare* (MAI; 7%), strongyloidiasis, giardiasis, cryptococcosis, histoplasmosis, campylobacter and cyclospora (Manatsathit *et al.*, 1996). The prevalence of cryptosporidiosis in a study of children and adults was 19% and 8%, respectively. The common features of cryptosporidiosis were chronic diarrhoea (85%), usually watery diarrhoea and weight loss or malnutrition (100%) (Moolasart *et al.*, 1995). Among African AIDS patients with diarrhoea, cryptosporidium was the causative organism in 6–59% across seven studies (Grant *et al.*, 1997).

HIV-related malignancies. In Thailand and India, the incidence of two HIV-related non-Hodgkin's lymphoma (NHL) and Kaposi's sarcoma (KS) is low (< 2%) (Sivayathorn *et al.*, 1995; Kumarasamy *et al.*, 1995). A higher incidence of KS (11%) was observed in a cohort of AIDS-related hospital inpatients in Jakarta (Samsuridjal *et al.*, 1997). However, the incidence and prevalence of KS is much higher in Africa and was considered to be the cause of death in 16% of 51 AIDS patients in Zaïre (Nelson *et al.*, 1993). NHL was present in 3% of AIDS autopsies in Côte d'Ivoire. Patients usually die of other opportunistic infections before NHL develops (Lucas *et al.*, 1994; Grant *et al.*, 1997).

Clinical evaluation of HIV in developing countries

Many patients in the developing world will progress to AIDS and often die before a diagnosis of HIV infection is made. The main objectives of evaluating a patient with definite or suspected HIV infection are the early diagnosis and treatment of opportunistic or other infections, the consideration of whether antiretroviral therapy (if available) or primary prophylaxis of opportunistic infection needs to be initiated, and for patient education to reduce transmission. As in all clinical environments, evaluation consists of clinical history, physical examination and laboratory evaluation if available. Special attention should be paid to the diagnosis of AIDS-defining conditions of high local prevalence, serious conditions with high mortality if untreated and easily treatable conditions such as bacterial pneumonia or diarrhoea (see Tables 36.1 and 36.4).

The time of estimated HIV seroconversion and first HIV serodiagnosis is often not available but should be elicited to estimate the duration of HIV infection. Details of past medical illnesses should be obtained, especially other sexually transmitted infections, constitutional symptoms (chronic fever, diarrhoea, weight loss), shingles, and any opportunistic or other infections found in late-stage HIV disease. History of drug allergy and an impression of the patient's ability to adhere to treatment is also important. The suspected route of acquired HIV infection should be included to complete the medical record and for future natural history studies, although this will not play a role in patient care.

The physical examination should include the oral cavity, lymph nodes, skin, lung, central nervous system (CNS), eye and abdomen. Common findings important for clinical staging and consideration of further treatment are summarized in Table 36.4. Examination of the oral cavity is crucial, as it can provide rapid informative clinical data for assessment of the immune status of the patient. OHL, oral candidiasis, herpetic or aphthous ulcers and severe gingivitis are common oral disorders among symptomatic HIV-infected patients, both in the developing world and in Western countries. Persistent generalized lymphadenopathy, with nodes usually less than 2 cm in diameter, is common. Patients with asymmetrical lymphadenopathy greater than 2 cm in diameter should be investigated for TB lymphadenitis, systemic mycosis and lymphoma. Particular attention should be given to the presence of the common dermatological disorders found in symptomatic HIV disease: old scars or new lesions of shingles, PPEs (see Figure 34.1), papulonecrotic or molluscum-like lesions suggesting systemic mycosis, and seborrhoeic dermatitis. Hepatomegaly and/or abdominal mass suggests mesenteric lymphadenopathy associated with disseminated tuberculosis, mycosis or lymphoma. Patients presenting with dry cough, tachypnoea or dyspnoea (especially on exertion), fever, with or without abnormal lung signs should be investigated for PCP if possible. The presence of fever with productive cough, with or without dyspnoea suggests tuberculosis. Empirical treatment for the most likely cause should be initiated if precise diagnosis may be delayed. Clinical symptoms and signs may suggest meningitis and increased intracranial pressure (fever, headache, vomiting) and possible localized neurological signs may suggest common CNS infections such as cryptococcal meningitis, toxoplasmosis or lymphoma. Symptoms and signs of peripheral neuropathy may also be present, due to HIV infection or from certain antiretroviral therapies. As in developed countries, fundoscopic examination is recommended at least every 3 months in patients with advanced HIV disease or with CD4 lymphocyte counts below 100 cells/μl, for the early diagnosis of CMV retinitis. However, the costly treatment and poor access to therapy for CMV infection for most HIV-infected patients in developing countries means that CMV disease will often remain untreated.

Laboratory monitoring of HIV

General laboratory assessments

Complete blood count and liver function tests (LFTs) (in particular, SGOT and SGPT) and serum amylase should be considered for patients on antiretroviral drugs or treatment for opportunistic infections, to monitor drug-related toxicity. Nevertheless, in a resource-poor setting, LFTs and serum amylase are usually omitted, unless hepatotoxicity or pancreatitis is clinically suspected. Anaemia is common in the developing world in people without HIV infection, usually due to poor diet and parasitic infestation. Therefore exclusion of anaemia is important, even in a resource-poor setting.

HIV prognostic markers

In asymptomatic patients, laboratory testing is required to assess immune function. CD4 lymphocyte counts and plasma HIV-1 RNA (or viral load) are two laboratory

Table 36.4 Common clinical findings in Thai and Indian patients with early symptomatic HIV-1 infection

Clinical manifestation	Frequency (%)	Usual CD4 lymphocyte count (per μl)	Comments
Shingles (reactivated herpes zoster)	16–17	300	Usually more than one dermatone involved
Oral hairy leukoplakia (OHL)	15–45	350	
Oral candidiasis	26–34	< 300	
Pruritic papular eruption (PPE)	27–33	< 200	No cause identified
Constitutional symptoms	10	< 300	If no other cause identified
Seborrhoeic dermatitis	6–21	< 200	More extensive, more atypical than non-HIV-infected patients

(Modified from Sivayathorn *et al.*, 1995; Ruxrungtham *et al.*, 1996.)

parameters that have been shown to be independent predictors for HIV disease progression and survival (Mellors *et al.*, 1997). CD4 lymphocyte counts should be performed if locally available at least every 6 months, primarily for consideration of initiation of prophylaxis for opportunistic infections, antiretroviral therapy if available and to monitor the response to therapy. The normal range of CD4 lymphocyte counts in the Thai population is 900 ± 300 cells/μl (Vithayasai *et al.*, 1997) and in Indian patients the range is 290–2600 (Speciality Ranbaxy Laboratory Services, Mumbai, India). However a comparative of HIV-infected adults in France and west Africa found the CD4 lymphocyte counts in the West African patients were one-third higher than in French patients. CD4 lymphocyte counts can be performed manually, and this is a cheaper alternative to the more expensive flow cytometry analysis. The assessment of total lymphocyte count or percentage can also be used as a cheap alternative to a CD4 lymphocyte count in developing countries, but the low sensitivity and specificity of this test may limit clinical application. A total lymphocyte count of less than 1000 cells/μl correlates approximately with a CD4 lymphocyte count of less than 200 cells/μl, when prophylaxis for opportunistic infections should be considered (Stewart *et al.*, 1996; Kumarasamy *et al.*, 1998a). It is essential that laboratories in each country establish their own reference ranges for T-lymphocyte subsets and total lymphocyte counts.

There are presently three commercially available HIV-1 viral load assays: Amplicor Monitor (RT-PCR, Roche Diagnostic Laboratories), Quantiplex (bDNA, Bayer Diagnostics) and NucliSens (NASBA, Organon Teknika), which cost on average US$130 per test – beyond the financial means of most patients or health budgets of developing countries. Interpretation of results may be problematic due to differences in assay performance with different subtypes of HIV-1 present in Asia and Africa (Ubolyam *et al.*, 1998). Viral load testing is therefore unavailable for the majority of HIV-infected persons in developing countries.

Assessment of latent or active opportunistic infections

There are a number of clinical and laboratory investigations that should be done to exclude latent infectious diseases, reactivation of latent infections or opportunistic diseases. These include the VDRL to exclude syphilis co-infection, chest X-ray, sputum smear for acid-fast bacilli and tuberculin skin test to exclude tuberculosis and chest X-ray and induced sputum examination to diagnose PCP. Early and appropriate prophylaxis and treatment of these infections are of major importance in the management of HIV-infected patients in resource-limited countries, where accessibility to antiretroviral therapy is poor.

Treatment

Prevention of perinatal transmission

The administration of antiretroviral drugs to women in the late stage of pregnancy has been shown to significantly reduce transmission of HIV from mothers to their babies (see also Chapters 8 and 9). In a large, randomized placebo-controlled study of 363 deliveries in HIV-infected pregnant women, the proportion of infants infected when zidovudine (ZDV) was given to mothers antipartum, during delivery and to the infants for 6 weeks was 8.3% compared to 25.5 % in the placebo group. This represents a 67.5% reduction in transmission (Connor *et al.*, 1994). A Thai study showed that a shorter regimen of oral ZDV from 36 weeks of gestation until delivery, with no neonatal treatment can reduce transmission by 50% (Centers for Disease Control and Prevention, 1998). Recently, another study has shown that shorter courses of perinatal treatment with ZDV may be just as effective, as the perinatal transmission rate where ZDV was commenced prepartum, intrapartum and within 2 days after delivery was 6.1%, 10.0% and 9.3%, respectively (Wade *et al.*, 1998). Antiretroviral therapy during the perinatal period is now considered the most cost-effective use of the limited drug budget (Stewart *et al.*, 1996; Colebunders *et al.*, 1997).

Primary prophylaxis of opportunistic infections (see Table 36.5)

In the developing world, primary prophylaxis of PCP is cheap and effective, due to the general availability and low cost of trimethoprim-sulfamethoxazole (co-trimoxazole; TMP-SMX) and also protection against toxoplasmosis. The usual dose is two standard tablets (80–400 mg) daily, administered to persons who have developed any opportunistic infection or HIV-related illness and also asymptomatic individuals with CD4 lymphocyte counts of less than 200 cells/μl. A study of 207 patients who had followed regular co-trimoxazole daily prophylaxis showed no PCP during the 2-year study period and also reductions in bacterial and diarrhoeal diseases (Kumarasamy *et al.*, 1998b). However, co-trimoxazole prophylaxis was relatively ineffective in a study in Senegal (Maynart *et al.*, 2001). In developing countries, co-trimoxazole prophylaxis will play a major role in delaying disease progression.

For prophylaxis against tuberculosis, primary prophylaxis with isoniazid 300 mg/day is cheap and readily available. Isoniazid prophylaxis is used in Thailand if the tuberculin skin test suggests latent tuberculosis, even if the chest X-ray is normal. The efficacy of this measure of TB prevention is under investigation. Prophylaxis of other opportunistic infections such as cryptococcosis, MAC and CMV infection is beyond the resources of most developing countries.

Treatment of opportunistic infections
Tuberculosis. The Thai CDC clinical management guidelines (Ministry of Public Health, Thailand, 1997) recommend a 6-month course of therapy including four drugs for the first 2 months – isoniazid, rifampicin, ethambutol and pyrazinamide – followed by two drugs for the next 4 months – isoniazid and rifampicin. In cases of extrapulmonary tuberculosis, parenteral streptomycin is used for 3 weeks, with administration of the other four drugs for a period of 12 months. Patients' adherence to treatment is the most important factor for the success of therapy. Therefore, directly supervised or observed therapy is highly recommended, in particular for patients where adherence may become a difficult issue.

The rates of resistance to antituberculous drugs in HIV-infected individuals are not different, except for streptomycin, which is higher in HIV-infected than uninfected patients. Between 1985 and 1990, the prevalence of multiple drug-resistant tuberculosis (MDR-TB) in Thailand was only 0.15–1.4%. Since then the prevalence rate has increased to 1.7–10% in different cohorts (Paliphat *et al.*, 1997b). Most of the large cohorts report a prevalence rate of MDR-TB of approximately 5% (Thanakitjaru *et al.*, 1996; Paliphat *et al.*, 1997b). The risk of developing MDR-TB is related to a history of previous TB therapy (odds ratio 2.8, 95% CI, 4.75–34.90), but not related to the presence of HIV infection (Hongthiamthong *et al.*, 1994; Thanakitjaru *et al.*, 1996).

Pneumocystis carinii pneumonia. PCP should be treated using standard regimens, as outlined in Chapter 25, with consideration given to oral high-dose TMP-SMX in patients with less severe presentations, to reduce hospitalization and the associated costs of intravenous therapy. However, these patients may need close outpatient monitoring.

Penicilliosis. In one Thai study, the observed response rates to amphotericin B (0.3–0.6 mg/kg/day for 8 weeks) itraconazole (400 mg/day), and fluconazole (400 mg/day) were 77 %, 75%, and 36%, respectively (Supparatpinyo *et al.*, 1993). Another Thai study showed that treatment with amphotericin B followed by itraconazole is generally well tolerated and successful, with a 97% response rate; therefore this is recommended as a cost-effective approach to shorten hospitalization (Sirisanthana *et al.*, 1998). However, in mild cases of penicilliosis with no respiratory failure or shock, itraconazole may be used as an initial treatment (Supparatpinyo *et al.*, 1992a). Clinical response will usually appear within 2 weeks of therapy (see Table 36.3 for recommended dosing and regimens). Ketoconazole following a parenteral course of amphotericin B has been shown anecdotally to be effective; nevertheless, further study is required (Peto *et al.*, 1998). Delayed diagnosis and treatment can lead to a high mortality.

Rhodococcus. Based on *in vitro* susceptibility, *Rhodococcus equi* is resistant to all penicillins and cephalosporin agents but is usually sensitive to erythromycin, rifampicin, vancomycin, gentamicin, amikacin, ciprofloxacin and ofloxacin. Treatment with antibiotics should be continued for at least 2 months and lifelong secondary prophylaxis is recommended.

Secondary prophylaxis of opportunistic infections (see Table 36.6)
The secondary prophylaxis of PCP presents no problems due to the low cost of TMP-SMX, but the cost of secondary prophylaxis of cryptococcosis is considerable. In one Bangkok hospital where 50% of inpatients had cryptococcal infection, the cost of secondary prophylaxis ranged from US$5 to 16/day/patient, too high for most countries with limited resources. The cost may even discourage the initial treatment of this infection (Stewart *et al.*, 1996).

In penicilliosis, 15% of patients relapsed within 6 months of cessation of treatment. Therefore lifelong secondary prophylaxis with oral itraconazole (100–200 mg/day) is recommended (Supparatpinyo *et al.*, 1993; Ministry of Public Health, Thailand, 1997). In a pediatric cohort, no relapse was observed in patients given ketoconazole as secondary prophylaxis (Sirisanthana *et al.*, 1995b).

Antiretroviral therapy
Although many antiretroviral drugs commonly used in the West are licensed and available in developing countries, few

Table 36.5 Primary prophylaxis for opportunistic diseases in Thailand.

Pathogen	Indication(s)	First Choice prophylactic regimens	Alternative prophylactic regimens	Comments
Pneumocystis carinii	CD4 lymphocyte count less than 200 cells/μl	Cotrimoxazole, 2 single-strength or	Dapsone 100 mg/day or	Most cost-effective widely implemented regimen in Thailand
	Oropharyngeal candidiasis	1 double-strength, p.o. daily	Aerosolized pentamidine 300 mg monthly via Respigard II™ nebulizer	For patients who develop skin rash, desensitization should be performed; high success rates have been shown
	Other AIDS-defining illness			
M. tuberculosis	TST reaction ≥ 5 mm	Isoniazid, 300 mg plus pyridoxine 50 mg p.o. daily for 12 months		Exclude active tuberculosis
	Prior positive result without treatment			Evaluate potential patient adherence to this long duration – if in doubt, avoid starting prophylaxis
	Contact with case of active tuberculosis			
Toxoplasma gondii	Toxoplasma IgG positive and CD4 lymphocyte count of less than 100 cells/μl	The same as PCP prophylaxis, as will cross-protect against toxoplasmosis	Dapsone 50 mg p.o./day plus pyrimethamine, 50 mg p.o., weekly	

TST: tuberculin skin test. PCP: *Pneumocyslis carinii* pneumonia.
(Modified from Centers for Disease Control and Prevention, 1997; Ministry of Public Health, Thailand, 1997.)

individual patients or public health departments can afford them. In sub-Saharan Africa, the provision of triple combination antiretroviral therapy would be estimated to cost more than 25% of the gross national product in several countries (Hogg *et al.*, 1997) and in some Asian countries, the annual health expenditure *per capita* is less than $10 per year (Arya, 1998). However, in some countries, such as Thailand, the cost of antiretroviral drugs can be reduced by local manufacture. Recent Thai National Guidelines (Ministry of Public Health, Thailand, 1997) have considered dual nucleoside reverse transcriptase inhibitors (NRTIs) as standard of care for treatment of HIV-infected persons in this setting. Although dual NRIT regimens have been shown to have clinical benefit over ZDV monotherapy (Delta Co-ordinating Committee, 1996; Hammer *et al.*, 1996), current evidence has shown that these are now considered suboptimal regimens, as significantly fewer patients experience durable virological responses with plasma HIV-1 RNA below the lower limit of detection, com-

pared with those receiving triple therapy (Hammer *et al.*, 1997).

As many patients in developing countries are smaller in body weight compared with Caucasians (60 ± 10 kg in Thailand), there is a need to evaluate whether dose reduction of antiretroviral regimens can be effective in HIV-infected patients in the developing world. However, a study of half-dose ZDV/zalcitabine revealed that the low dose in Thailand was significantly less effective than the full doses at 48 weeks and the percentage of patients with undetectable HIV RNA (below 400 copies/ml) in the half-dose and the full dose groups was 26% and 52%, respectively (Kroon *et al.*, 1998). In another Thai study of several stavudine/didanosine dose combinations, regimens containing the recommended dose of didanosine (ddI) showed a significant better antiviral activity in comparison to that of the low-dose ddI regimens (Ruxrungtham *et al.*, 1998). These studies indicate that although Asians have smaller body weights in general, there is a risk of giving suboptimal treatment regimens if one reduces the recommended dose to reduce cost.

There is no doubt that potent antiretroviral regimens should be recommended worldwide (Wadman, 2001). The WHO recommendation of dual nucleosides as first-line therapy was considered inappropriate by Western experts (Rhone et al., 1998). The real issue of antiretroviral therapy in the developing world is accessibility due to the high cost of the drugs, especially the protease inhibitors (PIs). Both local and worldwide efforts are needed to improve accessibility to antiretroviral treatment. Recent Thai guidelines for antiretroviral therapy considered dual NRTs as first-line therapy in resource-limited patients (Ministry of Public Health, Thailand, 1997). Arguments for and against this approach are listed in Table 36.7. Studies and our clinical observations suggest that patients at the inter-mediate stage of HIV infection with CD4 lymphocyte counts of 100–500 cells/μl and plasma HIV-1 RNA below 4.5 $\log_{10}$ copies/ml will have a good rate of both clinical and virological response to dual nucleoside therapy (Hammer et al., 1996; Kroon et al., 1998; Ruxrungtham et al., 1998). In countries where triple drug regimens cannot be implemented, studies evaluating the efficient use of a dual nucleoside regimens, including when to start, what to start with, when and what to switch to, are urgently needed, as are studies examining which markers can predict a beneficial outcome are required. It is likely that for many countries, Western standard guidelines can not be applied. The issues of education, prevention and surveillance of transmission of drug-resistant viruses are even more essential in a resource-limited environment, where less potent antiretroviral treatments form the standard of care.

Table 36.6 Secondary prophylaxis for opportunistic diseases recommended by Ministry of Public Health, Thailand

Pathogen	Indication	First choice	Alternative prophylactic regimens	Comments
Pneumocystis carinii	Prior PCP	Cotrimoxazole, two single-strength, p.o., or one double-strength p.o. daily; duration: for life	Dapsone 100 mg p.o., daily or aerosolized pentamidine 300 mg p.o., via Respigard II™ nebulizer; duration: for life	For patients who develop skin rash, densensitization should be performed; high success rate has been shown
Toxoplasma gondii	Prior toxoplasmic encephalitis	Sulfadiazine, 500 mg four times/day plus pyrimethamine 25 mg four times/day	If intolerance to sulfadiazine, clindamycin (150 mg) two or three tablets orally four times daily plus pyrimethamine, 25 mg four times daily, duration: for life	Haematological complications uncommon in Thai population
Cryptococcus neoformans	Documented systemic disease	Fluconazole, 200 mg/day Duration: for life.	Amphotericin B 1 mg/kg i.v., weekly for life	
Penicillium marneffei	Documented disease	Itraconazole, 200 mg p.o., daily		
MAC	Documented disease	Azithromycin, 1250 mg (five capsules) single-dose, weekly; duration: for life	Clarithromycin 500 mg twice daily; duration: for life	Some experts prefer to add ethambutol 15 mg/kg/day
CMV	Prior disease	Ganciclovir 5 mg/kg, i.v. 5 days/week	Foscarnet, 0.1 ml intravitreous weekly or foscarnet, 90 mg/kg/day i.v	Very few patients or health budgets in developing countries can afford this regimen

PCP: Pneumocystis carinii pneumonia; MAC: Mycobacterium avium complex; CMV: cytomegalovirus.

Table 36.7 Arguments for and against the provision of dual nucleoside antiretroviral therapy as a standard of care in developing countries

Arguments for use	Arguments against use
Less expensive and more affordable in intermediate income countries	Considered as a sub-optimal regimen; will compromise future options when virological failure occurs
Proven clinical benefit, both in reduction of AIDS progression and AIDS-related death in patients who are at intermediate stage of HIV disease[a]	Clinical benefit is only of short to intermediate duration
Less toxicity and drug interactions, compared to triple drug therapy	High risk of developing NRTI resistance and/or multidrug resistance

NRTI: Nucleoside reverse transcriptase inhibitor.
(From Delta Co-ordinating Committee, 1996; Hammer *et al.*, 1996.)

Treatment of coexistent sexually transmitted diseases

The early detection and treatment of other STDs should form part of an effective anti-HIV strategy, especially in the developing world (Centers for Disease Control and Prevention, 1998). One large, randomized study in Tanzania showed that the group with an effective STD intervention programme had a 38% reduction (1.2% versus 1.9%) in seroconversions to HIV over a 2-year period (Grosskurth *et al.*, 1996). In contrast, another study using a different design of intermittent, episodic versus continued enhanced treatment of symptomatic STDs found no difference in HIV incidence between the two groups (Wawer *et al.*, 1998). However, the two studies were in populations of differing HIV prevalence: 4% in the Tanzanian study versus 16% in the Ugandan study, which could explain the difference between these results (Centers for Disease Control and Prevention, 1998).

An integrated model of HIV care

The premises upon which an integrated care model should function are:

(1) Significant symptom control is attainable at low cost.

(2) The cost of patient care decreases with training and experience of doctors.

(3) The early detection of HIV optimizes opportunistic infection prophylaxis.

(4) Management should focus on common opportunistic infections and on reducing maternal–fetal transmission.

(5) Antiretrovirals should be used only if affordable and provision of antiretrovirals to prevent mother–child transmission is already in place.

(6) Provision of a continuum of care using a multidisciplinary team.

(7) Enhancement of universal infection control precautions at all medical establishments.

A model of care in resource-poor settings with interaction between self-help groups, voluntary counselling and testing, health-care facilities, community-based care and home care has been described (Osborne, 1996). Depending on a particular country's resources, different care levels can be provided in a hierarchy, from the provision of the most basic levels of HIV testing, counselling, education and access to support groups through to the delivery of basic care within existing services and some specific HIV clinical services through to the provision of specialized HIV care, including antiretroviral therapy and advanced diagnostic facilities (Gilks *et al.*, 1997).

Counselling

Social stigmatization may exacerbate feelings of depression and damage the self-esteem of HIV-infected people, with possible consequences for their physical health. Discrimination against people with HIV may also affect their health by denying them such things as employment or housing. Lack of social support from family and in the workplace adds greatly to the stress of their HIV-infected status. The family and carers of a person with HIV will be affected by the disease. Shock, denial, anger, depression and other psychological reactions may affect their health and have an impact upon their ability to care for the HIV-infected individual. It can help doctors if they see their HIV-infected patients as living with the disease, rather than dying of it. Certainly, a positive attitude to being HIV-infected will make the most of living with HIV.

In extreme cases of depression, suicidal tendencies will be more life-threatening than the HIV infection itself. In general, psychological state can affect quality of life above and beyond the impact of physical illness, either mastering or compounding the adversity of HIV disease. Doctors can achieve much by attention to the quality of life and the psychosocial conditions of their patients.

Nutrition

Good nutrition, especially fruit and vegetables, is especially important for HIV-infected patients. A high-calorie, high-protein diet is encouraged due to increased metabolism and muscle wasting. An adequate fluid intake of boiled cooled water is essential. Intake is best with frequent small quantities, avoiding excessive spices. Raw food or salads are best avoided. Vitamins and minerals (especially vitamins A to E and minerals like selenium, zinc and iron supplements) help to maintain good health in the HIV-infected patient. Smoking and excessive alcohol are harmful and it should be suggested to patients that such money can be better spent on nutritious food and essential medications.

Personal hygiene

A regular dental check-up every 3 months should be encouraged. The tongue should be cleaned and antifungal drops used to prevent candidiasis. The skin and scalp should be kept clean.

Stress reduction and general well-being

Patients should continue to do their regular job, as long as they can, as it can provide funds for good nutrition and medication, as well as helping to keep the mind off other problems. If the job is physically demanding, a change to a less stressful job or part-time work should be advised. Regular exercise is important for an improved sense of well-being, as well as increasing muscle mass and improving sleep, appetite and immune function. Adequate sleep is essential.

Summary

The management of the HIV-infected patient in developing countries provides an enormous challenge to health-care workers, health departments and the affected patients and their communities. An integrated care model based primarily on community, home care and outpatient medical services is essential, with close attention given to cost-effec-

tive therapeutic measures of prophylaxis of common opportunistic infections and if possible, antiretroviral therapy. However, the main focus must still be the prevention of new HIV infections by perinatal, sexual and intravenous drug use-related transmission.

References

Arya SC. (1998). Antiretroviral therapy in countries with low health expenditure [letter]. *Lancet* **351**: 1433–4.

Carr A, Cooper DA. (1997). Primary HIV infection. In: M Sande, P Volberding (eds.) *The medical management of AIDS*. Philadelphia, PA: WB Saunders, 89–106.

Centers for Disease Control and Prevention (CDC). (1997). USPHS/IDSA guidelines for the prevention of opportunistic infections in persons infected with the human immunodeficiency virus. *MMWR* **46**.

CDC. (1998). HIV prevention through early detection and treatment of other sexually transmitted diseases – United States. *MMWR* **47**: July.

Chariyalertsak S, Vanittanakom P, Nelson KE. (1996a). *Rhizomys sumatrensis* and *Cannomys badius*, new natural animal hosts of *Penicillium marneffei*. *J Med Vet Myco* **34**: 105–10.

Chariyalertsak S, Sirisanthana T, Supparatpinyo K *et al.* (1996b). Seasonal variation of disseminated *Penicillium marneffei* infections in northern Thailand: a clue to the reservoir? *J Infect Dis* **173**: 1490–3.

Chariyalertsak S, Nelson KE, Saengwonloey A *et al.* (1997). Comparison of AIDS-defining illnesses among different geographic areas in Thailand. *Fourth International Conference on AIDS in Asia and the Pacific*, Manila.

Chuchottharworn C. (1996). Tuberculosis and HIV infection. In: B Satapatayakul (ed.) *HIV/AIDS in Thailand 1996. Adults and Pediatrics*. Bangkok: Sawicha Karnpim; 30–42.

Colebunders R, Karita E, Taelman H *et al.* (1997). Antiretroviral treatment in Africa. *AIDS* **11**: S107–13.

Connor E, Sperling R, Gelber R *et al.* (1994). Reduction of maternal-infant transmission of human immunodeficiency virus type 1 with zidovudine treatment. *N Engl J Med* **331**: 1173–80.

Delta Coordinating Committee. (1996). Delta: a randomized double-blind controlled trial comparing combinations of zidovudine plus didanosine or zalcitabine with zidovudine alone in HIV-infected individuals. *Lancet* **348**: 283–91.

Deschamps MM, Fitzgerald DW, Pape JW, Johnson W (2000). HIV infection in Haiti: natural history and disease progression. *AIDS* **14**: 2515–21.

Fauci AS, Lane HC. (1998). HIV disease: AIDS and related disorders. In: AS Fauci, E Braunwald, KJ Isselbacher *et al.* (eds). *Harrison's principle of internal medicine*. 14th edition. New York: McGraw-Hill, 1856–971.

Gilks C, Katabira E, DeCock K. (1997). The challenge of providing effective care for HIV/AIDS in Africa. *AIDS* **11**: S99–106.

Golub B, Folk G, Spink WW. (1967). Lung abscess due to *Corynebacterium equi*. Report of first human infection. *Ann Intern Med* **66**: 1174–7.

Grant A, Djomand G, DeCock K. (1997). Natural history and spectrum of disease in adults with HIV/AIDS in Africa. *AIDS* **11**: S43–54.

Grosskurth H, Mosha F, Todd J *et al.* (1996). Impact of improved treatment of sexually transmitted diseases on HIV infection in rural Tanzania: randomised controlled trial. *Lancet* **346**: 530–6.

Hammer SM, Katzenstein DA, Hughes MD et al. (1996). A trial comparing nucleoside monotherapy with combination therapy in HIV-infected adults with CD4 cell counts from 200 to 500 per cubic millimeter. N Engl J Med 335: 1081–90.

Hammer SM, Squires KE, Hughes MD et al. (1997). A controlled trial of 2 nucleosides analogues plus indinavir in persons with human immunodeficiency virus infection and CD4 cell counts (200 per mm³ or less). N Engl J Med 337: 725–33.

Hilmarsdottir I, Meynard JL, Rogeaux O et al. (1993). M. Disseminated Penicillium marneffei infection associated with human immuno deficiency virus: a report of two cases and a review of 35 published cases. J Acquir Immune Defic Syndr Hum Retrovirol 6: 466–71.

Hira S, Dore G, Sirisanthana T. (1998). Clinical spectrum of HIV/AIDS in the Asia-Pacific region. AIDS 12: S145–54.

Hogg R, Anis A, Weber A. (1997). Triple combination therapy in sub-Saharan Africa [letter]. Lancet 350: 1406.

Hongthiamthong P, Riantawan P, Subhannachart P et al. (1994). Clinical aspects and treatment outcome in HIV-associated pulmonary tuberculosis: an experience from a Thai referral centre. J Med Assoc Thailand 77: 520–5.

Imwidthaya P. (1994). Update of Penicillosis marneffei in Thailand [Review article]. Mycopathologia 127: 135–7.

Julander I, Petrini B. (1997). Penicillium marneffei infection in a Swedish HIV-infected immunodeficient narcotic addict. Scand J Infect Dis 29: 320–2.

Kantipong P. (1996). Penicillosis marneffei. In: B Satapatayakul (ed.) HIV/AIDS in Thailand 1996: adult and pediatrics. Bangkok: Sawichs Karnpim, 58–62.

Kaufman L, Standard PG, Jalbert M et al. (1996). Diagnostic antigenemia tests for Penicillosis marneffei. J Clin Microbiol 34: 2503–5.

Kitayaporn D, Tansuphaswadikul S, Lohsomboon P et al. (1996). Survival of AIDS patients in the emerging epidemic in Bangkok, Thailand. J Acquir Immun Def Syndr Hum Retrovirol 11: 77–82.

Kroon E, Ungsedhapand C, Ruxrungtham K. (1998). Study HIV-NAT 001: a randomised double blind trial to evaluate the efficacy of combination antiviral therapy with ZDV 200 mg TID plus ddC 0.75 mg TID versus ZDV 100 mg TID plus ddC 0.375 mg TID for the treatment of HIV-1 infection in a Thai study population. Twelfth World AIDS Conference, Geneva, Switzerland.

Kumarasamy N, Solomon S, Jayaker S. (1995). Spectrum of opportunistic infection among AIDS patients in Tamilnadu, India. Int J STD AIDS 6: 447–9.

Kumarasamy N, Solomon S, Amalraj R et al. (1998a). Correlation between CD4/CD8 and total lymphocyte cell counts to opportunistic infections in persons with HIV/AIDS in Chennai (Madras), India. Twelfth World AIDS Conference, Geneva, Switzerland.

Kumarasamy N, Solomon S, Purnima M et al. (1998b). Effects of trimethoprim sulphamethoxazole prophylaxis in persons with HIV disease in South India. Fourth International Congress on HIV Drug Therapy, Glasgow, Scotland.

Kumarasamy N, Solomon S, Purnima M et al. (2000). Dermatalogical manifestations amony HIV patients in South India. Int J Dermatol 39: 1–4.

Limpakarnjanarat K, Tansuphasawadikul S, Mastro TD et al. (1996). Clinical presentation, risk category, and HIV-1 subtypes B and E in 1241 HIV/AIDS patients in Thailand. Int Conf AIDS, July 11: 235.

Lucas S, Diomande M, Hounnou A et al. (1994). HIV associated lymphoma in Africa: an autopsy study in Cote d'Ivoire. Int J Cancer 156: 202–4.

Manatsathit S, Tansupasawasdikul S, Wanachiwanawin D et al. (1996). Causes of chronic diarrhea in patients with AIDS in Thailand: a prospectiveclinical and microbiological study. J Gastroenterol 31: 533–7.

Mellors JW, Munoz A, Giorgi JV et al. (1997). Plasma viral load and CD4+ lymphocytes as prognostic markers of HIV-1 infection. Ann Intern Med 126: 946–54.

Ministry of Public Health, Thailand. (1997). Guidelines for the clinical management of HIV infection in children/adults. Fifth edition. Bangkok: Kansasana, 136–7.

Moolasart P, Eampokalap B, Ratanasrithong M et al. (1995). Cryptosporidiosis in HIV-infected patients in Thailand. Southeast Asian J Trop Med Pub Health 26: 335–8.

Morgan D, Whitworth J (2001). The natural history of HIV-1 infection in Africa. Nature Medicine 7: 143–5.

Munoz A, Sabine CA, Phillips AN. (1997). The incubation period of AIDS. AIDS 11: S69–76.

Nelson AM, Perriens JH, Kapita B et al. (1993). A clinical and pathological comparison of the WHO and CDC case definitions for AIDS in Kinshasa, Zaire: is passive surveillance valid? AIDS 7: 1241–5.

Nelson KE, Celentano DD, Eiumtrakol S et al. (1996). Changes in sexual behavior and a decline in HIV infection among young men in Thailand. N Engl J Med 335: 297–303.

O'Farrell N, Lau R, Yoganathan K et al. (1995). AIDS in Africans living in London. Genitourin Med 71: 358–62.

Osborne C. (1996). HIV/AIDS in resource poor settings: comprehensive care across a continuum. AIDS 10: S61–7.

Palella FJ, Delaney KM, Moorman AC et al. (1998). Declining morbidity and mortality among patients with advanced human immunodeficiency virus infection. N Engl J Med 338: 853–60.

Paliphat T, Thantives S, Keswit W et al. (1997a). Situation of tuberculosis in Thailand 1995. Thai Weekly Epidemiol Surv Rep 28: 313–26.

Paliphat T, Thantives S, Keswit W et al. (1997b). Situation of multiple drug-resistant tuberculosis in Thailand 1996. Thai Weekly Epidemiol Surv Rep 28: 169–79.

Peto TE, Bull R, Millard PR et al. (1998). Systemic mycosis due to Penicillium marneffei in a patient with antibody to human immunodeficiency virus. J Infect 16: 285–90.

Piot P, Aggleton P. (1998). The global epidemic. AIDS Care 10 (Suppl. 2): S201–8.

Pope M, Frankel SS, Mascola J et al. (1997). Human immunodeficiency virus type 1 strains of subtypes B and E replicate in cutaneous dendritic cell-T-cell mixtures without displaying subtype-specific tropism. J Virol 71: 8001–7.

Raviglione M, deHarries A, Msiska R. et al. (1997). Tuberculosis and HIV: current status in Africa. AIDS 11: S115–23.

Rhone S, Hogg R, Yip B et al. (1998). Do dual nucleoside analogue regimen have a role in an era of plasma viral load-driven antiretroviral therapy? J Infect Dis 178: 662–8.

Ruxrungtham K, Muller O, Sirivichayakul S et al. (1996). AIDS at a University Hospital in Bangkok, Thailand. AIDS 10: 1047–9.

Ruxrungtham K, Ungsedhaphan C, Teeratakulpisarn S et al. (1998). Study HIV-NAT 002: The safety and efficacy of didanosine (ddI) stavudine (d4T) in high/low dose combinations in an antiretroviral therapy naive Thai adult population with CD4 counts 150-350/mm3 and predominantly infected with HIV-1 clade E. Twelfth World AIDS Conference, Geneva, Switzerland.

Saenghirunvattana S. (1996). CD4 + T counts with a course of antituberculous therapy in healthy and HIV-infected patients. J Med Assoc Thai 79: 246–8.

Samsuridjal, Djoerban Z, Lydia A. (1997). HIV infection in Central Hospital Jakarta. *Ninth Annual Conference of the Australasian Society of HIV Medicine*, Adelaide, Australia.

Sathapatayakul B, Tansupsawasdikul S. (1996). *Mycobacterium avium complex (MAC) in patients with AIDS*. In: B Sathapatayakul (ed.) *HIV/AIDS in Thailand 1996: adult and pediatrics*. Bankok: Sawicha Karnpim, 13–19.

Seaton R, Wembri J, Armstrong P et al. (1996). Symptomatic human immunodeficiency virus (HIV) infection in Papua New Guinea. *Aust NZ J Med* **26**: 783–8.

Sirisanthana V. (1995). Opportunistic infections in HIV-infected children at Chiang Mai University Hospital, Chiang Mai Thailand. *J Infect Dis Antimicrob Agents* **12**: 59–62.

Sirisanthana T. (1996). In: B Satapatayakul (ed.) *Rhodococcosis. HIV/AIDS in Thailand: adult and pediatrics*. Bangkok: Sawicha Karnpim, 20–3.

Sirisanthana T. (1997). Infection due to *Penicillium marneffei*. *Ann Acad Med Singapore* **26**: 701–4.

Sirisanthana V, Sirisanthana T. (1995). Disseminated *Penicillium marneffei* infection in human immunodeficiency virus-infected children. *Ped Infect Dis J* **14**: 935–40.

Sirisanthana T, Supparatpinyo K, Perriens J et al. (1998). Amphotericin B and Itraconazole for treatment of disseminated *Penicillium marneffei* infection in human immunodeficiency virus-infected patients. *Clin Infect Dis* **26**: 1107–10.

Sirivichayakul S, Phanuphak P, Hanvanich M et al. (1992). Clinical correlation of the immunological markers of HIV infection in individuals from Thailand. *AIDS* 6: 393–7.

Sivayathorn A, Srihra B, Leesanguankul W. (1995). Prevalence of skin disease in patients infected with human immunodeficiency virus in Bangkok, Thailand. *Ann Acad Med Singapore* **24**: 528–33.

Soto-Ramirez LE, Renjifo B, McLane MF et al. (1996). HIV-1 Langerhans' cell tropism associated with heterosexual transmission of HIV. *Science* **271**: 1291–3.

Stewart G, Kunanusont C, Phanuphak P et al. (1996). Managing HIV with limited medical resources. *Med J Aust* **165**: 499–503.

Supparatpinyo K, Chiewchanvit S, Hirunsri P et al. (1992a). A efficacy study of itraconazole in the treatment of *Penicillium marneffei*. *J Med Assoc Thai* **75**: 688–91.

Supparatpinyo K, Chiewchanvit S, Hirunsri P et al. (1992b). *Penicillium marneffei* infection in patients infected with human immunodeficiency virus. *Clin Infect Dis* **14**: 871–4.

Supparatpinyo K, Sirisanthana T. (1994). Disseminated *Penicillium marneffei* infection diagnosed on examination of a peripheral blood smear of a patient with human immunodeficiency virus infection. *Clin Infect Dis* **18**: 246–7.

Supparatpinyo K, Nelson KE, Mera WG et al. (1993). Response to antifungal therapy by HIV-infected patients with disseminated *Penicillium marneffei* infection and *in vitro* susceptibility of isolates from clinical specimens. *Antimicrob Agents Chemother* **37**: 2407–11.

Supparatpinyo K, Khamwan C, Baosoung V et al. (1994). Disseminated *Penicillium marneffei* infection in southeast Asia. *Lancet* **344**: 110–13.

Suwanagool S, Chuenarom V, Pechthanon L et al. (1995). A comparative study of tuberculin skin test reactivity between asymptomatic HIV-1 seropositive subjects and healthy volunteers. *Asian Pacific J Allerg Immunol* **13**: 139–44.

Thanakitjaru S, Chareonphan P, Kiatboonsri S et al. (1996). Multiple drug-resistant (MDR) tuberculosis in Ramathibodhi hospital: Current status. *J Tuberculosis Chest* **17**: 209–15.

Tyndall M, Nasio J, Agoki E et al. (1995). Herpes zoster as the initial presentation of HIV type 1 infection in Kenya. *Clin Infect Dis* **21**: 1035–7.

Ubolyam S, Ruxrungtham, Weverling GJ et al. (1998). Comparative evaluation of Amplicor HIV-1 monitor with added primer set with Quantiplex v2.0 HIV RNA assay and the nuclisense for quantitation of HIV-1 RNA in a Thai study population, primarily infected with subtype E (abstract 41128). *Twelfth World AIDS Conference*, Geneva, Switzerland.

Ungsedhaphand C. (1998). *Penicillium marneffei* infection. In: K Ruxrungtham (ed.) *State of the art review 1998: clinical and clinical research*. Bangkok: Sahamitre Printing, 133–8.

Uthaivoravit W, Parlich V, Yanai H et al. (1994). Increasing HIV related tuberculosis burden in Chiangmai, Thailand (abstract 261c). *Tenth International Conference on AIDS*, Yokohama, Japan.

Verville TD, Huycke MM, Greenfield RA et al. (1994). *Rhodococcus equi* infection of human: 12 cases and review of literature. *Medicine* **73**: 119–32.

Vithayasai V, Sirisanthana T, Sakonwasun C et al. (1997). Flow cytometric analysis of T-lymphocytes subsets in adult Thais. *Asian Pacific J Allergy Immunol* **15**: 141–6.

Viviani MA, Tortorano AM, Rizzardini G et al. (1993). Treatment and serological studies of an Italian case of *penicilliosis marneffei* contracted in Thailand by a drug addict infected with the human immunodeficiency virus. *Eur J Epidemiol* **9**: 79–85.

Wade N, Birkhead G, Warren B et al. (1998). Abbreviated regimens of zidovudine ans perinatal transmission of the human immunodeficiency virus. *N Engl J Med* **339**: 1409–14.

Wadman M (2001). Experts clash over likely impact of cheap AIDS drugs in Africa. *Nature* **410**: 615–6.

Wannamethee SG, Sirivichayakul S, Phillips AN. (1998). Clinical and immunological features of human immunodeficiency virus infection in patients from Bangkok, Thailand. *Int J Epidemiol* **27**: 289–95.

Wawer WJ, Gray RH, Sewankanbo NK et al. (1998). A randomized community trial of intensive sexually transmitted disease control for AIDS prevention, Rakai, Uganda. **12**(10); 1211–25.

Yanai H, Uthaivoravit W, Mastro TD et al. (1997). Utility of tuberculin and anergy skin testing in predicting tuberculosis infection in human immunodeficiency virus-infected persons in Thailand. *Int J Tubercul Lung Dis* **1**: 427–34.

TILMAN RUFF AND DANIEL O'BRIEN

HIV-infected people commonly travel, with one study reporting up to 45% travelling within their own country for 1 week or more, and 20% travelling abroad over a 2-year period (Kemper *et al.*, 1997). However, travel, particularly to developing countries, also poses a number of risks and challenges. Some of these are similar to the issues and risks faced by all international travellers; others are increased, of different nature, or specific to HIV-infected travellers. A range of infections may be more frequent or severe in HIV-infected travellers, who may be less able to cope with certain environmental stresses than uninfected travellers. In addition, HIV-infected persons are more likely to develop adverse reactions to drugs used for prophylaxis and therapy. They may also face discrimination and accentuated legislative, bureaucratic, and social obstacles during travel abroad. Access to good medical care may be difficult, and the possibilities of disease progression, and new potentially serious problems unrelated to travel may be a constant source of concern. Immunosuppression related to HIV is associated with an increased risk of adverse events caused by live vaccines and reduced effectiveness of immunizations in those at greatest risk of the target diseases. Despite this, almost half of HIV-infected travellers do not consult a physician prior to travel, fewer (12%) receive health information specifically related to their HIV infection and only one in 18 international travellers consults a travel medicine expert (Kemper *et al.*, 1997).

The possibility of previously unrecognized HIV infection should be considered prior to travel, particularly when travel is planned to a developing country for an extended period. For those with advanced HIV disease and severe immunosuppression, overseas travel, for a prolonged period or to developing countries, may not be medically recommended. The criteria for medical advice for or against limitations on travel for HIV-infected persons should avoid discrimination and be similar to those applied to other patients with chronic and immunodeficiency conditions. The risks to health for HIV-infected travellers and available strategies to minimize these risks are discussed herein.

Travel-associated risks

Infections
Enteric infections
Pathogens that enter the human host via the gastrointestinal tract are a major cause of disease in HIV-infected persons, particularly those who travel. Traveller's diarrhoea affects at least 20%, and commonly 50%, of all travellers to developing countries, irrespective of duration of stay (Ericsson and DuPont, 1993; Steffen *et al.*, 1999). A number of the pathogens known to be important causes of travel-associated diarrhoea cause disease in HIV-infected persons that is severe, persistent, recurrent, or associated with extraintestinal complications. The increased susceptibility of HIV-infected persons to a range of bacterial and protozoan pathogens may be attributable to a number of factors. Reduced gastric acid production is common in patients with AIDS (Lake-Bakaar *et al.*, 1988), compromising an important barrier to gastrointestinal tract infection. In addition to systemic immunosuppression, HIV-infected persons often have reduced numbers of CD4-expressing cells in the lamina propria of the gastrointestinal tract; this results in impaired mucosal immune function (Ullrich *et al.*, 1989).

Campylobacter species cause an estimated 3–17% of episodes of traveller's diarrhoea, with considerable regional and seasonal fluctuation. HIV-infected patients have an increased susceptibility to infection (Angulo and Swerdlow, 1995) and the antibody response to *Campylobacter* sp. infection is severely impaired (Perlman *et al.*, 1988). This organism may cause bacteraemia, cholecystitis (Costel *et al.*, 1984), and chronic, relapsing disease (Perlman *et al.*, 1988;

Bernard *et al.*, 1989). Prophylactic use of fluoroquinolones is likely to reduce the risk of disease, but resistance is increasing (Hoge *et al.*, 1998).

Non-typhoidal *Salmonella* spp. account for up to 15% of traveller's diarrhoea (Black, 1990). AIDS patients are at higher risk of salmonellosis and this genus is more likely to cause severe invasive disease in these patients compared to the uninfected population. Non-typhoidal *Salmonella* spp. are an important cause of bacteraemic illness (Glaser *et al.*, 1985; Nadelman *et al.*, 1985; Fischl *et al.*, 1986; Sperber and Schleupner, 1987) and prolonged antimicrobial treatment is often necessary to prevent relapses (Jacobs *et al.*, 1985, Angulo and Swerdlow, 1995). Little has been documented about the relationship between typhoid fever and HIV infection, but infection is more common (Gotuzzo, 1991), and there is good reason to expect that more severe and complicated disease is likely in HIV-infected persons, compared with uninfected individuals.

Shigella species cause an estimated 5–15% of traveller's diarrhoea (Black, 1990), both dysenteric and non-dysenteric. In HIV-infected patients, shigellosis is more likely to be persistent, severe, bacteraemic, complicated by chronic gastrointestinal tract carriage (Mandell and Neu, 1986; Whimby *et al.*, 1986; Baskin *et al.*, 1987), and to require prolonged antibiotic treatment (Blaser *et al.*, 1989) than in uninfected persons.

AIDS patients would also be expected to have an increased susceptibility to cholera, as do other patients with reduced gastric acid; however, there are no published data to confirm this. There are reports of substantially increased mortality associated with cholera in HIV-infected persons, especially in children under 18 months of age (Rey *et al.*, 1995). Nevertheless, the low risk of cholera among travellers, the limitations of the injectable vaccine and limited availability of the killed oral vaccine, mitigate against their widespread use.

Escherichia coli, particularly enterotoxigenic strains, is the most common cause of traveller's diarrhoea. However, this species has not been documented to cause more severe disease in immnunocompromised than in non-compromised hosts.

Antibiotic treatment or prophylaxis, such as against *Pneumocystis carinii*, is associated with increased susceptibility to enteric colonization and disease caused by *Clostridium difficile*.

Cryptosporidial infection is thought to cause around 5% of traveller's diarrhoea. It is also the most commonly identi-

fied cause of chronic diarrhoea in AIDS patients (Malebranche *et al.*, 1983; Colebunders *et al.*, 1987). In healthy persons, *Cryptosporidium* spp. cause diarrhoea that commonly lasts some weeks but is self-limited, whereas in AIDS patients, chronic infection can lead to wasting and an increased susceptibility to other infections. In addition, there are some recent published data to suggest that travellers are at risk of infection with *Microsporidia*, another protozoan that causes chronic diarrhoea in patients with advanced HIV infection (Lopez-Velez *et al.*, 1999).

Isospora belli, another enteric protozoan that is endemic in developing countries, is present in 15–19% of AIDS patients with diarrhoea (DeHovitz *et al.*, 1986; Colebunders *et al.*, 1987). It may cause chronic, watery diarrhoea, with malabsorption and weight loss, with relapse being common if therapy is discontinued.

The recently identified coccidian protozoan parasite *Cyclospora cayatenensis* has been associated with sporadic cases and outbreaks of watery diarrhoea in a wide range of countries (Long *et al.*, 1990) and is increasingly recognized as a cause of traveller's diarrhoea. In immunocompetent hosts, diarrhoea is often associated with anorexia, fatigue, and weight loss, averaging between 3 and 6 weeks in duration. In HIV-infected persons, diarrhoea is often chronic and unremitting (Hart *et al.*, 1990; Wurtz, 1994). In both immunocompetent (Mudico *et al.*, 1993) and HIV-infected (Pape *et al.*, 1994) hosts, co-trimoxazole therapy results in both clinical and parasitological cure (Hoge *et al.*, 1995), although prevention of recurrences in HIV-infected persons requires long-term trimethoprim-sulfamethoxazole (TMP-SMX) prophylaxis.

Giardiasis is the most common cause of chronic traveller's diarrhoea. Amoebiasis, although found in only 2% of travellers with diarrhoea, is important because of its potential to cause dysentery, prolonged disease, and late liver abscesses. However, neither *Giardia lamblia* nor *Entamoeba histolytica* has been associated with more severe or complicated disease in HIV-infected persons.

Although major strides are being made in the control of poliomyelitis in most parts of the world, particularly the Americas and Western Pacific region (Hoge *et al.*, 1995; Jelinek *et al.*, 1997), the disease is still endemic in a number of developing countries, particularly in Africa, the Middle East and South Asia, and the potential for outbreaks in industrialized countries is still very real. For example, there was an outbreak in The Netherlands in 1992. Paralytic disease due to both wild and vaccine-strain virus is more frequent and severe in immunodeficient persons (Niko-wane et al., 1987; Onorato et al., 1988; Centres for Disease Control and Prevention [CDC], 1993) and a case of vaccine-associated paralytic poliomyelitis has been reported in a 26-month-old HIV-infected girl (Ion-Nedelcu et al., 1994). Whether this represents a chance occurrence or increased risk is uncertain.

Hepatitis A is the most common vaccine-preventable disease of travellers, but it has not been described as being more severe in HIV-infected persons. Outbreaks of hepatitis A have recently been described among male homosexuals in cities around the industrialized world (CDC, 1992).

A recent report from Brazil of 25 cases of strongyloidiasis in HIV-infected patients suggests an increased severity of this infection, with seven patients having hyperinfection syndrome, all of whom died (Ferreira et al., 1999). It is of note that only four patients in this series had eosinophilia.

Table 37.1 Selected enteric infections in travellers

Estimated incidence in travellers[a]	Disease/organism	Estimated morbidity and mortality in HIV-infected persons	Specific preventative measures[b]
Common			
	Campylobacteriosis	Increased	Fluoroquinolones are likely to reduce risk of disease but resistance is increasing (Hoge et al., 1998)[c]
	Escherichia coli	Possibly increased	None[c]
	Hepatitis A	Same	Vaccine and/or immune globulin
	Salmonellosis	Increased	None[c]
	Shigellosis	Increased	None[c]
	Giardiasis	Same or increased	None
	Viruses-rotavirus Norwalk-like agents	Probably same	None
Probably common, or common in some areas	Cryptosporidiosis	Increased	None
	Hepatitis E	No data	None
Uncommon, or probably uncommon in most areas	*Aeromonas* sp.	No data	None[c]
	Amebiasis	Same or increased	None
	Cyclosporiasis	Increased	TMP-SMX prophylaxis may decrease risk
	Isosporiasis	Increased	TMP-SMX prophylaxis may decrease risk
	Typhoid fever	Probably increased	Vaccine[c]
	Vibrio parahaemolyticus and other non-cholera vibrios	Probably increased	Avoid raw or undercooked seafood[c]
	Microsporidiosis	Increased	None
Rare			
	Cholera	Probably increased	Vaccine[c]
	Poliomyelitis	Probably increased	eIPV
	Yersiniosis	Insufficient data; bacteraemia reported	None[c]

[a]Common: reported to cause at least 5% of cases of diarrhoea in travellers in several studies in different geographical areas; for non-diarrhoeal illnesses, incidence in travellers is greater than 100/100 000/month.
Uncommon: reported in less than 5% of cases of traveller's diarrhoea in most studies in most areas; for non-diarrhoeal illnesses, incidence in travellers is 10–100/100 000/month.
Rare: not found as a case of diarrhoea in most studies; for non-diarrhoeal illnesses, incidence in travellers is less than 10/100 000/month.
[b]Avoidance of contaminated food and drink is likely to reduce the risk of most if not all causes of traveller's diarrhoea.
[c]Prophylactic antibiotic treatment is likely to reduce the risk.
TMP-SMX: trimethoprim-sulfamethoxazole; eIPV: enhanced inactivated polio vaccine.
(Adapted from Wilson et al., 1991 with permission.)

The risks of selected enteric infections in travellers are summarized in Table 37.1. The risks are compared for HIV-infected and non-infected hosts.

Respiratory infections

Travel-related respiratory infections are common. In Swiss travellers to developing countries, Steffen and associates (1987) estimated the incidence of acute respiratory infections accompanied by fever to be 1261/100 000 travellers/month. Although the course of influenza in HIV-infected persons has not been shown to be markedly different from that in HIV-uninfected persons, one study suggests longer duration of viral shedding in the former (Safrin *et al.*, 1990). Pneumonia due to bacterial pathogens that may cause secondary infections complicating influenza (particularly *Streptococcus pneumoniae*, *Hemophilus influenzae*, and *Staphylococcus aureus*) are common in HIV-infected persons. Influenza tends to be a winter or early spring disease in temperate zones, whereas it occurs year-round in the tropics. In addition, it is common; in our experience it was responsible for 5% of cases among 232 febrile returned travellers admitted to a tertiary hospital in Melbourne, Australia.

Measles is prevalent in many developing countries, is highly contagious and is more likely to be severe in HIV-infected persons (CDC, 1988). Recent outbreaks in a number of countries have affected previously immunized young adults and have provided impetus for the recommendation for two doses of measles–mumps–rubella vaccine. A number of countries have embarked on intensified measles control activities aiming for elimination, including mass immunization campaigns among children, adolescents and young adults. It is likely that measles will follow polio as a target for global eradication through immunization. Generally, all travellers to developing countries, particularly those travelling for extended periods and who anticipate contact with children, should be offered measles (or preferably, measles–mumps–rubella) vaccine unless they are known to be immune to measles or of an age when measles immunity can reasonably be assumed (see section on immunization below).

Some HIV-infected children who receive measles vaccine lose protective antibodies over time, sometimes resulting in fatal measles infection (Palumbo *et al.*, 1992). However, a cohort study of homosexual men in whom measles immunity was mostly naturally acquired did not demonstrate accelerated waning of immunity in HIV-infect-

ed compared with HIV-uninfected men (Zolopa *et al.*, 1994).

Tuberculosis, highly endemic in most developing countries, poses only a small risk to short-term travellers. Nevertheless, the probability of infection increases with longer stays and the risk of developing active disease is much higher for HIV-infected persons. A baseline, and if appropriate, periodic tuberculin skin tests and chest roentgenograms are indicated for HIV-infected who have recently travelled to developing countries. Anergy renders the tuberculin test unhelpful in the majority of those with advanced HIV-related immunosuppression.

A number of outbreaks of legionellosis have occurred in travellers staying in certain hotels and using spas. The frequency of this disease in AIDS patients has also been noted to be increased (Murray *et al.*, 1984). Melioidosis, due to infection with *Burkholderia pseudomallei*, a water and soil saprophyte, is a common cause of acute (focal and disseminated) and chronic sepsis in southeast Asia and northern Australia. Chronic disease and immunosuppression, including diabetes mellitus, alcoholism, chronic pulmonary disease, cirrhosis, and chronic renal failure, as well as age over 50 years, predispose to more severe acute disease, most commonly pneumonia, and to reactivation of latent infection. (The same risk factors apply to severe legionellosis.) Although it would appear possible that HIV-infected persons may be at increased risk of melioidosis, to date this has not been documented.

Meningococcal disease is found worldwide and is a rare disease in travellers except during epidemics, which occur annually during the dry season in much of sub-Saharan Africa and more erratically elsewhere. Data about the effect of HIV infection on meningococcal disease risk are limited. A study in Tanzania found that there was a statistically significant association between HIV infection and risk of meningococcal meningitis before but not during a meningococcal epidemic (Pallangyo *et al.*, 1992). In the same study, mortality from meningococcal meningitis in those with HIV infection was 3/6 (50%), significantly higher than the rate of 3/29 (10%) found in HIV-uninfected patients. On the other hand, no association was found in a study in Nairobi (Brindle *et al.*, 1991).

Histoplasmosis and coccidioidomycosis are fungal infections known to be more common and severe in HIV-infected persons (Graybill, 1988; Calgiani and Ampel, 1990; Wilson; 1991), either because of more severe disseminated primary infection or reactivation of past

Table 37.2 Selected respiratory infections in travellers

Estimated incidence in travellers[a]	Disease/organism	Estimated morbidity and mortality in HIV-infected persons	Specific preventative measures
Common	Influenza	Increased secondary infections	Vaccine, prophylactic amantadine
Uncommon	Measles	Increased	Consider vaccine (preferably or measles–mumps–rubella) if non-immune and not severely immunocompromised
Rare	Coccidioidomycosis	Increased	Avoid exposure to soil and dust in endemic areas
	Histoplasmosis	Increased	Avoid exposure to soil in endemic areas
	Melioidosis	No information	Wear shoes; avoid immersion, especially of skin lesions, in surface freshwater
	Penicillium marneffei	Increased	None
	Leprosy	Increased progression to lepromatous end of disease spectrum	Avoid prolonged exposure
Rare except during epidemics	Legionellosis	Possibly increased	Avoid spas and showers with potentially contaminated water
	Meningococcaemia	Possibly increased	Vaccine prior to travel to areas reporting epidemics
	Tuberculosis[b]	Increased	Preventive therapy (isoniazid) in asymptomatically infected and high exposure risk; BCG vaccine contraindicated

[a]Common: incidence in travellers is greater than 100/100 000/month.
Uncommon: incidence in travellers is 10 to 100/100 000/month.
Rare: incidence in travellers is less than 10/100 000/month.
[b]Incidence increases with duration of travel.
(Adapted from Wilson *et al.*, 1991 with permission.)

infection. Histoplasmosis occurs most often in central USA, although it has been described in most continents. In contrast, coccidioidomycosis is limited to parts of Mexico, Central and South America, and the southwestern USA.

Penicillium marneffei infection is an important opportunistic infection in some areas in southeast Asia, particularly Thailand, and has been identified in HIV-infected travellers (Hilmarsdottir *et al.*, 1993; Kok *et al.*, 1994). Clinical manifestations include fever, papular skin lesions and pulmonary infiltrates.

Table 37.2 summarizes the risks of selected respiratory disease for HIV-infected travellers. Comparison is made with the risks in non-HIV-infected hosts.

Vector-borne infections

Vector-borne diseases are a major cause of morbidity and mortality in tropical and subtropical areas and pose a considerable risk to travellers (Table 37.3). Malaria is by far the most important of these. Recently, there has been convincing evidence of an interaction between malaria and HIV in residents of an endemic area, where HIV was asso-

ciated with increased frequency of clinical malaria and parasitaemia, with this association becoming more pronounced with advancing immunosuppression (Whitworth *et al.*, 2000). In addition, in co-infected patients there is an increased prevalence of peripheral parasitemia and higher parasite densities in pregnant women (Sreketee *et al.*, 1998), and a possible increased rate of vertical transmission of HIV (Chandramohan and Greenwood, 1998). There are concerns that persistent malarial infection leads to increased HIV viral burden, and therefore accelerated HIV disease progression and facilitated HIV transmission (Hoffman *et al.*, 1998). However, no information is available on the relative morbidity of malaria in HIV-infected travellers from areas where malaria is not endemic.

Yellow fever is caused by a mosquito-borne flavivirus prevalent in the northern and Amazonian part of South America and in tropical Africa. Although the major reservoir is vertebrates in forest areas, the disease may occur in jungle, intermediate, and urban settings, often in the form of outbreaks. The case fatality rate in non-immune adults is over 60%. No specific information on incidence or outcome of yellow fever in HIV-infected persons is available.

Table 37.3 Selected vector-borne infections in travellers

Estimated incidence in travellers	Disease/organism	Estimated morbidity and mortality in HIV-infected persons	Specific preventative measures
Variable[a]	Malaria	Increased level of clinical malaria and parasitaemia. Placental malaria and possibly increased vertical transmission of HIV	Avoid mosquito bites, chemoprophlaxis, prompt diagnosis and treatment of febrile illness
Rare[b]	Dengue	Unknown	Avoid mosquito bites
	Babesiosis	Possibly increased	Avoid tick bites in endemic areas
	Trypanosomiasis (American)	Increased	Avoid reduviid bug bites in endemic areas
	Visceral leishmaniasis	Increased	Avoid sandfly bites in endemic areas
	Yellow fever	Unknown (high mortality in immunocompetent persons)	Avoid currently infected areas; avoid mosquito bites; consider immunization if not immunocompromised

[a]The risk of malaria in British visitors to West Africa was 2.4% (Phillips-Howard et al., 1990).
[b]Rare: incidence in travellers is less than 10/100 000/month.
(Adapted from Wilson et al., 1991 with permission.)

Immunization (with the live attenuated 17D vaccine) is required by many countries in the endemic zone, and by many more countries if travellers have visited endemic areas (WHO, 2000). Live attenuated vaccines should not be administered to HIV-infected individuals who are immunocompromised.

Visceral leishmaniasis (kala-azar) is prevalent in Africa, Latin America, the Mediterranean area, and central and south Asia. Persons infected with HIV and other immunocompromised persons with kala-azar are the subject of numerous reports (Clauvel et al., 1986; Berenguer et al., 1989; Montalban et al., 1989; Jeannel et al., 1991). Symptoms of infection often do not develop until months or years following exposure. Typical clinical manifestations such as fever, splenomegaly, pancytopenia and hypergammaglobulinaemia may be absent, and serological tests may be negative in the HIV-infected person, despite advanced infection. Treatment is not always successful, and the mortality rate tends to be high. Early diagnosis is likely to be important for successful outcomes. Leishmaniasis causes immunosuppression and theoretically could hasten the progression of HIV-related disease (Wilson et al., 1991).

Babesiosis (caused by *Babesia* species, protozoan parasites of red blood cells, that are endemic in Europe, Mexico, and the USA and transmitted by ticks) may be severe and recurrent in HIV-infected persons, both splenectomized (Ong et al., 1990) and non-splenectomized

(Benezra et al., 1987). The risk to travellers, however, appears to be very low.

Limited data are available on American trypanosomiasis (Chagas' disease) in HIV-infected persons. The risk of this disease is low in short-term travellers, but may be considerably higher in long-term residents in endemic areas. *Trypanosoma cruzi* is a protozoan transmitted by blood-sucking reduviid insects, or kissing bugs. A number of reports document cases of single or multiple tumor-like mass lesions and abscesses in the central nervous system (CNS) of patients with HIV infection, sometimes occurring years after exposure (Bouzas et al., 1989; Castillo et al., 1990; Gluckstein et al., 1992).

A wide range of other vector-borne diseases may occur in travellers, including arboviruses such as dengue (second only to malaria), viruses causing encephalitis such as Japanese encephalitis, viral haemorrhagic fevers, and rickettsial infections borne by fleas, lice, mites and ticks. Many of these are focal in geographical distribution. Plague is an extremely rare disease in travellers, with only one case being documented in a traveller in recent decades (CDC, 1991). Information on the risks of any of these diseases specific to HIV-infected travellers is not currently available.

Sexually transmitted infections

All HIV-infected persons should avoid sexual and any other activities that could transmit HIV to others, and not expose

Table 37.4 Selected sexually transmitted infections in travellers

Estimated incidence in travellers	Diseases/organism	Estimated morbidity and mortality in HIV-infected persons	Specific preventative measures
Common[a]	Gonorrhoea	Probably similar	None
Uncommon	Hepatitis B	Increased; in many areas, HIV-infected persons are more likely to be chronically infected or immune	Vaccine; postexposure hepatitis B immune globulin
	Hepatitis C	Increased progression to cirrhosis and increased vertical transmission of hepatitis C	None
	Syphilis	Increased	None

[a]Common: Incidence in travellers is greater than 100/100 000/month. Uncommon: incidence in travellers is 10–100/100 000/month.
(Adapted with permission from Wilson *et al.*, 1991.)

themselves to other sexually transmissible infections (Table 37.4). Ulcerative and inflammatory genital lesions increase the risk of HIV transmission. Syphilis, gonorrhoea, chancroid, lymphogranuloma venereum, and granuloma inguinale are common in many developing countries. The natural history and management of syphilis are altered in HIV-infected persons (Musher *et al.*, 1992).

Hepatitis B is one of the most common viral infections worldwide – 10–15% of the population of many developing countries, including sub-Saharan Africa, southeast and east Asia, and the Pacific islands, are chronic carriers of the virus. Although globally the common forms of transmission are by contact between young children and vertical transmission; sexual transmission also plays a major role, particularly in low-incidence areas. Long-term residents in highly endemic areas are at significantly greater risk than short-term travellers. Because of the similar modes of transmission between hepatitis B and HIV, HIV-infected persons are more likely to have been exposed to hepatitis B. The risks of chronic carriage and high levels of hepatitis B viral replication following hepatitis B infection are increased in HIV-infected persons (Hadler, 1988; Hadler *et al.*, 1991), although associated liver injury appears milder than in HIV-uninfected persons (Horvath and Raffanti, 1994). Progression to AIDS can result in re-activation of latent hepatitis B infection, or re-infection with another hepatitis B subtype (Horvath and Raffanti, 1994).

Although less easily transmitted than hepatitis B, hepatitis C is also sexually transmissible, and its transmissibility would appear to be increased in the setting of HIV infection (Eyster *et al.*, 1991), perhaps because of prolonged or increased viraemia (Horvath and Raffanti, 1994). HIV and hepatitis C co-infection results in more rapid progression to cirrhosis (Martin *et al.*, 1989; Soto *et al.*, 1997; Lesens *et al.*, 1999) and increased vertical transmission of hepatitis C virus (Chang, 1996). HIV infection may reduce the accuracy of diagnostic tests for hepatitis C (Horvath and Raffanti, 1994).

Many systemic infections, such as cytomegalovirus (CMV) infection, and many enteric pathogens, such as hepatitis A, amebiasis, and shigellosis may also be sexually transmitted. Although the effective use of barrier protection, particularly condoms, substantially reduces the risk of sexually transmitted disease, it does not wholly eliminate the risk.

Percutaneous infections

A number of worms, such as hookworms, *Strongyloides stercoralis*, and *Schistosoma* spp., infect humans by percutaneous penetration of infective larval forms. The latter two are important because of their potential for chronic infection with serious sequelae. Disseminated strongyloidiasis has been described in HIV-infected persons (Gompels *et al.*, 1991), but it appears that this association is uncommon. Whether or not HIV-infected persons are at any increased risk of rabies is not currently known.

Bloodborne infections

A number of sexually transmissible, vector-borne, and other infectious agents are also transmissible by blood, certain blood products, or unsterile instruments that pierce the skin or contact mucosal surfaces. Although HIV antibody screening of donated blood is now routine in central blood banks and transfusion facilities in virtually all countries, in many rural and smaller centres, particularly where donated blood is used immediately rather than stored, such screening is still performed inconsistently, if at all. Even fewer centres in developing countries screen donated blood for hepatitis B, and very few screen for hepatitis C. Routine screening for HIV antibodies does not guarantee the safety of blood supplies, particularly in areas where HIV infection is highly prevalent. Studies in Abidjan, Côte d'Ivoire, for example, suggest that the overall risk of HIV infection from a single unit of blood remains substantial (5.4–10.6/1000 units), even with routine testing for antibodies to HIV-1 and HIV-2 (Savarit et al., 1992). Many bloodborne pathogens pose an increased risk of severe or complicated disease to HIV-infected persons, including syphilis, cytomegalovirus (CMV), leishmaniasis, toxoplasmosis, hepatitis B and C and Chagas' disease. The natural history of human T-cell leukaemia/lymphoma virus-1 infection in HIV-infected persons has not been documented. Measures to reduce the risks of infection with bloodborne agents for travellers are summarized in Table 37.5.

Environmental hazards

Altitude and flying

The atmospheric pressure maintained in passenger aircraft cabins is equivalent to an altitude of 1700–2800 m, with a median of 1900 m. In healthy sea-level-adapted persons, haemoglobin saturation is maintained over 90% when arterial oxygen tension is greater than 60 mmHg. The critical point of saturation of 90%, below which reduction in arterial oxygen tension results in steeper falls in saturation, occurs at approximately 2400 m altitude. Those with underlying lung disease, however, may desaturate at altitudes much lower than this. HIV-infected persons with impaired lung function, such as may occur following *Pneumocystis carinii* pneumonia (PCP), may experience difficulties with flying or at high altitude, particularly if exposure to low ambient partial pressure of oxygen is combined with anaemia (common in HIV-infected patients, whether due to opportunistic disease such as disseminated *Mycobacterium avium* complex [MAC] or drugs such as zidovudine [ZOV]) and vigorous exercise, such as trekking. Predeparture exercise tolerance is the most useful clinical yardstick. Patients with significant activity limitations whose plans include unaccustomed exertion or travel to altitudes over 2400 m (8000 feet) should have lung function testing and be referred to a respiratory physician. This applies particularly to those unable to walk 50 m or climb 15 stairs without significant symptoms.

Sunlight

Levels of ambient ultraviolet radiation are considerably higher at tropical and subtropical latitudes than at higher latitudes, and are also increased at high altitude. High levels of exposure to ultraviolet radiation have measurable effects on cutaneous and systemic cell-mediated immune function and may precipitate reactivation of herpes simplex ulceration; for these reasons excessive sun exposure should be avoided.

In addition, a number of drugs that might be taken by an HIV-infected traveller, such as tetracyclines and sulfonamides, may cause photosensitive rashes. Travellers to sunny areas should be warned of this possibility.

Medication and health care abroad

All travellers with medical conditions that require ongoing therapy and regular review or that are associated with a risk of emergency should carry with them a recent letter from their treating physician that outlines their history, problem list, current status, physical findings, recent investigation results, treatment, and physician contact details. Such documentation is extremely valuable for medical personnel who may be consulted abroad. The more serious and unstable the patient's condition and the more intensive the patient's management, the more useful it is for the patient's physician to make prior contact with colleague(s) abroad who can continue the patient's care. All travellers

Table 37.5 Prevention of bloodborne infections

- Medical and dental check-up and performance of elective procedures before travel
- Avoidance of childbirth and elective procedures in areas where safety of blood supply and infection control practice may be inadequate
- Ensure that any medical or dental procedures abroad are necessary and performed according to good infection control practice (including universal body substance precautions)
- Avoid injuries, particularly motor vehicle injuries (use seatbelts); avoid alcohol and driving, motorcycles (especially without helmet), riding in the back of open vehicles, bald tyres, night driving, and excessive speed
- Avoid any potentially unsterile skin-piercing instrument, whether for medical injection, drugs, tattooing, acupuncture, ear piercing, or scarification
- Carry sterile needles and syringes; for expatriates suture materials and i.v. cannulae may be considered

should ensure that they either take supplies of regular medication ample for the planned duration of travel (preferably carried in hand luggage rather than check-in bags) or that they can be sure of access to additional supplies abroad.

HIV-infected travellers who are concerned that they may breach a country's entry restrictions for persons with HIV infection or AIDS often remove drugs from the original packaging so as not raise suspicion of their HIV status. For example, some travellers remove antiretroviral medications from their blister pack and place them in a vitamin capsule container.

For prolonged stays in the tropics, careful attention should be paid to appropriate storage of medication – many drugs undergo more rapid degradation in hot humid conditions, particularly if they are removed from their original packaging or if they are not kept away from insects, such as cockroaches.

Travel restrictions

A number of countries restrict the entry of travellers or immigrants with HIV infection or AIDS, despite the dubious public health rationale for such practices and the recommendations against restrictions based solely on a person's HIV status by the World Health Organization and other bodies (Gilmore et al., 1989; Gostlin et al., 1990; von Reyn et al., 1990; WHO, 2000). There is no convincing evidence that such restrictions have any effect in reducing the rate of HIV transmission.

Updated unofficial information compiled by the US Department of State on HIV testing requirements for various countries is available at the following address on the World Wide Web (http://travel.state.gov/HIVtestingregs.html). Because requirements for entry are subject to change, HIV-infected travellers should be advised to anonymously consult the embassy or consulate of each country they plan to visit. Restrictions vary from country to country and also within a country; for example, at the time of writing, the HIV testing requirement in China for those staying more than 6 months does not apply to Hong Kong, and a requirement for testing for those staying over 180 days applies in Bavaria but not elsewhere in Germany. At this time, no country requires proof of a negative HIV antibody test for tourists, but restrictions may apply if a person is already known to be HIV-infected. A number of countries require testing if a person intends to stay for longer than around 15 days–3 months. Testing is often necessary for immigrants

and longer-term temporary residents, such as students and workers. Some countries accept the documented result of a recent test performed in the traveller's home country, particularly at a World Health Organization collaborating laboratory; others do not. Enforcement of restrictions also varies; for example, a number of HIV-infected persons have travelled to the USA unimpeded by official restrictions prohibiting their entry.

Recommendations for HIV-infected travellers

Most recommendations for HIV-infected travellers are similar or identical to recommendations for other travellers. Reduction of risk of enteric, sexually-transmitted, and bloodborne infections, avoidance of insect (particularly mosquito) bites, avoidance of animal bites in areas endemic for rabies, injury prevention, appropriate immunizations and chemoprophylaxis, and adequate health insurance, including access to emergency assistance, are important issues for all travellers. Excellent sources of information on health advice for travellers are those published by the WHO (2000), Centres for Disease Control and Prevention (1999), Wilson (1995), DuPont and Steffen (1997), Dawood (1992), Bia (1992), and Yung and Ruff (1999). In addition, a variety of regularly updated health information sources are available by subscription, a number providing automated individualized health advice. These include Catis, Edisan, Macnet, Masta, Timatic, Travax, Tropimed, and others. Information about these can be obtained from travel health centres or The International Society of Travel Medicine (P.O. Box 871089, Stone Mountain, GA 30087-0028, USA, Tel: +1 770 736 7060, Fax: +1 770 736 6732, e-mail bcbistm@aol.com).

HIV-infected travellers should discuss their travel plans with their treating physician at an early date. Advice should be obtained from an expert in travel medicine for those planning high-risk travel – isolated, prolonged, or in settings of high infectious disease risk, such as exists in most developing countries. The general principles of travel health advice are summarized in Table 37.6; additional measures specific to HIV-infected travellers are summarized in Table 37.7.

Immunization

Publications by Wilson and associates (1991), Wilson (1992), Onorato and Markowitz (1992), the CDC (1999),

Van Gompel *et al.* (1997) and Yung and Ruff (1999) provide detailed information on immunization of HIV-infected persons, including travellers. CDC recommendations are available on the World Wide Web at http://www.cdc.gov/

Table 37.6   General principles of travel health advice

- Identify risk factors such as HIV infection, other immuno-compromising and chronic conditions, pregnancy
- Individualize advice: this trip for this person at this time
- Start early to allow for multidose schedules, possible vaccine interactions and possible adverse events. maximal immune response to immunization takes weeks to develop
- Give multimodal advice (at least verbal plus written, which the patient should take on their travels)
- Encourage personal responsibility
- Emphasize behaviour to reduce pathogen exposure:
  - eat well and freshly cooked steaming hot food (greater than 60°C), fruit that can be peeled; drink boiled, bottled, or canned fluids. If this is not possible, disinfect water with iodine (or less preferably chlorine) or filter through iodine-impregnated filter. Avoid raw or undercooked fish, shellfish, meat or eggs, raw unpeeled vegetables (particularly green leafy) and fruit, unpasteurized milk and milk products, tap water and ice made with unboiled water. Dry food, highly acidic citrus fruits, and hyperosmolar foods (e.g. jellies and syrup) are likely to be safe
  - avoid biting insects by using protective clothing, DEET-containing insect repellents, sleeping in screened accommodation or under a permethrin-impregnated mosquito net and avoiding outdoor exposure at times of high insect activity
  - avoid sexual intercourse, or use a high-quality latex condom every time from start to finish
  - reduce risk of injury (see Table 37.5)
  - avoid any unsterile instrument that pierces the skin, whether for drug use, medical or dental injections, acupuncture, ear-piercing, tattooing or scarification
- Provide written documentation of chronic illness and, if necessary, arrange continuing care abroad
- Assist patient to obtain adequate quantities of appropriate medication and equipment
- Administer indicated vaccines, document batch numbers, and complete patient-held immunization record
- Prescribe appropriate chemoprophylaxis, particularly for malaria
- Advise on appropriate medical kit. Common items include aspirin or paracetamol, simple first-aid equipment including dressings and antiseptic, insect repellent, sunscreen, oral rehydration salts, especially if travelling with children, medication for diarrhoea (usually loperamide plus a fluoroquinolone antibiotic) needles and syringes, and condoms
- Advise appropriate travel insurance, including provision for emergency assistance

Table 37.7   Specific measures for HIV-infected travellers

- Detailed assessment of current immune function (including CD4 lymphocyte count and viral load) and health status
- Take account of legal restrictions on travel for persons with HIV infection or AIDS
- Review travel plans with patient. For severely immuno-compromised patients, and those with active medical problems, the best advice may be not to travel at all, not to travel to developing countries, or to travel for only a short period. When appropriate, explore safer alternatives. A helpful travelling companion may be valuable.
- Arrange documentation, including list of current medications and recent test results, adequate supplies of medication, and if needed, continuing medical care during travel
- Educate patient regarding prompt medical attention and early treatment for infections, including early self-treatment of diarrhoeal disease with ciprofloxacin
- Individually tailor immunizations and prophylaxis,. tuberculin skin test if appropriate
- Local AIDS organizations and self-help groups may be able to provide useful information, such as on counterpart organizations in other countries
- Advise flexible, refundable ticket, health insurance and if appropriate, trip cancellation insurance

travel/hivtrav.htm. The morbidity and mortality of a number of infections that pose a risk to travellers can be reduced by immunization, and as has been outlined, a number of vaccine-preventable diseases, such as typhoid, hepatitis B and influenza are likely to be more frequent or are more severe in HIV-infected travellers. However, the immunogenicity of vaccines in HIV-infected persons is generally reduced in proportion to the degree of immunosuppression present, and live vaccines may be associated with an increased risk of adverse events. Thus, indicated vaccines are optimally given early in the course of HIV disease, or if late, preferably after commencement of highly active antiretroviral therapy (HAART). HIV-infected individuals of any age who are well controlled on combination antiretroviral therapy, with undetectable of low viral load and well-preserved CD4 lymphocyte counts are likely to respond well to vaccines (NHMRC, 2000). The most immunogenic regimen should be used, such as double usual-dose hepatitis B vaccine and intramuscular rather than intradermal administration of hepatitis B and rabies vaccines.

The combined hepatitis A and B vaccine (Twinrix, SmithKline Beecham Biologicals, Rixensart, Belgium) is not suitable as it contains only standard doses of hepatitis B surface antigen. It may be useful to measure post-immunization antibody levels, particularly for hepatitis B and rabies, for which post-exposure prophylaxis with specific immune globulin is available.

As with hepatitis B vaccine, hepatitis A vaccine given to HIV-infected individuals results in reduced seroconversion rates and antibody titres and faster decline in antibody levels (Santagostino *et al.*, 1994; Clemens *et al.*, 1995; Singer and Sax, 1996). Immune globulin should be used for prevention of hepatitis A if significant immunoparesis is present (Van Gompel, 1997).

Few efficacy studies of vaccines in HIV-infected patients are available: some important recent studies deserve comment. A randomized, double-blind, placebo-controlled efficacy trial of influenza vaccine was recently performed in 102 patients attending a military clinic in California (Tasker *et al.*, 1999). As the study was conducted in 1995/96, antiretroviral regimens were limited to reverse transcriptase inhibitors, and all patients had received at least one previous influenza immunization. No effects on HIV-1 RNA levels or CD4 cell counts were observed. Although over 80% of subjects had CD4 lymphocyte counts over 200 cells/μl, only 12–36% of vaccine recipients had a fourfold or greater antibody response to each of the three vaccine strains. Nevertheless, substantial efficacy was demonstrated: 16/55 (29%) of vaccine recipients reported respiratory symptoms over the 1995/96 autumn/winter, compared with 23/47 (49%) placebo recipients ($p = 0.04$). Ten placebo recipients but no vaccine recipients had laboratory-confirmed symptomatic influenza A (protective efficacy 100%, 95% CI, 73–100%, $p < 0.001$). This protection is comparable to the 70% efficacy typically described in immunocompetent adults. Although involving a relatively small number of participants, this study provides impressive evidence for efficacy of influenza vaccine in HIV-infected adults.

In relation to pneumococcal polysaccharide vaccine, the available data are less clearcut, and an important recent study suggests no benefit, and possible negative effect. This is noteworthy, since pneumococcus is currently the most important potentially vaccine-preventable HIV-associated pathogen. USA case–control studies have suggested some benefit of immunization (Gebo *et al.*, 1996), but not in black patients (Fedson and Watson, 2000), although the patient numbers in the latter group are relatively small and the confidence intervals wide.

In Uganda, however, a recently reported, double-blind, randomized, placebo-controlled trial, which appears to have been rigorously conducted, had quite different findings (French *et al.*, 2000). All 1392 HIV-1-infected adults (937 female) were equally randomized to well-matched vaccine and placebo groups. No significant differences were found in the incidence of first culture-proven invasive pneumococcal infection (hazard ratio 1.47; 95% CI, 0.7–3.3) or all pneumococcal events (HR 1.41; 0.7–2.8). However, all cause pneumonia was significantly more frequent in the vaccine group (40 *vs* 21; HR 1.89; 1.1–3.2). No effect was found on mortality in the trial, where patients had relatively easy access to good care. The authors suggest that the harmful effect of pneumococcal polysaccharides may be due to destruction of polysaccharide-responsive B cell clones, and this is supported by evidence of a decline in vaccine serotype-specific antibody avidity following administration of pneumococcal polysaccharide vaccine to HIV-1-infected children (Spoulou *et al.*, 2000).

However, over 40% of patients in the Ugandan study had CD4 counts of less than 200 cells/μl, whereas prospective cohort data from the USA CDC suggest a protective effect of 23-valent pneumococcal polysaccharide vaccine only in HIV-infected individuals with CD4 counts greater than 500 cells/μl.

While it is to be hoped that the new generation of conjugate pneumococcal vaccines will be substantially more effective in HIV-infected persons than polysaccharide vaccine, no efficacy data in this population are yet available. Comparative trials of the two vaccines in HIV-infected persons are indicated; in non-African settings continued use of the polysaccharide pneumococcal vaccine, particularly early in the course of HIV disease, seems justified.

Concerns about the safety of immunizing HIV-infected persons have centered around the safety of immunizations themselves and the possibility of adverse effects on the progression of HIV disease. No increase in adverse events, serious or otherwise, has been described for diphtheria–pertussis–tetanus, bacillus Calmette-Guerin, measles, or measles–mumps–rubella vaccines administered to HIV-infected children (Onorato *et al.*, 1988; Onorato and Markowitz, 1992; CDC, 1993). The only adverse effects reported in HIV-infected adults are a case of generalized vaccinia in a person with asymptomatic HIV infection (Redfield *et al.*, 1987), two cases of disseminated infection following bacillus Calmette-Guérin immunization of adults with symptomatic HIV infection (CDC, 1985; Armbruster *et al.*, 1990), fatal MMR-associated pneumonitis (CDC, 1996a), and an increased risk of chronic hepatitis B (HB) carriage among HIV-infected men who received hepatitis B vaccine at the time they were incubating hepatitis B infection (Hadler *et al.*, 1991).

No change in viral load was observed in HIV-infected individuals given typhoid Vi capsular polysaccharide vaccine (Kroon *et al.*, 1999); however, transient increases in HIV replication reflected by rises in plasma HIV RNA titre have been observed following immunization with influenza (Ho, 1992; O'Brien *et al.*, 1995; Hasheeve *et al.*, 1998; Vigano *et al.*, 1998), tetanus (Stanley *et al.*, 1996), pneumococcal (Brichacek *et al.*, 1996; Vigano *et al.*, 1998), hepatitis B (Cheeseman *et al.*, 1996), and rabies (Pancharoen *et al.*, 1998) vaccines. There is concern that this may lead to accelerated HIV disease progression. However, presently available clinical data show no evidence to support this, including a recent study that showed no significant changes in HIV viral load, CD4 lymphocyte counts or mortality 1 year following hepatitis A vaccination (Bodsworth *et al.*, 1997). In addition, similar and often more sustained rises in plasma HIV RNA titres occur upon development of the diseases the vaccines are designed to prevent (Ho, 1992; Stanley, 1996), and a number of recent studies have suggested that any effects on CD4 cell counts and HIV DNA titre are rare and transient (Fuller *et al.*, 1999; Keller *et al.*, 2000). As described, the diseases targeted by immunization are associated with significant morbidity and mortality. At present, the benefits of immunization appear to outweigh the above theoretical risks (Kroon *et al.*, 1996; Stanley, 1996; Van Gompel *et al.*, 1997). However, we believe that these concerns justify a policy not to use vaccines in HIV-infected individuals for which there are not strong reasons to support their use. The main vaccine that has been routinely recommended by some authorities for HIV-infected persons, which we believe is no longer justified in adults, is *Haemophilus influenzae* type b vaccine.

In general, HIV-infected persons should not receive live viral or bacterial vaccines. However, two exceptions are made. Because of the increased severity and occasional lethality of measles in HIV-infected persons, immunity is desirable. Previously, measles–mumps–rubella (MMR) was recommended for all those without prior natural measles infection, regardless of their HIV status. However a recent case of fatal MMR-associated measles pneumonitis in a 21-year-old man with AIDS (CDC, 1996a) has led to more conservative recommendations for children. The American Academy of Pediatrics (AAP) and the CDC now advise against MMR for severely immunocompromised children with HIV (i.e. CD4 lymphocyte count of less than 750

cells/μl for children aged less than 12 months, less than 500 cells/μl for ages 1–5, less than 200/μl for those 6 years or older, or CD4 lymphocyte counts of less than 15% of total), and the US Public Health Service suggests that measles-containing vaccine should not be given to adults with advanced disease (CD4 lymphocyte counts of less than 200 cells/μl). We feel it is important that long-term travellers and expatriates should be protected against measles. Testing for measles antibody is useful to identify those susceptible, as well as those who do not need immunization, particularly among those with significant immunoparesis (CD4 lymphocyte count less than 200 cells/μl). We would still recommend MMR vaccine to susceptible HIV-infected long-term travellers and expatriates with CD4 lymphocyte counts of less than 200 cells/μl who are able to make an informed choice. Most persons born before 1960 in industrialized countries, and before 1980 in developing countries, are likely to be naturally immune to measles. Immune globulin may provide a useful alternative means of protecting severely immunocompromised travellers against measles (as well as hepatitis A).

Yellow-fever vaccine has not been associated with an increased frequency or severity of adverse effects in HIV-infected persons (Wilson *et al.*, 1991; Goujon *et al.*, 1995; Receveur *et al.*, 2000) and may be given to asymptomatic HIV-infected persons with CD4 lymphocyte counts of greater than 200 cells/μl when the risk of exposure is significant. There is insufficient evidence to determine whether the vaccine poses a risk to symptomatic HIV-infected individuals (WHO, 2000). Therefore, in these persons, a waiver letter should be provided, along with advice regarding the risks of infection, and mosquito avoidance measures. A recent trial of CVD 103-HgR live oral cholera vaccine in Mali found no safety or tolerability differences in 38 HIV-infected individuals compared with 387 HIV-seronegative adults (Perry *et al.*, 1998).

Killed or inactivated vaccines do not represent an increased risk for immunocompromised, including HIV-infected, persons and should generally be administered as recommended for non-HIV-infected persons, using the most immunogenic route and schedule, with the recognition that their effectiveness may be reduced.

Because immune globulin can interfere with the immune response to measles vaccine, it should be given at least 3 months (and preferably 6 months) before, or at least 2 weeks after, a measles-containing vaccine. Immunizations recommended for HIV-infected travellers are outlined in Table 37.8.

Malaria chemoprophylaxis

Chloroquine is immunosuppressive *in vitro* (Wilson *et al.*, 1991) and has been shown to inhibit the antibody response to human diploid cell rabies vaccine (Pappaioanou *et al.*, 1986). It is therefore theoretically possible that it may contribute to HIV disease progression, but clinical data to assess this possibility are lacking. It is not known whether other antimalarial drugs such as mefloquine have a similar effect.

The most effective agents available for chloroquine-resistant malaria are mefloquine and doxycycline. Although there are no published reports that address the use of these drugs for malaria chemoprophylaxis in HIV-infected persons, their use in this setting is thought to be safe. The most important contraindication to mefloquine (apart from previous adverse experience with the drug) is neuropsychiatric disease (Steffen *et al.*, 1993), which is common in HIV-infected persons. It is also more likely that side-effects with mefloquine, which are commonly neuropsychological, may cause a diagnostic problem. This is less likely with doxycycline. In addition, mefloquine may have important interactions with the protease inhibitors (PIs) and non-nucleoside reverse transcriptase inhibitors (NNRTIs). These antiretroviral agents either inhibit or induce the hepatic cytochrome P450 3A4 enzymes, which also catalyze the metabolism of mefloquine. This could potentially result in either toxic or inadequate levels of mefloquine. However, interaction studies have been performed to date. Therefore, we recommend doxycycline for HIV-infected travellers to chloroquine-resistant areas.

The increased risk of adverse drug reactions in HIV-infected persons applies to a wide variety of agents.

Table 37.8 Immunizations recommended for HIV-infected travellers

Routine	• Diphtheria-tetanus (booster every 10 years) • Hepatitis B (three double-strength doses unless already infected or immune; assess antibody response) • Influenza (annual) • Pneumococcal (polysaccharide boost every 5 years); conjugate vaccine (two or three doses, depending on age) preferred, licensed up to 9 years, followed > 2 years of age by polysaccharide vaccine • *Haemophilus influenzae* type b (for children less than 5 years) • Varicella (consider in asymtomatic susceptible HIV-infected person with CD4 percentage ≥ 25% [CDC Class 1])
Travel to developing countries	• Hepatitis A vaccine (two doses, long-term protection likely) and/or immune globulin (up to 6 months dose-dependent passive immunity, can be combined with vaccine); use IG in significantly immunocompromised • Polio: enhanced inactivated (eIPV) (boosters every 10 years). • Typhoid: inactive injectable; Vi vaccine (one dose every 3 years) preferable to heat-killed vaccine (two doses with single booster every 3 years) • Measles–mumps–rubella (one dose for adults, two for children); care or avoidance in severely immunocompromised (see text); measles antibody testing useful to determine susceptibility
Selected circumstances	• Yellow fever (1 dose, booster every 10 years) if risk of infection high, asymptomatic, CD4 count over 200 cells/μl; otherwise waiver letter • Meningococcal polysaccharide (one dose for children over 2 years, two doses 3 months apart for children under 2 years, booster every 3 years); conjugate vaccine preferred if available, and risk principally Group C • Japanese encephalitis (three doses, booster after 3 years) • Rabies (three intramuscular doses, check antibody response, boosters at least every 2 years or according to antibody level) • Cholera: oral killed whole cell/B subunit (WC/BS) vaccine (three doses, boosters every year for children under 5 years, every 3 years for older persons); parenteral killed vaccine (two doses, single booster every 6 months), rarely indicated • Tick-borne encephalitis vaccine (inactivated): (three doses at 0, 1–3 and 9–12 months or rapid schedules: days 0, 7, 21 or 2 doses on day 0, booster on day 7; boost every 3 years) • Lyme disease, three doses at 0, 1, and 12 months (licensed ages 15–70 years)
Contraindicated	• Oral polio vaccine (WHO recommends for HIV-infected children in high incidence areas) • Oral live-attenuated Ty21a typhoid vaccine • Bacillus Calmette-Guerin (indicated for asymptomatic HIV-infected children in areas of high tuberculosis prevalence) • Yellow fever (if symptomatic, CD4 lymphocytes less than 200 cells/μl) • Oral live-attenuated (CVD 103HgR) cholera vaccine

Pyrimethamine-sulfadoxine is no longer recommended for malaria chemoprophylaxis because of the risk of potentially fatal Stevens-Johnson syndrome, as well as increasing malaria parasite resistance to the drug. The high risk of side-effects (particularly rash), declining antimalarial effectiveness, and the importance of sulfa agents in the treatment and prevention of PCP mean that pyrimethamine-dapsone and pyrimethamine-sulfadoxine should generally not be used as chemoprophylactic agents for malaria in HIV-infected persons. Few data exist on the use of proguanil in HIV-infected persons. Although safe, its utility is markedly limited by its lack of effectiveness, particularly outside Africa (Lobel et al., 1993; Steffen et al., 1993).

Whatever chemoprophylactic agent is used, avoidance of mosquito bites and prompt medical consultation (within 24–36 h of onset of symptoms) with blood-smear examination for febrile illnesses that occur during or after a period of malaria risk are of fundamental importance. Emergency self-treatment with atovaquone-proguanil, quinine, mefloquine, pyrimethamine-sulfadoxine (in areas where resistance to this agent is not yet widespread) or artemisinin derivatives is indicated for travellers at risk of malaria in areas where medical care is not accessible within 24 h (WHO, 1998). Atovaquone-proguanil is preferred as the emergency self-treatment drug of choice. It is highly effective, even against multidrug resistant *Plasmodium falciparum*, well tolerated, has a simple regimen, and can be used whatever antimalarial prophylaxis or therapy has preceded its use.

Rapid and simple immunochromatographic tests for detection of circulating falciparum histidine-rich protein-2 in whole blood have recently become available. They have a potentially useful role to help guide the management of fever in travellers (Yung and Ruff, 1998). These tests have shown a high sensitivity and specificity in hospital and laboratory settings. But experience to date, when used by travellers, indicates poor sensitivity and specificity. A negative test, particulary outside a laboratory setting, should not delay seeking medical care of emergency self-treatment in the face of a persistent, especially severe, or worsening, febrile illness.

Prophylaxis and management of traveller's diarrhoea

Fluid and electrolyte replacement is the cornerstone of treatment for severe diarrhoea, particularly if accompanied by volume depletion; in such cases an oral rehydration solution is valuable. For mild-to-moderate cases any non-alcoholic, non-dairy, and preferably non-caffeine-containing fluid generally suffices. Because of their high risk of diarrhoea and more severe and complicated disease, HIV-infected persons should take great care to reduce the risk of enteric infection by eating and drinking safely. Prophylactic antimicrobial therapy is highly effective in reducing the incidence of traveller's diarrhoea (Ericsson and Dupont, 1993). In HIV-infected travellers the risks of adverse reactions, alteration of faecal flora predisposing to enteric infection, partial treatment of infections, and selection of resistant organisms may be outweighed by the benefits. Prophylactic antibiotics should be offered to immunosuppressed HIV-infected persons who are likely to be at high risk of diarrhoea for a short time (less than 2–3 weeks) or who plan to perform some critical task abroad (e.g. a key public speech or diplomatic mission). Because of the frequency of adverse reactions to trimethoprim-sulfamethoxazole (TMP-SMX) and the prevalence of strains of *Salmonella* spp., *Shigella* spp., *Vibrio cholerae*, and *E. coli* in many parts of the world that are resistant to this drug combination, a fluoroquinolone is the preferred prophylactic agent, in half the usual treatment dose. TMP-SMX or azithromycin can be used for pregnant women or young children.

All HIV-infected travellers, particularly those who are immunocompromised who plan to travel in developing countries, should carry an antibiotic for prompt self-treatment of any diarrhoeal illness that is associated with three or more loose stools within 24 h, distressing or incapacitating symptoms, fever, or bloody stools. Fluoroquinolones are most effective for therapy and are the agents of choice. Ciprofloxacin, norfloxacin, ofloxacin, and fleroxacin generally seem equally effective for treatment of traveller's diarrhoea (DuPont and Ericsson, 1993; Ericsson and Dupont, 1993). However, because of the risk of bacteraemic disease in HIV-infected persons and the better systemic activity of ciprofloxacin, this agent is preferred in these patients. A 3-day course of ciprofloxacin is recommended; an initial double dose of 1 g followed by standard doses of 500 mg twice a day for 3 days may be more effective than standard dose alone (Ericsson and Dupont, 1993). Although there are no clear guidelines for this situation, those who develop diarrhoea while on a prophylactic antibiotic could be advised to initiate full treatment doses of a fluoroquinolone (preferably ciprofloxacin) and to seek medical advice if symptoms do not improve within 12–24 h.

Prophylaxis and treatment for respiratory disease

For severely immunocompromised HIV-infected persons (CD4 lymphocytes less than 200 cells/μl or symptomatic disease) spending a prolonged period in highly tuberculosis endemic areas, consideration may be given to offering prophylaxis with isoniazid 300 mg daily (Conlon, 1993; Yung and Ruff, 1998).

It has been found that almost half of HIV-infected people become ill while travelling, mainly with a respiratory focus such as otitis media, sinusitis, bronchitis or pneumonia (Kemper et al., 1997). It would seem advisable to begin a course of appropriate antibiotics early if symptoms of respiratory infection develop (Conlon, 1993).

Short-term prophylaxis against coccidioidomycosis with fluconazole or itraconazole has been suggested for those travelling to endemic areas (Mileno, 1998).

On return

HIV-infected travellers who experienced any illness during travel or who travelled for an extended period in developing countries should be reviewed by their treating physician, if necessary in consultation with a travel-medicine or infectious-disease physician, soon after return. Evaluation of such patients should err on the side of being comprehensive and include full blood and blood-smear examinations, liver function tests, stool examinations, appropriate serology, and chest roentgenograms, in addition to routine monitoring for HIV disease.

All travellers, HIV-infected or otherwise, should be aware of the importance of always informing their physician of their travel abroad and of seeking prompt medical attention for any febrile illness after travel, particularly to malarious areas. With appropriate care and precautions, for most HIV-infected persons travel can be an enriching and rewarding experience, without unduly compromising their health.

References

Angulo FJ, Swerdlow DL. (1995). Bacterial enteric infections in persons infected with human immunodeficiency virus. Clin Infect Dis 21: S84–93.

Armbruster C, Junker W, Vetter N et al. (1990). Disseminated bacille Calmette-Guerin infection in an AIDS patient 30 years after BCG vaccination. J Infect Dis 162: 1216.

Baskin DH, Lax JD, Barenberg D. (1987). Shigella bacteraemia in patients with the acquired immune deficiency syndrome. Am J Gastroenterol 82: 338–41.

Benezra D, Brown AE, Polsky B et al. (1987). Babesiosis and infection with human immunodeficiency virus. Ann Intern Med 107: 944.

Berenguer J, Moreno S, Cercenddado E et al. (1989). Visceral leishmaniasis in patients infected with human immunodeficiency virus (HIV). Ann Intern Med 111: 129–32.

Bernard E, Roger PM, Carles D et al. (1989). Diarrhoea and Campylobacter infections in patients infected with the human immunodeficiency virus. J Infect Dis 159: 142–4.

Bia FJ. (eds.). (1992). Travel medicine advisor. Atlanta: American Health Consultants.

Black RE. (1990). Epidemiology of travellers' diarrhoea and relative importance of various pathogens. Rev Infect Dis 12: S73–9.

Blaser MJ, Hale TL, Formal SB. (1989). Recurrent shigellosis complicating human immunodeficiency virus infection: failure of preexisting antibodies to confer protection. Am J Med 86: 105–7.

Bodsworth NJ, Neilsen GA, Donovan B. (1997). The effect of immunization with inactivated hepatitis A vaccine on the clinical course of HIV-1 infection: one-year follow-up. AIDS 11: 747–9.

Bouzas MB, Corral R, Muchinik C et al. (1989). HIV-infection and Chagas' disease in haemophiliacs in Argentina. Proceedings of the Fifth International Conference on AIDS, Montreal; Canada.

Brichacek B, Swindells S, Janoff EN et al. (1996). Increased plasma human immunodeficiency virus type 1 burden following antigenic challenge with pneumococcal vaccine. J Infect Dis 174: 1191–9.

Brindle R, Simani P, Newnham R et al. (1991). No association between meningococcal disease and human immunodeficiency virus in adults in Nairobi, Kenya. Trans R Soc Trop Med Hyg 83: 651.

Calgiani JN, Ampel NM. (1990). Coccidioidomycosis in human immunodeficiency virus-infected patients. J Infect Dis 162: 1165–9.

Castillo MD, Mendoza G, Oviedo J et al. (1990). AIDS and Chagas' disease with central nervous system tumor-like lesions. Am J Med 88: 693–4.

Centres for Disease Control and Prevention. (1985). Disseminated Mycobacterium bovis infection from BCG vaccination of a patient with acquired immunodeficiency syndrome. MMWR 34: 227–8.

Centres for Disease Control and Prevention (CDC). (1988). Measles in HIV-infected children, United States. MMWR 37: 183–6.

CDC. (1991). Imported bubonic plague – District of Colombia. MMWR 39: 895–6.

CDC. (1992). Hepatitis A among homosexual men – United States, Canada and Australia. MMWR 41: 161–4.

CDC. (1993). Recommendations of the Advisory Committee on Immunization Practices (ACIP): use of vaccines and immune globulins in persons with altered immunocompetence. MMWR 42: 1–18.

CDC (1996a). Measles pneumonitis following measles–mumps–rubella vaccination of a patient with HIV infection, 1993. MMWR 45: 603–6.

CDC (1999). Health information for international travel, 1999–2000. Atlanta: Centers for Disease Control and Prevention.

Chandramohan D, Greenwood BM. (1998). Is there an interaction between human immunodeficiency virus and Plasmodium falciparum? Int J Epidemiol 27: 296–301.

Chang MH. (1996). Mother-to-infant transmission of hepatitis C virus. Clin Invest Med 19: 368–72.

Cheeseman SH, Davaro RE, Ellison RT. (1996). Hepatitis B vaccination and plasma HIV-1 RNA. New Engl J Med 334: 1272.

Clauvel JP, Couderc LJ, Belmin J et al. (1986). Visceral leishmaniasis complicating acquired immunodeficiency syndrome (AIDS). Trans R Soc Trop Med Hyg **80**: 1010–11.

Clemens R, Safary A, Hepburn A et al. (1995). Clinical experience with an inactivated hepatitis A vaccine. J Infect Dis **171**: S44–9.

Colebunders R, Francis H, Mann JM et al. (1987). Persistent diarrhoea strongly associated with HIV infection in Kinshasa, Zaire. Am J Gastroenterol **82**: 859–64.

Conlon CP. (1993). The immunocompromised traveller. Br Med Bull **49**: 412–22.

Costel EE, Wheeler AP, Gregg CR. (1984). Campylobacter fetus spp fetus cholecystitis and relapsing bacteraemia in a patient with acquired immunodeficiency syndrome. South Med J **77**: 927–8.

Dawood R. (1992). Traveller's health. How to stay healthy abroad. 3rd edition. Oxford: Oxford University Press.

DeHovitz JA, Pape JW, Boney M et al. (1986). Clinical manifestations and therapy of Isospora belli infection in patients with the acquired immunodeficiency syndrome. N Engl J Med **315**: 87–90.

DuPont HL, Ericsson CD. (1993). Prevention and treatment of traveller's diarrhoea. N Engl J Med **25**: 1821–7.

DuPont HL, Steffen R (eds). (1997). Textbook of travel medicine and health. Hamilton, Ontario: BC Decker.

Ericsson CD, DuPont HL. (1993). Traveller's diarrhoea: approaches to prevention and treatment. Clin Infect Dis **16**: 616–26.

Eyster ME, Alter HJ, Alecdort LM et al. (1991). Heterosexual co-transmission of hepatitis C virus (HCV) and human immunodeficiency virus (HIV). Ann Intern Med **115**: 764–8.

Fedson DS, Watson M. (2000). Pneumococcal infection and HIV-1 infection. Lancet **356**: 1272.

Ferreira MS, Nishioka SdA, Borges AS et al. (1999). Strongyloidiasis and infection due to human immunodeficiency virus: 25 cases at a Brazilian teaching hospital, including seven cases of hyperinfection syndrome. Clin Infect Dis **28**: 154–5.

Fischl MA, Dickinson GM, Sinave C et al. (1986). Salmonella bacteraemia as manifestation of acquired immunodeficiency syndrome. Arch Intern Med **146**: 113–5.

French N, Nakiyingi J, Carpenter LM et al. (2000). 23-valent pneumococcal polysaccharide vaccine in HIV-1 infected Ugandan adults: double-blind, randomised and placebo-controlled trial. Lancet **355**: 2106–11.

Fuller JD, Craven DE, Steger KA et al. (1999). Influenza vaccination of human immunodeficiency virus (HIV) – infected adults: impact on plasma levels of HIV type 1 RNA and determinants of antibody response. Clin Infect Dis **28**: 541–7.

Gilmore N, Orkin AJ, Duckett M et al. (1989). International travel and AIDS. AIDS **3**: S225–30.

Gebo JA, Moore RD, Keruly JC, Chaisson RE. (1996). Risk factors for pneumococcal disease in human immunodeficiency virus-infected patients. J Infect Dis **173**: 857–62.

Glaser JB, Morton-Kute L, Berger SR et al. (1985). Recurrent Salmonella typhimurium bacteraemia associated with the acquired immunodeficiency syndrome. Ann Intern Med **102**: 189–93.

Gluckstein D, Ciferri F, Ruskin J. (1992). Chagas' disease: another cause of cerebral mass in the acquired immunodeficiency syndrome. Am J Med **92**: 429–32.

Gompels MM, Todd J, Peters BS et al. (1991). Disseminated strongyloidiasis in AIDS: uncommon but important. AIDS **5**: 3 29–32.

Gostlin LO, Cleary PD, Mayer KH et al. (1990). Screening immigrants and international travellers for the human immunodeficiency virus. N Engl J Med **322**: 1743–6.

Gotuzzo E, Frisancho O, Sanchez J et al. (1991). Association between the acquired immunodeficiency syndrome and infection with Salmonella typhi or Salmonella paratyphi in an endemic typhoid area. Arch Intern Med **151**: 381–2.

Goujon C, Tohr M, Feuillie V et al. (1995). Good tolerance and efficacy of yellow fever vaccine among carriers of human immunodeficiency virus. J Travel Med **2**: 145.

Graybill JR. (1988). Histoplasmosis and AIDS. J Infect Dis **158**: 623–6.

Hadler SC. (1988). Hepatitis B prevention and human immunodeficiency virus (HIV) infection. Ann Intern Med **109**: 92–3.

Hadler SC, Judson FN, O'Malley PM et al. (1991). Outcome of hepatitis B infection in homosexual men and its relation to prior human immunodeficiency virus infection. J Infect Dis **163**: 454–9.

Hart AS, Ridinger MT, Soundarajan R et al. (1990). Novel organism associated with chronic diarrhoea in AIDS. Lancet **335**: 169–70.

Hasheeve D, Thompson CE, Salvato PD. (1998). Effect of influenza vaccination on viral loads in HIV patients. Twelfth World AIDS Conference, Geneva, Switzerland.

Hilmarsdottir I, Meynard JL, Rogeaux O et al. (1993). Disseminated Penicillium marneffei infection associated with human immunodeficiency virus: a report of two cases and review of 35 published cases. J Acquir Immune Defic Syndr **6**: 466–71.

Ho DD. (1992). HIV-1 viraemia and influenza. Lancet **339**: 1549.

Hoffman I, Taylor TE, Jere C et al. (1998). The association between Plasmodium falciparum malaria illness and HIV-1 RNA viral burden. Twelfth World AIDS Conference, Geneva, Switzerland.

Hoge CW, Shlim DR, Ghimire M et al. (1995). Placebo-controlled trial of co-trimoxazole for cyclospora infections among travellers and foreign residents in Nepal. Lancet **345**: 691–3.

Hoge CW, Gambel JM, Srijan A et al. (1998). Trends in antibiotic resistance among diarrhoeal pathogens isolated in Thailand over 15 years. Clin Infect Dis **26**: 341–5.

Horvath J, Raffanti SP. (1994). Clinical aspects of the interactions between human immunodeficiency virus and the hepatotropic viruses. Clin Infect Dis **18**: 339–47.

Ion-Nedelcu N, Dobrescu A, Strebel PM et al. (1994). Vaccine-associated paralytic poliomyelitis and HIV infection. Lancet **343**: 51–2.

Jacobs JO, Gold JW, Murray HW et al. (1985). Salmonella infections in patients with the acquired immunodeficiency syndrome. Ann Intern Med **102**: 186–8.

Jeannel D, Tuppin P, Brucker G et al. (1991). Imported and autochthonous kala-azar in France. Br Med J **303**: 336–8.

Jelinek T, Lotze M, Eichenlaub S et al. (1997). Prevalence of infection with Cryptosporidium parvum and Cyclospora cayetanesis among international travellers. Gut **41**: 801–4.

Keller M, Deveikis A, Cutillar-Garcia M et al. (2000). Pneumococcal and influenza immunization and human immunodeficiency virus load in children. Pediatr Infect Dis J **19**: 613–18.

Kemper CA, Linett A, Kane C et al. (1997). Travels with HIV: the compliance and health of HIV-infected adults who travel. Int J STD AIDS 8: 44–9.

Kok I, Veenstra J, Rietra PJGM et al. (1994). Disseminated Penicillium marneffei infection as an imported disease in HIV-1 infected patients. Neth J Med 44: 18–22.

Kroon FP, van Dissel JT, Ravensbergen E et al. (1999). Impaired antibody response after immunization of HIV-infected individuals with the polysaccharide vaccine against Salmonella typhi (Typhim-Vi®). Vaccine 17: 2941–5.

Kroon CW, Van Furth, Bruisten SM. (1996). The effects of immunization in human immunodeficiency virus type 1 infection. N Engl J Med 335: 817–18.

Lake-Bakaar G, Quadros E, Beidas S et al. (1988). Gastric secretory failure in patients with the acquired immunodeficiency syndrome. Ann Intern Med 109: 502–4.

Lesens O, Deschenes M, Steben M et al. (1999). Hepatitis C virus is related to progressive liver disease in human immunodeficiency virus – positive hemophiliacs and should be treated as an opportunistic infection. J Infect Dis 179: 1254–8.

Lobel HO, Miani M, Eng T et al. (1993). Long-term malarial prophylaxis with weekly mefloquine. Lancet 341: 848–51.

Long EG, Ebrahimzadeh A, White EH et al. (1990). Alga associated with diarrhoea in patients with acquired immunodeficiency syndrome and in travellers. J Clin Microbiol 28: 1101.

Lopez-Velez E, Turrientes MC, Garron C et al. (1999). Microsporidiosis in travelers with diarrhea from the tropics. J Travel Med 6: 223–7.

Madico G, Gilman RH, Miranda E et al. (1993). Treatment of Cyclospora infection with co-trimoxazole. Lancet 342: 122–3.

Malebranche R, Arnoux E, Guerin JM et al. (1983). Acquired immunodeficiency syndrome with severe gastrointestinal manifestations in Haiti. Lancet 2: 873–7.

Mandell W, Neu H. (1986). Shigella bacteraemia in adults [letter]. JAMA 255: 3116–17.

Martin P, Di Bisceglie AM, Kassianides C et al. (1989). Rapidly progressive non-A, non-B hepatitis in patients with human immunodeficiency virus infection. Gastroenterology 197: 1559–61.

Mileno MD, Bia FJ. (1998). The compromised traveller. Infect Dis Clin N Am 12: 369–412.

Montalban C, Martinez-Fernandez R, Calleja JO et al. (1989). Visceral leishmaniasis (kala-azar) as an opportunistic infection in patients infected with the human immunodeficiency virus in Spain. Rev Infect Dis 11: 655–60.

Murray JF, Felton CP, Garay SM et al. (1984). Pulmonary complications of the acquired immunodeficiency syndrome. N Engl J Med 310: 1682–8.

Musher DM, Hamill RJ, Baughm RE. (1992). Effect of human immunodeficiency virus (HIV) infection on the course of syphilis and on the response to treatment. Ann Intern Med 113: 872–81.

Nadelman RB, Mathur-Wagh U, Yancovitz SR et al. (1985). Salmonella bacteraemia associated with the acquired immune deficiency syndrome (AIDS). Arch Intern Med 145: 1968–71.

National Health and Medical Research Council (NHMRC). (2000). The Australian immunisation handbook, 7th edition. Canberra: Australian Government Publishing Service, 32–4.

Nguyen-Dinh P, Greenberg AE, Mann JM et al. (1987). Absence of association between Plasmodium falciparum malaria and human immunodeficiency virus infection in children in Kinshasa, Zaire. Bull WHO 65: 607–13.

Nikowane BM, Wassilak SC, Orenstein WR et al. (1987). Vaccine-associated paralytic poliomyelitis. USA: 1973 through 1984. JAMA 257: 1335–40.

O'Brien WA, Grovit-Ferbas K, Namazi A et al. (1995). Human immunodeficiency virus-type 1 replication can be increased in peripheral blood of seropositive patients after influenza vaccination. Blood 86: 1082–9.

Ong KR, Stavropoulos C, Inada Y (1990). Babesiosis, asplenia and AIDS [letter]. Lancet 336: 112.

Onorato IM, Markowitz LE. (1992). Immunizations, vaccine-preventable diseases, and HIV infection. In: GP Wormser (ed.) AIDS and other manifestations of HIV infection. Second edition. New York: Raven Press, 671–81.

Onorato IM, Markowitz LE, Oxtoby MJ. (1988). Childhood immunization, vaccine-preventable diseases and infection with human immunodeficiency virus. Pediatr Infect Dis J 6: 588–95.

Pallangyo K, Hakanson A, Lema L et al. (1992). High HIV seroprevalence and increased HIV-associated mortality among hospitalized patients with deep bacterial infections in Dar es Salaam, Tanzania. AIDS 6: 971–6.

Palumbo P, Hoyt L, Demassio K et al. (1992). Population-based study of measles and measles immunization in human immunodeficiency virus-infected children. Pedatr Infect Dis J 11: 1008–14.

Pancharoen C, Thisyakorn U, Ruxrungtham K et al. (1998). Safety and immunogenicity of pre-exposure rabies immunization in HIV-infected children. Twelfth World AIDS Conference, Geneva, Switzerland.

Pappaioanou M, Fishbein DB, Dreesen DW. (1986). Antibody response to pre-exposure human diploid cell rabies vaccine given concurrently with chloroquine. N Engl J Med 314: 280–4.

Pape JW, Verdier RI, Boncy M et al. (1994). Cylclospora infection in adults infected with HIV: Clinical manifestations, treatment, prophylaxis. Ann Intern Med 121: 654–7.

Perlman DM, Ampel NM, Schifman RB et al. (1988). Persistent Campylobacter jejuni infection in patients with human immunodeficiency virus (HIV). Ann Intern Med 108: 540–6.

Perry RT, Plowe CV, Koumare B et al. (1998). A single dose of live oral cholera vaccine CVD 103-HgR is safe and immunogenic in HIV-infected and HIV-noninfected adults in Mali. Bull WHO 76: 63–71.

Phillips-Howard PA, Radalowicz A, Mitchell J et al. (1990). Risk of malaria in British residents returning from malarious areas. Br Med J 300: 499–503.

Receveur MC, Thiebaut R, Vedy S et al. (2000). Yellow fever vaccination of HIV-infected patients: report of 2 cases. Clin Infect Dis 31: E7–8.

Redfield RR, Wright DC, James WD et al. (1987). Disseminated vaccinia in a military recruit with human immunodeficiency virus disease. N Engl J Med 316: 673–6.

Rey J-L, Milleliri J-M, Soares J-L et al. (1995). HIV seropositivity and cholera in refugee children from Rwanda. AIDS 9: 1203–4.

Safrin S, Rush JD, Mills J. (1990). Influenza in patients with human immunodeficiency virus infection. *Chest* **98**: 33–7.

Santagostino E, Gringeri A, Rocino A *et al.* (1994). Patterns of immunogenicity of an inactivated hepatitis A vaccine in anti-HIV positive and negative hemophiliac patients. *Thromb Haemost* **72**: 508–10.

Savarit D, De Cock KM, Schutz R *et al.* (1992). Risk of HIV infection from transfusion with blood negative for HIV antibody in a West African city. *Br Med J* **305**: 498–501.

Singer M, Sax P. (1996). Routine immunization in HIV: helpful or harmful? *AIDS Clin Care* **8**: 13–15.

Soto B, Sanchez-Quijano A, Rodrigo L *et al.* (1997). Human immunodeficiency virus infection modifies the natural history of chronic parenterally-acquired hepatitis C with an unusually rapid progression to cirrhosis. *J Hepatol* **26**: 1–5.

Sperber SJ, Schleupner CJ. (1987). Salmonellosis during infection with human immunodeficiency virus. *Rev Infect Dis* **9**: 925–34.

Spoulou V, Theodoridou M, Papaevangelou VG *et al.* (2000). 23-Valent pneumococcal vaccination and HIV. *Lancet* **356**: 1027–8.

Sreketee R, Nahlen BD, Ayisi J *et al.* (1998). HIV and malaria overlap and do interact in sub-Saharan African pregnant women. *Twelfth World AIDS Conference*, Geneva, Switzerland.

Stanley SK, Ostrowski MA, Justement JS *et al.* (1996). Effect of immunization with a common recall antigen on viral expression in patients infected with human immunodeficiency virus type 1. *New Engl J Med* **334**: 1222–30.

Steffen R, Rickenbach M, Wilhelm U *et al.* (1987). Health problems after travel to developing countries. *J Infect Dis* **156**: 84–91.

Steffen R, Fuchs E, Schildknecht J *et al.* (1993). Mefloquine compared with other malaria chemoprophylactic regimens in tourists visiting East Africa. *Lancet* **341**: 1299–1303.

Steffen R, Collard F, Tornieporth N *et al.* (1999). Epidemiology, etiology, and impact of traveler's diarrhea in Jamaica. *JAMA* **281**: 811–17.

Tasker SA, Treanor JJ, Paxton WB, Wallace MR. (1999). Efficacy of influenza vaccination in HIV-infected persons. *Ann Intern Med* **131**: 430–3.

Ullrich R, Zeitz M, Heise W *et al.* (1989). Small intestinal structure and function in patients infected with human immunodeficiency virus (HIV): evidence for HIV-induced enteropathy. *Ann Intern Med* **111**: 15–21.

Van Gompel A, Kozarsky P, Colebunders R. (1997). Adult travellers with HIV infection. *J Travel Med* **4**: 136–43.

Vigano A, Bricalli D, Trabattoni D *et al.* (1998). Immunization with both T cell-dependent and T cell-independent vaccines augments HIV viral load secondarily to stimulation of tumour necrosis factor alpha. *AIDS Res Hum Retrovir* **14**: 727–34.

von Reyn CF, Mann JM, Chin J. (1990). International travel and HIV infection. *Bull WHO* **68**: 251–9.

Whimby E, Cold JW, Polsky B *et al.* (1986). Bacteraemia and fungemia in patients with the acquired immunodeficiency syndrome. *Ann Intern Med* **104**: 511–14.

Whitworth J, Morgan D, Quigley M *et al.* (2000). Effect of HIV-1 and increasing immunosuppression on malaria parasitaemia and clinical episodes in adults in rural Uganda: a cohort study. *Lancet* **356**: 1051–6.

Wilson ME. (1991). Geographically focal infections and the HIV-infected traveller. In: HO Lobel, R Steffen, PE Kozarsky (eds.) *Travel medicine 2*. Atlanta, GA: International Society of Travel Medicine. 218–19.

Wilson ME. (1992). Use of vaccines in the HIV-infected traveller. In: HO Lobel, R Steffen, PE Kozarsky (eds.) *Travel medicine 2*. Atlanta, GA: International Society of Travel Medicine. 216–17.

Wilson ME. (1995). Travel and HIV infection. In: ED Jong, R McMullen (eds.) *The travel and tropical medicine manual*. Second edition. Philadelphia: WB Saunders: 166–76.

Wilson ME, von Reyn F, Fineberg HV. (1991). Infections in HIV-infected travellers: risks and prevention. *Ann Intern Med* **114**: 582–92.

World Health Organization (WHO). (2000). *International travel and health*. Geneva: WHO.

Wurtz R. (1994). Cyclospora: a newly identified intestinal pathogen of humans. *Clin Infect Dis* **18**: 620–3.

Yung AP, Ruff TA. (1999). *Manual of travel medicine*. Melbourne: Victorian Infectious Diseases Service, Royal Melbourne Hospital.

Zolopa AR, Kemper CA, Shiboski S *et al.* (1994). Progressive immunodeficiency due to infection with human immunodeficiency virus does not lead to waning immunity to measles in a cohort of homosexual men. *Clin Infect Dis* **18**: 636–8.

Index